A COMPENDIUM OF NEUROPSYCHOLOGICAL TESTS

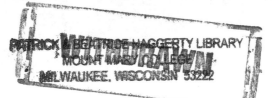
A COMPENDIUM OF NEUROPSYCHOLOGICAL TESTS

Administration, Norms, and Commentary

SECOND EDITION

OTFRIED SPREEN
ESTHER STRAUSS

Department of Psychology
University of Victoria
Victoria, B.C., Canada

New York   Oxford
OXFORD UNIVERSITY PRESS
1998

Oxford University Press

Oxford   New York
Athens   Auckland   Bangkok   Bogota
Bombay   Buenos Aires   Calcutta   Cape Town
Dar es Salaam   Delhi   Florence   Hong Kong
Istanbul   Karachi   Kuala Lumpur   Madras
Madrid   Melbourne   Mexico City   Nairobi
Paris   Singapore   Taipei   Tokyo
Toronto   Warsaw

and associated companies in
Berlin   Ibadan

Library of Congress Cataloging-in-Publication Data
Spreen, Otfried.
A compendium of neuropsychological tests :
administration, norms, and commentary /
Otfried, Spreen, Esther Strauss. — 2nd ed.
p.   cm.   Includes bibliographical references and index.
ISBN 0-19-510019-0
1. Neuropsychological tests—Handbooks, manuals, etc.
I. Strauss, Esther.   II. Title.
RC386.6.N48S67   1997   152—dc20   96-34724

9 8 7 6 5 4 3 2 1

Printed in the United States of America
on acid-free paper

Preface

This manual presents a compilation of the main neuropsychological tests currently used in the University of Victoria Psychology Laboratory and its associated facilities. The need for a manual of this type will be obvious to the practicing clinician: while neuropsychological tests have been developed in numerous laboratories, only a limited number of them have reached formal publication by commercial publishers—although that number has increased rapidly in recent years. As a result, photocopied manuals of administration and norms are passed along among clinicians or as in-house laboratory publications (e.g., Harley et al., 1980; Trites, 1977, 1985) like underground literature, and they may remain available only for short periods of time as authors move from place to place or in and out of the clinical field. Worse, in the process of exchanging manuals and normative data, inaccuracies and deliberate changes may slip in which modify the intent of the original investigator, as well as rendering previously developed norms useless. Information on reliability and validity is scattered across both well-known and less accessible journals and conference reports (frequently unpublished) or are hidden in studies where these topics are not the primary objective.

Exceptions to this generalization are a number of formally published tests and the "fixed" test batteries: Reitan's battery of tests is still available in its original form from Tucson, Arizona, but even this battery has been modified in many laboratories (e.g., Jarvis & Barth, 1994), and inter-laboratory differences in norms resulting from apparently minor changes are common. The Christensen-Luria battery, used relatively little in North America, and its North American amalgamation by Golden (1976, 1980) are other examples of fixed batteries. Also commercially available are a few specific batteries for the assessment of aphasia (Goodglass & Kaplan, 1983; Kertesz, 1982; Porch, 1967, 1973). Clinicians who are satisfied with a "fixed" battery approach to neuropsychological examinations may not need this book although normative data for some tests are included here.

Neuropsychological tests originate from several sources including (1) the clinical neurological examination, (2) experimental psychology, (3) neuropsychological research, and (4) clinical psychology; only a small number of tests were originally designed for the neuropsychological clinician. As a result, the original descriptions of many of the procedures included here had to be traced to scattered and often obscure sources. Commercial distribution of such information was often not practical.

In contrast to the neurological examination, which consists largely of checking the presence or absence of all-or-none effects or "signs," neuropsychological tests in general measure abilities distributed on a gradient, ranging from high above average to below average and severely impaired, taking into account the relationship of each measure with age, education, gender, and intelligence if such relation can be found in normative studies. For this reason we do not include instruments based on a "sign" approach, such as the "Mini Inventory of Right Brain Injury" (Pimental & Kingsbury, 1989), which provides pseudo-accuracy by summing a collection of 27 "signs," attaching point-values to some, and stakes a poorly substantiated claim for diagnostic validity. Moreover, many such "signs" in inventories are better investigated by more detailed neuropsychological testing.

We believe that with the growth of clinical neuropsychology as a discipline, a compendium of tests is essential, if only to guide the reader through the maze of published and unpublished tests and to form a common base of reference for the user and the researcher who wants to refer to available studies of validity, reliability, and norms.

For each test entry, information is provided under the following headings listed in the actual order of presentation: Test Name, Other Test Name(s), Purpose, Source, Description, Administration, Approximate Time for Administration, Scoring, Comment, Normative Data. Most neuropsychological tests have been developed primarily for the adult age range; however, we have included all available norms for pediatric and gerontological populations, as well as neuropsychological tests developed especially for children.

Because of the history of many of these tests, psychometric standards are not always met since procedures developed for a single experiment or a clinical routine are not necessarily backed up by a full psychometric development. Once the test is in use as a clinical instrument, however, such procedures should be adhered to. We have tried to provide as much documentation as was available at the time of writing. Notes on particular features, experiences with the test, and a comparison with similar tests are also frequently included. For unpublished tests, full descriptions of the test and test material as well as administration procedures, sample score sheets, norms, and data on reliability and validity are presented. Where copyrighted studies are used for the documentation, permission of the author and publisher has been obtained. The manual also includes a number of tests that are commercially available. These are described briefly, unless the administration manuals distributed with the test deviate from our use. Ordering information is provided, including prices most recently available to us. The user will have to

obtain the material from the publisher or distributor. However, we have furnished norms and data from other studies if they are not included in the published version of the test. We have also included the approximate time required for the administration of each test under normal conditions in order to allow the user to plan an estimated timetable for a given patient's evaluation. The time required may be considerably longer if a patient has comprehension problems or sensory or motor deficits.

A word of caution about the use of norms may be appropriate. Even if normative data have been meticulously collected for the general population, the use of such norms in populations with geographic and ethnic differences may be misleading, especially for verbal tests. Similarly, the application of such norms to special populations with suspected handicaps may lead to erroneous conclusions. For example, motor skill or motor speed in boxers with concussion may show no deficits, unless compared to norms from the same special population, i.e., other athletes.

The tests presented here constitute our most commonly used measures. Less frequently used tests are not included. Our selection of tests is deliberately eclectic: over the years, our laboratory has added and deleted many procedures, retaining what we hope is a useful selection for the practitioner. At the beginning of each section, we provide a rationale for our selections and indicate when a given test may be of particular use. Others may disagree with our selection. Nevertheless, we hope that this book will serve as a useful manual for neuropsychologists, whether they choose to use the book just for a few of the tests ancillary to their own battery, as a working manual supplementing details and norms of their own selection of tests, or as their main administration manual.

It should be explicitly stated that in our approach only a few tests are routinely used with most clients. Others are used rarely for the exploration of a specific problem. The selection presented here should not be mistakenly construed as a "battery." Our choice of tests is tailored to the specific questions raised in an individual's assessment.

Most tests allow administration by a psychometrician although we do not advocate "blind" interpretation: the psychometrician administers tests carefully selected by the clinician in light of the referral question after the initial interview. The test selection for a given patient is revised as the results of earlier tests are considered midway through the examination. Some tests are self-administered, some of them by desktop computer; however, the same principles of test selection apply.

For this second edition we have written new chapters on test selection, administration, and preparation of the client; report writing and informing the client; executive function; attention; occupational interest and aptitudes; and detection of malingering and symptom validity testing. Several tests have been added, others deleted, but all sections were carefully updated. We have included a note on tests for which computer administration or interpretation programs are available, but the reader should carefully consider our comments on computer use in the section on report writing. We have avoided the temptation to extend this volume into a general handbook or manual on neuropsychological assessment. These topics are well covered by Lezak (1995) and Puente and McCaffrey (1992). Since the publication of the first edition of this book, much additional normative data and many other studies have become available. Erickson et al. (1994) provide a list of references for normative studies of cognitive tests for older adults, and Heaton, Grant, and Matthews (1991) offer a collection of normative data for the Halstead-Reitan battery of tests.

We would like to express our gratitude to many colleagues in other institutions and to several former Victoria students who generously shared their published or unpublished data with us and frequently provided additional helpful comments. A special note of thanks goes to Maxine Stovel and our graduate students who helped us with a preliminary version of this second edition of the "Victoria Manual" and clarified many points of test administration and use of norms.

Victoria, B.C.   O.S.
Aug 1997   E.S.

References

Erickson, R.C., Eimon, P., & Hebben, N. (1994). A listing of references to cognitive test norms for older adults. In M. Storandt & G. R. VandenBos (Eds.), *Neuropsychological Assessment of Dementia and Depression*. Washington, D.C.: American Psychological Association.

Golden, C.J. (1980). *Luria-Nebraska Neuropsychological Battery—Children's Revision*. Los Angeles, CA: Western Psychological Services.

Golden, C.J., Hammeke, T.A., & Purisch, A.D. (1976). *Luria-Nebraska Neuropsychological Battery*. Los Angeles, CA: Western Psychological Services.

Goodglass, H., & Kaplan, E. (1983). *The Assessment of Aphasia and Related Disorders*. (2nd Ed.). Philadelphia: Lea & Febiger.

Harley, J.P., Leuthold, C.A., Matthews, C.G., & Bergs, L.E. (1980). *Wisconsin Neuropsychological Test Battery T-Score Norms for Older Veterans Administration Medical Center Patients*. Mimeo. Madison, WI: Department of Neurology, University of Wisconsin.

Heaton, R.K., Grant, I., & Matthews, C.G. (1991). *Comprehensive Norms for an Expanded Halstead-Reitan Battery: Demographic Corrections, Research Findings, and Clinical Applications*. Odessa, FL: Psychological Assessment Resources.

Jarvis, P.E., & Barth, J.T. (1994). *The Halstead-Reitan Neuropsychological Battery: A Guide to Interpretation and Clinical Applications*. Odessa, FL: Psychological Assessment Resources.

Kertesz, A. (1982). *Western Aphasia Battery Test. Manual*. New York: Grune & Stratton.

Lezak, M.D. (1995). *Neuropsychological Assessment* (3rd ed.). New York: Oxford University Press.

Pimental, P.A., & Kingsburg, N.A. (1989). *Mini Inventory of Right Brain Injury*. Austin, TX: Pro-Ed.

Porch, B. (1967, 1973). *The Porch Index of Communicative Ability, Vol. 1, 2*. Palo Alto: Consulting Psychologists Press.

Puente, A.E., & McCaffrey, R.J. (Eds.) (1992). *Handbook of Neuropsychological Assessment*. New York: Plenum Press.

Trites, R.L. (1977, 1985). *Neuropsychological Test Manual*. Ottawa, Ont.: Royal Ottawa Hospital.

Contents

List of Abbreviations

AAMD   American Association on Mental Deficiency
ABCD   Arizona Battery for Communication Disorders of Dementia
ACID   Arithmetic-Coding-Information-Digit Span WISC pattern
ACoA   Aneurysm of the anterior communicating artery
AD   Alzheimer's disease (see also DAT)
ADL   activities of daily living
AL   Associate Learning (WMS subtest)
AMI   Autobiographical Memory Interview
AMNART American New Adult Reading Test
APM   Advanced Progressive Matrices
AVLT   Auditory-Verbal Learning Test (= RAVLT)

BADS   Behavioral Assessment of the Dyexecutive Syndrome
BASA   Boston Assessment of Severe Aphasia
BDAE   Boston Diagnostic Aphasia Examination
BDI   Beck Depression Inventory
BNT   Boston Naming Test
BSID-II Bayley Scales of Infant Development
BTA   Brief Test of Attention
BVMT-R Brief Visuospatial Memory Test—Revised
BVRT-R Benton Visual Retention Test—Revised

CADL   Communication Abilities in Daily Living
CAI   Cancer Assessment Inventory
CBCL   Child Behavior Checklist
CCC   consonant trigrams
CCT   Children's Category Test
CDI   Children's Depression Inventory
CELF-3 Clinical Evaluation of Language Fundamentals—3
CET   Cognitive Estimation Test
CFT   Rey-Osterrieth Complex Figures Test (= CF)
CHI   closed head injury
CLTR   consistent long-term retrieval (Buschke)
CLTS   consistent long-term storage (Buschke)
CNT   Colorado Neuropsychology Tests
COWA   Controlled Oral Word Association (Word Fluency)
CPM   Colored Progressive Matrices

CPT	Continuous Performance Test
CRS	Conner's Rating Scale
CRVET	Comprehension and Expressive Vocabulary Test
CST	California Sorting Test
CTT	Color Trails Test
CVA	cerebrovascular accident
CVLT	California Verbal Learning Test
d2	Concentration Endurance Test
DAT	Dementia of the Alzheimer type (= AD)
DRS	Dementia Rating Scale
DSF	Digit Span, forward
DSR	Digit Span, reversed
DSM IV	Diagnostic and Statistical Manual of Mental Disorders, 4th ed.
DSp	Digit Span
EST	estimated
FAS	Controlled Oral Word Association (Word Fluency)
FIT	Fifteen Item Test
FSIQ	Full Scale IQ
FOT	Finger Oscillation Test (= FTT)
FP	Form Perception
FTT	Finger Tapping Test (= FOT)
GATB	General Aptitude Test Battery
GDS	Geriatric Depression Scale
GNDS	General Neuropsychological Deficit Scale
HCT	Halstead Category Test
HD	Huntington's disease
H-R	Halstead-Reitan
IBRS	Infant Behavior Rating Scale
IMC	Information Memory Concentration Test
ITPA	Illinois Test of Psycholinguistic Abilities
K-ABC	Kaufman Assessment Battery for Children
K-BIT	Kaufman Brief Intelligence Test
LAMB	Learning and Memory Battery
LM	Logical Memory (WMS subtest)
LTR	long-term retrieval (Buschke)
LTS	long-term storage (Buschke)
MAE	Multilingual Aphasia Examination
MC	Mental Control (WMS subtest)
MCDI	Minnesota Child Development Inventory
MDI	Mental Development Index (BSID Index)
MDRS	Mattis Dementia Rating Scale

MMPI-2	Minnesota Multiphasic Personality Inventory-2
MMSE	Mini-Mental State Examination
MOANS	Mayo's Older Americans Normative Studies
MPRI	Mayo Percent Retention Index
MQ	Memory Quotient (WMS)
MS	Memory Span (WMS subtest)
NAART	North-American Adult Reading Test
NART	National Adult Reading Test
NBAP	Neuropsychology Behavior and Affect Profile
NCCEA	Neurosensory Comprehensive Examination for Aphasia
NIS	Neuropsychological Impairment Scale
NRS	Neurobehavioral Rating Scale
OPIE	Oklahoma Premorbid Intelligence Estimate
OR	Orientation (WMS subtest)
PAI	Personality Assessment Inventory
PAL	Paired Associate Learning (WMS subtest)
PASAT	Paced Auditory Serial Addition Test
PCI	Personal and Current Information (WMS subtest)
PD	Parkinson's disease
PDI	Psychomotor Development Index
PET	positron emission tomography
PIAT-R	Peabody Individual Achievement Test—Revised
PIC	Personality Inventory for Children
PIQ	Performance IQ
POMS	Profile of Mood States
PPVT-R	Peabody Picture Vocabulary Test—Revised
PR	percentile rank
PTSD	Posttraumatic Stress Disorder
RAVLT	Rey Auditory-Verbal Learning Test
RBMT	Rivermead Behavioral Memory Test
RF	Rey Figure Test (= CF)
RLTR	random long-term retrieval (Buschke)
RMI	Relative Mastery Index (WJ-R ACH scoring system)
RMT	Recognition Memory Test
RPM	Raven's Progressive Matrices
SAS	standard age score (SBIS scoring system)
SBIS	Stanford-Binet Intelligence Scale
SBIS-R	Stanford-Binet Intelligence Scale-Revised
SCT	Short Category Test
SD	standard deviation
SDMT	Symbol Digit Modalities Test
SDRT	Stanford Diagnostic Reading Test
SEM	Standard Error of Measurement
SOMPA	System of Multicultural Pluralistic Assessment

SPM	Standard Progressive Matrices
SRT	Selective Reminding Test (Buschke)
STR	Short-Term Recall (Buschke)
TAT	Thematic Apperception Test
TBI	traumatic brain injury
TOMM	Test of Memory Malingering
3-D	Three-dimensional Block Construction
3-MS	Modified Mini-Mental State Examination
TOLD	Test of Language Development
TPT	Tactual Performance Test
TVPS	Test of Visual-Perceptual Skills
VIQ	Verbal IQ
VMI	Developmental Test of Visuo-Motor Integration (Beery Test)
VOT	Hooper Visual Organization Test
VR	Visual Reproduction (WMS subtest)
VRT	Visual Retention Test (= BVRT)
VSAT	Visual Search and Attention Test
WAIS-R	Wechsler Adult Intelligence Test—Revised
WAIS-R NI	Wechsler Adult Intelligence Scale—Revised as a Neuropsychological Instrument
WCST	Wisconsin Card Sorting Test
WHO	World Health Organization
WIAT	Wechsler Individual Achievement Test
WISC-III	Wechsler Intelligence Scale for Children, 3rd ed.
WJ-ACH	Woodcock-Johnson Psychoeducational Battery—Revised Tests of Achievement
WMS	Wechsler Memory Scale
WMS-R	Wechsler Memory Scale—Revised
WPPSI-III	Wechsler Primary and Preschool Scale of Intelligence, 3rd ed.
WPT	Wonderlic Personnel Test
WRAML	Wide Range Achievement of Memory and Learning
WRAT3	Wide Range Achievement Test-3

A COMPENDIUM OF
NEUROPSYCHOLOGICAL
TESTS

1

History Taking

The patient's account of the problem and the patient's behavior during the interview can provide a wealth of information regarding the presence, nature, and impact of cognitive disturbances. Consequently, taking a detailed history is essential to the neuropsychological evaluation and often invaluable since it may yield important clues to a correct diagnosis, to the effects of the disorder on daily life, and to decisions regarding rehabilitative interventions. Sometimes the patient's account must be supplemented by information from other people because the patient's statements may prove misleading with regard to both the gravity of the symptoms and the time course of their evolution. For example, patients with a memory disorder or who lack insight are likely to be poor informants.

Competent history taking is a skill that requires, in addition to a broad knowledge of neuropsychology, an awareness of interactions that may occur in interview situations. Often patients are tense and concerned about their symptoms. The clinician's job is to put the patient at ease and to convey that the assessment is a collaborative venture to determine the presence, nature, and impact of the problem. The patient should be encouraged to relate the history in an unhurried manner. Introductory questions such as "What brings you in? How can I help you? Tell me about your problem" may be useful.

History taking does not follow a fixed format. Rather, the choice of questions and their order of presentation are guided by the patient's account. During this account, the following information should be obtained: basic descriptive data (age, marital status, etc.), description of the illness (nature of onset, duration, physical, intellectual and emotional changes), relevant past medical history, relevant family history, educational and vocational history, and the effect of the disorder on daily life and personal relations. In addition, with a view toward future management and rehabilitation, the clinician should obtain information on the compensatory techniques that the patient uses to negotiate impairments, and to reduce or solve problems. Because compensatory strategies rely on functions that are relatively intact, the clinician should also identify the patient's resources and strengths. At the end of the history, the clinician may wish to go over the material with the patient to ensure that the details are correct and to check for additional information. Informal test questions about a patient's orientation and ability to recall current events, TV shows, local politics, or geography may be included in the interview.

We use two questionnaires, one designed for adult patients (Fig. 1–1) and the other (adapted from M. Ehrenberg) for use with parents when children are clients (Fig. 1–2). These questionnaires should be used only as guides, not as a substitute for the interview, although the child questionnaire may in some cases be filled out by the parent prior to the

PERSONAL HISTORY:

Name _____ Sex M _____ F _____

Address _____

Phone No. _____

Date of Birth _____ Age _____

Date tested _____

Referred by _____

Referral question _____

Reason for referral (as reported by patient) _____
_____
_____
_____

Family doctor _____

Other specialists _____

Place of birth _____ Native language _____

Handedness _____

Education _____

Special training _____

School problems (any failures) _____
_____
_____

Occupation _____

Current or last job _____

Previous work history _____

Marital status S _____ M _____ D _____ W _____

List all children and relatives living with the patient. (Indicate their names, sex, age, relation to patient, education, occupation, their health or other problems)

Name	Sex	Age	Relationship	Education	Occupation	Health	Other
____	____	____	____	____	____	____	____
____	____	____	____	____	____	____	____
____	____	____	____	____	____	____	____
____	____	____	____	____	____	____	____

List immediate family members not living in the home (e.g., child)

Name	Sex	Age	Relationship	Education	Occupation	Health	Other
____	____	____	____	____	____	____	____
____	____	____	____	____	____	____	____
____	____	____	____	____	____	____	____
____	____	____	____	____	____	____	____

MEDICAL HISTORY:

Previous hospitalizations/operations/acidents (Description, age, length of hospital stay) _____
_____

Serious illnesses _____

History of emotional disorder _____

Any medical problems currently affecting patient (explain) _____
_____

Family history of serious illness/neurological disease/emotional disorder (explain) _____
_____

Head injuries (provide description including length of loss of consciousness, retrograde/anterograde amnesia) _____
_____
_____
_____
_____

Other cerebral damage (CVA, hemorrhage, etc.) Provide description. _____
_____
_____

Medications (type & dose) _____

Recent changes in medication _____

Alcohol consumption _____

(continued)

Drug abuse _____
Food allergies _____
Drug allergies _____
List any special test patient has completed:

Test	Age	Where done	When	Results

Hearing _____
Vision _____
EEG _____
CT Scan _____
MRI _____
Psychological _____
Speech & language _____
Other _____
Medical findings & dx: _____

PHYSICAL SYMPTOMS & CHANGES:
Note (and describe) the symptoms that are of concern:
Weakness _____
Numbness _____
Muscle tics or twitches _____
Clumsiness _____
Headache _____
Pain _____
Dizziness _____
Nausea _____
Visual defects _____
Auditory defects _____
Hear or see things that others do not _____
Problems with taste _____
Problems with smell _____
Bladder/bowel control _____
Change in appetite/weight _____
Change in sleep pattern _____
Seizures _____
Fainting spells _____
Other _____

BEHAVIORAL CONCERNS:

Unusual fears	_____	High activity level	_____
Slowed response	_____	Sexual difficulties	_____
Destructiveness	_____	Aggressiveness	_____
Irritability	_____	Restlessness	_____
Excessive sadness	_____	Defiance	_____
Self-destructive	_____	Immature behavior	_____
Stubbornness	_____	Eating problems	_____
Sleep problems	_____	Mood swings	_____
Overly compliant	_____	Nightmares	_____
Suicidal thoughts	_____	Easily frustrated	_____
Isolated	_____	Withdrawn	_____

Problems in driving _____
Other _____

INTELLECTUAL CONCERNS:
General intellectual level _____
Difficulty with planning/organization _____
Difficulty completing an activity _____
Difficulty adapting to changes (rigid) _____
Inability to concentrate _____
Easily distracted _____
Impulsive _____
Difficulty learning or remembering _____
Difficulty with comprehension _____
Difficulty with expression _____
Gets lost easily _____
Difficulty with writing _____
Difficulty with reading _____
Difficulty with mathematics/handling money _____
Periods of confusion/disorientation _____
Slowed thought processes _____
Other _____

(continued)

5

PSYCHOSOCIAL CONCERNS:
Any change in mood/personality _____

Any change in ability to handle household chores or job _____

Any change in the way patient gets along with wife/husband/family members _____

Any change in social activities _____

ADDITIONAL DESCRIPTION:
Are symptoms/complaints static or getting worse _____

What is the patient's best guess as to why the symptoms/complaints are happening _____
CONSEQUENCES:
Has daily living at home, at work, or in social situations been affected by the complaints? How. _____

How does patient/caregiver get the problem(s) to stop or to be less intense/frequent/of shorter duration.
_____
_____
_____
_____

Figure 1—1. History questionnaire for adult patients.

This questionnaire was developed to obtain basic information about your *child* so that we can make the best use of our time together. You are not likely to remember every detail of your child's development, so it is not necessary to spend a lengthy period of time struggling with a particular point. Whatever information you may be able to provide will be helpful. If there are any specific questions that seem unclear, please mark them so that they can be clarified during our interview.

PERSONAL HISTORY:
Child's name _____ Sex M _____ F _____
Address _____
Date of Birth _____ Age _____
Date Tested _____
Phone No._____ Mo (wk) _____ Fa (wk) _____
Referred by _____
Family physician _____
Other specialists _____
Was this child adopted   Yes (when) _____ No _____
FAMILY COMPOSITION:
Please list all other children and relatives living with the child. Indicate their names, sex, age, relation to child, education, occupation, their health or other problems.

Name	Sex	Age	Relationship	Education	Occupation	Health	Other
____	___	___	_____	_____	_____	_____	_____
____	___	___	_____	_____	_____	_____	_____
____	___	___	_____	_____	_____	_____	_____

Please list immediate family members not living in the home (e.g., biological parent)

Name	Sex	Age	Relationship	Education	Occupation	Health	Other
____	___	___	_____	_____	_____	_____	_____
____	___	___	_____	_____	_____	_____	_____
____	___	___	_____	_____	_____	_____	_____

IDENTIFICATION OF PROBLEM:
Please describe in your own words the problem for which you are seeking advice:
_____
_____
_____

What do you think is the cause of this problem?
_____
_____
_____

(continued)

To date, what steps have been taken to deal with your concerns?
_____
_____

How has the problem affected your family?
_____
_____

One problem may be related to or influenced by another family problem. Has your family experienced any of the following circumstances in the past two years?

Separation _____   Illness of family member _____
Divorce _____   Change of residence _____
Change of school _____   Loss/Change of job _____
Addition to family _____   Financial stress _____
Legal problems _____   Other stress (specify) _____
How do you get the problem(s) to stop or to be less intense/frequent/shorter in duration _____
_____
_____
_____

MEDICAL HISTORY:
Pregnancy with this child:
Were there any complications with your pregnancy with the referred child (e.g., anemia, high blood pressure, toxemia, diabetes, infections, hospitalizations, etc.)?
_____
_____
_____

Were any medications/drugs used during pregnancy? If yes, please explain.
_____
Length of pregnancy. _____
Number of previous pregnancies: _____   Any complications? _____
_____

Birth History:
Length of labor. _____
Complications during birth:
Induced _____
C-Section _____
Forceps _____
Fetal distress _____
Breech (feet first) _____
Twins _____
Other (e.g., breathing problems, cord around neck).
_____
_____

Newborn:
Birth weight _____
Length of hospital stay _____
Following delivery, was the baby:
Blue at birth _____
Required oxygen _____
Had jaundice _____
Required phototherapy _____
Had seizures _____
Other. _____
Was medication used? _____ Yes   No   If yes, reason _____
_____

Were there problems with:

Sucking	_____	Colic	_____	Crying	_____	Sleeping _____
Feeding	_____	Vomiting	_____	Food refusal	_____	Apnea _____
Weight gain	_____					(stops breathing)

Childhood:
Has your child ever experienced:

Very high fever	_____	Polio	_____	Dizzy spells	_____
Measles	_____	Whooping Cough	_____	Frequent colds	_____
Mumps	_____	Chickenpox	_____	Scarlet Fever	_____
Seizures	_____	Asthma	_____	Freq. ear infect.	_____
Meningitis	_____	Encephalitis	_____	Head injuries	_____
Heart Disease	_____	Migraines	_____	Headaches	_____
AIDS	_____	Visual defects	_____	Hearing defects	_____
Other.	_____				

(continued)

Food allergies. _____

Drug allergies. _____

Are there any medical problems currently affecting your child? If yes, please explain.
_____
_____
_____

Is your child currently receiving medication (specify) _____

Does your child miss school frequently because of illness? How frequently in the past year? _____

Please indicate any hospitalizations/accidents/operations your child has experienced:

Description   Age   Length of hospital stay
_____
_____
_____

Please list any special tests your child has completed:

Test	Age	Where done	When	Results
Hearing				
Vision				
EEG				
CT scan				
MRI				
Allergies				
Psychological				
Speech & language				
Psycho-educational				
Other				

FAMILY MEDICAL HISTORY:

What serious physical, neurological, or psychiatric illnesses or accidents has your family had to deal with?

Name	Diagnosis	Year began	Duration of treatment	Present condition

Do any illnesses run in your family? (Please specify)
_____
_____

DEVELOPMENTAL

Please indicate your child's age when she/he achieved the following developmental milestones:

Milestone	Child's age
Sat alone	_____
Walked alone	_____
Toilet training	_____
Spoke 2 or 3 words together	_____

Do you have any early concerns about your child's development in any of the following skills?

	Yes	No
Gross motor (walking, running, physical activities)	____	____
Fine motor (use of pencil, manipulation of objects)	____	____
Speech & language (comprehension, expression)	____	____
Cognitive development (intelligence/ability to plan)	____	____
Social development (play, social skills, peer interaction)	____	____
Independent functioning (eating, dressing self)	____	____

Are any of these developmental areas still of concern to you now? _____

If so, please explain _____

PHYSICAL CONCERNS

Please note (and describe) only the symptoms that are **currently** of concern to you:

Weakness _____

Numbness _____

Clumsiness _____

Headache _____

Pain _____

Dizziness _____

Nausea _____

Visual defects _____

Auditory defects _____

Hear or see things others do not _____

Problems with taste _____

Problems with smell _____

Bladder/bowel control _____

Seizures _____

(continued)

Fainting spells _____
Other _____

BEHAVIORAL CONCERNS:

Please check only the behaviors that are **currently** of concern to you:

Temper tantrums	_____	Thumbsucking	_____
Sexual difficulties	_____	Breath holding	_____
Muscle tics	_____	Fear of separation	_____
Unusual fears	_____	High activity level	_____
Destructiveness	_____	Fire setting	_____
Aggressiveness	_____	Lying	_____
Restlessness	_____	Stealing	_____
Excessive sadness	_____	Defiance	_____
Cruelty to animals/children	_____	Self-destructive behavior	_____
Stubbornness	_____	Eating problems	_____
Sleep problems	_____	Mood swings	_____
Overly compliant	_____	Nightmares	_____
Night terrors	_____	Drug/alcohol use	_____
Immature behavior	_____	Truancy	_____
Suicidal thoughts	_____	Easily frustrated	_____
Isolated	_____	Withdrawn	_____
Slowed response	_____		

Others. _____

INTELLECTUAL CONCERNS:

Please check only the areas that are **currently** of concern to you:

General intellectual level	_____
Difficulty with planning/organization	_____
Difficulty completing an activity	_____
Difficulty adapting to changes (rigid)	_____
Inability to concentrate	_____
Easily distracted	_____
Impulsive	_____
Difficulty learning or remembering	_____
Difficulty with comprehension	_____
Difficulty with expression	_____
Gets lost easily	_____
Periods of confusion/disorientation	_____
Difficulty with writing	_____
Difficulty with reading	_____
Difficulty with math/handling money	_____

Other _____

CHILD MANAGEMENT:

Who ordinarily manages/disciplines your child? _____

What have you found to be the most effective methods for managing/disciplining your child (using rewards, taking away privileges, isolation, spanking, etc.)?

_____
_____

How does your child react to discipline? _____

SCHOOL EXPERIENCES:

Schools Attended	Location	Grades	Grade failures

Has your child received or been involved in any of the following?

	Grade/Age
Learning disabilities/special education class	_____
Behavior adjustment class	_____
Tutoring	_____
Summer school	_____
Enrichment gifted	_____
Language immersion	_____
Other	_____

Are you satisfied with your child's present school program? _____ Yes _____ No

Comments _____

(continued)

Does your child:
Like school _____ Yes _____ No
Like teachers _____ Yes _____ No
Get along with peers _____ Yes _____ No
List school problems that are of concern to you:

_____

ADDITIONAL COMMENTS:
Describe what you see as your child's personal strengths (strong points):

_____
_____

Please provide any additional information that you feel is relevant to this referral:

_____
_____
_____

This form was completed by:
    Mother _____ Father _____ Both _____ Other _____
Signature _____
Date completed _____

Figure 1—2. History questionnaire for parents of child patients.

interview. In this case, the interview can focus on the major questions concerning the child and need not touch on minor details already provided by the parent.

During the interview, additional, diagnostically valuable information can be gleaned from (1) general appearance (e.g., eye contact, modulation of face and voice, personal hygiene, habits of dress), (2) motor activity (e.g., hemiplegia, tics, tenseness, hyper- or hypokinesia), (3) mood, (4) degree of cooperation, and (5) abnormalities in language, prosody, or memory.

Questionnaires have been designed to screen patients for head injury (e.g., Philadelphia Head Injury Questionnaire). How-ever, these are not recommended because they lack information regarding reliability and validity (Albanese, 1994; Deardorff, 1994).

References

Albanese, M. (1994). Review of the Philadelphia Head Injury Questionnaire. In J.C. Conoley & J.C. Impara (Eds.), *Supplement to the Eleventh Mental Measurements Yearbook*. Lincoln, Nebraska: Buros Institute, pp. 177–178.

Deardorff, W.W. (1994). Review of the Philadelphia Head Injury Questionnaire. In J.C. Conoley & J.C. Impara (Eds.), *Supplement to the Eleventh Mental Measurements Yearbook*. Lincoln, Nebraska: Buros Institute, pp. 178–179.

2

Test Selection and Administration, and Preparation of the Client

Test Selection

To select tests for a given client, it is crucial that the neuropsychologist be fully familiar with the range of available tests and their purposes. McKinlay (1992) cites the case of an inexperienced psychologist who relied on only a measure of general intelligence and a memory test. The results of such a limited selection can be seriously misleading. On the other hand, a fixed test battery, such as the Halstead-Reitan battery, may be overly time-consuming and leaves little room for in-depth testing in areas of specific deficits. In our practice, the selection of tests for a given client is often open-ended, i.e., not all tests to be given in a particular case are determined in advance. Rather, some basic tests are given first, based on the information available about the client's problem. These usually include an intelligence test appropriate for the age of the client and several short screening tests in the areas of presumed deficit, i.e., tests of memory, concentration/attention, etc. Further tests are selected after a review of the results of the broad-band initial testing, of the client's complaints, and of behavior during testing. Occasionally, it is obvious that the client fatigues easily or is likely to fail more demanding tests. In that case, the selection of additional tests is critical and must focus directly on the target problems and the client's capacity to work with the examiner.

Our eclectic test selection usually precludes the use of "impairment indices" resulting from fixed test batteries (e.g., the General Neuropsychological Deficit Scale, Reitan & Wolfson, 1988; Oestreicher & O'Donnell, 1995). Such indices have become more and more obsolete as neuropsychology has moved away from the "organic or not organic" question, which is better answered by neuroradiologic and electrophysiologic techniques. Instead, neuropsychology has moved toward a detailed description of the nature of the deficit, its impact on daily living, and its rehabilitation. Sweet et al. (1996) report that, according to a survey of 184 neuropsychologists in 1984 and 279 neuropsychologists in 1994, the fixed battery use has dwindled from 18% to 14%, while all other clinicians preferred a "flexible approach."

A recent addition to the fixed batteries is the Mayo Cognitive Factor Scales, designed for elderly patients and including an empirically derived selection of 17 subtests from the WAIS-R, the Wechsler Memory Scale—Revised, and the Rey Auditory-Verbal Learning Test (Ivnik et al., 1994). The test battery targets reasonably stable factors of verbal comprehension, perceptual organization, attention/concentration, learning, and retention. Smith et al. (1994) present norms and corrections for education for the composite sum of the factor scales, which may be useful for screening elderly subjects, especially if detection of dementia is desired.

Although many neuropsychologists prefer to administer the tests personally, test administration by a well-trained psychometrician is widely accepted. Sweet et al.'s (1996) survey showed that between 59% and 69% of neuropsychologists use a psychometrician. However, almost all (97%) conducted the interview personally, and 78% observed the patient during all of the testing. The administration of projective tests like the Rorschach or the TAT, although never used by 33% of the sample of the survey, is usually conducted by the clinician.

Computer administration of tests is becoming popular. To start with, close supervision is needed for computer-administered tests in order to ensure that the patient is able to follow instructions properly to provide valid results. Note that computer-administered tests do not necessarily provide identical or even similar results as the same test administered by an examiner in person (Van Schijndel & Van der Vlugt, 1992). Hence, the existing normative data may not be applicable. A study by Beaumont and French (1987; French & Beaumont, 1987) compared automated and standard forms of eight tests in 367 subjects: While some tests, including Raven's Progressive Matrices, the Mill Hill Vocabulary Test, and Eysenck's Personality Questionnaire showed acceptable reliability, others, especially the Digit Span Test and the Differential Aptitude Test, produced quite low reliabilities. The authors concluded that some tests were not amenable to automation.

Neuropsychological Assessment and the Client

Relatively little attention has been paid to the consumer side of neuropsychological assessments. In order to get the maximum benefit to the client, however, the neuropsychologist should be prepared to follow some of the basic rules that emerged from a mail follow-up of 129 outpatients seen in five Australian cen-

ters. These rules would seem to apply equally to other geographic locations (Bennett-Levy et al., 1994):

1. Clients are usually not prepared for what to expect during an assessment. Sixty percent of the clients in the study had no information on what to expect or were unaware that the assessment could take up to 3 hours. This can be remedied by educating referring agents, by sending an informative letter prior to the assessment, and by providing a detailed introduction prior to the beginning of testing.

2. Clients should be given an adequate rationale for the tests so that they can see the relevance of the tests to their own situation in daily life.

3. Feedback on strengths and problem areas with suggestions about how to get around problem areas is essential.

4. Inviting a relative to accompany the client may be beneficial to alleviate anxiety, but may also help in history taking and in the informing interview. In most cases, the accompanying person should be interviewed separately to avoid embarrassment to both client and interviewee. Also, the discrepancies between statements made by the informant and the client may provide clues about the client's insight or awareness of deficits, and about the effects of such deficits on daily functioning.

5. Alleviate anxiety in the client as much as possible. The testing experience can have a significant impact on self-confidence. Reassurance that not all items of a test can be completed by most clients, or that on some tests (e.g., Rorschach, MMPI-2) there are no "correct" answers should be provided routinely. Most clients understand that a test contains high-difficulty items to avoid a ceiling effect for very bright subjects.

6. Provide a comfortable testing environment and ask the client how it can be made more comfortable. More than 90% of clients in the Bennett-Levy study mentioned that it was too hot, too cold, or too noisy. Some clients complain of backache; the availability of a back support may alleviate these complaints. Children should be provided with appropriately sized desks and chairs.

7. Provide adequate rest breaks and hot

and cold refreshments. Usually, a break after 1¹/₂ hours of testing is indicated.

8. Offer the client the choice of a one-session assessment, or a split one. Seventy-two per cent of clients in the Bennett-Levy study stated that, for a 3-hour assessment, they would have preferred two sessions instead of one.

In situations where the client is a third party, i.e., in forensic assessments where the psychologist works for the defendant or insurer, ostensibly "against" the client, the client should be assured that the aim of the assessment is to provide a valid picture of his or her strengths and weaknesses. The client should be encouraged to cooperate fully to avoid misleading results. There is some evidence (e.g., Johnson & Lesniak-Karpiak, 1997) that warning clients that it may be possible to detect exaggeration of deficits on neuropsychological tests may reduce malingering behavior.

We rarely encounter clients who refuse outright to collaborate, but occasionally they may show lack of effort, trying to "get it over with." In such cases, a repeated brief discussion of the purpose of the assessment and/or a break is indicated. If a client refuses to cooperate on a given test, switching to a very different test may be an option. General refusal to cooperate, though extremely rare, should be accepted by the examiner, who then discontinues the session. In such cases, offer the client a face-saving way out of the situation, by assuring him or her that the tests can be scheduled at another time when the client feels better.

When testing children or adolescents, it is especially important to establish good rapport. As with adults, an attitude of acceptance, understanding, and respect for the client is more important than entertaining tricks to create and maintain rapport. Older children may experience the testing as similar to a school test situation, which may evoke fear of failure and anxiety. Reassurance and encouragement for the effort may work better than praise for the results of the effort because most tests progress from easy to difficult items where failure is inevitable (Sattler, 1990). Younger children and children with behavior problems may try to manipulate the examiner

by asking questions, refusing to answer, getting up, constantly asking for breaks, or even exhibiting open hostility or leaving the testing room. This can be avoided by changing the test material to a different test or to tasks with which the client is more comfortable. The examiner should keep in mind that the behavior of the child does not reflect on the examiner, but shows a manner of "coping" that the child may use in similar situations. An examiner inexperienced with children may wish to call in a colleague who regularly works with children. Open confrontation ("Do you want to do this, or should I send you back to your parents?")—although it may work in some cases—should be avoided unless the examiner is convinced that the child is probably untestable. This may be the only course of action in children with marked deficit in attention and motivation, or with active psychosis.

Storandt (1994) discusses characteristics of elderly clients that may affect the progress and the results of the assessment. The overly loquacious client may frequently stray off-target and may relay long personal stories while being tested. For this type of client, Storandt recommends a pleasant but businesslike attitude on the part of the examiner, deferring all discussions to the end of the session, explaining that during testing there is much to be covered. In contrast, the depressed or despondent client may require considerable encouragement and patience from the examiner (and also more time). Other personality types frequently encountered in testing older adults are the "sage", the "matriarch/patriarch," and the "perfect grandparent." In all such cases, it is important that the examiner maintain a friendly, neutral attitude rather than submit to countertransference (viewing the elderly client as a parent).

Test Modifications and Testing Patients with English as a Second Language

With handicapped patients, it is often necessary to modify standard testing procedures, either by allowing more time or by using modifications of the response mode (e.g., pointing rather than giving a verbal response). Most modifications invalidate the existing norms although they may lead to valid inferences. This should be clearly stated in the report, and any conclusions should be qualified appropriately.

The client with English as a second language deserves specific considerations. Even though the client's English may appear fully fluent, some first-language habits, such as silent counting and spelling in the first language, frequently persist, and these habits may invalidate some test results that require related skills (e.g., digit repetition, recitation of the alphabet). Even more problems are posed by the patient with poor English and different cultural experiences; these conditions may invalidate not only verbal tests, but also so-called nonverbal tests with complex instructions. The psychologist may wish to resort to an interpreter, but good practice suggests that the client be referred to a colleague who is fully fluent in that language. Acculturation effects have been reported even for seemingly nonverbal tasks, such as the TPT, Seashore Rhythm, and Category Test (Arnold et al., 1994). It should be noted that a simple translation of English-language tests may distort the results, especially in the case of verbal tests that may be much more difficult or much easier in translation, thus invalidating the available norms. In addition, item and construct bias may be present: Van de Vijver and Hambleton (1996) developed a number of guidelines for this situation. This problem is particularly prominent when testing older adults (Loewenstein et al., 1994). The use of foreign-language versions of existing tests (e.g., the WAIS-R is available in a large number of foreign adaptations) may be appropriate, but this approach may also lead to problems: A test adapted and standardized for Spain or France may not contain items appropriate for Spanish-speaking American immigrants or for Quebec francophones, nor would the published norms for such tests be valid. Fortunately, some Spanish-language versions have been developed for the Hispanic U.S. population (WAIS-R, PPVT-R). These are listed together with foreign adaptations in the test descriptions of this book. A recent publication (Ponton et al., 1996) also offers a Neuropsychological Screening Battery for Hispanics, including Spanish adaptations for

10 neuropsychological tests available from the author (Harbor–UCLA Medical Center, Bld. F–9, 1000 W. Carson Street, Torrance, CA 90509). For a full discussion of testing Hispanic clients, see Ardila et al. (1994) and Geisinger (1992).

References

Ardila, A., Rosselli, M., & Puente, A.E. (1994). *Neuropsychological Evaluation of the Spanish Speaker*. New York: Plenum.

Arnold, B.R., Montgomery, G.T., Castaneda, I., et al. (1994). Acculturation and performance of Hispanics on selected Halstead-Reitan neuropsychological tests. *Assessment*, *1*, 239–248.

Beaumont, J.G. & French, C.C. (1987). A clinical field study of eight automated psychometric procedures: The Leicester/DHS project. *International Journal of Man-Machine Studies*, *26*, 661–682.

Bennett-Levy, J., Klein-Boonschate, M.A., Batchelor, J., McCarter, R., & Walton, N. (1994). Encounters with Anna Thompson: The consumer's experience of neuropsychological assessments. *Clinical Neuropsychologist*, *8*, 219–238.

French, C.C. & Beaumont, J.G. (1987). The reaction of psychiatric patients to computerized assessment. *British Journal of Clinical Psychology*, *26*, 267–278.

Geisinger, K.F. (Ed.) (1992). *Psychological Testing of Hispanics*. Washington, D.C.: American Psychological Association.

Ivnik, R.J., Smith, G.E., Malec, J.F., Kokmen, E., & Tangalos, E.G. (1994). Mayo Cognitive Factor Scales: Distinguishing normal and clinical samples by profile variability. *Neuropsychology*, *8*, 203–209.

Johnson, J.L. & Lesniak-Karpiak, K. (1997). The effect of warning on malingering on memory and motor tasks in college samples. *Archives of Clinical Neuropsychology*, *12*, 231–238.

Loewenstein, D.A., Arguelles, T., Arguelles, S., & Lynn-Fuente, P. (1994). Potential cultural bias in the neuropsychological assessment of the older adult. *Journal of Clinical and Experimental Neuropsychology*, *16*, 623–629.

McKinlay, W.W. (1992). Assessment of the head-injured for compensation. In J.R. Crawford, D.M. Parker & W.M. McKinlay (Eds.), *A Handbook of Neuropsychological Assessment*. Hillsdale, NJ: Lawrence Erlbaum, pp. 381–392.

Oestreicher, J.M. & O'Donnell, J.P. (1995). Validation of the General Neuropsychological Deficit Scale with nondisabled, learning-disabled, and head-injured young adults. *Archives of Clinical Neuropsychology, 10*, 185–191.

Ponton, M.O., Satz, P., Herpara, L., et al. (1996). Normative data stratified by age and education for the Neuropsychological Screening Battery for Hispanics (NeSBHS). *Journal of the International Neuropsychological Society, 2*, 96–104.

Reitan, R.M., & Wolfson, D. (1988). *Traumatic Brain Injury: Recovery and Rehabilitation*. Tucson, AZ: Neuropsychology Press.

Sattler, J.M. (1990). *Assessment of Children* (3rd ed.). San Diego: J.M. Sattler.

Smith, G.E., Ivnik, R.J., Malec, J.F., Petersen, R.C., Kokmen, E., & Tangalos, E.G. (1994). Mayo Cognitive Factor Scales: Derivation of a short battery and norms for factor scores. *Neuropsychology, 8*, 194–202.

Storandt, M. (1994). General principles of assessment of older adults. In M. Storandt & G.R. VandenBos (Eds.), *Neuropsychological Assessment of Dementia and Depression*. Washington, D.C.: American Psychological Association.

Sweet, J.J., Moberg, P.J., & Westergaard, C.K. (1996). Five year follow-up survey of practices and beliefs of clinical neuropsychologists. *The Clinical Neuropsychologist, 10*, 202–221.

Van de Vijver, F. & Hambleton, R.K. (1996). Translating tests: Some practical guidelines. *European Psychologist, 1*, 89–99.

Van Schijndel, F.A.A. & van der Vlugt, H. (1992). Equivalence between classical neuropsychological tests and their computer version: Four neuropsychological tests put to the test. *Journal of Clinical and Experimental Neuropsychology, 14*, 45 (abstract).

3

Profile of Test Results
and Meaning of Scores

For the purpose of interpretation, most clinicians prepare a summary or profile sheet of the test results obtained during the neuropsychological examination. It should be stressed that such a summary is no substitute for careful analysis of the patient's problem-solving approach, actual answers, and behavior on a given test, which may reveal particular characteristics of psychopathology. However, a profile of test results can be the starting point of interpretative considerations for diagnostic and intervention and rehabilitation purposes.

For the convenience of the user, it is preferable to translate all test raw scores into standard scores, z-scores, T-scores, or percentile ranks. Our profile (Fig. 3–1, Fig. 3–2 for children), which we offer only as an example, uses percentile ranks, grouping tests by area. The test descriptions in this book or the original test manuals frequently provide age-appropriate percentile ranks. Ideally, percentile ranks are based on the actual score distributions (which may be quite skewed). Where these are not provided, deviations from the age-appropriate mean (z-scores: $\bar{X} - X / SD$) can be converted into percentile ranks by using Table 3–1, which shows the percentile ranks that correspond to portions or multiples of the standard deviation as they would be expected by the area under the normal curve (see Fig. 3–3). Suggested qualitative descriptors are also provided. If test manuals

transcribe test scores into T-scores (T = 50 + 10 z), or standard scores ($S = 100 \pm 15 [\bar{X} - X] / SD$; $z = [\bar{X} - X] / SD$), a similar conversion can be made using Table 3–1. It should be noted that such conversions are based on the assumption of a normal distribution of the ability measured, and the conversions are inappropriate if this assumption is not met. Few neuropsychological tests contain information about score distributions in a normal population. In fact, some tests are deliberately designed to measure deficit; these have a concentration of items in the low and very low range of abilities with a ceiling score appropriate for a healthy person with average abilities. Such score distributions must be considered in the interpretation of any of the tests. Since few personality tests yield scores that can be expressed in percentiles and others provide their own specially designed profile sheet, a check mark or a brief mark on the appropriate line in the profile sheet is usually sufficient.

Sensitivity and Specificity, the Meaning of Test Scores

Using the profile sheet, a score can be defined as "abnormal" (i.e., below the major part of the normal distribution of test scores) by using portions or multiples of the standard deviation or, as suggested above, by using percentile ranks. Considering the lower end of the distri-

Name _____ D.O.B. _____ Age _____ Sex _____
Education _____ Handedness _____ Tested by _____
Test Date(s) _____ Previous Testing _____

CONCEPTUAL

	Score	Age Adj.	z	%ile	z	−2 −1 ___ 0 ___ +1 +2 10 20 30 40 50 60 70 80 90
WAIS-R						
Information	____	____	____	____		
Digit Span F ____ B ____	____	____	____	____		
Vocabulary	____	____	____	____		
Arithmetic	____	____	____	____		
Comprehension	____	____	____	____		
Similarities	____	____	____	____		
Picture Completion	____	____	____	____		
Picture Arrangement	____	____	____	____		
Block Design	____	____	____	____		
Object assembly	____	____	____	____		
Digit-symbol	____	____	____	____		
Mazes	____					
V.I.Q.	____		____	____		
P.I.Q.	____		____	____		
F.S.I.Q.	____		____	____		
V.I.Q. - P.I.Q.	____		____	____		
V.I.Q. Scatter	____		____	____		
P.I.Q. Scatter	____		____	____		
F.S.I.Q. Scatter	____		____	____		
V.C.	____		____	____		
P.O.	____		____	____		
F.F.D.	____		____	____		
MMSE	____		____	____		
MDRS						
Attention	____		____	____		
Initiation/Perseveration	____		____	____		
Construction	____		____	____		
Conceptualization	____		____	____		
Memory	____		____	____		
Total	____		____	____		
Ravens Matrices (____)	____		____	____		
NAART						
V.I.Q.	____		____	____		
P.I.Q.	____		____	____		
F.S.I.Q.	____		____	____		

EXECUTIVE

WCST					
Categories	____		____	____	
Perseverative Errors	____		____	____	
F.M.S.	____		____	____	
Design Fluency (____)					
Total	____		____	____	
Perseverations	____		____	____	
HCT	____		____	____	
Stroop (form ____)	Time	Errors			
I	____	____	____	____	
II	____	____	____	____	
III	____	____	____	____	
Interference Score	____		____	____	
SOPT	____		____	____	
Other _____	____		____	____	

(continued)

ATTENTION / CONCENTRATION

	Score	Errors	z	%ile	z	-2 -1		0		$+1$ $+2$
						10 20 30 40	50	60 70	80 90	

PASAT
  2.4 sec. ____ ____ ____ ____
  2.0 sec. ____ ____ ____ ____
  1.6 sec. ____ ____ ____ ____
  1.2 sec. ____ ____ ____ ____

Trails
  A ____ ____ ____ ____
  B ____ ____ ____ ____

d2 Cancellation Test
  Total Score ____ ____ ____ ____
  Error Percentage ____ ____ ____ ____

Symbol-Digit ____ ____ ____ ____

CPT ____ ____ ____ ____

BTA ____ ____ ____ ____

Other _____ ____ ____ ____ ____

MEMORY

WMS-R
  General Memory Index ____ ____ ____
  Verbal Memory Index ____ ____ ____
  Visual memory Index ____ ____ ____
  Attention/Conc. Index ____ ____ ____
  Delayed Recall Index ____ ____ ____
  Digit Span Forward ____ ____
  Digit Span Backward ____ ____
  Visual Span Forward ____ ____
  Visual Span Backward ____ ____
  Logical Memory I ____ ____
  Logical Memory II ____ ____
  % Savings ____ ____
  Visual Reproduction I ____ ____
  Visual Reproduction II ____ ____
  % Savings ____ ____

B.V.R.T. ____ ____ ____
  Correct ____ ____ ____
  Expected Correct ____ ____ ____
  Expected Errors ____ ____ ____
  Multiple Choice ____ ____ ____

CVLT
  List A Trials 1-5 Total ____ ____ ____
  List A Trial 1 ____ ____ ____
  List A Trial 5 ____ ____ ____
  List B ____ ____ ____
  List A Short-Delay Free Recall ____ ____ ____
  List A Short-Delay Cued Recall ____ ____ ____
  List A Long-Delay Free Recall ____ ____ ____
  List A long-Delay Cued Recall ____ ____ ____
  A1 - B ____ ____ ____
  A5 - Short-Delay ____ ____ ____
  Short-Delay - Long Delay ____ ____ ____
  Recognition - A5 ____ ____ ____
  Learning Slope ____ ____ ____
  Semantic Cluster Ratio ____ ____ ____
  Serial Cluster Ratio ____ ____ ____
  Recall Consistency ____ ____ ____
  % Primacy ____ ____ ____

(continued)

	Score	Errors	z	%ile	z	−2 −1		0		+1 +2
						10 20 30 40		50 60 70 80 90		
% Middle	___		___	___						
% Recency	___		___	___						
Perseverations Total	___		___	___						
Free Recall Intrusions	___		___	___						
Recognition Hits	___		___	___						
False Positives	___		___	___						
Bias	___		___	___						
Complex Figure (Rey / Taylor)										
Copy	___		___	___						
3 min Delay	___		___	___						
30 min Delay	___		___	___						
Recognition	___			___						
Brief Visuospatial Memory Test-R										
T1	___		___	___						
T2	___		___	___						
T3	___		___	___						
T4	___		___	___						
Total Recall	___		___	___						
Learning	___		___	___						
Discrim. Index	___		___	___						
Percent Retained	___		___	___						
Other	___		___	___						

MEMORY / MOTIVATION

	Score					
Rey 15 Item	___					
VSVT						
Easy Correct	/ 24		z=	p<		
Difficult Correct	/ 24		z=	p<		
Easy Time	___		sd=			
Difficult Time	___		sd=			
Other	___					

LANGUAGE

	Score	Age Eq.	z	%ile		
Word Fluency						
F.A.S.	___		___	___		
Animals	___		___	___		
Token Test	___		___	___		
Boston Naming Test	___		___	___		
Sentence Repetition	___		___	___		
Dichotic Listening						
L. Ear	___		___	___		
R. Ear	___		___	___		
Total	___		___	___		
PPVT-R	___	___	___	___		
Other _____	___		___	___		
Other _____	___		___	___		

AUDITORY

	Score					
Reaction Time						
L. Hand	___		___	___		
R. Hand	___		___	___		

(continued)

VISUAL / VISUOSPATIAL / VISUOMOTOR

	Score	z	%ile	z	−2 −1		0		+1 +2
					10 20 30	40 50	60 70	80 90	

Reaction Time
L. Hand _____ _____ _____
R. Hand _____ _____ _____

Embedded Figures _____ _____ _____

Right-Left Orientation
Total Correct _____ _____ _____
Reversal Score _____ _____ _____

Hooper VOT _____ _____ _____

Beery   V.M.I. _____ _____ _____ _____

MOTOR

Purdue Pegboard
L   /25 _____ _____
R   /25 _____ _____
Both   /25 _____ _____
Assembly /100 _____ _____

Finger Tapping
L _____ _____ _____
R _____ _____ _____

Dynamometer
L _____ _____ _____
R _____ _____ _____

Other _____ _____ _____ _____

Other _____ _____ _____ _____

SOMESTHESIS

Finger Localization
L /30 _____ _____
R /30 _____ _____

Benton 2-D Stereognosis
L _____ _____ _____
R _____ _____ _____

Tactile Naming
L _____ _____ _____
R _____ _____ _____

Von Frey Hairs
L _____ _____ _____
R _____ _____ _____

2-Pt Aesthesiometer
L _____ _____ _____
R _____ _____ _____

T.P.T.
L   _____ _____ _____
R   _____ _____ _____
Both   _____ _____ _____
Memory   _____ _____ _____
Location _____ _____ _____

Other _____ _____ _____ _____

Other _____ _____ _____ _____

(continued)

ACHIEVEMENT

	Score	Grade	z	%ile	z	-2 -1	0	+1 +2
						10 20 30 40	50 60 70	80 90

WRAT-3
  Reading
  Spelling
  Arithmetic

W-J Achievement
  Letter/Word Identification
  Passage Comprehension
  Word Attack
  Reading Vocabulary
  Calculation
  Applied Problems
  Quantitative Concepts
  Dictation
  Writing Samples
  Writing Fluency
  Spelling
  Usage
  Handwriting
  Punct. & Capitalization

Stanford Reading (_____)
  Literal Comprehension
  Inferential Comprehension
  Reading Rate

PIAT-R - Reading Comp

Other _____

Other _____

PERSONALITY

MMPI-2 _____

M.C.M.I. _____

Beck _____

G.D.I. _____

Penn. Inventory _____

Figure 3—1. University of Victoria Psychology Clinic adult test profile form.

Name _____ D.O.B. _____ Age _____ Sex _____
Education _____ Handedness _____ Tested by _____
Test Date(s) _____ Previous Testing _____

CONCEPTUAL

	Score	z	%ile	z −2 −1 0 +1 +2
				10 20 30 40 50 60 70 80 90
WISC-III				
Information	_____	_____	_____	
Similarities	_____	_____	_____	
Arithmetic	_____	_____	_____	
Vocabulary	_____	_____	_____	
Comprehension	_____	_____	_____	
Digit Span	_____	_____	_____	
Picture Completion	_____	_____	_____	
Coding	_____	_____	_____	
Picture Arrangement	_____	_____	_____	
Block Design	_____	_____	_____	
Object Assembly	_____	_____	_____	
Symbol Search	_____	_____	_____	
Mazes	_____	_____	_____	
V.I.Q.	_____	_____	_____	
P.I.Q.	_____	_____	_____	
F.S.I.Q.	_____	_____	_____	
V.I.Q. - P.I.Q.	_____	_____	_____	
V.I.Q. Scatter	_____	_____	_____	
P.I.Q. Scatter	_____	_____	_____	
F.S.I.Q. Scatter	_____	_____	_____	
V.C.	_____	_____	_____	
P.O.	_____	_____	_____	
F.F.D.	_____	_____	_____	
P.S.	_____	_____	_____	
Raven's Matrices				
Coloured	_____	_____	_____	
Standard	_____	_____	_____	

EXECUTIVE

WCST				
Categories	_____	_____	_____	
Perseverative Errors	_____	_____	_____	
F.M.S.	_____	_____	_____	
HCT (Child / Adolescent)	_____	_____	_____	
Design Fluency (_____)				
Total	_____	_____	_____	
Perseverations	_____	_____	_____	
SOPT _____	_____	_____	_____	
Other _____	_____	_____	_____	

ATTENTION / CONCENTRATION

Trails - Intermediate				
A	_____	_____	_____	
B	_____	_____	_____	
d2 Cancellation Test				
Total Score	_____	_____	_____	
Error Percentage	_____	_____	_____	
CPT	_____	_____	_____	
Symbol-Digit	_____	_____	_____	
Other _____	_____	_____		

(continued)

22

MEMORY

	Score	z	%ile	z −2 −1 0 +1 +2 / 10 20 30 40 50 60 70 80 90

WRAML
Story Memory ____ ____ ____
Sentence memory ____ ____ ____
Number-Letter ____ ____ ____
Picture Memory ____ ____ ____
Design Memory ____ ____ ____
Fingers Windows ____ ____ ____
Verbal Learning ____ ____ ____
Sound Symbol ____ ____ ____
Visual Learning ____ ____ ____
Verbal Memory Index ____ ____ ____
Visual Memory Index ____ ____ ____
Learning Index ____ ____ ____
General Memory Index ____ ____ ____

Complex Figure (Rey / Taylor)
Copy ____ ____ ____
Recall ____ ____ ____
% Savings ____ ____ ____

B.V.R.T.
Correct ____ ____ ____
Expected Correct ____ ____ ____
Expected Errors ____ ____ ____
Multiple Choice ____ ____ ____

RAVLT TOT
Trial 1 ____ ____ ____
Trial 5 ____ ____ ____
List B ____ ____ ____
A6 ____ ____ ____
A7 ____ ____ ____
List A Recognition ____ ____ ____
List B Recognition ____ ____ ____

CVLT - Children's
List A Trials 1-5 Total ____ ____ ____
List A Trial 1 ____ ____ ____
List A Trial 5 ____ ____ ____
List B ____ ____ ____
List A Short-Delay Free Recall ____ ____ ____
List A Short-Delay Cued Recall ____ ____ ____
List A Long-Delay Free Recall ____ ____ ____
List A Long-Delay Cued Recall ____ ____ ____
Semantic Cluster Ratio ____ ____ ____
Serial Cluster Ratio ____ ____ ____
Percent Recall Consistency ____ ____ ____
Perseverations Total ____ ____ ____
Intrusions Total ____ ____ ____
Recognition Hits ____ ____ ____
False Positives ____ ____ ____
Discriminability ____ ____ ____
Bias ____ ____ ____

Other _____ ____ ____ ____

LANGUAGE

Word Fluency
F.A.S. ____ ____ ____
Animals ____ ____ ____
Foods ____ ____ ____
Sh ____ ____ ____

Token Test ____ ____ ____

(continued)

	Score	z	%ile	z	−2 −1 0 +1 +2
					10 20 30 40 50 60 70 80 90
Boston Naming Test	———	———	———		
Sentence Repetition	———	———	———		
Dichotic Listening					
L. Ear	———	———	———		
R. Ear	———	———	———		
Total	———	———	———		
PPVT-R	———	———	———		
Other ———————	———	———	———		
Other ———————	———	———	———		

AUDITORY

	Score	z	%ile		
Reaction Time					
L. Hand	———	———	———		
R. Hand	———	———	———		
Other ———————	———	———	———		
Other ———————	———	———	———		

VISUAL / VISUOMOTOR

	Score	z	%ile		
Reaction Time					
L	———	———	———		
R	———	———	———		
Embedded Figures	———	———	———		
Right-Left Orientation					
Total Correct	———	———	———		
Reversal Score	———	———	———		
Hooper VOT	———	———	———		
Beery V.M.I.	———	———	———		
Other ———————	———	———	———		
Other ———————	———	———	———		

SOMESTHESIS

	Score	z	%ile		
Finger Localization					
L	/30	———	———		
R	/30	———	———		
Benton 2-D Stereognosis					
L	———	———	———		
R	———	———	———		
Tactile Naming					
L	———	———	———		
R	———	———	———		
Von Frey Hairs					
L	———	———	———		
R	———	———	———		
2-Pt. Aesthesiometer					
L	———	———	———		
R	———	———	———		

(continued)

	Score	z	%ile	z	-2 -1	0	$+1$ $+2$
					10 20 30 40	50	60 70 80 90

T.P.T.
- L
- R
- Both
- Memory
- Location
- Other _____
- Other _____

	Score	z	%ile
T.P.T. L	___	___	___
R	___	___	___
Both	___	___	___
Memory	___	___	___
Location	___	___	___
Other _____	___	___	___
Other _____	___	___	___

MOTOR

	Score	z	%ile
Purdue Pegboard			
L	/25	___	___
R	/25	___	___
Both	/25	___	___
Assembly	/100	___	___
Finger Tapping			
L	___	___	___
R	___	___	___
Dynamometer			
L	___	___	___
R	___	___	___
Other _____	___	___	___
Other _____	___	___	___
Other _____	___	___	___

ACHIEVEMENT

	Age	Grade	%ile
WIAT			
Basic Reading	___	___	___
Math Reasoning	___	___	___
Spelling	___	___	___
Reading Comprehension	___	___	___
Numerical Operations	___	___	___
Listening Comprehension	___	___	___
Oral Expression	___	___	___
Written Expression	___	___	___
Reading	___	___	___
Mathematics	___	___	___
Language	___	___	___
Writing	___	___	___
Total Composite	___	___	___
WRAT-3			
Reading	___	___	___
Spelling	___	___	___
Arithmetic	___	___	___
W-J Achievement			
Letter/Word Identification	___	___	___
Passage Comprehension	___	___	___
Word Attack	___	___	___
Reading Vocabulary	___	___	___
Calculation	___	___	___
Applied Problems	___	___	___
Quantitative Concepts	___	___	___
Dictation	___	___	___
Writing Samples	___	___	___
Writing Fluency	___	___	___
Spelling	___	___	___
Usage	___	___	___
Handwriting	___	___	___
Punct. & Capitalization	___	___	___

(continued)

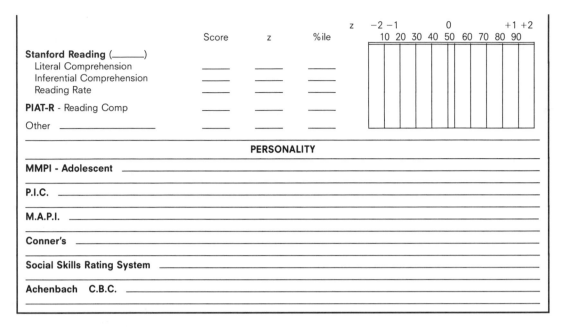

	Score	z	%ile	z	−2 −1	0	+1 +2
					10 20 30 40 50 60 70 80 90		
Stanford Reading (_____)							
Literal Comprehension	____	____	____				
Inferential Comprehension	____	____	____				
Reading Rate	____	____	____				
PIAT-R - Reading Comp	____	____	____				
Other _____	____	____	____				

PERSONALITY

MMPI - Adolescent _____

P.I.C. _____

M.A.P.I. _____

Conner's _____

Social Skills Rating System _____

Achenbach   C.B.C. _____

Figure 3—2. University of Victoria Psychology Clinic child or adolescent test profile form, for ages 6–16.

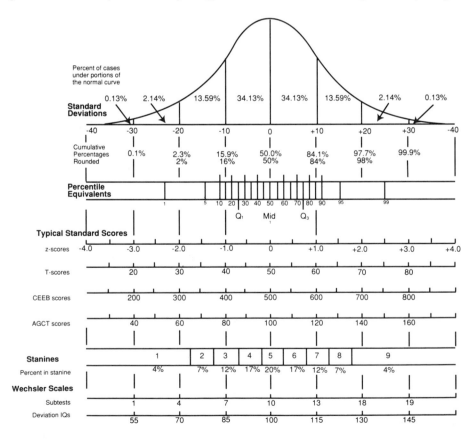

Figure 3—3. The relationship of some commonly used test scores to the normal curve and to one another. (*Test Service Bulletin* of the Psychological Corporation, No. 48, 1955) Note: This chart cannot be used to equate scores on one test to scores on another test. For example, both 600 on the CEEB and 120 on the AGCT are one standard deviation above their respective means, but they do not represent "equal" standings because the scores were obtained from different groups.

26

Table 3—1. Conversion of Standard Deviations and T-Scores into Percentile Ranks

Percentile	SD (z-score)	T-score	Descriptor
>99.9	4.0	90	very superior
99.9	3.0	80	
99	2.5	75	superior
98	2.0	70	
97	1.9	69	
96	1.7	67	
95	1.6	66	
93	1.5	65	
92	1.4	64	
90	1.3	63	above average
88	1.2	62	
86	1.1	61	
84	1.0	60	
82	0.9	59	
79	0.8	58	
76	0.7	57	
73	0.6	56	average
69	0.5	55	
66	0.4	54	
62	0.3	53	
58	0.2	52	
54	0.1	51	
50	0.0	50	
46	−0.1	49	
42	−0.2	48	
38	−0.3	47	
34	−0.4	46	
31	−0.5	45	
27	−0.6	44	
24	−0.7	43	low average
21	−0.8	42	
18	−0.9	41	
16	−1.0	40	
14	−1.1	39	
12	−1.2	38	
10	−1.3	37	
8	−1.4	36	borderline
7	−1.5	35	
5	−1.6	34	
4	−1.7	33	
4	−1.8	32	
3	−1.9	31	
2	−2.0	30	very poor
2	−2.1	29	
1	−2.2	27	
0.8	−2.3	26	
0.6	−2.5	25	
0.5	−2.6	24	
0.4	−2.7	23	
0.3	−2.8	22	
0.2	−2.9	21	
0.1	−3.0	20	

bution, a score lower than 1 to 2 SD below the mean (16th to 3rd percentile) is considered borderline abnormal, a score 2 to 3 SD below the mean (2nd to .01 percentile) abnormal, and scores 3 or more SD below the mean abnormal at a high level of confidence.

While this interpretation is based on the distribution of scores under the normal curve, other interpretations have been developed based on the comparison of scores found in actual samples of normal subjects and abnormal groups (e.g., groups of brain-damaged subjects). When two such groups are compared, an overlap in scores is almost invariably found. The optimal separation between such groups is achieved at the point of minimal misclassification in both groups, i.e., subjects correctly classified as brain-damaged (the *true positive rate*) and normal subjects correctly classified as unimpaired (the *true negative rate*). The true positive rate is also described as defining the *sensitivity* of a test, and the true negative rate as defining the *specificity* of the test. Some test authors have designated a *cut-off score* as defining this point of minimal overlap. However, such cut-off scores may be misleading because they are often based on the comparison of normal people with an unspecified population of people with "brain damage" with a 100 percent base rate. If, for example, normal people drawn from the general population or hospital staff are compared with severely brain-damaged subjects, little if any overlap is to be expected. As Lezak (1995) points out, even the ability to use a can opener could be used to classify each of these two groups correctly. However, if milder or specific cases of brain damage are compared with normal patients hospitalized for nonneurologic disorders and matched for estimated premorbid IQ, the overlap may be considerable. In addition, cut-off points appropriate for younger adults may misclassify 51 to 100 percent of elderly normal controls (Bornstein, Paniak, & O'Brian, 1987). Hence, age (and education) corrections are essential for most tests.

As Lindeboom (1989) and Elwood (1993) have pointed out, the probability values attached to each point of scoring, based on Bayes' theorem (Ingelfinger et al., 1983), provide better guidelines for interpretation and

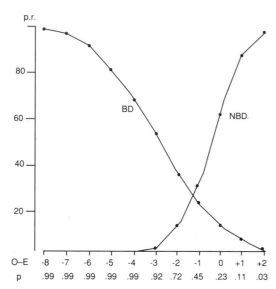

$$p(A) = \frac{p'.LR_x}{1 - p' + (p'.LR_x)}$$

where p(A) is the estimated confidence of classification as A, p' the prior probability or base rate, and LR the likelihood ratio of score X.

As pointed out in the section on report writing, each test score contributes only its own probabilities of correct classification and should be used only in conjunction with other test results. The significance of an isolated single deviant score may be questionable if multiple comparisons have been made. The process of clinical interpretation takes into account not only the probabilities of individual test results, but also the combination of many test results, the observations during the process of testing, the question posed for the examiner, and the characteristics of a specific disorder.

Figure 3—4. Normative Data of the Revised Visual Retention Test (O-E = observed minus expected number correct) converted to percentile ranks (p.r.) in descending order for brain damaged subjects and in ascending order for controls. The estimated confidence classification as brain-damaged (p) is given below the score values. Source: J. Lindeboom (1989).

do not make the assumption of a normal distribution of test scores. As shown in Fig. 3–4, each scorepoint carries its own probability of correct classification, which can be used to estimate the confidence with which a judgment of group membership can be made. It should be noted that the base rate of the occurrence of brain damage in the population may be less than 50 percent. For example, the population referred to a neuropsychology clinic may contain only 25 percent of truly brain-damaged cases while others have other neuropsychiatric disorders. In that case, the prior probability (base rate) of brain damage (.25) must be entered into the formula.

References

Bornstein, R.A., Paniak, C., & O'Brien, W. (1987). Preliminary data on classification of normal and brain-damaged elderly subjects. *The Clinical Neuropsychologist, 1*, 315–323.

Elwood, R.A. (1993). Clinical discrimination and neuropsychological tests: An appeal to Bayes' theorem. *The Clinical Neuropsychologist, 7*, 224–233.

Ingelfinger, J.A., Mosteller, F., Thibodeau, L.A., & Ware, J.H. (1983). *Biostatistics in Clinical Medicine*. New York: McMillan.

Lezak, M.D. (1995). *Neuropsychological Assessment* (3rd ed.). New York: Oxford University Press.

Lindeboom, J. (1989). Who needs cutting points? *Journal of Clinical Psychology, 45*, 679–683.

4

Report Writing and Informing the Client

The purpose of neuropsychological assessment is to help the client in many different ways: to advise and counsel directly, to provide information for the diagnostic process, to gain data essential for therapy, and to measure progress or decline of function over time. At times, this information is gathered to assist in deciding forensic issues. In all cases, a report is prepared that reflects test findings, observations, and other relevant material. It is clear from this brief listing that neuropsychological assessment reports vary greatly in format, content, and language, depending on the purpose of the assessment. No fixed format is appropriate for all purposes. Nevertheless, the steps in preparing the report are similar and will be outlined in this chapter (for general guides to report writing see Ownby [1997] and Tallent [1993]). In addition, we will comment briefly on questions of content, confidentiality, computer use, and other relevant issues in report writing.

Content of the Report: The Basic Shell

Most neuropsychological assessment reports contain certain basic information. It is useful to prepare the report in thirteen steps, organizing the information gathered during the assessment into the following basic "shell":*

1. Client data

*Several data management and storage, "report build-

2. Reason for referral
3. Relevant history
4. Review of relevant previous reports
5. Client's current concerns
6. Report of informant(s)
7. Observations during history taking and testing
8. Test results

>General intellectual status
>
>Achievement
>
>Executive function
>
>Attention/Concentration
>
>Learning/Memory
>
>Language
>
>Visuospatial ability
>
>Motor function
>
>Sensory function
>
>Personality/Mood

9. Interpretation of test results and observations
10. Diagnostic summary
11. Recommendations
12. Vocational implications
13. Appendix: Tests administered

---

ing", and report writing computer programs are available (Psychological Corporation, Psychological Assessment Resources), with options ranging from organizing inputted test scores to providing outlines and fully written reports. We have not checked the usefulness or quality of such programs.

Client Data. To avoid confusion in the transmission of the report and filing, the full name, birthdate, and address of the patient, as well as the date of testing and the referral source should be listed at the top of the report. Whether the report is written on a standard form provided by the hospital or agency or in letter form, this information is best listed separately at the beginning of the report. The identity of the person writing the report can be indicated by the letterhead or by the signature. In reports written for forensic purposes, the qualifications of the psychologist (registration or license, Board certification, area of specialization, years of experience) are required and usually form the first sentence of the report ("I am a psychologist registered to practice in _____. Attached is my curriculum vitae outlining some of my qualifications"). Test-user competencies and qualifications for test purchasers should be carefully observed and documented (Moreland et al., 1995).

Depending on the recipient of the report, a *preface sentence* outlining the limited validity of a report over time should be inserted at the beginning, especially when the patient is a child. Usually, for children, a one-year limit of the use of the report is indicated. While old reports may be useful for comparison purposes, all too often old reports in school files are cited again and again rather than replaced by a new assessment; this leads to prejudicial judgments long after a problem has been successfully overcome by the client. Recognizing this problem, some school boards have removed references to assessment reports, the reports themselves, and even achievement test results obtained by classroom teachers from the permanent school record. However, this information is valuable in determining the premorbid ability.

Reason for Referral. It is essential to state briefly the purpose of the report right at the beginning in order to focus the report and to clarify the relationship of the writer with the recipient of the report. Since the reason for referral often guides the selection of tests, citing it helps clarify why certain tests were given as well as the thrust of the subsequent inquiry. In cases referred by a physician or other psychologist, a lawyer, and even in the case of a self-referred patient, a sentence or two confirms that you have understood the request and are addressing relevant questions ("referred because of possible mental deterioration . . . , because of learning and memory problems") rather than giving an unsolicited general opinion. This does not preclude addressing other problems in your report; in fact, the recipient will be grateful to find other information in the report of which he or she has not been aware. Some referrals are made without a clear statement of purpose ("request neuropsychological assessment," "query organicity"); in such cases, a phone call or further correspondence is needed to clarify the reason for the referral. A referral form with specific questions should be used, whenever possible, to "educate" the referring agent.

Relevant History. This section is based on the history taking outlined in Chapter 1 and typically includes information regarding the client's place of birth, relevant personal and family medical history, educational attainment, occupational history, contact with chemicals at work, alcohol and drug use, family and living situation, hobbies, and interpersonal relationships.

The emphasis in this section is on information that is relevant to the purpose of the report. Include information only if it contributes to an understanding of the referral question. For example, if cognitive deterioration is suspected, this section of the report lays the groundwork for determining the type of disorder by detailing any genetic contributions as well as the course of the disorder (e.g., abrupt or insidious). It allows an estimate of premorbid functioning to be derived by describing highlights of educational and occupational achievement. It also contributes to an understanding of the impact of the disorder on the client's social and occupational situation. Information that is true and interesting but not relevant to the referral question, however, should be omitted. Duplication of information readily available from other sources should also be avoided. This only adds bulk to the report and wastes both the writer's and the reader's time.

Omitting irrelevant information throughout the report is also mandated by principle 5A of the APA Ethical Principles of Psychologists and Code of Conduct (1992). According to this principle the psychologist must not write into the report statements that are not germane to the evaluation or that are an undue invasion of privacy. Other items of the Ethics Code of specific concern to the neuropsychologist (e.g., documentation of assessment results, competence, multiple relationships) are outlined by Binder and Thompson (1995).

Review of Relevant Previous Reports. This section provides information from other sources, such as medical reports, school reports, and prior psychological test data. While some neuropsychologists merely list the reports received, others provide a brief summary of the relevant reports. Again, duplication of information readily available from other sources should be avoided. The guiding principle for inclusion should be whether the information contributes to a clearer understanding of the current test findings, interpretations, and recommendations. For example, if a client has undergone previous psychological examination, then highlighting briefly the major findings may be useful since the writer may wish to contrast current with previous test results. It may be important in cases of traumatic brain injury to report information from the medical history regarding the length of alteration of consciousness, extent of memory loss, etc., since this information may have bearing on the diagnosis and prognosis. Similarly, it might be useful to review the client's medications since this may have implications regarding the validity of the test findings.

Client's Current Concerns. It is important to include a description of the client's complaints and concerns. Note that these may be quite different from those of the referral source (e.g., neurologist, employer). In addition to physical and cognitive concerns, this section should also include information about the patient's emotional state (e.g., stress, anxiety, depression) and the impact of symptoms or complaints on daily living since this may affect

the interpretation of the test results as well as the recommendations. We recommend that each area (physical, cognitive, emotional) be dealt with in a deliberate fashion (e.g., "In terms of physical complaints, the patient reported nausea, dizziness, etc.").

Report of Informant(s). This section includes information from other people (spouse, relative, teacher) that contributes to an understanding of the client's performance. Such information may highlight additional concerns and symptoms as well as uncover client statements that are misleading with regard to both the gravity of the symptoms and the time course of their evolution.

Observations during History Taking and Testing. Since testing frequently extends over several hours or days, the patient's behavior during that period provides valuable information about day-to-day functioning. Competence as a historian, personal appearance, punctuality, cooperativeness, rapport with the examiner, approach to novel or routine tasks, comprehension of instructions, response to encouragement, reaction to failure, and degree of effort can all be judged by an experienced examiner. Rated cooperativeness has been estimated to correlate as high as .64 with test results in geriatric outpatients; such correlations include, of course, not only the willingness, but also the ability to cooperate. The behavior at the beginning and toward the end of the session, or the effect of breaks during testing on subsequent motivation, allow conclusions about persistence, fatigue, speed of response, and emotional control; in fact, substantial changes during the course of the assessment should be carefully documented because they may affect the validity of the test results. Any concerns that assessment findings may not be reliable or valid indicators of an individual's ability should be stated clearly in this section along with reasons for the concerns ("The test results may underestimate the client's abilities because he had a severe cold on the day of testing").

Again, this section of the report should be kept to a minimum of relevant details. There is no need to overload the report with general observations not pertinent to the purpose of the assessment.

Test Results. This section of the report contains a description of the results in terms of level of performance, usually expressed in percentile ranks as described in Chapter 3 (Fig. 3–1). Other authors may prefer T-scores. The section should be prefaced with an explanation of the scoring system used (i.e., "a percentile rank of 60 indicates that the estimated performance was better than 60 percent of the general population of the client's age based on a comparison with a normative sample") unless the recipient of the report can be expected to be fully familiar with the system used.

The reporting of raw scores, scaled scores, or IQ scores is still recommended by authors like Freides (1993, 1995) or Tallent (1993). Naugle and McSweeny (1995) point out that this practice may lead to misinterpretations and contravenes the Ethical Principles of Psychologists (APA, 1992).* There is an emerging consensus that the use of percentile ranks or T-scores in a report addressed to other health professionals or to the patient and relatives is preferable: It avoids the myths often attached to IQ scores, and it provides the reader with a single, easily comprehensible scoring system across tests. However, one drawback of percentile-rank reporting is the pseudoaccuracy implied in such scores. Basically, percentile ranks represent the number of people covered by the normal distribution curve as expressed in standard deviations. (See Fig. 3–3) One-half of a standard deviation from the mean changes the percentile ranks from 50 to 69 (or 31). With computer calculations, even small fractions of a standard deviation can be translated into percentile points that are meaningless (and nonsignificant) in reality, but may seem to reflect differences to the reader unfamiliar with basic psychometrics.

*A recent "Statement on the Disclosure of Test Data" (American Psychological Association, 1996) is consistent with our practice and elaborates further on rules of disclosure and consent of the client.

An Iowa State law of 1994 prohibits the release of "psychological test data" to anyone but a licensed psychologist.

Moreover, some test scores are not normally distributed, and norms for other tests allow only a very limited range of scores (see Chapter 3); in such cases it is more appropriate to describe the test results not in percentile ranks, but in terms of very superior, superior, above average, average, low average, mildly impaired, moderately impaired, or severely impaired, following the traditional terminology used in IQ testing (within 1 SD = normal range, between 1 and 2 SD = mild or suggested ("questionable") impairment, between 2 and 3 SD = moderate impairment, etc.).

Such guidelines following SD ranges must, however, consider the premorbid abilities of the client. "Average" or "normal range" scores in a previously gifted individual may very well indicate considerable loss of abilities. On the other hand, for a person with borderline premorbid intelligence, impairment can only be inferred from scores 2 or 3 SD below the mean. Considerable judgment and information is required for the interpretation of scores for people with nonaverage premorbid abilities. Moreover, each score must be interpreted in the context of scores on other tests of related abilities. A single "deviant" score may be the result of one of several error sources: misunderstanding of instructions, inattention, distraction, momentary lapse of effort, etc.

While some neuropsychologists describe test scores test-by-test, a good report writer organizes the information into domains (general intellectual level, achievement, executive function, attention/concentration, learning/memory, language, visuospatial ability, motor function, sensory function, personality/mood, etc.) that may vary depending on the purpose of the assessment. Noncontributory results are omitted or summed up briefly. Our typical report includes separate sections for each domain (with subtitles). Topic sentences integrate the information from different tests that are relevant to interpreting the client's functioning within that domain. This is followed by a report of the data that led to the interpretation. Our usual practice is to substantiate statements by providing the supporting data and referencing in brackets the relevant tests (e.g., "Language: Verbal comprehension appeared intact. She was well able to follow complex commands [Token Test—90th percentile]. By contrast, expressive functions were poor. Her ability to generate words to command within a fixed time period [Verbal Fluency] was poor, below the 10th percentile. She also had considerable difficulty naming pictured objects [Boston Naming Test], her score falling below the 5th percentile. Some paraphasias [substitution of sounds] were apparent on naming tasks [e.g., acorn—aircorn]. The provision of phonemic cues facilitated naming").

It is also useful to keep in mind that most tests provide results for several different domains. For example, the WAIS-R subtest scores need not all be referenced under "intellectual ability"; rather, digit span may be considered under "attention," vocabulary under "language," block design under "constructional praxis," etc. Similarly, the Trail Making Test may be considered under "executive function," "attention," and under "visuomotor ability."

Interpretation of Test Results and Observations. The interpretation should never follow a test-by-test order, but should present a logical and coherent picture of all relevant findings. In cases of suspected deficits after brain damage, it is useful to start by establishing the premorbid abilities first, and then to proceed to the referral questions. These questions can now be phrased in the context of a more detailed evaluation and should not simply repeat test results ("While no actual decline in general intellectual status was found, some rigidity in response strategies and perseveration was observed in several tests as well as in the client's interaction during the interview"; "Memory for verbal material was average, but tests of visual memory showed a significant deficit").

It is important to list areas of strength as well as weaknesses of the client in the interpretation part of the report. Strengths in certain cognitive or other areas provide the main basis for intervention strategies. We wish to stress that the discussion of strengths and weaknesses refers to functional components and not to tests.

When reviewing the test results, it is useful to highlight both the best and the poorest results indicated on the profile sheet. These may be from one or more areas of psychological functioning and will generate several hypothetical psychological "syndromes." The neuropsychologist must then proceed by reviewing other tests that measure functions similar to each of these "syndromes" as well as other information (e.g., behavioral observations, informant reports, etc.) and verify, modify, refute, or explicate them and discuss their neurological significance as the preparation of the report progresses. The interpretation, based on quantitative and qualitative information, must respect what is known about brain–behavior relations, i.e., it must make sense from a neurological and neuropsychological point of view and must also take into account information regarding test reliability and validity.

Leckliter and Matarazzo (1989) caution that age, education, IQ, ethnic, and gender effects may be large enough to cause false-positive errors when inferences about adequacy of brain function are made based on uncorrected norms. In addition, life history and medical findings must be considered when judgments about cognitive impairment are made (Matarazzo, 1990). Leckliter and Forster (1994) show similar problems for the Halstead-Reitan battery for older children.

Recently, Reitan and Wolfson (1995) have argued that age and education corrections are appropriate for normal, healthy individuals, but that they are not needed for brain-damaged subjects. This contention was based on a study of the General Neuropsychological Deficit Scale (GNDS), a revision of the Halstead-Reitan Impairment Index, which is a summary score resulting from 42 individual variables in the Halstead-Reitan battery for 50 normal and 50 brain-damaged subjects. While the GNDS differed substantially between well-educated and less-educated and between younger and older normal people, it showed only a minor trend in the same direction for brain-damaged subjects.

Aside from the somewhat obsolete goal of obtaining a single cutoff score to determine the presence or absence of brain damage, the study remains unconvincing: The small number of subjects, the failure to include older subjects (the age for both groups ranged from 22 to 50 years), the failure to include subjects with mild brain damage, and the trends of actually obtained differences all argue against the contention of the authors. Moreover, a conscientious clinician would wish to compare the obtained test scores with the score expected according to age- and education-corrected norms for each test individually. The argument "against adjusting scores for brain-damaged subjects according to age and education norms for normal *children*" (Reitan & Wolfson, 1995, 1996) is even less justified because it was based on a comparison of only 35 brain-damaged and 35 normal children, ages 9 to 14 years, split into two age groups at the age of 11:5. The reported correlation coefficient of $-.49$ with education is, in fact, significant, and the correlation of $-.13$ with age would most likely be significant if a larger n were used.

Bengtson et al. (1996) raise another important question about the use of test norms: It has been accepted for some time that average IQ scores have increased by approximately 14 points during the period between 1932 and 1978. Such a gradual increase, often ascribed to educational and cultural, rather than intellectual improvement, was also observed in a meta-analysis of the Halstead-Reitan test norms published in 69 studies during the last 20 years, and were as high as 1.3 SD for the Category Test, and 1.0 SD for the Location score of the Tactual Performance Test. The authors warn that for clinical use, current, rather than dated normative standards should be used.

Normative data are often based on samples of healthy volunteers drawn from the community. Even though such samples may be representative of the U.S. census, it should be kept in mind that patients are often tested in a hospital setting with the attendant anxiety about an ongoing illness and with less than optimal attention and motivation; dependent on the type of hospital, such patients may also be far from representative for the general population. Lichtenberg et al. (1995) and Ross and Lichtenberg (1997) found, for example, that norms for elderly inner-city inpatients with

non-neurological disorders on the Boston Naming Test and other tests (Fuld Object Memory, Logical Memory of the WMS, Visual Form Discrimination, Hooper Visual Organization Test) were considerably lower than other published norms, based on "community-dwelling volunteers," and showed considerably larger SDs. In fact, some "norms" exceeded the recommended cut-off points for brain-damaged subjects. The clinician should scrutinize published norms carefully in order to determine whether they should be applied to a given patient.

Special care should be taken when the patient shows indications of depression. As Sweet et al. (1992) point out, the customary cutoffs to determine impairment on tests known to be strongly influenced by depression (e.g., Trails, WAIS-R Digit Symbol) cannot be used. "Instead, use a more stringent criterion, such as a cutoff that is an additional standard deviation away from normal performance . . . . The presence of patterns of impairment that are not associated with depression carries much more weight. For example, signs of aphasia, a true 'Stroop' effect as opposed to slowness on all three Stroop Color-Word pages, impaired recall *and* recognition, impaired incidental *and* intentional learning, and impaired recall of both easy *and* difficult word pairs are not common findings in depressed patients" (p. 40).

Intraindividual variability of test scores is only rarely addressed in cognitive neuropsychology, although it has been noted in personality assessment by the development of "state" vs. "trait" inventory contents. An individual's scores on many tests may vary considerably from one test session to another as a result of changes in attention, mood, health, and environmental factors. Such changes are referred to as "state"-dependent, whereas structural changes of abilities or personality changes of a more permanent nature are described as "traits." Dixon et al. (1993) tested normal elderly subjects and one Alzheimer's disease patient weekly for up to 90 weeks with 25 versions of a story-recall test similar to the Wechsler Logical Memory subtest. They observed that short-story recall in one of their normal elderly subjects ranged from 14 percent on one occasion to 64 percent on another. Such intraindividual variability tends to lower test–retest correlations, although it does not necessarily affect other measures of test reliability, i.e., split-half or internal consistency measures. Unfortunately, little information about the size of this variability is available for most tests. If it remains within the range of one standard deviation, it may be considered a minor nuisance factor, but if it exceeds these limits, repeat testing on multiple occasions or testing the function with several different measures may be the only recourse for the examiner who suspects that a particular test result is especially affected by such "state" factors. The examiner should also be aware of which tests are subject to high intraindividual variability.

In addition to test scores, many authors recommend a "process" (as opposed to achievement) approach to testing, i.e., a qualitative exploration of how the patient attained the test scores, how he or she succeeds or fails at a task (Goldstein & Scheerer, 1941; Kaplan, 1988; Lezak, 1995; Milberg et al., 1986). Such procedural differences have been especially pointed out for older subjects (Albert & Kaplan, 1980; Erickson et al., 1992) and for children. A process approach requires careful observation of the patient during each task and a follow-up of unusual approaches or errors by questioning or by the use of *ad hoc* tasks, including test modifications that are administered to clarify why this particular approach was used by the patient or how the error occurred. The discussion by Milberg et al. (1986) provides many illustrations of this process.

The Boston Process approach has led to test modifications including the WAIS-R-NI described elsewhere in this book. Caplan and Shechter (1994) have argued strongly in favor of nonstandard neuropsychological testing with clients who have motor impairment of the upper limbs, or who have limited vision, hearing, or speech. They present procedural modifications for a number of tests, including substitution of reading for spoken instructions, multiple-choice pointing for such tests as the Block Design, and similar changes for Maze Learning, Raven Matrices, and the Hooper VOT. For example, to avoid effects of visual neglect, the six choices of the Raven Matrices can be arranged in vertical order rather than in a three by two matrix. One already standardized method is the multiple-choice version of the Visual Retention Test described elsewhere, but most of the suggested modifications are not standardized and cannot be interpreted following published norms. Substantiable conclusions are therefore difficult to draw. It should also be noted that such modifications may change the purpose of the test, i.e., the modified test may measure an ability that may be substantially different from that measured in the standard administration. Moreover, the use of a modification may seriously affect the subsequent administration of the standard form. For example, Slick et al. (1996) found that a substantial minority of normal subjects obtained lower scores on some multiple-choice items of the WAIS-NI than on the standard administration of the WAIS-R.

Diagnostic Summary. A brief summary concludes the formal portion of the assessment report. It can be done in point form. It includes a brief restatement of the client's history (e.g., (1) This is a 54-year-old right-handed psychologist with no previous history of neurological disorder. (2) She was in a motor vehicle accident on Dec. 12, 1992, and suffered a severe head injury; she was comatose for two weeks. (3) On current examination, . . .), the major findings together with a diagnostic statement that includes the presumed origin of the deficit. The diagnostic statement should be couched in terms that do not overstate the psychological nature of the findings ("The findings of a verbal memory deficit are consistent with a left temporal lobe lesion"); the neurological examination and radiological and other techniques may provide more definite indications of a specific disorder. A prognostic statement is also expected ("Verbal deficits have persisted for a considerable period of time, at least five years, and further significant improvement is unlikely").

Recommendations. Over the years, the value of neuropsychological assessment has shifted away from purely diagnostic purposes toward remediation and psychological treatment. Such recommendations should be both practical and realistic. The neuropsychologist preparing the assessment report should be fully familiar with remedial techniques, therapies, and basic management procedures in his or her field of expertise as well as with the available local resources that provide such assistance. Names and phone numbers for specific treatment, training, or support facilities should be included.

Other recommendations include practical hints for the patient and the caregiver for the management of particular problems in daily living, educational and occupational implications, and frequently the time when a reassessment should be scheduled to measure future progress or decline.

The ability to drive a motor vehicle is often an issue of concern for the patient, the caregiver, and the referring psychologist or physician. Neuropsychological tests do not provide direct information about the ability to drive safely, although in instances of severe impairment it is obvious that the driver's license should be suspended. Hartje et al. (1991) found that driving ability could not be reliably judged from test results; presence of aphasia in brain-damaged patients, especially those of higher age, was more frequently associated with failure on an on-road driving test. The referring physician can recommend suspension to the issuing authorities. In case of doubt, an on-road driving test is recommended.

Appendix: Tests Administered. Some neuropsychologists include a full listing of all tests administered in the course of the assessment. Such a list is of interest only to a reader thoroughly familiar with neuropsychological assessment. It should not be part of the report but should be appended.

General Comments on Report Writing and Oral Reporting

Style and Length. The style of report writing should be kept as clear and simple as possible regardless of who the recipient of the report is. In particular, psychological jargon should

be avoided and technical terms, if necessary, should be explained. Keep in mind that in many cases the clients will read the report (see Informing Interview). A clinician's thesaurus for wording psychological reports (American Psychological Association, 1997; Zuckerman, 1995) may be useful for the choice of appropriate, precise, and comprehensible wording.

It has become the policy of many journals to use "person first language," i.e., the patient should not be described as "a 43-year-old hemiplegic," but rather as "a 43-year-old man with hemiplegia"; not as "a crippled child," but as "a child who walks with crutches." Such policies should apply also to psychological report writing.

The report should contribute to positive changes for the patient. Appelbaum (1970) has argued that reports are "political, diplomatic, strategic persuasions in a complex socio-psychological context" (p. 349). While this may be overstating the case, especially for a neuropsychological report, the report writer should be aware that he or she is writing to convince the report recipient about the "ecological" validity of findings for a specific individual living in a specific set of circumstances; the findings may not apply to another individual or at another time, depending on available resources, the individual's personal background, habits, living arrangements, emotional state, and personal goals and expectations, as well as society's current thinking. Heaton and Pendleton (1981) raised similar questions specifically for neuropsychological tests, and Sbordone and Long (1995) present a full discussion of the ecological validity of neuropsychological testing. Wilson (1993) made concrete suggestions for including tests designed to measure everyday behavior relevant to the patient, the caregiver, and the rehabilitation worker, (e.g., the Rivermead Behavioral Battery and other tests) and recently published a new Behavioral Assessment of the Dysexecutive Syndrome (Wilson et al., 1996), based on the same principles. Many neuropsychological tests are poor predictors of functional behavior. For example, Loewenstein et al. (1992) compared the performance of 33 AD patients on the BNT, the MMSE, the Fuld Object Memory Test, the COWA, and

Block Design, Object Assembly, and Similarities of the WAIS-R with eight functional tasks (reading a clock, telephone skills, preparing a letter for mailing, counting currency, writing a check, balancing a checkbook, shopping with a written list); only the MMSE, COWA, Object Assembly, Similarities, and Fuld Retrieval Score contributed to a stepwise regression analysis of predicting functional competence. All tests combined accounted for less than 50 percent of the explained variance. Heaton and Chelune (1988) performed a stepwise discriminant function analysis between 360 employed and unemployed neuropsychological referrals tested with the Halstead-Reitan (H-R) Battery, the WAIS, the PIAT, and the MMPI and found that only measures of current adaptive abilities (H-R, MMPI, and WAIS-R) contributed to group discrimination; measures of past experience and education (WAIS-V, PIAT, years of education) did not contribute to group discrimination. A recent study by Richardson et al. (1995) found that the prediction of performance-based activity of daily living ratings showed a significant canonical correlation of .43 with the performance on five neuropsychological tests in a geriatric population, accounting for only 14 to 32 per cent of the variance. The best predictors were tests of visuospatial ability (Hooper Visual Organization Test), followed by memory tests (Wechsler Visual Reproductions I, Wechsler Logical Memory). In contrast, Bau et al. (1996) found canonical correlations of .92 and .75 between memory, mental control, and learning tests and measures of manual apraxia, kitchen tasks, and activities of daily living in 126 AD patients between 65 and 85 years. They concluded that, with the exception of highly routinized activities like sitting and climbing stairs, both functional tasks and neuropsychological tests assess the same global deterioration which characterizes Alzheimer's disease.

The length of a report depends, of course, on the purpose and on the complexity of the findings. However, the report should be kept as brief as possible by avoiding irrelevant or redundant information. As pointed out above, the report should be problem-oriented and should not use a shotgun approach; normal test results can be covered in a single sentence ("All other test results were in the normal range"; "Motor and sensory testing showed average results without significant side differences"). In many cases, a single-page report is perfectly adequate. Lengthy and wordy reports are less likely to be read in full by the recipient: A busy physician may read no more than the summary statement.

Confidentiality. The confidentiality of assessment reports is frequently misunderstood. Confidentiality exists between the person conducting the assessment and the client or patient, not the neuropsychologist and the referring physician (or lawyer). Even if the report is not directly shared with the patient, he or she has the right to see the report through the Freedom of Information Act. It is good practice to allow the patient to read the report before it is mailed out (see Informing Interview) and to clarify with the patient in writing who should receive a copy.

Confidentiality does exist with respect to all third parties including relatives, agencies, research staff, etc., unless specifically waived by the patient. Specific attention to the protection of confidentiality should be exercised if the report is stored on a computer base, and security of data storage facilities should be maintained. The standard informed consent form we use states that test results can be used anonymously for research purposes and allows for listing names of people who should receive a copy of the report.

Informing Interview. Psychological assessment results are of direct interest to the patient, who is usually concerned about his or her mental or emotional problems. Therefore, it is good practice to schedule an informing interview with the client and, if desired, with the spouse or other caregiver soon after the assessment. The informing interview usually starts with a review of the purpose of the assessment as stated by the client. Other questions raised by the referring agent should then be introduced. Test results can be summarized briefly and should be explained in language suitable for the client. Be explicit and use examples: For instance, if "acting out behavior" is found, explain how severe it is and how it may be stopped; if "perseverative tendencies" are found, explain how this impacts upon the client's occupational status. To prevent the impression that test results are kept "secret" from the client, it is often appropriate to show some of the test results directly to him or her to explain why the psychologist came to a certain conclusion ("You remember that list of words that you had to repeat: You got only two out of 10 while most people your age get at least 6"). While it is true that few clients have the training and sophistication to fully understand test scores, terms like "average" or "seriously below average for your age" do make sense to most people.

The most important parts of the informing interview, however, are the conclusions reached and the recommendations. The patient wants to know whether she or he has a serious problem, whether it is progressive or not, and what can be done about it. This should be discussed at some length and repeated as necessary. Most clients retain only a small portion of the information given during the informing interview. Make sure that the client remembers the recommendations and provide her or him with written instructions when appropriate (i.e., phone and address of therapist, training group, or rehabilitation facility).

It is good practice to allow clients to read a draft of your assessment report at the end of the interview and to take a copy home if desired. Providing written as well as oral feedback is one of the recommendations resulting from a study of consumers of neuropsychological assessment (Bennett-Levy et al., 1994; Gass and Brown, 1992); 74 percent of the clients in the study complained that they did not receive written feedback. Frequently, however, the psychologist may gain additional information during the informing interview; occasionally, the client may dispute the accuracy of statements attributed to her or him in the report. This may lead to a revision of the draft report. This should be explained to the client, and a copy of the report can be mailed later.

Forensic Assessment Reports. Forensic assessment is a specialty in itself, but any clinician may be subpoenaed to testify in court in a case that leads to litigation at a later time. Forensic reports by neuropsychologists are most frequently concerned with questions of compensation, wills and estate, guardianship as to estate and person, and diminished criminal responsibility. Such reports are written for lawyers on both sides of the issue and should be couched in clear language that cannot be misinterpreted. Statements of probability are appropriate, but statements that a certain deficit is "possible" or "likely" are not. The report may address questions of the existence of brain damage, cause of brain injury, degree of impairment, and prognosis. The question of admissibility of testimony by neuropsychologists in various states is reviewed by Richardson and Adams (1992). If the report is used in court, the report writer will be sworn in, and give direct testimony in answer to questions by the lawyer introducing the material, and is subject to cross-examination by the opposing lawyer.

Due to the adversarial nature of court proceedings, the testifying neuropsychologist can expect extremely critical questioning. Well-prepared lawyers are familiar with many of the tests and their weaknesses, based on books specifically written for that purpose (Doerr & Carlin, 1991; Faust, Ziskin, & Hiers, 1991; Hall & Pritchard, 1996; Sbordone, 1995; Melton et al., 1997; Ziskin & Faust, 1988). Attacks may be expected, particularly on results based on personality tests like the MMPI or the Rorschach Test. Authors like Brodsky (1991), Hall & Pritchard (1996), Shapiro (1991), and Milton et al. (1987) provide detailed guidance for the psychologist. Pope et al. (1993) focus their book primarily on the MMPI, the MMPI-2, and the MMPI-A.

A particularly difficult aspect of forensic reports is the question of symptom validity: Was the patient cooperating fully? Are some or all of the symptoms valid or are they influenced by a tendency to exaggerate or even to malinger? Many tests, especially the MMPI and other personality tests, have developed scales or indices that can assist in the detection of malingering. In addition, special testing for symptom validity has been developed (described in Chapter 17 of this book). Such information is crucial for the interpretation of test results. However, the problem is complicated by the fact that these tests can at best only indicate that motivational or emotional factors (e.g., depression, anxiety, lack of effort) may be influencing task performance. Even in cases where financial or other incentives exist, and the patient's performance is suspect, the patient may be impaired and/or acting without conscious intent. Accurate diagnosis requires examination of both test and extra-test behavior as well as a thorough evaluation of the patient's history and pertinent reports, including injury characteristics. Communication of findings can be problematic, given the difficulty in diagnosing malingering and the complexity of an individual's motivations. The report should be written in a factual manner, providing a detailed description of the patient's behavior, and should acknowledge any limitations in the assessment. In some cases, the clinician may merely comment that the invalidity of the testing precludes a firm diagnosis.

Another complicating factor is the possible presence of post-traumatic stress disorder (PTSD), a recognized neuropsychiatric syndrome that is acceptable for compensation in many courts. The separation of PTSD from other disorders, such as head injury, can only be based on a thorough study of the behavior, the personality, and the performance of the client.

Computer-Generated Scores and Reports. Computer scoring programs are fairly common, and the sophistication of interpretative programs has increased over time. Krug (1993) provides a regularly updated, nonevaluative compilation and description of most commercially available programs, including sample printouts. The clinician, however, remains responsible for what goes into the report. For this reason, she or he should be thoroughly familiar with all material used in such programs.

Computer scoring can save time and often avoids computation errors. However, the translation of raw scores into standardized scores must be scrutinized by the psychologist to check which normative data base is used and to assure that proper corrections for age, education, and other factors are applied.

Computer interpretation has been offered for some time for the MMPI as well as for other tests, and attempts have been made to provide computer interpretation and even brain-diagram scattergrams for the Halstead-Reitan battery of neuropsychological tests (Adams & Heaton, 1985; Gur et al., 1988; Russell et al., 1970; Russell & Starkey, 1993; Bracy, 1992) and similar fixed or semi-flexible batteries (Dougherty & Bortnick, 1990; Hammainen, 1994). Some of them are commercially available (Integrated Professional Systems, 5211 Mahoning Ave., Suite 135, Youngstown, OH 44515; Psychological Assessment Resources, P.O. Box 998, Odessa, FL 33556). However, the value of such computer-generated interpretations has been disputed. Goldstein et al. (1996) report a sensitivity of only 58% for acute, and of 78% for static stroke cases with the "key" approach. The American Psychological Association (1986) has issued firm guidelines for their use: "Computer-generated interpretative reports should be used only in conjunction with professional judgment. The user should judge for each test taker the validity of the computerized test report based on the user's professional knowledge of the total context of testing and the test taker's performance and characteristics" (p. 12).

One reason for such warning is that clinicians may be tempted to use the computer as a "cheap consultant" and take the validity of the computer-generated report for granted. The other reason is that computer-generated reports by their very nature use a gunshot rather than a problem-oriented approach, and they address a hypothetical, "typical" individual, based on averages of certain test scores, not the particular client who is the subject of a specific report. "With almost no exception, today's software produces only a single, typically very lengthy, clinical narrative" (Matarazzo, 1986). Butcher (1987) comments that such reports "give you everything you could possibly tell about a person from the test." It follows then, that a computer-generated report can only be used selectively and with modifications required by the referral questions and the specific circumstances of a specific client.

Test Modifications and Foreign-Language and Bilingual Clients. Test modifications for the handicapped client and problems related to testing clients for whom English is a second language, as discussed in Chapter 2, should be clearly stated and restrictions on the use of published norms and consequent limitations in interpretation should be explained in the report.

References

Adams, K.M., & Heaton, R.K. (1985). Automated interpretation of neuropsychological test data. *Journal of Consulting and Clinical Psychology*, *53*, 790–802.

Albert, M.S., & Kaplan, E. (1980). Organic implications of neuropsychological deficits in the elderly. In L.W. Poon, J.L. Fozard & L.S. Cermak (Eds.), *New Directions in Memory and Aging*, pp. 403–432. Hillsdale, NY: Erlbaum.

American Psychological Association. (1992). Ethical principles of psychologists and code of conduct. *American Psychologist*, *47*, 1597–1611.

American Psychological Association. (1986). *Guidelines for Computer-Based Tests and Interpretations*. Washington, D.C.

American Psychological Association. (1996). Statement on the disclosure of test data. *American Psychologist*, *51*, 644–648.

American Psychological Association (1997). Thesaurus of Psychological Index Terms (8th ed.). Washington, D.C.

Appelbaum, S.A. (1970). Science and persuasion in the psychological test report. *Journal of Consulting and Clinical Psychology*, *35*, 349–355.

Bau, C., Edwards, D., Yonan, C., & Storandt, M. (1996). The relationship of neuropsychological test performance to performance on functional tasks in dementia of the Alzheimer type. *Archives of Clinical Neuropsychology*, *11*, 69–75.

Beaumont, J.G., & French, C.C. (1987). A clinical field study of eight automated psychometric procedures: The Leicester/DHS project. *International Journal of Man-Machine Studies*, *26*, 661–682.

Bengtson, M.L., Mittenberg, W., Schneider, B., & Seller, A. (1996). An assessment of Halstead-Reitan test score changes over 20 years. *Archives of Clinical Neuropsychology*, *11*, 368 (abstract).

Bennett-Levy, J., Klein-Boonschate, M.A., Batchelor, J. et al. (1994). Encounters with Anna Thompson: The consumer's Experience of neuropsychological assessment. *The Clinical Neuropsychologist*, *8*, 219–238.

Binder, L.M., & Thompson, L.L. (1995). The ethics code and neuropsychological assessment practices. *Archives of Clinical Neuropsychology*, *10*, 27–46.

Bracy, O.L. (1992). *Impairment Scattergram ISG HR (Halstead-Reitan Version)*. Indianapolis, IN: Psychological Software Services.

Brodsky, S.L. (1991). *Testifying in Court: Guidelines and Maxims for the Expert Witness*. Washington, D.C.: American Psychological Association.

Butcher, J.N. (Ed.) (1987). *Computerized Psychological Assessment: A Practitioner's Guide*. New York: Basic Books.

Caplan, B., & Shechter, J. (1994). The role of nonstandard neuropsychological assessment in rehabilitation: History, rationale, and examples. In L.A. Cushman & M.J. Scherer (Eds.), *Psychological Assessment in Medical Rehabilitation*. Boston, MA: Allyn & Bacon.

Dixon, R.A., Hertzog, C., Friesen, I., & Hultsch, D.F. (1993). Assessment of intraindividual change in text recall of elderly adults. In H.H. Brownell & Y. Joanette (Eds.), *Narrative Discourse in Neurologically Impaired and Normal Aging Adults*. San Diego, CA: Singular Publishing Group.

Doerr, H.O., & Carlin, A.S. (Eds.) (1991). *Forensic Neuropsychology: Legal and Scientific Bases*. Odessa, FL: Psychological Assessment Resources.

Dougherty, E., & Bortnick, D.M. (1990). *Report Writer: Adult's Intellectual Achievement, and Neuropsychological Screening Tests*. Toronto, Ont.: Multi-Health Systems.

Erickson, R.C., Eimon, P., & Hebben, N. (1992). A bibliography of normative articles on cognition tests for older adults. *The Clinical Neuropsychologist*, *6*, 98–102.

Faust, D., Ziskin, J., & Hiers, J.B. (1991). *Brain Damage Claims: Coping with Neuropsychological Evidence*. 2 Vol. Odessa, FL: Psychological Assessment Resources.

Freides, D. (1993). Proposed standard of professional practice: Neuropsychological reports display all quantitative data. *The Clinical Neuropsychologist*, *7*, 234–235.

Freides, D. (1995). Interpretations are more benign than data? *The Clinical Neuropsychologist*, *9*, 248.

French, C.C., & Beaumont, J.G. (1987). The reaction of psychiatric patients to computerized assessment. *British Journal of Clinical Psychology*, *26*, 267–278.

Gass, C.S., & Brown, M.C. (1992). Neuropsychological test feedback to patients with brain dysfunction. *Psychological Assessment*, *4*, 272–277.

Goldstein, G., Shemansky, W.J., Beers, S.R., George, T. & Roberts, K. (1996). A clarification of the Russell, Neuringer, and Goldstein process key: Implications for outcome. *Archives of Clinical Neuropsychology, 11*, 581–587.

Goldstein, K.H., & Scheerer, M. (1941). Abstract and concrete behavior: An experimental study with special tests. *Psychological Monographs, 53*, No. 2 (Whole No. 239).

Gur, R.C., Trivedi, S.S., Saykin, A.J., & Gur, R.E. (1988). "Behavioral Imaging"—A procedure for analysis and display of neurobehavioral test scores: I. Construction of algorithm and initial clinical evaluation. *Neuropsychiatry, Neuropsychology, and Behavioral Neurology, 1*, 53–60.

Hall, H.V. (1993). *Disorders of Executive Functions: Civil and Criminal Law Applications.* Delray Beach, FL: St. Lucie Press.

Hall, H.V., & Pritchard, D.A. (1996). *Detecting Malingering and Deception. Forensic Decision Analysis.* Delray Beach, FL: St. Lucie Press.

Hammainen, L. (1994). Computerized support for neuropsychological test interpretation in clinical situations. *The Clinical Neuropsychologist, 8*, 167–185.

Hartje, W., Willmes, K., Pach, R., & Hannen, P. (1991). Driving ability of aphasic and non-aphasic brain-damaged patients. *Neuropsychological Rehabilitation, 1*, 161–174.

Heaton, R.K., & Chelune, J.G. (1988). Neuropsychological and personality tests to assess the likelihood of patient employment. *Journal of Nervous and Mental Disease, 166*, 408–416.

Heaton, R.K., & Pendleton, M.G. (1981). Use of neuropsychological tests to predict adult patients' everyday functioning. *Journal of Consulting and Clinical Psychology, 49*, 807–810.

Kaplan, E. (1988). A process approach to neuropsychological assessment. In T. Boll & B.K. Bryant (Eds.), *Clinical Neuropsychology and Brain Function: Research, Measurement, and Practice*, pp. 127–167. Washington, D.C.: American Psychological Association.

Krug, S.E. (1993). *Psychware Sourcebook* (4th ed.). Champaign, IL: Metritech.

Leckliter, I.N., & Forster, A.A. (1994). The Halstead-Reitan Neuropsychological Test Battery for older children: A need for a new standardization. *Developmental Neuropsychology, 10*, 455–471.

Leckliter, I.N., & Matarazzo, J.D. (1989). The influence of age, education, IQ, gender, and alcohol abuse on Halstead-Reitan neuropsychological test battery performance. *Journal of Clinical Psychology, 45*, 484–512.

Lezak, M.D. (1995). *Neuropsychological Assessment* (3rd ed.). New York: Oxford University Press.

Lichtenberg, P.A., Manning, C.A., Vangel, S.J., & Ross, T.P. (1995). Normative and ecological validity data in older urban medical patients: A program of neuropsychological research. *Advances in Medical Psychotherapy, 8*, 121–136.

Loewenstein, D.A., Rupert, M.P., Berkowitz-Zimmer, N., Guterman, A., Morgan, R., & Hayden, S. (1992). Neuropsychological test performance and prediction of functional capacities in dementia. *Behavior, Health, and Aging, 2*, 149–158.

Matarazzo, J.D. (1986). Computerized psychological test interpretations: Unvalidated plus all mean and no sigma. *American Psychologist, 41*, 14–24.

Matarazzo, J.D. (1990). Psychological assessment versus psychological testing: Validation from Binet to the school, clinic, and courtroom. *American Psychologist, 45*, 999–1017.

Melton, G.B., Petrila, J., Poythress, N.G. & Slobogin, C. (1997). *Psychological Evaluations for the Courts* (2nd ed.). New York: Guilford.

Milberg, W.P., Hebben, N., & Kaplan, E. (1986). The Boston process approach to neuropsychological assessment. In I. Grant & K.M. Adams (Eds.), *Neuropsychological Assessment of Neuropsychiatric Disorders*, pp. 65–86. New York: Oxford University Press.

Milton, G.B., Petrila, J., Poythress, N.G., & Slobogin, C. (1987). *Psychological Evaluations for the Courts*. New York: Guilford.

Moreland, K.L., Eyde, L.D., Robertson, G.J., Primoff, E.S., & Most, R.B. (1995). Assessment of test user qualifications. *American Psychologist, 50*, 14–23.

Naugle, R.I., & McSweeny, A.J. (1995). On the practice of routinely appending neuropsychological data to reports. *The Clinical Neuropsychologist, 9*, 245–247.

Ownby, R.L. (1997). Psychological Reports. 3rd ed. New York: Wiley.

Pope, K.S., Butcher, J.N., & Seelen, J. (1993). *The MMPI, MMPI-2, and MMPI-A in Court: A Practical Guide for Expert Witnesses and Attorneys*. Washington, D.C.: American Psychological Association.

Reitan, R.M., & Wolfson, D. (1995). Influence of age and education on neuropsychological test results. *The Clinical Neuropsychologist, 9*, 151–158.

Reitan, R.M., & Wolfson, D. (1996). The influence of age and education on the neuropsychological test performance of older children. *Child Neuropsychology, 1,* 165–169.

Richardson, E.D., Nadler, J.D., & Malloy, P.F. (1995). Neuropsychologic prediction of daily living skills in geriatric patients. *Neuropsychology, 9,* 565–572.

Richardson, R.E.L., & Adams, R.L. (1992). Neuropsychologists as expert witnesses: Issues of admissability. *The Clinical Neuropsychologist, 6,* 295–308.

Ross, T.P., & Lichtenberg, P.A. (1997). Expanded normative data for the Boston Naming Test in an urban medical sample of elderly adults. Paper presented at the Meeting of the International Neuropsychological Society, Orlando, FL.

Russell, E.W., Neuringer, C., & Goldstein, G. (1970). *Assessment of Brain Damage: A neuropsychological key approach.* New York: Wiley.

Russell, E.W., & Starkey, R.I. (1993). *Halstead Russell Neuropsychological Evaluation System.* Los Angeles: Western Psychological Services.

Sbordone, R.J. (1995). *Neuropsychology for the Attorney.* Delray Beach, FL: St. Lucie Press.

Sbordone, R.J., & Long, C.J. (Eds.) (1995). *Ecological Validity of Neuropsychological Testing.* Delray Beach, FL: St. Lucie Press.

Shapiro, D.L. (1991). *Psychological Evaluation and Expert Testimony.* New York: Van Norstrand Reinhold.

Slick, D., Hopp, G., Strauss, E., Fox, D., Pinch, D., & Stickgold, K. (1996). Effects of prior testing with the WAIS-NI on subsequent retest with the WAIS-R. *The Clinical Neuropsychologist, 11,* 123–130.

Sweet, J.J., Newman, P., & Bell, B. (1992). Significance of depression in clinical neuropsychological assessment. *Clinical Psychology Review, 12,* 21–45.

Tallent, N. (1993). *Psychological Report Writing* (4th Ed.). Englewood Cliffs, NJ: Prentice Hall.

Van Schijndel, F.A.A., & van der Vlugt, H. (1992). Equivalence between classical neuropsychological tests and their computer version: Four neuropsychological tests put to the test. *Journal of Clinical and Experimental Neuropsychology, 14,* 45 (abstract).

Wilson, B.A. (1993). Ecological validity of neuropsychological assessment: Do neuropsychological indexes predict performance in everyday activities? *Applied and Preventive Psychology, 2,* 209–215.

Wilson, B.A., Alderman, N., Burgess, P., Emslie, H., & Evans, J.J. (1996). *Behavioral Assessment of the Dysexecutive Syndrome.* Gaylord, MI: National Rehabilitation Services.

Ziskin, J., & Faust, D. (1988). *Coping with Psychiatric and Psychological Testimony* (4th ed.) Vol. 1–3. Marina Del Rey, CA: Law & Psychology Press.

Zuckerman, E.L. (1995). *The Clinician's Thesaurus: A Guidebook for Wording Psychological Reports and other Evaluations* (4th ed.). Toronto, Ont.: Mental Health Systems.

5

General Intellectual Ability and Assessment of Premorbid Intelligence

Although early psychologists treated intelligence as a unitary concept, subsequent work has suggested that intelligence is best considered as a multiplicity of abilities (Neisser et al., 1996), and therefore best evaluated with multifaceted instruments. There are, however, diverse contemporary conceptions of intelligence and how it should be measured (Neisser et al., 1996). These include: process views (e.g., Sternberg, 1985; Das et al., 1994); hierarchical descriptions that support a general factor (g) at the highest level (e.g., Vernon, 1950; Gustafsson, 1984) or two types of intelligence (Horn and Cattell, 1967); and the multiple intelligences perspective (e.g., Gardner, 1983; Guilford, 1988). A wide variety of techniques are used to assess intelligence (Neisser et al., 1996, for a recent review). Some use only a single type of item (e.g., the Peabody Picture Vocabulary Test, Raven's Progressive Matrices) although the more common measures of general intelligence (the Wechsler Tests and the Stanford-Binet) include many different types of items, both verbal and nonverbal. Test-takers may be asked to give the meaning of words, to complete a series of pictures, to construct block patterns, etc. Their performance can then be scored to yield several subscores and an overall score. Typically, intelligence test scores are converted to a scale in which the mean is 100 and the standard deviation (a measure of variability of the distribution of scores) is 15. About 95 per cent of the population has scores within two standard deviations of the mean, that is, between 70 and 130.

It is worth bearing in mind that a wide range of human abilities are outside the domain of standard intelligence tests (Neisser et al., 1996). Obvious facets include wisdom, creativity, practical knowledge, and social skills. Standard intelligence tests do predict certain forms of achievement—especially school achievement—quite effectively. The correlations between IQ scores and grades is about .50. In this context, the skills measured by intelligence tests are clearly important. Note, however, that correlations of this magnitude account for only about 25% of the overall variance. Other individual characteristics (e.g., persistence, interest) are probably of equal or greater importance.

We present here the Wechsler Intelligence Scales (Wechsler 1981, 1989, 1991), which are composed of a variety of subtests and are the most popular measures of general intellectual ability. We tend to give the Wechsler test early in the course of the assessment because it allows the examiner to observe how the patient behaves on a wide array of tasks. In this way, the examiner can develop hypotheses about the patient's spared and impaired abilities that can then be tested more thoroughly during the course of the assessment. We also consider the recent modification of the WAIS-R, the WAIS-R NI (Kaplan et al., 1991), designed to provide quantified process information for each of the subtests of the WAIS-R. When adults are familiar with the Wechsler test and/or when time constraints preclude the administration of this test, the examiner may wish to consider measures such as the Wonderlic Personnel Test (1972) or the K-BIT (Kaufman & Kaufman, 1990). We prefer the K-BIT since it appears to have better agreement with the Wechsler test. It is relatively motor-free and takes only about 15 to 30 minutes to give. Wechsler Intelligence Scale short forms (see Wechsler Test), however, are somewhat better at predicting WAIS-R Full Scale IQ, and have the advantage that, should there be a need for a complete Wechsler profile, the non-administered subtests can be administered at a later date (Eisenstein & Engelhart, 1997).

The Raven's Progressive Matrices (Raven, 1938, 1947, 1965) may be the instrument of choice in patients who have trouble understanding English. MicroCog (Powell et al., 1993), a computer-administered and computer-scored test, provides broad screening of neuropsychological functioning. Batteries developed specifically for children (as opposed to downward extensions of adult measures) are considered in the next section. Measures such as the Category Test and Wisconsin Card Sorting Test are considered in the section entitled Executive Function.

When adults generate very few responses on the Wechsler Adult Intelligence Scale, making it difficult to rank them according to the extent of their cognitive deficits, tests such as the Mattis Dementia Rating Scale (DRS; Mattis, 1976) or the Mini-Mental State Exam (MMSE; Folstein et al., 1975) may be preferred in order to provide gross estimates of cognitive functioning. We tend to use the DRS more than the MMSE since the DRS provides for a broader coverage of cognitive functions, more accurately tracks progression of decline, and is better able to discriminate among patients with dementia. Nonetheless, the clinician may prefer the MMSE, particularly with those individuals who have difficulty concentrating longer than 5 to 10 minutes.

There are a number of clinical, medicolegal, and research situations where knowledge of premorbid IQ is important. Since data on premorbid testing are rarely available, it becomes necessary to estimate an individual's premorbid level of functioning. There are four general methods used to estimate premorbid IQ.

1. The best performance method which consists of identifying the highest test score (e.g., on the WAIS-R) or highest level of functioning in everyday tasks, and using this level as the "standard against which all other aspects of the patient's current performance are compared" (Lezak, 1983);

2. The subject's performance on WAIS-R subtests that are thought to be relatively insensitive to the effects of brain damage (e.g., Vocabulary, Information);

3. Tests of overlearned skills such as reading which are highly correlated with intelligence (e.g., NART, NAART, WRAT3);

4. Actuarial methods that use demographic data such as age, sex, race, education, and occupation to estimate premorbid IQ (e.g., Barona Index, Barona et al., 1984).

The best performance method has been criticized because it does not take into account the normal variability among tests and has been shown to overestimate premorbid IQ. Thus, the final result will be a systematic overestimation of intellectual impairment or deficits (Mortensen et al., 1991).

Many investigators have relied on the Vocabulary and Information subtest scores of the Wechsler Scales as the best indicators of premorbid intelligence. Although Vocabulary is among the most resistant of the Wechsler subtests, performance on the test is markedly impaired in a range of clinical conditions. It is therefore likely to seriously underestimate premorbid intelligence (Crawford, 1989; Lezak, 1995). The Information subtest score reflects a person's general fund of knowledge. However, this score may be misleading in clients with poor educational opportunities. Information scores may also be affected by a number of clinical conditions.

Nelson and her colleagues (Nelson, 1982; Nelson & O'Connell, 1978) have proposed that a reading test for irregularly spelled words would be a better indicator of premorbid ability since it assesses the level of reading achieved before the onset of brain impairment. They developed in Britain a test called the National Adult Reading Test (NART). The NART consists of 50 irregular words (e.g., debt, naive) and does indeed provide a better estimate of WAIS-R IQ than Vocabulary subtest scores (Crawford, 1989). The NART has recently been standardized against the WAIS-R (Crawford, 1992; Ryan & Paolo, 1992). Blair and Spreen (1989) have adapted the NART for use with a North American population (North American Adult Reading Test or NAART or NART-R). A similar version (AMNART) has recently been developed by Grober and Sliwinski (1991).

It is worth bearing in mind, however, that deterioration in NART performance does occur in some patients with cerebral dysfunction; for example, in cases of moderate to severe levels of dementia (Patterson et al., 1994; Stebbins et al., 1988, 1990a). The NART also appears to underestimate IQ in patients with mild dementia who have accompanying linguistic deficits (Stebbins et al., 1990b). Thus the NART is not insensitive to cerebral dysfunction. Nonetheless, it may prove useful in providing a lower limit to the estimate of premorbid IQ (Stebbins et al., 1990a,b). One should also note that the NART cannot be used with aphasic or dyslexic patients, nor in patients with significant articulatory or visual acuity problems (Crawford, 1989, 1992). Finally, there is evidence that the NART overestimates FSIQ at the lower end of the IQ range and underestimates it at the higher end (Ryan & Paolo, 1992; Wiens et al., 1993).

Some have suggested using the Reading subtest of the Wide Range Achievement Test (WRAT) as an indicator of premorbid intellectual status (Johnstone et al., 1996; Kareken et al., 1995). NART (NAART) and WRAT-R scores are highly correlated (about .8) and both show a moderate relation with WAIS-R IQ (r = .45 to .62) (Johnstone et al., 1996;

Wiens et al., 1993). In normal individuals, Wiens et al. (1993) reported that WRAT-R Reading scores underestimate FSIQ in the higher IQ ranges to an even greater degree than the NART/NAART. At the lower end of the IQ range (80 to 89), the WRAT-R may, however, be more appropriate than the NART/NAART. Johnstone et al. (1996) reported that in a neurologically impaired population, the WRAT-R and NAART were equivalent and accurate estimates of average VIQ levels, the WRAT-R and NAART were equivalent but underestimates of higher intelligence ranges, and the WRAT-R is a more accurace estimate of lower IQ ranges, although both are overestimates. Johnstone et al. (1996) prefer the WRAT-R because it has superior normative data than the NAART, has a less restricted range (46 to 150), and standard deviations equal to that of the WAIS-R (15). Kremen et al. (1996) reported that WRAT-R Reading and Spelling scores are relatively unaffected in schizophrenic patients and provide a better estimate of expected ability than parental education (see also Kareken et al., 1995). As with other cognitive tasks (e.g., NART), Reading or Spelling are likely to underestimate substantially premorbid ability in those with verbal deficits.

The use of demographic measures to estimate premorbid IQ has also shown some promise, with education, race, and occupation being the most powerful predictors. A number of investigators (e.g., Barona et al., 1984; Crawford & Allan, 1997; Reynolds & Gutkin, 1979; Wilson et al., 1978) have developed regression equations to calculate premorbid IQ. Wilson and colleagues regressed WAIS IQs on five demographic variables (age, sex, race, education and occupation) with moderately favorable results. Barona and colleagues updated the formulae for the WAIS-R, again with promising results, although the standard errors of estimate for the regression equations were rather large (e.g., 12.14 for Full Scale WAIS-R IQ). The complete Barona Index equations and demographic variable weights are given in Table 5–1. A sample worksheet (Table 5–2) is provided to facilitate the calculation of predicted IQs. These indices should be considered as rough estimates

Table 5—1. Barona Index Equations and Variable Weights

Estimated VIQ = 54.23 + 0.49(age) + 1.92(sex) + 4.24(race) + 5.25(education) + 1.89(occupation) + 1.24(urban–rural residence). Standard error of estimate of VIQ = 11.79; R = .62.

Estimated PIQ = 61.58 + 0.31(age) + 1.09(sex) + 4.95(race) + 3.75(education) + 1.54(occupation) + .82(region). Standard error of estimate of PIQ = 13.23; R = .49.

Estimated FSIQ = 54.96 + 0.47(age) + 1.76(sex) + 4.71(race) + 5.02(education) + 1.89(occupation) + .59(region). Standard error of estimate of FSIQ = 12.14; R = .60.

Variables take the following values:
Sex
Female = 1   Male = 2

Race
White = 3   Black = 2   Other = 1

Occupation
Professional/Technical = 6
Managerial/Official/Clerical/Sales = 5
Craftsmen/Foremen (Skilled labor) = 4
Not in labor force = 3
Operatives/Service workers/Farmers and farm managers (Semiskilled labor) = 2
Farm laborers, Farm foremen, and laborers (Unskilled labor) = 1

Region (U.S.)
Southern = 1   North central = 2
Western = 3   Northeast = 4

Residence
Rural (<2,500) = 1   Urban (>2,500) = 2

Age

16–17 = 1	25–34 = 4	55–64 = 7	75–79 = 10	90–94 = 13
18–19 = 2	35–44 = 5	65–69 = 8	80–84 = 11	95–99 = 14
20–24 = 3	45–54 = 6	70–74 = 9	85–89 = 12	>100 = 15

Education (years of school)

0–7 = 1	8 = 2	9–11 = 3
12 = 4	13–15 = 5	16+ = 6

Note: VIQ = Verbal IQ; PIQ = Performance IQ, and FSIQ = Full Scale IQ.

Source: Barona et al. (1984). Copyright by the APA. Reprinted with permission. Helmes (1996) has extended the age coding to permit use with individuals over the age of 74. Reprinted with permission Swets & Zeitlinger.

of premorbid functioning, rather than exact indicators, accounting for 38 per cent, 24 per cent, and 36 percent of VIQ, PIQ, and FSIQ scores, respectively. Crawford and Allan (1997) have recently used the demographic approach to predict WAIS-R IQ in the U.K. Their regression equations predicted 53, 53, and 32 per cent of the variance in FSIQ, VIQ and PIQ and are given in Table 5–3. Less than five per cent of the healthy sample exhibited a positive discrepancy (predicted minus observed IQ) of 17 or greater in the case of VIQ and FSIQ and of 19 or greater in the case of PIQ. In general, prediction is better for VIQ and FSIQ, than for PIQ (see also Perez et al., 1996). Note that the band of error associated with these various demographic equations is considerable. In addition, in cases where the premorbid Full Scale IQ is above 120 or below 69, use of these formulas may result in serious under- or overestimation, respectively (Barona et al., 1984; Sweet et al., 1990). It is recommended that the demographic indices be used with considerable caution in the individual case. They should not be used to estimate the premorbid ability of exceptional individuals such as the gifted, mentally retarded, or even slow learners from special education pro-

Table 5—2. Computational Worksheet for Barona Index

	VIQ	PIQ	FSIQ
Age			
16–17	.49	.31	.47
18–19	.98	.62	.97
20–24	1.47	.93	1.41
25–34	1.96	1.24	1.88
35–44	2.45	1.55	2.35
45–54	2.94	1.86	2.82
55–64	3.43	2.17	3.29
65–69	3.92	2.48	3.76
70–74	4.41	2.79	4.23
75–79	4.90	3.10	4.70
80–84	5.39	3.41	5.17
85–89	5.88	3.72	5.64
90–94	6.37	4.03	6.11
95–99	6.86	4.34	6.58
>100	7.35	4.65	7.05
Sex			
Female	1.92	1.09	1.76
Male	3.84	2.18	3.52
Race			
White	12.72	14.85	14.13
Black	8.48	9.90	9.42
Other	4.24	4.95	4.71
Education			
0–7	5.25	3.75	5.02
8	10.50	7.50	10.04
9–11	15.75	11.25	15.06
12	21.00	15.00	20.08
13–15	26.25	18.75	25.10
16+	31.50	22.50	30.12
Occupation			
Professional, Technical	11.34	9.24	11.34
Managerial/Office/Clerical/Sales	9.45	7.70	9.45
Skilled Labor	7.56	6.16	7.56
Not in Labor Force	5.67	4.62	5.67
Semiskilled Labor	3.78	3.08	3.78
Unskilled Labor	1.89	1.54	1.89
Region			
Urban	2.48	1.64	1.18
Rural	1.24	.82	.59
Add	54.23	61.58	54.96
Predicted Score	_____	_____	_____
15% Confidence Interval			
Add: Pred. Score ± 1 (SEE)	11.79	13.23	12.13
	__ to __	__ to __	__ to __
5% Confidence Interval			
Add: Pred. Score ± 2 (SEE)	23.58	26.46	24.28
	__ to __	__ to __	__ to __

Table 5—3. Crawford Index Equations and Variable Weights

Predicted FSIQ = 87.14 − (5.21 × occupation) + (1.78 × education) + (.18 × age).
Standard error of estimate = 9.11

Predicted VIQ = 87.42 − (5.08 × occupation) + (1.77 × education) + (.17 × age).
Standard error of estimate = 8.83

Predicted PIQ = 90.89 − (4.34 × occupation) + (1.33 × education + (.16 × age).
Standard error of estimate = 11.2

Source: Crawford & Allan, (1997). In recording years of education, credit with 0.5 of a year for every year spent in part-time education. Part-time education is defined as day-release courses and evening classes provided they lead to qualification. Occupation is coded as follows: 1 = professional, 2 = intermediate, 3 = skilled, 4 = semi-skilled, 5 = unskilled. Retired individuals, and those describing themselves as househus-bands/housewives, are coded by their previous occupations as are those who are currently unemployed. Those who have never worked are coded as unskilled.

grams (Ryan & Prifitera, 1990). They should also not be used to infer lateralized damage (Perez et al., 1996). Recently, Paolo et al. (1996) have developed demographically-based regression equations to predict Wechsler subtest scaled scores. Like other demographically based indices, the equations to predict subtest scores tend to underestimate ability at the high end and overestimate ability at the low end. The available evidence suggests that the NART (or NAART) is a more powerful predictor of IQ (at least VIQ and FSIQ) than demographic indices (Blair & Spreen, 1989; Crawford, 1992). On the other hand, demographic methods have the advantage of being applicable to a wide variety of patients and, unlike performance on cognitive tests (e.g., Vocabulary and Information subtests, NART, NAART), they are not subject to decline in clinical conditions (e.g., dementia).

Pairing test behavior (e.g., Vocabulary, Information, Picture Completion, NART, NAART, AMNART, MMPI) or other information (school or military records, level of functioning of immediate family members) with data from demographic variables seems to increase the power of prediction (Crawford, 1992; Grober & Sliwinski, 1991; Krull et al., 1995; Raguet et al., 1996; Sweet et al., 1990; Vanderploeg & Schinka, 1995; Vanderploeg et al., 1996; Willshire, Kinsella, & Prior, 1991; Wrobel & Wrobel, 1996). Such attempts are superior to the individual methods and appear promising. For example, Raguet et al. (1996)

recommend simple averaging of NAART and Barona estimates. Clinicians may also refer to the Oklahoma Premorbid Intelligence Estimate (OPIE), a linear prediction algorithm, developed on the WAIS-R standardization sample, designed to combine either verbal and/or nonverbal current performance measures (Vocabulary and Picture Completion from the WAIS-R) with demographic information (age, education, race, and occupation) to predict premorbid IQ (Krull, Scott, & Sherer, 1995). The OPIE equations provide reasonable estimates of IQ (accounting for 76 percent, 63 percent, and 75 percent of VIQ, PIQ, FSIQ, respectively) without the severe degree of range restriction that is found in purely demographically derived algorithms. Note, however, that some restriction of range also occurs with the OPIE. The OPIE prediction equations and demographic variable weights are given in Table 5–4. Some notes of caution are in order. First, using the OPIE formulas on young adults may influence the accuracy of prediction by underestimating potential educational and occupational attainment. The use of the occupational rating of the parent may be a viable alternative. Second, the prediction equations should not be used with children under the age of 16 years, since the validity of such use has not been established. Third, additional research is needed to examine the performance of the OPIE relative to other methods of premorbid IQ estimation (e.g., combining NART with demographic data).

Table 5—4. OPIE Equations and Variable Weights

Estimated FSIQ = 53.80 + .10(age) + .64(education) − 1.73(race) − .51(occupation) + .57(Vocabulary raw score) + 1.33(Picture Completion raw score); Standard error of the estimate = 6.41

Estimated FSIQv = 69.43 + .85(educ) − 2.68(race) − .66(occup) + .76 (Voc raw score); Standard error of the estimate = 7.10

Estimated FSIQp = 52.76 + .24 (age) + 3.10(educ) − 3.73(race) − .71(occup) + 2.30(Picture Completion raw score); Standard error of the estimate = 7.45

Estimated VIQ = 65.87 + .87(education) − 1.53(race) − .50(occupation) + .79(Vocabulary raw score); Standard error of the estimate = 6.29

Estimated PIQ = 52.45 + .23(age) + 1.34(education) − 3.14(race) − .62(occupation) + 2.77(Picture Completion raw score); Standard error of the estimate = 7.41

Age
Calculate in years

Race
1 = caucasian
2 = non-caucasian

Education
1 = 0–7 years
2 = 8 years
3 = 9–11 years
4 = 12 years
5 = 13–15 years
6 = 16 years

Occupation
1 = Professional/Technical
2 = Manager/Administrator/Clerical/Sales
3 = Craftsman/Foreman
4 = Operators/Service/Domestic/Farmers
5 = Laborers
6 = Unemployed

Summary Worksheet

	Obtained	Predicted	95% Confidence Interval (Pred. Score ± 2(SEE)	Discrepancy
FSIQ	_____	_____	_____	_____
VIQ	_____	_____	_____	_____
PIQ	_____	_____	_____	_____

Source: Krull et al. 1995. Reprinted with permission Swets & Zeitlinger.

Fourth, in those patients where a lateralized lesion is suspected, either from a large disparity between verbal and nonverbal cognitive functioning or the results of biomedical tests, the use of alternate formulas (see Table 5–4) utilizing only Vocabulary or Picture Completion in predicting Full Scale IQs may yield a more accurate estimate of premorbid IQ. If Vocabulary and Picture Completion non-age-corrected scaled scores are equal or Vocabulary is higher, estimate FSIQ using only Vocabulary; if Picture Completion is higher, estimate FSIQ using only Picture Completion (Scott et al., 1997). Fifth, Krull and colleagues (1995) chose the Vocabulary and Picture Completion subtests because of their reliability and relative resistence to neurological insult. Vanderploeg and Schinka (1995) developed 33 regression formulas, each combining one of the 11 WAIS-R subtests with demographic variables, to predict IQ scores. When there is no a priori knowledge on which to base selection of hold (or preserved) measures, they too recommend equations using Vocabulary, Information, and Picture Completion for prediction purposes since they are highly correlated with actual ability (Vanderploeg et al., 1996). Finally, demographic indices alone may be preferred for estimating premorbid IQ in patients for whom reliance on cognitive performance (e.g., Vocabulary, Picture Completion, NART, NAART, WRAT3) would be inappropriate (e.g., patients with moderate or advanced dementia or aphasia). Alternatively, clinicians may correct test behavior (e.g., NART) with information regarding dementia severity, using specially derived correction factors (Taylor et al., 1996).

In addition to detecting decline in patients with neurological disorders, neuropsychologists are also asked to assess brain dysfunction in patients with psychiatric disturbances. Wrobel and Wrobel (1996) have recently paired demographic (Barona IQ) and MMPI variables to determine what the patient's IQ would be, given the effects of their current psychiatric condition but without any identifiable brain insult. The equations account for about 40 per cent, 26 per cent and 34 per cent of VIQ, PIQ, and FSIQ, respectively. The authors noted that application of the Barona equation alone tended to overestimate current functioning. Consistent with other research described above, the inclusion of the MMPI variables to the Barona formulae enhanced the accuracy of prediction of current functioning.

References

Barona, A., Reynolds, C.R., & Chastain, R. (1984). A demographically based index of pre-morbid intelligence for the WAIS-R. *Journal of Consulting and Clinical Psychology*, 52, 885–887.

Blair, J.R., & Spreen, O. (1989). Predicting premorbid IQ: A revision of the National Adult Reading Test. *The Clinical Neuropsychologist*, 3, 129–136.

Crawford, J.R. (1989). Estimation of premorbid intelligence: a review of recent developments. In J.R. Crawford & D.M. Parker (Eds.), *Developments in Clinical and Experimental Neuropsychology*. London: Plenum.

Crawford, J.R. (1992). Current and premorbid intelligence measures in neuropsychological assessment. In J.R. Crawford, D.M. Parker, and W.M. McKinlay (Eds.), *A Handbook of Neuropsychological Assessment*. West Sussex: LEA.

Crawford, J.R., & Allan, K.M. (1997). Estimating premorbid WAIS-R IQ with demographic variables: Regression equation derived from a U.K. sample. *The Clinical Neuropsychologist*, 11, 192–197.

Das, J.P., Naglieri, J.A., Kirby, J.R. (1994). *Assessment of Cognitive Processes: The PASS Theory of Intelligence*. Needham, MA: Allyn and Bacon.

Eisenstein, N., & Engelhart, C.I. (1997). Comparison of the K-BIT with short forms of the WAIS-R in a neuropsychological population. *Psychological Assessment*, 9, 57–62.

Folstein, M.F., Folstein, S.E., & McHugh, P.R. (1975). "Mini-Mental State": A practical method for grading the cognitive state of outpatients for the clinician. *The Journal of Psychiatric Research*, 12, 189–198.

Gardner, H. (1983). *Frames of mind: The theory of multiple intelligences*. New York: Basic Books.

Grober, E., & Sliwinski, M. (1991). Development and validation of a model for estimating premorbid verbal intelligence in the elderly. *Journal of Clinical and Experimental Neuropsychology*, 13, 933–949.

Guilford, J.P. (1988). Some changes in the structure-of-intellect model. *Education and Psychological Measurement*, 48, 1–4.

Gustafsson, J.E. (1984). A unifying model for the structure of intellectual abilities. *Intelligence*, 8, 179–203.

Helmes, E. (1996). Use of the Barona method to predict premorbid intelligence in the elderly. *The Clinical Neuropsychologist*, 10, 255–261.

Horn, J.L., & Cattell, R.B. (1967). Age difference in fluid and crystallized intelligence. *Acta Psychologica*, 26, 107–129.

Johnstone, B., Callahan, C.D., Kapila, C.J., & Bouman, D.E. (1996). The comparability of the WRAT-R reading test and NAART as estimates of premorbid intelligence in neurologically impaired patients. *Archives of Clinical Neuropsychology*, 11, 513–519.

Kaplan, E., Fein, D., Morris, R., & Delis, D.C. (1991). *WAIS-R NI Manual*. San Antonio: Psychological Corporation.

Kareken, D.A., Gur, R.C., & Saykin, A.J. (1995). Reading on the Wide Range Achievement Test—Revised and parental education as predictors of IQ: Comparison with the Barona formula. *Archives of Clinical Neuropsychology*, 10, 147–157.

Kaufman, A.S., & Kaufman, N.L. (1990). *Kaufman*

Brief Intelligence Test. Circle Pines, MN: American Guidance Service.

Kremen, W.S., Seidman, I.J., Faraone, S.V., Pepple, J.R., Lyons, M.J., & Tsuang, M.T. (1996). The "3Rs" and neuropsychological function in schizophrenia: An empirical test of the matching fallacy. *Neuropsychology, 1,* 22–31.

Krull, K.R., Scott, J.G., & Sherer, M. (1995). Estimation of premorbid intelligence from combined performance and demographic variables. *The Clinical Neuropsychologist, 9,* 83–88.

Lezak, M.D. (1983). *Neuropsychological Assessment* (2nd ed.). New York: Oxford University Press.

Lezak, M.D. (1995). *Neuropsychological Assessment* (3rd ed.). New York: Oxford University Press.

Mattis, S. (1976). Mental status examination for organic mental syndrome in the elderly patient. In L. Bellak & T.B. Karasu (Eds.), *Geriatric Psychiatry.* New York: Grune & Stratton.

Mortensen, E.L., Gade, A., & Reinisch, J.M. (1991). A critical note on Lezak's "Best performance method" in clinical neuropsychology. *Journal of Clinical and Experimental Neuropsychology, 13,* 361–371.

Neisser, U., Boodoo, G., Bouchard, T.J., Boykin, A.W., Brody, N., Ceci, S.J., Halpern, D.F., Loehlin, J.C., Perloff, R., Sternberg, R.J., & Urbina, S. (1996). Intelligence: Knowns and unknowns. *American Psychologist, 51,* 77–101.

Nelson, H.E. (1982). *National Adult Reading Test (NART): Test Manual.* Windsor, England: NFER Nelson.

Nelson, H.E., & O'Connell, A. (1978). Dementia: The estimation of pre-morbid intelligence levels using the new adult reading test. *Cortex, 14,* 234–244.

Paolo, A.M., Ryan, J.J., & Troster, A.I. (1996). Demographically based regression equations to estimate WAIS-R subtest scaled scores. *The Clinical Neuropsychologist, 10,* 130–140.

Patterson, K., Graham, N., & Hodges, J.R. (1994). Reading in dementia of the Alzheimer type: A preserved ability? *Neuropsychology, 8,* 395–407.

Perez, S.A., Schlottmann, R.S., Holloway, J.A., & Ozolins, M.S. (1996). Measurement of premorbid intellectual ability following brain injury. *Archives of Clinical Neuropsychology, 11,* 491–501.

Powell, D.H., Kaplan, E.F., Whitla, D., Weintraub, S., Catlin, R., & Funkenstein, H.H. (1993). *MicroCog Manual: Assessment of Cognitive Functioning.* San Antonio: The Psychological Corporation.

Raguet, M.L., Campbell, D.A., Berry, D.T.R., Schmitt, F.A., & Smith, G.T. (1996). Stability of intelligence and intellectual predictors in older persons. *Psychological Assessment, 8,* 154–160.

Raven, J.C. (1938). *Progressive Matrices: A Perceptual Test of Intelligence.* London: H.K. Lewis.

Raven, J.C. (1947). *Colored Progressive Matrices Sets A, Ab, B.* London: H.K. Lewis.

Raven, J.C. (1965). *Advanced Progressive Matrices Sets I and II.* London: H.K. Lewis.

Reynolds, C.R., & Gutkin, T.B. (1979). Predicting the premorbid intellectual status of children using demographic data. *Clinical Neuropsychology, 1,* 36–38.

Ryan, J.J., & Paolo, A.M. (1992). A screening procedure for estimating premorbid intelligence in the elderly. *The Clinical Neuropsychologist, 6,* 53–62.

Ryan, J.J., & Prifitera, A. (1990). The WAIS-R index for estimating premorbid intelligence: accuracy in predicting short form IQ. *International Journal of Clinical Neuropsychology, 12,* 20–23.

Scott, J.G., Krull, K.R., Williamson, D.J.G., & Adams, R.L. (1997). Oklahoma Premorbid Intelligence Estimation (OPIE): Utilization in clinical samples. *The Clinical Neuropsychologist, 11,* 146–154.

Stebbins, G.T., Wilson, R.S., Gilley, D.W., Bernard, B.A., & Fox, J.H. (1988). Estimation of premorbid intelligence in dementia. *Journal of Clinical and Experimental Neuropsychology, 10,* 63–64.

Stebbins, G.T., Wilson, R.S., Gilley, D.W., Bernard, B.A., & Fox, J.H. (1990a). Use of the National Adult Reading Test to estimate premorbid IQ in dementia. *The Clinical Neuropsychologist, 4,* 18–24.

Stebbins, G.T., Gilley, D.W., Wilson, R.S., Bernard, B.A., & Fox, J.H. (1990b). Effects of language disturbances on premorbid estimates of IQ in mild dementia. *The Clinical Neuropsychologist, 4,* 64–68.

Sternberg, R.J. (1985). *Beyond I.Q.: A Triarchic Theory of Human Intelligence.* New York: Cambridge University Press.

Sweet, J., Moberg, P., & Tovian, S. (1990). Evaluation of Wechsler Adult Intelligence Scale—Revised premorbid IQ clinical formulas in clinical populations. *Psychological Assessment, 2,* 41–44.

Taylor, K.I., Salmon, D.P., Rice, V.A., Bondi, M.W., Hill, L.R., Ernesto, C.R., & Butters, N. (1996). A longitudinal examination of American National Adult Reading Test (AMNART) performance in dementia of the Alzheimer Type (DAT):

Validation and correction based on rate of cognitive decline. *Journal of Clinical and Experimental Neuropsychology, 18*, 883–891.

Vanderploeg, R.D., & Schinka, J.A. (1995). Predicting WAIS-R premorbid ability: Combining subtest performance and demographic variable predictors. *Archives of Clinical Neuropsychology, 10*, 225–239.

Vanderploeg, R.D., Schinka, J.A., & Axelrod, B.N. (1996). Estimation of WAIS-R premorbid intelligence: Current ability and demographic data used in a best-performance fashion. *Psychological Assessment, 8*, 404–411.

Vernon, P.E. (1950). *The Structure of Human Abilities*. New York: Wiley.

Wechsler, D. (1989). *Manual for the WPPSI*. New York: Psychological Corporation.

Wechsler, D. (1991). *Manual for the WISC III*. New York: Psychological Corporation.

Wechsler, D. (1981). *Manual for the WAIS-R*. New York: Psychological Corporation.

Wechsler, D. (1996). *WISC-III Manual Canadian Supplement*. Toronto: The Psychological Corporation.

Wiens, A.N., Bryan, J.E., & Crossen, J.R. (1993). Estimating WAIS-R FSIQ from the National Adult Reading Test—Revised in normal subjects. *The Clinical Neuropsychologist, 8*, 70–84.

Wilson, R.S., Rosenbaum, G., Brown, G., Rourke, D., Whitman, D., & Grisell, J. (1978). An index of premorbid intelligence. *Journal of Consulting and Clinical Psychology, 46*, 1554–1555.

Willshire, D., Kinsella, G., & Prior, M. (1991). Estimating WAIS-R IQ from the National Adult Reading Test: A cross-validation. *Journal of Clinical and Experimental Neuropsychology, 13*, 204–216.

Wrobel, N.H., & Wrobel, T.A. (1996). The problem of assessing brain damage in psychiatric samples: Use of personality variables in prediction of WAIS-R scores. *Archives of Clinical Neuropsychology, 11*, 625–635.

DEMENTIA RATING SCALE (DRS)

Purpose

The purpose of this scale is to provide an index of cognitive function in subjects with known or suspected dementia.

Source

The test can be ordered from Psychological Assessment Resources, Inc., P.O. Box 998, Odessa, Florida, at a cost of $69 US.

Description

Some patients, such as the elderly with profound cognitive impairments, may generate very few responses on such standard tests as the Wechsler Adult Intelligence Scale—Revised or Wechsler Memory Scale—Revised, making it difficult to assess the magnitude of their mental impairments. The Dementia Rating Scale (DRS) was developed to quantify the mental status of such patients (Coblentz et al., 1973; Mattis, 1976, 1988). Items are similar to those employed by neurologists in bed-side mental status examinations. They are arranged hierarchically so that adequate performance on an initial item allows the examiner to discontinue testing within that section and assume that credit can be given for adequate performance on the subsequent tasks. A global measure of dementia is derived from subscores of specific cognitive capacities. The subtests include measures of attention (e.g., digit span), initiation and perseveration (e.g., performing alternating movements), construction (e.g., copying designs), conceptualization (e.g., similarities), and verbal and nonverbal short-term memory (e.g., sentence recall, design recognition).

Administration

See source. Briefly, the examiner asks questions or gives instructions in each area (e.g., "In what way are an apple and a banana alike?" "The same?") and records responses. Based on factor analysis of data from patients with Alzheimer's Disease (AD), Colantonio et al. (1993) developed a short version of the DRS, to be used for screening purposes. This consists of the sum of the individual scores of priming inductive reasoning, similarities and differences, identities and oddities, graphomotor, construction, alternating movements, attention, sentence recall, and orientation. The maximum total score for the short form is 86 points.

Approximate Time for Administration

The time required is approximately 10–15 minutes for normal elderly subjects. With a demented patient, administration may take 30–45 minutes.

Scoring

See source. One point is given for each item performed correctly. Maximum score is 144.

Comment

Gardner et al. (1981) reported a split-half reliability of .90 for the Total scale in a sample of nursing home patients with neurological disorders. Smith et al. (1994) found mixed support for the reliability of DRS scales in a sample of 274 older patients with cognitive impairment. Internal consistency (Crohnbach's alpha) was greater than .7 for Construction, Conceptualization, Memory, and Total score, greater than .65 for Attention, and only about .45 for Initiation and Perseveration. Interpretation of the Initiation and Perseveration scale is, therefore, somewhat hazardous. When patients with provisional diagnoses of AD were retested following a one-week interval, the correlation for the DRS Total score was .97, whereas subscale correlations ranged from .61 to .94 (Coblentz et al., 1973). Smith et al. (1994) retested a sample of 154 older normal individuals following an interval of about one year and found that DRS Total score declines of 10 points or greater occurred in less than 5 percent of normals. Not surprisingly, over this comparable interval, 61 percent of 110 dementia patients displayed a decline in DRS Total scores of 10 or more points.

With regard to validity, the test correlates with the Wechsler Memory Scale Memory Quotient (.70), the WAIS Full Scale IQ (.67), and cortical metabolism (.59) as determined by positron emission tomography (PET) (Chase et al., 1984). Smith et al. (1994) found that in older adults who were cognitively impaired, DRS Total score shared 54 percent of its variance with FSIQ and 57 percent with VIQ, as assessed in the MAYO Older Americans Normative Studies. In retarded individuals, the test loaded on the same factor as the Peabody

Picture Vocabulary Test—Revised (Das et al., 1995). Moreover, the test correlates highly with other commonly used standardized mental status examinations, such as the Mini-Mental-State Exam (MMSE) and the Information-Memory-Concentration test (IMC) (Salmon et al., 1990).

In designing the test, Mattis grouped the tasks according to their face validity into five subsets: memory, construction, initiation and perseveration, conceptualization, and attention. Smith et al. (1994) provided evidence of convergent validity for some of the DRS scales. In a sample of 234 elderly patients with cognitive impairment, DRS subscale scores for Memory, Attention, and Conceptualization were significantly correlated with appropriate indices (GMI, ACI and VIQ, respectively) from the WAIS-R and Wechsler Memory Scale–Revised, as assessed in the Mayo Older Americans Normative Studies. Support for the convergent validity of the Construction scale was more problematic. Smith et al. found that this scale correlated more highly with VIQ and ACI scales than with PIQ, raising the concern that it may provide a better index of attention and general cognitive status than of visuoperceptual/visuoconstructional skills *per se*. Marson et al. (1997) reported that in a sample of fifty patients with mild to moderate AD, four of the five DRS subscales correlated most strongly with their assigned criterion variables (Attention with WMS-R Attention, Initiation-Perseveration with COWA, Conceptualization with WAIS Similarities, Memory with WMS-R Verbal Memory). Again, the Construction scale correlated as highly with Block Design as WMS-R Attention.

Further, factor analytic studies suggest that the five subsets do not reflect exclusively the constructs with which they are labeled (Colantonio et al., 1993; Kessler et al., 1994; Woodard et al., 1996). Kessler et al. (1994) found a two-factor model, measuring separate verbal and nonverbal functions, fit the data best in a heterogeneous sample, approximately one-third of which carried psychiatric diagnoses. In a study by Colantonio et al. (1993) on a sample of patients with probable AD, three factors emerged: (1) *conceptualiza-*

tion/organization, containing items consisting of priming inductive reasoning, similarities, differences, identities and oddities, and sentence generation; (2) *visuospatial*, containing items assessing graphomotor, construction, attention, alternating movements, and word and design recognition memory; and (3) *memory*, consisting of sentence recall and orientation. Similar results have recently been reported by Woodard et al. (1996) in a sample of patients with probable AD for both the standard and abbreviated DRS. Moderate correlations were also found between these factors and supplementary neuropsychological measures, supporting the validity of these factors. The contrasting results (Kessler et al., 1994, versus Colantonio et al., 1993; Woodard et al., 1996) highlight the fact that the resulting factor structure depends critically on the characteristics of the population studied.

Recent data suggest that the DRS may be useful in determining cognitive dysfunction relating to HIV infection (Kovner et al., 1992). The DRS can also differentiate brain-damaged patients clearly from normal elderly subjects, is sensitive to early stages of dementia (Vitaliano et al., 1984) even in retarded individuals, and is useful in identifying stages (severity) of impairment (Shay et al., 1991). Further, the DRS has demonstrated ability to accurately track progression of cognitive decline, even in the later stages of AD (Salmon et al., 1990). Although the DRS is highly correlated with other mental status exams, such as the Information Memory Cencentration (IMC) test and MMSE, it shows much greater sensitivity to change in severely demented patients, perhaps because it includes more easy items (Salmon et al., 1990). Therefore, to follow progression in severely demented patients, the DRS is clearly the instrument of choice.

Unlike other standardized mental status examinations that were developed as screening instruments (e.g., MMSE), the DRS was designed with the intention of discriminating among patients with dementia. Recently, it has been demonstrated that pattern analysis of the DRS can effectively distinguish the dementias associated with AD from those associated with Huntington's Disease (HD) or Parkinson's Disease (PD) (Salmon et al., 1989;

Paolo et al., 1994). Patients with dementia of AD display more severe memory impairment; patients with HD are more severely impaired on items that involve the programming of motor sequences (Initiation subtest) while patients with PD display more severe constructional problems. These distinctions were made even when the subjects were similar in terms of overall level of cognitive impairment.

Further, DRS scores show modest correlations with measures of functional competence (ability to perform activities of daily living as well as engage in complex recreational activities) (Lemsky et al., 1996; Loewenstein et al., 1992; Smith et al., 1994; Vitaliano et al., 1984). Nadler and her colleagues (1993) found that the Initiation/Perseveration and Memory subtests were the best predictors of everyday functioning in geriatric patients referred for neuropsychological evaluation. In addition, the DRS may be useful in predicting functional decline (Hochberg et al., 1989) and survival (Smith et al., 1994). Smith et al. (1994) reported that in a sample of 274 persons over age 55 with cognitive impairment, DRS Total scores supplemented age information and provided a better basis for estimating survival than did gender or duration of disease. Median survival for those with DRS Total scores below 100 was 3.7 years.

In short, the summary score appears to have relatively good convergent and predictive validity. Given that the DRS may also be helpful in distinguishing among dementing disorders, the focus should also be on specific cognitive dimensions. In this context, it is worth recalling that the Conceptualization and Memory subscales appear fairly reliable and seem to represent discrete constructs. Construction, Attention, and Initiation and Perseveration items should also be administered (e.g., to derive valid DRS Total scores), but their interpretation may be more problematic. It is also important to note that the test is a screening device, and the clinician should follow up with more in-depth investigation.

Normative Data

Mattis (cited in Montgomery, 1982; Mattis, 1976) recommends a cutoff of 137. However,

Table 5—5. Mean Scores and Standard Deviations on the Dementia Rating Scale for Subjects Ages 62–95

| | Vangel and Lichtenberg | | | | Montgomery Age 65–89 | |
| | Age 62–79 | | Age 80–95 | | | |
	M	SD	M	SD	M	SD
Total score	133.8	6.3	128.2	8.2	137.28	6.94
Attention	35.3	1.3	35.1	2.0	35.47	1.59
Initiation & Perseveration	33.9	3.3	31.7	4.9	35.50	3.02
Construction	5.5	1.3	5.1	1.8	5.80	0.61
Conceptualization	35.5	2.8	34.7	2.8	37.25	2.58
Memory	23.4	1.8	20.7	3.5	23.28	2.12

Source: Vangel & Lichtenberg (1995). The 73 inpatients in the younger group had a mean age of 72.3 (SD = 4.0), and a mean education of 10.6 (SD = 3.7). The 17 patients in the older group had a mean age of 83.5 (SD = 2.9) and a mean education of 10.3 (SD = 3.1). Reprinted with permission of Swets and Zeitlinger. Montgomery (1982). Data based on 85 volunteers, mean age of 74.04 and mean educational level of 12.4 years. Reprinted with permission of author.

Table 5—6. Mattis Dementia Rating Scale Score by Educational Level and Age

| | Age Ranges | | | |
Educational Level	50–59	60–69	70–80	Total
4–9 years				
n	119	161	37	317
Mean	140.7	140.0	139.0	140.2
SD	4.8	3.8	3.7	4.2
Lowest quintile	135	133	130	134
10–13 years or high school diploma				
n	245	282	50	577
Mean	142.1	141.3	140.7	141.6
SD	2.1	3.0	2.4	2.6
Lowest quintile	137	135	135	137
College experience or higher degree				
n	33	58	16	107
Mean	143.1	142.2	141.3	142.3
SD	1.9	1.7	1.7	1.7
Lowest quintile	140	139	138	139
Total				
n	397	501	103	1,001
Mean	141.8	141.0	140.1	141.2
SD	3.2	3.2	3.0	3.2
Lowest quintile	137	135	134	135

Source: Schmidt et al., 1994. The sample consisted of 1,001 randomly selected, elderly, healthy volunteers in the setting of a population-based stroke prevention study. Reprinted by permission of Little, Brown and Company, Inc.

his data are of limited value since the sample sizes on which scores are based (Coblentz et al., 1973) were extremely small (i.e., 20 brain-damaged subjects, 11 normals).

Montgomery (1982; also see Table 5-5 and DRS professional manual) compiled data on 85 normal volunteers (60 women, 25 men), ranging in age from 65 to 89 (mean = 74.04), with an average educational level of 12.4 years and a mean scaled score of 13.5 on the Vocabulary subtest of the WAIS. Her data suggest a cutoff of 123 (based upon the mean ± 2 SD). Montgomery's sample is not truly representative of the elderly population since her sample is better educated, of higher socioeconomic status, and probably healthier than most elderly. Moreover, sample sizes for all age groups, especially those above age 80, are small. Consequently, one must be cautious in interpreting low scores of people with more advanced age, reduced education, and low verbal ability.

Slightly different cutoff scores have been provided by Shay et al., (1991). According to these researchers, patients can be classed as mild or moderately demented according to their DRS total score: mild dementia (total: 103 to 130) and moderate to severe dementia (total: <103). The clinical utility of these scores is limited, however, because the sample size was small and the subjects were relatively well-educated.

Schmidt et al. (1994) derived norms from 1,001 Austrian subjects, aged 50 to 80 years, who were free of neuropsychiatric or severe general diseases. The data are shown in Table 5–6 stratified by age and education. They also present their data in the form of percentile points and recommend referring to the lowest quintile percentile value as a cutoff point when screening for cognitive dysfunction.

Vangel and Lichtenberg (1995) recently provided norms based on a sample of 90 cognitively intact inpatients (aged 62 to 95 years) at a large midwestern university medical center. The majority of participants were African-American. Vangel and Lichtenberg (1995) reported that a cutoff score of 125 correctly classified 87 percent of their sample as cognitively intact vs. impaired. The data are somewhat lower than those provided by Montgomery

(1982) and Schmidt et al. (1994) yet higher than those reported by Marcopulos et al. (1997), perhaps reflecting differences in health status and/or cultural factors. They may, however, be appropriate for use with African-American patients and are applicable to a wider age range. The data are shown in Table 5–5.

Age affects performance, with younger subjects obtaining higher scores than older ones. Some (Marcopulos et al., 1997; Schmidt et al., 1994, Smith et al., 1994) have reported that performance varied not only by age, but also by education and IQ. Vangel and Lichtenberg (1995), however, found that the effects of gender, race, and education were negligible once the influence of age was partialed out. Cerebrovascular risk factors (e.g., history of arterial hypertension, coronary heart disease, diabetes, smoking, obesity, hypercholesterolemia) do not affect performance (Schmidt et al., 1994).

References

Chase, T.N., Foster, N.L., Fedio, P., Brooks, R., Mansi, L., & Di Chiro, G. (1984). Regional cortical dysfunction in Alzheimer's disease as determined by positron emission tomography. *Annals of Neurology, 15*, S170–S174.

Coblentz, J.M., Mattis, S., Zingesser, L.H., Kasoff, S.S., Wisniewski, H.M., & Katzman, R. (1973). Presenile dementia. *Archives of Neurology, 29*, 299–308.

Colantonio, A., Becker, J.T., & Huff, F.J. (1993). Factor structure of the Mattis Dementia Rating Scale among patients with probable Alzheimer's Disease. *The Clinical Neuropsychologist, 7*, 313–318.

Das, J.P., Mishra, R.K., Davison, M., & Naglieri, J.A. (1995). Measurement of dementia in individuals with mental retardation: Comparison based on PPVT and Dementia Rating Scale. *The Clinical Neuropsychologist, 9*, 32–37.

Gardner, R., Oliver-Munoz, S., Fisher, L., & Empting, L. (1981). Mattis Dementia Rating Scale: Internal reliability study using a diffusely impaired population. *Journal of Clinical Neuropsychology, 3*, 271–275.

Hochberg, M.G., Russo, J., Vitaliano, P.P., Prinz, P.N., Vitiello, M.V., & Yi, S. (1989). Initiation and perseveration as a subscale of the Dementia Rating Scale. *Clinical Gerontologist, 8*, 27–41.

Kessler, H.R., Roth, D.L., Kaplan, R.F., & Goode, K.T. (1994). Confirmatory factor analysis of the Mattis Dementia Rating Scale. *The Clinical Neuropsychologist, 8*, 451–461.

Kovner, R., Lazar, J.W., Lesser, M., Perecman, E., Kaplan, M.H., Hainline, B., & Napolitano, B. (1992). Use of the Dementia Rating Scale as a test for neuropsychological dysfunction in HIV-positive IV drug abusers. *Journal of Substance Abuse Treatment, 9*, 133–137.

Lemsky, C.M., Smith, G., Malec, J.F., & Ivnik, R.J. (1996). Identifying risk for functional impairment using cognitive measures: An application of CART modeling. *Neuropsychology, 10*, 368–375.

Loewenstein, D.A., Rupert, M.P., Berkowitz-Zimmer, N., Guterman, A., Morgan, R., & Hayden, S. (1992). Neuropsychological test performance and prediction of functional capacities in dementia. *Behavior, Health, and Aging, 2*, 149–158.

Marcopulos, B.A., McLain, C.A., & Giuliano, A.J. (1997). Cognitive impairment or inadequate norms? A study of healthy, rural, older adults with limited education. *The Clinical Neuropsychologist, 11*, 111–131.

Marson, D.C., Dymek, M.P., Duke, L.W., & Harrell, L.E. (1997). Subscale Validity of the Mattis Dementia Rating Scale. *Archives of Clinical Neuropsychology, 12*, 269–275.

Mattis, S. (1976). Mental status examination for organic mental syndrome in the elderly patient. In L. Bellak & T.B. Karasu (Eds.), *Geriatric Psychiatry*. New York: Grune and Stratton.

Mattis, S. (1988). *Dementia Rating Scale: Professional Manual*. Odessa, FL: Psychological Assessment Resources.

Montgomery, K.M. (1982). A normative study of neuropsychological test performance of a normal elderly sample. Unpublished master's thesis. University of Victoria, Victoria, British Columbia.

Nadler, J.D., Richardson, E.D., Malloy, P.F., Marran, M.E., & Hostetler Brinson, M.E. (1993). The ability of the Dementia Rating Scale to predict everyday functioning. *Archives of Clinical Neuropsychology, 8*, 449–460.

Paolo, A.M., Troster, A.I., Glatt, S.L., Hubble, J.P., & Koller, W.C. (1994). Utility of the Dementia Rating Scale to differentiate the dementias of Alzheimer's and Parkinson's Disease. Paper presented to the International Neuropsychological Society, Cincinnati, OH.

Salmon, D.P., Kwo-on-Yuen, P.F., Heindel, W.C., Butters, N., & Thal, L.J. (1989). Differentiation of Alzheimer's disease and Huntington's disease with the Dementia Rating Scale. *Archives of Neurology, 46*, 1204–1208.

Salmon, D.P., Thal, L.J., Butters, N., & Heindel, W.C. (1990). Longitudinal evaluation of dementia of the Alzheimer's type: A comparison of 3 standardized mental status examinations. *Neurology, 40*, 1225–1230.

Schmidt, R., Freidl, W., Fazekas, F., Reinhart, P., Greishofer, P., Koch, M., Eber, B., Schumacher, M., Polmin, K., & Lechner, H. (1994). The Mattis Dementia Rating Scale: Normative data from 1,001 healthy volunteers. *Neurology, 44*, 964–966.

Shay, K.A., Duke, L.W., Conboy, T., Harrell, L.E., Callaway, R., & Folks, D.G. (1991). The clinical validity of the Mattis Dementia Rating Scale in staging Alzheimer's dementia. *Journal of Geriatric Psychiatry and Neurology, 4*, 18–25.

Smith, G.E., Ivnik, R.J., Malec, J.F., Kokmen, E., Tangalos, E., & Petersen, R.C. (1994). Psychometric properties of the Mattis Dementia Rating Scale. *Assessment, 1*, 123–131.

Vangel Jr., S.J., & Lichtenberg, P.A. (1995). Mattis Dementia Rating Scale: Clinical utility and relationship with demographic variables. *The Clinical Neuropsychologist, 9*, 209–213.

Vitaliano, P.P., Breen, A.R., Russo, J., Albert, M., Vitiello, M., & Prinz, P.N. (1984). The clinical utility of the Dementia Rating Scale for assessing Alzheimer's patients. *Journal of Chronic Disabilities, 37* (9/10), 743–753.

Woodard, J.L., Salthouse, T.A., Godsall, R.E., & Green, R.C. (1996). Confirmatory factor analysis of the Mattis Dementia Rating Scale in patients with Alzheimer's disease. *Psychological Assessment, 8*, 85–91.

KAUFMAN BRIEF INTELLIGENCE TEST (K-BIT)

Purpose

The aim of this individually administered test is to provide a brief estimate of intelligence for screening and related purposes.

Source

The kit (including manual, easel, and record forms) can be ordered from the American Guidance Service, Circle Pines, Minnesota 55014-1796 at a cost of $105.95 US.

Description

The test (Kaufman & Kaufman, 1990) is suitable for the age range of 4–90 years and is based on the measurement of both verbal and nonverbal abilities. It consists of two subtests, Vocabulary and Matrices, that are presented in an easel format. The Vocabulary subtest provides an estimated Verbal IQ; the Matrices subtest was designed to yield a Nonverbal IQ estimate; the scores from both measures provide a Composite IQ.

Subtest 1, Vocabulary, is an 82-item measure of verbal ability that demands oral responses for all items. Part A, Expressive Vocabulary (45 items), administered to individuals of all ages, requires the person to provide the name of a pictured object such as a lamp or calendar. Part B, Definitions (37 items), administered to individuals 8 years and older, requires the person to provide the word that best fits two clues (a phrase description and a partial spelling of the word). For example, a dark color; BR—W—. Performance on the Vocabulary subtest measures word knowledge and verbal concept formation and is thought to assess crystallized intelligence.

Subtest 2, Matrices, is a 48-item nonverbal measure composed of several types of items involving visual stimuli, both meaningful (people and objects) and abstract (designs and symbols). All items require understanding of relations among stimuli, and all are multiple choice, requiring the patient either to point to the correct response or to say the letter corresponding to the position of the item. For the easiest items, the patient selects which one of five items goes best with a stimulus picture (e.g., a car goes with a truck). For the next set of items, the patient must choose which one of six or eight pictures completes a 2 × 2 or 3 × 3 matrix. Abstract matrices were popularized by Raven (1956, 1960) as a method of assessing intelligence in a more "culture-fair" manner. The ability to solve visual analogies, especially those with abstract stimuli, is considered an excellent measure of general intelligence and fluid thinking (that is, the ability to be flexible when encountering novel problem-solving situations).

Administration

Directions for administering the items, the correct responses, and examples of typical responses that should be queried appear on the easel facing the examiner. The only task that requires timing is Definitions. Patients are allowed 30 seconds to respond to each item. Starting points for each task are tailored to the patient's age. Items are organized in units, and the examiner discontinues the task if the patient fails every item in one unit. The order of K-BIT tasks is fixed but not inviolable. The inclusion of both verbal and nonverbal subtests in the K-BIT allows the examiner flexibility when testing a patient with special needs (e.g., patients with aphasic disorders can be given only the Matrices subtest).

Approximate Time for Administration

The test can be administered in about 15–30 minutes, depending in part on the age of the patient.

Scoring

The examiner records scores on each task and converts, by means of tables provided in the K-BIT manual, raw scores to standard scores (mean of 100, SD = 15) for the separate subtests (Vocabulary and Matrices) and the total scale (the K-BIT IQ Composite). Space is also provided on the record form to record confidence intervals (a 90 percent confidence interval is recommended), percentile ranks, descriptive categories (e.g., average, below average, etc.), normal curve equivalents, and stanines, using tables provided in the K-BIT manual. Examiners can also compare the patient's performance on the two K-BIT subtests to determine if the difference is significant and unusual by referring to tables in the manual.

Comment

Split-half reliability coefficients for Vocabulary are excellent, ranging from .89 to .98 (mean = .92) depending upon the age range. Matrices split-half coefficients range from .74 to .95 (mean = .87). Matrices coefficients for very young children, ages 4–6 years, are acceptable (mean = .78) but improve with older age groups. The split-half reliability of the K-BIT IQ composite is excellent, with values ranging from .88 to .98 (mean = .93) (see source).

Test–retest reliability was evaluated by administering the K-BIT twice to 232 normal children and adults ages 5–89. The interval between tests ranged from 12 to 145 days, with a mean of 21 days. Reliability coefficients are high for all age groups. Slight practice effects emerge following such short retest periods. One can expect increases of about 3 standard score points on the K-BIT IQ Composite and about 2 to 4 standard score points on the Vocabulary and Matrices subtests on retest. These small increases caused by practice apply equally to all age groups.

The K-BIT IQ Composite and Vocabulary standard scores have average standard errors of measurement of about 4 points across the entire age range, whereas Matrices standard scores have an average SEM of about 5.5 points. The correlations between Vocabulary and Matrices subtests range from .38 to .75 (mean = .59), depending upon the age group. Correlations tend to increase with age (see source).

As might be expected (Horn, 1985), average raw scores on the Expressive Vocabulary task increase steadily from ages 4 to 15 years, peak at about age 16, and maintain that same high level through age 74 before declining for the oldest age group. Mean raw scores on the Definitions task increase steadily to 44 years and then decline gradually. Average raw scores on the Matrices subtest increase up to 17 years, peak at ages 17 to 19 years, and decline stead-

ily across the rest of the adult age range (see source).

K-BIT IQ scores correlate moderately well with other measures of intelligence such as the Wechsler (WISC-R, WISC-III, WAIS-R), the Stanford-Binet, the Kaufman Assessment Battery for Children, the Slosson, and the Test of Nonverbal Intelligence (see source; Eisenstein & Engelhart, 1997; Naugle et al., 1993; Prewett, 1992a, 1992b, Prewett & McCaffery, 1993; Prewett, 1995). Correlations ranging from .61 to .88 have been reported between K-BIT Composite and Wechsler Full-Scale IQ scores. In a heterogeneous group of patients referred for neuropsychological assessment, Naugle et al. (1993) reported that correlations between the Verbal, Nonverbal, and Composite scales of the two measures were .83, .77, and .88, respectively. K-BIT scores tend to be about five points higher than their WAIS-R or WISC-III counterparts (Eisenstein & Engelhart, 1997; Naugle et al., 1993; Prewett, 1995). On the other hand, K-BIT IQ composite scores are on average about five points lower than the mean Stanford-Binet Test Composite (Prewett & McCaffery, 1993).

Like longer tests of intelligence (e.g., the Wechsler tests), the K-BIT includes measures of both verbal and nonverbal intelligence. For this reason, the K-BIT has an advantage over alternative screening measures such as the Peabody Picture Vocabulary Test–III, the Test of Nonverbal Intelligence, or the Raven Progressive Matrices which tap primarily one type of ability (Naugle et al., 1993). Although the verbal–nonverbal dichotomy invites the user to contrast the two, the discrepancy derived from the K-BIT tends to correlate only modestly (.23 to .59) with that of the WAIS-R (Naugle et al., 1993). Structural equation analysis of the K-BIT and the WAIS-R in a sample of neurologically impaired adults revealed that the K-BIT Vocabulary subtest had a significant visual-spatial component (Burton et al., 1995). That is, the K-BIT appears to provide less of a differentiation between verbal and nonverbal intellectual functions than the WAIS-R. Given this substantial visual-spatial component on the Vocabulary subtest, the K-BIT Verbal IQ may give a spuriously low estimate of verbal intelligence and consequently may obscure performance discrepancies between K-BIT Verbal and Matrices IQs (Burton et al., 1995).

K-BIT scores correlate moderately well with measures of achievement, such as the WRAT-R and the Kaufman Test of Educational Achievement (see Source; Prewett & McCaffery, 1993).

In short, the K-BIT appears to be a promising screening measure of verbal, nonverbal, and general intellectual ability when time constraints or functional abilities of the patient preclude the use of a longer measure or when the patient is familiar with standard tests such as the Wechsler. It covers a wide age range, ages 4–90. The findings, however, should be considered tentatively when making clinical decisions, particularly with regard to Verbal IQ and differences between verbal and nonverbal performance. Test results need to be supported by a more comprehensive assessment. Despite the finding that K-BIT scores are highly correlated with IQ scores from other standardized tests, K-BIT scores can differ markedly from their counterparts. For example, Naugle et al. (1993) reported that K-BIT composite scores ranged from 12 points lower to 22 points higher than WAIS-R FSIQ; 5 percent of the differences between tests exceeded 15 points, or one standard deviation. Eisenstein and Engelhart (1997) reported that in a sample of clinic referrals, Wechsler four-subtest short forms did better than the K-BIT in predicting WAIS-R FSIQ. Difference scores between the K-BIT and FSIQ were 16 points or less for 95 percent of the cases. Difference scores for the four-subtest short forms were 12 points or less for about 95% of the cases. Further, the limited response alternatives that make the K-BIT easy to administer and score preclude an assessment of the diversity of behavior required for a process or qualitative approach (Naugle et al., 1993).

Normative Data

The K-BIT was normed on a nationwide standardization sample of 2,022 people, ages 4–90 years (age 4–6: n = 327; age 7–19: n = 1, 195; age 20–44: n = 320; age 45–90: n = 180), stratified according to recent U.S. census data on four background variables: gender, geographic region, socioeconomic status, and race or ethnic group.

Age affects performance, and age-based norm tables are provided in the K-BIT manual (see source). In clinical populations, K-BIT scores show a moderate relation with educational attainment (r = .44) (Naugle et al., 1993).

References

Burton, D.B., Naugle, R.I., & Schuster, J.M. (1995). A structural equation analysis of the Kaufman Brief Intelligence Test and the Wechsler Intelligence Scale—Revised. *Psychological Assessment, 7*, 538–540.

Eisenstein, N., & Engelhart, C.I. (1997). Comparison of the K-BIT with short forms of the WAIS-R in a neuropsychological population. *Psychological Assessment, 9*, 57–62.

Horn, J.L. (1985). Remodeling old models of intelligence. In B.B. Wolman (Ed.), *Handbook of Intelligence*. New York: Wiley.

Kaufman, A.S., & Kaufman, N.L. (1990). Kaufman Brief Intelligence Test Manual. Circle Pines, MN: American Guidance Service.

Naugle, R.I., Chelune, G.J., & Tucker, G.D. (1993). Validity of the Kaufman Brief Intelligence Test. *Psychological Assessment, 5*, 182–186.

Prewett, P.N. (1992a). The relationship between the K-BIT and the Wechsler Intelligence Scale for Children—Revised (WISC-R). *Psychology in the Schools, 29*, 25–27.

Prewett, P.N. (1992b). The relationship between the Kaufman Brief Intelligence Test (K-BIT) and the WISC-R with incarcerated juvenile delinquents. *Educational and Psychological Measurement, 52*, 977–982.

Prewett, P.N., & McCaffery, L.K. (1993). A comparison of the Kaufman Brief Intelligence Test (K-BIT) with the Stanford-Binet, a two subtest short form, and the Kaufman Test of Educational Achievement (K-TEA Brief Form). *Psychology in the Schools, 30*, 299–304.

Prewett, P.N. (1995). A comparison of two screening tests (the Matrix Analogies Test—Short Form and the Kaufman Brief Intelligence Test) with the WISC-III. *Psychological Assessment, 7*, 69–72.

Raven, J.C. (1956). *Guide to Using the Coloured Progressive Matrices (rev. ed.)* London: H.K. Lewis.

Raven, J.C. (1960). *Guide to Using the Standard Progressive Matrices (rev. ed.)* London: H.K. Lewis.

MICROCOG: ASSESSMENT OF COGNITIVE FUNCTIONING

Purpose

The purpose of this computer-administered and computer-scored test is to screen for and diagnose mental impairment in adults.

Source

The kit (including user's guide, technical manual, 3 ½" high-density diskettes, and ten report credits) can be ordered from The Psychological Corporation, 555 Academic Court, San Antonio, TX 78204-2498 at a cost of $150 US, or from The Psychological Corporation, 55 Horner Ave., Toronto, ON M8Z 4X6, for $200 Cdn. Additional report credits can be ordered from the Psychological Corporation (e.g., 10 report credits cost $100 US or $140 Cdn). Note that a DOS based PC is required, 286 or higher, to run the program.

Description

The test (Powell et al., 1993) is suitable for individuals aged 18–89 years. Two forms of MicroCog are available: The Standard Form consists of 18 subtests; the Short Form contains 12 of these subtests (denoted below by an asterisk). The subtests are organized into five domains: Attention/Mental Control, Memory, Reasoning/Calculation, Spatial Processing, and Reaction Time.

Four subtests were selected to assess Attention/Mental Control. Numbers Forward* and Numbers Reversed are visual digit span tasks that require the patient to reproduce strings of digits using the numeric keypad. The Alphabet subtest is a continuous performance task in which letters of the alphabet (A to O) are presented, embedded in a random series of letters. The patient responds to the letters in sequence (A, B, C, etc.). The Wordlist subtests involve presentation of a list of categorized words. In Wordlist 1,* sixteen words, containing five groups of category-related items, are presented four times. Each time, the patient is instructed to respond to words that are members of one of four categories. A response is not requested for the fifth category. In Wordlist 2,* a list of 36 words, including the 16 from Wordlist 1, is presented, and the

patient must indicate which words were previously presented, including the four that were learned incidentally.

The second domain, Memory, includes five subtests that measure immediate and delayed recognition of the content of two stories (Story 1* and Story 2*) as well as the delayed recall of a name and address.*

The third domain, Reasoning/Calculation, consists of three subtests. In the Analogies* subtest, pairs of verbal analogies are presented and answered by choosing from a multiple choice array. In Object Match, the subject is presented with four stimuli for abstraction and conceptual flexibility. For example, there may be three green circles and a red circle. Two of the green circles are the same size as the red circle. The patient is then required to identify the figure that does not match the other three (e.g., the size of figure 2 is too small). Then the patient is asked to group the figures according to a different principle. The Math* subtest assesses the ability to solve addition, subtraction, multiplication, and division problems. Responses are made using the numeric keyboard.

Two subtests are used to sample the domain of Spatial Processing. In Tic Tac 1, a 3 × 3 block matrix is presented in which three to five blocks contain a colored square. Immediately after presentation, the examinee reproduces the pattern using the numeric keypad. Tic Tac 2 involves a second presentation of images with different configurations later on in the test. The Clocks* subtest displays analog clock faces indicating the time with and without associated hour markings. The patient is presented with five digital choices from which the correct time is chosen.

The fifth domain, Reaction Time, consists of the Timers 1* and 2 subtests which assess simple reaction time in both auditory and visual modalities. Timers 1 is administered at the beginning of MicroCog and Timers 2 at the close of the session.

MicroCog's subtest scores contribute to three levels of index scores. Level 1 index scores represent the five content domains described above. Level 2 index scores (Information Processing Speed and Information Processing Accuracy) are based on factor analytic studies and consist of respective speed and accuracy scores; they are not domain specific. Level 3 index scores represent measures of global functioning (General Cognitive Functioning and General Cognitive Proficiency). The General Cognitive Functioning Index score consists of the Information Processing Speed and Information Processing Accuracy Indices. The General Cognitive Proficiency Index consists of the individual subtest proficiency (i.e., the interaction of accuracy and speed) scores.

Administration

MicroCog is essentially self-administered; the instructions for each subtest are shown on the screen. The examiner's role is to orient the patient to the computer, answer the patient's questions related to keyboard operation or subtest instructions, and to provide encouragement and reassurance. In our experience, the examiner should remain in close proximity with the patient during the testing session in order to ensure that the patient understands instructions. A pause function is built into most subtests to enable patients to take time out from testing when they choose. Patients are not penalized for pausing. In addition to the pause function, one can stop or discontinue a subtest. Patients, however, cannot repeat a subtest without taking the entire test over again. The order of test administration is fixed.

Approximate Time for Administration

The Standard Form can be administered in 60 minutes, and the Short Form takes about 30 minutes.

Scoring

Potential problems with ceiling performance are addressed by evaluating both accuracy and speed of performance. Accuracy, response times, and proficiency raw scores are recorded and calculated by computer (Proficiency score = accuracy × speed, where accuracy reflects a dichotomously scored item and

speed equals an exponential weighting of correct response speed). MicroCog software calculates standard scores (mean of 10, SD of 3) for each subtest. Index scores are also computed (mean of 100, SD of 15) by summing the standard scores on the relevant subtests or indices. The standard error of measurement for all subtests and index scores is automatically calculated, and the confidence intervals are displayed in MicroCog's test report. Test scores and confidence bands are plotted on a scale that places the score in one of four categories: above average, average, low average, or below average. Additionally, for each subtest, the start time, end time, and the resultant elapsed time is recorded on the subtest test report. The data printout also provides information pertaining to the speed and accuracy of the subject's responses on an item-by-item basis.

Comment

Moderate to high estimates of internal consistency are reported (see source). Reliability coefficients are higher for the composite (.78 and above) than the individual subtest scores—an expected pattern because the composite scores are based on a broader sample of behaviors than the individual subtests. Test–retest reliability estimates (following an interval of about seven months) are moderate to high, with scores remaining relatively stable over such a time period. Percentage agreement for index score classification decisions ranges from 73 to 99 percent for the Standard Form and 73 to 96 percent for the Short Form, depending upon the age range. The authors of MicroCog warn that shorter test–retest intervals would likely show some degree of practice effects.

Evidence of construct validity is provided by the pattern of intercorrelations of subtests and indices (see source). The relationship of the Standard with the Short Form is reported to be very strong. In general, correlations were above .9, except for the Spatial Processing Index, which was .78. Exploratory factor analyses revealed two factors. The first factor was labeled Information Processing Accuracy and consisted of the subtest total scores. It appears to tap overall cognitive ability and shows a moderate correlation (.54) with WAIS-R Full Scale IQ. The second factor was labeled Information Processing Speed and consisted of the average response time scores. It shows modest relations with Full Scale IQ (.29) and the Digit Symbol Substitution task (.29), but is unrelated to the Finger Tapping test (<.10).

Correlations between individual MicroCog scores show modest correlations with corresponding functions assessed on tests such as the Dementia Rating Scale, WAIS-R, Shipley Institute of Living Scale, Wechsler Memory Scale–Revised, Trail Making Test, the Benton Visual Form Discrimination Test, and the Rey Auditory Verbal Learning Test. MicroCog's memory measures, however, appear to be unrelated to the Rey-Osterrieth Complex Figure test immediate and delayed recall conditions (see source). Further, the Computation subtest is not valid as a test of arithmetic computational skills. Devivo et al. (1997) gave three subjects who scored below the first percentile on the MicroCog calculation test the WRAT-3 Arithmetic. All achieved scores on the latter test well above their results on the MicroCog Math. Powell (1997) views this subtest not as an achievement test, but as a measure of working memory. He reports that Math Calculations has often factored with Numbers Forward and Backward and Immediate Delayed Story Recall, as well as Tic Tac.

The authors report that MicroCog is a reasonable predictor of the presence of neurological impairment, even in mild forms of dementia (see source). The correct total classification rates for groups with known or suspected organic etiology range from 65 percent (Lupus group) to 92 percent (dementia group). Sensitivity classifications (percentages of clinical groups accurately identified) range from 65 to 89 percent, and the specificity classifications (percentages in nonclinical groups accurately identified) range from 65 to 94 percent. The test, however, may be less than ideal when psychiatric patients are included in the discrimination. MicroCog does appear to be relatively insensitive to depression, suggesting that the test may provide useful information for decisions that clinicians are commonly required to make (e.g.,

to distinguish dementia versus depression). However, independent validity studies are not yet available.

Chapter 6 of the MicroCog Manual provides clinicians with guidelines for interpreting test profiles and item-errors. The chapter also includes a rich source of hypotheses about the etiology of certain patterns of deficits. It is important to bear in mind that these hypotheses, while based on considerable clinical experience and some research data, require extensive additional investigation. Further, no information is yet available on MicroCog's relations with measures of functional capacity (e.g., cooking, caring for finances), mortality, histopathological findings (e.g., plaque counts), its sensitivity to cognitive change, or its ability to provide useful information in differentiating among patient groups.

It is also worth bearing in mind that Micro-Cog provides only a limited view of the patient's functioning. It does not sample all aspects of cognition (e.g., naming, spontaneous recall, motor function, divided attention) and therefore does not replace a complete clinical appraisal. The examiner needs to follow up suspicions of impairment with an in-depth evaluation. While MicroCog may serve as a beginning point for differential diagnosis, the presence and nature of cognitive impairment should not be diagnosed on the basis of Micro-Cog scores alone.

Note too that while computerized testing has numerous advantages (e.g., standardized administration, speed of scoring), the computer also has potential limitations. These include a restriction in the choice of item types, anxiety in those unfamiliar with computers, and a reduction or even lack of qualitative data. The disadvantages of computerized testing may be overcome by the addition of items during the interview or by supplemental testing (see source). Elderly patients do not appear to be especially computer phobic, although the fact that different keys are used for different MicroCog tasks may be confusing to some patients. Motor difficulties, however, may invalidate test results. The examiner should also note that MicroCog's method of timing is only accurate to approximately $1/10$ second (Kane, 1995).

Normative Data

The standardization sample ($n = 810$) for MicroCog was chosen to be representative of the U.S. population of adults 18 to 89 years of age. The sample was stratified in terms of age (90 Ss in each of nine age groups: 18–24, 25–34, 35–44, 45–54, 55–64, 65–69, 70–74, 75–79, 80–89), gender (half male, half female in each age group), race/ethnicity (African American, Hispanic, White), geographic region, and education (less than high school, high school, greater than high school). This method of sampling, while traditional and representative, produces cell sizes that vary in size and may be, in some instances, quite small (Kane, 1995). For example, according to the U.S. sample, 13.8 percent of the population between the ages of 18 to 24 have less than a high school education. In the MicroCog sample, this produced a cell size of 13 (Kane, 1995).

Two sets of normative scores were derived for the subtest and index scores. One set is from a reference group between the ages of 18 and 34 who generally achieved the highest scores in the sample. Standard scores for the subtests (mean of 10, SD of 3) and indices (mean of 100, SD of 15), based on this reference group, are automatically calculated in the MicroCog software for both the Standard and Short Forms. Use of these norms is appropriate when the examiner must answer questions about performance relative to optimal adult performance. A second set of normative scores, consisting of age- and education-corrected subtest scores, is also automatically calculated in the MicroCog software. When clinical decisions must be made about the presence or absence of cognitive deficits relative to cognitive changes expected as part of normal aging, the age- and education-adjusted norms are appropriate. Note that norms are not broken down by gender since this variable apparently accounts for little in the variance of scores (see source).

In addition, the software program (see also tables provided in the MicroCog manual) allows the examiner to determine whether significant scatter exists within a domain (indicated by Y = yes or N = no on the report summary), whether meaningful differences exist between particular subtest standard scores or between Index standard scores, and whether these discrepancies are unusual in the normal population according to base rates.

One should keep in mind that the large number of comparisons made possible with MicroCog leads to an increasing likelihood of spurious results. The values are more accurate when comparisons are made between indices of subtests selected *a priori* and when base rate data are also considered (see source).

References

DeVivo, K., Rothland, J., Price, L., & Fein, G. (1997). Computerized assessment of arithmetic computation skills with MicroCog. *Journal of the International Neuropsychological Society, 3,* 199–200.

Kane, R.L. (1995). MicroCog: A review. *NAN Bulletin, 11,* 13–16.

Powell, D.H. (1997). Comment on computerized assessment of arithmetic computational skills with MicroCog. *Journal of the International Neuropsychological Society, 3,* 200.

Powell, D.H., Kaplan, E.F., Whitla, D., Weintraub, S., Catlin, R., & Funkenstein, H.H. (1993). *Manual for MicroCog: Assessment of Cognitive Functioning.* San Antonio: The Psychological Corporation.

MINI-MENTAL STATE EXAMINATION (MMSE)

Purpose

The purpose of this test is to screen for mental impairment, particularly in the elderly.

Source

There is no commercial source. Users may refer to the following description in order to design their own material.

Description

The MMSE is a popular measure to screen for cognitive impairment, to document intellectual changes that occur with time, and to as- sess the effects of potential therapeutic agents on cognitive functioning. It is attractive because it is brief, easily administered, and easily scored. Many of the items were used routinely by neurologists to screen mental ability informally. The items were formalized by Folstein, Folstein, and McHugh (1975) in order to distinguish neurologic from psychiatric patients. The test consists of a variety of items that assess orientation to time and place, attention/concentration, language, constructional ability, and immediate and delayed recall. The items are shown in Fig. 5–1. A Spanish-language version is also available (Taussig et al., 1996).

	Max. Points
1. What is the: Year? Season? Date? Day? Month?	5
2. Where are we: State (Country)? County (Province)? Town or City? Hospital (Place)? Floor (Street)?	5
3. Name three objects (Apple, Penny, Table), taking one second to say each. Then ask patient to tell you the three words. Repeat the answers until the patient learns all three, up to 6 trials. The score is based on the first trial.	3
4. Serial 7s. Subtract 7 from 100. Then subtract 7 from that number, etc. Stop after five subtractions (93, 86, 79, 72, 65). Score the total number of correct answers. Alternate: Spell WORLD backwards. The score is the number of letters in correct order. E.G. dlrow = 5, dlorw = 3	
5. Ask for the names of the three objects learned in # 3.	3
6. Point to a pencil and watch. Have the patient name them as you point.	2
7. Have the patient repeat "No ifs, and, or buts". Only one trial.	1
8. Have the patient follow a three-stage command: "Take the paper in your right hand. Fold the paper in half. Put the paper on the floor". Patient should carry out commands only after all three instructions have been given. Score 1 point for each part correctly executed.	3
9. Have the patient read and obey the following: "CLOSE YOUR EYES". (Write in large letters).	1
10. Have the patient write a sentence of his or her own choice.	1
11. Have the patient copy the following design (overlapping pentagons).	1

Figure 5–1. Mini-Mental State Examination. Reprinted from Tombaugh and McIntyre, 1992. Note that the choice of words used to test a person's ability to learn and retain three words was left originally to the discretion of the examiner. Most studies however, have adopted the words *apple, penny,* and *table.* Folstein et al. (1975) routinely administered the serial 7s task. However, patients were permitted to spell the word WORLD backward if they could not or would not perform the serial 7s task. Some authors use WORLD as an alternative; others use only the serial 7s task; others use only WORLD; others routinely include both tasks and score in one of the following ways: (1) the higher of the two scores is used (the recommended procedure); (2) the two scores are combined, or (3) each task is analyzed separately. For the purpose of testing Canadian patients, the orientation item is modified by replacing state and county with country and province (Lamarre & Patten, 1991). Copyright Williams & Wilkins.

Administration

The examiner asks questions and records responses. Questions are asked in the order listed (see Fig. 5–1) and are scored immediately. In addition, the following suggestions are offered:

1. The test should not be given unless the person has at least an eighth-grade education and is fluent in English (Tombaugh & McIntyre, 1992).

2. A written version of the test may be preferable for hearing-impaired individuals (Uhlmann et al., 1989).

3. Serial 7s and WORLD should not be considered equivalent items. Both items should be given, and the higher of the two should be used. WORLD should be spelled forward (and corrected) prior to spelling it backward (Tombaugh & McIntyre, 1992).

4. The "country" and "where are you" orientation-to-place questions should be modified. The name of the county (province) where the person lives should be asked rather than the name of the county where the test site is given. The name of the street where the individual lives should be asked rather than the name of the floor where the testing takes place (Tombaugh & McIntyre, 1992).

5. The words *apple*, *penny*, and *table* should be used for registration and recall. If necessary, the words may be administered up to three times in order to obtain perfect registration, but the score is based on the first trial (Tombaugh & McIntyre, 1992).

Approximate Time for Administration

The task can be administered in 5–10 minutes.

Scoring

The MMSE score is the total number of correct answers. The maximum score is 30 points. Failures to respond should be scored as errors (Fillenbaum et al., 1988).

Comment

Estimates of internal consistency range from .31 for community-based samples to .96 for a mixed group of medical patients (Foreman, 1987; Jorm et al., 1988; Hopp et al., in press; Tombaugh et al., 1996). Scoring of some items (e.g., overlapping polygons) is subjective, and there is no suggested time limit for any item. Inter-rater reliability is nonetheless good (above .65) (Folstein et al., 1975; Foster et al., 1988) but can be enhanced with more precise administration and scoring criteria (Molloy et al., 1991; Olin & Zelinski, 1991). Additionally, test–retest reliability estimates for intervals of less than two months generally fall between .80 and .95 (see Folstein et al., 1975; O'Connor et al., 1989; Tombaugh & McIntyre, 1992, for a recent review). With lengthier retest intervals (e.g., 1–2 years), normal subjects typically show a small amount of change (about 2 points), and retest correlations are lower (<.80) (Hopp et al., in press; Mitrushina & Satz, 1991; Olin & Zelinski, 1991). Recall and Attention subtests tend to be the least reliable (Olin & Zelinski, 1991). The implication of these findings is that clinicians monitoring change in older adults should be cautious in interpreting small declines in scores. It is worth noting in this regard that a number of investigators report an *average* annual rate of decline of about 2–3 points on the MMSE for patients with probable dementia of the Alzheimer type (AD) (Becker et al., 1988; Salmon et al., 1990; Small et al., 1997a).

Most studies report that the MMSE is sensitive to the presence of dementia, particularly in those with moderate to severe forms of cognitive impairment. The test, however, is less than ideal when those with mild cognitive impairment are evaluated, when focal neurological deficits are present, or when psychiatric patients are included (Benedict & Brandt, 1992; Feher et al., 1992; Grut et al., 1993; Kupke et al., 1993; O'Connor et al., 1989; Tombaugh & McIntyre, 1992; Shah et al., 1992; Van Der Cammen et al., 1992; Wells et al., 1992; for recent reviews). There are a number of possible explanations for this decreased sensitivity (ability to identify those who are impaired) and specificity (ability to identify those who are *not* affected). One possibility rests on the fact that the MMSE is biased toward verbal items and does not adequately measure other functions such as ability to attend to relevant input, ability to solve abstract problems, ability to retain information over prolonged time intervals, visuospatial ability, constructional praxis, and mood. Accordingly, it may overestimate dementia in aphasic patients. At the same time, it may be relatively insensitive to various amnestic syndromes as well as disturbances of the right hemisphere, resulting in an increase in false negatives. In addition, the language items are very simple, and mild impairments may go undetected.

The MMSE is useful in predicting who will develop AD. Small et al. (1997b) found that lower baseline scores on the MMSE (but nonetheless above 23) were associated with an increased risk of AD after a 3-year follow-up period. The MMSE is also sensitive to cognitive decline although as the disorder becomes more severe, the test loses its sensitivity (Salmon et al., 1990; Tombaugh & McIntyre, 1992). In such cases, other tests are preferred, such as the DRS, which includes more easy items.

The MMSE shows modest-to-high correlations with other brief screening tests such as the Blessed Test, the Dementia Rating Scale, Spanish versions of the Mental Status Questionnaire, Information-Memory-Concentration Test, and Orientation-Memory-Concentration Test (e.g., Fillenbaum et al., 1987; Foreman, 1987; Salmon et al., 1990; Taussig et al., 1996). Modest-to-high correlations have also been reported between total MMSE score and measures of intelligence, memory, attention/concentration, and executive function (Axelrod et al., 1992; Feher et al., 1992; Folstein et al., 1975; Giordani et al., 1990; Mitrushina & Satz, 1991; Tombaugh & McIntyre, 1992), although concordance rates between individual MMSE tasks and neuropsychological tests addressing corresponding cognitive domains are quite low (Benedict & Brandt, 1992; Giordani et al., 1990; Mitrushina & Satz, 1994). Further, MMSE scores show modest correlations with measures of functional capacity (e.g., cooking, caring for finances) and measures of mortality, as well as with histopathological findings (plaque counts) (Burns et al., 1991; Fillenbaum et al., 1988; Lemsky et al., 1996; Marcopulos et al., 1997; Martin et al., 1987;

Taussig et al., 1996). For example, Lemsky et al. (1996) advise that a MMSE score less than or equal to 26 raises the concern of functional impairment. If the MMSE score is greater than 26, but the individual is under 85 years of age, and the Mattis DRS Memory scale is less than 20, functional impairment should also be suspected. MMSE scores also correlate with CT abnormality, cerebral ventricular size, perfusion deficits on SPECT, and long-latency, event-related potentials (Aylward et al., 1996; Colohan et al., 1989; DeKoskey et al., 1990; Finley et al., 1985; Pearlson & Tune, 1989; Tsai & Tsuang, 1979).

Because the MMSE is organized into discrete subsections (e.g., orientation, registration, attention and concentration, recall, language, copy), the user may be tempted to use subsection scores or individual items as indicators of specific cognitive impairment. The literature suggests, however, that MMSE subsections and individual items cannot be viewed as measures of specific aspects of cognition (Giordani et al., 1990; Mitrushina & Satz, 1994). Factor analytic studies of the MMSE typically yield a two-factor solution, although the items contained in each factor tend to vary somewhat among studies (Braekhus et al., 1992; Giordani et al., 1990; Tombaugh & McIntyre, 1992). The results from these factor analytic studies imply that the set of cognitive domains sampled by the MMSE are less than the seven categories into which the questions are usually grouped (Tombaugh & McIntyre, 1992). Because of the nonspecific nature of the individual subsection scores of the MMSE, they should not be used in lieu of more comprehensive assessments if a detailed diagnostic profile is desired (Giordani et al., 1990). This does not mean that the MMSE cannot provide useful information in differentiating among patients with dementia. Brandt et al. (1988) showed different profiles on the MMSE in patients with AD and patients with Huntington's disease. The differences between the groups rested on different scores on the memory and attention-concentration items. Patients with AD did worse on the memory items whereas patients with Huntington's disease did worse on the attention-concentration items.

Table 5—7. Mini-Mental State Examination Score by Age and Education Level, Number of Participants, Mean, SD, and Selected percentiles[a]

								Age, in Years								
	18–24	25–29	30–34	35–39	40–44	45–49	50–54	55–59	60–64	65–69	70–74	75–79	80–84	≥85	Total
0–4 years education															
n	17	23	41	33	36	28	34	49	88	126	139	112	105	61	892
Mean	22	25	25	23	23	23	23	22	23	22	22	21	20	19	22
SD	2.9	2.0	2.4	2.5	2.6	3.7	2.6	2.7	1.9	1.9	1.7	2.0	2.2	2.9	2.3
Lower quartile	21	23	23	20	20	20	20	20	19	19	19	18	16	15	19
Median	23	25	26	24	23	23	22	22	22	22	21	21	19	20	22
Upper quartile	25	27	28	27	27	26	25	26	26	25	24	24	23	23	25
5–8 years education															
n	94	83	74	101	100	121	154	208	310	633	533	437	241	134	3223
Mean	27	27	26	26	27	26	27	26	26	26	26	25	25	23	26
SD	2.7	2.5	1.8	2.8	1.8	2.5	2.4	2.9	2.3	1.7	1.8	2.1	1.9	3.3	2.2
Lower quartile	24	25	24	23	25	24	25	25	24	24	24	22	22	21	23
Median	28	27	26	27	27	27	27	27	27	27	26	26	25	24	26
Upper quartile	29	29	28	29	29	29	29	29	29	29	28	28	27	27	28
9 to 12 years education or high school diploma															
n	1326	958	822	668	489	423	462	525	626	814	550	315	163	99	8240
Mean	29	29	29	28	28	28	28	28	28	28	27	27	25	26	28
SD	2.2	1.3	1.3	1.8	1.9	2.4	2.2	2.2	1.7	1.4	1.6	1.5	2.3	2.0	1.9
Lower quartile	28	28	28	28	28	27	27	27	27	27	26	25	23	23	27
Mean	29	29	29	29	29	29	29	29	28	28	28	27	26	26	29
Upper quartile	30	30	30	30	30	30	30	30	30	29	29	29	28	28	30

College experience or higher degree

n	783	1012	989	641	354	259	220	231	270	358	255	181	96	52	5701
Mean	29	29	29	29	29	29	29	29	29	29	28	28	27	27	29
SD	1.3	0.9	1.0	1.0	1.7	1.6	1.9	1.5	1.3	1.0	1.6	1.6	0.9	1.3	1.3
Lower quartile	29	29	29	29	29	29	28	28	28	28	27	27	26	25	29
Median	30	30	30	30	30	30	30	29	29	29	29	28	28	28	29
Upper quartile	30	30	30	30	30	30	30	30	30	30	29	29	29	29	30

Total

n	2220	2076	1926	1443	979	831	870	1013	1294	1931	1477	1045	605	346	18056
Mean	29	29	29	29	28	28	28	28	28	27	27	26	25	24	28
SD	2.0	1.3	1.3	1.8	2.0	2.5	2.4	2.5	2.0	1.6	1.8	2.1	2.2	2.9	2.0
Lower quartile	28	28	28	28	27	27	27	26	26	26	24	23	21	21	27
Median	29	29	29	29	29	29	29	29	28	28	27	26	25	25	29
Upper quartile	30	30	30	30	30	30	30	30	29	29	29	28	28	28	30

[a]Data from the Epidemiologic Catchment Area household surveys in New Haven, Conn; Baltimore, MD; St. Louis, MO; Durham, NC; and Los Angeles, Calif, between 1980 and 1984. The data are weighted based on the 1980 U.S. population census by age, sex, and race.

Source: Crum et al. 1993. Copyright, American Medical Association.

Analyses of individual items reveal that errors rarely occur on questions related to orientation to place and language; for both normal and dementing individuals, most errors occur for the recall of three words, serial 7s/WORLD, pentagon, and orientation to time. In short, these latter items are the most sensitive to both normal aging and dementing processes (Tombaugh & McIntyre, 1992; Tombaugh et al., 1996; Wells et al., 1992). Further, there is evidence that serial 7s and reverse spelling of WORLD represent different tasks. Spelling WORLD backward consistently produces higher scores than does counting backward by sevens (Tombaugh & McIntyre, 1992).

Several attempts have been made to improve the utility of the MMSE by omitting items of limited diagnostic utility and/or adding items or tests known to be sensitive to cognitive impairment. For example, the Modified Mini-Mental State Examination (3MS) by Teng et al. (1987) added four additional items (date and place of birth, word fluency, similarities, and delayed recall of words). The maximum score was increased from 30 to 100 points. A recent study by Tombaugh et al. (1996) found, however, that the MMSE and 3MS were not differentially sensitive to AD. Although the two tests produce comparable effects, the inclusion of a verbal fluency test is recommended to increase the sensitivity of the MMSE. The various revisions have not gained widespread use.

It is worth bearing in mind that the MMSE is fundamentally a screening test and does not replace a complete clinical appraisal of the patient. The examiner needs to follow up suspicions of impairment with a more in-depth evaluation. Presence and nature of cognitive impairment should not be diagnosed on the basis of MMSE scores alone.

Normative Data

MMSE scores are related to premorbid intelligence and educational attainment: Individuals with higher premorbid ability and/or more education tend to score higher than those of lower IQ and/or with few years of schooling (Anthony et al., 1982; Christensen & Jorm,

1992; Crum et al., 1993; Jorm et al., 1988; Marcopulos et al., 1997; O'Connor et al., 1989; Olin & Zelinski, 1991; Starr et al., 1992; Taussig et al., 1996; Tombaugh et al., 1996; Van Der Cammen et al., 1992). There is evidence that low educational or intelligence levels increase the likelihood of misclassifying normal subjects as cognitively impaired while higher ability and educational levels may mask mild impairment. Education and premorbid ability, however, may also reflect etiological factors (e.g., hypertension, obesity) critical in the process that eventually results in some form of dementia (e.g., multi-infarct dementia). In short, education may represent a psychometric bias and/or a risk factor (for further discussion see Crum et al., 1993; Jorm et al., 1988; Tombaugh & McIntyre, 1992).

MMSE scores decrease with advancing age (Bleecker et al., 1988; Crum et al., 1993; Jorm et al., 1988; O'Connor et al., 1989; Olin & Zelinski, 1991; Starr et al., 1992; Tombaugh & McIntyre, 1992; Tombaugh et al., 1996). Most of the age-related change begins at about age 55–60 and then dramatically accelerates at the age of 75–80. These age effects persist even when subjects are stratified by educational level.

There is some evidence that MMSE scores are also affected by race/ethnicity and social class; gender and depression, however, have little impact (Bleecker et al., 1988; George et al., 1991; O'Connor et al., 1989; Olin & Zelinski, 1991; Taussig et al., 1996; Wells et al., 1992). MMSE scores tend to be decreased in individuals of nonwhite ethnicity (but see Marcopulos et al., 1997) and lower social class.

In short, the MMSE, like most measures of cognitive ability, is affected by demographic factors. There have been attempts to alter the cutoff scores in order to compensate for various age and/or educational levels. In general, however, changing the cutoff points alters the sensitivity and specificity of the test, increasing one while decreasing the other (Anthony et al., 1982; Bleecker et al., 1988; Galasko et al., 1990; Grut et al., 1993; O'Connor et al., 1989; Tombaugh & McIntyre, 1992; Uhlmann and Larson, 1991). The solution may not lie with a change in cutoff score, but in the use of a

Table 5—8. MMSE Norms (Percentile Scores) Stratified for Age and Years of Education for Participants Diagnosed As No Cognitive Impairment

MMSE Score	Age 65–79		Age 80–89	
	0–8 Years of education ($n = 58$)	9+ Years of education ($n = 168$)	0–8 Years of education ($n = 65$)	9+ Years of education ($n = 115$)
30	98	86	100	93
29	88	62	97	77
28	76	41	89	57
27	98	29	83	37
26	48	21	66	30
25	36	14	58	18
24	26	9	49	11
23	19	6	35	6
22	16	5	23	4
21	10	4	14	3
20	5	4	8	1
19	5	3	5	<1
18	4	1	<5	
17	4	<1		
16	3			
<16	<3			

Note: MMSE = Mini-Mental State Examination

Source: Tombaugh et al. 1996. Copyright American Psychological Association. Reprinted with permission.

more comprehensive assessment (Olin & Zelinski, 1991).

Recently, extensive norms by age ($18 \geq 85$) and education (no formal schooling to one or more college degrees) have been reported (Crum et al., 1993), based on probability sampling of more than 18,000 community-dwelling adults. The sample includes individuals, regardless of their physical or mental health status, from five metropolitan areas: New Haven, Baltimore, Durham, St. Louis, and Los Angeles. The data are presented in Table 5–7. Note that the MMSE scores were based on either the response to serial sevens or spelling *world* backwards, whichever yielded the higher score. Also note the wider range of scores in the lowest educational groups and at the oldest ages. MMSE scores ranged from a median of 29 for those aged 18–24 years, to 25 for individuals aged 80 years and older. The median MMSE score was 29 for individuals with at least 9 years of schooling, 26 for those with 5–8 years of schooling, and 22 for those with 0–4 years of schooling. Tombaugh et al. (1996) have recently reported

similar data for the MMSE and the 3MS based on a sample of 406 healthy, community-dwelling participants drawn from five geographical regions in Canada. On the basis of a series of medical, laboratory, and neuropsychological tests, they were deemed to be cognitively intact. The percentile equivalents are shown in Table 5–8. Sensitivity, specificity, positive predictive power (PPP) and negative predictive power (NPP) values are given in Table 5–9. Note that PPP and NPP values are very sensitive to baseline rates of illness and should be interpreted with caution (Tombaugh et al., 1996). For example, a PPP of 76% is excellent if 30% of all patients in a given setting (e.g., general geriatric ward) have AD, but it is less than adequate if, in another setting (e.g., AD and related disease ward), 85% have AD. Thus, the clinical usefulness of the PPP and NPP values varies among clinical settings and the prevalence of the specific illness. Similarly, the calculation of the values reported here reflect the prevalence of dementia in the various age and educational groupings found in that sample (Tombaugh et al., 1996).

Table 5—9. Sensitivity, Specificity, Positive Predictive Power, and Negative Predictive Power for the MMSE

MMSE Criterion Score	0–8 Years Education				9+ Years Education			
	SEN	SPE	PPP	NPP	SEN	SPE	PPP	NPP
Ages 65–69								
27	100	24	29	100	96	59	23	98
26	100	38	33	100	93	71	30	98
25	100	52	39	100	91	79	36	99
24	100	64	46	100	82	86	46	97
23	100	74	55	100	68	91	55	96
22	89	81	59	96	59	94	60	95
21	83	84	63	94	52	95	62	93
20	67	90	67	90	46	96	59	93
19	33	95	67	82	36	96	59	92
18	28	95	63	81	27	98	62	91
17	24	96	60	79	25	99	86	91
Ages 80–89								
27	100	10	41	100	100	43	37	100
26	100	17	43	100	100	63	48	100
25	98	34	48	96	97	70	52	99
24	93	42	49	90	95	82	63	98
23	88	51	52	87	82	89	71	94
22	70	65	55	78	69	94	79	90
21	63	77	63	77	44	96	77	83
20	50	86	69	74	39	97	83	82
19	48	92	79	74	36	98	93	82
18	45	95	86	74	28	98	100	80
17	35	96	82	71	26	100	100	80

Note: All results are given in percentages. For the age 65–79 category, n = 58 for no cognitive impairment (NCI) participants and n = 18 for AD participants with 0–8 years education, and n = 22 for AD participants and n = 168 for NCI participants with 9+ years education. For the age 80–89 category, n = 40 for AD participants and n = 65 for NCI participants with 0–8 years education, and n = 39 for AD participants and n = 115 for NCI participants with 9+ years education. MMSE = Mini-Mental State Examination; SEN = sensitivity (number of AD participants correctly identified by the score to have AD divided by total number of AD participants); SPE = specificity (number of NCI participants correctly identified by the score to be "normal" divided by total number of NCI participants); PPP = positive predictive power (number of participants correctly identified by the score to have AD divided by the total number of participants correctly and incorrectly identified with AD); NPP = negative predictive power (number of participants correctly identified by the score to be "normal" divided by the total number of participants correctly and incorrectly identified as "normal").

Source: Tombaugh et al., 1996. Copyright American Psychological Association.

References

Anthony, J.C., LeResche, L., Niaz, U., Von Korff, M.R., & Folstein, M.F. (1982). Limits of the 'Mini-Mental State' as a screening test for dementia and delirium among hospital patients. *Psychological Medicine, 12*, 397–408.

Axelrod, B.N., Goldman, R.S., & Henry, R.R. (1992). Sensitivity of the Mini-Mental State Examination to frontal lobe dysfunction in normal aging. *Journal of Clinical Psychology, 48*, 68–71.

Aylward, E.H., Rasmussen, D.X., Brandt, J.,

Raimundo, L., Folstein, M., and Pearlson, G.D. (1996). CT measurement of supracellar cistern predicts rate of cognitive decline in Alzheimer's disease. *Journal of the International Neuropsychological Society, 2*, 89–95.

Becker, J.T., Huff, F.J., Nebes, R.D., Holland, A., & Boller, F. (1988). Neuropsychological function in Alzheimer's disease: Pattern of impairment and rate of progression. *Archives of Neurology, 45*, 263–268.

Benedict, R.H.B., & Brandt, J. (1992). Limitation of the Mini-Mental State Examination for the detection of amnesia. *Journal of Geriatric Psychiatry and Neurology*, 5233–5237.

Bleecker, M.L., Bolla-Wilson, K., Kawas, C., and Agnew, J. (1988). Age-specific norms for the Mini-Mental State Exam. *Neurology, 33,* 1565–1568.

Braekhus, A., Laake, K., & Engedal, K. (1992). The Mini-Mental State Examination: Identifying the most efficient variables for detecting cognitive impairment in the elderly. *Journal of the American Geriatrics Society, 40,* 1139–1145.

Brandt, J., Folstein, S.E., & Folstein, M.F. (1988). Differential cognitive impairment in Alzheimer's disease and Huntington's disease. *Annals of Neurology, 23,* 555–561.

Burns, A., Jacoby, R., & Levy, R. (1991). Progression of cognitive impairment in Alzheimer's disease. *Journal of the American Geriatric Society, 39,* 39–45.

Christensen, H., & Jorm, A.F. (1992). Effect of premorbid intelligence on the Mini-Mental State and IQCODE. *International Journal of Geriatric Psychiatry, 7,* 159–160.

Colohan, H., O'Callaghan, E., Larkin, C., Waddington, J.L. (1989). An evaluation of cranial CT scanning in clinical psychiatry. *Irish Journal of Medical Science, 158,* 178–181.

Crum, R.M., Anthony, J.C., Bassett, S.S., & Folstein, M.F. (1993). Population-based norms for the Mini-Mental State Examination by age and educational level. *Journal of the American Medical Association, 269,* 2386–2391.

DeKosky, S.T., Shih, W.J., Schmitt, F.A., Coupal, J., & Kirkpatrick, C. (1990). Assessing utility of single photon emission computed tomography (SPECT) scan in Alzheimer disease: Correlation with cognitive severity. *Alzheimer Disease and Associated Disorders, 4,* 14–23.

Feher, E.P., Mahurin, R.K., Doody, R.S., Cooke, N., Sims, J., & Pirozzolo, F.J. (1992). Establishing the limits of the Mini-Mental State. *Archives of Neurology, 49,* 87–92.

Fillenbaum, G.G., Heyman, A., Wilkinson, W.E., et al. (1987). Comparison of two screening tests in Alzheimer's disease. *Archives of Neurology, 44,* 924–927.

Fillenbaum, G.G., Hughes, D.C., Heyman, A., et al. (1988). Relationship of health and demographic characteristics to Mini-Mental State Examination Scores among community residents. *Psychological Medicine, 18,* 719–726.

Fillenbaum, G.G., George, L.K., & Blazer, D.G. (1988). Scoring nonresponse on the Mini-Mental State Examination. *Psychological Medicine, 18,* 1021–1025.

Finley, W.W., Faux, S.F., Hutcheson, J., & Amstutz, L. (1985). Long-latency event-related potentials in the evaluation of cognitive function in children. *Neurology, 35,* 323–327.

Folstein, M.F., Folstein, S.E., & McHugh, P.R. (1975). 'Mini-mental State'. A practical method for grading the cognitive state of patients for the clinician. *Journal of Psychiatric Research, 12,* 189–198.

Foreman, M.D. (1987). Reliability and validity of mental status questionnaires in elderly hospitalized patients. *Nursing Research, 36,* 216–220.

Foster, J.R., Sclan, S., Welkowitz, J., Boksay, I., & Seeland, I. (1988). Psychiatric assessment in medical long-term care facilities: Reliability of commonly used rating scales. *International Journal of Geriatric Psychiatry, 3,* 229–233.

Galasko, D., Klauber, M.R., Hofstetter, C.R., et al. (1990). The Mini Mental State Examination in the early diagnosis of Alzheimer's dementia. *Archives of Neurology, 47,* 49–52.

George, L.K., Landerman, R., Blazer, D.G. (1991). Cognitive impairment. In L.N. Robbins & D.A. Regier (eds.), *Psychiatric Disorders in America.* New York: Free Press, pp. 291–327.

Giordani, B., Boivin, M.J., Hall, A.L., Foster, N.L., Lehtinen, S.J., Bluemlein, M.S., & Berent, S. (1990). The utility and generality of Mini-Mental State Examination scores in Alzheimer's disease. *Neurology, 40,* 1894–1896.

Grut, M., Fraiglioni, L., Viitanen, M., & Winblad, B. (1993). Accuracy of the Mini-Mental Status Examination as a screening test for dementia in a Swedish elderly population. *Acta Neurologica Scandinavica, 87,* 312–317.

Hopp, G.A., Dixon, R.A., Backman, I., & Grut, M. (in press). Stability of two measures of cognitive functioning in nondemented old-old adults. *Journal of Clinical Psychology.*

Jorm, A.F., Scott, R., Henderson, A.S., et al. (1988). Educational level differences on the Mini-Mental State. *Psychological Medicine, 18,* 727–788.

Kupke, T., Revis, E.S., & Gantner, A.B. (1993). Hemispheric bias of the Mini-Mental State Examination in elderly males. *The Clinical Neuropsychologist, 7,* 210–214.

Lamarre, C.J., & Patten, S.B. (1991). Evaluation of the modified Mini-Mental State Examination in a general psychiatric population. *Canadian Journal of Psychiatry, 36,* 507–511.

Lemsky, C.M., Smith, G., Malec, J.R., & Ivnik, R.J. (1996). Identifying risk for functional impairment using cognitive measures: An application of CART modeling. *Neuropsychology, 10,* 368–375.

Marcopulos, B.A., McLain, C.A., & Giuliano, A.J. (1997). Cognitive impairment or inadequate norms? A study of healthy, rural, older adults with limited education. *The Clinical Neuropsychologist, 11*, 111–131.

Martin, E.M., Wilson, R.S., & Penn, R. D., et al. (1987). Cortical biopsy results in Alzheimer's Disease: Correlation with cognitive deficits. *Neurology, 37*, 1201–1204.

Mitrushina, M., & Satz, P. (1991). Reliability and validity of the Mini-Mental State Exam in neurologically intact elderly. *Journal of Clinical Psychology, 47*, 537–543.

Mitrushina, M., & Satz, P. (1994). Utility of Mini-Mental State Examination in assessing cognition in the elderly. Paper presented to the *International Neuropsychological Society*, Cincinnati, Ohio.

Molloy, D.W., Alemayehu, E., & Roberts, R. (1991). Reliability of a standardized Mini-Mental State Examination compared with the traditional Mini-Mental State Examination. *American Journal of Psychiatry, 148*, 102–105.

O'Connor, D.W., Pollitt, P.A., Treasure, F.P., Brook, C.P.B., & Reiss, B.B. (1989). The influence of education, social class and sex on Mini-Mental State scores. *Psychological Medicine, 19*, 771–776.

Olin, J.T., & Zelinski, E.M. (1991). The 12-month stability of the Mini-Mental State Examination. *Psychological Assessment, 3*, 427–432.

Pearlson, G.D., & Tune, L.E. (1986). Cerebral ventricular size and cerebrospinal fluid acetylcholinesterase levels in senile dementia of the Alzheimer type. *Psychiatry Research, 17*, 23–29.

Salmon, D.P., Thal, L.J., Butters, N., & Heindel, W.C. (1990). Longitudinal evaluation of dementia of the Alzheimer type: A comparison of 3 standardized mental status examinations. *Neurology, 40*, 1225–1230.

Shah, A., Phongsathorn, V., George, C., Bielawska, C., & Katona, C. (1992). Psychiatric morbidity among continuing care geriatric inpatients. *International Journal of Geriatric Psychiatry, 7*, 517–525.

Small, B.J., Viitanen, M., Winblad, B., & Bäckman, L. (1997a). Cognitive changes in very old persons with dementia: The influence of demographic, psychometric, and biological variables. *Journal of Clinical and Experimental Neuropsychology, 19*, 245–260.

Small, B.J., Herlitz, A., Fratiglioni, L., Almkvist, O., & Bäckman, L. (1997b). Cognitive predictors of incident Alzheimer's Disease: A prospective longitudinal study. *Neuropsychology, 11*, 413–420.

Starr, J.M., Whalley, L.J., Inch, S., & Shering, P.A. (1992). The quantification of the relative effects of age and NART-predicted IQ on cognitive function in healthy old people. *International Journal of Geriatric Psychiatry, 7*, 153–157.

Taussig, I.M., Mack, W.J., & Henderson, V.W. (1996). Concurrent validity of Spanish-language versions of the Mini-Mental State Examination, Mental Status Questionnaire, Information-Concentration Test, and Orientation-Memory-Concentration Test: Alzheimer's disease patients and non-demented elderly comparison subjects. *Journal of the International Neuropsychological Society, 2*, 286–298.

Teng, E.L., Chiu, H.C., Schneider, L.S., and Metzger, L.E. (1987). Alzheimer's dementia: Performance on the Mini-Mental State Examination. *Journal of Consulting and Clinical Psychology, 55*, 96–100.

Tombaugh, T.N., & McIntyre, N.J. (1992). The Mini-Mental State Examination: A comprehensive review. *Journal of American Geriatric Society, 40*, 922–935.

Tombaugh, T.N., McDowell, I., Krisjansson, B., & Hubley, A.M. (1996). Mini-Mental State Examination (MMSE) and the Modified MMSE (3MS): A psychometric comparison and normative data. *Psychological Assessment, 8*, 48–59.

Tsai, L., & Tsuang, M.T. (1979). The Mini-Mental State Test and computerized tomography. *American Journal of Psychiatry, 136*, 436–439.

Uhlmann, R.F., Teri, L., Rees, T.S., Mozlowski, K.J., & Larson, E.B. (1989). Impact of mild to moderate hearing loss on mental status testing. *Journal of the American Geriatrics Society, 37*, 223–228.

Uhlmann, R.F., & Larson, E.B. (1991). Effect of education on the Mini-Mental State Examination as a screening test for dementia. *Journal of the American Geriatric Society, 39*, 876–880.

Van Der Cammen, T.J.M., Van Harskamp, F., Stronks, D.L., Passchier, J., & Schudel, W.J. (1992). Value of the Mini-Mental State Examination and informants' data for the detection of dementia in geriatric outpatients. *Psychological Reports, 71*, 1003–1009.

Wells, J.C., Keyl, P.M., Aboraya, A., Folstein, M.F., & Anthony, J.C. (1992). Discriminant validity of a reduced set of Mini-Mental State Examination items for dementia and Alzheimer's disease. *Acta Psychiatrica Scandinavica, 86*, 23–31.

NATIONAL ADULT READING TEST (NART)

Other Test Name

The test has been adapted for use in the United States (Grober & Sliwinski, 1991) and in the United States and Canada (Blair & Spreen, 1989). The second edition of the original version (NART: Nelson, 1982; NART-2: Nelson & Willison, 1991) and the North American Adult Reading Test (NAART or NART-R), developed by Blair and Spreen (1989 are presented here.

Purpose

The purpose of the test is to provide an estimate of premorbid intellectual ability.

Source

The NART-2 (word card and booklet, manual including pronunciation guide (2nd edition), and scoring forms) can be purchased from NFER-Nelson, Darville House, 2 Oxford Road East, Windsor, Berkshire, SL4 1DF, at a cost of 59.25 pounds sterling. There is no commercial source for the NAART. Users may refer to the following text in order to design their own material.

Description

There are a number of clinical, medico-legal or research situations where knowledge of premorbid IQ is essential. Since premorbid test data are rarely available, methods of estimation are needed. The National Adult Reading Test or NART-2 (Nelson, 1982; Nelson & O'Connell, 1978; Nelson & Willison, 1991), a reading test of 50 irregularly spelled words (e.g., ache, naive, thyme), has promise as an assessment tool for the determination of premorbid intellectual function (Fig. 5–2). Assuming that the subject is familiar with the word, accuracy of pronunciation is used to predict IQ. As the words are short, subjects do not have to analyze a complex visual stimulus and because they are irregular, intelligent guesswork will not provide the correct pronunciation. Therefore, it has been argued that performance depends more on previous knowledge than on current cognitive capacity (Nelson & O'Connell, 1978). The value of the test lies in the high correlation between reading ability and intelligence in the normal population (Crawford et al., 1989a), the fact that word-reading tends to produce a fairly accurate estimate of pre-injury IQ (Moss & Dowd, 1991), and the fact that the ability to pronounce irregular words is generally retained in mild and moderately demented individuals (Crawford et al., 1988a; Fromm et al., 1991; Sharpe & O'Carroll, 1991; Stebbins et al., 1990a; see Comment section).

Nelson developed the test in England for use with the WAIS. Recently, Nelson & Willison (1991) restandardized the test on a British sample so that it is possible to convert NART-2 scores directly to WAIS-R scores. Ryan and Paolo (1992) also standardized the NART/NART-2 for the WAIS-R, using an American sample of people 75 years and older. Blair and Spreen (1989) modified the test for use with North American populations (NAART) and validated it against the WAIS-R. The NAART consists of a list of 61 words printed in two columns on both sides of an 8 ½" × 11" card which is given to the subject to read. The examiner records errors on a

Ache	Procreate	Leviathan
Debt	Quadruped	Aeon
Psalm	Catacomb	Detente
Depot	Superfluous	Gauche
Chord	Radix	Drachm
Bouquet	Assignate	Idyll
Deny	Gist	Beatify
Capon	Hiatus	Banal
Heir	Simile	Sidereal
Aisle	Rarefy	Puerperal
Subtle	Cellist	Topiary
Nausea	Zealot	Demesne
Equivocal	Abstemious	Campanile
Naive	Gouge	Labile
Thyme	Placebo	Syncope
Courteous	Facade	Prelate
Gaoled	Aver	

Figure 5–2. The New Adult Reading Test. Source: Extract from the National Adult Reading Test. Hazel S. Nelson, 1991, by permission of the publishers, NFER-Nelson.

```
                                    NAART
                            Sample Scoring Sheet
     Page 1
       DEBT    det                        SUBPOENA   sə·pē'·nə
       DEBRIS  də·brē, dā·brē', dā'·brē   PLACEBO   plə·sē'·bō
       AISLE   īl                         PROCREATE  prō'·krē·āt
       REIGN   rān                        PSALM   säm, sälm*
       DEPOT   dē,·pō, de'·pō             BANAL   bə·nál', bā·nal', bān'·əl
       SIMILE  sim'·ə·lē                  RAREFY  rár'·ə·fī
       LINGERIE  lan'·zhə·rē', lon'·zhə·rā'   GIST  jist
       RECIPE  res'·ə·pē                  CORPS   kor, korz
       GOUGE   gauj                       HORS D'OEUVRE  òr' dərv(r)'
       HEIR    ār                         SIEVE   siv
       SUBTLE  sət'·əl                    HIATUS  hī·ā·təs
       CATACOMB  kat'·ə·kōm               GAUCHE  gōsh
       BOUQUET  bō·kā', bü·kā'            ZEALOT  zel'·ət
       GAUGE   gāj                        PARADIGM  par'·ə·dīm, par'·ə·dim
       COLONEL  kərn'·əl                  FACADE  fə·säd'

     Page 2
       CELLIST  chel'·əst                 LEVIATHAN  li·vī'·ə·thən
       INDICT  in·dīt'                    PRELATE  prel'·ət, prē'·lāt*
       DETENTE  dā·tä(n)t                 QUADRUPED  kwäd'·rə·ped
       IMPUGN  im·pyün'                   SIDEREAL  sī·dir'·ē·al, sə·dir'·ē·al
       CAPON   kā'·pən, kā'·pon           ABSTEMIOUS  ab·stē'·mē·əs
       RADIX   rād'·iks                   BEATIFY  bē·at'·ə·fī
       AEON    ē'·ən, e'·an               GAOLED  jāld
       EPITOME  i·pit'·ə·mē               DEMESNE  di·mān', di·mēn'
       EQUIVOCAL  i·kwiv'·ə·kəl           SYNCOPE  sing'·kə·pē, sin'·k'rrn·pē
       REIFY   rā'·ə·fī, rē'·ə·fi         ENNUI  an·wē'
       INDICES  in'·də·sēz               DRACHM  dram
       ASSIGNATE  as'·ig·nāt'             CIDEVANT  sēd·ə·vä(n)'
       TOPIARY  tō·pē·er'·ē               EPERGNE  i·pərn', ā·pərn'
       CAVEAT  kav'·ē·at, kāv'·ē·at,      VIVACE  vē·väch'·ā, vē·väch'·ē
                 kā·vē·at'**              TALIPES  tal'·ə·pēz
       SUPERFLUOUS  sù·pėr'·flü·əs        SYNECDOCHE  sə·nek'·də·kē
```

Figure 5–3. North American Reading Test sample scoring sheet. Pronunciation symbols follow Webster's. Single asterisk indicates correct U.S. pronunciation only. Double asterisks indicate correct Canadian pronunciation only.

scoring sheet. A sample scoring sheet along with the correct pronunciations is given in Fig. 5–3.

Administration

For the NART-2, see Source. Briefly, the patient is presented with the word card and is instructed to read each word. Because the reading of words in a list format may be confusing for some subjects, the NART-2 is available in booklet format with each word displayed in large print on a separate card. The reading of words is paced by requiring the patient to pause between words until the examiner calls, "next."

An optional criterion for discontinuation of the NART (14 incorrect in 15 consecutive re-

sponses) is presented in the test manual. However, Beardsall and Brayne (1990) have reported that, in a sample of elderly subjects, this criterion was rarely met. In order to reduce anxiety or distress in subjects with poor reading skills, they developed an equation that estimates a subject's score on the second half of the NART (items 26–50) from the first half (the Short NART). If a client scores less than 12 correct on the Short NART, this is taken as the total correct score since Beardsall and Brayne (1990) showed that subjects who score 0–11 correct are unlikely to add to their score by completing the second half of the test. For subjects scoring between 12–20, a conversion table (Table 5–10) is used to predict the full error score. For subjects scoring more than 20 correct, the complete NART is

Table 5—10. Conversion Table for Predicted Full
NART Error Score from Short NART Score

Short NART Correct Score	Conversion to Full NART Error Score
0–11	As in Full NART (50 minus correct)
12	38
13	36
14	34
15	33
16	31
17	30
18	28
19	26
20	24
21 +	As in Full NART (50 minus correct)

Source: Beardsall and Brayne, 1990 (p. 89). Compute the
number of correct words in the Short NART. If 0 to 20 correct, then do not continue to Full NART. If 21 to 25 correct, then continue to Full NART. These scores can then be converted to predicted IQ scores using appropriate equations. Copyright Swets Zeitlinger. Reprinted with permission.

administered. The accuracy of the Short NART in estimating premorbid IQ has been found to be virtually equivalent to the full NART in a cross-validation study (Crawford et al., 1991).

Another useful modification is to place the words into sentences (Beardsall & Huppert, 1994) since the provision of semantic and syntactic cues (context) results in a larger number of words being read correctly and, hence, in a higher estimate of IQ, particularly among demented subjects and poor-to-average readers.

For the NAART, the following instructions are given:

"I want you to read slowly down this list of words starting here (indicate 'debt') *and continuing down this column and on to the next. When you have finished reading the words on the page, turn the page over and begin here* (indicate top of second page). *After each word please wait until I say 'Next' before reading the next word. I must warn you that there are many words that you probably won't recognize, in fact,* most *people don't know them, so just guess at these, O.K.? Go ahead."*

The subject should be encouraged to guess, and all responses should be reinforced

("good," "that's fine," etc.). The subject may change a response if he or she wishes to do so but if more than one version is given, the subject must decide on the final choice. No time limit is imposed.

Approximate Time for Administration

The approximate time required is 10 minutes.

Scoring

The use of a tape recorder is recommended in order to facilitate scoring. Each incorrectly pronounced word counts as one error. Slight variations in pronunciation are acceptable when these are due to regional accents. The total number of errors is tabulated.

NART-2 scores can be converted to WAIS-R VIQ, PIQ, and FSIQ using a table provided in the manual (Nelson & Willison, 1991). Note that Short NART scores must be converted to full NART scores. An additional table is provided in the test manual in order to evaluate whether the predicted–obtained discrepancy is unusual. Alternatively, examiners working with American clients can use Ryan and Paolo's (1992) equations to predict WAIS-R IQ:

$$\text{Estimated VIQ} = 132.3893 + (\text{NART errors}) \; (-1.164)$$

$$\text{Estimated PIQ} = 123.0684 + (\text{NART errors}) \; (-0.823)$$

$$\text{Estimated FSIQ} = 131.3845 + (\text{NART errors}) \; (-1.124)$$

The standard errors of estimate are 7.70, 12.08, and 8.83, for WAIS-R VIQ, PIQ, and FSIQ, respectively. Note that the regression equations were developed on a sample of normal, community-dwelling subjects, 75 years and older. The equations will likely be most effective in estimating the premorbid intelligence of elderly persons who have mild cognitive loss and who do not require custodial care. The inclusion of education (plus NART errors) in the equation did not significantly improve prediction.

Willshire et al. (1991), however, included demographic variables with the NART and provided a substantially better estimate of premorbid cognitive functioning than that given by the NART or by demographic information alone. The equation (appropriate for subjects between the ages of 55 and 69 years) is as follows:

$$\text{Estimated IQ} = 123.7 - 0.8\,(\text{NART errors}) + 3.8\,\text{education} - 7.4\,\text{sex}$$

To use this equation, note that educational level comprised the following five categories: (1) some primary school; (2) some secondary school; (3) some secondary school plus trade qualifications; (4) secondary school completed; (5) tertiary education begun. Sex was assigned as males = 1 and females = 2.

NAART equations (Blair and Spreen, 1989) to predict WAIS-R VIQ, PIQ, and FSIQ are as follow:

$$\text{Estimated VIQ} = 128.7 - .89\,(\text{NAART errors})$$
$$\text{Estimated PIQ} = 119.4 - .42\,(\text{NAART errors})$$
$$\text{Estimated FSIQ} = 127.8 - .78\,(\text{NAART errors})$$

The standard errors of estimate for VIQ, PIQ, and FSIQ are 6.56, 10.67, and 7.63, respectively.

Comment

The NART/NART-2 is among the most reliable tests in clinical use. When internal consistency is considered, reliability estimates are above .90 (Crawford et al., 1988b). A test–retest reliability of .98 has been reported (Crawford et al., 1989b). Practice effects do emerge over the short term (10 days). However, the mean decrease is less than one NART error, suggesting that practice effects are of little clinical significance. The NART also has high inter-rater reliability (above .88) (O'Carroll, 1987; Crawford et al., 1989b; Sharpe & O'Carroll, 1991). Some NART words, however, have a disproportionately high rate of inter-rater disagreement (aeon, puerperal, aver, sidereal and prelate) and particular care should be taken when scoring these words (Crawford et al., 1989b).

Blair and Spreen (1989) report that a measure of interscorer reliability for the NAART was .99 (p < .001). Coefficient alpha, a measure of internal consistency, was .94. Raguet et al. (1996) gave the NAART to 51 normal adults on two separate occasions, separated by about one year. NAART estimates were highly reliable, with a coefficient of .92.

Researchers generally report moderate to high correlations (.4 to .8) between NART (or NAART) performance and measures of general intellectual ability (Blair & Spreen, 1989; Crawford et al., 1989b; Johnstone et al., 1996; Nelson & O'Connell, 1978; Raguet et al., 1996; Sharpe & O'Carroll, 1991; Wiens et al., 1993; Willshire et al., 1991) and education (Maddrey et al., 1996). The test has good accuracy even in the retrospective estimation of Wechsler IQ (Berry et al., 1994; Moss & Dowd, 1991; Raguet et al., 1996). In the standardization sample, the NART predicted 55, 60, and 30 percent of the variance in prorated WAIS Full Scale, Verbal, and Performance IQ respectively (Nelson, 1982). Similar results have recently been reported by others (e.g., Blair & Spreen, 1989; Crawford et al., 1989b; Ryan & Paolo, 1992; Wiens et al., 1993). In short, the test is a good predictor of VIQ and FSIQ, but is relatively poor at predicting PIQ. Among verbal subtests, NART (NAART) errors correlate most highly with Vocabulary and Information (Wiens et al., 1993). Combined factor analysis of the NART and WAIS (Crawford et al., 1989a) has revealed that the NART has a very high loading (.85) on the first unrotated principal component, which is regarded as representing general intelligence (g). NART scores have been found to be normally distributed in a study of over 300 normal community-dwelling adults (Brayne & Beardsall, 1990).

Prediction of IQs, at least in normal people, is more accurate with equations based on NART (or NAART) scores than with the Wechsler Vocabulary subtest or with demographic prediction equations developed by Barona et al. (1984) (Blair & Spreen, 1989; Crawford et al., 1988; Ryan & Paolo, 1992; Sharpe & O'Carroll, 1991). Combining Barona and NAART estimates, however, appears to increase predictive accuracy. Raguet et al. (1996) recommend averaging estimates from the Barona and NAART. Willshire et al. (1991)

report that in a sample of residents in Melbourne, Australia, 56 percent of the variance in WAIS-R IQ scores could be predicted on the basis of a formula that includes NART error score, education and sex. This was 24 percent more than could be predicted on the basis of education alone and 18 percent more than on the basis of NART error score alone (see Scoring).

In short, the NART (or NAART) does provide a useful measure of intelligence. It also correlates highly (.82) with WRAT-R Reading (Johnstone et al., 1993; Wiens et al., 1993). The test is generally resistant to depression (Crawford et al., 1987) and provides a reasonable estimate of premorbid ability in acutely ill, unmedicated schizophrenic patients (O'Carroll et al., 1992). However, as indicated earlier, the test is not insensitive to cerebral damage, and deterioration in reading test performance does occur in patients with cerebral dysfunction; for example, in patients with moderate to severe levels of dementia (Fromm et al., 1991; Stebbins et al., 1988; Stebbins et al., 1990a), in patients with mild dementia who have accompanying linguistic deficits (Stebbins et al., 1990b), and in patients with executive dysfunction who fail to check their errors prior to response production (O'Carroll et al., 1992). Patterson et al. (1994) found a dramatic decrease in NART performance as a function of AD severity and reported a correlation of .56 between MMSE and NART scores. They attributed the specific reading deficit manifested on the NART to the deterioration of semantic memory in AD and to an impaired ability to perform specific phonological manipulations. Paque and Warrington (1995) compared the performance of 57 dementing patients on the NART and the WAIS-R. Patients were examined on two occasions spaced at least 10 months apart. Although NART performance declined over time, the deterioration on VIQ and PIQ was more rapid and severe. Patients whose reading declined tended to have a lower VIQ than PIQ, raising the concern that verbal skills may have already been compromised by disease. Taylor et al. (1996) tested a sample of AD patients on three or four occasions each separated by about one year. AMNART performance declined with increasing dementia

severity as measured by the Mini Mental State Examination (MMSE). In order to take increasing dementia into account, they derived an MMSE-based correction factor to estimate IQ.

Although the NART may not be entirely insensitive to cerebral damage, the available evidence suggests that it may be less sensitive than many other cognitive measures (Berry et al., 1994; Christensen et al., 1991; Maddrey et al., 1996). Thus, although far from perfect, it may be the instrument of choice. The test, however, should not be used with aphasic or dyslexic patients, with those who have VIQ less than PIQ, nor with patients who have significant articulatory or visual acuity problems.

It is also important to bear in mind that use of regression procedures has some limitations, including regression toward the mean and limited range of scores. These limitations suggest that two types of errors may occur when the equations are applied to individuals with suspected dementia (Boekamp et al., 1995; Ryan & Paolo, 1992; Wiens et al., 1993). In the case of superior premorbid ability, the predicted IQ will represent an underestimate of the amount of cognitive deterioration present. However, since patients with dementia are rarely referred for psychological assessment when their intelligence levels remain in the superior range, this ceiling effect should not invalidate the clinical utility of the test (Ryan & Paolo, 1992). On the other hand, in individuals whose premorbid abilities were relatively low, the estimated IQ might suggest cognitive deterioration when, in actuality, it had not occurred.

These limitations underscore the need to supplement NART (NAART) estimates of premorbid functioning with clinical observations as well as information about a patient's educational and occupational accomplishments (Ryan & Paolo, 1992). Combining the NART with demographic information or other performance-based data (e.g., MMSE) may also increase predictive accuracy (see the introduction). The majority of research on the NART has focussed on estimating premorbid intelligence and has employed the Wechsler Intelligence Scale as the criterion variable. NART equations are, however, also available for estimating premorbid performance on the FAS verbal fluency task (Crawford et al., 1992) and the PASAT (Crawford et al., in press) (See COWA and PASAT in this book). In addition, some (Schlosser & Ivison, 1989) have suggested that NART equations based on memory test performance may be capable of assessing dementia earlier than the NART/ WAIS-R combination.

Normative Data

NART-2 (NAART) performance is correlated with years of education and social class. Age and sex have little effect on performance (Crawford et al., 1988b; Graf & Uttl, 1995; Ivnik et al., 1996: Nelson, 1982; Nelson & Willison, 1991; Starr et al., 1992; Wiens et al., 1993) although when a wide age range is studied (well-educated healthy individuals aged 16–84 years), an age-related increase in *correct* NAART scores appears to emerge (See Table 5–11) (Graf & Uttl, 1995; Uttl & Graf, submitted). As might be expected, NART (NAART) errors systematically decrease with increasing FSIQ (Wiens et al., 1993).

For the NART-2, Nelson and Willison have provided a discrepancy table to determine the probability of a chance occurrence of a discrepancy in favor of NART-2 estimated IQ over observed WAIS-R IQ. The equations are based on a British sample. For North American samples, Ryan and Paolo (1992) developed regression equations to predict WAIS-R IQs from NART error scores (see Scoring), but they did not provide corresponding discrepancy tables.

Willshire and colleagues (1991) have developed regression equations to predict WAIS-R IQs for use with adults, aged 55–69 years, based on a combination of NART errors and demographic variables. The equation (see Scoring) is based on an Australian sample. However, standard errors of the estimate and discrepancy tables are not provided. Crawford and his colleagues (1989c) have also developed regression equations that combine NART errors and demographic variables to predict premorbid IQ. These researchers (Crawford et al., 1990) developed a regression equation to predict the number of NART errors made on the basis of demographic variables. Unfortunately, these equations are based on the WAIS, not the WAIS-R.

For the NAART, Blair and Spreen (1989) recommended that for PIQ, a positive discrepancy of at least 21 points between estimated and actual IQs indicates the possibility of deterioration. For VIQ and FSIQ, a positive discrepancy of 15 or more points between estimated and actual IQ scores indicates the possibility of intellectual deterioration or impairment (based on the calculation of 95 per cent confidence levels). Wiens et al. (1993) reported that only about 10 per cent of normal individuals have predicted–obtained FSIQ differences as large as 15 points. Thus, a difference of this size is infrequent enough among healthy people to merit clinical attention (see also Berry et al., 1994).

It is important to note the ranges of possible predicted WAIS-R scores. The range of possible NAART-predicted IQs is 129–74 for the Verbal Scale, 119–94 for the Performance Scale, and 128–80 for the Full Scale (Wiens et al., 1993). The range of possible NART predicted IQs is 132–74 for the Verbal Scale, 123–82 for the Performance Scale, and 131–75 for the Full Scale (Ryan & Paolo, 1992). Thus, there is truncation of the spread of predicted IQs on either end of the distribution,

Table 5—11. NAART Mean Number Correct by Age Group

	Age in Years					
	16–29	30–39	40–49	50–59	60–69	70+
n	19	23	30	31	29	31
Mean	36.68	40.07	43.13	43.78	43.06	45.81
SD	6.70	9.46	8.79	8.17	10.78	8.43

Source: Graf & Uttl, 1995. Reprinted with permission of Swiss Journal of Psychology.

leading to unreliable estimates for individuals at other than average levels of ability (Ryan & Paolo, 1992; Wiens et al., 1993).

References

Barona, A., Reynolds, C.R., & Chastain, R. (1984). A demographically based index of pre-morbid intelligence for the WAIS-R. *Journal of Consulting and Clinical Psychology, 52,* 885–887.

Beardsall, L., & Brayne, C. (1990). Estimation of verbal intelligence in an elderly community: A prediction analysis using a shortened NART. *British Journal of Clinical Psychology, 29,* 83–90.

Beardsall, L., & Huppert, F.A. (1994). Improvement in NART word reading in demented and normal older persons using the Cambridge Contextual Reading Test. *Journal of Clinical and Experimental Neuropsychology, 16,* 232–242.

Berry, D.T.R., Carpenter, G.S., Campbell, D.A., Schmitt, F.A., Helton, K., & Lipke-Molby, T. (1994). The New Adult Reading Test–Revised: Accuracy in estimating WAIS-R IQ scores obtained 3.5 years earlier from normal older persons. *Archives of Clinical Neuropsychology, 9,* 239–250.

Blair, J.R., & Spreen, O. (1989). Predicting premorbid IQ: A revision of the National Adult Reading Test. *The Clinical Neuropsychologist, 3,* 129–136.

Boekamp, J.R., Strauss, M.E., & Adams, N. (1995). Estimating premorbid intelligence in African-American and white elderly veterans using the American version of the National Adult Reading Test. *Journal of Clinical and Experimental Neuropsychology, 17,* 645–653.

Brayne, C., & Beardsall, L. (1990). Estimation of verbal intelligence in an elderly community: An epidemiological study using the NART. *British Journal of Clinical Psychology, 29,* 217–223.

Christensen, H., Hadzi-Pavlovic, D., & Jacomb, P. (1991). The psychometric differentiation of dementia from normal aging: a meta-analysis. *Psychological Assessment, 3,* 147–155.

Crawford, J.R., Besson, J.A.O., Parker, D.M., Sutherland, K.M., & Keen, P.L. (1987). Estimation of premorbid intellectual status in depression. *British Journal of Clinical Psychology, 26,* 313–314.

Crawford, J.R., Parker, D.M., & Besson, J.A.O. (1988a). Estimation of premorbid intelligence in organic conditions. *British Journal of Psychiatry, 153,* 178–181.

Crawford, J.R., Stewart, L.E., Garthwaite, P.H., Parker, D.M., and Besson, J.A.O. (1988b). The relationship between demographic variables and NART performance in normal subjects. *British Journal of Clinical Psychology, 27,* 181–182.

Crawford, J.R., Stewart, L.E., Cochrane, R.H.B., Parker, D.M., & Besson, J.A.O. (1989a). Construct validity of the National Adult Reading Test: A factor analytic study. *Personality and Individual Differences, 10,* 585–587.

Crawford, J.R., Stewart, L.E., Besson, J.A.O., Parker, D.M., & De Lacey, G. (1989b). Prediction of WAIS IQ with the National Adult Reading Test: Cross-validation and extension. *British Journal of Clinical Psychology, 28,* 267–273.

Crawford, J.R., Stewart, L.E., Parker, D.M., Besson, J.A.O., & Cochrane, R.H.B. (1989c). Estimation of premorbid intelligence: Combining psychometric and demographic approaches improves predictive accuracy. *Personality and Individual Differences, 10,* 793–796.

Crawford, J.R., Allan, K.M., Cochrane, R.H.B., & Parker, D.M. (1990). Assessing the validity of NART-estimated premorbid IQs in the individual case. *British Journal of Clinical Psychology, 29,* 435–436.

Crawford, J.R., Parker, D.M., Allan, K.M., Jack, A.M., & Morrison, F.M. (1991). The Short NART: Cross-validation, relationship to IQ and some practical considerations. *British Journal of Clinical Psychology, 30,* 223–229.

Crawford, J.R., Obansawin, M.C., & Allan, K.M. (in press). PASAT and components of WAIS-R performance: convergent and discriminant validity. *Neuropsychological Rehabilitation.*

Fromm, D., Holland, A.L., Nebes, R.D., & Oakley, M.A. (1991). A longitudinal study of word-reading ability in Alzheimer's disease: Evidence from the National Adult Reading Test. *Cortex, 27,* 367–376.

Graf, P., & Uttl, B. (1995). Component processes of memory: Changes across the adult lifespan. *Swiss Journal of Psychology, 54,* 113–130.

Grober, E., & Sliwinski, M. (1991). Development and validation of a model for estimating premorbid verbal intelligence in the elderly. *Journal of Clinical and Experimental Neuropsychology, 13,* 933–949.

Ivnik, R.J., Malec, J.F., Smith, G.E., Tangalos, E.G., & Petersen, R.C. (1996). Neuropsychological tests norms above age 55: COWAT, BNT, Token, WRAT-R Reading, AMNART, Stroop, TMT, JLO. *The Clinical Neuropsychologist, 10,* 262–278.

Johnstone, B., Callahan, C.D., Kapila, C.J., &

Bouman, D.E. (1996). The comparability of the WRAT-R Reading test and NAART as estimates of premorbid intelligence in neurologically impaired patients. *Archives of Clinical Neuropsychology*, *11*, 513–519.

Maddrey, A.M., Cullum, C.M., Weiner, M.F., & Filley, C.M. (1996). Premorbid intelligence estimation and level of dementia in Alzheimer's disease. *Journal of the International Neuropsychological Society*, *2*, 551–555.

Moss, A.R., & Dowd, T. (1991). Does the NART hold after head injury: A case report. *British Journal of Clinical Psychology*, *30*, 179–180.

Nelson, H.E. (1982). *National Adult Reading Test (NART): Test Manual*. Windsor, UK: NFER Nelson.

Nelson, H.E., & O'Connell, A. (1978). Dementia: The estimation of pre-morbid intelligence levels using the new adult reading test. *Cortex*, *14*, 234–244.

Nelson, H.E., & Willison, J. (1991). *National Adult Reading Test (NART): Test Manual*. Second Edition. Windsor, UK: NFER Nelson.

O'Carroll, R.E. (1987). The inter-rater reliability of the National Adult Reading Test (NART): A pilot study. *British Journal of Clinical Psychology*, *26*, 229–230.

O'Carroll, R.E., Walker, M., Dunan, J., Murray, C., Blackwood, D., Ebmeier, K.P., & Goodwin, G.M. (1992). Selecting controls for Schizophrenia research studies: The use of the national adult reading test (NART) as a measure of premorbid ability. *Schizophrenia Research*, *8*, 137–141.

O'Carroll, R.E., Moffoot, A., Ebmeier, K.P., & Goodwin, G.M. (1992). Estimating pre-morbid intellectual ability in the Alcoholic Korsakoff Syndrome. *Psychological Medicine*, *22*, 903–909.

Paque, L., & Warrington, E.K. (1995). A longitudinal study of reading ability in patients suffering from dementia. *Journal of the International Neuropsychological Society*, *1*, 517–524.

Patterson, K., Graham, N., & Hodges, J.R. (1994). Reading in dementia of the Alzheimer type: A preserved ability? *Neuropsychology*, *8*, 395–407.

Raguet, M.L., Campbell, D.A., Berry, D.T.R., Schmitt, F.A., & Smith, G.T. (1996). Stability of intelligence and intellectual predictors in older persons. *Psychological Assessment*, *8*, 154–160.

Ryan, J.J., & Paolo, A.M. (1992). A screening procedure for estimating premorbid intelligence in the elderly. *The Clinical Neuropsychologist*, *6*, 53–62.

Schlosser, D., & Ivison, D. (1989). Assessing memory deterioration with the Wechsler Memory Scale, the National Adult Reading Test, and the Schonell Graded Word Reading Test. *Journal of Clinical and Experimental Neuropsychology*, *11*, 785–792.

Sharpe, K., & O'Carroll, R. (1991). Estimating premorbid intellectual level in dementia using the National Adult Reading Test: A Canadian study. *British Journal of Clinical Psychology*, *30*, 381–384.

Starr, J.M., Whalley, L.J., Inch, S., & Shering, P.A. (1992). The quantification of the relative effects of age and NART-predicted IQ on cognitive function in healthy old people. *International Journal of Geriatric Psychiatry*, *7*, 153–157.

Stebbins, G.T., Wilson, R.S., Gilley, D.W., Bernard, B.A., & Fox, J.H. (1988). Estimation of premorbid intelligence in dementia. *Journal of Clinical and Experimental Neuropsychology*, *10*, 63–64.

Stebbins, G.T., Gilley, D.W., Wilson, R.S., Bernard, B.A., & Fox, J.H. (1990a). Effects of language disturbances on premorbid estimates of IQ in mild dementia. *The Clinical Neuropsychologist*, *4*, 64–68.

Stebbins, G.T., Wilson, R.S., Gilley, D.W., Bernard, B.A., & Fox, J.H. (1990b). Use of the National Adult Reading Test to estimate premorbid IQ in dementia. *The Clinical Neuropsychologist*, *4*, 18–24.

Taylor, K.I., Salmon, D.P., Rice, V.A., Bondi, M.W., Hill, L.R., Ernesto, C.R., & Butters, N. (1996). A longitudinal examination of American National Adult Reading Test (AMNART) performance in dementia of the Alzheimer Type (DAT): Validation and correction based on rate of cognitive decline. *Journal of Clinical and Experimental Neuropsychology*, *18*, 883–891.

Uttl, B., & Graf, P. (submitted). Color word Stroop test performance across the life span. *Journal of Clinical and Experimental Neuropsychology*.

Wiens, A.N., Bryan, J.E., & Crossen, J.R. (1993). Estimating WAIS-R FSIQ from the National Adult Reading Test–Revised in normal subjects. *The Clinical Neuropsychologist*, *7*, 70–84.

Willshire, D., Kinsella, G., & Prior, M. (1991). Estimating WAIS-R from the National Adult Reading Test: A cross-validation. *Journal of Clinical and Experimental Neuropsychology*, *13*, 204–216.

RAVEN'S PROGRESSIVE MATRICES (RPM)

Purpose

The purpose of Raven's Progressive Matrices is to assess reasoning in the visual modality.

Source

The test, including all levels, can be ordered from The Psychological Corporation, P.O. Box 9954, San Antonio, Texas 78204-0954, for approximately $549 US or from The Psychological Corporation, 55 Horner Avenue, Toronto, Ontario M5Z 4X6, for about $733.50 Cdn. Research supplements (containing normative data) are also available for purchase from The Psychological Corporation. Each supplement costs about $53 US or $70 Cdn.

Description

Raven's Progressive Matrices is consensually accepted as the quintessential test of inductive reasoning (Alderton & Larson, 1990). Test items require the examinee to infer a rule relating to a collection of elements, and then to use the rule to generate the next items in a series, or to verify that a presented element is legitimate relative to the rule (Alderton & Larson, 1990). Problems become progressively more difficult, the easier items serving as a learning experience for later and more difficult items. Thus, the test has been used to assess intellectual efficiency or the ability to become more efficient by learning from immediate experience with the problems (Mills et al., 1993). The test is a popular measure of conceptual ability because responses require neither verbalization, skilled manipulative ability, or subtle differentiation of visuospatial information. In addition, verbal instruction is kept to a minimum (Zaidel et al., 1981). Three forms of this test have been developed.

The Standard Progressive Matrices (SPM) (Raven, 1938, 1996) consist of 60 items grouped into five sets (A to E), each set containing 12 items. Each item contains a pattern problem with one part removed and 6–8 pictured inserts, one of which contains the correct pattern. Each set involves different principles of matrix transformation, and within each set the items become increasingly more difficult. The scale is intended for the entire range of intellectual development starting with the time a child is able to grasp the idea of finding a missing piece to complete a pattern. Young children, mentally defective people, and very old individuals, however, are not expected to solve more than the problems in Sets A and B of the scale and the easier problems of Sets C and D, where reasoning by analogy is not essential.

The Colored Progressive Matrices (CPM) (Raven, 1947, 1995) provide a shorter and simpler form of the test. The test consists of 36 items, grouped into three sets (A, Ab, B) of 12 items each. It was developed for use with children (age 5.5+) and old people, for anthropological studies, and for clinical work. The test can be used with people who, for any reason, cannot understand English; people who suffer from physical disabilities, aphasias, cerebral palsy or deafness; and with people who are intellectually subnormal. The problems are printed on colored backgrounds in order to attract the subject's attention. The scale is arranged so that it can be presented in the form of illustrations in a book or as boards with movable pieces. The test covers the cognitive processes of which children under the age of 11 years are usually capable. Once the intellectual capacity to reason by analogy has developed, the SPM is the more suitable scale to use.

The Advanced Progressive Matrices (APM) (Raven, 1965, 1994) were constructed as a test of intellectual efficiency that could be used with people of more than average intellectual ability and that could differentiate clearly between people of even superior ability. It is intended for those for whom the SPM are too easy; i.e., for persons obtaining a raw score above about 50 on the SPM. With highly able children beyond the age of 10 years, the APM may be the most appropriate level to ensure an adequate ceiling (Mills et al., 1993). It consists of two sets of items. In Set I, there are 12 problems designed to introduce a person to the method of working and to cover the intellectual processes assessed by the SPM. It can be used as a short 10-minute test or as a practice test before starting Set II. The 36 items in Set II are identical in presentation and reasoning with those in Set I. They increase in difficulty more steadily and become considerably more complex.

Administration

See source. Briefly, the subject points to the pattern piece he or she selects as correct or writes its number on an answer sheet. There is some evidence that computerized forms can produce the same results as paper and pencil forms (Raven, 1996). Raven cautions that, in order to obtain equivalence, the answer selected by respondents be shown on the screen and be alterable, and that the respondents should be required to make a second, separate response to move the display to the next item.

Approximate Time for Administration

Both the SPM and CPM are untimed tests. The SPM takes about 40 minutes and the CPM requires about 25 minutes. Set II of the APM can be used without a time limit in order to assess a person's total reasoning capacity. In that case, the subject should be shown the problems of Set I as examples to explain the principles of the test. Allow about one hour to complete the task. To assess a person's intellectual efficiency, Set I can be given as a short practice test followed by Set II as a speed test. The most common time limit for Set II is 40 minutes.

Scoring

Record the total number correct.

Comment

Test–retest reliability data are acceptable (above .8), although for young children (CPM—less than age 8; APM—less than age 11) the Raven is somewhat less reliable (see source). The median test–retest value is about .8, with somewhat lower values for retest intervals over one year. A single brief training session (with the examiner verbalizing problem-solving strategy) is sufficient to improve performance on the RPM (Denney &

Heidrich, 1990). In view of these practice effects, retesting after short intervals should be avoided. When internal consistency is considered, reliability estimates are acceptable (above .70) (Burke, 1985; Powers et al., 1986).

The RPM is not homogeneous with regard to its problem-solving requirements. In many instances, an item may be solved using several different rules, or the specific solution steps may be ordered differently. However, underlying this medley of diverse items is a singular ability construct—g, or general intellectual functioning—along which individuals can be ordered (Alderton & Larson, 1990; Arthur & Woehr, 1993). Although not strictly a pure measure of Spearman's g, the RPM comes as close as many consider possible (Llabre, 1984). Concurrent validity studies show a modest correlation (about .7) between Raven and conventional tests of intelligence such as the Wechsler and Stanford-Binet scales (Burke, 1985; Jensen et al., 1988; O'Leary et al., 1991; also see Source), suggesting that the underlying processes may be general rather than specific to this one test. When the Wechsler subtests are considered, the strongest relationship is found with Block Design, which involves visuospatial skills and is considered a good measure of fluid intelligence (Mills et al., 1993). The RPM is considered more culture-fair than the Wechsler test for measuring IQ (O'Leary et al., 1991). It has relatively low correlations with tests of academic achievement (Esquivel, 1984; Llabre, 1984), consistent with the notion that it is a fairer measure than most intelligence tests or specific ability measures (Mills et al., 1993; Raven, 1990). The RPM, however, is not culture-blind (Owen, 1992).

Raven (1995) argues that the qualitatively different items of which the test is composed form part of a common continuum and are absolutely dependent on the abilities required to solve the easier items.

It has been suggested that the core abilities tapped by the RPM include an incremental, reiterative strategy for encoding and inducing the regularities in each problem, the ability to induce abstract relations, and the ability to dynamically manage a large set of problem-solving goals in working memory (Carpenter et al., 1990).

The bulk of the evidence suggests that brain damage depresses the total score on the CPM (see Court and Drebing in Raven et al., 1990, for a recent review of the RPM in various neurological populations). The literature suggests that there is no significant difference between average scores of right and left brain-damaged individuals (e.g., Costa et al., 1969; Denes et al., 1978; Villardita, 1985). This may reflect a lack of homogeneity of items composing the CPM (e.g., Burke, 1958; Costa, 1976). There is some evidence that left–right hemispheric differences emerge when the items of the CPM are categorized on the basis of the cognitive ability presumed to underlie their solution (Denes et al., 1978; Villardita, 1985; Zaidel et al., 1981). Some have suggested that Subtest A performance tends to be associated with the functions of the right (visuospatial) hemisphere, and Subtest B performance with the functions of the left hemisphere (analogic reasoning) (Costa 1976; Cronin-Golomb & Braun, 1997; Denes et al., 1978; Zaidel, 1981).

Recently, Gainotti et al. (1992) found that qualitative analysis of responses on the RCM can increase the diagnostic accuracy with regard to AD. The tendency to give globalistic (reproducing on a reduced scale the whole shape of the model instead of completing it) and odd (completely different from the missing part and from the general form of the model) responses are good markers of dementia and point more to AD than to a vascular form of dementia.

The RPM is often described as a measure of nonverbal intelligence. The question arises whether language plays a central role in mediating performance on the task. While the literature suggests that aphasic patients perform worse than normal controls on the RPM, findings are less consistent when aphasic patients are compared to other nonaphasic patients with left-hemisphere damage (Court and Drebing in Raven et al., 1990).

Unlike the findings with respect to aphasia, the findings with regard to RPM performance in the presence of constructional apraxia are quite consistent. Constructional apraxia is associated with lower RPM scores (Court and Drebing in Raven et al., 1990).

Costa et al. (1969) developed criteria for assessing the presence of unilateral spatial inattention from CPM protocols. The number of answers chosen from the right side of the page (alternatives 3 and 6) is subtracted from the number of answers from the left side of the page (alternatives 1 and 4). The probability of this score, called the 'position preference score' (PP), being 7 or greater, or −7 or less, is less than .01 in a normal population. A positive score of 7 or greater suggests right-sided neglect whereas a negative score of 7 or less suggests left-sided neglect. The measure appears more sensitive than copying and drawing tasks to unilateral spatial inattention (Campbell & Oxbury, 1976). In order to reduce the influence that neglect for left-sided alternatives may have on the performance of right-brain-damaged patients, the response array for each item on the CPM can be arranged vertically (Caltagirone et al., 1977; Villardita, 1985).

In short, the simplicity, the nonverbal nature of the RPM and the culture-fairness of the task are distinct advantages for certain patients. However, it provides little information about an individual's strengths or weaknesses. Thus, the RPM may provide additional information but alternative measures are needed to gain a true picture of an individual's abilities (Mills et al., 1993). It is also important to note that performance is affected by factors such as visual field defects, unilateral neglect, and aphasia. Accordingly, interpretation may be difficult in the presence of these factors (Court & Drebing in Raven et al., 1990). Further, the task is not particularly useful with regard to questions of localization of lesion, although there is some evidence that posterior brain regions play an important role. Studies using cerebral blood flow or Positron Emission Tomography suggest that performance on the RPM is associated with increased blood flow or glucose metabolism in the posterior half of the brain, that is, in parieto-temporal-occipital regions (Haier et al., 1988; Risberg et al., 1977).

Normative Data

Score conversion is to percentiles. Raven scores show a significant increase with increasing years of education and socioeconomic status (Burke, 1985; Marcopulos et

Table 5—12. Standard Progressive Matrices: Smoothed Summary Norms for North American Children,

Percentile Rank	Age in Years									
	6.03–6.08	6.09–7.02	7.03–7.08	7.09–8.02	8.03–8.08	8.09–9.02	9.03–9.08	9.09–10.02	10.03–10.09	10.09–11.02
95	30	33	36	38	40	42	44	46	47	48
90	27	30	33	36	38	40	42	44	45	46
75	21	25	28	31	34	36	38	40	41	43
50	14	17	20	23	26	29	32	34	36	37
25	12	13	14	16	18	21	24	26	28	30
10	9	10	11	13	14	16	17	19	21	23
5	7	8	9	10	11	12	13	15	17	18

Source: Data are reprinted with permission of J.C. Raven Ltd. and derived from Raven et al. (1995a). Based on a series of systematic random samples of North American school children.

Table 5—13. Standard Progressive Matrices: Smoothed Summary Norms for Adults in The United States of America

Percentile Rank	Age in Years										
	18–22	23–27	28–32	33–37	38–42	43–47	48–52	53–57	58–62	63–67	68+
95	59	59	59	59	59	59	59	58	57	56	55
90	58	58	58	58	58	58	58	57	56	55	53
75	56	56	56	56	56	56	56	55	54	53	51
50	52	52	52	52	52	52	51	50	49	47	45
25	47	47	47	47	47	47	47	45	43	39	35
10	41	41	41	41	41	41	41	39	35	31	27
5	35	35	35	35	35	35	35	31	27	23	18
n	28	54	72	77	121	69	33	36	28	33	55

Based on the 1993 standardization of the SPM in Des Moines, Iowa. Tests completed at leisure.

Source: Data are reprinted with permission of J. C. Raven Ltd. and derived from Raven et al., 1995a.

Table 5—14. Colored Progressive Matrices: Smoothed Summary Norms for North Americans, Ages 5.5 to 11.5

Percentile Rank	Age in Years											
	5.03–5.08	5.09–6.03	6.04–6.08	6.09–7.02	7.03–7.08	7.09–8.02	8.03–8.08	8.09–9.02	9.03–9.08	9.09–10.02	10.03–10.08	10.09–11.02	11.03–11.09
95	23	25	28	30	31	32	33	34	35	35	35	35	35
90	21	23	25	27	29	30	31	32	33	33	34	34	35
75	17	19	21	23	25	27	29	30	31	32	32	33	34
50	12	14	16	18	20	22	24	26	27	28	29	30	31
25	11	12	13	14	15	17	19	21	22	23	24	25	26
10	9	10	11	12	13	14	15	16	17	18	19	20	21
5	8	9	9	10	11	12	12	13	14	15	16	17	18

Source: Reprinted with permission of J. C. Raven Ltd. and derived from Raven et al. (1990). Based on a series of systematic random samples of schoolchildren.

Ages 6.5 to 16.5

					Age in Years					
11.03– 11.08	11.09– 12.02	12.03– 12.08	12.09– 13.02	13.03– 13.08	13.09– 14.02	14.03– 14.08	14.09– 15.02	15.03– 15.08	15.09– 16.02	16.03– 16.08
49	50	51	52	53	54	55	56	56	57	57
47	48	49	50	51	52	52	53	54	55	56
44	45	46	47	48	49	49	50	51	52	53
38	39	40	41	42	43	44	45	46	47	48
32	33	34	35	36	37	38	39	40	41	42
25	27	28	30	31	32	33	35	35	36	37
19	21	22	24	26	27	28	29	29	30	31

al., 1997; O'Leary et al., 1991; also see Source). Further, scores on the Raven are correlated with the subject's age. There appears to be an increase of ability through childhood, a period of maximum ability from adolescence to adulthood, and then—perhaps—a decline with extreme age. However, what had previously been thought to be a decline with advancing age appears to be an increase with date of birth (Raven et al., 1995a). Numerous reports of normative data have appeared in the literature (see source). Many norms are derived from studies conducted in the 1930s and 1940s. Since that time, there appears to have been an upward shift in levels of performance. Consequently, more recent normative data are preferred. International and local norms are available from the source. In addition, given the evidence of some cultural bias, the use of local norms may be desirable. Local norms appear preferable for use for clinical purposes but are problematic when used to make comparative judgements across populations (Mills et al., 1993). Tables giving detailed percentages are also available (Peck, 1970; also see source). Although conversion of percentages to IQ scores is possible (see Table 47 under Wechsler test for general comparisons), the practice is discouraged. Progressive Matrices scores are not interchangeable with those obtained from intelligence tests, which sample a wider range of abilities.

For the SPM, summary North American norms for ages 6.5–16.5 are given by Raven et al. (1995a). These data are derived from a series of systematic random samples of school-children and are shown in Table 5–12. American norms for ages 18+ have been developed by Raven et al (1995a) and are given in Table 5–13.

For the CPM, summary North American norms for ages 5.5–11.5 are presented by Raven et al. (1990). These data are derived from a series of norming studies with schoolchildren and are shown in Table 5–14. Yeudall et al. (1986) tested 225 normal Canadian men and women, ages 15–40, with the CPM. At each age-group interval (e.g., 15–20, 21–25, etc.), there were few if any errors. The mean number correct for the combined group (ages 15–40) was 34.9 (SD = 1.25). Norms for the elderly, ages 55–85, are provided by Raven et al. (1995a,b) and are given in Table 5–15. Educa-

Table 5—15. Colored Progressive Matrices: Estimated Norms for 1994 for Elderly People in The Netherlands

	Age in Years		
Percentile Rank	55–64 (n = 958)	65–74 (n = 899)	75–85 (n = 964)
95	35	34	33
90	34	33	31
75	33	31	28
50	30	28	23
25	26	23	19
10	21	18	13
5	18	15	12

Calculated from norms for Sets A & B in Smits (1994) using Table CPM8.

Source: Reprinted from Raven et al. (1995b). Reprinted with permission of J. C. Raven Ltd.

Table 5—16. Advanced Progressive Matrices Set II: Occupational Norms for Various Groups

Percentile Rank	UK General Popn 23 yr olds Untimed (n = 71)	US Navy 25–28 yr olds 40 mins (n = 195)	UK TA Officer Applicants 40 min (n = 104)	UK Retail Managers 40 mins (n = 104)	UK Police Officers (reconst.) (n = 157)	UK Senior Mngs (Hotels) 40 min (n = 49)	UK Accountancy Staff 40 min (n = 52)	UK Oxford Undergrads. 40 min (n = 104)	UK Local Authority Jun/Mid Mgt 40 min (n = 61)	UK Research Scientist 40 min (n = 34)
95	33	29	34	30	34	28	32	34	30	33
90	31	27	32	28	32	26	31	32	28	31
75	27	23	29	25	30	22	28	30	25	28
50	22	18	25	22	27	19	25	27	21	24
25	17	13	21	19	25	15	23	25	17	21
10	12	10	18	16	22	12	20	22	13	18
5	9	8	16	14	21	10	19	21	11	16

UK general population data derived from the 1992 Standardization of the SPM and APM (TABLE APM XIII).

US Navy data extracted from data supplied by Alderton (see Knapp & Court, 1992) (TABLE APM XVII).

UK Police Officers' data extracted from Feltham (1988) (TABLE APM XXVI).

Other data collected by Oxford Psychologists Press. Reprinted with permission from J. Raven (1994).

Table 5—17. Advanced Progressive Matrices Set II (Untimed) Smoothed Summary Norms for the USA

Percentile Rank	Age in Years										
	18–22 (n = 28)	23–27 (n = 53)	28–32 (n = 72)	33–37 (n = 77)	38–42 (n = 121)	43–47 (n = 69)	48–52 (n = 33)	53–57 (n = 36)	58–62 (n = 27)	63–67 (n = 33)	68+ (n = 54)
95	32	32	32	32	32	32	31	30	29	27	25
90	30	30	30	30	30	30	29	28	27	25	23
75	27	27	27	26	26	26	26	25	24	22	19
50	20	20	20	19	19	19	19	18	16	14	12
25	15	15	15	15	15	14	14	13	12	10	8
10	10	10	10	10	10	10	9	8	7	6	4
5	7	7	7	7	7	7	6	5	4	3	1

Based on the 1993 standardization of the APM in Des Moines, Iowa.

Tests completed at leisure. Reprinted with permission from J. Raven (1994)

tion is a significant predictor of test scores. Marcopulos et al. (1997) report a mean of 17.5 (SD = 6.0) for 110 community-dwelling older adults (mean age = 76.48, SD = 7.87) with an average educational level of 6.65 years (SD = 2.14).

For the APM (Set II), Raven (1994) provides norms for adults from various occupational groupings (Table 5–16). The scores are generally based on an administration where working time is limited to 40 minutes. Norms for the untimed version have been compiled by Raven (1994) and are shown in Table 5–17.

References

Alderton, D.L., & Larson, G.E. (1990). Dimensionality of Raven's Advanced Progressive Matrices items. *Educational and Psychological Measurement, 50*, 887–900.

Arthur, W., & Woehr, D.J. (1993). A confirmatory factor analytic study examining the dimensionality of the Raven's Advanced Progressive Matrices. *Educational and Psychological Measurement, 53*, 471–478.

Burke, H.R. (1958). Raven's Progressive Matrices: Validity, reliability, and norms. *Journal of Psychology, 22*, 252–257.

Burke, H.R. (1985). Raven's Progressive Matrices: More on norms, reliability, and validity. *Journal of Clinical Psychology, 41*, 231–235.

Caltagirone, C., Gainotti, G., & Miceli, G. (1977). A new version of Raven's Colored Matrices designed for patients with focal hemispherical lesion. *Minerva Psichiatrica, 18*, 9–16.

Campbell, D., & Oxbury, J. (1976). Recovery from unilateral visuo-spatial neglect? *Cortex, 12*, 303–312.

Carpenter, P.A., Just, M.A., & Shell, P. (1990). What one intelligence test measures: A theoretical account of the processing in the Raven Progressive Matrices Test. *Psychological Review, 97*, 404–431.

Costa, L.D. (1976). Interset variability on the Raven Colored Progressive Matrices as an indicator of specific ability deficit in brain-lesioned patients. *Cortex, 12*, 31–40.

Costa, L.D., Vaughan, H.G., Horwitz, M., & Ritter, W. (1969). Patterns of behavioral deficit associated with visual spatial neglect. *Cortex, 5*, 242–263.

Cronin-Golomb, A., & Braun, A.E. (1997). Visuo-spatial dysfunction and problem-solving in Parkinson's Disease. *Neuropsychology, 11*, 44–52.

Court, J.H. (1983). Sex differences on Raven's Progressive Matrices: A review. *The Alberta Journal of Educational Research, 29*, 54–74.

Denes, F., Semenza, C., & Stoppa, E. (1978). Selective improvement by unilateral brain-damaged patients on Raven Coloured matrices. *Neuropsychologia, 16*, 749–752.

Denney, N.W., & Heidrich, S.M. (1990). Training effects on Raven's Progressive Matrices in young, middle-aged, and elderly adults. *Psychology and Aging, 5*, 144–145.

Esquivel, G.B. (1984). Coloured Progressive Matrices. In D.J. Keyser & R.C. Sweetland (Eds.), *Test Critiques*, Vol. 1. Missouri: Test Corporation of America, pp. 206–213.

Gainotti, G., Parlato, V., Monteleone, D., & Carlomagno, S. (1992). Neuropsychological markers of dementia on visual-spatial tasks: A comparison between Alzheimer's type and vascular forms of dementia. *Journal of Clinical and Experimental Neuropsychology, 14*, 239–252.

Haier, R., Seigel, B., Nuechterlein, K., et al. (1988). Cortical glucose metabolic rate correlates of abstract reasoning and attention studied with positron emission tomography. *Intelligence, 12*, 199–217.

Jensen, A.R., Saccuzzo, D.P., & Larsen, G.E. (1988). Equating the standard and advanced forms of the Raven Progressive Matrices. *Educational and Psychological Measurement, 48*, 1091–1095.

Llabre, M.M. (1984). Standard Progressive Matrices. In D.J. Keyser & R.C. Sweetland (Eds.), *Test Critiques*. Vol. 1. Missouri: Test Corporation of America, pp. 595–602.

Marcopulos, B.A., McLain, C.A., & Giuliano, A.J. (1997). Cognitive impairment or inadequate norms? A study of healthy, rural, older adults with limited education. *The Clinical Neuropsychologist, 11*, 111–131.

Mills, C.J., Ablard, K.E., & Brody, L.E. (1993). The Raven's Progressive Matrices: Its usefulness for identifying gifted/talented students. *Roeper Review, 15*, 183–186.

O'Leary, U-M., Rusch, K.M., & Guastello, S.J. (1991). Estimating age-stratified WAIS-R IQs from scores on the Raven's Standard Progressive Matrices. *Journal of Clinical Psychology, 47*, 277–284.

Owen, K. (1992). The suitability of Raven's Standard Progressive Matrices for various groups in South Africa. *Personality and Individual Differences, 13*, 149–159.

Peck, D.F. (1970). The conversion of Progressive Matrices and Mill Hill Vocabulary raw scores into deviation IQs. *Journal of Clinical Psychology*, *26*, 67–70.

Powers, S., Barkan, J.H., & Jones, P.B. (1986). Reliability of the Standard Progressive Matrices Test for Hispanic and Anglo-American children. *Perceptual and Motor Skills*, *62*, 348–350.

Raven, J.C. (1938, 1996). *Progressive Matrices: A Perceptual Test of Intelligence*. Individual Form. Oxford: Oxford Psychologists Press Ltd.

Raven, J.C. (1947, 1995). *Colored Progressive Matrices Sets A, Ab, B*. Oxford: Oxford Psychologists Press Ltd.

Raven, J.C. (1965, 1994). *Advanced Progressive Matrices Sets I and II*. Oxford: Oxford Psychologists Press Ltd.

Raven, J., Summers, B., Birchfield, M., et al. (1990). *Manual for Raven's Progressive Matrices and Vocabulary Scales*. Research Supplement No. 3: A Compendium of North American Normative and Validity Studies. Oxford: Oxford Psychologists Press Ltd.

Raven, J., Raven, J.C., & Court, J.H. (1995a). General Overview (1995 Edition). Oxford: Oxford Psychologists Press Ltd.

Raven, J., Court, J.H., et al. (1995b). Summary of normative, reliability and validity studies. *Raven Manual Research Supplement 4*. Oxford: Oxford Psychologists Press Ltd.

Risberg, J., Maximilian, A., & Prohovnik, I. (1977). Changes of cortical activity patterns during habituation to a reasoning test. *Neuropsychologia*, *15*, 793–798.

Villardita, C. (1985). Raven's Colored Progressive Matrices and intellectual impairment in patients with focal brain damage. *Cortex*, *21*, 627–634.

Yeudall, L.T., Fromm, D., Reddon, J.R., & Stefanyuk, W.O. (1986). Normative data stratified by age and sex for 12 neuropsychological tests. *Journal of Clinical Psychology*, *42*, 920–946.

Zaidel, E., Zaidel, D.W., & Sperry, R.W. (1981). Left and right intelligence: Case studies of Raven's Progressive Matrices following brain bisection and hemidecortication. *Cortex*, *17*, 167–186.

WECHSLER INTELLIGENCE TESTS (WAIS-R, WISC-III, WPPSI-III)

Other Test Names

There are three scales: the Wechsler Adult Intelligence Scale–Revised (WAIS-R), the Wechsler Intelligence Scale for Children–III (WISC-III), and the Wechsler Preschool and Primary Scale of Intelligence–Revised (WPPSI-III). Previous versions with similar content were the Wechsler-Bellevue Scale, the Wechsler Adult Intelligence Scale, the Wechsler Intelligence Scale for Children, the Wechsler Intelligence Scale for Children–Revised, and the Wechsler Preschool and Primary Scale of Intelligence. A new edition of the WAIS-R (WAIS-III) is due out in 1997 (see Description).

Purpose

The purpose of the Wechsler Scales is to provide measures of general intellectual function.

Source

The Wechsler Scales can be obtained from The Psychological Corporation, P.O. Box 9954, San Antonio, Texas 78204-0954. Each scale (WAIS-R, WISC-III, WPPSI-R) costs about $500 US. Each Scale can also be ordered from The Psychological Corporation, 55 Horner Avenue, Toronto, Ontario M5Z 4X6, for about $800 Cdn each. The Psychological Corporation provides a computer scoring system that gives age-extended normative standard score transformations for subtests and indices for the WAIS-R. The program also computes the MAYO cognitive factor scale scores (MCFS) if the WMS-R and RAVLT have also been given. The cost is $67 US or $75 Cdn for the disk.

Description

The Wechsler test is one of the most frequently used measures in neuropsychological batteries (Lees-Haley et al., 1996). It is often considered "the gold standard" in intelligence testing (Ivnik et al., 1992). It is a core instrument, giving information about the overall level of intellectual functioning and the presence or absence of significant intellectual disability, and providing clues to altered functions (Lezak, 1995). The test materials for each scale (WAIS-R, WISC-III, WPPSI-R) are conveniently packaged in a case about the size of a briefcase. The complete kit contains the manual, record form booklets, cards, puzzles, and blocks that are used in the subtests.

The WAIS-R (Wechsler, 1981) covers the age range 16–74 years. It is composed of 11 subtests, 6 verbal- and 5 performance-oriented. The verbal and performance tests can be administered separately or together to yield, respectively, a Verbal (VIQ), a Performance (PIQ), and a Full Scale IQ (FSIQ). The Verbal subtests are Information, Digit Span, Vocabulary, Arithmetic, Comprehension, and Similarities. The Performance subtests are Picture Completion, Picture Arrangement, Block Design, Object Assembly, and Digit Symbol. The items on the Information subtest assess general knowledge. Digit Span consists of two parts: Digits Forward requires the subject to repeat sequences of three to nine digits; Digits Backward sequences are two to eight numbers long, and the subject must say them in reverse order. The Vocabulary subtest requires the subject to provide definitions of words. The Arithmetic subtest ranges from the simple counting of blocks to the more complex comprehension of verbally presented mathematical problems. Items on the Comprehension subtest assess acquired knowledge, practical reasoning, and the meaning of proverbs. On the Similarities subtest, the subject must explain in what way two things are alike. On the Picture Completion subtest, the subject is shown pictures in which there is an important part missing; the subject must indicate the part that is missing. Picture Arrangement consists of sets of cartoon-like pictures in a mixed-up order. The subject is asked to arrange them in an order that tells a sensible story. On the Block Design subtest, the subject is presented with red and white blocks and is asked to construct replicas of constructions made by the examiner or of designs printed in smaller scale. Object Assembly consists of cut-up figures of common objects, and the subject's task is to put the pieces of the puzzles together. The Digit Symbol substitution task consists of rows of blank squares; each has a randomly assigned number (1 to 9) printed above. A key is printed above these rows showing each number paired with a different nonsense symbol. The subject's task is to fill the blanks with the corresponding symbols as rapidly as possible.

A simpler version of the WAIS-R, the WISC-III (Wechsler, 1991), is available for children, ranging in age from 6 years to 16 years 11 months. The IQs are calculated on the basis of 5 verbal and 5 performance tests: Information, Similarities, Arithmetic, Vocabulary, Comprehension, (Digit Span), Picture Completion, Picture Arrangement, Block Design, Object Assembly, Coding (or Symbol Search), (Mazes). Coding (called Digit Symbol on the WAIS-R) has two forms: Coding A is for children ages 6–7, and Coding B is for children 8 years and older. The Maze task has no counterpart on the WAIS-R and requires the subject to draw paths through mazes within time limits. In the Symbol Search subtest, the child scans two groups of symbols and indicates whether the target symbol appears in the search group. Digit Span on the Verbal Scale and Mazes and Symbol Search on the Performance Scale are supplementary tests that provide a richer picture of the child's abilities. They are to be administered when time permits, or they may serve as a substitute if a regularly administered test cannot properly be given or is invalidated. If the supplementary subtests are administered in addition to the standard subtests, their scores are not entered into the FSIQ, VIQ, and PIQ score computations. In addition to the Verbal, Performance, and Full Scale IQ scores, four factor-based index scores can be calculated: Verbal Comprehension (Information, Similarities, Vocabulary, Comprehension); Perceptual Organization (Picture Completion, Picture Arrangement, Block Design, Object Assembly); Freedom from Distractibility (Arithmetic, Digit Span); and Processing Speed (Coding, Symbol Search). Thus, in order to calculate all four factor-based index scores, the supplementary subtests of Digit Span and Symbol Search must be given.

The WPPSI-R (Wechsler, 1989) is available for children ranging in age from 3 years to 7 years 3 months. Although the materials, test items, and directions were selected for their suitability for young children, some of the concepts may be difficult for low functioning individuals to understand (Kaufman, 1992). In such cases, other tests (e.g., Stanford-Binet, Kaufman-ABC) may be preferred. The Verbal Scale consists of a simpler version of the subtests found on the WISC-R. The Sentences test is a supplementary task that substitutes for Digit Span as the test of immediate memory. The Performance Scale includes Object Assembly, Picture Completion, Mazes, and Block Design. Animal pegs (formerly Animal House) is an optional subtest that is similar in format to Digit Symbol or Coding. The child has to put colored pegs into holes under animal pictures according to the pairing of animals and colored pegs displayed in a model at the top of the pegboard. Geometric Design has two parts: part 1 requires the identification of target stimuli from an array of four designs; part 2 requires the copying of figures.

On all three tests, IQ scores compare the performance of an individual with the average scores attained by members of that person's age group. Identical IQ scores obtained by a 60-year-old and a 20-year-old reflect the same relative standing among people of the subject's age group. In one sense, however, IQ scores at different ages are not identical because test scores change with age, typically rising to a peak during young adulthood, then falling off later on. Consequently, a lower level of test performance is needed to obtain a given IQ at 60 than at 20 years of age.

The WAIS-R is currently being updated. The WAIS-III (due out in 1997) includes up-to-date norms, an extension of the normative sample to include older adults (e.g., 74–89), supplemental normative data that allow adjustment for both age and educational level, factor-based composite scores (e.g., Verbal Comprehension, Perceptual Organization, Attention/Working Memory, and Speed of Information Processing), and new subtests (e.g., Matrix Reasoning, Letter–Number Span, Symbol Search). In addition, the WAIS-III standardization sample was co-normed with the Wechsler Memory Scale (WMS-III), the revision of the WMS-R, allowing clinicians to better assess IQ/MQ discrepancy scores and multiple domains of cognitive functioning.

Administration

See source. Briefly, the examiner asks test questions, displays pictures or puzzles to the patient, and records the patient's responses in an individual response booklet. There is a suggested order of subtest administration; however, the examiner can depart from the standard order. Completion of all subtests in one session is preferable, but not obligatory. The examiner can call a recess at the end of a subtest. If a subtest must be stopped in the middle, the test can usually be resumed where it had been stopped. However, the easy items on Similarities, Block Design, and Picture Arrangement provide subjects with the practice they need to succeed at more difficult items. Lezak (1995) suggests that if the examination must be stopped in the middle of any of these three subtests, the first few items should be repeated at the next session so that the patient can reestablish the skills necessary to pass the harder items.

The WISC-III overlaps with the WPPSI-R for the age range 6 years to 7 years 3 months and overlaps with the WAIS-R for the age period 16 years to 16 years 11 months. Kaufman (1994) recommends the WISC-III over the WPPSI-R, in part because of its greater reliability and lesser emphasis on speed. Some of the WPPSI-R subtests also have less than ideal ceilings and therefore are not appropriate for high functioning children. Sattler (1992) points out that a more thorough sampling of ability can be obtained from the WPPSI-R than from the WISC-III and from the WISC-III than from the WAIS-R in their overlapping age ranges. Thus, a child 16 years 8 months old needs more successes on the WISC-III than on the WAIS-R to obtain the same scaled score. To illustrate, 14 correct WISC-III Information items but only 6 correct WAIS-R Information items are needed to obtain a scaled score of 5. In addition, the Verbal and Performance IQ scores on the WAIS-R extend to 54 and 49 at the lower end, respectively, whereas on the WISC-III these IQ scores each extend to 46. The WISC-III is also recommended at age 16 because the WAIS-R has peculiar norms for that age group. Kaufman (1990) suggests that the WAIS-R norms for 16- to 19-year-olds are too "easy" because the reference group performed more poorly than 16- to 19-year-olds really perform. In general, WAIS-R IQ scores tend to be greater than WISC-III scores, and the latter tend to

Item	Recommended Item	Acceptable Answer
1.	What are the colours of the Canadian flag?	Red and White
6.	Name 2 people who have been Prime Ministers of Canada since 1950.	Any two from St. Laurent to the present
8.	Who is Gordon Lightfoot?	Singer, composer, writer
9.	In what direction would you travel if you went from Winnipeg to Panama?	South, SW, SE
13.	Who was the first Prime Minister of Canada?	John A. MacDonald or MacDonald
14.	What are W.O. Mitchell and Margaret Atwood famous for?	Famous Canadian writers or authors
17.	Who was Louis Riel?	Metis Leader
22.	Name two houses in the Canadian parliament	House of Commons and the Senate
23.	How far is it from Montreal to Vancouver?	2500–3500 mi or 4000–5700 km
27.	What is the population of Canada?	Within ± 5% of Cdn population (28 million)

Figure 5–4. Recommended items for substitution on the Information Subtest of the WAIS-R for Canadian subjects, Adapted from Pugh and Boer, 1991. Copyright 1991. Canadian Psychological Association. Reprinted with permission.

be greater than WPPSI-R IQ scores. The average difference between tests (WISC-III and WAIS-R or WPPSI-R) for FSIQ scores is about 4 points, although the differences are greater at the extremes of the distribution (Wechsler, 1991).

The Wechsler Scales contain an Information subtest that can be troublesome for subjects from other English-speaking countries because of items with U.S.-biased content. Several psychometric studies have been carried out with Canadian versions of the Information subtest (Bornstein et al., 1983; Crawford and Boer, 1985; Marx, 1984; Pugh and Boer, 1991; Vernon, 1977; Violato, 1984, 1986). Some changes have been recommended so that Canadians are not unduly penalized by the American items and in order to achieve a gain in face validity (Violato, 1986; Pugh and Boer, 1991). Fig. 5–4 shows the recommended items for substitution on the WAIS-R. A cautionary statement is in order: For the WAIS-R, item 8 is disproportionately difficult for Canadians. WISC-III Information items do not appear to be unduly difficult for Canadians (but see Scoring).

There have been numerous attempts to develop abbreviated forms of the Wechsler scales (see Banken & Banken, 1987; Crawford, Allan, & Jack, 1992; Kaufman, 1990; LoBello, 1991; Sattler, 1992; Silverstein, 1990a; Ward & Ryan, 1996; Ward & Ryan, 1997; for review). Some procedures involve administering parts of each subtest (e.g., Satz & Mogel, 1962), while others have relied on

administering specific subtests (e.g., Short Form 2: Vocabulary, Block Design; Short Form 4: Vocabulary, Block Design, Arithmetic, Picture Arrangement; Short Form 7: Information, Digit Span, Arithmetic, Similarities, Picture Completion, Block Design, Digit Symbol) and transforming results by means of a formula or referring to special tables to obtain estimated IQ scores (see Sattler, 1988). Reducing the number of items within subtests (e.g., Satz-Mogel short form) rather than the number of subtests exacts a steep price in terms of reliability (Silverstein, 1990a). Moreover, the alternate item approach virtually precludes subsequent administration of the full test should the more precise information provided by a full administration be required (Ehrenreich, 1996). Further, it represents a dramatic departure from the standard administration. Because half of the items are excluded, the difficulty slope of the items increases much more rapidly than under standard conditions, while the opportunity for practice decreases equally rapidly (Sattler, 1992). The dyad, Vocabulary and Block Design, is a popular short form that has good psychometric properties (mean reliability = .94, mean validity = .91). It has an average administration time of about 20 minutes and provides information about how an individual copes with less-structured situations (Sattler, 1992). Table 5–18 shows estimated Wechsler Full Scale IQ equivalents for the sum of scaled scores on Vocabulary and Block Design.

Table 5—18. Estimated Wechsler Full Scale IQ Equivalents for Sum of Scaled Scores, Vocabulary and Block Design

Vocabulary plus Block Design Scaled Score	WISC III	WAIS-R (broken down into age groups)		
		16–17 25–44 65–74	18–24	45–64
1	—	—	—	—
2	48	50	46	48
3	51	52	49	51
4	54	55	52	54
5	56	58	55	57
6	59	61	58	59
7	62	64	61	62
8	65	66	64	65
9	68	69	67	68
10	71	72	70	71
11	74	75	73	74
12	77	78	76	77
13	80	80	79	80
14	83	83	82	83
15	85	86	85	86
16	88	89	88	88
17	91	92	91	91
18	94	94	94	94
19	97	97	97	97
20	100	100	100	100
21	103	103	103	103
22	106	106	106	106
23	109	108	109	109
24	112	111	112	112
25	115	114	115	115
26	117	117	118	117
27	112	120	121	120
28	123	122	124	123
29	126	125	127	126
30	129	128	130	129
31	132	131	133	132
32	135	134	136	135
33	138	136	139	138
34	141	139	142	141
35	144	142	145	144
36	146	145	148	146
37	149	148	151	149
38	152	150	154	152

Source: Estimated WAIS-R Full Scale IQ equivalents are reprinted with permission of the publisher and authors from B.H. Brooker and J.J. Cyr. 1986. Estimated WISC-III full scale IQ equivalents from Sattler 1992 and reprinted with permission of J. Sattler.

Note: Use age-corrected scaled scores for the WAIS-R.

Miller et al. (1996) report that the number and combination of subtests that are used to predict FSIQ scores do not make much practical difference, so long as a reasonable number of them are used in combination. Four or more yield reasonable predictive accuracy. Fewer than four subtests yield respectable results, but the predictive accuracy is sufficiently low that they should be used only for rapid screening purposes (but see Ehrenreich (1996), who found no difference between a two- and a four-subtest form). A similar situation exists when predicting Verbal or Performance IQ scores. Here the choice of subtests is more limited, but any three or more subtest combinations will provide very good estimates of Verbal or Performance IQs.

As a rule, estimation may be better accomplished by selecting more subtests that are quick to administer than by choosing fewer, longer subtests (Ward & Ryan, 1996). A particularly useful combination is Ward's 7-subtest short form that takes about 35 minutes to administer. It consists of Information, Digit Span, Arithmetic, Similarities, Picture Completion, Block Design, and Digit Symbol. Benedict et al. (1992) studied 304 psychiatric inpatients whose mean full-scale IQ was 94.6 ± 15.1 and reported a Pearson correlation coefficient between the seven-subtest form and actual full scale IQ scores of .98. The mean difference in absolute value, between the seven-subtest form prorated and actual full-scale IQ scores was 2.4 ± 2.1 points, and 91 per cent of the patients' score pairs differed by ≤5 points. The seven-subtest short form can also be used to prorate MAYO VIQ, PIQ and FSIQ scores of elderly adults with good concurrent validity (Schretlen & Ivnik, 1996). Schretlen et al. (1994) found virtually identical reliability and standard error of measurement statistics as the full WAIS-R when assessed on the original standardization sample. Axelrod et al. (1996) corrected some computation errors and have provided more accurate reliability and standard error of measurement information for both the complete and seven-subtest short forms of the WAIS-R. Ryan et al. (1996) reported that in patients with lateralized or diffuse lesions, the correlation between the Verbal–Performance IQ discrepancies on the standard WAIS-R and the short form was .91. Seventy-five percent of the sample ($n = 95$) obtained IQ differences on the short form that fell within ±5 points of the WAIS-R discrepancy score. There was relatively good agreement between the WAIS-R and short form in terms of detecting reliable IQ differences (a discrepancy of 9 points or larger) and adequate agreement for the detection of abnormal discrepancies (18 points or larger). Iverson et al. (1996) found that, in patients with closed head injuries, the average short-form IQ score was within 1 point of VIQ, PIQ and FSIQ, and the validity coefficients for the patients ranged from .90 to .95. In patients with presumed dementia, the short form underestimated the average VIQ by nearly 5 points and the average FSIQ by 3.5 points. Validity coefficients were high (above .90). There was also relatively good agreement in detecting reliable VIQ-PIQ differences. However, a substantial percentage of patients (10–30%), with either a head injury or presumed dementia, had IQ estimates that were clinically significantly different (estimated IQ greater than 2 SEMs and in a different IQ classification) from their actual IQs (especially the VIQs of persons with presumed dementia).

Two algorithms are used to prorate the weighted sums of scaled scores so that Verbal, Performance, and Full Scale IQs can be derived using Table 20 of the WAIS-R manual. The sum of Verbal scaled scores is based on the algorithm

Verbal Score = [2(Information + Similarities) + (Digit Span + Arithmetic)]

and the sum of Performance scaled scores is based on

Performance Score = [2(Picture Completion + Block Design) + (Digit Symbol)]

With regard to the WISC-III, Donders (1997b) suggests the use of eight subtests (Vocabulary, Similarities, Block Design, Picture Completion, Arithmetic, Digit Span, Coding and Symbol Search). For the FD and PS factors, Table A.7 of the WISC-III manual can be used. Donders (1997b) provides tables that allow derivation of deviation quotients for VC, PO, and FSIQ estimates. Reliability and validity coefficients of these deviation quotients equaled or exceeded .85 and the values of SEM and SEE were within 1 standard score point of those for the respective full-length scales.

In general, the two- or four-subtest short forms are most appropriate for situations in which only rough estimates of IQ are required. These short forms might also be indicated when the subject's mental status precludes the administration of the full IQ scale, for brief reassessment, for screening purposes, or in research settings where the intellectual level of various groups of subjects is required and the IQ of any single individual is less of a consideration (Banken & Banken, 1989; Ehrenreich, 1996; Silverstein, 1990b). The seven/ eight-subtest form, or preferably, the long form, is recommended in situations that require a comprehensive assessment of intelligence, the classification of an individual according to level of intelligence, or when making clinical inferences about a person's strengths and weaknesses. Bear in mind that when using a short form, even the the seven-subtest form, relatively large errors in IQ estimation (i.e., over 10 points) do occur (see also Ward & Ryan, 1997). Whenever computing a short-form estimate of IQ, append the abbreviation EST next to the value (Kaufman, Ishikuma, & Kaufman-Packer, 1991).

Some clinicians adapt the Digit Symbol (or Coding) subtest not only to provide the standard performance but also as a measure of incidental learning. Edith Kaplan's procedure (see Lezak, 1983) for the Digit Symbol test on the WAIS-R involves noting the number of boxes completed by the patient in the allotted time (90 sec.), but allowing the patient to continue until the end of the next-to-last row. Then without prior mention, the test sheet is folded so that only the last row shows and the patient is asked to fill in from memory as many of the symbols as he or she can recall. Kaplan reports that remembering 7 of 9 symbols is low average for normal adults. Collaer and Evans (1982) use a slightly different procedure for Coding B on the WISC-R. The Coding test is completed in standard fashion and

Table 5—19. Mean Performance of Children on Coding Incidental Recall Task

Age	Males			Females		
	n	M	SD	n	M	SD
8	20	5.3	2.3	30	6.3	1.8
9	45	6.2	1.5	3	6.1	1.8
10	37	6.3	1.6	37	6.2	2.2
11	32	6.5	1.7	35	7.1	1.6
12	18	7.2	1.6	15	7.7	1.1

Source: Collaer & Evans, (1982). Norms are based on a population of U.S. schoolchildren.

the form is removed from view. Within 10 to 20 seconds of finishing the Coding subtest, and without prior warning, the child is provided with another sheet of paper containing the digits 1 to 9 and is told to fill in the associated symbols. The recall is scored as follows: 1 point is given for each accurately drawn *and* associated symbol, and ½ point is given for any accurately drawn but misassociated symbol. Coding recall norms for ages 8–12 are shown in Table 5–19. These data are derived from 305 elementary school children in the United States. The values should be treated with some caution because of the small number of subjects in some of the age/sex categories. Hultsch, Dixon and Hertzog (personal communication, 1997) use yet a different technique with the WAIS-R. The Digit Symbol subtest is completed in the standard manner and then removed from view. Upon finishing the subtest, and without prior warning, the individual is provided with another sheet

of paper containing the symbols and is told to fill in the associated numbers. One point is given for each correctly associated number. Digit Symbol and incidental recall norms for adults, aged 55 to 84, are given in Table 5–20. These data are based on 506 community-dwelling volunteers (mean age = 67.84, SD = 7.09; mean education = 14.76 years, SD = 3.35) living in Victoria, Canada.

Approximate Time for Administration

About 1–2 hours are required.

Scoring

See source. The Record Form provides space to record and score the subject's responses, to draw a profile of subtest scores, and to summarize information about the patient's behavior in the test situation. In order that scoring and qualitative features of the performance can be reviewed later, examiners should record responses to verbal subtests verbatim, or at least record each significant idea expressed by the subject. Atypical solutions on the Performance subtests should also be documented. Supplementary scoring sheets are available from the publisher in order to detail performance on the Block Design and Object Assembly subtests. For the WISC-III, a supplementary scoring guide is available for unique Canadian responses.

All of the timed tests, except for Digit Symbol, can yield two scores: the score for the patient's response within the time limit, and the

Table 5—20. Mean Performance of Adults on Digit Symbol and Incidental Recall Task (SD in Parentheses)

Age	Males			Females		
	n	Digit Symbol	Recall	n	Digit Symbol	Recall
55–64	59	52.81 (10.11)	7.32 (1.87)	126	56.04 (10.92)	6.98 (2.08)
65–74	80	46.04 (10.47)	5.98 (2.28)	140	50.16 (9.18)	6.56 (2.13)
75–84	24	42.58 (13.38)	4.96 (2.84)	77	42.04 (10.85)	5.84 (2.35)

Source: D. Hultsch, R. Dixon & C. Hertzog. Unpublished data, 1997.

score for his or her performance regardless of time. In order to describe different aspects of the patient's capacities, the examiner can change the standard procedures and give the patient an opportunity to solve problems failed under standard (timed) conditions. Usually, this means waiting an extra 1–2 minutes beyond the allotted time. The examiner should then use a dual scoring system, noting both the timed and untimed scores (Edith Kaplan, personal communication; Lezak, 1983). The WAIS-R NI (Kaplan et al., 1991), described in the subsequent section, provides a method for documenting performance.

It is worth noting that both students and professional examiners make numerous scoring errors on the Wechsler tests (Slate & Jones, 1990). Most errors tend to occur on verbal subtests (Vocabulary, Comprehension, and Similarities) where examiners are likely to award too much credit, fail to record responses verbatim (especially on Digit Span), or question inappropriately (do not question when required, or question when prohibited). Such examiner errors decrease the reliability and validity of Wechsler IQ scores.

Comment

Reliability. Across the Wechsler tests, split-half reliability (with speeded tests excluded) is high (above .88) for Verbal, Performance, and Full Scale IQs (see source). With the notable exceptions of Object Assembly and Mazes, the subtests generally have very good to excellent split-half and test–retest reliability. Test–retest reliability data are also high for Verbal, Performance, and Full Scale IQs as well as other indices, such as factor scores (see source; Bowden et al., 1995; Ivnik et al., 1995; Lowe et al., 1987; Matarazzo & Herman, 1984; Moore et al., 1990; Snow et al., 1989). Note that high test–retest correlations, even those as high as .90, can conceal large changes over time in individual scores (Ballard, 1984; Ivnik et al., 1995; Matarazzo & Herman, 1984; Moore et al., 1990). For example, scores of some children can fluctuate by as much as 25 IQ points over the school years (Richards, 1951; Sarazin & Spreen, 1986; Sontag et al., 1958). For persons aged 55 and older, verbal

intellectual skills are most stable over a span of about 1–5 years; nonverbal intellect, attention, and concentration are less stable (Ivnik et al., 1995). Scatter indices in the elderly are also not very stable. Snow et al. (1989) evaluated normal elderly and reported a stability coefficient of .69 for the VIQ-PIQ discrepancy over a 1-year period. Paolo and Ryan (1996) examined normal elderly following a four-month interval and found a test–retest coefficient of .76 for VIQ-PIQ discrepancy. About 56 per cent of subjects maintained a similar magnitude and direction of meaningful VIQ-PIQ differences from test to retest. Classification of subtest strengths and weakness from test to retest was generally poor with an average disagreement of 52 per cent from the first to the second assessment. Intrasubtest scatter also showed poor clinical stability, with 25 to 50 per cent of subjects demonstrating meaningful changes on retest. Such a situation makes diagnostic and predictive decisions hazardous, and the clinician must be mindful that considerable variability exists even among cognitively normal individuals. Some base-rate data on long-term stability is provided in Ivnik et al. (1995) and Paolo and Ryan (1996) for elderly individuals. In order to use the data by Ivnik et al., the WMS-R and RAVLT must also be given, and the Mayo Cognitive Factor Scales must be computed (Smith et al., 1994).

Moreover, after relatively short time intervals (less than 1 year), there are modest practice effects, with gains of about 4–10 IQ points (see source; Bowden et al., 1995; Moore et al., 1990; Rawlings & Crewe, 1992). The gains tend to be greater for the Performance scale than for the Verbal scale (Moore et al., 1990; Rawlings & Crewe, 1992; Sattler, 1982), and in particular the Comprehension and Picture Completion subtests (Rawlings & Crewe, 1992). One should note, however, that practice effects typically seen in middle-aged people (Wechsler, 1981; 3, 8, and 6 points, respectively, on the VIQ, PIQ, and FSIQ) may not occur as reliably or in as robust a fashion in older populations, aged 75 and above, retested following an interval of about 2 months (Ryan et al., 1992; 2, 3, and 2 points, respectively, on VIQ, PIQ, and FSIQ). The smaller practice effects in the elderly may reflect an age-related decline in the capacity for incidental learning, a component of fluid intelligence that declines with age (Ryan et al., 1992). The magnitude of gain or loss appears unrelated to initial level of intelligence or educational level. Ryan et al. (1992) suggest that in persons 75 years and older, a retest decline of 7 points or more in IQ or 3 or more scaled score points on a subtest should be cause for additional investigation.

Although practice effects for elderly individuals are less than those demonstrated for younger persons, effects are larger for PIQ than for VIQ. A trivial PIQ > VIQ on initial testing may become meaningful on retest simply because of practice effects that lead to greater improvement in PIQ relative to VIQ (Kaufman, 1990; Paolo & Ryan, 1996). Similarly, a relatively large VIQ > PIQ on initial testing may become trivial on retest. Thus, clinicians examining VIQ-PIQ discrepancies for repeat assessments should take into account predictable practice effects.

Validity. In terms of validity, there is a substantial correlation (about .5 to .8) between Wechsler IQs and other measures of intelligence and academic achievement (e.g., Carvajal et al., 1987, 1993; Faust & Hollingsworth, 1991; Gerken & Hodapp, 1992; Lowe et al., 1987; Matarazzo, 1972; Sattler, 1988; Spruill, 1984; Vernon, 1984). Typically, VIQs and FSIQs are better predictors of scholastic achievement than are PIQs. As might be expected, WAIS-R verbal subtests are more highly correlated with basic language skills than are performance subtests (Lincoln et al., 1994). Neurological dysfunction affects performance. For example, Zillmer et al. (1992) reported that on the WAIS-R, stroke patients perform below normative standards. Moreover, there is evidence that summary measures, such as FSIQ, are related to activities of daily living in patients with probable Alzheimer's Disease (AD) (Baum et al., 1995; Mahurin et al., 1991).

Factor Analysis. Several factor-analytic studies of the Wechsler Scales have been conducted. Two basic factors have been identi-

fied: a *verbal comprehension* factor and a *perceptual organization* factor (Kaufman, 1979, 1990, 1992; Little, 1992; Sattler, 1988; Spruill, 1984). The verbal comprehension factor measures verbal knowledge and comprehension, knowledge obtained partially from formal education, and reflecting the application of verbal skills to novel situations. In general, the verbal subtests (Information, Similarities, Vocabulary, and Comprehension) make up this factor. In a recent study of 260 adults with suspected head injury, Sherman et al. (1995) found that the Verbal Comprehension factor was moderately related to neuropsychological measures of verbal ability/memory (e.g., Boston Naming Test, Buschke) and executive function (WCST). The perceptual organization factor involves perceptual and organizational dimensions and reflects the ability to interpret and organize visually perceived material within a time limit. The factor appears to measure a variable common to the Performance subtests (Picture Completion, Picture Arrangement, Block Design, and Object Assembly). Sherman et al. (1995) reported that this factor correlated with visuospatial ability/memory (Hooper, Rey Copy, Rey Delay), visual attention (d2, Trails) and executive ability (WCST). Weaker support has been found for a third factor, *memory/freedom from distractibility* (Blaha & Wallbrown, 1996; Burton et al., 1994; Sherman et al., 1995; Waller & Waldman, 1990). Arithmetic and Digit Span are the major subtests for this factor. It is assumed to measure processes related to attention, concentration, and memory. Sherman et al. (1995) found that in head-injured adults, memory measures (e.g., Buschke Test) did not correlate with the freedom from distractibility factor. Results, however, supported the factor as a measure of attention as reflected by moderate correlations with the Trail Making Test and the PASAT. Wielkiewicz (1990) has recently suggested that the factor may reflect executive and short-term memory processes involved in planning, monitoring, and evaluating task performance, although Sherman et al. (1995) found little support for this view. Scores form the WCST were unrelated to this factor, although the Stroop showed a modest correlation with it ($r = .29$). This third factor has also been thought to be highly sensitive to adverse impact by high anxiety levels (Reynolds & Ford, 1994). Some have suggested that this factor may be useful in detecting brain damage (Scott et al., 1995). A weak fourth factor, *processing speed* (Coding and Symbol Search) has also emerged for the WISC-III (see also Blaha & Wallbrown, 1996). Donders (1997a) has recently reported that both Perceptual Organization and Processing Speed are related to head injury severity in children. Because of somewhat inconclusive results in the literature as well as a dearth of validity studies (e.g., Naglieri, 1993; Waller & Waldman, 1990), these latter two factors (freedom from distractibility, processing speed) should be interpreted with caution. More than two factors may be interpreted for a person, but it is possible that only two factors will be necessary to explain the test performance of some individuals (Kaufman, 1990). That is, examiners may choose to interpret two or three (four in the case of the WISC-III) factors, depending on the profile obtained. The decision rests on whether the small third (or fourth) dimension is interpretable for a given person (Kaufman, 1990). In deciding whether a factor is interpretable, the scores of subtests comprising that factor should be fairly consistent. Bear in mind, however, that when making multiple comparisons between indices, the probability of obtaining a significant difference by chance is increased (Naglieri, 1993). There is some evidence that a two-factor solution composed of verbal and perceptual-organization factors may best explain the WAIS-R test scores of persons at the lower end of the ability spectrum (i.e., FSIQ <85 or <12 years of schooling), whereas a three-factor solution (verbal comprehension, perceptual organization, freedom from distractibility) is most parsimonious for persons with average or higher levels of ability (i.e., FSIQ of 85+ or 12 or more years of schooling) (Paolo & Ryan, 1994).

The factor scores can be used to generate initial hypotheses about an individual's strengths and weaknesses (Donders, 1996; Kaufman, 1979, 1990; Sattler, 1988). For the WISC-III, tables are provided in the Manual to derive factor index scores (but see Parker & Atkinson, 1994; Reynolds & Ford, 1994; for different methods). Data are also provided regarding the statistical significance of a difference between scores and about the rarity of the difference in the general population. One way to obtain the three factor scores (verbal comprehension, perceptual organization, freedom from distractibility) for the WAIS-R (Sattler, 1988) is to find the sums of the respective age-corrected subtest scaled scores, which are then converted into Deviation IQs (M = 100, SD = 15). Table 5–21 provides for a rapid conversion of the three factor scores into Deviation IQs for the average of nine age groups (16–74). Note that for these calculations, Perceptual Organization includes Picture Completion, Block Design, and Object Assembly, but not Picture Arrangement. Table 5–22 provides the differences required for significance at the .05 and .01 levels between the three factors. Atkinson (1991) has also prepared tables for a statistically based interpretation of WAIS-R factor scores. Based on a combined administration of the WAIS-R, WMS-R, and RAVLT, Ivnik and colleagues (Ivnik et al., 1994, 1995; Smith, Ivnik et al., 1994) developed factor scores for use with older adults. They found that five factors underlie these three tests: Verbal Comprehension (Vocabulary, Information), Perceptual Organization (Block Design, Picture Completion, Picture Arrangement, and WMS-R Visual Reproduction), Attention/Concentration (Arithmetic, Digit Span, WMS-R Mental Control), Learning (WMS-R Verbal Paired Associates I, Visual Associates I and II, RAVLT learning over trials), and Retention (RAVLT delayed percent retention, WMR-R Logical Memory delayed percent retention, WMS-R Visual Reproduction delayed percent retention).

Another "rough" way to examine factor scores is to compare factor means (not IQs) to determine whether or not there is a meaningful discrepancy. Kaufman (1990) suggested that, as a rule of thumb, the means for the groupings should differ by 3 or more age-corrected scaled score points. Consider the following example (after Sattler, 1982): A subject obtains age-scaled scores of 8, 10, 11, 11 on the Information, Comprehension, Similarities, and Vocabulary subtests (mean = 10);

Table 5—21. Estimating WAIS-R Deviation IQs for Verbal
Comprehension (VC), Perceptual Organization (P) and Freedom
from Distractibility (FD) for the Average of Nine Age Groups Using
Age-Corrected Scores

Sum	VC	PO	FD	Sum	VC	PO	FD
2	–	–	49	40	100	121	–
3	–	–	51	41	101	123	–
4	–	49	54	42	103	125	–
5	51	51	57	43	104	127	–
6	52	53	60	44	106	129	–
7	54	55	63	45	107	131	–
8	55	57	65	46	108	133	–
9	57	59	68	47	110	135	–
10	58	61	71	48	111	137	–
11	59	63	74	49	113	139	–
12	61	65	77	50	114	141	–
13	62	67	79	51	115	143	–
14	64	69	82	52	117	145	–
15	65	70	85	53	118	147	–
16	66	73	88	54	120	149	–
17	68	75	91	55	121	151	–
18	69	77	93	56	122	153	–
19	71	79	96	57	124	–	–
20	72	81	99	58	125	–	–
21	73	83	102	59	127	–	–
22	75	85	105	60	128	–	–
23	76	87	107	61	129	–	–
24	78	89	110	62	131	–	–
25	79	90	113	63	132	–	–
26	80	93	116	64	134	–	–
27	82	95	119	65	135	–	–
28	83	97	121	66	136	–	–
29	85	99	124	67	138	–	–
30	86	101	127	68	139	–	–
31	87	103	130	69	141	–	–
32	89	105	133	70	142	–	–
33	90	107	135	71	143	–	–
34	92	109	138	72	145	–	–
35	93	110	141	73	146	–	–
36	94	113	144	74	148	–	–
37	96	115	147	75	149	–	–
38	97	117	149	76	150	–	–
39	99	119	–				

Source: Adapted from Sattler (1988), pp. 842–843.

Verbal Comprehension = Information, Similarities, Vocabulary and Comprehension.

Perceptual Organization = Picture Completion, Block Design and Object Assembly.

Freedom from Distractibility = Digit Span, Arithmetic.

age-scaled scores of 4, 5, 6, and 9 on the
Picture Completion, Picture Arrangement,
Block Design, and Object Assembly subtests
(mean = 6); and age-scaled scores of 6 and 8 on
Arithmetic and Digit Span (mean = 7). Using
Kaufman's rule of thumb, there is a meaningful discrepancy between "freedom from distractibility" and "verbal comprehension" (10
− 7 = 3) but not between "freedom from distractibility" and "perceptual organization" (7

Table 5—22. Significant Differences Between WAIS-R Factor Scores (.05/.01 Significance Levels)

	VCIQ	POIQ
POIQ	11/14	
FDIQ	11/15	13/17

Source: Sattler, 1988, p. 841.

VCIQ = Verbal Comprehension IQ

POIQ = Perceptual Organization IQ

FDIQ = Freedom from Distractibility IQ

− 6 = 1). Subtest scores composing a factor should be fairly consistent. If performance is inconsistent, then the factor score may be difficult to interpret.

VIQ–PIQ Discrepancies. Although Wechsler's assignment of subtests to the Verbal and Performance scales does not match exactly with each subtest's primary factor loading on verbal comprehension or perceptual organization, the match is sufficiently close to conclude that Wechsler's Verbal and Performance IQs have construct validity (Kaufman, 1990). Consequently, it is legitimate to explore differences between the two IQs. Interpretation of a VIQ-PIQ discrepancy first requires the determination of the significance of the difference (see Wechsler manuals). Once the difference has been found to be meaningful, it is necessary to determine how unusual the difference is in the normal population (see Normative Data: Tables 5–41 to 5–45). Only unusually large discrepancies can be used to support a diagnosis of abnormality. In this context it is important to bear in mind that it is very common for normal individuals to demonstrate significant VIQ–PIQ differences (Matarazzo & Herman, 1985). Further, large VIQ–PIQ discrepancies are more typical for individuals with high Full Scale IQs (or high educational level) than for those with relatively low IQs (or low educational level) (Kaufman, 1990; Matarazzo & Hermann, 1985).

Pattern Analysis in Neuropsychology. For many years, clinicians have attempted to identify patterns of test performance typical of specific brain-damaged groups. The identification of characteristic profiles, however, has proved to be difficult, and there are no firm rules. For example, investigators have examined whether laterality of the damage (left or right hemisphere) is linked to VIQ–PIQ differences. In general, patients with unilateral left hemisphere disease obtain lower VIQ than PIQ scores, whereas patients with unilateral right hemisphere or bilateral disease obtain lower PIQ than VIQ scores. However, these patterns do not occur regularly enough for clinical reliability (Bornstein, 1984; Kluger & Goldberg, 1990; Lezak, 1995; Paniak et al., 1992; Ryan et al., 1996a; Zilmer et al., 1992). Moreover, as noted above, significant differences between VIQ and PIQ are quite common among normal people, and these discrepancies vary as a function of education and FSIQ (Grossman, 1983; Kaufman, 1976a, 1990; Matarazzo & Herman, 1985; McDermott et al., 1989a; Reynolds & Gutkin, 1981; Ryan & Paolo, 1992; Sattler, 1988; see below). For example, the size of an abnormal VIQ–PIQ difference, occurring less than 5 percent of the time, may be as little as 14 points for adults with Full Scale IQs below 80, or as much as 27 points for adults with superior ability. When such base-rate data are used, the frequency of abnormally large VIQ–PIQ splits is found to occur rarely even among patients with verified brain damage (Ryan et al., 1996a; Ryan, Paolo, & Van Fleet, 1994; see Ryan, Paolo & Smith, 1992 for a similar view regarding the validity of intersubtest scatter as an indication of cognitive impairment due to brain damage). Further, it is worth bearing in mind that VIQ–PIQ discrepancies, due to reduced PIQ (even when the WAIS-R is given under unlimited time conditions), are characteristic of patients with major depressive disorder (Sackeim et al., 1992).

Researchers have also been interested in determining a WAIS-R marker for AD. Fuld (1984) reported a profile defined by the following formula: A > B > C ≤ D, A > D, in which A is the mean of the Information and Vocabulary subtest scores, B of the Similarities and Digit Span subtest scores, C of the Digit Symbol and Block Design subtest scores, and D is the Object Assembly subtest score. All subtest scores are age-corrected. The occurrence of this profile, however, does not seem specific to AD (Logsdon et al., 1989; Satz et al., 1987; Yamashita et al., 1997).

Investigators have also tried to determine whether or not various Wechsler patterns can identify learning-disabled children. One such pattern consists of depressed scores on four subtests—the ACID pattern, an acronym for Arithmetic, Coding, Information, and Digit Span. This pattern seems to be associated with a subsample, but not a majority, of learning-disabled children. Moreover, learning-disabled children who do exhibit the ACID pattern do not all have the same type of information-processing deficit (Joschko & Rourke, 1985). Similarly, while a significantly low freedom from distractibility factor may characterize some children with attention-deficit hyperactivity disorder, such a finding does not emerge in a substantial number of children with this disorder (Anastopoulos et al., 1994).

In short, while there are a few performance patterns that may occur in specific types of clinical disorders, there are no fixed rules. In order to identify a profile as unique, one must demonstrate that the profile is not common-place in the general population (see Normative Data). One must keep in mind, however, that pattern analysis can only provide clues about strengths and weaknesses. These ideas must then be checked against other information about the subject and must be considered in light of what is neurobehaviorally plausible. Any descriptions derived from pattern analysis should be treated as initial hypotheses, not the final conclusion. Discussions of pattern (and profile) analysis are available in Kaufman (1990), Lezak (1995), Sattler (1988), and Ryan and Bohac (1994).

Malingering. Qualitative analyses related to poor effort on the Wechsler scales have focused on scatter (excessive failures on easy items), absurd or grossly illogical responses, and approximate answers (e.g., Rawling & Brooks, 1990). The sensitivity and specificity of such qualitative indices are, however, somewhat disappointing (Milanovitch et al., 1996). There is some evidence (Trueblood, 1994) that such qualitative analyses are less effective at detecting poor effort than examina-tion of overall level of performance. Excessive levels of impairment raise the concern of malingering, at least in cases of mild traumatic brain injury. Recently, Iverson and Franzen (1996) reported that individuals instructed to malinger suppressed their Digit Span scores. An age-corrected scaled score of 4 correctly classified 77.5 percent of their malingerers and 100 percent of memory-impaired patients. Mittenberg et al. (1995) suggested that malingerers could be identified by exaggerated reductions of Digit Span relative to Vocabulary. They suggested that a Vocabulary–Digit Span difference score of 9 corresponded to a 95 percent probability of malingering.

Summary. The Wechsler test should be given early in the course of the assessment because it allows the examiner to observe how the patient negotiates a wide array of tasks. In this way, the examiner can begin to develop hypotheses about the patient's spared and impaired functions that can then be tested more thoroughly during the course of the assessment. One should bear in mind, however, that studies evaluating the intercorrelations among measures of verbal and nonverbal intellect, attention and concentration, and learning and memory reveal considerable variability even in cognitively normal individuals (e.g., Ivnik et al., 1995). It is therefore hazardous to suggest cognitive impairment when variability is seen across tests of different cognitive abilities. Diagnostic accuracy requires referral to base-rate information as well as converging evidence from multiple sources (e.g., clinical history, laboratory and imaging studies, etc.).

Normative Data

Norms are presented in the Wechsler manuals and are based on large groups representative of the U.S. population. Canadians outperform American children on all Index scores (Wechsler, 1996). The largest difference is in the Performance section, where Canadian children tend to score about 5 points higher than their American counterparts. The increased average performance of Canadian children likely reflects the differing demographic patterns of

Table 5—23. Conversion Table for Calculating Performance IQ When Symbol Search is Substituted for Coding on the WISC-III

Sum of Scaled Scores	IQ	Percentile Rank	Confidence Intervals 90%	95%	Sum of Scaled Scores	IQ	Percentile Rank	Confidence Intervals 90%	95%
5	44		42–56	41–57	51	102	55	95–109	94–110
6	46	< 0.1	44–58	43–59	52	103	58	95–109	95–111
7	47	< 0.1	45–58	44–60	53	104	61	97–110	96–112
8	48	< 0.1	46–59	45–61	54	105	66	98–111	96–112
9	49	< 0.1	47–60	45–62	55	107	68	100–113	98–114
10	51	0.1	49–62	47–63	56	108	70	101–114	99–115
11	52	0.1	49–63	48–65	57	109	75	101–115	100–116
12	53	0.1	50–64	49–65	58	110	77	102–116	101–117
13	54	0.1	51–65	50–66	59	112	79	104–118	103–119
14	56	0.2	53–67	52–68	60	113	81	105–119	104–120
15	57	0.3	54–68	53–69	61	114	84	106–119	105–121
16	58	0.3	55–68	54–70	62	115	86	107–120	106–122
17	59	0.4	56–69	55–71	63	116	87	108–121	106–122
18	61	1	58–71	56–72	64	118	90	110–123	108–124
19	62	1	59–72	57–73	65	119	91	110–124	109–125
20	63	1	60–73	58–74	66	120	92	111–125	110–126
21	64	1	60–74	59–75	67	121	94	113–127	112–128
22	66	1	62–76	61–77	68	123	95	114–127	112–129
23	67	2	63–77	62–78	69	124	96	115–128	114–130
24	68	2	64–78	63–79	70	125	96	116–129	115–131
25	69	2	65–78	64–80	71	126	97	117–130	115–131
26	71	3	67–80	66–82	72	128	98	119–132	117–132
27	72	3	68–81	66–83	73	129	98	119–133	118–134
28	73	4	69–82	67–83	74	130	98	120–134	119–135
29	74	4	70–83	68–84	75	131	99	121–135	120–136
30	76	5	72–85	70–86	76	133	99	123–137	122–138
31	77	6	72–86	71–87	77	134	99	124–137	123–139
32	78	7	73–87	72–88	78	135	99	125–138	124–140
33	79	8	74–88	73–89	79	136	99.5	126–139	124–141
34	80	9	75–89	74–90	80	138	99.6	128–141	126–142
35	82	10	77–90	76–92	81	139	99.7	129–142	127–143
36	82	12	78–91	77–93	82	140	99.7	129–143	128–144
37	83	13	79–92	78–94	83	141	99.8	130–144	129–145
38	84	14	80–93	78–94	84	143	99.9	132–146	131–147
39	85	18	82–95	80–96	85	144	99.9	133–147	132–148
40	87	19	82–96	81–97	86	145	99.9	134–148	133–149
41	89	23	83–97	82–98	87	146	99.9	135–148	134–150
42	90	25	84–98	83–99	88	147	> 99.9	136–149	134–151
43	92	27	86–100	85–101	89	149	> 99.9	138–151	136–152
44	93	32	87–100	86–102	90	150	> 99.9	139–152	137–153
45	94	34	88–101	87–103	91	151	> 99.9	139–153	138–154
46	95	37	89–102	87–103	92	152	> 99.9	140–154	139–155
47	97	39	91–104	88–104	93	154	> 99.9	142–156	141–157
48	98	45	91–105	90–106	94	155	> 99.9	143–157	142–158
49	99	47	92–106	91–107	95	156	> 99.9	144–159	143–159
50	100	50	93–107	92–108					

Note: WISC-III = Wechsler Intelligence Scale for Children—III. Copyright American Psychological Association. Reprinted with permission.

Table 5—24. Conversion Table for Calculating Full Scale IQ When Symbol Search is Substituted for Coding on the WISC-III

Sum of Scaled Scores	IQ	Percentile Rank	Confidence Intervals 90%	95%	Sum of Scaled Scores	IQ	Percentile Rank	Confidence Intervals 90%	95%
10	41	< 0.1	39–48	38–49	55	71	3	67–77	67–78
11	42	< 0.1	40–49	39–50	56	71	3	67–77	66–78
12	42	< 0.1	40–49	39–50	57	72	4	68–78	67–79
13	43	< 0.1	40–50	40–51	58	73	4	69–79	68–80
14	44	< 0.1	41–51	41–52	59	73	4	69–79	68–80
15	44	< 0.1	41–51	41–52	60	74	5	70–80	69–81
16	45	< 0.1	42–52	41–53	61	75	5	71–81	70–82
17	46	< 0.1	43–53	42–54	62	75	5	71–81	70–82
18	46	< 0.1	43–53	42–54	63	76	5	72–82	71–83
19	47	< 0.1	44–54	43–55	64	77	6	73–83	72–84
20	48	< 0.1	45–55	44–56	65	77	6	73–83	72–84
21	48	< 0.1	45–55	44–56	66	78	7	74–84	73–85
22	49	< 0.1	46–56	45–57	67	79	7	75–85	74–86
23	50	< 0.1	47–57	46–58	68	79	8	75–85	74–85
24	50	0.1	47–57	46–58	69	80	9	76–86	75–86
25	51	0.1	48–58	47–59	70	81	10	77–86	76–87
26	52	0.1	49–59	48–60	71	81	10	77–86	76–87
27	52	0.1	49–59	48–60	72	82	12	78–87	77–88
28	53	0.1	50–60	49–60	73	82	13	78–87	77–88
29	54	0.1	51–61	50–61	74	83	13	79–88	78–89
30	54	0.1	51–61	50–61	75	84	14	80–89	79–90
31	55	0.2	52–61	51–62	76	84	14	80–89	79–90
32	56	0.2	53–62	52–63	77	85	16	81–90	80–91
33	56	0.2	53–62	52–63	78	86	18	82–91	81–92
34	57	0.3	54–63	53–64	79	86	18	82–91	81–92
35	58	0.3	55–64	54–65	80	87	19	83–92	82–93
36	58	0.4	55–64	54–65	81	88	19	84–93	83–94
37	59	0.4	56–65	55–66	82	88	21	84–93	83–94
38	59	0.5	56–65	55–66	83	89	23	85–94	84–95
39	60	1	57–66	56–67	84	90	25	86–95	85–96
40	61	1	58–67	57–68	85	90	25	86–95	85–96
41	61	1	58–67	57–68	86	91	27	87–96	86–97
42	62	1	59–68	58–69	87	92	30	88–97	87–98
43	63	1	60–69	59–70	88	92	30	88–97	87–98
44	63	1	60–69	59–70	89	93	32	89–98	88–99
45	64	1	61–70	60–71	90	94	32	90–99	89–100
46	65	1	62–71	61–72	91	94	34	90–99	89–100
47	65	1	62–71	61–72	92	95	37	90–100	90–101
48	66	2	63–72	62–73	93	96	37	91–101	91–102
49	67	2	64–73	63–74	94	96	39	91–101	91–102
50	67	2	64–73	63–74	95	97	42	92–102	91–103
51	68	2	65–74	64–75	96	98	42	93–103	92–104
52	69	2	65–75	65–76	97	98	45	93–103	92–104
53	69	2	65–75	65–76	98	99	47	94–104	93–105
54	70	3	66–76	66–77	99	100	47	95–105	94–106

(continued)

Table 5—24. (*Continued*)

Sum of Scaled Scores	IQ	Percentile Rank	Confidence Intervals 90%	Confidence Intervals 95%	Sum of Scaled Scores	IQ	Percentile Rank	Confidence Intervals 90%	Confidence Intervals 95%
100	100	50	95–105	94–106	146	130	98	124–133	123–134
101	101	53	96–106	95–107	147	131	98	125–134	124–135
102	102	53	97–107	96–108	148	132	99	126–135	125–136
103	102	55	97–107	96–108	149	132	99	126–135	125–136
104	103	58	98–108	97–109	150	133	99	127–136	126–137
105	104	61	99–109	98–109	151	134	99	128–137	127–138
106	104	61	99–109	98–109	152	134	99	128–137	127–138
107	105	63	100–110	99–110	153	135	99	129–138	128–139
108	105	66	100–109	99–110	154	136	99	130–139	129–140
109	106	66	101–110	100–111	155	136	99	130–139	129–140
110	107	68	102–111	101–112	156	137	99.5	131–140	130–141
111	107	68	102–111	101–112	157	138	99.6	132–141	131–142
112	108	70	103–112	102–113	158	138	99.6	132–141	131–142
113	109	73	104–113	103–114	159	139	99.7	133–142	132–143
114	109	73	104–113	103–114	160	140	99.7	134–143	133–144
115	110	75	105–114	104–115	161	140	99.7	134–143	133–144
116	111	77	106–115	105–116	162	141	99.8	135–144	134–145
117	111	79	106–115	105–116	163	142	99.8	136–145	135–146
118	112	79	107–116	106–117	164	142	99.8	136–145	135–146
119	113	81	108–117	107–118	165	143	99.9	137–146	136–147
120	113	81	108–117	107–118	166	144	99.9	137–147	137–148
121	114	82	109–118	108–119	167	144	99.9	137–147	137–148
122	115	84	110–119	109–120	168	145	99.9	138–148	138–149
123	115	86	110–119	109–120	169	146	99.9	139–149	138–150
124	116	86	111–120	110–121	170	146	99.9	139–149	138–150
125	117	87	112–121	111–122	171	147	>99.9	140–150	139–151
126	117	88	112–121	111–122	172	148	>99.9	141–151	140–152
127	118	90	113–122	112–123	173	148	>99.9	141–151	140–152
128	119	91	113–123	113–124	174	149	>99.9	142–152	141–153
129	119	92	113–123	113–124	175	150	>99.9	143–153	142–154
130	120	92	114–124	114–125	176	150	>99.9	143–153	142–154
131	121	93	115–125	114–126	177	151	>99.9	144–154	143–155
132	121	93	115–125	114–126	178	152	>99.9	145–155	144–156
133	122	94	116–126	115–127	179	152	>99.9	145–155	144–156
134	123	94	117–127	116–128	180	153	>99.9	146–156	145–156
135	123	95	117–127	116–128	181	153	>99.9	146–156	145–156
136	124	95	118–128	117–129	182	154	>99.9	147–157	146–157
137	125	96	119–129	118–130	183	155	>99.9	148–157	147–158
138	125	96	119–129	118–130	184	155	>99.9	148–157	147–158
139	126	96	120–130	119–131	185	156	>99.9	149–158	148–159
140	127	96	121–131	120–132	186	157	>99.9	150–159	149–160
141	127	97	121–131	120–132	187	157	>99.9	150–159	149–160
142	128	97	122–132	121–132	188	158	>99.9	151–160	150–161
143	129	98	123–133	122–133	189	159	>99.9	152–161	151–162
144	129	98	123–133	122–133	190	159	>99.9	152–161	151–162
145	130	98	124–133	123–134					

Note. WISC-III = Wechsler Intelligence Scale for Children—III.

the two countries. Canadian norms have recently been developed for the WISC-III and can be obtained through The Psychological Corporation. The Canadian norms tend to yield lower IQs, especially at the high and low ends of the range, and as a result are very likely to impact placement decisions. Accessing Canadian norms is also critical for accurate profile analysis because of differences in index and subtest scores. If the examiner, however, wishes to use WISC-III/WIAT for ability-achievement comparisons, the American norms must be used until there are linking studies with a Canadian sample. Use of U.S. norms is also recommended when interpreting change on re-test between the WISC-R and WISC-III, as tables exist in the standard WISC-III manual to facilitate this type of comparison.

For the WPPSI-R or WISC-III subtests, scaled score equivalents of raw scores are provided in the test manuals for each age interval covered by the scale (3 month intervals for the WPPSI-R, 4 month intervals for the WISC-III). The sums of scaled scores are converted to Verbal, Performance and Full Scale IQs by means of a table that is used for all ages covered by the scale. In the case of the WISC-III, factor index scores (Verbal Comprehension, VCIQ; Perceptual Organization, POIQ; Freedom from Distractibility, FDIQ) are also derived (but see Parker and Atkinson, 1994, for a different method). The IQ distributions each have a mean of 100 and an SD of 15. In interpreting WPPSI-R or WISC-III scores for adults, the examiner can calculate test–age equivalents for any of the subtests using the tables provided in the manuals. A test–age ("mental age") represents the chronological age at which a given level of test performance is the average in a representative sample of the population.

Symbol Search is a better measure of the Performance and Full Scale IQ than is Coding, a subtest used to derive the Performance and Full Scale IQs. Symbol Search has a much higher correlation with the Performance IQ (.58 across age vs. 32 for Coding), a higher factor loading on the perceptual organization factor (.54 vs. .39), and a higher g loading (.56 vs. .41). Accordingly, Kaufman (1994) has recommended that clinicians substitute Symbol Search for Coding when calculating Performance and Full Scale IQs on the WISC-III. Reynolds et al. (1996) have provided tables (Tables 5–23 and 5–24) for accurate derivation of IQs, percentile ranks, and confidence intervals when this substitution is made.

The WAIS-R takes account of age differences when computing the IQ scores, but not in the conversion of raw scores to scaled scores. The scaled scores, located on the front of the Record Form as well as in the test manual, are based on the performance of a reference group of young adults between 20 and 34 years of age. This particular age range was selected because performance on most tests reaches a peak during this age span (Wechsler, 1981). These scaled scores enable the examiner to compare the performance of a person of any age with that of a young segment of the working population, and are useful for questions of disability and vocational or educational planning. Age-graded subtest scaled scores are also provided in the WAIS-R manual, but are *not* to be used for computing an individual's IQ. These age-scaled scores permit a subject's score on any single subtest to be interpreted in relation to the performance of the subject's age peers. In general, with increasing age, additional scaled-score points are awarded primarily to the Performance Scale subtests, especially the Digit Symbol test. These additional points actually reflect a decline in performance as a function of age. This age-related decline cannot fully be accounted for by a general age-related psychomotor slowing. Rather, there appear to be decrements in cognitive abilities beyond those attributable to motor slowing (Troyer et al., 1994). Below age 20 and above age 35, age-graded scaled scores should be used when making subtest comparisons, since it is difficult to interpret many of the subtests and to perform factor or pattern analyses unless the age-graded scores are computed. To facilitate inter- as well as intraindividual comparisons, our standard practice is to evaluate and report both scaled and age-corrected scaled scores (see also Binder, 1987; Lezak, 1995).

When working with scaled scores, it is often helpful to translate them to percentile ranks

Table 5—25. Percentile Ranks and Suggested Qualitative Descriptions for Scaled Scores on the WPPSI-R, WISC-III, and WAIS-R

Scaled Score	Percentile Rank	Qualitative Description	Educational Description
19	99	very superior	superior
18	99	very superior	superior
17	99	very superior	superior
16	98	very superior	superior
15	95	superior	superior
14	90	superior	superior
13	84	high average	bright average
12	75	high average	bright average
11	63	average/normal	average
10	50	average/normal	average
9	37	average/normal	average
8	25	low average	low average
7	16	low average	low average
6	9	borderline	slow learner
5	5	borderline	slow learner
4	2	mentally retarded	educable mentally retarded
3	1	mentally retarded	educable mentally retarded
2	1	mentally retarded	trainable mentally retarded
1	1	mentally retarded	trainable mentally retarded

Source: Sattler (1988).

(Sattler, 1988). Table 5–25 shows the estimated percentile ranks for each Wechsler scaled score. Scaled scores can also receive a qualitative description and these too are shown in Table 5–25. IQs, however, should *never* be estimated on the basis of a single subtest score (Sattler, 1988).

Unfortunately, the WAIS-R lacks norms for individuals aged 75 years and above. Recently, Ryan et al. (1990a) and Ivnik et al. (1992) extended the norms above age 74. Ryan et al. (1990a) published norms based on a sample of 130 healthy volunteers ranging in age from 75 to 96 years. The subjects were chosen to be representative of elderly individuals in the United States in terms of age, education, race, and gender. Thus the majority of subjects had less than 12 years of education (69.2 percent), and the sample included 10.8 percent African-Americans. IQ and age-corrected subtest scores were developed according to the methods described in the WAIS-R manual. Ivnik et al. (1992) generated WAIS-R normative tables based on a sample of 512 persons between the ages of 56 and 97 years, with 222 subjects aged 75 years and older. The data were obtained

through Mayo's Older Americans Normative Studies (MOANS). Because the sample reflects higher functioning than the general population of the United States (the vast majority had 12 or more years of education and 99.6 percent were white), MAYO IQ estimates have been corrected using regression equations to approximate corresponding Wechsler measures. Although there is excellent concordance between Mayo IQs and WAIS-R IQs in the age range (≤74 years) in which both can be calculated, concordance declines at lower IQ values or when IQ scores are based on prorated protocols (Ivnik et al., 1992). The normative data presented by Ivnik and colleagues yield scores similar to those of Ryan (Paolo & Ryan, 1995). Ryan and Mayo tables, however, are not interchangeable, and comparable scores may not necessarily be generated when individual cases are examined (Paolo & Ryan, 1995). Selection of which norms to use for a particular client may depend upon how closely the patient matches the demographic characteristics of the normative group. Note too that while Ivnik and colleagues have developed norms for factor scores, they are

Table 5—26. Verbal IQ Equivalents of Sums of WAIS-R Scaled Scores
for Age Group 75–79 Years ($n = 60$)

Sum of Scaled Scores	IQ	Sum of Scaled Scores	IQ	Sum of Scaled Scores	IQ	Sum of Scaled Scores	IQ	Sum of Scaled Scores	IQ
114	> 150	92	146	70	121	48	101	26	75
113	> 150	91	144	69	120	47	100	25	73
112	> 150	90	142	68	118	46	99	24	72
111	> 150	89	141	67	118	45	98	23	71
110	> 150	88	140	66	117	44	96	22	70
109	> 150	87	138	65	116	43	95	21	69
108	> 150	86	136	64	115	42	94	20	68
107	> 150	85	136	63	113	41	93	19	68
106	> 150	84	135	62	112	40	91	18	67
105	> 150	83	133	61	112	39	89	17	66
104	> 150	82	132	60	111	38	87	16	65
103	> 150	81	131	59	111	37	85	15	64
102	> 150	80	129	58	110	36	84	14	63
101	> 150	79	128	57	109	35	84	13	62
100	> 150	78	127	56	109	34	83	12	61
99	> 150	77	126	55	107	33	83	11	60
98	> 150	76	125	54	106	32	82	10	59
97	> 150	75	125	53	105	31	80	9	58
96	> 150	74	123	52	105	30	79	8	57
95	> 150	73	123	51	104	29	78	7	56
94	150	72	122	50	103	28	76	6	55
93	148	71	121	49	102	27	75		

Source: Ryan et al., 1990. Copyright American Psychological Association. Reprinted with permission.

based on an administration that includes not only the WAIS-R, but also the WMS-R, and the RAVLT (Smith et al., 1994).

When the Ryan norms are employed, the subject's raw subtest scores are converted to scaled scores using the 20- to 34-year-old reference group provided by Wechsler (1981). Tables 5–26, 5–27, and 5–28 present the Verbal, Performance, and Full Scale IQ equivalents for sums of scaled scores of persons age 75–79 years. The standard errors of measurement in IQ units for this group were VIQ = 2.46, PIQ = 3.85, and FSIQ = 2.56. The IQ equivalents for sums of scaled scores of subjects 80 years and older are given in Tables 5–29, 5–30, and 5–31. The standard errors of measurement are 3.06, 3.71, and 2.53 for the Verbal, Performance, and Full Scale IQs, respectively. Conversion tables for age-corrected subtest scores (mean = 10, SD = 3) were constructed for subjects between the ages of 75–79 years (Table 5–32) and 80 years and older (Table 5–33).

Recently, Ryan et al. (1996b) have evaluated Digit Span performance in their sample of normal elderly. For persons aged 75 years and older, means on Digits Forward (DF), Digits Backward (DB), and DF-DB were 5.79 (SD = 1.21), 4.18 (SD = 1.2), and 1.62 (SD = 1.2), respectively. Education was related to DF; education and preretirement occupation were associated with DB. With 11 or fewer years of education, normal achievement was 4 for DF; with 12 or more years of schooling, normal DF was 5. Persons with ≤11 years of education who were previously laborers/operatives or craftsmen/homemakers repeated 3 digits on DB; those with ≥12 years of education and professional/managerial backgrounds repeated 4 digits on DB. A DF-DB ≥4 was atypical.

When using the Mayo norms, Tables 5–34 to 5–37 convert the raw scores earned on each WAIS-R subtest to percentile ranks and age-specific scaled scores. Tables 5–38, 5–39, and 5–40 convert the sums of MOANS Scaled

Table 5—27. Performance IQ Equivalents of Sums of WAIS-R Scaled Scores
for Age Group 75–79 Years ($n = 60$)

Sum of Scaled Scores	IQ	Sum of Scaled Scores	IQ	Sum of Scaled Scores	IQ	Sum of Scaled Scores	IQ	Sum of Scaled Scores	IQ
92	> 150	74	> 150	56	148	38	121	20	83
91	> 150	73	> 150	55	146	37	120	19	81
90	> 150	72	> 150	54	145	36	117	18	79
89	> 150	71	> 150	53	144	35	114	17	79
88	> 150	70	> 150	52	142	34	112	16	78
87	> 150	69	> 150	51	141	33	110	15	77
86	> 150	68	> 150	50	140	32	108	14	75
85	> 150	67	> 150	49	139	31	106	13	74
84	> 150	66	> 150	48	137	30	104	12	73
83	> 150	65	> 150	47	135	29	102	11	77
82	> 150	64	> 150	46	134	28	100	10	70
81	> 150	63	> 150	45	133	27	98	9	68
80	> 150	62	> 150	44	131	26	96	8	67
79	> 150	61	> 150	43	128	25	93	7	66
78	> 150	60	> 150	42	126	24	92	6	65
77	> 150	59	> 150	41	125	23	91	5	64
76	> 150	58	150	40	124	22	89		
75	> 150	57	149	39	122	21	86		

Source: Ryan et al., 1990. copyright American Psychological Association.

Scores to MAYO IQs. These IQ scores can be corrected for level of education using tables provided in Malec et al. (1992). Since MAYO IQs are based almost exclusively on Caucasians who live in an economically stable region, the validity of MAYO IQs computed for persons of other ethnic, cultural, and economic backgrounds may be different.

Evaluation of Test Scatter. Examination of test scatter on the Wechsler Scales can provide valuable information about the subject's cognitive strengths and weaknesses, along with suggestions for possible remediation. It is important to note, however, that the individual subtests are associated with adequate, but less than perfect, test–retest reliability and with standard errors of measurement of varying magnitude. Information, Vocabulary, and Block Design, which are among the most reliable of the subtests, have the smallest standard errors of measurement; Object Assembly, Picture Arrangement, Mazes and Symbol Search are among the least reliable of the tests, and have the largest standard errors of measurement. It follows then that the clinician should be cautious in interpreting relative cognitive strength or weakness on the basis of a single subtest that has relatively poor reliability (e.g., Object Assembly, Picture Arrangement, Mazes, Symbol Search), since the result could be due to chance. In addition, change on retest may reflect alteration in neuropsychological status, practice effects, or imperfect test reliability.

Further, within-test variability is characteristic of many normally functioning people and therefore may not be associated with possible pathology. One frequently used scatter index is the discrepancy between Verbal and Performance IQs. Wechsler (1974, 1981) stated that a difference of 15 or more points is important (statistically significant) and merits further investigation. However, a discrepancy may be reliable in that it is unlikely to have happened by chance but it may occur with some frequency in the normal population. Table 5–41 shows the frequency of VIQ–PIQ difference scores, regardless of direction, for the WAIS-R and WISC-III. A Verbal–Performance discrepancy of 15 points is found in about 20 to 25 percent of the normal population (Grossman, 1983; Kauffman, 1976a, 1976b; Matarazzo & Herman, 1984; Reynolds

Table 5—28. Full Scale IQ Equivalents of Sums of WAIS-R Scaled Scores
for Age Group 75–79 Years ($n = 60$)

Sum of Scaled Scores	IQ	Sum of Scaled Scores	IQ	Sum of Scaled Scores	IQ	Sum of Scaled Scores	IQ	Sum of Scaled Scores	IQ
208	> 150	168	> 150	128	141	88	110	48	80
207	> 150	167	> 150	127	140	87	109	47	79
206	> 150	166	> 150	126	140	86	109	46	78
205	> 150	165	> 150	125	139	85	108	45	78
204	> 150	164	> 150	124	138	84	108	44	77
203	> 150	163	> 150	123	137	83	107	43	76
202	> 150	162	> 150	122	135	82	107	42	75
201	> 150	161	> 150	121	133	81	106	41	74
200	> 150	160	> 150	120	132	80	106	40	74
199	> 150	159	> 150	119	131	79	105	39	73
198	> 150	158	> 150	118	130	78	103	38	73
197	> 150	157	> 150	117	129	77	102	37	72
196	> 150	156	> 150	116	126	76	101	36	72
195	> 150	155	> 150	115	126	75	100	35	71
194	> 150	154	> 150	114	125	74	98	34	71
193	> 150	153	> 150	113	125	73	96	33	70
192	> 150	152	> 150	112	124	72	94	32	69
191	> 150	151	> 150	111	124	71	93	31	69
190	> 150	150	> 150	110	123	70	93	30	68
189	> 150	149	> 150	109	123	69	92	29	68
188	> 150	148	> 150	108	122	68	92	28	67
187	> 150	147	> 150	107	121	67	91	27	66
186	> 150	146	> 150	106	121	66	90	26	66
185	> 150	145	> 150	105	120	65	90	25	65
184	> 150	144	> 150	104	120	64	89	24	65
183	> 150	143	> 150	103	119	63	89	23	64
182	> 150	142	> 150	102	119	62	88	22	63
181	> 150	141	> 150	101	118	61	87	21	62
180	> 150	140	150	100	118	60	87	20	61
179	> 150	139	149	99	117	59	86	19	60
178	> 150	138	148	98	117	58	85	18	59
177	> 150	137	148	97	116	57	85	17	58
176	> 150	136	147	96	115	56	84	16	57
175	> 150	135	146	95	113	55	83	15	56
174	> 150	134	145	94	113	54	83	14	55
173	> 150	133	144	93	112	53	82	13	54
172	> 150	132	144	92	112	52	82	12	53
171	> 150	131	143	91	111	51	81	11	52
170	> 150	130	142	90	111	50	81		
169	> 150	129	142	89	110	49	80		

Source: Ryan et al., 1990. Copyright American Psychological Association.

& Gutkin, 1981; Sattler, 1992; Seashore, 1951). The finding that a person functions significantly better verbally than nonverbally (or vice versa) has practical significance, but the pattern may not be useful in supporting a diagnosis of exceptionality. Only when the discrepancy is rare (e.g., occurring in less than 5 percent of the population) can abnormality be inferred. Analyses of other scatter indices show similar results. For example, a 5- to 9-point scaled score range (highest minus lowest scaled score) is about average on the WISC-III or WPPSI (Kaufman, 1976b; Reynolds & Gutkin, 1981; Wechsler, 1991). Similar differences (mean = 7 points) between highest and lowest scaled scores are the norm

Table 5—29. Verbal IQ Equivalents of Sums of WAIS-R Scaled Scores
for Age Group 80 Years and Older ($n = 70$)

Sum of Scaled Scores	IQ	Sum of Scaled Scores	IQ	Sum of Scaled Scores	IQ	Sum of Scaled Scores	IQ	Sum of Scaled Scores	IQ
114	> 150	92	148	70	127	48	104	26	76
113	> 150	91	146	69	126	47	103	25	75
112	> 150	90	144	68	125	46	102	24	74
111	> 150	89	142	67	125	45	100	23	73
110	> 150	88	141	66	124	44	99	22	72
109	> 150	87	140	65	124	43	97	21	71
108	> 150	86	139	64	123	42	95	20	70
107	> 150	85	138	63	122	41	94	19	69
106	> 150	84	137	62	122	40	92	18	68
105	> 150	83	136	61	121	39	91	17	67
104	> 150	82	136	60	121	38	91	16	66
103	> 150	81	135	59	119	37	89	15	65
102	> 150	80	134	58	117	36	87	14	64
101	> 150	79	133	57	115	35	85	13	63
100	> 150	78	133	56	113	34	84	12	62
99	> 150	77	132	55	112	33	84	11	61
98	> 150	76	131	54	110	32	83	10	60
97	> 150	75	130	53	108	31	81	9	59
96	> 150	74	129	52	108	30	80	8	58
95	> 150	73	129	51	107	29	79	7	57
94	> 150	72	128	50	105	28	78	6	56
93	> 150	71	127	49	104	27	77		

Source: Ryan et al., 1990. Copyright American Psychological Association

Table 5—30. Performance IQ Equivalents of Sums of Scaled Scores
for Age Group 80 Years and Older ($n = 70$)

Sum of Scaled Scores	IQ	Sum of Scaled Scores	IQ	Sum of Scaled Scores	IQ	Sum of Scaled Scores	IQ	Sum of Scaled Scores	IQ
92	> 150	74	> 150	56	> 150	38	124	20	89
91	> 150	73	> 150	55	150	37	123	19	87
90	> 150	72	> 150	54	148	36	120	18	85
89	> 150	71	> 150	53	147	35	119	17	82
88	> 150	70	> 150	52	146	34	117	16	80
87	> 150	69	> 150	51	144	33	116	15	78
86	> 150	68	> 150	50	143	32	115	14	77
85	> 150	67	> 150	49	141	31	114	13	76
84	> 150	66	> 150	48	139	30	111	12	74
83	> 150	65	> 150	47	138	29	109	11	73
82	> 150	64	> 150	46	137	28	107	10	71
81	> 150	63	> 150	45	135	27	105	9	70
80	> 150	62	> 150	44	133	26	102	8	68
79	> 150	61	> 150	43	131	25	100	7	67
78	> 150	60	> 150	42	129	24	98	6	66
77	> 150	59	> 150	41	127	23	96	5	65
76	> 150	58	> 150	40	126	22	94		
75	> 150	57	> 150	39	125	21	92		

Source: Ryan et al., 1990. Copyright American Psychological Association.

Table 5—31. Full Scale IQ Equivalents of Sums of WAIS-R Scaled Scores for Age Group 80 Years and Older ($n = 70$)

Sum	IQ	Sum	IQ	Sum	IQ	Sum	IQ	Sum	IQ
208	> 150	168	> 150	128	144	88	115	48	81
207	> 150	167	> 150	127	143	87	114	47	80
206	> 150	166	> 150	126	142	86	113	46	80
205	> 150	165	> 150	125	140	85	112	45	79
204	> 150	164	> 150	124	139	84	112	44	78
203	> 150	163	> 150	123	138	83	111	43	78
202	> 150	162	> 150	122	137	82	111	42	77
201	> 150	161	> 150	121	136	81	109	41	76
200	> 150	160	> 150	120	136	80	108	40	75
199	> 150	159	> 150	119	135	79	107	39	75
198	> 150	158	> 150	118	135	78	105	38	74
197	> 150	157	> 150	117	134	77	105	37	74
196	> 150	156	> 150	116	133	76	104	36	73
195	> 150	155	> 150	115	133	75	104	35	72
194	> 150	154	> 150	114	132	74	103	34	72
193	> 150	153	> 150	113	131	73	103	33	71
192	> 150	152	> 150	112	130	72	102	32	70
191	> 150	151	> 150	111	129	71	102	31	69
190	> 150	150	> 150	110	129	70	101	30	69
189	> 150	149	> 150	109	128	69	101	29	68
188	> 150	148	> 150	108	128	68	99	28	68
187	> 150	147	> 150	107	127	67	98	27	67
186	> 150	146	> 150	106	126	66	97	26	66
185	> 150	145	> 150	105	125	65	96	25	66
184	> 150	144	> 150	104	125	64	94	24	65
183	> 150	143	> 150	103	124	63	92	23	64
182	> 150	142	> 150	102	124	62	92	22	63
181	> 150	141	> 150	101	123	61	91	21	63
180	> 150	140	> 150	100	123	60	91	20	62
179	> 150	139	> 150	99	122	59	89	19	61
178	> 150	138	> 150	98	122	58	88	18	60
177	> 150	137	150	97	121	57	87	17	59
176	> 150	136	149	96	121	56	86	16	58
175	> 150	135	148	95	120	55	86	15	57
174	> 150	134	148	94	120	54	85	14	56
173	> 150	133	147	93	119	53	84	13	55
172	> 150	132	146	92	118	52	83	12	54
171	> 150	131	146	91	118	51	83	11	53
170	> 150	130	145	90	117	59	82		
169	> 150	129	145	89	116	49	81		

Source: Ryan et al., 1990. Copyright American Psychological Association

for adults (Crawford & Allan, 1996; Matarazzo & Prifitera, 1989; McLean, Kaufman, & Reynolds, 1989). Intra-subtest scatter (clusters of zero-point scores appearing abruptly in a string of 1- or 2-point responses) is also quite common in the normal population (Mittenberg et al., 1989). There is also evidence that the inter- and intrasubtest differences vary at different points of the intelligence distribution (Matarazzo & Prifitera, 1989; McLean, Kaufman, & Reynolds, 1989; Mittenberg et al., 1989; Ryan & Paolo, 1992), in part a function of the potential range of scatter (Schinka et al., 1994; Schinka et al. 1997). In short, it is typical for the normal person, particularly a high IQ (generally more educated) individual, to demonstrate quite a bit of intertest scatter. An examination of frequency data should be a routine procedure when interpreting scatter scores, both when assessing an individual pa-

Table 5—32. Age-Corrected WAIS-R Subtest Scores for Persons 75 to 79 Years

Scaled Score	Verbal						Performance				
	I	DSp	V	A	C	S	PC	PA	BD	OA	DSy
19	29	24–28	68–70	—	31–32	27–28	20	18–20	41–51	38–41	70–93
18	28	23	67	—	29–30	26	18–19	13–17	38–40	36–37	63–69
17	27	22	66	19	—	25	17	12	35–37	33–35	58–62
16	26	19–21	65	18	28	23–24	16	11	33–34	32	51–57
15	25	18	63–64	17	27	22	—	10	31–32	31	48–50
14	23–24	16–17	56–62	16	25–26	21	15	9	28–30	30	44–47
13	21–22	15	53–55	14–15	23–24	19–20	14	8	24–27	28–29	41–43
12	19–20	14	47–52	12–13	21–22	17–18	12–13	7	21–23	25–27	38–40
11	17–18	13	45–46	10–11	19–20	15–16	11	6	19–20	23–24	34–37
10	14–16	12	39–44	9	17–18	12–14	9–10	4–5	14–18	21–22	29–33
9	12–13	11	32–38	8	15–16	10–11	7–8	3	12–13	19–20	25–28
8	10–11	10	26–31	6–7	13–14	7–9	6	—	9–11	15–18	20–24
7	9	9	19–25	5	10–12	5–6	4–5	2	6–8	11–14	18–19
6	7–8	8	13–18	4	7–9	3–4	3	1	3–5	9–10	12–17
5	5–6	7	10–12	3	5–6	1–2	2	—	1–2	4–8	8–11
4	4	5–6	7–9	2	4	0	1	0	0	2–3	6–7
3	2–3	2–4	5–6	0–1	3	—	0	—	—	1	3–5
2	0–1	1	2–4	—	1–2	—	—	—	—	0	1–2
1	—	0	0–1	—	0	—	—	—	—	—	0

Note: WAIS-R = Wechsler Adult Intelligence Scale—Revised (Wechsler, 1981); I = Information; DSp = Digit Span; V = Vocabulary; A = Arithmetic; C = Comprehension; S = Similarities; PC = Picture Completion; PA = Picture Arrangement; BD = Block Design; OA = Object Assembly; DSy = Digit Symbol.

Source: Ryan et al., 1990. Copyright American Psychological Association.

Table 5—33. Age-Corrected WAIS-R Subtest Scores for Persons 80 Years and Older

Scaled Score	Verbal						Performance				
	I	DSp	V	A	C	S	PC	PA	BD	OA	DSy
19	28–29	24–28	67–70		30–32	27–28	19–20	17–20	41–51	37–41	69–93
18	27	23	66	19	29	25–26	18	13–16	38–40	33–36	61–68
17	26	22	64–65	18	28	24	17	12	35–37	32	52–60
16	24–25	19–21	61–63	17	26–27	23	16	10–11	33–34	31	49–51
15	22–23	17–18	57–60	15–16	25	22	15	8–9	30–32	30	47–48
14	21	16	51–56	13–14	24	20–21	14	6–7	27–29	29	41–46
13	19–20	15	48–50	12	22–23	18–19	13	5	24–26	25–28	36–40
12	17–18	14	45–47	10–11	20–21	16–17	11–12	4	20–23	22–24	32–35
11	16	13	42–44	9	19	14–15	10	—	17–19	20–21	28–31
10	14–15	11–12	37–41	8	17–18	11–13	8–9	3	13–16	16–19	25–27
9	12–13	10	31–36	7	15–16	9–10	6–7	2	10–12	14–15	20–24
8	10–11	9	25–30	6	13–14	7–8	4–5	—	8–9	12–13	15–19
7	8–9	8	19–24	5	10–12	5–6	3	—	4–7	10–11	13–14
6	6–7	7	12–18	3–4	6–9	3–4	2	1	2–3	8–9	10–12
5	4–5	6	9–11	2	5	1–2	1	0	0–1	4–7	7–9
4	3	4–5	6–8	1	4	0	0	—	—	2–3	4–6
3	1–2	2–3	4–5	0	2–3	—	—	—	—	0–1	2–3
2	0	0–1	2–3	—	1	—	—	—	—	—	0–1
1	—	—	0–1	—	0	—	—	—	—	—	—

Note: WAIS-R = Wechsler Adult Intelligence Scale—Revised (Wechsler, 1981); I = Information; DSp = Digit Span; V = Vocabulary; A = Arithmetic; C = Comprehension; S = Similarities; PC = Picture Completion; PA = Picture Arrangement; BD = Block Design; OA = Object Assembly; DSy = Digit Symbol.

Source: Ryan et al., 1990. Copyright American Psychological Association.

Table 5—34. MOANS Scaled Scores: Midpoint Age = 79 (Age Range = 74–84, n = 179)

Scaled Scores	WAIS-R Subtests											Percentile Ranges
	Info.	D.Span	Vocab.	Arith.	Comp.	Simil.	P.C.	P.A.	B.D.	O.A.	D.Sym	
2	0–6	0–5	0–16	0–3	0	0	0	0	0–4	0–10	0–7	<1
3	7	6	17–18	4	1–3	1	1	—	5	11	8–16	1
4	8	7	19	—	4	2–3	2	—	6	12	17	2
5	9	8	20–23	—	5–6	4	—	1	7	13–14	18–20	3–5
6	10–11	—	24–28	5	7–12	5–8	3–4	—	8–9	15	21–24	6–10
7	12–13	9	29–36	6–7	13–14	9–10	5–6	2	10–11	16–18	25–27	11–18
8	14–15	10	37–40	8	15	11–12	7–8	3	12–14	19–20	28–30	19–28
9	16–17	11	41–45	9	16	13–14	9–10	—	15–18	21–22	31–34	29–40
10	18–20	12–13	46–50	10–11	17–19	15–17	11	4–5	19–22	23–26	35–39	41–59
11	21	14	51–53	12	20	18–19	12–13	6	23	27–28	40–42	60–71
12	22	15	54–56	13	21	20	—	7–8	24–27	—	43–46	72–81
13	23–24	16	57–58	14	22–23	21	14	9–10	28–29	29–30	47–49	82–89
14	—	17	59–60	15	24	22	15	11–12	30–32	—	50–52	90–94
15	25–26	18–19	61–62	16	25	23	16	13–14	33–35	31–32	53–56	95–97
16	27	—	63	17	—	24	—	15	36	33	57–58	98
17	28	20–21	64	18	26–27	25	17	16–17	37–38	34	59–65	99
18	29	22+	65+	19	28+	26+	18+	18+	39+	35+	66+	>99

Note: MOANS Scaled Scores are corrected for age influences. MOANS = Mayo's Older Americans Normative Studies, WAIS-R = Wechsler Adult Intelligence Scale—Revised, Info = Information subtest, D.Span = Digit Span subtest, Vocab. = Vocabulary subtest, Arith. = Arithmetic subtest, Simil. = Similarities subtest, P.C. = Picture Completion subtest, P.A. = Picture Arrangement subtest, B.D. = Block Design subtest, O.A. = Object Assembly subtest, D.Sym = Digit Symbol subtest.

Source: Ivnik et al., 1992. Copyright Mayo Clinic. Reprinted with permission.

Table 5—35. MOANS Scaled Scores: Midpoint Age = 82 (Age Range = 77–87, n = 149)

Scaled Scores	WAIS-R Subtests											Percentile Ranges
	Info.	D.Span	Vocab.	Arith.	Comp.	Simil.	P.C.	P.A.	B.D.	O.A.	D.Sym	
2	0–5	0–6	0–17	0–3	0	—	0	0	0–1	0–5	0–7	<1
3	6	7	18	4	1–3	0	—	—	2	6	8–16	1
4	7	—	19–20	—	—	—	1	—	3	7–8	17	2
5	8–9	8	21–24	—	4–6	1	2	—	4–6	9–11	18–19	3–5
6	10–11	—	25–28	5	7–9	2–6	—	1	7	12–13	20	6–10
7	12	9	29–33	6	10–13	7–9	3–4	—	8–10	14–15	21–25	11–18
8	13–14	10	34–38	7–8	14	10–11	5–6	2	11–12	16–18	26–28	19–28
9	15–16	11	39–43	9	15–16	12–13	7–8	3	13–15	19–20	29–31	29–40
10	17–18	12	44–49	10–11	17–18	14–16	9–10	4–5	16–20	21–24	32–36	41–59
11	19–20	13–14	50–52	12	19–20	17–18	11	—	21	25–26	37–40	60–71
12	21–22	—	53–55	13	21	19	12–13	6–7	22–23	27–28	41–44	72–81
13	23	15–16	56–58	14	22–23	20–21	14	8–9	24–27	29	45–46	82–89
14	24	17	59	15	24	22	15	10	28–30	30	47–50	90–94
15	25	—	60–61	16	25	—	—	11–14	31–33	31–32	51–53	95–97
16	26	18	62	—	26	23	16	—	34	33	—	98
17	27	19–21	63–64	17	27	24–25	17	15	35–38	34	54–57	99
18	28+	22+	65+	18+	28+	26+	18+	16+	39+	35+	58+	>99

Note: MOANS Scaled Scores are corrected for age influences. MOANS = Mayo's Older Americans Normative Studies, WAIS-R = Wechsler Adult Intelligence Scale—Revised, Info = Information subtest, D.Span = Digit Span subtest, Vocab. = Vocabulary subtest, Arith. = Arithmetic subtest, Simil. = Similarities subtest, P.C. = Picture Completion subtest, P.A. = Picture Arrangement subtest, B.D. = Block Design subtest, O.A. = Object Assembly subtest, D.Sym = Digit Symbol subtest.

Source: Ivnik et al., 1992.

Table 5—36. MOANS Scaled Scores: Midpoint Age = 85 (Age Range = 80–90, n = 113)

Scaled Scores	WAIS-R Subtests											Percentile Ranges
	Info.	D.Span	Vocab.	Arith.	Comp.	Simil.	P.C.	P.A.	B.D.	O.A.	D.Sym	
2	—	0–7	0–17	0	0	—	0	0	0	0–3	0–7	<1
3	0–5	—	—	1–3	—	0	1	—	1	4	8–12	1
4	6	—	18	4	1–3	—	—	—	2	5	13–16	2
5	7–9	—	19–23	—	4–6	1	2	—	3–5	6–9	17–18	3–5
6	10	8	24–28	5	7–9	2–5	—	—	6	10	19	6–10
7	11–12	—	29–33	6	10–13	6–8	3	—	7	11–14	20–22	11–18
8	13	9–10	34–37	7–8	14	9–10	4–5	1	8–10	15–17	23–26	19–28
9	14–15	—	38–42	—	15–16	11–12	6	2–3	11–13	18–19	27–29	29–40
10	16–18	11–12	43–48	9–11	17–18	13–16	7–9	—	14–18	20–22	30–34	41–59
11	19–20	13	49–51	12	19	17–18	10	4–5	19–20	23–25	35–37	60–71
12	21	14	52–56	13	20–22	19	11	6	21–22	26	38–42	72–81
13	22	15	57–58	14	23	20	12–13	7	23	27–28	43–45	82–89
14	23	16–17	59	15	24	21	14	8–9	24–27	29	46–47	90–94
15	24–25	18–20	60–62	16	25–26	22	—	10–14	28–32	30	48–51	95–97
16	26	21	63	—	—	—	15	15	—	31–32	52–53	98
17	27	22–23	64–65	17	27	23	16	15	33	33	54–55	99
18	28+	24+	66+	18+	28+	24+	17+	16+	34+	34+	56+	>99

Note: MOANS Scaled Scores are corrected for age influences. MOANS = Mayo's Older Americans Normative Studies, WAIS-R = Wechsler Adult Intelligence Scale—Revised, Info = Information subtest, D.Span = Digit Span subtest, Vocab. = Vocabulary subtest, Arith. = Arithmetic subtest, Simil. = Similarities subtest, P.C. = Picture Completion subtest, P.A. = Picture Arrangement subtest, B.D. = Block Design subtest, O.A. = Object Assembly subtest, D.Sym = Digit Symbol subtest.

Source: Ivnik et al., 1992.

Table 5—37. MOANS Scaled Scores: Midpoint Age = 88 and above (Age Range = 83 and above, n = 81)

Scaled Scores	Info.	D.Span	Vocab.	Arith.	Comp.	Simil.	P.C.	P.A.	B.D.	O.A.	D.Sym	Percentile Ranges
2	0–5	0	0–13	0–2	0–3	—	0	0	0	0–2	0–6	<1
3	6	—	14	3	4	0	1	—	—	3	7–12	1
4	7	1–6	15–18	—	5	—	—	—	1	4–5	13–16	2
5	8–9	7	19–26	4	6–7	1–3	—	—	2	6–8	17	3–5
6	10–11	8	27–29	5	8–9	4–6	—	—	3–6	9	18–19	6–10
7	12–13	9	30–34	6	10–12	7–9	2	—	7	10–11	20–21	11–18
8	14	10	35–40	7–8	13–15	10–11	3	—	8–9	12–13	22–24	19–28
9	15–16	—	41–44	9	16	12–13	4	1	10–12	14–17	25–27	29–40
10	17–18	11–12	45–50	10–11	17–18	14–15	5–8	2–3	13–17	18–21	28–31	41–59
11	19–20	13	51–53	—	19	16–18	9	4–5	18–20	22–25	32–35	60–71
12	21	14	54–56	12–13	20–22	19	10–11	—	21	26	36–37	72–81
13	22	15	57–58	14	23–24	20–21	12–13	6–7	22–23	27–28	38–43	82–89
14	23	16–17	59	15	25	—	14	8	24	—	44	90–94
15	24–25	18–20	60–61	16	26	22	15	9	25–26	29	45–46	95–97
16	26	21	62	17	—	—	—	10	27–30	30	47	98
17	27	22	63	—	27	23	16	11–15	31–32	31–32	48–49	99
18	28+	23+	64+	18+	28+	24+	17+	16+	33+	33+	50+	>99

Note: MOANS Scaled Scores are corrected for age influences. MOANS = Mayo's Older Americans Normative Studies, WAIS-R = Wechsler Adult Intelligence Scale—Revised, Info. = Information subtest, D.Span = Digit Span subtest, Vocab. = Vocabulary subtest, Arith. = Arithmetic subtest, Simil. = Similarities subtest, P.C. = Picture Completion subtest, P.A. = Picture Arrangement subtest, B.D. = Block Design subtest, O.A. = Object Assembly subtest, D.Sym = Digit Symbol subtest.

Source: Ivnik et al., 1992.

Table 5—38. Table for Converting Verbal Sum of MOANS Scaled Scores
to MAYO Verbal IQ

Verbal Sum of MOANS[a] Scaled Scores	MAYO[b] Verbal IQ	Verbal Sum of MOANS Scaled Scores	MAYO Verbal IQ	Verbal Sum of MOANS Scaled Scores	MAYO Verbal IQ	Verbal Sum of MOANS Scaled Scores	MAYO[b] Verbal IQ
≤12	≤64	35	83	58	101	81	120
13	65	36	84	59	102	82	121
14	66	37	84	60	103	83	122
15	67	38	85	61	104	84	122
16	68	39	86	62	105	85	123
17	68	40	87	63	105	86	124
18	69	41	88	64	106	87	125
19	70	42	88	65	107	88	126
20	71	43	89	66	108	89	126
21	72	44	90	67	109	90	127
22	72	45	91	68	109	91	128
23	73	46	92	69	110	92	129
24	74	47	93	70	111	93	130
25	75	48	93	71	112	94	130
26	76	49	94	72	113	95	131
27	76	50	95	73	113	96	132
28	77	51	96	74	114	97	133
29	78	52	97	75	115	98	134
30	79	53	97	76	116	99	134
31	80	54	98	77	117	100	135
32	80	55	99	78	118	≥101	≥136
33	81	56	100	79	118		
34	82	57	101	80	119		

[a]MOANS = Mayo's Older Americans Normative Studies

[b]IQ scores below 79 (Verbal Sum of MSS < 31) are extrapolated since no one in the MOANS normative project actually scored that low.

Source: Ivnick et al., 1992.

tient and when interpreting group data (Atkinson, 1992; Ivnik et al., 1994; Kaufman, 1990; Matarazzo & Prifitera, 1989; McDermott et al., 1989a, 1989b; Mittenberg et al., 1989). Tables for evaluating scatter are provided in the WISC-III manual (see also Sattler, 1992; Schinka etal., 1997). For the WAIS-R, Table 5–42 presents the size of the scaled score range that is needed to be abnormal for five different categories of Full Scale IQ, which range from "79 or less" to "120+." Alternatively, one can evaluate subtest scatter based on the value of the highest subtest scaled score (see Schinka et al., 1994). Silverstein (1984) has developed a method to determine if there are abnormal discrepancies between each subtest and the individual's mean subtest score. Table 5–43 records the esti-

mated discrepancy in age-scaled scores necessary to exceed that shown by various percentages of the healthy population. For example, a discrepancy of 4.6 between Digit Symbol and an individual's mean subtest score is estimated to occur in less than 5 percent of the healthy population. Similar data have been provided for use in the U.K. for the full-length WAIS-R (Crawford & Allan, 1996) as well as for various short-forms (Crawford et al., in press). Crawford and colleagues (Crawford & Allan, in press; Crawford et al., in press) found that the presence of at least one abnormal deviation is not uncommon. However, it is rare (occurring in less than 10 percent of their healthy sample) to exhibit two or more abnormal deviations. Sattler (1992) reports that differences of about 2.94 to 4.96 points between

Table 5—39. Table for Converting Sum of Performance Sum of MOANS Scaled Scores to MAYO Performance IQ

Performance Sum of MOANS[a] Scaled Scores	MAYO Performance IQ[b]	Performance Sum of MOANS Scaled Scores	MAYO Performance IQ	Performance Sum of MOANS Scaled Scores	MAYO Performance IQ	Performance Sum of MOANS Scaled Scores	MAYO Performance IQ
≤16	≤64	32	83	48	102	64	121
17	65	33	84	49	103	65	122
18	66	34	85	50	105	66	124
19	67	35	87	51	106	67	125
20	69	36	88	52	107	68	126
21	70	37	89	53	108	69	127
22	71	38	90	54	109	70	128
23	72	39	91	55	110	71	130
24	73	40	93	56	112	72	131
25	75	41	94	57	113	73	132
26	76	42	95	58	114	74	133
27	77	43	96	59	115	75	134
28	78	44	97	60	116	≥76	≥136
29	79	45	99	61	118		
30	81	46	100	62	119		
31	82	47	101	63	120		

[a]MOANS = Mayo's Older Americans Normative Studies

[b]IQ scores below 79 (Performance Sum of MSS < 29) are extrapolated since no one in the MOANS normative project actually scored that low.

Source: Ivnik et al., 1992.

each subtest scaled score and the respective average Verbal or Performance Scale were obtained by five percent of the WISC-III standardization sample. Table 5–44 shows the size of the WAIS-R VIQ–PIQ discrepancy (regardless of direction) required to be abnormal at various levels of occurrence, by IQ category. Table 5–45 presents data on expected WAIS-R VIQ–PIQ discrepancies as a function of educational level. The data are broken down by age, gender, and race. Significant scatter should alert the clinician to the possible presence of cognitive inefficiency and the need for further neuropsychological/ neurological examination.

Some clinicians use, in isolation, an individual's highest WAIS-R subtest score as a measure of that person's supposedly higher level of premorbid intelligence, and/or interpret the individual's lowest WAIS-R subtest scores as indices of impairment in brain-behavior function presumably reflected by these low subtest scores. Such a practice is risky (Matarazzo & Prifitera, 1989) and almost certainly

invalid, given the high degree of subtest scatter found in the normal population, the less than perfect test–retest reliabilities, and the magnitudes of the standard errors of measurement of each of the subtests (see above).

Mazes. Some neuropsychologists use the Mazes (WISC-III) subtest to provide a measure of planning. Recently, we collected normative data on a sample of healthy adults (60 men, 60 women), aged 20–79. The age groups did not differ in terms of their educational achievement (mean education of 14.9 years). Age, but not gender, affected performance on the Mazes, with scores declining with advancing age. Table 5–46 presents the mean raw score and standard deviation for each of six age groups.

Revisions. The periodic revisions of the Wechsler Scales present problems for investigators and clinicians since every Wechsler standardization sample from 1932 to the present established norms of a higher standard

Table 5—40. Table for Converting Full Scale Sum of MOANS Scaled Scores to MAYO Full Scale IQ

Full Scale Sum of MOANS[a] Scaled Scores	MAYO Full Scale IQ[b]	Full Scale Sum of MOANS Scaled Scores	MAYO Full Scale IQ	Full Scale Sum of MOANS Scaled Scores	MAYO Full Scale IQ	Full Scale Sum of MOANS Scaled Scores	MAYO Full Scale IQ
≤36	≤64	70	82	104	100	138	119
37	65	71	83	105	101	139	119
38	65	72	83	106	102	140	120
39	66	73	84	107	102	141	120
40	66	74	84	108	103	142	121
41	67	75	85	109	103	143	121
42	67	76	86	110	104	144	122
43	68	77	86	111	104	145	122
44	68	78	87	112	105	146	123
45	69	79	87	113	105	147	124
46	69	80	88	114	106	148	124
47	70	81	88	115	106	149	125
48	71	82	89	116	107	150	125
49	71	83	89	117	107	151	126
50	72	84	90	118	108	153	126
51	72	85	90	119	109	153	127
52	73	86	91	120	109	154	127
53	73	87	91	121	110	155	128
54	74	88	92	122	110	156	128
55	74	89	92	123	111	157	129
56	75	90	93	124	111	158	129
57	75	91	94	125	112	159	130
58	76	92	94	126	112	160	130
59	76	93	95	127	113	161	131
60	77	94	95	128	113	162	132
61	77	95	96	129	114	163	132
62	78	96	96	130	114	164	133
63	79	97	97	131	115	165	133
64	79	98	97	132	115	166	134
65	80	99	98	133	116	167	134
66	80	100	98	134	117	168	135
67	81	101	99	135	117	169	135
68	81	102	99	136	118	≥170	≥136
69	82	103	100	137	118		

[a]MOANS = Mayo's Older Americans Normative Studies

[b]IQ scores below 79 (Full Scale Sum of MSS < 65) are extrapolated since no one in the MOANS normative project actually scored that low.

Source: Ivnik et al., 1992.

than its predecessor (Flynn, 1984). As a result, the Wechsler tests get successively harder in order to compensate for the increased average performance of individuals over time. This means that the older the test, the greater the overestimation of the participant's IQ (Parker, 1986). A related implication is that one cannot directly equate performances on earlier and later versions of the test (Reitan & Wolfson, 1990). On average, IQ increases of 6–8 points

have been reported (Wechsler, 1974, 1981, 1991; Weiss, 1995) for successive versions of a scale (e.g., WAIS and WAIS-R; WISC-R and WISC-III). The larger differences are in the Performance scale norms, with less change in the Verbal scale norms (Weiss, 1995). One way to equate performances between early (e.g., WAIS) and later (WAIS-R) versions is simply to subtract the mean differences between the tests (Russell, 1992). It is important to recog-

Table 5—41. Percentage of Normal Population Obtaining VIQ–PIQ Differences (Regardless of Direction) on the WAIS-R and WISC-III

% in Population Obtaining Given or Greater Difference	Discrepancy Scores	
	WAIS-R Total Sample[a]	WISC-III Total Sample[b]
50	7	9
25	12	15
20	14	17
10	18	22
5	21	25
2	25	30
1	28	32
0.1	36	40

[a]*Source:* Grossman (1983).

[b]*Source:* Wechsler (1991).

nize, however, that the amount of difference between earlier and later versions of the test may vary with respect to a subject's age and ability (Feingold, 1984; Oscar-Berman et al., 1993; Ryan et al., 1987; Wechsler, 1981). In children, there is considerable variability across studies. The smallest difference between WISC-R and WISC-III FSIQ scores found was −1.35 points (WISC-III lower than WISC-R scores) in a sample of children with learning disabilities; the largest difference obtained was −18.09 points in a sample of gifted children (Weiss, 1995). In adults, the WAIS FSIQ tends to be about 5 points higher than the WAIS-R FSIQ in persons with high-average to superior intelligence and approximately 9 points greater in persons with average intelligence; conversely, WAIS-R IQs may be slightly higher than corresponding WAIS

IQs in mildly to moderately retarded individuals (Ryan et al., 1987). Oscar-Berman and colleagues (1993) note that the WAIS-R yields lower scores than the WAIS, particularly in older individuals aged 50 and above. Further, substantial differences in content are present, and at the level of profile analysis, different versions of the scale may produce different subtest patterns for a given subject (Wolfson & Reitan, 1990). Consequently, any attempt to apply decision rules derived from a consideration of subtest patterns on one version may not be applicable when using a different version (Chelune et al., 1987). One can also not assume that patterns of performance established between other neuropsychological tests and previous editions of the Wechsler test hold for the WAIS-R (Bornstein, 1987; Paniak et al., 1992). Additional studies are needed to address this issue.

Reporting IQ Data. Our usual practice is to translate IQ scores to percentile ranks. Table 5–47 is provided for ease of conversion. Note, however, that there is a moderate relation between FSIQ and educational attainment, suggesting that the examiner may wish to take years of formal schooling into account when interpreting WAIS-R scores for individual patients (Marcopulos et al., 1997; Ryan, Paolo, & Findley, 1991). Thus, a FSIQ of 90 carries different implications if earned by a university graduate as opposed to a high school dropout. One might speculate that the university graduate had sustained cognitive deterioration and suggest additional investigation to clarify the picture. To facilitate interpretation the examiner can refer to Table 5–48 which presents

Table 5—42. Size of Scaled-Score Range[a] on the WAIS-R Verbal, Performance, and Full Scales Required for Abnormality at Several Frequencies of Occurrence in the Normal Population, by Full Scale IQ

Frequency of Occurrence	≤79			80–89			90–109			110–119			120+		
	V	P	FS	V	P	FS	V	P	FS	V	P	FS	V	P	FS
< 5%	7	7	9	8	8	10	9	9	11	10	10	12	10	10	12
< 1%	8	9	10	10	10	12	11	12	13	11	12	14	11	12	14

[a]When referring to the above base rate table, note that scatter computations utilize the regular scaled scores, not the age scaled scores.

Source: McLean, Kaufman and Reynolds, 1989.

Table 5—43. Estimates of the Differences Obtained by Various Percentages of the WAIS-R Standardization Sample between Each Subtest Score and an Average Subtest Score

Subtest	Verbal Average 5%	Verbal Average 1%	Performance Average 5%	Performance Average 1%	Overall Average 5%	Overall Average 1%
Information	3.1	4.0			3.5	4.7
Digit Span	4.3	5.7			4.5	5.9
Vocabulary	2.7	3.5			3.3	4.3
Arithmetic	3.6	4.7			3.8	5.0
Comprehension	3.3	4.3			3.7	4.8
Similarities	3.4	4.4			3.6	4.7
Picture Completion			3.7	4.8	4.1	5.3
Picture Arrangement			4.1	5.4	4.3	5.7
Block Design			3.5	4.5	3.9	5.2
Object Assembly			3.8	5.0	4.5	6.0
Digit Symbol			4.3	5.6	4.5	5.9

Note: Tabled differences refer to age scaled scores, not to the scaled scores based on the reference group, ages 20–34, that are used for determining a subject's IQ.

Source: Silverstein, 1984. Copyright American Psychological Association. Reprinted with permission.

Table 5—44. Size of WAIS-R V-P IQ Discrepancy (Regardless of Direction) Required to Be Abnormal at Various Levels of Occurrence in Normal Population, by IQ Category

Frequency of Occurrence	≤79	80–89	90–109	110–119	120+
< 5%	14	20	24	24	27
< 1%	20	24	30+	30+	30+

Source: Adapted from Kaufman, 1990.

Table 5—45. Mean WAIS-R V-P IQ Discrepancy for Normals Differing in Educational Level, Separately by Age, Gender, and Race

	Years of education 0–8	9–11	12	13+
Age				
16–19	−4.7	−.6	+1.7	+3.0
20–34	−4.1	−3.1	−1.1	+1.9
35–44	−3.7	−3.6	−1.2	+2.4
45–54	−0.7	−3.7	−0.2	+5.7
55–64	−0.4	−1.3	−0.9	+4.8
65–74	−3.0	−2.2	+2.9	+7.2
Gender				
Male	−2.3	−1.4	+0.4	+3.8
Female	−2.9	−2.0	−0.4	+2.9
Race				
White	−3.1	−2.1	−0.1	+3.6
Black	−0.1	+1.4	+1.0	−1.7
Total	−2.6	−1.7	0.0	+3.4

Source: Kaufman, 1990, p. 339.

Table 5—46. Means by Age for the Mazes Subtest

Age	n	M	SD
20–29	20	21.30	3.83
30–39	20	20.35	4.40
40–49	20	20.50	2.78
50–59	20	18.65	4.93
60–69	20	17.60	8.64
70–79	20	14.05	6.84

Source: Strauss and Spreen, unpublished data, 1994.

Table 5—47. Conversion of Wechsler IQ Scores to Percentile Ranks

IQ	Percentile	IQ	Percentile	IQ	Percentile	IQ	Percentile
155	99.9	117	87	101	53	85	16
144	99.8	116	86	100	50	84	14
142	99.7	115	84	99	47	83	13
140	99.6	114	82	98	45	82	12
139	99.5	113	81	97	42	81	10
138	99	112	79	96	39	80	9
132	98	111	77	95	37	79	8
129	97	110	75	94	34	78	7
127	96	109	73	93	32	77	6
125	96	108	70	92	30	76	5
123	94	107	68	91	27	74	4
122	93	106	66	90	25	71	3
121	92	105	61	89	23	70	2
120	91	104	61	88	21	67	1
119	90	103	58	87	19	61	<1
118	88	102	55	86	18		

Table 5—48. Percentile Ranks by Educational Level

	Years of Education					
Percentile	0–7	8	9–11	12	13–15	16+
VIQ						
95th	105	108	119	120	126	135
75th	91	98	105	108	115	123
50th	82	90	96	100	108	116
25th	73	83	87	92	100	108
5th	60	72	73	80	90	97
PIQ						
95th	109	117	122	122	125	132
75th	95	103	108	109	113	120
50th	84	93	98	100	105	111
25th	74	83	88	91	97	102
5th	60	69	73	78	86	90
FSIQ						
95th	106	111	120	121	126	135
75th	92	99	106	108	115	123
50th	82	91	96	100	107	115
25th	73	83	87	92	100	107
5th	59	71	73	79	89	95

Source: Adapted from Ryan et al., 1991. Copyright by the American Psychological Association. Reprinted with permission.

estimated percentile ranks for VIQ, PIQ, and FSIQ at six different educational levels (Ryan et al., 1991).

Finally, it is important to emphasize that there is some variability in all testing and it is unlikely that a person would obtain exactly the same score if retested. Rather, the IQ score is best thought of as falling within a range of ±2 standard errors of measurement (SEM). This defines the interval within which the true score will fall 95 percent of the time. If one prefers the 68 percent confidence limits, simply use ±1 SEM. One way to communicate such information in a psychological report is as follows: "The patient's Full Scale IQ score on the WAIS-R falls at about the __ percentile. There is some variability in all testing and it is unlikely that a person would obtain exactly the same score on retest. Rather, the IQ score is best thought of as falling within a range. The chances that the range of scores from the __ to __ percentile includes her/his true IQ are about 95 (or 68) out of 100." Tables in the Wechsler manuals provide the standard errors of measurement of the IQ scores and of the scaled scores (See also Kramer, 1993, for interpretation of individual subtest scores on the WISC-III and Ryan et al., 1990b, for individuals aged 75 years and above).

References

Anastopoulos, A.D., Spisto, M.A., & Maher, M.C. (1994). The WISC-III freedom from distractibility factor: Its utility in identifying children with attention deficit hyperactivity disorder. *Psychological Assessment, 6*, 368–371.

Atkinson, L. (1991). Some tables for statistically based interpretation of WAIS-R factor scores. *Psychological Assessment, 3*, 288–291.

Atkinson, L. (1991). On WAIS-R difference scores in the standardization sample. *Psychological Assessment, 3*, 292–294.

Atkinson, L. (1992). Mental retardation and WAIS-R scatter analysis. *Journal of Intellectual Disability, 36*, 443–448.

Axelrod, B.N., Woodard, J.L., Schretlen, D., & Benedict, R.H.B. (1996). Corrected estimates of WAIS-R short form reliability and standard error of measurement. *Psychological Assessment, 8*, 222–223.

Ballard, K. (1984). Interpreting Stanford-Binet and WISC-R IQs in New Zealand: The need for more than caution. *New Zealand Journal of Psychology, 13*, 25–31.

Banken, J.A., & Banken, C.H. (1987). Investigation of Wechsler Adult Intelligence Scale–Revised short forms in a sample of vocational rehabilitation applicants. *Journal of Psychoeducational Assessment, 5*, 281–286.

Baum, C., Edwards, D., Yonan, C., & Storandt, M. (1995). The relation of neuropsychological test performance to performance of functional tasks in Dementia of the Alzheimer Type. *Archives of Clinical Neuropsychology, 11*, 69–75.

Benedict, R.H., Schretlen, D., & Bobholz, J.H. (1992). Concurrent validity of three WAIS-R short forms in psychiatric populations. *Psychological Assessment, 4*, 322–328.

Binder, L.M. (1987). Appropriate reporting of Wechsler IQ and subtest scores in assessments for disability. *Journal of Clinical Psychology, 43*, 144–145.

Blaha, J., & Wallbrown, F.H. (1996). Hierarchical factor structure of the Wechsler Intelligence Scale for Children - III. *Psychological Assessment, 8*, 214–218.

Bowden, S.C., Whelan, G., Long, C.M., & Clifford, C.C. (1995). Temporal stability of the WAIS-R and WMS-R in a heterogeneous sample of alcohol dependent clients. *The Clinical Neuropsychologist, 9*, 194–197.

Brooker, B.H., & Cyr, J.J. (1986). Tables for clinicians to use to convert WAIS-R short forms. *Journal of Clinical Psychology, 42*, 982–986.

Bornstein, R.A., McLeod, J., McClung, E., & Hutchison, B. (1983). Item difficulty and content bias on the WAIS-R Information subtest. *Canadian Journal of Behavioral Science, 15*, 27–34.

Bornstein, R.A. (1984). Unilateral lesions and the Wechsler Adult Intelligence Scale–Revised: no sex differences. *Journal of Consulting and Clinical Psychology, 52*, 604–608.

Bornstein, R.A. (1987). The WAIS-R in neuropsychological practice: Boon or bust? *The Clinical Neuropsychologist, 1*, 185–190.

Burton, D.B., Ryan, J.J., Paolo, A.M., & Mittenberg, W. (1994). Structural equation analysis of WAIS-R in a normal elderly sample. *Psychological Assessment, 6*, 380–385.

Carvajal, H., Gerber, J., Hewes, P., & Weaver, K.A. (1987). Correlations between scores on Stanford-Binet IV and Wechsler Adult Intelligence Scale–Revised. *Psychological Reports, 61*, 83–86.

Carvajal, H., Hayes, J.E., Miller, H.R., Wiebe, D.A., & Weaver, K.A. (1993). Comparisons of the vocabulary scores and IQs on the Wechsler Intelligence Scale for Children—III and the Peabody Picture Vocabulary Test–Revised. *Perceptual and Motor Skills*, 76, 28–30.

Chelune, G.J., Eversole, C., Kane, M., & Talbott, R. (1987). WAIS versus WAIS-R subtest patterns: A problem of generalization. *The Clinical Neuropsychologist*, 1, 235–242.

Collaer, M.L., & Evans, J.R. (1982). A measure of short-term visual memory based on the WISC-R Coding subtest. *Journal of Clinical Psychology*, 38, 641–644.

Crawford, J.R., Allan, K.M., McGeorge, P., & Kelly, S.M. (in press). Base rate data on the abnormality of subtest scatter for WAIS-R short-terms. *British Journal of Clinical Psychology*.

Crawford, J.R., & Allan, K.M. (1996). WAIS-R subtest scatter: Base-rate data from a healthy UK sample. *British Journal of Clinical Psychology*, 35, 235–247.

Crawford, J.R., Allan, K.M., & Jack, A.M. (1992). Short-forms of the UK WAIS-R: Regression equations and their predictive validity in a general population sample. *British Journal of Clinical Psychology*, 31, 191–202.

Crawford, M.S., & Boer, D.P. (1985). Content bias in the WAIS-R Information subtest and some Canadian alternatives. *Canadian Journal of Behavioral Science*, 17, 79–86.

Donders, J. (1996). Cluster subtypes in the WISC-III standardization sample: Analysis of factor index scores. *Psychological Assessment*, 8, 312–318.

Donders, J. (1997a). Sensitivity of the WISC-III to injury severity in children with traumatic head injury. *Assessment*, 4, 107–109.

Donders, J. (1997b). A short form of the WISC-III for clinical use. *Psychological Assessment*, 9, 15–20.

Ehrenreich, J.H. (1996). Clinical use of short forms of the WAIS-R. *Assessment*, 3, 193–200.

Faust, D.S., & Hollingsworth, J.O. (1991). Concurrent validation of the Wechsler Preschool and Primary Scale of Intelligence–Revised (WPPSI-R) with two criteria of cognitive abilities. *Journal of Psychoeducational Assessment*, 9, 224–229.

Feingold, A. (1984). The effects of differential age adjustment between the WAIS and WAIS-R on the comparability of the two scales. *Educational and Psychological Measurement*, 44, 569–573.

Flynn, J.R. (1984). The mean IQ of Americans: Massive gains 1932–1978. *Psychological Bulletin*, 95, 29–51.

Fuld, P.A. (1984). Test profile of cholinergic dysfunction and of Alzheimer-type dementia. *Journal of Clinical Neuropsychology*, 6, 380–392.

Gerken, K.C., & Hodapp, A.L. (1992). Assessment of preschoolers at risk with the WPPSI-R and the Stanford-Binet L-M. *Psychological Reports*, 71, 659–664.

Grossman, F.M. (1983). Percentage of WAIS-R standardization sample obtaining verbal–performance discrepancies. *Journal of Consulting and Clinical Psychology*, 51, 641–642.

Iverson, G.L., Myers, B., Bengston, M.L., & Adams, R.L. (1996). Concurrent validity of a WAIS-R seven-subtest short form in patients with brain impairment. *Psychological Assessment*, 8, 319–323.

Iverson, G.L., & Franzen, M.D. (1996). Using multiple object memory procedures to detect simulated malingering. *Journal of Clinical and Experimental Neuropsychology*, 18, 1–14.

Ivnik, R.J., Malec, J.F., Smith, G.E., Tangalos, E.G., Peterson, R.C., Kokmen, E., & Kurland, L.T. (1992). Mayo's Older American Normative Studies: WAIS-R norms for ages 56 to 97. *The Clinical Neuropsychologist*, 6,Supplement, 1–30.

Ivnik, R.J., Smith, G.E., Malec, J.F., Kokmen, E., & Tangalos, E.G. (1994). Mayo cognitive factor scales: Distinguishing normal and clinical samples by profile variability. *Neuropsychology*, 8, 203–209.

Ivnik, R.J., Smith, G.E., Malec, J.F., Petersen, R.C., & Tangalos, E.G. (1995). Long-term stability and intercorrelations of cognitive abilities in older persons. *Psychological Assessment*, 7, 155–161.

Joschko, M., & Rourke, B.P. (1985). Neuropsychological subtypes of learning-disabled children who exhibit the ACID pattern on the WISC. In B.P. Rourke (Ed.), *Neuropsychology of Learning Disabilities*. New York: Guilford Press, pp. 65–88.

Kaplan, E., Fein, D., Morris, R., & Delis, D.C. (1991). *WAIS-R NI Manual*. San Antonio, TX: Psychological Corporation.

Kaufman, A.S. (1976a). Verbal–Performance IQ discrepancies on the WISC-R. *Journal of Consulting and Clinical Psychology*, 44, 739–744.

Kaufman, A.S. (1976b). A new approach to the interpretation of test scatter on the WISC-R. *Journal of Learning Disabilities*, 9, 160–168.

Kaufman, A.S. (1979). *Intelligent Testing with the WISC-R*. New York: John Wiley and Sons.

Kaufman, A.S. (1994). *Intelligent Testing with the WISC-III*. New York: Wiley-Interscience.

Kaufman, A.S. (1990). *Assessing Adolescent and Adult Intelligence*. Boston: Allyn and Bacon.

Kaufman, A.S. (1992). Evaluation of the WISC-III

and WPPSI-R for gifted children. *Roeper Review, 14,* 154–158.

Kaufman, A.S., Ishikuma, T., & Kaufman-Parker, J.L. (1991). Amazingly short forms of the WAIS-R. *Journal of Psychoeducational Assessment, 9,* 4–15.

Kaufman, A.S. (1994). *Intelligent Testing with the WISC-III.* New York: Wiley-Interscience.

Kluger, A., & Goldberg, E. (1990). IQ patterns in affective disorder, lateralized and diffuse brain damage. *Journal of Clinical and Experimental Neuropsychology, 12,* 182–194.

Kramer, J.H. (1993). Interpretation of individual subtest scores on the WISC-III. *Psychological Assessment, 5,* 193–196.

Lees-Haley, P.R., Smith, H.H., Williams, C.W., & Dunn, J.T. (1996). Forensic neuropsychological test usage: An empirical survey. *Archives of Clinical Neuropsychology, 11,* 45–51.

Lezak, M.D. (1983). *Neuropsychological Assessment* (2nd ed.). New York: Oxford University Press.

Lezak, M.D. (1995). *Neuropsychological Assessment* (3rd ed.). New York: Oxford University Press.

Lincoln, R.K., Crosson, B., Bauer, R.M., Cooper, P.V., & Velozo, C.A. (1994). Relationship between WAIS-R subtests and language measures after blunt head injury. *The Clinical Neuropsychologist, 8,* 140–152.

Little, S.G. (1992). The WISC-III: Everything old is new again. *School Psychology Quarterly, 7,* 136–142.

LoBello, S.G. (1991). A short form of the Wechsler Preschool and Primary Scale of Intelligence–Revised. *Journal of School Psychology, 29,* 229–236.

Logsdon, R.G., Teri, L., Williams, D.E., Vitiello, M.V., & Prinz, P.N. (1989). The WAIS-R profile: A diagnostic tool for Alzheimer's disease? *Journal of Clinical and Experimental Neuropsychology, 11,* 892–898.

Lowe, J.D., Anderson, H.N., Williams, A., & Currie, B.B. (1987). Long-term predictive validity of the WPPSI and the WISC-R with black school children. *Personality and Individual Differences, 8,* 551–559.

Mahurin, R.K., DeBettignies, B.H., & Pirozzolo, F.J. (1991). Structured assessment of independent living skills: Preliminary report of a performance measure of functional abilities in dementia. *Journal of Gerontology: Psychological Sciences, 46,* 58–66.

Malec, J.F., Ivnik, R.J., Smith, G.E., Tangalos, E.G., Petersen, R.C., Kokmen, E., & Kurland, L.T. (1992). Mayo's Older American Normative Studies: Utility of corrections for age and education for the WAIS-R. *The Clinical Neuropsychologist, 6,* 31–47.

Marcopulos, B.A., McLain, C.A., & Giuliano, A.J. (1997). Cognitive impairment or inadequate norms? A study of healthy, rural, older adults with limited education. *The Clinical Neuropsychologist, 11,* 111–131.

Marx, R.W. (1984). Canadian content and the WISC-R information subtest. *Canadian Journal of Behavioral Science, 16,* 30–35.

Matarazzo, J.D. (1972). *Wechsler's Measurement and Appraisal of Adult Intelligence* (5th ed.). Baltimore: Williams and Wilkins.

Matarazzo, J.D., & Herman, D.O. (1984). Base rate data for the WAIS-R: Test–retest stability and VIQ–PIQ differences. *Journal of Clinical Neuropsychology, 6,* 351–366.

Matarazzo, J.D., & Herman, D.O. (1985). Clinical uses of the WAIS-R: Base rates of differences between VIQ and PIQ in the WAIS-R standardization sample. In B.B. Wolman (Ed.), *Handbook of Intelligence: Theories, Measurements, and Application.* New York: John Wiley and Sons.

Matarazzo, J.D., & Prifitera, A. (1989). Subtest scatter and premorbid intelligence: Lessons from the WAIS-R standardization sample. *Psychological Assessment, 1,* 186–191.

McDermott, P.A., Glutting, J.J., Jones, J.N., & Noonan, J.V. (1989a). Typology and prevailing composition of core profiles in the WAIS-R standardization sample. *Psychological Assessment, 1,* 118–125.

McDermott, P.A., Glutting, J.J., Jones, J.N., & Kush, J. (1989b). Core profile types in the WISC-R national sample: Structure, membership, and applications. *Psychological Assessment, 1,* 292–299.

McLean, J.E., Kaufman, A.S., & Reynolds, C.R. (1989). Base rates of WAIS-R subtest scatter as a guide for clinical and neuropsychological assessment. *Journal of Clinical Psychology, 45,* 919–926.

Milanovich, J.R., Axelrod, B.N., & Millis, S.R. (1996). Validation of the Simulation Index–Revised with a mixed clinical population. *Archives of Clinical Neuropsychology, 11,* 53–59.

Miller, H.R., Streiner, D.L., & Goldberg, J.O. (1996). Short, shorter, shortest: The efficacy of WAIS-R short forms with mixed psychiatric patients. *Assessment, 3,* 165–169.

Mittenberg, W., Hammeke, T.A., & Rao, S.M. (1989). Intrasubtest scatter on the WAIS-R as a pathognomic sign of brain injury. *Psychological Assessment, 1*, 273–276.

Mittenberg, W., Theroux-Fichera, S., Heilbronner, R.L., & Zielinski, R.E. (1995). Identification of malingered head injury on the Wechsler Adult Intelligence Scale–Revised. *Professional Psychology: Research and Practice, 26*, 491–498.

Moore, A.D., Stambrook, M., Hawryluk, G.A., Peters, L.C., Gill, D.D., & Hymans, M.M. (1990). Test–retest stability of the Wechsler Adult Intelligence Scale–Revised in the assessment of head-injured patients. *Psychological Assessment, 2*, 98–100.

Naglieri, J. (1993). Pairwise and ipsative comparisons of WISC-III IQ and Index scores. *Psychological Assessment, 5*, 113–116.

Oscar-Berman, M., Clancy, J.P., & Altman Weber, D. (1993). Discrepancies between IQ and memory scores in alcoholism and aging. *The Clinical Neuropsychologist, 7*, 281–296.

Paniak, C.E., Silver, K., Finlayson, M.A.J., & Tuff, L.P. (1992). How useful is the WAIS-R in closed head injury assessment? *Journal of Clinical Psychology, 48*, 219–225.

Paolo, A.M., & Ryan, J.J. (1994). Factor structure of the WAIS-R by educational level: An examination of elderly persons. *Archives of Clinical Neuropsychology, 9*, 259–264.

Paolo, A.M., & Ryan, J.J. (1995). Selecting WAIS-R norms for persons 75 years and older. *The Clinical Neuropsychologist, 9*, 44–49.

Paolo, A.M., & Ryan, J.J. (1996). Stability of WAIS-R scatter indices in the elderly. *Archives of Clinical Neuropsychology, 11*, 503–511.

Parker, K.C.H. (1986). Changes with age, year-of-birth cohort, age by year-of-birth cohort interaction, and standardization of the Wechsler Intelligence Tests. *Human Development, 29*, 209–222.

Parker, K.C.H., & Atkinson, L. (1994). Factor space of the Wechsler Intelligence Scale for Children—Third Edition: Critical thoughts and recommendations. *Psychological Assessment, 6*, 201–208.

Pugh, G.M., & Boer, D.P. (1991). Normative data on the validity of Canadian substitute items for the WAIS-R Information subtest. *Canadian Journal of Behavioral Science, 23*, 149–158.

Rawling, P.J., & Brooks, D.N. (1990). Simulation Index: A method for detecting factitious errors on the WAIS-R and WMS. *Neuropsychology, 4*, 223–238.

Rawlings, D.B., & Crewe, N.M. (1992). Test–retest practice effects and test score changes of the WAIS-R in recovering traumatically brain-injured survivors. *The Clinical Neuropsychologist, 6*, 415–430.

Reitan, R.M., & Wolfson, D. (1990). A consideration of the comparability of the WAIS and WAIS-R. *The Clinical Neuropsychologist, 4*, 80–85.

Reynolds, C.R., & Gutkin, T.B. (1981). Test scatter on the WPPSI: Normative analyses of the standardization sample. *Journal of Learning Disabilities, 14*, 460–464.

Reynolds, C.R., & Ford, L. (1994). Comparative three-factor solutions of the WISC-III and WISC-R at 11 age levels between 6 1/2 and 16 1/2 years. *Archives of Clinical Neuropsychology, 9*, 553–570.

Reynolds, C.R., Sanchez, S., & Willson, V.L. (1996). Normative tables for calculating the WISC-III Performance and Full Scale IQs when Symbol Search is substituted for Coding. *Psychological Assessment, 8*, 378–382.

Richards, T.W. (1951). Mental test performance as a reflection of the child's current life situation—a methodological study. *Child Development, 22*, 221–233.

Russell, E.W. (1992). Comparison of two methods of converting the WAIS to the WAIS-R. *Journal of Clinical Psychology, 48*, 355–359.

Ryan, J.J., Abraham, E., Axelrod, B.N., & Paolo, A.M. (1996a). WAIS-R Verbal–Performance IQ discrepancies in persons with lateralized lesions: Utility of a seven-subtest short form. *Archives of Clinical Neuropsychology, 11*, 207–213.

Ryan, J.J., & Bohac, D.L. (1994). Neurodiagnostic implications of unique profiles of the Wechsler Adult Intelligence Scale–Revised. *Psychological Assessment, 6* 360–363.

Ryan, J.J., Lopez, S.J., & Paolo, A.M. (1996b). Digit span performance of persons 75–96 years of age: Base rates and associations with selected demographic variables. *Psychological Assessment, 8*, 324–327.

Ryan, J.J., Nowak, T.J., & Geisser, M.E. (1987). On the comparability of the WAIS and WAIS-R: Review of the research and implications for clinical practice. *Journal of Psychoeducational Assessment, 5*, 15–30.

Ryan, J.J., & Paolo, A.M. (1992). Base rates of intersubtest scatter in the old age standardization sample of the WAIS-R. *Archives of Clinical Neuropsychology, 7*, 515–522.

Ryan, J.J., Paolo, A.M., & Brungardt, T.M. (1990a). Standardization of the Wechsler Adult Intelligence Scale–Revised for persons 75 years and older. *Psychological Assessment, 2*, 404–411.

Ryan, J.J., Paolo, A.M., & Brungardt, T.M. (1990b). WAIS-R reliability and standard errors for persons 75 to 79, 80 to 84, and 85 and older. *Journal of Psychoeducational Assessment, 8*, 9–14.

Ryan, J.J., Paolo, A.M., & Brungardt, T.M. (1992). WAIS-R test–retest stability in normal persons 75 years and older. *The Clinical Neuropsychologist, 6*, 3–8.

Ryan, J.J., Paolo, A.M., & Findley, G. (1991). Percentile rank conversion tables for WAIS-R IQs at six educational levels. *Journal of Clinical Psychology, 47*, 104–107.

Ryan, J.J., Paolo, A.M., & Smith, A.J. (1992). Wechsler Adult Intelligence Scale–Revised intersubtest scatter in brain-damaged patients: A comparison with the standardization sample. *Psychological Assessment, 4*, 63–66.

Ryan, J.J., Paolo, A.M., & Van Fleet, J.N. (1994). Neurodiagnostic implication of abnormal verbal–performance IQ discrepancies on the WAIS-R: A comparison with the standardization sample. *Archives of Clinical Neuropsychology, 9*, 251–258.

Sackeim, H.A., Freeman, J., McElhiney, M., Coleman, E., Prudic, J., & Devanand, D.P. (1992). Effects of major depression on estimates of intelligence. *Journal of Clinical and Experimental Neuropsychology, 14*, 268–288.

Sarazin, F.A., & Spreen, O. (1986). Fifteen-year stability of some neuropsychological tests in learning-disabled subjects with and without neurological impairment. *Journal of Clinical and Experimental Neuropsychology, 8*, 190–200.

Sattler, J. (1982). Age effects on Wechsler Adult Intelligence Scale–Revised tests. *Journal of Consulting and Clinical Psychology, 50*, 785–786.

Sattler, J. (1982). *Assessment of Children's Intelligence and Special Abilities*. Boston: Allyn and Bacon, Inc.

Sattler, J.M. (1988). *Assessment of Children* (3rd ed.). San Diego, CA: Sattler.

Sattler, J.M. (1992). *Assessment of Children*. WISC-III and WPPSI-R supplement. San Diego: Sattler.

Satz, P., & Mogel, S. (1962). An abbreviation of the WAIS for clinical use. *Journal of Clinical Psychology, 18*, 77–79.

Satz, P., Van Gorp, W.G., Soper, H.V., & Mitrushina, M. (1987). WAIS-R marker for dementia of the Alzheimer type? An empirical and statistical induction test. *Journal of Clinical and Experimental Neuropsychology, 9*, 767–774.

Schinka, J.A., Vanderploeg, R.D., and Curtiss, G. (1997). WISC-III subtest scatter as a function of highest subtest scaled score. *Psychological Assessment, 9*, 83–88.

Schinka, J.A., Vanderploeg, R.D., & Curtiss, G. (1994). Wechsler Adult Intelligence Scale–Revised subtest scatter as a function of maximum subtest scaled score. *Psychological Assessment, 6*, 364–367.

Schretlen, D., Benedict, R.H.B., & Bobholz, H. (1994). Composite reliability and standard errors of measurement for a seven-subtest short form of the Wechsler Adult Intelligence Scale–Revised. *Psychological Assessment, 6*, 188–190.

Schretlen, D., & Ivnik, R.J. (1996). Prorating IQ scores for older adults: Validation of a seven-subtest WAIS-R with the Mayo Older Americans Normative Sample. *Assessment, 3*, 411–416.

Scott, J.C., Sherer, M., & Adams, R.L. (1995). Clinical utility of WAIS-R factor-derived standard scores in assessing brain injury. *The Clinical Neuropsychologist, 9*, 93–97.

Seashore, H.G. (1951). Differences between Verbal and Performance IQs on the Wechsler Intelligence Scale for Children. *Journal of Consulting Psychology, 125*, 62–67.

Sherman, E., Strauss, E., Spellacy, F., & Hunter, M. (1995). Construct validity of WAIS-R factors: Neuropsychological test correlates in litigating head-injured adults. *Psychological Assessment, 7*, 440–444.

Silverstein, A.B. (1984). Pattern analysis: The question of abnormality. *Journal of Consulting and Clinical Psychology, 52*, 936–939.

Silverstein, A.B. (1990a). Short forms of individual intelligence tests. *Psychological Assessment, 2*, 3–11.

Silverstein, A.B. (1990b). Notes on the reliability of Wechsler short forms. *Journal of Clinical Psychology, 46*, 194–196.

Slate, J.R., & Jones, C.H. (1990). Examiner errors on the WAIS-R: A source of concern. *The Journal of Psychology, 124*, 343–345.

Smith, G.E., Ivnik, R.J., Malec, J.F., Petersen, R.C., Kokmen, E., & Tangalos, E.G. (1994). Mayo cognitive factor scales: Derivation of a short battery and norms for factor scores. *Neuropsychology, 8*, 194–202.

Snow, W.G., Tierney, M.C., Zorzitto, M.L., Fisher, R.H., & Reid, D.W. (1989). WAIS-R test–retest reliability in a normal elderly sample. *Journal of Clinical and Experimental Neuropsychology, 11*, 423–428.

Sontag, L.W., Baker, L.T., & Nelson, V.O. (1958). Mental growth and personality development: A longitudinal study. *Monograph of the Society for Research in Child Development, 23*, No. 2.

Spruill, J. (1984). Wechsler Adult Intelligence Scale–Revised. In D. Keyser & R. Sweetland (Eds.), *Test Critiques*. Kansas City, Missouri: Test Corporation of America.

Troyer, A.K., Cullum, C.M., Smernoff, E.N., & Kozora, E. (1994). Age effects on block design:

Qualitative performance features and extended-time effects. *Neuropsychology, 8,* 95–99.

Trueblood, W. (1994). Qualitative and quantitative characteristics of malingered and other invalid WAIS-R and clinical memory data. *Journal of Clinical and Experimental Neuropsychology, 16,* 597–607.

Vernon, P.E. (1977). Final report on modification of WISC-R for Canadian use. *Canadian Psychological Association Bulletin, 5,* 5–7.

Vernon, P.A. (1984). Wechsler Intelligence Scale for Children–Revised. In D. Keyser & R. Sweetland (Eds.), *Test Critiques.* Kansas City, Missouri: Test Corporation of America.

Violato, C. (1984). Effects of Canadianization of American biased items on the WAIS and WAIS-R Information subtests. *Canadian Journal of Behavioral Science, 16,* 36–41.

Violato, C. (1986). Canadian version of the Information subtests of the Wechsler Tests of Intelligence. *Canadian Psychology, 27,* 69–74.

Waller, N.G., & Waldman, I.D. (1990). A reexamination of the WAIS-R factor structure. *Psychological Assessment, 2,* 139–144.

Ward, L.C., & Ryan, J.J. (1996). Validity and time saving in the selection of short forms of the Wechsler Adult Intelligence Scale–Revised. *Psychological Assessment, 8,* 69–72.

Ward, L.C., & Ryan, J.J. (1997). Validity of quick short forms of the Wechsler Adult Intelligence Scale—Revised with brain-damaged patients. *Archives of Clinical Neuropsychology, 12,* 63–69.

Wechsler, D. (1989). *Wechsler Preschool and Primary Scale of Intelligence–Revised.* New York: Psychological Corporation.

Wechsler, D. (1974). *Wechsler Intelligence Scale for Children–Revised.* New York: Psychological Corporation.

Wechsler, D. (1981). *Wechsler Adult Intelligence Scale–Revised.* New York: Psychological Corporation.

Wechsler, D. (1991). *Wechsler Adult Intelligence Scale–III.* New York: Psychological Corporation.

Wechsler, D. (1996). *WISC-III Manual. Canadian Supplement.* Toronto: Psychological Corporation.

Weiss, L.G. (1995). WISC-III IQs: New norms raise queries. *Assessment Focus, 1,* 1–6.

Wielkiewicz, R.M. (1990). Interpreting low scores on the WISC-R third factor: It's more than distractibility. *Psychological Assessment, 2,* 91–97.

Yamashita, H., Hirono, N., Ikeda, M., Ikejiri, Y., Imamura, T., Shimomura, T., & Mori, E. (1997). Examining the diagnostic utility of the Fuld cholinergic deficit profile on the Japanese WAIS-R. *Journal of Clinical and Experimental Neuropsychology, 19,* 300–304.

Zillmer, E.A., Waechtler, C., Harris, B., & Khan, F. (1992). The effects of unilateral and multifocal lesions on the WAIS-R: A factor analytic study of stroke patients. *Archives of Clinical Neuropsychology, 7,* 29–40.

WAIS-R NI

Other Test Names

This measure is also called the WAIS-R as a Neuropsychological Instrument.

Purpose

The purpose of this supplement is to provide quantified process information in the form of additional scores for each of the standard subtests of the WAIS-R.

Source

This supplement to the WAIS-R is available from The Psychological Corporation, 555 Academic Court, San Antonio, TX 78204-2498, at a cost of $331 US. In Canada, the kit can be ordered from The Psychological Corporation, 55 Horner Avenue, Toronto, Ontario, M5Z 4X6, at a cost of $525 Cdn. Note that it is nec-essary to have the WAIS-R Complete Set in order to administer the WAIS-R NI.

Description

The WAIS-R NI (Kaplan, Fein, Morris, & Delis, 1991) was designed to provide a quantified method of documenting qualitative aspects of performance on the WAIS-R. The underlying rationale is that such a method would allow a more subtle and sensitive differentiation among clinical conditions and would provide for more effective therapeutic interventions. In order to identify problem-solving strategies and particular cognitive deficits, the authors found it necessary to alter the standard administration and scoring of most of the WAIS-R subtests. The authors indicate that, wherever possible, standard administration and scoring of the WAIS-R have been pre-

Subtest	Modification
Information	Discontinue rule is not followed; multiple-choice version administered later.
Picture Completion	Time limit not observed; discontinue rule need not be followed.
Digit Span	Discontinue rule is not followed. Sequencing, perseverations, substitutions, additions, and omissions may be scored.
Picture Arrangement	In Method 1, time limit is not observed; discontinue rule need not be followed. In Method 2, client is asked to tell a story for each of his or her arrangements. Sequencing is scored.
Vocabulary	Vocabulary Multiple Choice pages in WAIS-R NI Stimulus Booklet may be used; discontinue rule need not be followed. Multiple-choice version administered later.
Block Design	Extra blocks provided; discontinue rule is not followed. Client is asked to judge correctness of his or her constructions. Client is then presented with WAIS-R NI Stimulus Booklet (grid) version of each failed design.
	Order of construction is recorded. Single-block and configurational errors are scored. Percentage of total possible blocks correct is calculated.
Arithmetic	Time limit is not observed; discontinue rule need not be followed. Client is presented with WAIS-R NI Booklet (printed) version of failed itmes; for items then failed, paper and pencil are provided. Items still failed are presented in computational form found in WAIS-R NI Response Booklet.
Object Assembly	Three extra items have been added. In Method 1 time limit is not observed. In Method 2 time limit is not observed, and client is asked to identify object as soon as it is recognized. Order and strategy of assembly are recorded.
Comprehension	Items 12 and 14–15 are administered regardless of performance on other Comprehension items; multiple-choice version for each of these three items is administered later.
Digit Symbol	Client is asked to complete third row if it is not completed at the end of the time limit; Digit Symbol A (incidental learning: paired-and free-recall) is then administered.
Similarities	Discontinue rule need not be followed; multiple choice version is administered later.

Figure 5–5. Summary of subtest administration modifications. Adapted from Kaplan et al., 1991 (page 5) and D. Slick (personal communication, April 1992).

served so that scaled scores can be obtained in the customary manner. Fig. 5–5, adapted from Kaplan et al. (1991), provides a summary of the modifications to each of the WAIS-R subtests. Not all modifications need be used. The decision of whether or not to use the modification(s) for a given subtest depends upon the clinical picture, hypotheses, and questions concerning a particular client.

In addition, three new subtests may be given: Sentence Arrangement, Spatial Span, and Symbol Copy. Each item in Sentence Arrangement consists of a group of cards, with a single word on each card. The cards are presented in a given mixed-up order and the client is asked to arrange them in an order that makes good sense. The Spatial Span subtest (similar to the Corsi block test described by Milner, 1971) features 10 cubes randomly arranged on each half of a board. The client must touch blocks tapped by the examiner in the same order. Sequences of increasing length are given both forward and backward until the client's span is exceeded. Symbol Copy requires the client to copy as quickly as possible symbols into the boxes below them. The subtest features the same symbols found in the

WAIS-R Digit Symbol subtest and assesses perceptual and graphomotor speed.

Administration

See source. Briefly, the examiner asks test questions, displays the pictures or puzzles to the client, and records the client's responses in an individual response booklet. There is a suggested order of subtest administration; however, the examiner can depart from the standard order. Also, completion of all subtests in one session is not obligatory.

Scoring

In order to examine how a particular score is achieved, the client's oral responses are recorded verbatim. For the WAIS-R Performance subtests, the client's path toward solution of an item is recorded as well as response latency and time to completion. A quantified notation system is used to record the client's performance. This system includes noting sequencing processes, substitutions, intrusions and perseverations, overtime scores, and recording performance on multiple-choice versions. In addition, intrasubtest scatter is determined.

The authors state that scaled scores for most subtests can be derived. For example, the discontinue rules need not be followed and the client can be allowed to attempt additional items. In such a case, the subtest responses can be scored as if the discontinue rule had been followed with the successes achieved after the discontinue criterion not credited for purposes of computing scaled scores. Similarly, on timed subtests, the client can continue working on an item past the time limit, but the status of the response at the end of the time limit is used to obtain the scaled score. Kaplan et al. state that if Verbal and Performance IQ scores are needed, they can be derived from those subtests for which modifications in administration do not invalidate the score. A Verbal IQ score can be derived by using all the WAIS-R Verbal subtests. For a Performance IQ score, Picture Completion, Object Assembly (using Method 1; See Fig. 5–5), Picture Arrangement (using Method 1; See Fig. 5–5), and Digit Symbol Scores are recommended.

Comment

An important feature of the WAIS-R NI is that it allows clinicians the option of employing the process modifications on a subtest-by-subtest basis, following up specific hunches generated from observations of client performance on an as-needed basis. The manual is well-written. Instructions are clear and concise. The manual also provides useful clues or hypotheses regarding the presence of suspected cognitive dysfunction, the particular cognitive components affected, and the possible etiology associated with certain deficits.

The main problem with the WAIS-R NI is the lack of normative data (Slick et al., 1996). No data are provided on validity or reliability for any of the new subtests (i.e., Sentence Arrangement, Spatial Span, and Symbol Copy). Nor are normative data given for any of the modifications. In fact, the only norms that are provided are for intrasubtest scatter. These were derived from the original WAIS-R normative sample based upon standard discontinuation rules and therefore should not be

applied to overtime scores. In short, while the WAIS-R NI allows clinicians to systematically quantify both finer-grained aspects of client performance, it leaves them with little basis for meaningful interpretation of their data (Slick et al., 1996).

Another concern relates to the derivation of standard scores. For example, allowing a client to go over the time limit on Picture Completion items may affect performance on later items. The normative sample did not benefit from such a procedure, and therefore derivation of a standard score is questionable.

Of concern also is the possible enhancement of practice effects that may result from additional learning opportunities provided by new procedures (e.g., overtime, multiple choice) when clients are retested with the WAIS-R after they have been given the WAIS-R NI. No test–retest data are currently available for brain-damaged populations. Slick et al. (1996) gave the WAIS-R NI to normal subjects and retested them with the WAIS-R three to four weeks later. No significant differences were found between Wechsler's subjects and those in the Slick et al. study in terms of amount of scaled score gain at retest. On the other hand, normal subjects performed more poorly on many multiple-choice items than on corresponding standard items, suggesting that the multiple-choice items may need to be revised, or that caution should be exercised in viewing the multiple-choice items as easier than the standard ones.

Kaplan et al. (1991) hypothesized that elderly people display a "warming-up" pattern on the Digit Symbol subtest when performance is recorded at 30, 60, and 90 seconds. Paolo et al. (1994), however, reported that while some elderly people display the "warming-up" pattern, it is not the most frequent pattern and cannot be considered characteristic of persons 75 years and older.

In short, the WAIS-R NI is potentially of great clinical value. Additional studies are, however, required. In particular, it requires its own comprehensive norms.

Normative Data

Table 5–49 provides some normative data (Slick et al., 1996). The values are based on a

Table 5—49. Raw Scores for WAIS-R NI Subtests (SD in Parentheses)

Information	20.90 (4.55)
Information Raw Scatter	7.90 (4.02)
Information Multiple Choice	21.45 (4.51)
Block Design	38.35 (7.16)
Block Design Scatter	8.79 (5.16)
Object Assembly[a]	32.70 (4.84)
Object Assembly New Items	18.00 (.00)
Picture Arrangement	15.80 (2.61)
Picture Arrangement Scatter	5.80 (3.46)
Similarities	23.85 (1.79)
Similarities Multiple Choice	26.10 (1.80)
Similarities Multiple Choice Scatter	3.10 (2.95)
Vocabulary	56.30 (6.94)
Vocabulary Scatter	14.35 (5.57)
Vocabulary Multiple Choice	51.95 (5.52)
Vocabulary Multiple Choice Scatter	20.20 (4.43)

Source: Slick et al., 1996.

[a] New items were not included.

small sample ($n = 20$) of university students (mean education = 15.8 years), ages 20–44 years (mean age = 25.95 years). Discontinue rules were not followed for the subtests. For timed tasks, the values noted in Table 5–49 reflect scores obtained at standard time cutoffs.

References

Kaplan, E., Fein, D., Morris, R., & Delis, D.C. (1991). *WAIS-R NI Manual.* San Antonio, TX: Psychological Corporation.

Milner, B. (1971). Interhemispheric differences in the localization of psychological processes in man. *British Medical Bulletin, 27,* 272–277.

Paolo, A.M., & Ryan, J.J. (1994). WAIS-R Digit Symbol patterns for persons 75 years and older. Paper presented to the International Neuropsychological Society, Cincinnati, Ohio.

Slick, D., Hopp, G., Strauss, E., Fox, D., Pinch, D., & Stickgold, K. (1996). Effects of prior testing with the WAIS-R NI on subsequent retest with the WAIS-R. *Archives of Neurology, 11,* 123–130.

WONDERLIC PERSONNEL TEST

Purpose

The purpose of this test is to obtain a brief measure of intellectual functioning.

Source

The test (manual and 25 test forms) can be obtained from Wonderlic Personnel Test, Inc., 1509 N. Milwaukee Ave., Libertyville, IL 60048, at a cost of $65 US. The test has been translated into a number of different languages, including French and Spanish. Large-print versions of the test are available from the publisher for administration to visually impaired subjects. Braille and audio versions are also available.

Description

The Wonderlic Personnel Test (WPT) is a brief, 50-item, pencil-and-paper test of "problem-solving ability" used primarily by business and governmental organizations to evaluate job applicants for employment and occupational training (Wonderlic, 1992). It can be viewed as a measure of general intelligence since its items are based on the original Otis Test of Mental Ability and since scores correlate well with measures of aptitude and intelligence (see Comment section). There are 12 alternate forms of the WPT.

The questions include word comparisons, disarranged sentences, following of directions, number comparisons, number series, analysis of geometric figures, and story problems requiring either math or logic solutions. Questions are arranged in order of increasing difficulty.

Administration

The test can be given individually or in a group situation. Clients need approximately a 6th-grade reading level to take the test. Clients are asked to read the test instructions and complete the sample questions provided on the cover of the test booklet. A 12-minute period is provided for the client to write, underline, or circle the answer to the test question.

Although the test was designed to be administered as a timed test, the Wonderlic can also be administered as an untimed test. In this case, the examiner begins testing as if it were a regular, timed test. At the end of the timed 12-minute period, the examiner collects the client's pencil and gives the client a new one of a different color. In this way, the examiner can compute both a timed and an untimed score.

Approximate Time for Administration

The test takes 12 minutes to administer.

Scoring

The test score is the total number of questions answered correctly in the 12-minute period. Scoring is accomplished by matching the answers on the test sheet with the answers on a scoring key. Scores are then adjusted for the age of the applicant by adding points to the number of raw scores (the total number of correct answers) according to a table provided in the Wonderlic manual. There is some evidence that the age correction fails to adequately correct for age differences (Edinger et al., 1985; Rosenstein & Glickman, 1994).

Comment

Estimates of internal consistency (odd–even, KR-20) are high (.87–.94) (McKelvie, 1989; Wheeless & Serpento, cited in Wonderlic, 1992). Test–retest reliability, both over the short and long term, is also reported to be high (above .8) (Dodrill, 1983; McKelvie, 1992; Wonderlic, 1992). There are slight differences in difficulty level across forms. Alternate form reliabilities, when corrected for level of difficulty, range from .72 to .95 (Wonderlic, 1992).

Scores on the WPT correlate fairly well (.56–.80) with the cognitive or Aptitude G scale of the General Aptitude Battery (GATB) and very highly (.75 to .96) with Full Scale IQ scores from the Wechsler Intelligence Scale (see Wonderlic, 1992, for a recent review).

The Wonderlic appears to provide as good an estimate of Wechsler FSIQ as an estimation based on an addition of Block Design and Vocabulary subtest scores, at least in psychiatric populations (Hawkins et al., 1990). In patients referred for evaluation of possible traumatic brain injury, the Block Design/Vocabulary short form appears more suitable (Saltzman et al., submitted). Although the correlations between the Wonderlic and WAIS/WAIS-R Full Scale IQ are relatively high, the correlations may not be sufficiently high to conclude that it is an adequate substitute measure of intelligence. Clinically, the utility for the Wonderlic has been evaluated by examining the proportion of the participant sample for which the Wonderlic predicted WAIS/WAIS-R FSIQ within 10 IQ points. Dodrill (1981) considered that a discrepancy of more than 10 IQ points between Wonderlic predicted IQ and obtained WAIS/WAIS-R FSIQs constituted a significant error. Classification rates for the proportion of Wonderlic IQ scores that have predicted Wechsler FSIQs within 10 IQ points have ranged from 94 percent of the participants (psychiatric inpatients; Dodrill and Warner, 1988) to 71 percent of the participant sample (psychiatric inpatients; Edinger et al., 1985). Carswell and Snow (1996) reported that in eighty individuals with known or suspected head injury, Wonderlic IQs (adjusted for the WAIS-R by subtracting seven points) predicted WAIS-R FSIQs within ten points for 78 percent of the sample. That is, more than 20 percent of participants had a discrepancy of at least 10 IQ points between Wonderlic IQ and WAIS-R FSIQ. Similar results were obtained by Saltzman et al. (submitted) in a sample of 129 individuals with suspected head injury.

Correlations are quite low with personality tests, suggesting that the Wonderlic Test does not measure personality variables. Correlations between test scores and academic or job performance are modest in size, suggesting that the Wonderlic measures, at least to a limited extent, the characteristics necessary for either classroom performance or employment.

The Wonderlic is often used when adults are familiar with the Wechsler test or when time constraints are a concern. One should note, however, that while the Wonderlic Personnel Test does provide a gross estimate of IQ, it does not provide a sufficiently adequate substitute for the WAIS-R in a clinical setting. Furthermore, it does not direct itself to various types of intelligence or functional deficiencies, such as verbal or visuospatial abilities. An additional disadvantage of this test is that it does not provide for the detailed observations that can be made during the administration of a test such as the WAIS-R. If such information is required, other tests should be administered (Dodrill, 1981; Hawkins et al., 1990; Saltzman et al., submitted).

Several other points deserve mention. First, the test should not be given to individuals with poor reading or visuospatial skills (Hawkins et al., 1990; Dodrill, 1981). Second, because various neurological conditions tend to reduce speed, both the timed and untimed scores should be evaluated. Third, the Wonderlic may be somewhat more reflective of a person's habitual motivational status since it requires the client to complete the test alone without the constant prompting given in such measures as the Wechsler test (Dodrill, 1981). Thus, the Wonderlic may be a more pertinent measure of the ability to respond to the unstructured demands of everyday living (Hawkins et al., 1990). It may also be the measure of choice when the presence of an examiner may elicit significant anxiety, distractability, or withdrawal (Hawkins et al., 1990). Further, the existence of several alternate forms makes it a potentially useful instrument for serial evaluations. Because it is brief, however, the test should not be used to pinpoint specific deficiencies or sources of change (Hawkins et al., 1990). Finally, although limited in its ability to accurately estimate FSIQ on a case-by-case basis, the test may prove an adequate screening measure for research purposes.

Normative Data

Normative data were derived from a large group (n = 118,549) of job applicants. Timed scores are age-adjusted since speed of cognitive processing is believed to be reduced with advancing age. Because there is no limit on untimed scores, there is no age adjustment for

these values. Untimed scores tend to be about 6 points higher than timed scores for those individuals who score under 30 (Wonderlic, 1992). Thus, the untimed score less six points can be used to estimate the client's cognitive level.

Scores are evaluated with reference to the entire normative sample or against established averages that have been identified for most occupations and for all levels of education (see source). Age-corrected WAIS-R equivalent scores can also be computed by using Dodrill's (1981) Wonderlic-to-WAIS conversion table (provided in the Wonderlic manual) and then subtracting 8 points from this result (Frisch & Jessop, 1989). The subtraction is based on Wechsler's (1981) finding that WAIS-R Full Scale IQ scores are, on the average, about 8 points lower than WAIS FSIQs. Unfortunately, adequate Wonderlic-to-WAIS-R conversion tables are not available. Although some have found that Wechsler/Wonderlic scores tend to be within 10 points of each other (Dodrill and Warner, 1988) others report that Wonderlic scores misclassify about 30 per cent of participants using Dodrill's criterion of ± 10 IQ points (Edinger et al., 1985; Carswell & Snow, 1996; Saltzman et al., submitted). This may be less of a problem when only gross estimates of IQ are necessary.

References

Carswell, L.M., & Snow, W.G. (1996). An examination of potential alternative measures of WAIS-R FSIQ. Paper presented to the American Psychological Association, Toronto, Canada.

Dodrill, C.B. (1981). An economical method of evaluation of general intelligence. *Journal of Consulting and Clinical Psychology*, 49, 668–673.

Dodrill, C.B. (1983). Long-term reliability of the Wonderlic Personnel Test. *Journal of Consulting and Clinical Psychology*, 51, 316–317.

Dodrill, C.B., & Warner, M.H. (1988). Further studies of the Wonderlic Personnel Test as a brief measure of intelligence. *Journal of Consulting and Clinical Psychology*, 56, 145–147.

Edinger, J.D., Shipley, R.H., Watkins, C.E., & Hammett, E.B. (1985). Validity of the Wonderlic Personnel Test as a brief IQ measure in psychiatric patients. *Journal of Consulting and Clinical Psychology*, 53, 937–939.

Frisch, M.B., & Jessop, N.S. (1989). Improving WAIS-R estimates with the Shipley-Hartford and Wonderlic Personnel Tests: Need to control for reading ability. *Psychological Reports*, 65, 923–928.

Hawkins, K.A., Faraone, S.V., Pepple, J.R., Seidman, L.J., & Tsuang, M.T. (1990). WAIS-R validation of the Wonderlic Personnel Test as a brief intelligence measure in a psychiatric sample. *Psychological Assessment*, 2, 198–201.

McKelvie, S.J. (1989). The Wonderlic Personnel Test: Reliability and validity in an academic setting. *Psychological Reports*, 65, 161–162.

McKelvie, S.J. (1992). Does memory contaminate test–retest reliability? *Journal of General Psychology*, 119, 59–72.

Rosenstein, R., & Glickman, A.S. (1994). Type size and performance of the elderly on the Wonderlic Personnel Test. *Journal of Applied Gerontology*, 13, 185–192.

Saltzman, J., Strauss, E., Hunter, M., & Spellacy, F. (submitted). Validity of the Wonderlic Personnel Test as a brief measure of intelligence in individuals referred for evaluation of head injury.

Wechsler, D. (1981). *The Wechsler Adult Intelligence Scale–Revised*. New York: The Psychological Corporation.

Wonderlic, E.F. (1992). *Manual of the Wonderlic Personnel Test and Scholastic Level Exam* II: Libertyville, IL: Wonderlic Personnel Test, Inc.

6

Cognitive Tests for Children

The neuropsychological examination of children has only recently been fully developed (Holmes-Bernstein & Waber, 1990; Tramontana & Hooper, 1988). For the most part, downward extensions of the adult examination have been common; e. g., Reitan's "intermediate" battery for age 9 to 14, and his "children's" battery for ages 5–8; the Luria-Nebraska Neuropsychological Battery for Children for ages 8–12 (adapted from Christensen & Munksgaard, 1981; Golden, 1987); Wechsler's WISC-III and WPPSI-R; the Kaufman Brief Test of Intelligence for the age range of 4–90 years. A new addition is the Kaufman Adolescent and Adult Intelligence Test, suitable for age 11 to 85+ years (Kaufman and Kaufman, 1997). Such extensions are included in the general section of each test if described in this manual.

Downward extensions are not always appropriate because item pools designed for adults may not be appropriate for children, and because the test may make different requirements on a child versus an adult; for example, a cognitive test may pose primary visual, reading, or constructional problems for the child. For these reasons, even a highly simplified version of a test designed for adults may not be measuring similar functions. As a result, the functional significance of clusters of tests developed for adults and their interpretation may be different and needs to be explored for each age (Rourke & Adams, 1984). The construction of tests specifically designed for children would be preferable, but this has been accomplished only for a few tests.

Even more serious is the lack of neuropsychological tests suitable for children under the age of 5 years. The behavioral repertoire of the younger child is, of course, more limited, and the test-taking attitude less developed the younger the child is. As a result, traditional "developmental" or intelligence tests are usually the only ones available for that age, although parts of such tests could well serve as tests of specific neuropsychological functions if they were further developed psychometrically (Aylward, 1988). For such development, newborn assessment methods such as the Dubowitz (Dubowitz et al., 1970) and the Brazelton (1973) scale, and infant and child tests such as the Bayley, the Uzgiris-Hunt (1975; Dunst, 1980), and the Gesell (Knobloch et al., 1980) scales may provide a good starting point.

Our selection of tests specifically designed for children includes three general measures of developmental assessment: the Bayley Scale (Bayley, 1993), primarily designed for the age range from 2 months to 2 years; the Stanford-Binet Scale (Thorndike, Hagen, & Sattler, 1986), covering the age from 2 to 5 years (although it extends up to 18 years); and the Kaufman ABC (Kaufman & Kaufman, 1983), designed for ages 2 years, 6 months, to 12 years, 6 months, which is included because it offers a selection of tests designed along a neuropsychological theoretical model. A newcomer, the NEPSY (Korkman et al., 1997), specifically designed for the neuropsychological evaluation of children aged 3 to 12 years and based on Luria's clinical investigations, has been developed in Finland and Sweden for some time (Korkman, 1988), but is only now becoming available in English, and is as yet not available for review.

Readers working with children who have school problems may also wish to consider the Woodcock-Johnson Test of Cognitive Ability (Woodcock & Mather, 1989) which has an age range from 2 to 90 years, but so far has been used only with school-age populations without a specific neuropsychological approach, supplementing the Woodcock-Johnson Achievement test battery described elsewhere in this volume.

References

Aylward, G.P. (1988). Infant and early childhood assessment. In M.G. Tramontana & Hooper (Eds.), *Assessment Issues in Child Neuropsychology.* New York: Plenum, pp. 225–248.

Bayley, N. (1993). *Bayley Scales of Infant Development* (2nd ed.). San Antonio, TX: Psychological Corporation.

Brazelton, T.B. (1973). Neonatal Behavioral Assessment Scale. *Clinics in Developmental Medicine, #50.* Philadelphia: Lippincott.

Christensen, A., & Munksgaard, F. (1981). *Luria's Neuropsychological Investigations.* Copenhagen: Aalborg Stiftsbogtrykkeri.

Dubowitz, L.M.S., Dubowitz, V., & Goldberg, C. (1970). Clinical assessment of gestational age in the newborn infant. *Journal of Pediatrics, 77,* 1.

Dunst, C.J. (1980). *A Clinical and Educational Manual for Use with the Uzgiris and Hunt Scales of Infant Psychological Development.* Baltimore: University Park Press.

Golden, C.J. (1987). *Luria-Nebraska Neuropsy-*

chological Battery: Children's Revision. Los Angeles: Western Psychological Services.

Holmes-Bernstein, J., & Waber, D.P. (1990). Developmental neuropsychological assessment. In A. Boulton, G.B. Baker, & M. Hiscock (Eds.), *Neuromethods, Vol. 17: Neuropsychology.* Clifton, NJ: Humana Press.

Kaufman, A.S. & Kaufman, N.L. (1983). *K-ABC: Kaufman Assessment Battery for Children.* Circle Pines, MN: American Guidance Service.

Kaufman, A.S. & Kaufman, N.L. (1997). *KAIT: Kaufman Adolescent and Adult Intelligence Test.* Circle Pines, MN: American Guidance Service.

Knobloch, H., Stevens, F., & Malone, A.F. (1980). *Manual of Developmental Diagnosis.* New York: Harper & Row.

Korkman, M. (1988). NEPSY—An adaptation of Luria's investigation for young children. *The Clinical Neuropsychologist, 2,* 375–392.

Korkman, M., Kirk, U., & Kamp, S. (1997). *NEPSY.* San Antonio, TX: Psychological Corporation.

Rourke, B.P., & Adams, K.M. (1984). Quantitative approaches to the neuropsychological assessment of children. In R.E. Tarter & G. Goldstein (Eds.), *Advances in Clinical Neuropsychology,* Vol. 2. New York: Plenum.

Thorndike, R.L., Hagen, E. P., & Sattler, J.M. (1986). *Stanford-Binet Intelligence Scale* (4th ed.). Chicago: Riverside Publishing Company.

Tramontana, M.G., & Hooper, S.R. (eds.) (1988). *Assessment Issues in Child Neuropsychology.* New York: Plenum.

Uzgiris, I.C., & Hunt, J.McV. (1975). *Assessment in Infancy: Ordinal Scales of Psychological Development.* Urbana, Ill.: University of Illinois Press.

Woodcock, R.W., & Mather, N. (1989). *Tests of Cognitive Ability: Standard and Supplemental Batteries.* Allen, TX: DLM Teaching Resources.

BAYLEY SCALES OF INFANT DEVELOPMENT—SECOND EDITION (BSID-II)

Purpose

The purpose is the assessment of mental, motor, and behavioral development of children between the age of 1 month and 2½ years.

Source

The Bayley Scales of Infant Development–II can be ordered from the Psychological Corporation, P.O. Box 9954, San Antonio, TX 78204-0354. A complete kit with manual, 25

Record Forms, Motor Scale Forms, and Behavior Rating Scale Forms, Stimulus Cards, and other necessary manipulatives costs $760 US. In Canada, it can be ordered from 55 Horner Ave., Toronto, Ont. M8Z 4X6, for $1140 Cdn.

Description

This test (Bayley, 1969; 2nd ed., 1993) is an offshoot of the Gesell scales developed originally in 1933, which has gone through several revisions and appears to be the most popular and well-established infant test for placement purposes (Damarin, 1978, Lehr et al., 1987). The age range of the BSID-II has been expanded down to 1 month and up to 2½ years. The BSID consists of three parts:

1. The mental development scale assessing sensory-perceptual acuity, discrimination and ability to respond, object constancy, memory, learning, problem solving, vocalization, early verbal communication, the beginnings of abstract thinking (generalizations and classifications), habituation, complex language, and mathematical concept formation; for each 1- or 2-month age level between 20 and 30 items are provided;
2. The motor development scale, measuring degree of body control, coordination of larger muscles, hand and finger manipulative skills, dynamic movement and praxis, postural imitation, and stereognosis (between 15 and 18 items for each age level);
3. The 30-item infant behavior rating scale (IBRS), including behavior ratings of the child's motor quality, attention/arousal, orientation/engagement, and emotional regulation.

Administration

For details, see manual. Items for both development scales are numbered according to difficulty level corresponding to basal and ceiling age expectations. They are coded to alert the examiner to previous items in the series requiring similar skills or using the same objects; for example, item 7 requires that the child respond to and then habituate to the sound of the rattle; item 8 requires that the child show discrimination between the sound of a bell and a rattle.

As in the Binet method, items are organized according to age level. A "basal level," i.e., the level at which five or more items of a given age are passed, and a "ceiling level" at which three consecutive items are missed, are established, and all items between these two levels are tested. Experienced examiners may observe and score many responses incidentally without formal testing.

Testing is conducted under optimal condi-

tions, that is, when the infant is fully alert, in the presence of the mother, and with constant encouragement (see manual). The first set of items is administered with the child lying in a crib or on a comfortable supporting surface. If the child loses interest, the examiner may switch to other novel items, although as a rule the mental development scale is administered first.

The Behavior Rating Scale is filled in immediately after completion of the test and uses a 5-point rating for each item appropriate for the age of the child. Items range from parental assessments of the test session and test adequacy, to ratings of arousal, affect, persistence, fearfulness, and hyperactivity.

Approximate Time for Administration

The test takes an average of 45 minutes. This may vary considerably depending on the experience of the examiner, the choice of an appropriate basal level, and the variability of the child's responses.

Scoring

The raw score for each scale is the number of items passed between basal and ceiling level, plus all items below the basal level. This score is converted into a mental (MDI) and psychomotor (PDI) developmental index based on the child's exact age (corrected for prematurity if necessary) by using the appropriate tables in the manual. Scoring of specific clusters (e.g., five clusters, Kohen-Raz, 1967; seven clusters, Yarrow et al. 1982) has been described for the old Bayley, but has not yet been replicated with the Bayley-II.

Testing and scoring requires considerable experience with the test and with the age group of children, but can be done by a psychometrist under supervision.

Comment

The BSID-II has been improved by the age extensions described above, the addition of many items, and the deletion of some nonworking items to meet some of the criticisms leveled against the earlier version (LeTendre et al., 1992). Administration and scoring techniques follow the pattern of previous editions of the test. They have been well documented in the manual, and standardized on a new sample of 1,700 normal children. Coefficient alpha reliability is reported as .88 for the MDI and .84 for the PDI. The two scales correlate .44 with each other (not surprisingly since item assignment to one or the other of the two scales was based on the judgment of nine experts). Test–retest agreements after 6 months were reported as .83 for the mental scale, and as .77 for the motor scale; Cook et al. (1989) found reliability values of .71 and .69 at 6 and 12 months in high-risk infants.

Concurrent, construct, and discriminant validity for the MDI and PDI are good (based partly on studies with the old Bayley Scale). Concurrent validity of the new edition with various other scales (e.g., WPPSI-R, McCarthy Scales of Children's Ability, Preschool Language Scale) were tested with small samples and found satisfactory (.49 for Preschool Language Scales, .79 with McCarthy Scales, and .73 with WPPSI for the MDI). The new edition also provides studies with small clinical samples for premature, HIV-infected, prenatally drug-exposed children, and children with asphyxia at birth, developmental delay, chronic otitis media, autism, and Down syndrome: Both the MDI and the PDI showed the expected impairment (e.g., Down syndrome 58.6 and 55.2), except otitis media for which such impairment has not been found consistently (Spreen, Risser, & Edgell, 1995). These data may be helpful for clinicians looking for a particular syndrome, although the restriction of results to MDI and PDI scores is not as informative as might be expected. A new study, investigating differences between three age groups of Haitian, Vietnamese, and Quebecois infants (Pomerleau et al., 1994) found only one difference on the motor scale between the three cultural groups, while scoring with the Kohen-Raz cluster detected two differences between boys and girls, and scoring with the Yarrow clusters detected cultural differences in all three age groups. The authors conclude that the Yarrow's cluster scoring is more sensitive than the Bayley scoring. Unfortunately, the cluster scoring has not been extended to the Bayley-II as yet.

In general, predictive validity with infant tests for later IQ scores has been shown to be poor, but increasing with age (Bayley, 1970). Ramey et al. (1973) found for children in a relatively constant environment (i.e., attending the same day-care center) that the MDI became more predictive with age (i.e., the MDI at age 6–8, 9–12, and 13–16 months correlated with Stanford-Binet IQ at 3 years at a level of .49, .71, and .90 respectively, and with the Illinois Test of Psycholinguistic Abilities (ITPA) at a level of .21, .68, and .81) while the PDI decreased in predictive power (.77, .56, and .43, respectively, for the Stanford-Binet, and .73, .74, and .48 for the ITPA, respectively). A follow-up of a cohort of 200 children (Shapiro et al., 1989) from age 13 months to 7 1/2 years indicated poor sensitivity and specificity for predicting giftedness.

The usefulness of the IBRS, on the other hand, is limited because of its brevity, based only on observations during testing. Factor analytic studies with the older version have found test affect, test attention, and arousal factors (Kaplan et al. 1991). According to the 1993 manual, concurrent validity studies with other infant rating scales have been inconsistent. As the IBRS reflects optimal behavioral functioning during the test session, a modest but positive relationship between IBRS and MDI has been observed (Braungart et al., 1992). A modest predictive validity of the task orientation factor of the IBRS with infant IQ has also been found (DiLalla et al. 1990). High-risk and neurologically impaired infants typically score lower on the IBRS.

The author stresses that only the MDI and PDI summary scores should be used in interpreting test results, and that failure on a particular cluster of items (e.g., language) "should not be used as a measure of deficit in a specific skill area" (p. 4). This is a regrettable limitation of the Bayley, but the construction of the test in the Binet fashion does not provide for a similar cluster of items to appear at every age level, a prerequisite for the measurement of particular strengths and weaknesses.

Normative Data

Detailed normative data, based on a new sample of 1,700 normal children, representative of the geographic, ethnic, and socioeconomic characteristics of the 1991–92 U.S. census, are available in the manual. These are welcome because the norms for the old Bayley were seriously outdated (Campbell et al., 1986). Unfortunately, no breakdown by gender, socioeconomic level of parents, and geographic or ethnic origin is provided. Consistent with the re-standardization of other test revisions, the BSID-II produced scores about 12 points lower than the older form of the test, as shown on a sample of 200 children who were examined with both tests.

Atkinson (1990) provided tables of significant differences between the BSID-II and the Vineland Scales of adaptive behavior that may contribute in deciding whether discrepancies between the two tests are due to chance or whether they represent real differences.

References

Atkinson, L. (1990). Intellectual and adaptive functioning: Some tables for interpreting the Vineland in combination with intelligence tests. *American Journal of Mental Retardation, 95,* 198–203.

Bayley, N. (1969). *Bayley Scales of Infant Development.* Manual. New York: Psychological Corporation.

Bayley, N. (1970). Development of mental abilities. In P.H. Mussen (Ed.), *Carmichael's Manual of Child Psychology* (3rd ed.). New York: Wiley.

Bayley, N. (1993). *Bayley Scales of Infant Development* (2nd ed.) (Bayley-II). San Antonio, TX: Psychological Corporation.

Braungart, J.M., Plomin, R., DeFries, J.C., & Fulker, D.W. (1992). Genetic influence on tester-rated infant temperament as assessed by Bayley's Infant Behavior Record: Nonadoptive and adoptive siblings and twins. *Developmental Psychology, 28,* 40–47.

Campbell, S.K., Siegel, E., & Parr, C.A. (1986). Evidence for the need to renorm the Bayley Scales of Infant Development based on the performance of a population-based sample of 12-month-old infants. *Topics in Early Childhood Special Education, 6,* 83–96.

Cook, M.J., Holder-Brown, L., Johnson, L.J., & Kilgo, J.L. (1989). An examination of the stability of the Bayley Scales of Infant Development with high-risk infants. *Journal of Early Intervention, 13,* 45–49.

Damarin, F. (1978). Bayley Scales of Infant Development. In O.K. Buros (Ed.), *The Eighth Mental Measurement Yearbook.* Vol. 1, pp. 290–293. Highland Park, NJ: Gryphon.

DiLalla, L.F., Thompson, L.A., Plomin, R., Phillips, K., Fagan, J.F., Haith, M.M., Cyphers, L.H., & Fulker, D.W. (1990). Infant predictors of preschool and adult IQ: A study of infant twins and their parents. *Developmental Psychology, 26,* 759–769.

Kaplan, M.G., Jacobson, S.W., & Jacobson, J.L. (1991). Alternative approaches to clustering and scoring the Bayley Infant Behavior Record at 13 months. Paper presented at the meeting of the Society for Research in Child Development. Seattle, WA.

Kohen-Raz, R. (1967). Scalogram analysis of some developmental sequences of infant behavior as measured by the Bayley infant scales of mental development. *Genetic Psychology Monographs, 76,* 3–21.

Lehr, C.A., Ysseldyke, J.E., & Thurlow, M.L. (1987). Assessment practices in model early childhood special education programs. *Psychology in the Schools, 24,* 390–399.

LeTendre, D., Spiker, D., Scott, D.T., & Constantine, N.A. (1992). Establishing the "ceiling" on the Bayley Scales of Infant Development at 25 months. *Advances in Infancy Research, 7,* 187–198.

Pomerleau, A., Leahey, L., & Mulcuit, G. (1994). Evaluation du developpement de l'enfant au cours de la premiere annee: l'utilisation de regroupements d'items du Bayley. *Canadian Journal of Behavioural Science, 26,* 85–103.

Ramey, C.T., Campbell, F.A., & Nicholson, J.E. (1973). The predictive power of the Bayley Scales of Infant Development and the Stanford-Binet Intelligence Test in a relatively constant environment. *Child Development, 44,* 790–795.

Shapiro, B.K., Palmer, F.B., Antell, S.E., Bilker, S., Ross, A., & Capute, A.J. (1989). Giftedness: Can it be predicted in infancy? *Clinical Pediatrics, 28,* 205–209.

Spreen, O., Risser, A.H., & Edgell, D. (1995). *Developmental Neuropsychology.* New York, NY: Oxford University Press.

Yarrow, L.J., Morgan, G.A., Jennings, K.D., et al. (1982). Infants' persistence at tasks: Relationship to cognitive functioning and early experience. *Infant Behavior and Development, 5,* 131–141.

KAUFMAN ASSESSMENT BATTERY FOR CHILDREN (K–ABC)

Purpose

This is an intelligence test for children between 2½ and 12½ years of age.

Source

The complete K–ABC kit (regular edition) can be ordered from American Guidance Service, Circle Pines, MN 55014 for $395.00 US, or from Psycan Corporation, P.O. Box 290, Station V, Toronto, Ont., M6R 3A5 for $620 Cdn., with plastic carrying case $745 Cdn. Administration videotape costs $95 US, $155 Cdn. The K–ABC ASSIST computer scoring manual and software cost $180 US, $295.00 Cdn.

Description

The Kaufman and Kaufman (1983) battery covers the age range from 2 years, 6 months to 12 years, 6 months and is the most recently developed intelligence test which, compared to the Stanford-Binet and the Wechsler Scales, follows a different theoretical model, and also incorporate six achievement subtests. Of the ten "mental processing" subtests (the core of the battery), seven are labeled "simultaneous" and three "sequential." Six (one sequential and four simultaneous subtests) are considered "nonverbal" and therefore especially suited for children with communication handicaps. The theoretical model adopted for the construction of this test is based on Das et al.'s (1979) notion of a sequential and simultaneous information processing dichotomy, which is claimed to be related to Luria's theoretical framework. A brief description of each of the subtests, the type of scale to which it belongs, and the age range for which it is used follows:

1. *Magic Window* (15 items, simultaneous): This subtest measures the ability of the child to identify and name an object (e.g., car, girl, snake) rotated behind a narrow slit, which allows only partial exposure of the picture at any time. It is essentially a vocabulary test for young children (Goldstein et al., 1986)

(age range: 2 years, 6 months to 4 years, 11 months).

2. *Face Recognition* (15 items, simultaneous): A face is exposed briefly, and the child must select the same face in a different pose from a group photograph (age range: 2 years, 6 months to 4 years, 11 months).

3. *Hand Movements* (21 items, sequential): The child must copy the exact sequence of taps on the table with the fist, palm, or side of hand as demonstrated by the examiner. The test is adapted from Luria (1980) (all ages).

4. *Gestalt Closure* (25 items, simultaneous): The child must name or describe an ink drawing that is only partially complete (similar to the Gestalt Completion Test by Street, 1931) (all ages).

5. *Number Recall* (19 items, sequential): This subtest is identical to other digit repetition tasks (all ages).

6. *Triangles* (18 items, simultaneous): The child must assemble several identical rubber triangles (blue on one side, yellow on the other) to match a picture of abstract design. The test is similar to Kohs' Block Design (age range 4 years to 12 years, 6 months).

7. *Word Order* (20 items, sequential): The child must point to silhouettes of common objects in the same order as the objects were named by the examiner. The test is similar to McCarthy's (1972) serial recall (age range 4 years to 12 years, 6 months).

8. *Matrix Analogies* (20 items, simultaneous): The child must select from an array the picture or design that best completes a 2 × 2 visual analogy. The test is similar to Raven's (1938) progressive matrices (age range 5 years to 12 years, 6 months).

9. *Spatial Memory* (21 items, simultaneous): The child must recall the location of pictures arranged randomly on a page (age range 5 years to 12 years, 6 months).

10. *Photo Series* (17 items, simultaneous): The child must arrange a series of photographs in proper time sequence. The test is similar to the Wechsler Picture Arrangement (age range 6 years to 12 years, 6 months).

11. *Expressive Vocabulary* (24 items, achievement): The child must name photo-

graphed objects correctly. The test is similar to the Peabody Picture Vocabulary Test (age range 2 years, 6 months to 4 years, 11 months).

12. *Faces and Places* (35 items, achievement): The child must name fictional characters, famous persons, or well-known places (e.g., Santa Claus, pyramids, liberty bell, Fidel Castro) (all ages). For non-U.S. users it should be noted that some items may be easier for children growing up in the United States.

13. *Arithmetic* (38 items, achievement): The task begins with simple counting, recognition of shapes (e.g., triangle), numbers, comparison of two counts, verbally enclosed arithmetic ("If four of the elephants walked away, how many would be left?"), including time concepts, centered around a family visit to the zoo (age range 3 years to 12 years, 6 months).

14. *Riddles* (32 items, achievement): The child must infer the name of a concrete or abstract concept from several given characteristics (e.g., "What has fur, wags its tail, and barks?", "What was used by ancient Egyptians, is carved in stone, and is a form of writing?") (age range 3 years to 12 years, 6 months).

15. *Reading/Decoding* (38 items, achievement): The test indicates the child's ability to identify letters and to read and pronounce words (age range 5 years to 12 years, 6 months).

16. *Reading/Understanding* (24 items, achievement): Reading comprehension is tested by acting out commands printed on plates (age range 7 years to 12 years, 6 months).

Not all tests are given to children of all ages; only seven subtests are administered to children 2 years, 6 months old, whereas 13 subtests are given to children from 7 years old to 12 years, 6 months old. With progressing age, some tests are phased out and others are added. The test comes in a durable box or carrying case. The test material is mounted on easels and consists of pages that can be flipped over by the examiner to move on to the next item to be shown to the subject, and which allow the examiner to read instructions on the

back of the page facing him or her. The test manual includes correct answers in English and Spanish; oral instructions are given in English.

Administration

See administration and scoring manual. The usual caution of extensive training in test administration applies. The "Individual Test Record" of 12 pages assists in both administration and scoring while the battery is administered. Teaching items are included in all mental processing subtests. Items for each age are arranged in units. As with the "basal level" in the Stanford-Binet, a starting age for each subtest is determined by the chronological age of the child, but may require going back to easier items. The examiner then proceeds until the "stopping point" (ceiling level) or the last item of a subtest is reached. Subtests are administered in a prearranged order, but flexibility is allowed if a child shows resistance or fatigue.

Approximate Time for Administration

The time required varies from 30 minutes for children 2 years, 6 months old to 75 minutes for children 7 years to 12 years, 6 months old.

Scoring

As with the Stanford-Binet, the raw score consists of the number of the ceiling item minus errors. This score can be translated into a scaled score with a mean of 10 and a standard deviation (SD) of 3 for mental processing subtests, and into standard scores with a mean of 100 and SD of 15 for achievement subtests. The sums of scaled scores for the sequential and the simultaneous sets of subtests, and the sum of both ("Mental Processing Composite") as well as the sum of achievement subtest standard scores can be converted into age-appropriate standard scores by using tables (at 2-month intervals up to age 6 years, 11 months). A special feature of this battery is the possibility of converting the sum of "nonverbal scales" (for children with communication impairment) into standard scores. Confidence levels for each subtest standard score and summary score can be entered into the scoring page of the test record. National percentile ranks and "sociocultural percentile ranks" (separate for blacks and whites) are also provided. Finally, age equivalents for the scaled score of each of the subtests can be obtained from the tables in the manual. Significant differences between subtests indicating strengths and weaknesses of the child can also be read directly from the appended table.

Comment

Split-half reliabilities range from .62 for Gestalt Closure for 7-year-olds to .92 for Triangles in 5-year-olds; internal consistency ranges from .84 to .97; 6-month retest reliability ranges from .72 to .95 (see source). Internal consistency for K-ABC composite and subtest scores were equivalent for 311 black and 1,450 white children aged 2 years, 6 months to 12 years, 6 months (Matazow et al., 1991). Matazow et al.'s study also reported reliability coefficients between .84 and .95; no significant difference between black and white children was found.

Validity has been investigated in 43 studies cited in the interpretive manual and in many additional studies (Kamphaus & Reynolds, 1987) and is based on factor-analytic, convergent, and discriminant validation (e.g., Hooper, 1986) and correlational studies, with generally positive results. Gridley et al. (1990) were unable to demonstrate separate simultaneous and sequential factors in a group of 122 at-risk preschoolers, although a general g-factor emerged in that study.

Correlations of the individual subtests with the Wechsler Intelligence Scale for Children (WISC-R) ranged from .27 to .66 (with the highest correlations for the achievement subtests), and with the Stanford-Binet IQ from .10 (for Gestalt Closure) to .68 (for Riddles). The three Global Scale scores correlated with the Stanford-Binet from .15 (for Simultaneous Processing in normal preschoolers) to .79 (for Achievement in normal kindergarten children), whereas high-risk preschoolers and gifted referrals showed somewhat lower correlations. The Test Composite/Mental Processing correlated .74 and the Achievement Composite .85 with the Stanford-Binet Fourth Edition in children with learning disabilities (Smith et al., 1989). Discriminant validity for hyperactivity was $-.51$ but was negligible in size for a child anxiety scale (Cooley & Ayres, 1985).

Hooper et al. (1988) reported a modest but significant correlation of .50 between the arithmetic achievement subtest and the corresponding part of the Woodcock-Johnson (W-J) Achievement Clusters in 80 children referred for special education evaluation; the correlations between reading–decoding and W-J reading was .88, between reading–understanding and W-J reading .80, and between riddles and W-J knowledge .58. Correlation between K-ABC Achievement and the Metropolitan Readiness Test in 99 preschool children was .49 (Zucker & Riordan, 1990), although the K-ABC was found to be significantly more difficult; the same study found that the K-ABC ACH predicted scores on the PPVT and the Boehm Test of Basic Concepts and its extension into preschool age one year later significantly ($r = .55, .64,$ and .61, respectively). Convergent validity of the mental processing scale with the Peabody Individual Achievement Test reading recognition and comprehension was .59 and .69, respectively (Cooley & Ayres, 1985).

Predictive validity for standard school achievement tests 12 months later was between .21 and .70 for the mental processing composite score in various groups, and between .34 and .84 for the achievement subtests. Worthington and Bening (1988) also noted that the Mental Processing Composite score predicted school achievement test scores more poorly in females than in males. Kline et al. (1992) investigated subtest scatter (shape and variability) and found that it did not show incremental validity over general elevation in predicting school achievement. K-ABC processing subtypes did not predict unique reading–spelling profiles in learning-disabled children (Kampa et al., 1988).

In addition to subtests familiar to most psychologists from other intelligence tests, the K-ABC strikes out into new territory by adding novel subtests (some adapted from the work of Das et al., 1979) and by using a new theoretical orientation along Das's formulations, forcing the clinician to rethink the concept of intelligence and the implications of this theory for educational and therapeutic practice. This has led to a "mixed" critical reception of the test as well as to numerous studies evaluating its merits. Salvia and Ysseldyke (1985) consider the orientation "quite revolutionary," ask for a "considerably larger base of research support" (p. 458), and recommend patience and skepticism. Jensen (1984) claims that the test does not measure anything different from the WISC-R or the Stanford-Binet.

Neuropsychologists may appreciate the theoretical orientation better, because the battery claims to have been constructed on the basis of neuropsychological theory (interpretative manual, p. 21) and is purported to break down into left (analytic-sequential) and right (gestalt-holistic-simultaneous) hemisphere functions, (Kaufman & Kaufman, 1983, pp. 28, 29, 232), and because it includes several subtests that are similar to specific neuropsychological tests. However, little evidence has been supplied so far that actually validates the neuropsychological implications of the sequential–simultaneous (left–right hemisphere) dimension. For example, Morris and Bigler (1987) found that K-ABC dimensions from 79 neurologically impaired children correlated with lesion localization inferred from other neuropsychological tests presumed to measure right- vs. left-hemisphere function rather than neurological and radiological data, although this approach relies on circular reasoning. Generally, the validity of this dimension rests on factor-analytic research, and even that has been questioned in replication studies that include other tests (Goetz & Hall, 1984; Goldstein et al., 1986; Strommen, 1988). The dichotomy has little if any foundation in Luria's theories about brain function, which speculated that the sequential–simultaneous dichotomy may also be related to the anterior–posterior dimensions of the brain (Luria, 1980); Sternberg (1984) accuses the test authors of misrepresenting Luria's work, and Donders (1992) warns that, while the K-ABC is "an attractive measure of g," caution is necessary when attributing specific

neuropsychological significance to this test; in his sample of 43 children with traumatic brain injury, the test did not discriminate these children better than the WISC-R from healthy controls. Sternberg also notes that all three sequential processing subtests and some of the simultaneous subtests contain an "overemphasis on rote learning" (p. 275), which he feels is inappropriate in an intelligence test and which most other tests avoid. Sternberg also suggests that the strong rote-learning component of the battery is a major reason for the lack of differences between ethnic groups reported in the manual and elsewhere (e.g., Whitworth & Chrisman, 1987).

Applegate and Kaufman (1989) suggested a short-form estimation of the sequential and simultaneous processing dimensions "for research and screening" purposes: Best predictors for the simultaneous dimension were Gestalt Closure, Triangles, and Matrix Analogies; for the sequential dimension, Number Recall and Word Order.

The addition of six achievement subtests to an intelligence test battery is also novel. Kaufman and Kaufman claim that the mental processing subtests measure fluid and the achievement subtests crystallized intelligence. Although this claim remains to be examined, the addition seems to create a "double-duty" test, replacing standard achievement tests to some extent. However, the limited number of items in the achievement subtests and the modest correlations with standard achievement tests would suggest that one cannot expect more than a superficial screening of the academic achievement level of the child. Hopkins and Hodge (1984) also point out that the achievement tests do not correspond to most other achievement tests because they are not closely related to the school curriculum.

Positive features of the construction of this test include the measurement of the ability to deal with novelty, the attempt to integrate an information-processing paradigm into basically psychometric testing approaches, the attempt to achieve culture-fairness by sampling minority and handicapped populations, and the attempt to ensure the subjects' task comprehension by including teaching items and explicit instructions (Sternberg, 1984). Attention level does influence the performce on this test, as indicated by correlations of .44 between the Mental Processing Score and the Continuous Performance Test (corresponding correlations of .49 with Sequential, .29 with Simultaneous, and .42 with Achievement Standard Scores) (Gordon et al., 1990).

For use in neuropsychological practice, it should be remembered that the K-ABC is not equivalent to the WPPSI-R, the WISC-III, or the Stanford-Binet-Fourth Edition. In fact, results may be quite different, as indicated by some of the studies of concurrent validity. Nor should the construction of the test along a two-factor dimension be translated into a simple right–left hemisphere dichotomy. This is also specifically stated in the interpretative manual (p. 21). Nevertheless, the test does offer a new approach to the testing of young children, so that the comparison of K-ABC results with those of other tests may provide additional insights. Alternatively, individual subtests may be used to supplement other tests. A single-subject-design study (Barry & Riley, 1987) demonstrated how one single subtest (fist-edge-palm test, i.e., Hand Movements) can be used for rehabilitation in adult acute head injury rehabilitation patients. The interpretative manual (pp. 36–57) provides a thoughtful discussion of each test, its background (including remarks on neuropsychological significance), and a "psychological analysis" listing specific abilities that are tapped by each subtest; reading this discussion may provide the clinician with a better understanding of how each subtest may contribute to the overall clinical profile of the client. The interpretative manual also contains useful comments on remediation in children with learning problems.

Normative Data

See interpretative and scoring manuals. The battery is well standardized, based on 1,981 children representing the 1980 U.S. census in terms of geographic region, sex, socioeconomic status, race or ethnic group, and community size, with samples of approximately 200 children for each year of age.

Table 6—1. Adult Norms for the Hand Movements Subtest

	Age (decade)				
	20s	30s	40s	50s	Total
Women					
M	17.7	17.1	15.3	13.4	15.9
SD	1.25	2.81	3.65	4.12	3.47
n	10	10	10	10	40
Men					
M	15.7	15.8	14.7	13.8	15.0
SD	3.27	2.66	3.13	1.87	2.80
n	10	10	10	10	40

Source: Barry & Riley, 1987.

Compared to the WISC-R, the K-ABC tends to overestimate IQ scores by about 3–5 points in the average range (Naglieri & Haddad, 1984) and by inference 4–13 points for the WISC-III; by 8 points in a Navajo children sample (Naglieri, 1984), and by 7 points in the mentally retarded range (Naglieri, 1985). For the Hand Movement subtest only, Barry and Riley (1987) presented adult norms (Table 6–1); both age and gender effects were significant. The obtained mean scores of 17 and 15 in the younger groups correspond to scaled scores of 10 and 12 in 12-year-olds, suggesting that no further improvement with age occurs on this subtest.

References

Applegate, B., & Kaufman, A.S. (1989). Short form estimation of the K-ABC sequential and simultaneous processing for research and screening. *Journal of Clinical Child Psychology, 18,* 305–313.

Barry, P., & Riley, J.M. (1987). Adult norms for the Kaufman Hand Movements Test and a single-subject design for acute brain injury rehabilitation. *Journal of Clinical and Experimental Neuropsychology, 9,* 449–455.

Cooley, E.J., & Ayres, R. (1985). Convergent and discriminant validity of the Mental Processing Scales of the Kaufman Assessment Battery for Children. *Psychology in the Schools, 22,* 373–377.

Das, J.P., Kirby, J.R., & Jarman, R.F. (1979). *Simultaneous and Successive Cognitive Processes.* New York: Academic Press.

Donders, J. (1992). Validity of the Kaufman Assessment Battery for Children when employed with children with traumatic brain injury. *Journal of Clinical Psychology, 48,* 225–230.

Goetz, E.T., & Hall, R.J. (1984). Evaluation of the Kaufman Assessment Battery for Children from an information-processing perspective. *Journal of Special Education, 18,* 281–296.

Goldstein, D.J., Smith, K.B., & Waldrep, E.E. (1986). Factor analytic study of the Kaufman Assessment Battery for Children. *Journal of Clinical Psychology, 42,* 890–894.

Gordon, M., Thomason, D., & Cooper, S. (1990). To what extent does attention affect K-ABC scores? *Psychology in the Schools, 27,* 144–147.

Gridley, B.E., Miller, G., Barke, C., & Fisher, W. (1990). Construct validity of the K-ABC with an at-risk preschool population. *Journal of School Psychology, 28,* 39–49.

Hooper, S.R. (1986). Performance of normal and dyslexic readers on the K-ABC: a discriminant analysis. *Journal of Learning Disability, 19,* 206–210.

Hooper, S.R., Brown, L.A., & Elia, F.A. (1988). A comparison of the K-ABC with the Woodcock-Johnson Test of Academic Achievement in a referred population. *Journal of Psychoeducational Assessment, 6,* 67–77.

Hopkins, K.D., & Hodge, S.E. (1984). Review of the Kaufman Assessment Battery (K-ABC) for Children. *Journal of Counselling and Development, 63,* 105–107.

Jensen, A.R. (1984). The Black-white difference on the K-ABC: Implications for future testing. *Journal of Special Education, 18,* 255–268.

Kampa, L., Humphries, T., & Kershner, J. (1988). Processing styles of learning-disabled children on the Kaufman Assessment Battery for Children (K-ABC) and their relationship to reading and spelling performance. *Journal of Psychoeducational Assessment, 6,* 242–252.

Kamphaus, R.W., & Reynolds, C.R. (1987). *Clinical and Research Applications of the K-ABC.* Circle Pines, MN: American Guidance Service.

Kaufman, A.S., & Kaufman, N.L. (1983). *K-ABC: Kaufman Assessment Battery for Children.* Circle Pines, MN: American Guidance Service.

Kline, R.B., Snyder, J., Guilmette, S., & Castellanos, M. (1992). Relative usefulness of elevation, variability, and shape information from WISC-R, K-ABC, and Fourth Edition Stanford-Binet profiles in predicting achievement. *Psychological Assessment, 4,* 426–432.

Luria, A. (1980). *Higher Cortical Functions in Man* (2nd ed.). New York: Basic Books.

Matazow, G.S., Kamphaus, R.W., Stanton, H.C., & Reynolds, C.R. (1991). Reliability of the Kaufman Assessment Battery for Children for black and white students. *Journal of School Psychology, 29,* 37–41.

McCarthy, D. (1972). *McCarthy Scales of Children's Abilities.* San Antonio, TX: The Psychological Corporation.

Morris, J.M., & Bigler, E.D. (1987). Hemispheric functioning and the Kaufman Assessment Battery for Children: Results in the neurologically impaired. *Developmental Neuropsychology, 3,* 67–79.

Naglieri, J.A. (1986). Concurrent and predictive validity of the Kaufman Assessment Battery for Children with a Navajo sample. *Journal of School Psychology, 22,* 373–379.

Naglieri, J.A. (1985). Use of the WISC-R and the K-ABC with learning disabled, borderline mentally retarded, and normal children. *Psychology in the Schools, 22,* 133–141.

Naglieri, J.A., & Haddad, F.A. (1984). Learning disabled children's performance on the Kaufman Assessment Battery for Children: A concurrent validation study. *Journal of Psychoeducational Assessment, 2,* 49–56.

Raven, J.C. (1938). *Progressive Matrices: A Perceptual Test of Intelligence.* Individual Form. Oxford: Psychologists Press Ltd.

Salvia, J., & Ysseldyke, J.E. (1985). *Assessment in Special and Remedial Education.* Boston: Houghton Mifflin.

Smith, D.K., St. Martin, M.E., & Lyon, M.A. (1989). A validity study of the Stanford-Binet: Fourth Edition with students with learning disabilities. *Journal of Learning Disabilities. 22,* 260–262.

Sternberg, R.J. (1984). The Kaufman Assessment Battery for Children: An information-processing analysis and critique. *Journal of Special Education, 18,* 269–279.

Street, R.F. (1931). *A Gestalt Completion Test.* Contributions to Education No. 481. New York: Teachers College, Columbia University.

Strommen, E. (1988). Confirmatory factor analysis of the Kaufman Assessment Battery for Children: A reevaluation. *Journal of School Psychology, 26,* 13–23.

Whitworth, R.H., & Chrisman, S.M. (1987). Validation of the Kaufman Assessment Battery for Children comparing Anglo and Mexican-American preschoolers. *Educational and Psychological Measurement, 47,* 695–702.

Worthington, G.B., & Bening, M.E. (1988). Use of the Kaufman Assessment Battery for Children in predicting achievement in students referred for special education services. *Journal of Learning Disabilities, 21,* 370–374.

Zucker, S., & Rirodan, J. (1990). One-year predic-

tive validity of new and revised conceptual language measurement. *Journal of Psychoeducational Assessment, 8,* 4–8.

STANFORD-BINET INTELLIGENCE SCALE—REVISED (SBIS-R)

Purpose

The SBIS is an intelligence test for children between 2 and 18 years of age.

Source

The Stanford-Binet Intelligence Scale (SBIS), 4th ed., can be ordered from Riverside Publishing Company, 8420 Bryn Mawr Ave., Chicago, IL. 60631, for $420 US, or from Nelson Canada, 1120 Birchmount Rd., Scarborough, Ont. M1K 4G4 for $974.45 Cdn.

Description

This scale (Thorndike et al., 1986a) is the most recent revision of Terman's first North American edition in 1916 of the test developed by Binet in France in 1905. The second and third editions in 1937 and 1960 included further development; new norms for the third edition were published in 1973 (Terman & Merrill, 1973); the current edition provides a substantial revision by grouping items into 15 subtests covering four broad areas—verbal reasoning, abstract/visual reasoning, quantitative reasoning, and short-term memory—and by providing new normative data for each. Nine of these tests evolved from the previous edition of the test, and six were added. The test is designed for the age range from 2 to 18 years and provides intelligence estimates up to 23 years of age. While previous editions were based primarily on the pragmatic stance of the original Binet-Simon test, the new edition follows the theoretical model of a *g*-factor and these second-level factors: "crystallyzed abilities," "fluid-analytic abilities" (Cattell, 1971), and "short-term memory". Within the "crystallized abilities," a distinction is made between third-level factors of verbal reasoning (including tests of vocabulary, comprehension, absurdities, and verbal relations) and quantitative reasoning (including quantitative

tasks, number series, and equation building); the "fluid-analytic abilities" comprise only one third-level factor (including tests of pattern analysis, copying, matrices, and paper folding and cutting); "short-term memory" includes bead memory, memory for sentences, memory for digits, and memory for objects. Another difference from previous editions is that vocabulary and chronological age are used to determine the "entry level" for testing, but the subject must still pass all items at that level to establish the "basal level" (see Bayley Scales). The scales are packed in a small suitcase; much of the material is mounted on easels that allow pages to be turned over to move on to the next item facing the subject, and the back page contains instructions for the examiner.

A short description of the 15 tests follows:

1. *Vocabulary:* Picture naming (to item 14), definition vocabulary (items 15 to 46).

2. *Comprehension:* 42 questions (example: "Give two reasons why children should not handle firearms").

3. *Absurdities:* 32 pictures with incongruous content ("What is wrong with this picture"; example: girl eating from plate with scissors).

4. *Verbal Relations:* 18 items with three words and a fourth word that does not fit, presented on cards and read aloud by the examiner. Subject must find how the first three words are alike, but different from the fourth (example: box, carton, bag, not apples).

5. *Pattern Analysis:* The first 10 items require correct block placement into holes (similar to the formboard test), items 11 to 42 are block design tasks with up to 9 blocks (similar to the Wechsler Block Design).

6. *Copying:* For the first 12 items, examiner arranges up to four blocks in a pattern and asks subject to copy the arrangement. For items 13 to 28 copying of simple geometric shapes shown on cards is required.

7. *Matrices:* A 2 × 2 matrix is presented on a card with three of the boxes filled with geometric designs; below are three choices. Subject must indicate which of the three best fits into the empty box. The test increases after two items to a 3 × 3 matrix with up to five choices. Items 23 to 26 contain letter patterns instead of geometric designs.

8. *Paper Folding and Cutting:* Three line drawings of paper patterns are presented on the top of a card. Beneath are five choices of patterns with folding marks. Subject must indicate which of the choices looks like one of the patterns when it is unfolded. A folded sample is used to demonstrate the task if subject does not respond correctly.

9. *Quantitative:* This test proceeds from placing blocks with varying numbers of dots correctly on a tray (12 items) to counting the number of children, pencils, etc. on cards, including simple subtraction (items 13, 14), to relations ("between," item 15), to arithmetic illustrated with pictures (items 16 to 23), to verbally enclosed arithmetic questions (items 24 to 40).

10. *Number Series:* Subject must find the subsequent two numbers in a series printed on cards (26 items).

11. *Equation Building:* Subject must rearrange numbers and basic arithmetic symbols to find the correct equation (18 items). Example: 1 2 7 3 × + = , subject must find the equation $(2 \times 3) + 1 = 7$.

12. *Bead Memory:* This test proceeds from pointing out the correct colored and shaped bead in a box (as shown on a card) to arranging beads on a stick with base after the pictured pattern has been exposed for five seconds (42 items).

13. *Memory for Sentences:* Repetition of sentences ranging from 2 to 22 words (42 items).

14. *Memory for Digits:* Repetition ranging from three to nine digits; repetition in reverse order is also required (14 and 12 items).

15. *Memory for Objects:* Subject must find in correct sequence 2 to 8 objects shown previously on a multiple-choice card with distractor items.

For Canadian children, the use of metric equivalents for imperial measures and the substitution of Canadian coins in the quantitative subtest are recommended (Wersh & Thomas, 1990).

Administration

See manual. Full familiarity and considerable practice are needed to administer this test. The examiner's handbook (Delaney & Hopkins, 1987) should be consulted since it clarifies a number of administration problems, e.g., the use of introductory explanations and/or training items when shifting to a new set of items or a different task in the determination of basal levels (Wersh & Thomas, 1990). Briefly, vocabulary is given first as a "routing test" that determines the items to begin with on each test. A "basal level" is then established for each test (passing two consecutive items), and testing is continued until the ceiling level (four consecutive failures on each test) is reached.

The test items are presented in a standardized manner, but some flexibility is acceptable; for example, the examiner may shift to another test if the subject shows fatigue or resistance to a given test. Ambiguous responses are clarified during testing or on follow-up questioning.

Of the 15 tests, only pattern analysis has definite time limits, while for all other tests it is left to the examiner to determine whether a satisfactory response can be elicited by allowing more time.

Approximate Time for Administration

The time required is 60–90 minutes.

Scoring

A detailed scoring guide including examples of "pass," "query," and "fail" responses is included in the manual. The extensive (39 pp.) record booklet provides information for the examiner on item presentation and helpful guides for scoring so that the manual does not have to be constantly consulted. Raw scores for each test are converted into Standard Age Scores (SAS) by reference to the tables in the manual. The sums of raw scores for each of the four areas are converted into area SASs, based on additional tables in the manual. Finally, a composite SAS is derived from the manual by entering the sum of area SASs. The conversion tables make allowance for the possibility that some tests were not appropriate for the age of the child or may have been omitted for other reasons by providing area SASs for one, two, three, or four tests administered. Similarly, the composite SAS may be based on one, two, three, or four area scores.

Comment

Although many of the SBIS subtests may seem similar or identical to those used in other intelligence tests or in other tests like the Raven's or the Tactual Performance Test, it should be remembered that it was the SBIS that first developed these procedures and that tests like the WISC or WAIS were the "upstarts."

Although the use of 15 tests seemingly provides a fixed set of tasks for all ages (a serious problem of previous editions), only six of them are actually appropriate for all age levels, while others cover only 7 to 13 years of the age span. Hence the SAS in the age range 2 to 6 years is based on only eight tests (with the possibility of obtaining an "estimated" SAS for an additional four tests). In addition, vocabulary switches from picture naming to definition vocabulary after item 14; the task requirements for pattern analysis, copying, and quantification also change after the first set of items.

It should be noted that the limited number of items for the younger age range leads to a floor effect which truncates results at the low end for 2- to 5-year-olds: mental retardation of even mild degree cannot be assessed in 2-year-olds (lowest possible IQ is 95), and more severe retardation cannot be measured in 3- or 4- and 5-year-olds (lowest IQ 73, 55, and 44, respectively, Wilson 1992). Robinson (1992) points out that there is a similar ceiling effect which makes assessment of gifted children above the 5- to 11-year-old range questionable.

While the standardization of the previous edition of the SBIS has been severely criticized (Waddell, 1980), the new edition comes with a good technical manual (Thorndike et al. 1986b) that documents the development of the test, field trials for the new edition, standardization, and descriptive statistics, scaling, reliability, and validity. The standardization of this edition was accomplished on a carefully selected sample of over 5,000 children, adolescents, and young adults representative of the U.S. census in terms of gender, race, geographic distribution, and parental occupation and education. Test–retest reliability after an average of 16 weeks ranged from .71 and .51 (quantitative reasoning) to .91 and .90 for the composite score in preschoolers and elementary school children respectively. Subtest reliability ranged from .28 (quantitative) to .86 (comprehension). It should be noted that retesting resulted in an overall gain of 7–8 points on the composite score. Atkinson (1989) warned that the standard errors of estimation and prediction for the composite score range from 3.49 and 5.00, respectively, at age 2 to 1.59 and 2.26, respectively, at age 17–23, and the error range is even higher if 2-, 4-, or 6-subtest estimates are used. Hence the 95 and 99 percent confidence level for this score ranges from 1.96 to 2.58 times the standard errors of estimation and prediction as with all test scores; these values should be used to show the possible variance of the "true score" in interpreting SAS.

Construct validity of the SBIS, as assessed by factor analysis, has generated much debate. The technical manual of the test proposes a g-factor and three second-level factors (verbal and quantitative reasoning [crystallized abilities], abstract/visual reasoning [fluid analytic abilities], and short-term memory). McCallum (1990) argues that factor-analytic construct validity must be confirmed by confirmatory, hypothesis-testing analyses. Keith et al. (1988) point out that these factors have not been established for the age span from 2 to 6 years, and that there is little support so far for the distinction of the crystallized vs. fluid intelligence as a second-level factor dimension. Molfese et al. (1992) confirm that factor structure changes with age; they found two factors in 3-year-old children, one verbal and one nonverbal factor. The verbal factor corresponded partially to the verbal score of the McCarthy (1972) scales. Thorndike (1990) agrees with the two-factor structure in young children, but maintains that above age 7 three correlated factors can be found (verbal, abstract/spatial, and memory), and that the intercorrelation between factors forms the basis for a general g-factor. Further criticism about the validity of the factor structure was raised by Laurent et al. (1992), and Vernon (1987) questioned the claim to measure differential abilities as well as general intelligence. Questions were also raised about psychometric limitations of the four-area-score factorial composition, especially at younger age levels (Vernon 1987). Wersh and Thomas (1990) report problems in the determination of basal and ceiling levels on subtests with changed item content and the interpretation of Quantitative Reasoning and Short-Term Memory areas due to the limited data provided in the technical manual.

According to the manual, concurrent validity with the previous edition is .81, with the WPPSI .80, with the WISC-R .83, with the WAIS-R .79 to .91, and with the Kaufman-ABC .89. Correlation with the Test of Cognitive Skills is only .41 (Robinson & Nagle, 1992), and correlation with the WIPPSI-R in preschool to grade 2 children was reported as .61 (Carvajal et al., 1991). The correlations with the WISC-R and WAIS-R for gifted, learning-disabled, and mentally retarded populations ranged from .66 to .79. In 32 younger (<24 years) and 38 older (>24 years) mentally retarded adults, the correlation between SBIS standard age scores and WAIS-R was low, though significant, with the SBIS producing significantly lower scores than the WAIS-R (Spruill, 1991). Sattler (1992) concludes that the SB produces scores comparable to the Wechsler in the average range, but that, with gifted and mentally handicapped subjects, the SB may yield lower scores (about 10 points) than the WAIS-R or WISC-R. Johnson and McGowan (1984) also report that the SBIS significantly predicted school grades at age 7–9 in low-income Mexican-American children. The correlation with the Woodcock-Johnson reading test is .54, with the reading composite of the Kaufman Test of Educational

Achievement .49, and with the total reading score of the Peabody Individual Achievement Test .46 (Prewett & Giannuli 1991).

Other researchers (Canter, 1990) have questioned the utility of the test for daily assessment practices in the schools because of "lack of treatment utility," i.e., the failure to address specific referral concerns or the impact of educational intervention. In contrast, N.M. Robinson (1992) considers the SBIS the "test of choice for bright children over a wide age range" (p. 33). Brown and Morgan (1991) studied 80 learning-disabled children assigned to an auditory-linguistic, a visuospatial, and a mixed type, based on WISC-R verbal-performance scale differences. Twelve of the SBIS subtests contributed to a 75 percent correct classification rate, but correlations between SBIS subtests and corresponding WISC-R subtests were only low to moderate for this group. Smith et al. (1989) compared the SBIS with the K-ABC and conclude that in learning-disabled children both tests show strength in the assessment of verbal and abstract reasoning, but a relative weakness in achievement and memory/sequential processing.

In the context of the neuropsychological assessment of children, the SBIS fills an age gap not covered by the Bayley scale (ages 2–4), although the Kaufman-ABC is also designed to cover this age range. The choice between the SBIS and the K-ABC depends on the theoretical orientation of the examiner. The WPPSI-R covers age 3 but tends to show floor effects that are undesirable in children of less than average intelligence. In clinical practice, the user may also wish to utilize some of the subtests that are similar in content to some neuropsychological tests used in clinical practice with adults: for example, sentence memory, matrices, copying pattern analysis, absurdities, and comprehension. Such tests may allow confirmation and a more detailed exploration of areas of deficit, or they may be substituted for these tests in more severely impaired patients who cannot perform on the adult tests.

Normative Data

As previously mentioned, the standardization of this edition has been exemplary. Weighting

Table 6—2. Differences Between SBIS Subtest Scores Required for Statistical Significance at the .01 and .05 Levels of Confidence for 6- to 10-year-olds

	Voc	Comp	Abs	PA	Copy	Mat	Quan	NS	B-M	MemS	MemD	MemO
Voc		12	13	11	12	11	12	11	12	12	12	14
Comp	9		13	11	12	11	12	11	12	12	12	14
Abs	10	10		11	12	12	13	12	12	12	13	14
PA	8	8	9		10	9	11	9	10	10	11	12
Copy	9	9	9	7		10	12	10	11	11	11	13
Mat	8	8	9	7	8		11	9	10	10	11	13
Quant	9	9	10	8	9	8		11	12	12	12	14
NS	8	8	9	7	8	7	8		10	10	11	13
B-Mem	9	9	9	8	8	8	9	8		11	12	13
MemS	9	9	9	7	8	8	9	8	8		11	13
MemD	9	9	10	8	9	8	9	8	9	9		14
MemO	11	11	11	9	10	10	11	10	10	10	10	

Note: Values above the diagonal are at the .01 level; values below the diagonal are at the .05 level. Voc = Vocabulary, Comp = Comprehension, Abs = Absurdities, PA = Pattern Analysis, Copy = Copying, Mat = Matrices, Quant = Quantitative, NS = Number Series, B-Mem = Bead Memory, MemS = Memory for Sentences, MemD = Memory for Designs, MemO = Memory for Objectives.

Source: Rosenthal and Kamphaus, 1988.

procedures were used to simulate the U.S. census as closely as possible. This body of normative data has been used in constructing the tables for conversion of raw scores into SAS for each test, area SASs, and composite SAS. The composite SAS, of course, functions similarly to IQ scores in comparable tests. It should be noted, however, that the SBIS uses a standard deviation of 16 (as in previous editions of this test), whereas most other intelligence tests use a standard deviation of 15. Hence, if a definition of 2 SD below the mean is used to designate the mentally retarded range, the subject should obtain a score of less than 68 (not 70, as in other tests).

Vincent (1991) noted that even after renorming, a 1 SD difference between black and white adults remains, although the IQ differences in children are declining.

As for the WISC-III and the WPPSI-R, "profile interpretation," i.e., the interpretation of differences between subtests and between area scores in a given individual, has stimulated considerable interest. Kline et al. (1992) found that subtest profile shape had virtually no incremental validity over elevation when compared to the WISC-R or the K-ABC. Rosenthal and Kamphaus (1988) computed differences between subtest scores required for statistical significance at the .01 and .05 level of confidence. Table 6–2 shows these

values for 6- to 10-year-olds; the values for 2- to 5-year-olds and for 11- to 14-year-olds are similar; for 15- to 23-year-olds the respective values are about 3 points lower. Table F.1 in the technical manual shows the differences between area scores significant at the .01 and .05 level of significance. However, Spruill (1988) points out that this table is appropriate only for a single comparison, and that, for multiple comparisons of several area scores at the .05 level of significance, the values should be approximately 3–4 points higher than shown in the table. Smaller difference can and should be used for the generation of hypotheses, which can be confirmed by results from other tests, but not as significant findings.

References

Atkinson, L. (1989). Three standard errors of measurement and the Stanford-Binet Intelligence Scale, fourth edition. *Psychological Assessment, 1,* 242–244.

Brown, T.L., & Morgan, S.B. (1991). Concurrent validity of the Stanford-Binet, 4th edition, in classifying learning disabled children. *Psychological Assessment, 3,* 247–253.

Canter, A. (1990). A new Binet, and old premise: A mismatch between technology and evolving practice. *Journal of Psychoeducational Assessment, 8,* 443–450.

Carvajal, H.H., Parks, J.P., Bays, K.J., & Logan,

R.A. (1991). Relationships between scores on Wechsler Preschool and Primary Scale of Intelligence—Revised and Stanford-Binet IV. *Psychological Reports, 69,* 23–26.

Cattell, R.B. (1971). *Abilities: Their structure, Growth and Action.* New York: Harcourt, Brace & Janovich.

Delaney, E.A., & Hopkins, T.F. (1987). *Examiner's Handbook: The Stanford-Binet Intelligence Scale: Fourth Edition.* Chicago: Riverside Publishing.

Johnson, D.L., & McGowan, R.J. (1984). Comparison of three intelligence tests as predictors of academic achievement and classroom behaviors of Mexican-American children. *Journal of Psychoeducational Assessment, 2,* 345–352.

Keith, T.Z., Cool, V.A., Novak, C.G., White, L.J., & Pottebaum, S.M. (1988). Confirmatory factor analysis of the Stanford-Binet Fourth Edition: Testing the theory-test match. *Journal of School Psychology, 26,* 253–274.

Kline, R.B., Snyder, J., Guilmette, S., & Castellanos, M. (1992). Relative usefulness of elevation, variability, and shape information from WISC-R, K-ABC, and Fourth Edition Stanford-Binet profiles in predicting achievement. *Psychological Assessment, 4,* 426–432.

Laurent, J., Swerdlik, M., & Ryburn, M. (1992). Review of validity research on the Stanford-Binet Intelligence Scale: Fourth Edition. *Psychological Assessment, 4,* 102–112.

McCarthy, D.A. (1972). *Manual for the McCarthy Scales of Children's Abilities.* San Antonio, TX: Psychological Corporation.

McCallum, R.S. (1990). Determining the factor structure of the Stanford-Binet: Fourth edition—the right choice. *Journal of Psychoeducational Assessment, 8,* 436–442.

Molfese, V., Yaple, K., Helwig, S., Harris, L., & Connell, S. (1992). Stanford-Binet Intelligence Scale (Fourth edition): Factor structure and verbal subscale scores for three-year-olds. *Journal of Psychoeducational Assessment, 10,* 47–58.

Prewett, P.N., & Giannuli, M.M. (1991). Correlations of the WISC-R, Stanford-Binet Intelligence Scale: Fourth Edition, and the reading subtests of three popular achievement tests. *Psychological Reports, 69,* 1232–1234.

Robinson, E.L., & Nagle, R.J. (1992). The comparability of the Test of Cognitive Skills with the Wechsler Intelligence Scale for Children–Revised and the Stanford-Binet Fourth Edition with gifted children. *Psychology in the Schools, 29,* 107–112.

Robinson, N.M. (1992). Stanford-Binet, of course! Time marches on! *Roeper Review, 15,* 32–34.

Rosenthal, B.L., & Kamphaus, R.W. (1988). Interpretive tables for test scatter on the Stanford-Binet Intelligence Scale: Fourth Edition. *Journal of Psychoeducational Assessment, 6,* 359–370.

Sattler, J. (1992). *Assessment of Intelligence* (3rd ed.). San Diego: Sattler Publisher.

Smith, D.K., St. Martin, M.E., & Lyon, M.A. (1989). A validity study of the Stanford-Binet: Fourth Edition with students with learning disabilities. *Journal of Learning Disabilities, 22,* 260–262.

Spruill, J. (1988). Two types of tables for use with the Stanford-Binet Intelligence Scale: Fourth edition. *Journal of Psychoeducational Assessment, 6,* 78–86.

Spruill, J. (1991). A comparison of the Wechsler Adult Intelligence Scale—Revised with the Stanford-Binet Intelligence Scale (4th Edition). *Psychological Assessment, 3,* 133–135.

Terman, L.M., & Merrill, M.A. (1973). *Stanford-Binet Intelligence Test: 1972 Norms Edition.* Boston: Houghton Mifflin.

Thorndike, R.M. (1990). Would the real factors of the Stanford-Binet fourth edition please come forward? *Journal of Psychoeducational Assessment, 8,* 412–435.

Thorndike, R.L., Hagen, E.P., & Sattler, J.M. (1986a). *Stanford-Binet Intelligence Scale* (4th ed.). Chicago: Riverside Publishing.

Thorndike, R.L., Hagen, E.P., & Sattler, J.M. (1986b). *Technical Manual: Stanford-Binet Intelligence Scale: Fourth Edition.* Chicago: Riverside Publishing.

Vernon, P.E. (1987). The demise of the Stanford-Binet Scale. *Canadian Psychology, 28,* 251–258.

Vincent, K.R. (1991). Black-white IQ differences: Does age make a difference? *Journal of Clinical Psychology, 47,* 266–270.

Waddell, D.D. (1980). The Stanford-Binet: An evaluation of the technical data available since the 1972 restandardization. *Journal of School Psychology, 18,* 203–209.

Wersh, J., & Thomas, M.R. (1990). The Stanford-Binet Intelligence Scale: Fourth Edition; observations, comments and concerns. *Canadian Psychology, 31,* 190–193.

Wilson, W.M. (1992). The Stanford-Binet: Fourth Edition and Form L-M in assessment of young children with mental retardation. *Mental Retardation, 30,* 81–84.

7

Achievement Tests

This chapter considers a selection of commonly used measures of scholastic attainment. Tests such as the Peabody Individual Achievement Test (Markwardt, 1989), Wide Range Achievement Test (Wilkinson, 1993), the Wechsler Individual Achievement Test (WIAT, 1992) and the Woodcock-Johnson Psychoeducational Battery (Woodcock & Mather, 1989), sample a large number of abilities that have neuropsychological and educational implications: sight reading, reading comprehension, mathematics, spelling, writing, and general knowledge. The Woodcock-Johnson is the more comprehensive measure, both in terms of the domains assessed and the age range covered. The WIAT, however, is particularly suitable for investigating ability–achievement discrepancies in children because its normative base is linked to that of the WISC-III.

It is worth noting that these achievement tests do not assess any of these abilities in great depth. The value of these tests (Hessler, 1984) is that they provide a comparison of the subject's level of development or deterioration with normative populations in the areas that they assess. These general screening measures permit the examiner to determine whether a person is in need of and qualifies for special instruction in a particular domain. Further, the progress of a person and the effectiveness of an instructional program can be assessed. The results of these tests also permit the examiner to develop hypotheses about an individual's strengths and weaknesses. However, more detailed, in-depth information is needed in order to evaluate these hypotheses and to develop instructional plans. The Stanford Diagnostic Reading Test (Karlsen and Gardner, 1995) may be the test of choice since technical aspects are fairly adequate and it offers measures of comprehension and scanning. The Key-Math Test (Connolly, 1991) can be used to provide a more in-depth assessment of skills in mathematics.

It is important to bear in mind that normative data are usually based on a representative U.S. sample. Local or regional norms and norms for minority populations may have to be considered in the interpretation of the tests. Note, too, that achievement test results provide only a limited view of the individual. Learning difficulties need to be determined in the context of information gained from direct observation (e.g., teacher report), the individual's family history, and the particular instructional environment (e.g., local curricula).

References

Connolly, A.J. (1991). *KeyMath Diagnostic Arithmetic Test—Revised*. Toronto: Psycan.

Hessler, G.L. (1984). *Use and interpretation of the Woodcock-Johnson Psychoeducational Battery*. Allen, TX: DLM Teaching Resources.

Karlsen, B., & Gardner, E.F. (1995). *Stanford Diagnostic Reading Test*. New York: The Psychological Corporation.

Markwardt, F.C. (1989). *Peabody Individual Achievement Test—Revised*. Circle Pines, Minn: American Guidance Service.

Wechsler Individual Achievement Test (1992). San Antonio, TX: The Psychological Corporation.

Wilkinson, G. (1993). *The Wide Range Achievement Test 3*. Delaware: Wide Range.

Woodcock, R.W., & Mather, N. (1989). *Woodcock-Johnson Psycho-Educational Battery—Revised*. Allen, TX: DLM Teaching Resources.

KEYMATH DIAGNOSTIC ARITHMETIC TEST—REVISED

Purpose

The purpose of the KeyMath-R is to assess strengths and weaknesses in several areas of mathematics.

Source

The test (including two parallel forms, A and B) can be ordered from the American Guidance Service, Publishers' Building, Circle Pines, MN 55014, at a cost of $374.95 US. A separate Canadian edition is available from Psycan, P.O. Box 290, Station V, Toronto, Ontario M6R 3A5, for $500.00 Cdn. A computer scoring and profiling system is also available at a cost of $189.95 US or $250 Cdn.

Description

The KeyMath-R (Connolly, 1991) is a popular diagnostic measure, designed primarily for use from kindergarten through grade 9, or ages 5 years, 6 months to 15 years, 5 months. There are two forms of the test, Forms A and B, that are matched statistically and by content. The test consists of 13 subtests (called "strands") that are organized into three major areas. The Basic Concepts area measures foundations of mathematical knowledge and is composed of three subtests: numeration, rational numbers, and geometry. The Operations area stresses computational processes and contains five subtests: addition, subtraction, multiplication, division, and mental computation. The Applications area contains problems involving the use of mathematics in everyday life. There are five subtests: measurement, time and money, estimation, interpreting data, and problem solving. Each subtest within the KeyMath-R contains three or four domains represented by a set of six test items. For example, Numerations consists of four domains: numbers 0 to 9, numbers 0 to 99, numbers 0 to 999, multi-digit numbers and advanced numeration topics. Rational numbers contains three domains: fractions, decimals, and percents.

The materials include the test plates bound into an easel, a manual, a diagnostic record form, and a report to parents. The easel presents the stimulus material to the subject and at the same time provides the examiner with instructions, test items, and the acceptable answers on the reverse side. Most items require the subject to respond verbally to open-ended questions presented orally by the examiner. Some items, however, require written computation. Within a subtest, the items are identified by their domain affiliation in an easy-to-follow columnar display.

Four levels of diagnostic information are available: total test, area, subtest, and domain. In addition, the analysis of subject performance at the item level is made possible through the use of a table (Appendix A in the KeyMath-R manual) that describes the skill sampled by each item.

Administration

See source. Briefly, the examiner displays a test plate to the subject, asks a test question, and records the subject's response on a record form. The client's performance on the Numeration subtest will establish a basal item that guides the selection of starting points on all other subtests, which must be administered in order until the subject reaches the ceiling level (three consecutive errors).

Approximate Time for Administration

Typically, children in the primary grades will complete the test in 30–40 minutes. Older students may take 40–50 minutes.

Scoring

See source. Briefly, to calculate the subject's raw score, count all items below the basal level as correct whether or not they were administered. To that number add one point for each additional item correctly answered before reaching the ceiling level.

The Record Form provides space to record and score the subject's responses, to draw a profile of subtest and area scores, to indicate confidence intervals, to evaluate domain performance, and to note information about the subject's behavior in the test situation.

Comment

Split-half subtest reliability coefficients fall mostly in the .70s and .80s; for the areas and total test, values cluster in the .90s (see source). Another reliability estimate, based on item response theory and the Rasch model, is reported to be high (see source). Alternate form reliability coefficients computed from grade-based scaled scores range from the .50s to the .70s for the subtests, fall in the low .80s for the areas, and average .90 for the total test (see source). When subjects are retested 2–4 weeks after the initial testing, practice effects do emerge. For subtests, average gains of .2 to 1.3 scaled score points were found; for areas, average gains ranged from 1 to 5.9 standard score points; and on the total test, average gains of 2.2 to 5.8 standard score points were observed. The area and total-test scores exhibited a consistently greater practice effect for Form B followed by Form A than for Form A followed by Form B. Similar results emerge when age-based scaled scores are considered.

As might be expected (see source), mean performance on the KeyMath-R increases with grade level. Support for the content validity of subtests is given through intercorrelation data that demonstrate expected relationships between subtests and areas (see source). The KeyMath-R is related to its predecessor, the KeyMath, with correlation coefficients in the moderate range at the subtest level, and higher correlations (above .8) at the total-score level. The KeyMath-R is also related to other measures of arithmetic achievement; however, the correlation coefficients, while significant, tend to be modest (Eaves et al., 1990; also see Source).

The interpretation of errors may be facilitated by referring to the list of behavioral objectives in Appendix A and the domain affiliation in Appendix B of the KeyMath manual. This information can be used to guide teachers in the selection of appropriate procedures for remediation of arithmetic deficiencies.

The relative lack of reading and writing requirements makes the KeyMath-R attractive for individuals with poor reading skills. However, people with receptive or expressive language deficits may not be reliably assessed by the KeyMath-R (Price, 1984).

Normative Data

The test was standardized separately in the United States ($n = 1,798$ students) and Canada ($n = 742$ students). In each case, the norms are based on a relatively large sample of school children considered representative of the country in terms of grade, gender, and geographical region. In the U.S. standardization, race/ethnic group and level of parental education were also controlled. Performance of Canadian and U.S. students are most similar at the early grades and on operations throughout the grades. By about fifth grade, Canadian students begin to slightly outperform the American students on basic concepts and on the test overall.

The KeyMath-R provides a set of derived scores to which the raw scores may be converted: scaled scores (for subtests) with a mean of 10 and standard deviation of 3, standard scores (for areas and total-test) with a mean of 100 and standard deviation of 15, percentile ranks, and grade and age equivalents (for area and total-test performance). The manual also provides information that allows the examiner to determine whether there are significant discrepancies between areas and between subtest scores. In addition, performance within a subtest domain can be analyzed with reference to the standardization sample.

References

Connolly, A.J. (1991). *KeyMath Revised: A diagnostic inventory of essential mathematics*. Toronto: PsyCan Corporation.

Eaves, R.C., Vance, R.H., Mann, L., & Parker-Bohannon, A. (1990). Cognition and academic achievement: The relationship of the Cognitive

Levels Test, the KeyMath Revised, and the Woodcock Reading Mastery Tests–Revised. *Psychology in the Schools, 27,* 311–318.

Price, P. A. (1984). A comparative study of the California Achievement Test (Forms C and D) and the KeyMath Diagnostic Arithmetic Test with secondary DH students. *Journal of Learning Disabilities, 17,* 392–396.

PEABODY INDIVIDUAL ACHIEVEMENT TEST—REVISED (PIAT-R)

Purpose

The purpose of this test is to provide a wide-range screening measure of achievement in the areas of mathematics, reading recognition, reading comprehension, spelling, and general information.

Source

The test can be ordered from the American Guidance Service, Inc., Publishers' Building, Circle Pines, MN 55014, at a cost of $269.95 US, or from Psycan Corporation, P.O. Box 290, Station V, Toronto, Ontario M6R 3A5, at a cost of $520 Cdn.

Description

The PIAT-R (Dunn & Markwardt, 1970; Markwardt, 1989) is a popular screening measure of achievement, appropriate for children in kindergarten through grade 12 or ages 5 years through 18 years, 11 months. It is often administered to determine whether a more detailed diagnostic test should be given. The PIAT-R test materials include four volumes of test plates. These contain the demonstration and training exercises, the test items, and the instructions for administering the six subtests. A Written Expression Response Booklet is used by the subject for his or her responses to the Written Expression subtest. The Test Record booklet provides space for recording and scoring other test responses and plotting the profiles.

The test consists of six subtests and uses two item formats: multiple-choice and free response. The General Information subtest contains 100 open-ended questions that are read aloud by the examiner and answered orally by the subject. The items measure general encyclopedic knowledge in the content areas of science, social studies, fine arts, humanities, and recreation. The Reading Recognition subtest consists of 100 items and is an oral test of single-word reading. The initial prereading items measure the subject's ability to recognize the sounds associated with printed letters; in the following items, the subject reads words aloud. The Reading Comprehension subtest consists of 82 items that measure a subject's ability to derive meaning from printed words. For each item, the subject reads a sentence silently, and on the next page the subject chooses the one picture out of four that best illustrates the sentence. The Mathematics subtest contains 100 multiple-choice items that range in difficulty from discriminating and matching tasks to geometry and trigonometry content. The examiner reads each item aloud while displaying the response choices to the subject. The Spelling subtest consists of 100 multiple-choice items. The first few items measure the subject's ability to recognize letters from their names or sounds. In subsequent items, the examiner reads a word aloud and uses it in a sentence, and the subject then selects the correct spelling for the word. The Written Expression subtest assesses the subject's written language skills at two levels: Level I tests prewriting skills—copying and writing letters, words, and sentences from dictation; Level II requires the subject to write a story in response to a picture prompt.

Administration

See PIAT-R Manual. Briefly, the examiner displays a test plate to the subject, asks a test question, and records the subject's responses on the record form. There is a standard order of subtest administration: General Information, Reading Recognition, Reading Comprehension, Mathematics, Spelling, Written Expression (Level I or Level II).

The starting point for the first subtest, General Information, is based on grade level. For all subsequent subtests, starting points are determined by the subject's raw score on the preceding test. Such a practice, however, may be problematic for children who have uneven skill development (Costenbader & Adams, 1991). The recommended dropping-back procedure provides some safeguard, however, that the student is not tested at an inappropriately high level (Allinder & Fuchs, 1992).

Approximate Time for Administration

The PIAT-R is an untimed test, with the exception of the supplemental Written Expression subtest, and takes approximately 60 minutes.

Scoring

See PIAT-R Manual. The scoring criteria for the items are clearly stated with examples of correct and incorrect responses given on the examiner's side of the book of test plates. To obtain the raw score for each subtest, the errors are subtracted from the number of the ceiling items. Thus, the raw score for a subtest is the number of actual and assumed correct responses up to the ceiling item. A basal level is determined below which all items are assumed correct. Items above the ceiling item are assumed incorrect. Raw scores for each of the subtests are recorded on the test record. Composite scores summarize the subject's achievement. The Total Reading score is the sum of the Reading Recognition and Reading Comprehension raw scores and is an overall measure of reading ability. The Total Test composite raw score is the sum of the General Information, Reading Recognition, Reading Comprehension, Mathematics, and Spelling subtest raw scores. An optional Written Language composite, formed by the written Expression and Spelling subtests, can also be computed.

The Scores page in the test record provides space for recording raw scores, derived scores, and confidence intervals for the first five PIAT-R subtests and the two composites. There is a separate section on the page for recording scores for Written Expression.

The test record includes two profiles for graphic representation of the PIAT-R results (except Written Expression): The Developmental Score Profile is used for plotting either grade equivalents or age equivalents; the Standard Score Profile is used for plotting standard scores.

Comment

Markwardt (1989) reports that the PIAT-R subtests and composites show a high degree of internal consistency, with reliability coefficients above .90. Test–retest reliability coefficients are also high, above .90, at least after intervals of about 2–4 weeks. Other reliability coefficients, based on item response theory and the Rasch model, are also high.

Reliabilities for each of the two Written Expression subtests were reported separately and were in the moderate range. Markwardt suggests that the written expression subtests (for Level II) be scored by a second person and that the results should be interpreted with caution. Given the low reliabilities associated with these subtests, their use for other than qualitative data is not recommended (Costenbader & Adams, 1991; Luther, 1992).

As might be expected, PIAT-R subtest and composite raw score means increase with age and grade. Further support for the content validity of each specific subtest is given through intercorrelation data provided by Markwardt (1989) that demonstrate expected relationships between subtests based on similar constructs. There is a substantial overlap between the PIAT-R and the PIAT, with correlations between scores on the two tests ranging from .46 to .97. Correlations between the PIAT-R and the Peabody Picture Vocabulary Test—Revised are modest and range from .50 to .72 (Markwardt, 1989). Scores on the PIAT-R correlate highly (above .8) with those of other achievement tests, such as the K-ABC, Woodcock-Johnson Psychoeducational Battery—Revised, WRAT-R, and Stanford Diagnostic Mathematic Test (Goh & McElheron, 1992; McClosky cited in Costenbader & Adams, 1991; Prewett & Giannulli, 1991). Correlations with intelligence tests are moderate to high (Goh & McElheron, 1992; McClosky cited in Costenbader & Adams, 1991).

Factor analysis of the PIAT-R suggests three basic factors (Markwardt, 1989). Factor I represents a general verbal–educational ability factor that has high loadings on General Information, Reading Comprehension, and Mathematics. Factor II has the highest loadings on Reading Recognition and Spelling and appears to define a narrower verbal factor that is more dependent on knowledge of letter–sound correspondences. Factor III has the highest loadings on Reading Comprehension and Written Expression and seems to place a premium on knowledge of grammatical and syntactical structures.

Both the PIAT-R and Woodcock-Johnson Psychoeducational Battery (WJ-R) provide a broad overview of scholastic attainment. Although scores are highly intercorrelated, the two tests do not necessarily yield similar standard scores when administered concurrently to the same student. This raises the concern that diagnosis may depend on which achievement test is given. For example, Prewett and Giannuli (1991) report that PIAT-R reading scores tend to be lower than the WJ-R reading scores. Of the two tests, the WJ-R is the more comprehensive measure. However, the PIAT-R may be more appropriate when the subject's verbal skills are limited. The multiple-choice pointing format on some of the subtests (Reading Comprehension, Mathematics, Spelling) makes it possible to obtain an achievement measure for individuals who otherwise might be impossible to test because of their poor verbal abilities (Costenbader & Adams, 1991; Sattler, 1982). One should bear in mind, however, that the type of information gained from these multiple-choice tests may be similar, but not identical, to information gained from other tests in which a response must be produced by the student. Tests that have a production response format may be more sensitive to and representative of academic problems manifested in classrooms, where production tasks are common (Allinder & Fuchs, 1992; Costenbader & Adams, 1991).

Clinicians should also note that the PIAT-R is fundamentally a screening device. It will help to spot problem areas, but it is not a diagnostic instrument. Nor should it be used in the development of individual educational programs (Allinder & Fuchs, 1992; Costenbader & Adams, 1991). Further, some of the arithmetic items will be problematic for subjects taught with the metric system.

Normative Data

The PIAT-R standardization sample consisted of about 1,500 children (half males, half females), having a similar proportional distribution as the U.S. population in terms of geographic region, socioeconomic status, and race or ethnic group. Because the norms are based solely on U.S. children, caution should be taken in interpreting scores of people who reside outside the United States.

For the first five PIAT-R subtests (General Information, Reading Recognition, Reading Comprehension, Mathematics, Spelling) and the two composite scores (Total Reading, Total Test), the following types of derived scores are provided in the PIAT-R manual: grade and age equivalents, standard scores by grade or age, percentile ranks, normal curve equivalents, and stanines. Standard scores and percentile ranks by grade are provided for fall, winter, and spring administration. For Levels I and II of the Written Expression subtest, grade-based stanines are given; for Level II, a developmental scaled score is also provided that permits comparison with the entire standardization sample. Confidence intervals can be calculated for raw and derived scores.

The PIAT-R has an inadequate floor for very young children and an inadequate ceiling at the highest age and grade levels (Costenbader & Adams, 1991). For example, for the 5 years to 5 years, 2 months age group, a total test raw score of 0 yields a standard score of 77. For the 18 years, 9 months to 18 years, 11 months age group, a perfect total test score of 55 yields a standard score of 117. In short, the PIAT is not recommended for individuals at the extremes of the age and grade distribution.

References

Allinder, R.M., & Fuchs, L.S. (1992). Screening academic achievement: Review of the Peabody

Individual Achievement Test—Revised. *Learning Disabilities Research and Practice, 7,* 45–47.

Costenbader, V.K., & Adams, J.W. (1991). A review of the psychometric and administrative features of the PIAT-R: Implications for the practitioner. *Journal of School Psychology, 29,* 219–228.

Dunn, L.M., & Markwardt, F.C. (1970). *Peabody Individual Achievement Test Manual.* Circle Pines, MN: American Guidance Service.

Goh, D.S., & McElheron, D. (1992). Another look at the aptitude–achievement distinction. *Psychological Reports, 70,* 833–834.

Luther, J.B. (1992). Review of the Peabody Individual Achievement Test—Revised. *Journal of School Psychology, 30,* 31–39.

Markwardt, F.C. (1989). *Peabody Individual Achievement Test—Revised.* Circle Pines, MN: American Guidance Service.

Prewett, P.N., & Giannuli, M.M. (1991). The relationships among the reading subtests of the WJ-R, PIAT-R, K-TEA, and WRAT-R. *Journal of Psychoeducational Assessment, 9,* 166–174.

Sattler, J.M. (1982). *Assessment of Children's Intelligence and Special Abilities* (2nd ed.). Boston: Allyn and Bacon.

STANFORD DIAGNOSTIC READING TEST (SDRT)

Purpose

The purpose of this test is to assess strengths and weaknesses in reading.

Source

The materials include test booklets, answer sheets and scoring keys, norms booklet, manual for interpretation. The six levels can be ordered from the Psychological Corporation, P.O. Box 9954, San Antonio, TX 78204, at a cost of about $150 US or from the Psychological Corporation, 55 Horner Ave, Toronto, Ontario, M8Z 4X6, at a cost of about $200 Cdn.

Description

The SDRT 4th Edition (Karlsen & Gardner, 1995) was designed to provide assessment of reading, particularly for low-achieving students. It consists of six levels (Red, Orange, Green, Purple, Brown, Blue), with two parallel forms (J and K) at each of the three upper levels (Purple, Brown, Blue). Although some skills are measured at all levels, the ways in which these skills are measured changes from level to level.

The Red Level is intended for use at the end of grade 1 and first half of grade 2. It measures skills in phonetic analysis ("Identify the letter or letter combination that matches initial or final sounds of words"), auditory vocabulary ("Select the picture or word that best fits the word tested or the meaning of sentences"), word recognition ("Identify words that describe a particular picture"), and reading comprehension ("Identify a picture that illustrates the meaning of a printed sentence and answer questions in a multiple-choice format after reading short passages").

The Orange level is intended for use in the second half of grade 2 and the first half of grade 3. It measures prereading skills of phonetic analysis and auditory vocabulary. It also assesses reading vocabulary and comprehension of informational, recreational and functional text.

The Green Level is intended for use in grades 3 and 4. It measures skills in phonetic analysis, reading vocabulary and comprehension ("Answer questions after reading of short passages").

The Purple Level can be used in grades 4 through 6. It measures skills in reading vocabulary and comprehension of different types of text. A scanning subtest is also included in which subjects are presented with a set of questions and are asked to find the answers in the accompanying article, without reading the article through completely.

The Brown level is intended for students in grades 6 to 8. It measures reading vocabulary, comprehension and scanning.

The Blue level is intended for use in grades 9 through 12 and first year of college. This level also measures skills in reading vocabulary, comprehension of textual, functional, and recreational reading material, and scanning.

Administration

The test can be group-administered or given individually. Not all subtests must be given.

Procedures for administration are clearly described in the SDRT manuals. Briefly, the examiner reads the instructions and the subject responds in the test booklet or answer folder.

Approximate Time for Administration

The time required is about 1½–2 hours if all subtests are given.

Scoring

The test booklets or answer folders can be hand-scored using stencil keys. Alternatively, they may be processed by machine through the Psychological Corporation.

Comment

Internal consistency and alternate-form reliability are adequate, with coefficients generally above .7 (see source). No test–retest information is available.

The test appears to be fairly comparable to the previous third edition of the test (see Source). Both editions were given to about 3000 children per grade in grades 2–5, 7, and 10. Correlations between the two editions were high (.8 and above for total battery scores). Students in the standardization sample also took the Otis-Lennon School Ability Test, 6th Edition. Moderate to high correlations obtained between tests. In addition, about 2500 students in grades 3–5, 7 and 9 were given two adjacent levels, the on-grade level and one level lower on the SDRT. Correlations between corresponding subtests and totals at adjacent levels were moderate to high (above .6).

One advantage of the test is that it was designed to be most useful with individuals who are experiencing reading difficulty. It was developed specifically to include very easy items at each level, so that even very low achievers would experience some success. Consequently, the SDRT may be less appropriate to assess the strengths and weaknesses of average-to-above average readers or to monitor program gains for such individuals.

Another advantage of the test is that it provides coverage of a number of different aspects of reading, including inferential comprehension. Many brain-damaged patients have difficulty handling abstract concepts, and the inclusion of measures of high-level conceptual abilities may be particularly revealing.

One other feature of the SDRT warrants some comment. The SDRT reflects a U.S. national consensus curriculum. Therefore, it may be inappropriate for non-U.S. individuals.

Normative Data

The authors state that the test was standardized on a large number of students (more than 50,000), in grades 1 to 12, considered representative of the U.S. school population. The stratification variables were geographic region, socio-economic status, urbanicity and ethnicity. Type of school, public versus private, was also a stratification variable. In addition, 2,000 college freshmen were given the Blue level, resulting in grade 13 norms. A variety of different transformed scores can be obtained including percentile ranks, stanines, grade equivalents and scaled scores.

In addition to the norm-referenced scores, the test manual also includes tables of Progress Indicators. These are criterion-referenced scores that describe an individual's performance on the various content clusters of the SDRT (e.g., comprehension of type of text: recreational, textual, functional; mode of comprehension: the capacity to make inferences, capacity for critical analysis).

References

Karlsen, B. & Gardner, E.F. (1995). *Stanford Diagnostic Reading Test* (4th Ed.). New York: The Psychological Corporation.

WECHSLER INDIVIDUAL ACHIEVEMENT TEST

Purpose

The purpose of this test is to measure oral expression, listening comprehension, reading, spelling, arithmetic, and writing.

Source

The test, including the manual, stimulus booklets, and 25 record forms and response booklets can be ordered from The Psychological Corporation, P. O. Box 9954, San Antonio, Texas 78204-0954, at a cost of approximately $238.50 US. or from The Psychological Corporation, 55 Horner Avenue, Toronto, ON M8Z 4X6 for about $360.00 Cdn.

Description

The Wechsler Individual Achievement Test (WIAT) is a comprehensive individually administered measure designed to assess individuals aged 5 years to 19 years, 11 months. It is particularly suitable for investigating ability–achievement discrepancies in children aged 6 years to 16 years, 11 months because its normative sample is linked to that of the WISC-III.

The Stimulus Booklets are in an easel format and contain all the necessary administration and response information. The Comprehensive Battery consists of eight subtests. The Basic Reading subtest consists of a series of pictures and printed words for assessing decoding and word-reading ability. The client responds by pointing to the response item or orally. The Mathematics Reasoning subtest examines problem solving, geometry, measurement, and statistics. The items are presented orally and visually, and the client responds orally or by pointing to a response. The Spelling subtest requires the individual to write letters, sounds, and words that are dictated. Reading Comprehension consists of a series of printed passages and orally presented questions designed to tap skills such as recognizing details and making inferences. The subject responds orally to the questions. In Numerical Operations, the client writes responses involving all basic operations (addi-

tion, subtraction, multiplication, and division). Listening Comprehension requires the subject to point to the picture that corresponds to an orally presented word or to answer questions regarding an orally presented passage. The Oral Expression subtest consists of a series of items focusing on the ability to express words, describe scenes, give directions, and explain steps. Items consist of pictures accompanied by orally presented instructions to which the client responds orally. The Written Expression subtest is for grades 3 to 12 only and evaluates skills such as the development and organization of ideas, capitalization, and punctuation.

In addition to providing information at the subtest level, five composite scores can be computed from the sum of the scores on the relevant subtests: Reading (Basic Reading plus Reading Comprehension), Mathematics (Mathematics Reasoning plus Numerical Operations), Language (Listening Comprehension plus Oral Expression), Writing (Spelling plus Written Expression), and Total Composite (Reading, Mathematics, Language, and Writing).

A brief overview, the Screener, can be administered and consists of the Basic Reading, Mathematics Reasoning, and Spelling subtests. A Screener Composite score can be determined from the sum of these three subtests. The examiner can then follow up with the more comprehensive examination if time permits.

Administration

See source. Briefly, the examiner presents a stimulus card, reads aloud words and sentences, asks test questions and records responses. The subtests should be administered in the sequence indicated in the Stimulus Booklets. To facilitate administration, start points, reverse rules, discontinue rules, and time guidelines are provided not only in the manual but also in the Stimulus Booklets and Record Forms. For all subtests except Written Expression, which has a 15-minute time limit, the time information is intended only as a guideline because these subtests are untimed. The purpose of including general time guidelines is to provide an even administration pace. For most subtests, items and instructions may be repeated once if the client asks or misunderstands them.

Approximate Time for Administration

The test takes about 30–50 minutes for children in grades K–2 and about 55–60 minutes, excluding the time for Written Expression, for children in grades 3–12. Administration of the Screener requires approximately 10 minutes for children in kindergarten and approximately 15 to 18 minutes for children in grades 1–12.

Scoring

All subtests except Oral Expression and Written Expression have reverse and discontinue rules that necessitate scoring responses as items are given. Scoring procedures for Basic Reading, Mathematics Reasoning, Spelling, and Numerical Operations are straightforward since items are scored dichotomously (1 = correct, 0 = incorrect) using the answers provided in the Stimulus Booklets. Scoring of the items for Reading Comprehension, Listening Comprehension, Oral Expression, and Written Expression is more subjective. Guidelines for scoring these subtests are provided in the WIAT manual. After all desired subtests have been given, raw scores are recorded on the Record Form.

Derived scores are obtained for subtests and composites, and these are recorded on the Record Form. The Record Form pages also contain sections and information that can be used in conducting a skills analysis. For example, on the Mathematics Reasoning page, space is given to note whether the client used an appropriate strategy but made computational errors, used an inappropriate strategy, guessed, or made no attempt.

Comment

Split-half reliability coefficients are provided for the subtest and composite standard scores

at each age and range (see source). Coefficients are moderate to high (.69 to .98) and are generally greater for the composite than for individual subtest scores. Stability of scores on the WIAT was assessed in 367 children (grades 1, 3, 5, 8, and 10) who were tested twice with a median retest interval of 17 days. Test–retest correlations are moderate to high (see source). The differences between testings tend to be small, usually between 1 and 3 standard score points. The exceptions are on Oral Expression and the Language Composite, both of which have differences between 4 and 9 standard score points. Interscorer agreement is high (above .79) for all subtests (see source).

Support for the construct validity of the WIAT comes from the pattern of intercorrelations among subtests (see source). The mathematics subtests correlate more highly with each other than with the reading subtests, and the reading subtests correlate more highly with each other than with the mathematics subtests. Moreover, the raw-score averages at each age and each grade show the expected group differences.

Scores on the WIAT correlate moderately with Wechsler IQ scores. Most of the correlations range from .30 to .70 for the FSIQ scores (see source). As might be expected, there is substantial correlation (generally above .70) between scores on the WIAT and other individually administered achievement tests such as the Basic Skills Individual Screener, the Kaufman Test of Educational Achievement, the Wide Range Achievement Test—Revised, the Woodcock-Johnson Psycho-Educational Battery—Revised, and the Differential Ability Scales. Correlations between the WIAT and group-administered achievement tests, such as the Metropolitan Achievement Test and the Comprehensive Test of Basic Skills, are somewhat lower and generally fall in the moderate range. Modest correlations (.17 to .46) are found between WIAT scores and teacher-assigned grades (see source). Data on special groups (e.g., learning disabled, ADHD) are provided in the WIAT manual and show the expected patterns of mean scores and predicted–actual discrepancies, although the samples are relatively small.

The WIAT manual is well-written and includes a section containing useful information regarding the skills addressed by particular test items and specific deficits that may underlie low scores. Such an analysis can help focus the direction of subsequent evaluation.

Although the WIAT item content encompasses a wide range of skills and concepts, few rudimentary and advanced items were included in the design of the test. Therefore, for 5-year-olds and 19-year olds, achievement and ability–achievement discrepancies must be viewed cautiously due to floor and ceiling effects. Supplementary testing is necessary at the extremes of the WIAT age range. Because of the restriction in item range, the test should also not be used as a measure of academic giftedness (see source). Further, the WIAT represents a composite of the curricula found across the United States. Accordingly, there may be a lack of correspondence with curricula in Canada and other English-speaking countries.

It is worth bearing in mind that the Screener Composite and Total Composite scores provide broad levels of achievement. These scores reflect many facets of an individual's achievement, within which there may be great variation. Accordingly, these general scores should be interpreted with caution and are not recommended for use in computing ability–achievement discrepancies (see source).

Normative Data

The WIAT was standardized on a large American sample ($n = 4,252$), stratified according to age (5 years through 19 years), regional residence, gender, race/ethnicity, and parental education. A subset of the WIAT standardization sample ($n = 1,284$) was also administered the Wechsler Intelligence scales. In this way, ability–achievement discrepancy statistics could be computed.

The WIAT manual provides norm tables containing standard scores (mean = 100, SD = 15) for both age and grade (with separate fall, winter, and spring tables); tables for determining confidence intervals, percentile ranks, stanines, age and grade equivalents, and normal curve equivalents; tables to be used in calculating standard score differences (between subtests as well as between composites), ability–achievement discrepancies, and their significance and frequency in the normal population. Note that one must use age-based standard scores to calculate ability–achievement discrepancies. The relationship of the ability standard score to the WIAT standard score can also be plotted on the Record Form.

WIAT standard scores can be compared to other intellectual ability instruments (e.g., the Stanford-Binet). Such a practice, however, requires caution. The examiner must evaluate the psychometric characteristics of each test and the comparability of the years in which the tests were standardized, bearing in mind that, by definition, standard scores derive their meaning from the performance of individuals in the standardization sample (see source). One may need to convert the scores from the alternative test to the WIAT standard metric, with a mean of 100 and a standard deviation of 15.

References

Wechsler Individual Achievement Test. (1992). San Antonio, TX: The Psychological Corporation.

WIDE RANGE ACHIEVEMENT TEST 3 (WRAT3)

Purpose

The purpose of this test is to measure reading (word recognition and pronunciation), spelling, and arithmetic.

Source

The test, including the two equivalent alternate forms, manual, and reading/spelling cards, can be ordered from The Psychological Corporation, P.O. Box 9954, San Antonio, Texas 78204-0954, at a cost of approximately $105 US or from the Psychological Corporation, 55 Horner Avenue, Toronto, ON M8Z 4X6 for about $185 Cdn.

Description

The WRAT is one of the most frequently used measures of academic achievement (Sheehan, 1983) because it is quick, easy to administer, and assesses three different ability areas: reading, spelling, and arithmetic. It was originally published in 1936. Revisions appeared in 1946, 1965, 1976, 1978, 1984, and 1993. The latest revision, the WRAT3 (Wilkinson, 1993), differs only slightly in item content from its predecessors. In addition, two equivalent forms were designed and new record forms and norms have been provided. The complete kit consists of the administration and scoring manual, the test forms, and plastic cards containing the reading and spelling word lists.

The 1993 edition of the WRAT has returned to a single-level format for use with all individuals aged 5–75 years. Two alternate test forms (Blue and Tan) provide the three subtests: reading, spelling, and arithmetic. The reading skills measured are letter and word recognition. The spelling skills include copying marks, writing one's name, and writing single words from dictation. The arithmetic skills cover counting, reading number symbols, solving oral problems, and performing written computations. If desired, an examiner can administer both forms (Combined Form) to a client at a single examination session.

Administration

See source. Briefly, the examiner presents a test card, reads aloud words and sentences, asks test questions, and records responses. The three subtests can be given in any order.

The "5/10 Rules" notation on the test forms pertains to the Spelling and Reading subtests of the WRAT3. The "5" represents the rule that if an individual 8 years or older is able to successfully respond to five or more of the formal Spelling or Reading items, then the preliminary section need not be given in the respective subtest. All clients 7 years and younger must be administered the preliminary sections. Individuals who do not respond correctly to five of the formal items on these subtests must be given the respective preliminary sections. The "10" rule concerns the discontinuance of the respective subtests. After 10 consecutive errors on the Spelling and/or the Reading subtest, the examiner should terminate the administration of the formal items of the subtest.

Approximate Time for Administration

The test is timed and takes about 15–30 minutes. Note that the WRAT3 arithmetic subtests have been extended to 15 minutes rather than the 10 minutes used with the WRAT-R.

Scoring

For each test, the total number correct is recorded. Raw scores can be converted to derived scores.

Comment

Reliability estimates, based on item and person separation indices, are reported to be high (see source). Coefficient alphas range from .85 to .95 over the nine WRAT3 tests. With regard to the alternate forms, the Blue and Tan forms are made up mostly of items that were used on previous editions of the WRAT. There are however, several new items on each test. Alternate form reliability is reported to be high (above .8) (see source). When healthy individuals aged 6–16 years are retested with the WRAT3 about one month later, test–retest correlations range from .91 to .98.

As might be expected (see source), the mean test scores show a steady increase until the 45–54 year-old age group. After this age, scores begin to decline. The various skills measured by the WRAT3 show moderate-to-high intercorrelations (.54 to .91). Further, scores on the WRAT3 correlate moderately (.5 to .6) with WISC-III Full Scale IQ scores. The tests tend to have a somewhat higher correlation with the Verbal than the Performance Scale. Similarly, scores on the WRAT3 are reported to correlate highly (.79 to .99) with the WRAT-R. Moderate-to-high correlations are found between the WRAT3 and relevant subtests of the California Test of Basic Skills—4th Edition, California Achievement Test Form E, and the Stanford Achievement Test. Finally, the WRAT3 also appears moderately sensitive to differences of academic skill. The test was given to gifted, learning-disabled, educable mentally retarded, and normal students and was able to distinguish group membership at a 68 percent correct discrimination level.

One problem for non-U.S. users is a lack of correspondence with curricula in Canada and other English-speaking countries. The Arithmetic subtest in particular is of questionable use since students may not have been exposed to the teaching of some of the skills. Canada has adopted the metric system, and there is much less emphasis on fractions, with more stress on decimals (Sheehan, 1983). Canadian normative data for the WRAT3 are not available.

The WRAT3 provides only a limited amount of information about reading, arithmetic, and spelling (Sattler, 1982). For example, reading comprehension is not assessed, only letter or word recognition. In addition, no specific breakdowns are provided to enable the user to determine the specific types of reading, arithmetic, or spelling difficulties (Sattler, 1982). Because of these issues, the test should not be used as a diagnostic measure of academic difficulties. The test, however, may be useful as a quick, but gross, screening device. Our own view is that better tests are available

(e.g., Woodcock-Johnson, WIAT, PIAT-R), but that clinicians should be familiar with the WRAT-3, given its wide-spread use. If used, the formula-type arithmetic subtest should be compared with the Applied Problems subtest of the Woodcock-Johnson or WIAT, and the reading recognition subtest should be supplemented with the Reading or Passage Comprehension subtest of the WIAT, PIAT-R, or Woodcock-Johnson.

Reading tests are sometimes used as estimates of premorbid intelligence to determine the existence and extent of cognitive decline following brain damage (Johnstone et al., 1996; Kareken et al., 1995; Wiens et al. 1993). WRAT-R scores show a moderate relation with WAIS-R IQ (r = 0.45 to 0.62) and provide a reasonable estimate of average IQ levels. However, WRAT scores tend to underestimate at the higher IQ ranges and overestimate at the lower IQ ranges. Johnstone and Wilhelm (1996) recently evaluated the longitudinal stability of reading (WRAT-R/3) and intelligence (WAIS-R FSIQ) for a mixed group of neurological and psychiatric patients. The average time between test-retest was about 28 months. They found that reading scores may be appropriate estimates of premorbid intelligence for individuals demonstrating intellectual decline/stability but not for those showing significant intellectual improvement. Additionally, significant variability in reading score decline or improvement (−8 to +22) in this sample suggests that caution must be used in estimating premorbid intelligence from WRAT-R/WRAT3 Reading scores.

Normative Data

The WRAT3 was standardized on a large American sample (n = 4,433) stratified according to age (5 years to 74 years, 11 months), regional residence, gender, ethnicity, and socioeconomic level. Norm tables, broken down by age, are found in the WRAT3 manual for each of the Blue, Tan, and Combined forms. These tables provide raw scores, standard scores (mean of 100 and standard deviation of 15), absolute scores, grade scores, percentiles, stanines, scaled scores, T-scores, and normal curve equivalents.

Care should be taken when comparing test scores between current and previous editions. The standard scores for the WRAT-R are about 8–11 points lower than the corresponding WRAT (1978) scores (Spruill & Beck, 1986). WRAT3 raw scores are lower than those of the WRAT-R because there are fewer items on the WRAT3. Standard scores, however, are comparable between the WRAT3 and WRAT-R (G. Wilkinson, personal communication, December 1994).

References

Johnstone, B., & Wilhelm, K.L. (1996). The longitudinal stability of the WRAT-R Reading subtest: Is it an appropriate estimate of premorbid intelligence? *Journal of the International Neuropsychological Society, 2*, 282–285.

Johnstone, B., Callahan, C.D., Kapila, C.J., & Bouman, D.E. (1996). The comparability of the WRAT-R reading test and NAART as estimates of premorbid intelligence in neurologically impaired patients. *Archives of Clinical Neuropsychology, 11*, 513–519.

Kareken, D.A., Gur, R.C., & Saykin, A.J. (1995). Reading on the Wide Range Achievement Test-Revised and parental education as predictors of IQ: Comparison with the Barona formula. *Archives of Clinical Neuropsychology 10*, 147–157.

Sattler, J.M. (1982). *Assessment of Children's Intelligence and Special Abilities* (2nd ed.). Boston: Allyn and Bacon.

Sheehan, T.D. (1983). Re-norming the WRAT: An urban Ontario sample. *Ontario Psychologist, 15*, 16–33.

Spruill, J., & Beck, B. (1986). Relationship between the WRAT and WRAT-R. *Psychology in the Schools, 23*, 357–360.

Wiens, A.N., Bryan, J.E., & Crossen, J.R. (1993). Estimating WAIS-R FSIQ from the National Adult Reading Test-Revised in normal subjects. *The Clinical Neuropsychologist, 7*, 70–84.0

Wilkinson, G.S. (1993). *WRAT3 Administration Manual*. Delaware: Wide Range.

WOODCOCK-JOHNSON PSYCHOEDUCATIONAL BATTERY—REVISED: TESTS OF ACHIEVEMENT (WJ-R ACH)

Purpose

This is a wide-range test that includes measures of achievement in the areas of reading, mathematics, written language, and knowledge of science, social studies, and humanities.

Source

The achievement section of the battery can be ordered from Riverside Publishing Company, 425 Spring Lake Drive, Itasca, Illinois 60143, or from Nelson Canada, 1120 Birchmont Road, Scarborough, Ontario M1K 5G4. There are two alternate forms (A and B) and each can be had for $323 US or about $532.95 Cdn. Computer scoring programs (Compuscore) are also available at an additional cost of $220 US or about $385 Cdn.

Description

The WJ-R (Woodcock & Mather, 1989) is a revised and expanded version of the 1977 Woodcock-Johnson battery developed as a comprehensive, individually administered measure of cognitive ability, academic achievement, scholastic aptitude, scholastic/nonscholastic interests, and independent function. It is intended for both handicapped and nonhandicapped populations from ages 2 to 90. Our focus here is on the Tests of Achievement (WJ-R ACH), which has two separate forms (Form A and Form B), each of which must be purchased separately. The WJ-R ACH is subdivided into a Standard Battery and a Supplemental Battery and allows for analysis of four curriculum areas: reading, mathematics, written language, and knowledge. The subtests are presented in two flip-page easel books, one for the Standard and one for the Supplemental Battery, designed to stand on the table during administration. The books contain the items for each subtest and the instructions for administration. Separate manuals provide instructions for scoring, instructions for administration, and the tables necessary for score interpretation. Response booklets are provided to record, summarize, and interpret test performance. Most of the subtests are untimed and have basal and ceiling levels established by six consecutive correct and six consecutive failed items, respectively.

The Standard Battery of the WJ-R ACH consists of nine subtests, each of which measures different aspects of scholastic achievement:

Letter-Word Identification: measures the ability to identify letters and words.

Passage Comprehension: measures the subject's skill in supplying the appropriate word to complete a short passage after silently reading the passage.

Calculation: tests the subject's ability to perform calculations ranging from simple addition and subtraction to those involving trigonomic, logarithmic, geometric, and calculus operations. Procedures are specified and no application skills are required. Items are completed in a special Subject Response Booklet.

Applied Problems: measures the subject's ability to solve practical problems. The subject must recognize the correct procedure, identify the relevant data, and perform relatively simple calculations. Problems are presented visually or are read to the subject to minimize the effect of reading ability. The use of note paper is permitted.

Dictation: tests the subject's ability to respond in writing to a variety of questions requiring knowledge of punctuation, capitalization, spelling, and word usage (e.g., contractions, abbreviations, plurals).

Writing Samples: measures the subject's skill in writing responses to a variety of demands. The subject must phrase and present written sentences that are evaluated with respect to the quality of expression. The subject is not penalized for errors in basic orthography such as spelling or punctuation.

Science: tests the subject's knowledge in the biological and physical sciences. Items are read aloud by the examiner.

Social Studies: tests the subject's knowledge in geography, government, economics, and other aspects of broad social studies. Items are read aloud by the examiner.

Humanities: measures the subject's knowledge in various areas of art, music, and literature. The subject responds orally to questions read by the examiner.

Six tests from the Standard Battery are suitable for use as early development measures: Letter-Word Identification, Applied Problems, Dictation, Science, Social Studies, and Humanities. In addition to preschool children, this set of tests may be administered to low-functioning individuals of any age.

The WJ-R ACH Supplemental Battery can provide a more comprehensive assessment of a subject's achievement in reading, mathematics, and written language. It consists of five tests:

Word Attack: requires the subject to read nonsense words and assesses phonic and structural analysis skills.

Reading Vocabulary: measures the subject's skill in reading words and applying appropriate meanings. In Part A, Synonyms, the subject must state a word similar in meaning to the word presented. In Part B, Antonyms, the subject must state a word that is opposite in meaning to the word presented.

Quantitative Concepts: measures the subject's knowledge of mathematical concepts and vocabulary. The test does not require the subject to perform any calculations or to make any application decisions.

Proofing: tests the subject's ability to read a short passage that is known to contain one and only one error. The error may be one of punctuation, capitalization, spelling, or usage. The subject's task is to identify the error and to indicate how it should be corrected.

Writing Fluency: measures the subject's skill in formulating and writing simple sentences quickly. Each sentence must relate to a given stimulus picture and use a set of three words. This test has a 7-minute time limit.

In addition to these five subtests, four test scores, identified by letter names, may be derived. Scores for Punctuation and Capitalization (P), Spelling (S), and Usage (U) are determined from the analysis of performance on the

Dictation test in the Standard Battery and the Proofing test in the Supplemental Battery. The score for Handwriting (H) is determined from an analysis of the subject's handwriting produced during the Writing Samples test in the Standard Battery.

Although subtests are the basic components of the battery, clusters of scores (Reading, Mathematics, Written Language, Knowledge, Skills) can be derived from certain combinations of subtests. Five cluster scores can be calculated from the Standard Battery. The Broad Reading Cluster is a combination of the Letter-Word Identification and Passage Comprehension tests and provides a broad measure of reading achievement. The Broad Mathematics Cluster is a combination of the Calculation and Applied Problems tests and provides a broad measure of mathematical achievement. The Broad Written Language Cluster is a combination of the Dictation and Writing Samples tests and provides a broad measure of written language achievement, including both production of single-word responses and production of sentences embedded in context. The Broad Knowledge Cluster is a combination of the Science, Social Studies, and Humanities tests. The Skills cluster is a combination of the Letter-Word Identification, Applied Problems, and Dictation tests and provides a quick screening of broad achievement. It may be used as an early development measure.

In addition to the cluster scores derived from the Standard Battery, six additional cluster scores can be derived using tests from the Standard and Supplemental Batteries. The Basic Reading Skills cluster is a combination of Letter-Word Identification and Word Attack and provides a measure of basic reading skills that includes both sight vocabulary and the ability to apply phonic and structural analysis skills. The Reading Comprehension cluster is a combination of Passage Comprehension and Reading Vocabulary and provides a measure of reading comprehension skills that includes both comprehension of single-word stimuli and context-embedded stimuli. The Basic Mathematics Skills cluster is a combination of the Calculation and Quantitative Concepts tests and provides a measure of basic mathe-

matical skills, including computation skills and knowledge of mathematical concepts and vocabulary. The Mathematics Reasoning Cluster consists only of the Applied Problems test and provides a measure of the ability to analyze and solve practical math problems. The Basic Writing Skills cluster is a combination of Dictation and Proofing and provides a measure of basic writing skills, including both writing single-word responses and identifying errors in spelling, punctuation, capitalization, and word usage. Finally, the Written Expression cluster is a combination of Writing Samples and Writing Fluency and provides a measure of written expression skills, including production of simple written sentences with ease and of increasingly complex sentences to meet special requirements.

Administration

See WJ-R Manual. The easel format facilitates administration. The notation of basal and ceiling rules directly on the Test Record and the uniformity of the basal (six consecutive correct responses) and ceiling (six consecutive incorrect responses) rules for most subtests also contribute to the ease of administration. Further, the use of basal and ceiling rules makes it possible to match the difficulty level of subtests to the ability of the individual being tested. Not all subtests need to be given (principle of selective testing), and the subtests may be given in any order.

Approximate Time for Administration

Approximately 50–60 minutes are needed to give the nine tests of the Standard Battery. The Writing Samples test requires about 15 minutes to administer, while the other eight tests require an average of 5 minutes each. The four tests in the Supplemental Battery take an additional 30 minutes to give.

Scoring

See WJ-R ACH Manual. The scoring criteria for the items are clear. Examples of correct and incorrect responses are presented on the examiner's side of the easel and in the examiner's manual. Various derived scores are available, including age equivalents, grade equivalents, relative mastery indices (RMI), test or cluster difference scores, percentile ranks, standard scores, T-scores, stanines, and normal curve equivalents. RMIs are statements describing mastery or quality of performance. This score allows statements to be made about a subject's expected level of performance on tasks similar to the ones tested. It indicates the percent of mastery predicted for a given subject when the reference group would perform with 90 percent mastery. RMIs are also interpreted by functioning levels ranging from "very advanced" to "severely deficient."

The process of obtaining derived scores is somewhat lengthy, complex, and prone to error but may be simplified by using the Compuscore for the WJ-R. Briefly, the raw score for each subtest is associated by a table in the Test Record with the W score (which is an intermediate score needed to complete the calculations), the standard error of measurement of the W score, the age equivalent, and the grade equivalent. The Age/Grade Profiles, located on the front and back covers of the Test Record, are then completed by transferring the W scores for each subtest and cluster into the appropriate box on the front or back cover. Expected test and cluster W scores (REF W) for age (Table B) or grade (Table C) and the standard error of measurement (SEM) for the standard scores are then entered on the Test Record, and the difference is calculated between the observed and expected scores. After difference scores have been determined, RMIs, standard scores (mean = 100, SD = 15) and percentile ranks (PR) may be obtained from norm Table D in the manual. Confidence bands for the standard scores and percentile ranks are then obtained, either directly from the Test Record (for standard scores) or from Table E in the manual (for PR). The bars on the Standard Score/Percentile Rank Profiles, found on the Test Record, are completed next and are based on one standard error of measurement. The degree of overlap between the confidence bands can be used to provide clues about a subject's strengths and weaknesses.

Once the scores have been derived, one can evaluate whether subjects with a significant intra-achievement discrepancy exhibit specific achievement deficits using tables F to H in the manual.

Comment

Woodcock and Mather (1989) report impressive split-half reliability coefficients. Reliabilities are generally in the high .80s and low .90s for the tests and in the mid .90s for the clusters. Data on test–retest reliability are available only for the Writing Fluency test (.76). Interrater reliability for the Writing Samples test is high (above .88; Mather et al., 1991).

The concurrent validity of the WJ-R ACH, using a variety of achievement tests (e.g., KABC, PPVT, PIAT, WRAT-R, TOWL), is moderate, with correlations typically in the .50 to .70 range (see source; Mather et al., 1991). When the tests and clusters are grouped by curriculum areas, the tests and clusters within the same area correlate more highly with each other than with tests and clusters belonging to other curricular areas. Finally, Woodcock and Mather (1989) note that the test yields the expected pattern of scores with different populations: namely, scores show a progressive increase going from the mentally retarded, learning-disabled, normal, to gifted populations, and there is an increase in scores with age for each type of sample.

One should note that the Reading cluster primarily measures word recognition skills, with reading comprehension only minimally assessed. Further, the reading comprehension that is evaluated is literal rather than a higher type of comprehension, such as critical or inferential reading (Hessler, 1984).

The WJ-R ACH is a technically excellent instrument and provides a more comprehensive measure of written language, mathematics, and content knowledge than other individually administered survey instruments (e.g., PIAT-R, WRAT-3, WIAT). The PIAT-R, however, may be more appropriate when the subject's verbal skills are limited. The WIAT has the advantage of being co-normed with the WISC-III. One should also note that the WJ-

R ACH is fundamentally a screening device, not a diagnostic instrument. Further testing with other instruments (e.g., KeyMath, Stanford Diagnostic Reading Test) may be necessary to provide in-depth information about a subject's skills. Further, some of the items contain typical U.S. content and may be troublesome for other English-speaking populations.

Normative Data

Data provided in the WJ-R ACH manual were derived from a large sample ($n = 6,359$) of normal people, ranging in age from 24 months to 95 years, residing in the United States. The norms can be considered representative in terms of U.S. census data. Since the norms are derived solely from U.S. samples, caution should be used when interpreting scores of people residing outside the United States.

References

Hessler, G.L. (1984). *Use and interpretation of the Woodcock-Johnson Psycho-Educational Battery.* Allen, TX: DLM Teaching Resources.

Mather, N., Vogel, S.A., Spodak, R.B., & McGrew, K.S. (1991). Use of the Woodcock-Johnson—Revised writing tests with students with learning disabilities. *Journal of Psychoeducational Assessment, 9,* 296–307.

Woodcock, R.W., & Mather, N. (1989). *Woodcock-Johnson Tests of Achievement.* Allen, TX: DLM Teaching Resources.

8

Executive Functions

The term *executive function* has only recently been added to the neuropsychological terminology (Lezak, 1982) as a shorthand description of a multidimensional construct referring to a variety of loosely related higher-order cognitive processes including initiation, planning, hypothesis generation, cognitive flexibility, decision making, regulation, judgment, feedback utilization, and self-perception that are necessary for effective and contextually appropriate behavior. It comprises numerous subordinate component cognitive operations, with working memory perhaps the most important of these (Tranel et al., 1994). It is important to note that it is quite possible to find impairment of executive functions such as planning, flexibility of thought, and judgment without major change in general intellectual status (Kolb & Whishaw, 1995). Further, while executive disturbances often arise following damage to prefrontal regions, they may also occur in the context of dysfunction to other brain regions (Lezak, 1995; Luria, 1966; Tranel et al., 1994).

Interviews with the patient, the family, or other persons familiar with the patient may bring some of these executive problems to light. The major difficulty in examining executive dysfunction within formal examinations is that this format typically allows the patient little room for discretionary behavior. The challenge for the clinician, therefore, is how to transfer initiation, planning, and judgment from the examiner to the patient within the structured testing situation (Lezak, 1995).

Some techniques (e.g., WISC-III Mazes to assess planning; Trail Making Test to measure shifting of perceptual set; Consonant Trigrams for working memory) have been presented elsewhere in this book. We describe here a number of additional tests that may allow the patient to demonstrate some components of the executive system.

Cognitive flexibility refers to the ability to look at objects/events from many vantage points, particularly when dealing with a novel context. It can be divided into reactive and spontaneous components (Eslinger & Grattan, 1993). Spontaneous flexibility, or fluency, requires the intrinsic generation of responses or alternatives, typically within a set of constraints, and can be assessed by measures of verbal (see Controlled Oral Word Association in the section on Language Tests) and nonverbal (Design Fluency, Five-Point Test) fluency.

Reactive flexibility, on the other hand, reflects the ability to realign a behavioral predisposition to altered contingencies; it can be assessed with the Category Test, the Wisconsin Card Sorting Test, the California Sorting Test, and the Stroop Test. It is important to bear in mind that these various tests appear to tap somewhat different abilities, and use of one or more of these tests depends upon the diagnostic question. The Category Test, a measure of abstraction, has the disadvantage of providing only a single summary score and therefore may provide little information about why patients perform poorly. The Wisconsin Card

Sorting Test provides several different measures of behavior, including problem solving and some aspect of attention. However, performance on the global measure of problem solving (categories achieved) is highly and negatively correlated with perseverative responding. The California Sorting Test provides separate assessments of concept generation, concept identification, and concept execution, as well as several different measures of perseveration. Measures of concept attainment do not appear to be strongly correlated with measures of perseveration, suggesting that any increased perseverative tendencies are not simply the result of poor overall problem-solving performance. A pencil and paper version of the task has recently been described by Levine et al. (1995). Finally, the Stroop Test places demands on cognitive flexibility by requiring shifting of perceptual set in accordance with changing external demands, as well as the inhibition of a habitual response in favor of a novel one.

Executive functioning also involves the ability to make judgments in dealing with unfamiliar situations. The Cognitive Estimation Test evaluates the ability to make reasonable estimates, to monitor, and to self-correct.

Additional tests can also be used to examine goal-directed behavior. The Self-Ordered Pointing Test (Petrides & Milner, 1982) requires individuals to organize information, maintain a record, and monitor responses. Maze tracing tasks can provide information involving planning and foresight. We typically use the WISC III mazes (for some preliminary data for adults, see normative section under Wechsler Intelligence Scale), although clinicians might also refer to the Porteus Maze Test. The Tower of Hanoi (London or Toronto) is thought to measure planning (Shallice, 1982) and requires patients to rearrange colored balls on pegs of varying height to match a presented goal configuration, using a set of simple rules governing acceptable moves. Davis et al. (1995) have provided a software package, the Colorado Neuropsychology Tests, that includes these puzzles (see section on Memory). The Tinker Toy Test (Lezak, 1995), not considered here, allows examination of purposive behavior in a fairly unstructured setting. The patient is provided with 50 pieces of a standard Tinker Toy set and told to make whatever the patient wishes during a 5-minute minimum time limit.

Most neuropsychological tests give the patient an explicit, brief task to solve. Typically, task initiation is prompted by the examiner and task success is well-defined. Rarely are patients required to organize or plan their behavior over longer time periods or to set priorities in the face of two or more competing tasks. It is, however, these sorts of executive abilities that are a large component of everyday activities. We include here a description of the BADS (Wilson et al. 1996), a collection of six tests (Rule Shift Cards, Action Program Test, Key Search Test, Temporal Judgement Test, Zoo Map, Modified Six Elements Test) that appear to capture aspects of everyday problems that may pose difficulty for some patients with executive dysfunction. In addition, a questionnaire given to both the patient and rater is also included.

Characterization and measurement of executive function deficits remains a major challenge for neuropsychologists. Although numerous clinical and experimental techniques have been developed, it is important to bear in mind that very few have been shown to have a high degree of sensitivity and specificity with regard to characterizing executive function defects and, relatedly, frontal lobe dysfunction (Tranel et al., 1994). Clinicians have tended to choose executive function tests for their face validity rather than their psychometric properties, and some tests purporting to measure executive functions lack adequate normative data. Recently, Kafer and Hunter (1997) gave 130 normal adults four tests purporting to measure planning/problem-solving. Tests included the Tower of London, the Six Elements Test, the 20 Questions Test, and the Rey Complex Figure (Copy). A structural equation modeling approach suggested that the four tests are measuring different, unrelated constructs, begging the question as to what clinicians are measuring when they administer these tests to clinical populations.

References

Davis, H.P., Bajszar, G.M., & Squire, L.R. (1995). *Colorado Neuropsychology Tests*. Colorado

Springs, CO: Colorado Neuropsychology Tests Co.

Eslinger, P.J., & Grattan, L.M. (1993). Frontal lobe and frontal striatal substrates for different forms of human cognitive flexibility. *Neuropsychologia, 31,* 17–28.

Kafer, K.L., & Hunter, M. (1997). On testing the face validity of planning/problem-solving tasks in a normal population. *Journal of the International Neuropsychological Society, 3,* 108–119.

Kolb, B., & Whishaw, I.Q. (1995). *Fundamentals of Human Neuropsychology.* New York: Freeman Press.

Levine. B., Stuss, D.T., & Milberg, W.P. (1995). Concept generation: Validation of a test of executive functioning in a normal aging population. *Journal of Clinical and Experimental Neuropsychology, 17,* 740–758.

Lezak, M.D. (1982). The problems of assessing executive functions. *International Journal of Psychology, 17,* 281–297.

Lezak, M. (1995). *Neuropsychological Assessment* (3rd ed.). New York: Oxford University Press.

Luria, A.R. (1966). *Higher Cortical Functions in Man.* New York: Basic Books.

Petrides, M., & Milner, B. (1982). Deficits on subject-ordered tasks after frontal- and temporal-lobe lesions in man. *Neuropsychologia, 20,* 249–262.

Shallice, T. (1982). Specific impairments of planning. *Philosophical Transactions of the Royal Society of London, 298,* 199–209.

Tranel, D., Anderson, S.W., & Benton, A. (1994). Development of the concept of "executive function" and its relationship to the frontal lobes. In *Handbook of Neuropsychology,* F. Boller & J. Grafman, (Eds.). New York: Elsevier, 9, 125–148.

Wilson, B.A., Alderman, N., Burgess, P.W., Emslie, H., & Evans, J.J. (1996). *Behavioral Assessment of the Dysexecutive Syndrome.* Bury St. Edmunds, England: Thames Valley Test Company.

BEHAVIORAL ASSESSMENT OF THE DYSEXECUTIVE SYSTEM (BADS)

Purpose

The purpose of this battery is to predict everyday problems arising from executive disturbances.

Source

The kit includes manual, test materials, and 25 scoring and rating sheets and can be ordered from Northern Speech Services, Inc., 117 N. Elm, P.O. Box 1247, Gaylord MI 49735, at a cost of $398 US.

Description

The authors (Wilson et al., 1996) note that most neuropsychological tests give the patient an explicit task to solve, with a short trial, task initiation prompted by the examiner, and task success well-defined. Rarely are patients required to organize or plan their behavior over longer time periods or to set priorities in the face of two or more competing tasks despite the fact that these sorts of executive abilities are a large component of everyday activities. BADS presents a collection of six new tests that are similar to real-life activities and could cause difficulty for some patients with Dys-

executive Syndrome (DES). In addition, a questionnaire given to both the patient and a rater are also included.

1. The Rule Shift Cards Test uses 21 spiral-bound non-picture playing cards and examines the subject's ability to respond correctly to a rule and to shift from one rule to another. In the first part of the test, the subject is asked to say "Yes" to a red card and "No" to a black card. This rule, typed on a card, is left in full view throughout to reduce memory constraints. In the second part of the test, the subject must 'forget' the first rule and concentrate on applying a new rule. The subject is asked to respond "Yes" if the card that has just been turned over is the same color as the previously turned card and "No" if it is a different color. This new, typed rule is left in full view of the subject. The test, therefore, is a measure of the ability to shift from one rule to another and to keep track of the color of the previous card and the current rule. The measures are time taken and number of errors on the second trial.

2. The Action Program Test was adapted from a task originally described by Klosowaska (1976) and requires five steps to its solution. The subject is presented with a rectangular

stand into one end of which is set a large transparent beaker with a removable lid that has a small central hole in it. Into the other end of the stand is set a thin transparent tube at the bottom of which is a small piece of cork. The beaker is two-thirds full of water. To the left of the stand is placed an L-shaped metal rod, which is not long enough to reach the cork, and a small screw top container on one side, with its top unscrewed and lying beside it. Subjects are asked to get the cork out of the tube using any of the objects in front of them but without lifting up the stand, the tube, or the beaker, and without touching the lid with their fingers. To solve the problem subjects must work out that the key to the problem is to use the water to make the cork float to the top of the tall tube and then work out how to get the water out of the beaker and into this tube. This involves removing the lid with the metal hook, screwing the top onto the small container, filling the small container with water from the beaker, pouring it into the tube, and repeating this at least once until the cork floats to the top of the tube. There is no time limit, and prompts may be given if a subject is unable to progress through any one of the five stages. A profile score is obtained according to the number of stages completed independently.

3. In the Key Search Test, subjects are presented with a piece of paper with a 100 mm square in the middle and a small black dot 50 mm below it. The subjects are told to imagine that the square is a large field in which they have lost their keys. They are asked to draw a line, starting on the black dot, to show where they would walk to search the field to make absolutely certain that they would find their keys. The efficiency of the strategy is evaluated.

4. The Temporal Judgement Test comprises four short questions concerning commonplace events which take a few seconds (e.g., how long does it take to blow up a party balloon?) to several years (how long do most dogs live?). The authors note that some of the questions and answers may prove culturally specific to subjects in the United Kingdom, and American users may wish to leave out this task and prorate on the other five tests in the

battery. Each of the four questions is scored 0 or 1.

5. The Zoo Map Test requires subjects to show how they would visit a series of designated locations on a map of a zoo. Certain rules must be followed which include, starting at the entrance and finishing at a designated picnic area, and using designated paths in the zoo just once. The map and rules have been constructed so that there are only four variations on route that can be followed in order that none of the rules are infringed. There are two trials. In both trials, the subject is required to visit six out of twelve possible location (e.g., the cafe, the bears, the elephants). The first trial consists of a high demand version of the task in which the planning abilities of the subject are rigorously tested. To minimize errors, the subject must plan in advance the order in which the designated locations will be visited. Errors will be incurred if the subject simply visits the locations in the order given in the instruction. Scrupulously following the instructions in the high demand version will maximise the total error. In the second, low demand trial, the subject is simply required to follow the instructions to produce an error-free performance. In both versions, the ability of the subject to minimise errors by modifying performance on the basis of feedback, once a rule is broken, is assessed. It is envisaged that comparison of performance on the two trials will permit quantitative evaluation of a subject's spontaneous planning ability when structure is minimal, versus ability to follow a concrete externally imposed strategy when structure is high. The profile score reflects the sequence produced, the number of errors made, and the time to task completion.

6. The Modified Six Elements Test is modeled after a task developed by Shallice and Burgess (1991). The subject is given instructions to do three tasks (dictation, arithmetic, and picture naming) each of which is divided into two parts, called A and B. The subject is required to attempt at least something from each of the six subtasks within a ten minute period. In addition, the subject is told that there is one rule which must not be broken: Subjects are not allowed to do the two parts of

the same task consecutively. So, for example, if they were naming one set of pictures they could not switch to naming the other set of pictures. They would have to do one of the arithmetic or one of the dictation subtasks first and return to the other set of pictures later. It is not important how well the subject performs the individual components; rather, the point of the test is how well subjects organize themselves. The profile score is based on the number of tasks completed, the number of tasks where rule breaks were made and the time spent on any one task.

7. The Dysexecutive Questionnaire (DEX) is a 20-item questionnaire that samples four broad areas of likely changes: emotional or personality changes, motivational changes, behavioral changes, and cognitive changes. Items include statements such as: 'I act without thinking, doing the first thing that comes to mind' or 'I have difficulty thinking ahead and planning for the future.' Each item is scored on a 5-point (0–4) Likert scale, ranging from 'Never' to 'Very Often.'" The questionnaire compares responses in two versions, one of which is designed to be completed by the subject and another by a relative or a caregiver who has close, preferably daily, contact with the subject.

Administration

Instructions for administration are given in the BADS manual. Some items have timed components. The scoring sheet prompts the examiner about various aspects of the administration and scoring procedures.

Approximate Time for Administration

The entire test can be given in about one-half hour.

Scoring

Scoring guidelines are found in the BADS manual. In addition, the scoring sheet prompts the examiner to record various aspects of the subject's performance for each of the six tests. The method of scoring was devised so that a 'profile' score, ranging from 0 to 4, is calculated for each test. An overall profile score for the whole battery is obtained by adding together the individual profile scores for each test. The DEX, however, is not formally part of the BADS in the sense that it is not used in the calculation of the profile score for the battery. Rather, it is used to supplement information obtained on the battery, through the provision of additional qualitative information. Therefore, any subject who completes the whole battery will obtain a BADS profile score within the range of 0 to 24. Although it is recommended that all six tests of the BADS be administered to obtain the total BADS profile score, it is possible to prorate on the basis of 5 tests.

Comment

The authors report that twenty-five normal individuals were tested with a second tester present. Inter-rater reliability was high (above .88). Twenty-nine normals were retested on the battery as well as three other executive tasks (Modified Card Sorting Test, Cognitive Estimation Task, FAS) after an interval of 6 to 12 months. Test-retest correlations for the BADS tests ranged from −.08 (Rule Shift Cards) to .71 (Key Search). Low to moderate correlations between testing occasions were also found for the other executive tasks. In general, there was a tendency for improvement on repeat testing. The authors suggest that the test-retest correlations may not be high on these tests because they are no longer assessing novelty, a critical aspect of the dysexecutive syndrome. Reliability in patient populations remains to be evaluated.

Wilson et al. (1996) report that the overall BADS profile score differentiated the performance of healthy controls from a group of 78 patients with neurological disorders, most with closed head injury. In addition, the performance of neurological patients was poorer than that of controls on all six of the individual tests making up the BADS. Patients, as a group, rated themselves as having fewer problems than their significant others reported—a pattern expected following brain injury where problems of reduced insight are evident. Further, there were moderate negative correlations between the ratings of others and performance on the six individual tests; that is, satisfactory performance on each BADS test indicated low ratings regarding the presence or severity of everyday executive problems by significant others who knew the patients well. There was also a moderate correlation between WAIS-R FSIQ and others' rating although the magnitude of this correlation ($-.42$) was less than that of the BADS total Profile score ($-.62$). None of the BADS tests, the total Profile score or FSIQ correlated with the patients' ratings of their perception of the presence of everyday executive problems. In short, performance on the BADS appears to be associated with objective ratings of everyday executive problems among brain-injured people. While WAIS-R IQ is moderately correlated with these ratings, the BADS profile score appears more highly correlated with the objective ratings.

Preliminary analysis of others' ratings on the DEX suggested that the questionnaire measures change in at least three areas, representing behavioral, cognitive and emotional components. The only significant predictor of each of the factors was the BADS Profile score. Performance on the Cognitive Estimation Test, the WCST (Nelson version), NART FSIQ, WAIS-R FSIQ and age did not enter into the equation.

In summary, the evidence suggests that the BADS may be a useful tool for picking up subtle difficulties in planning and organization, particularly in those people who appear to be cognitively well preserved and functioning well in structured settings. The battery, however, is relatively new, and in need of further study. The rationale for choosing the six tests needs to be clarified. Future work should include additional studies of reliability (e.g., the internal consistency of the various tasks and test-retest reliability in patients) and validity (e.g., the relation of the different tasks to each other, their relation to other executive, and non-executive function tasks, as well as their relation to measures of intellectual level). Since several tasks require good spatial orientation, correlation with tests of spatial abilities would also be desirable. In addition, large scale studies of normals and diverse patient populations are needed. Currently, there is no way to evaluate individual subtest performance.

Normative Data

Wilson et al. normed the test on a group of 216 healthy individuals (mean age = 46.6, SD = 19.8), in each of three ability bands (below average, average, above average according to the NART; mean NART FSIQ = 102.7, SD = 16.2, range, 69–129) and balanced to have approximately equal numbers of men and women in each of these bands from each of four age groups (16–31, 32–47, 48–63 and 64+; mean age = 58.93, SD = 15.35; mean educational level of 13.83 years, SD = 2.70).

The profile score can be converted (using Table 5 in BADS manual) into a standardized score with a mean of 100 and a standard deviation of 15. In this way, it is possible to classify BADS performance as either being impaired, borderline, low average, average, high average, or superior. Age affects task performance, with poorer overall scores for subjects aged 65 years and above. The overall profile score is evaluated with reference to three age groups (40 or less, 41 to 65, 65 to 87). However, age-based data on the individual tasks are not provided. The authors also do not report on the potential influences of gender, education, or intelligence.

References

Klosowaska, D. (1976). Relation between ability to program actions and location of brain damage. *Polish Psychological Bulletin, 7,* 245–255.

Shallice, T., & Burgess, P. (1991). Deficits in strategy application following frontal lobe damage in man. *Brain, 114,* 727–741.

Wilson, B.A., Alderman, N., Burgess, P.W., Emslie, H., & Evans, J.J. (1996). *Behavioral Assessment of the Dysexecutive Syndrome.* Bury St. Edmunds, England: Thames Valley Test Company.

CALIFORNIA SORTING TEST (CST)

Purpose

The purpose of this test is to differentiate various components of problem solving.

Source

The test (D. Delis, E. Kaplan, & J. Kramer) will be published by the Psychological Corporation in 1998. A research edition can be ordered from Dean Delis, Ph.D., Psychology Service 116B, V.A. Medical Center, 3350 La Jolla Village Drive, San Diego, CA 92161.

Description

This test was originally developed by Delis et al. (1992) to provide separate assessments of concept generation, concept identification, and concept execution, as well as several measures of verbal and nonverbal perseveration. The original version of the test consisted of three conditions: Subjects were asked (1) to sort six cards spontaneously into two groups of three each, according to as many different rules as possible (maximum = 8), and to report the rule after each sort; (2) to report the rules for correct sorts performed by the examiner; and (3) to sort the cards according to abstract cues or explicit information provided by the examiner.

The current version of the task consists of two alternate forms, each with two sets of six stimulus cards with a single word (e.g., butterfly) printed on each card. The cards in both sets can be sorted into two groups of three cards, each based on eight different sorting rules. The specific rules differ from set to set. Within each set, three rules involve verbal properties of the words and five involve nonverbal properties of the cards (e.g., Verbal Domain: Land objects vs. air objects; Nonverbal Domain: Big cards vs. small cards). Further, subjects are tested under two different conditions within each set. In the first condition, Free Sorting, the subject sorts the cards and states the rule upon which each sort is based. In the second condition, Structured Sorting, the examiner sorts the cards according to each rule and the subject is asked to ver-

bally describe the rule. This sequence is completed for each of the two sets of stimulus cards. Note that the current version has eliminated the cued sorting condition.

Administration

See source. For the Free Sorting (FS) condition, the six cards are arranged randomly on the table in front of the subject, who is instructed to sort the cards in as many different ways as possible. Each time, the subject is told to make two piles with three cards in each pile and to describe the sorting rule after each sort. Three minutes are allowed for this phase.

In the second condition, Structured Sorting (SS), the examiner sorts the cards according to each rule, and the subject is given 60 seconds to verbally describe the rule after each sort.

One deterrent to the widespread use of the original CST was the time required to administer the complete version, 45–60 minutes (Beatty et al. 1994). The revised version is much shorter.

Approximate Time for Administration

The time required is about 25 minutes.

Scoring

Multiple measures of performance can be derived from the CST. For the Free Sorting condition, the total number of sorts attempted provides a measure of initiation. This total score is broken down into three additional measures: (1) the number of correct sorts, (2) the number of perseverative sorts (i.e., sorting the cards according to the same rule a second or third time), and (3) the number of other errors (e.g., sorting the cards into piles with unequal numbers of cards). The quality of the verbal explanations for the sorts correctly achieved is scored as follows: Two points are assigned if the subject verbalizes the sorting principle that applies to both piles (e.g., "Color of the cards" or "These are green and these are yellow"); one point is assigned if the subject verbalizes the rule as it applies to only one of the piles (e.g., "These are green and these are not"); zero points are assigned for "don't know" responses and for responses that are clearly incorrect. The number of verbal perseverations (i.e., restating a previously given rule) is also counted. The Structured Sorting condition is scored exactly as the verbal portion of the Free Sorting phase.

Comment

Information regarding test reliability is currently not available.

Factor analysis of the original version of CST scores of healthy young adults (Greve et al., 1995) revealed four factors. Factor 1, labeled "Accuracy," consisted of FS nontarget sorts, FS total sorts, FS incorrect descriptions, and Total perseverations. FS correct sorts and nonverbal descriptions loaded highly on Factor 2 and was labeled the "Nonverbal Domain Factor." Factor 3 contained four structured and cued sort scores. Finally, Factor 4 contained FS correct sorts and descriptions for the verbal domain and was called the "Verbal Domain Factor."

Greve et al. (1995) also factor analyzed the factor scores derived from the CST along with scores from several commonly used tests of executive function, including the Shipley Scale, Trails A and B, the Category Test, and the WCST. Factor 1 consisted entirely of scores from the WCST. Factor 2 consisted of Shipley scores although CST errors had a modest loading (−.39) on this factor. Factor 3 consisted of the remaining CST scores and also had a modest loading from Trails B (−.31) and Total errors on the Category Test (−.57). Factor 4 contained WCST Total Correct and failure to maintain set as well as Trails A. The implication is that the CST is a measure of concept formation that is tapping abilities different from those assessed by various other standard measures.

Delis et al. (1992) reported that patients with acquired lesions to the frontal lobe and patients with Korsakoff's syndrome generated, identified, and executed fewer correct concepts and made more perseverative responses than did normal controls. Although non-Korsakoff amnesic patients performed similarly to normal subjects on most mea-

sures, a finer analysis suggested that successful performance was also dependent to some extent on memory function.

The CST has been used successfully to describe the problem-solving deficits in a number of other conditions including Parkinson's Disease (Beatty & Monson, 1990; Bondi et al., 1993), multiple sclerosis (MS) (Beatty & Monson, 1996), chronic alcoholism (Beatty et al., 1993), and schizophrenia or schizoaffective illness (Beatty et al., 1994). The CST appears more sensitive than the Wisconsin Card Sorting Test in detecting deficits, at least among patients with Parkinson's Disease (PD) (Beatty & Monson, 1990). Moreover, the test appears better able than the WCST to characterize the different problem-solving capacities of various patient populations. Whereas patients with PD, MS, and chronic alcoholism exhibit qualitatively similar patterns of performance on the WCST (fewer categories and more perseverative responses), they exhibit dissimilar profiles of impairment on the CST (Beatty et al., 1994). For example, Beatty and Monson (1990) have shown that a subgroup of PD patients (those with generalized cognitive disturbances) display an increased tendency to respond perseveratively as well as an impairment in identifying and generating concepts even when explicit cues are provided. The major difficulty for MS patients, however, is in identifying concepts. They generate and identify fewer concepts, but perform normally when sorting is cued by the examiner and make no more perseverations than controls (Beatty & Monson, 1996). Alcoholics appear to have a disproportionately severe difficulty in accounting (verbally explaining) for correct sorting performance (Beatty et al., 1993).

The CST has a number of advantages over other measures of complex problem-solving ability. First, it distinguishes verbal and nonverbal concept formation abilities (Greve et al., 1995). Second, by design, it allows the clinician to test the limits of the patient's problem-solving abilities (Delis et al., 1992). Third, although the WCST may be adequate to detect impairment, the CST may provide more information about which cognitive processes underlie the deficit. Fourth, the WCST performance on the global measure of problem solving (that is, the number of categories achieved) is so highly and negatively correlated with perseverative responding that it is doubtful that these measures are independent (Beatty & Monson, 1990). On the CST, in contrast, measures of concept attainment (number of correct free sorts, number of points achieved during structured sorting) are highly and positively correlated with one another but are only weakly and inconsistently related to measures of perseveration, suggesting that any increased perseverative tendencies are not simply the result of poor overall problem-solving performance (Beatty & Monson, 1990, 1996; Beatty et al., 1993; Beatty et al., 1994). Finally, the CST is a sorting task with little negative feedback. As a result, it may be easier to maintain good rapport with patients, an important consideration particularly when assessing children.

Normative Data

When the test is published, normative data will be available for subjects aged 8–89 years. For preliminary normative data, see D. Delis (see source). The test is sensitive to the effect of age. Beatty (1993) reported that healthy individuals aged 60 and older generated and identified fewer correct concepts and executed concepts less accurately when guided by abstract cues, but they showed increased perseveration on only one of three measures. Gender also affects performance. Greve et al. (1995) reported that females scored lower than males in the verbal domain of the Free Sort condition. Education appears to have little impact on performance (Beatty, 1993).

References

Beatty, W.W. (1993). Age differences on the California Card Sorting Test: Implications for the assessment of problem solving by the elderly. *Bulletin of the Psychonomic Society, 31,* 511–514.

Beatty, W.W., Jocic, Z., Monson, N., & Katzung, V.M. (1994). Problem solving by schizophrenic and schizoaffective patients on the Wisconsin and California Card Sorting Test. *Neuropsychology, 8,* 49–54.

Beatty, W.W., Katzung, V.M., Nixon, S.J., & Moreland, V.J. (1993). Problem-solving deficits in alcoholics: Evidence from the California Card Sorting Test. *Journal of Studies on Alcohol, 54,* 687–692.

Beatty, W.W., & Monson, N. (1990). Problem solving in Parkinson's disease: Comparison of performance on the Wisconsin and California Card Sorting Test. *Journal of Geriatric Psychiatry and Neurology, 3,* 163–171.

Beatty, W.W., & Monson, N. (1996). Problem solving by patients with Multiple Sclerosis: Comparison of performance on the Wisconsin and California Card Sorting Test. *International Journal of Clinical Neuropsychology, 2,* 132–140.

Bondi, M.W., Kaszniak, A.W., Bayles, K.A., & Vance, K.T. (1993). Contributions of frontal system dysfunction to memory and perceptual abilities in Parkinson's Disease. *Neuropsychology, 7,* 89–102.

Delis, D.C., Squire, L.R., Bihrle, A., & Massman, P. (1992). Componential analysis of problem-solving ability: Performance of patients with frontal lobe damage and amnesic patients on a new sorting test. *Neuropsychologia, 30,* 683–697.

Greve, K.W., Farrwell, J.F., Besson, P.S., & Crouch, J.A. (1995). A psychometric analysis of the California Card Sorting Test. *Archives of Clinical Neuropsychology, 10,* 265–278.

CATEGORY TEST

Purpose

This test measures a patient's abstraction or concept formation ability, flexibility in the face of complex and novel problem solving, and capacity to learn from experience.

Source

Original Version. The Halstead-Reitan version of the test can be obtained from Reitan Neuropsychology Lab, 2920 S 4th Ave., Tucson, AZ 85775. The projection box, examiner's control panel, and projector cost $665 US and the test slides (for adults, children aged 9–14 and young children, aged 5–8) cost $410 US. Recording forms are $20 US per package (100/pkg).

Booklet Version. The booklet versions of the Adult and Intermediate forms of the test are portable and can be ordered from Psychological Assessment Resources (PAR), PO Box 998, Odessa, FL 33556, for about $230 US. A booklet version of the Short Category Test is available through Western Psychological Services, 12031 Wilshire Blvd., Los Angeles, CA 90025-1251, for $160 US. A booklet form of the Children's Category Test, appropriate for ages 5 years through 16 years, 11 months, can be ordered from the Psychological Corporation, 555 Academic Court, San Antonio, TX 78204-2498, at a cost of $249 US.

Computer Version. A number of different versions (e.g., standard, Russell's Short Form, Intermediate) are available through MHS, 65 Overlea Blvd., Suite 210, Toronto Ontario, M4H 1P1, at a cost of $450 Cdn. PAR also offers computer versions of the Category Test. The computer program allows the examiner to give any of three versions of the test: the standard 208-item version and two short-form versions. The price from PAR is $395 US.

Description

The Category Test, developed by Halstead (1947), is also part of the Reitan test battery (Reitan & Davison, 1974). The original version involves the projection of seven sets of items, with a total of 208 items. Each set is organized on the basis of a different principle, such as number of objects, ordinal position of an odd stimulus, etc. Subjects must use feedback they receive from their correct and incorrect guesses on the series of items in each subtest to infer the rule behind the subtest. No clues are given as to what the rule might be. The adult version covers the age range 15 years, 6 months and up. An intermediate version (Reed, Reitan, & Klove, 1965) covers the age range 9 years to 15 years, 6 months and includes 168 items, divided into six subtests. A children's version (Reed, Reitan, & Klove, 1965) consisting of 80 items, arranged into five subtests, is available for ages 5–8 years or for individuals suspected of being mentally retarded.

One problem with the original slide version of the test is that it relies on expensive and unwieldy equipment that may break down and is difficult to use at bedside examinations. Booklet (DeFilippis & McCampbell, 1979, 1991) and computer forms of the test are available (see source), and preliminary evidence suggests that these forms yield results that are equivalent to the original version (Choca & Morris, 1992; DeFilippis & McCampbell, 1979, 1991; Holz et al., 1996; Mercer et al., 1997). The advantages of a computer version include error-free test administration as well as the collection of additional data, such as reaction time and number of perseverations.

Another problem is that impaired subjects take a long time (up to 2 hours) to complete the test. Short forms of the adult version of the Category Test have been developed (e.g., Boyle, 1986; Caslyn et al., 1980; Charter et al., 1997; Gregory et al., 1979; Russell & Levy, 1987; Labreche, 1983; Wetzel & Boll, 1987). The Short Category Test, Booklet Format (SCT) developed by Wetzel and Boll (1987) consists of 100 items and appears to be a good alternative to the original form since a growing body of literature suggests that the SCT functions in a similar fashion as the original Category Test in terms of its psychometric properties, discriminative ability, and relation to standard neuropsychological tests (Gelowitz & Paniak, 1992). Recently, a similar attempt has been made to shorten the forms given to adolescents. The Children's Category Test (CCT; Boll, 1993) is also available in booklet format and consists of two levels: Level 2 is given to children aged 9–16 years and consists of 83 items as opposed to 168 items in the original version; Level 1 is given to children 5–8 years of age and consists of 80 items, the same number as in the original version. The internal structure of the test was not changed by Boll, although the administration method is different because the stimuli are presented in booklet format. Also, the colors white and black have been substituted for the original red and green in order to avoid problems for children who are color blind. Boll (1993) contends that scores on the original and CCT versions are highly correlated (.88) and that therefore the versions are parallel forms.

The SCT and the CCT are very attractive for general clinical use given their relatively short administration time and good predictive accuracy (see also Donders, 1996). The SCT and the CCT have the added advantage of being relatively inexpensive and highly portable.

Administration: Manual Versions

Briefly, the apparatus for presenting the test items to the subject consists of a slide projector, a console with a viewing screen for rearview projection, and the examiner's control board. The idea of the test as a whole is to find the underlying principle by choosing one out of four presented stimuli. The subject responds by pressing one of four levers, numbered 1,2,3,4 (colored knobs for children), from left to right, and placed on the apparatus immediately below the screen. A correct response produces a chime; an incorrect response produces a buzzer sound.

The purpose for presenting the Category Test is usually to determine the subject's ability in abstraction or concept formation. To achieve this purpose, it is necessary that the examiner elicit the best performance of which the subject is capable. We insist that each subject observe each item carefully before making a response. Usually the subject reacts to the test with interest and makes an obvious effort to answer correctly. Occasionally a patient will answer apparently at random, and in such instances the examiner must attempt to get the patient to make a serious effort (or, if this is not possible, declare the test results invalid). Since the main purpose is to measure the patient's concept formation ability rather than motivation for doing well, a variety of techniques may be used as necessary. Some patients need to be told repeatedly to observe the items carefully (in some instances they must be asked to describe the figures before being permitted to respond), or to state the reason for selecting a particular response. A patient who says only that he was "just guessing" must be encouraged not to "just guess" but to "try to figure out the principle."

As a general rule, any part of the instructions may be repeated when the examiner believes it necessary. Our purpose is to give the subject a clear understanding of the problem he or she is facing and the rules involved in its solution. The principles themselves are never given to a subject, but when working with subjects who are extremely impaired in their ability to form concepts, it may become necessary to urge them to study the picture carefully; to ask for their descriptions of the stimulus material which are then followed by examiner questions such as, "Does that give you any idea of what might be the right answer?"; to urge them to try to notice and remember how the pictures change, since this often provides clues to the underlying principle; and to try to think of the reason when they answer correctly. Subjects rarely ask the examiner to state the principle, but it is possible that in conversations as described above, an unwary examiner may give unwarranted reinforcement to the patient's hypotheses. Examiners should always remember that their questions and advice should be consistent with the aims of the formal instructions and should not provide information relevant to the solution of the problems presented by the test. The only information of this kind comes from the bell or buzzer following each response.

Most subjects are able to take the Category test with little additional information or direction than is provided in the formal instructions. Impaired subjects sometimes find the test trying and frustrating. The examiner should make every effort to encourage the subject to continue working at the task. If a subject shows no sign of making progress on the first 20 items of any one of subtests III through VI and *also* gives evidence of extreme frustration with the task, it is better to discontinue the subtest at this point and prorate the error scores (linear extrapolation) than run the risk of not being able to complete the test.

The apparatus, as a whole, constitutes in effect a multiple-choice situation. The subject's keyboard on the front of the projection cabinet enables the subject to indicate his or her choices objectively. The examiner's control board is set each time for the "correct" response and controls the presentation of successive items.

The test items are projected from the slide projector. The slides begin with eight Roman numeral items varying from I to IV. The keys on the subject's board are numbered, so this first subtest serves to associate the items on the screen with the subject's keys, as well as to acquaint the subject with the test procedure and to relieve test anxiety. Between each subtest or group there is one blank frame.

The master off–on switch is located on the left of the examiner's control board. When this switch is turned on, the screen and examiner's control board are ready for use.

A hand control switch that causes the successive items to appear on the screen is located at the right of the examiner's control board. When this switch is depressed once quickly, a new item will replace the previous item on the screen. Do *not* keep the switch depressed.

A four-way control switch that corresponds to the subject's four response keys is located in the center of the examiner's control board. To set any key on the subject's board as correct (sound the chime), set the handle into the appropriate numbered slot. A prepared record blank tells the examiner the proper setting of this switch for each item.

Always set the answer key before changing the slide. Some additional points should be mentioned briefly:

1. Although speed is not a factor and subjects should not be hurried, neither should they be permitted to sit and daydream or to take an unduly long time to respond. Some subjects would impair the continuity of the test if not encouraged to make reasonably prompt decisions and thus would impair their prospect of making better scores.

2. The examiner should always be alert to the slide on the screen, not only to keep in touch with the subject's performance, but also to note if a slide has somehow gotten out of order, necessitating a quick change of the answer switch.

3. The testing room should be somewhat darkened, yet light enough for the examiner to record errors.

4. The subject should sit directly in front of the screen. The colors particularly may be difficult to see from an angle.

Adult Manual Version—Standard (Original) Version. The adult version covers the age from range 15 years, 6 month and up. Say to the patient: "*On this screen you are going to see different geometrical figures and designs. Something about the pattern on the screen will remind you of a number between 1 and 4. On the keyboard in front of you* (pointing) *the keys are numbered 1, 2, 3 and 4. You are to press down on the key which is the same number that the pattern on the screen reminds you of. That is, if the picture on the screen reminds you of the number 1, pull key number 1. If the pictures on the screen remind you of the number 2, pull key number 2. And so on. For example, what number does this remind you of?*"

Put on the first slide. If the subject says "one," ask the subject which key he or she should press. After the subject has pressed the number 1 key, say: "*The bell you have just heard tells you that you got the right answer. Every time you have the right answer you will hear the bell ring.*" Instruct the subject to try one of the other keys in order to find out what happens when an incorrect key is pressed. Then say: "*The buzzer is what you hear when you have the wrong answer. In this way, you will know each time whether you have the right or wrong answer. However, for each picture on the screen you get only one choice. If you make a mistake we just go right on to the next picture.*"

Proceed with Subtest I. Say: "*Now which key would you pick for this picture?*" After Subtest 1, say: "*That was the end of the first subtest. This test is divided into seven subtests. In each subtest there is one idea or principle that runs throughout the entire subtest. Once you have figured out what the idea or principle in the subtest is, by using this idea you will get the right answer each time. Now we are going to begin the second subtest. The idea in it may be the same as in the practice set, or it may be different. We want you to figure it out.*"

Proceed with Subtest II. After Subtest II, say: "*That was the end of the second subtest and, as you probably noticed, you don't necessarily have to see a number to have a number suggested to you. You saw squares, circles, and other figures. Also, as you may or may not have noticed, in each of these subtests, there is* one idea or principle that runs throughout. Once you figure out the idea, you continue to apply it to get the right answer. Now we are going to start the third subtest. The idea may be the same as the last one or it may be different. I want to see if you can figure out what the idea is and then use it to get the right answer. Remember, the idea remains the same throughout the subtest. I will tell you when we complete one subtest and are ready to begin a new one."

Proceed with Subtest III. In Subtest IV, after slide #6 (the first slide without numbers), say: "This is still the same group, but now the numbers are missing. The principle is still the same. After Subtests III, IV, and V, say: "That was the end of that subtest. Now we are going to begin the next one. The idea in it may be the same as the last one or it may be different. We want you to figure it out."

After Subtest VI, say: "In the last subtest there is no one idea or principle that runs throughout the group because it is made up of items you have already seen in preceding subtests. Try to remember what the right answer was the last time you saw the pattern and give that same answer again."

Intermediate Manual Version—Standard Form. This version is designed for children aged 9–15 years. The instructions for the standard versions are similar to those given above. Note, however, that the task consists of 6 subtests. Following Subtest 5, say: "That was the end of the fifth subtest and now we are going to begin the last one. In this last subtest, there is no one idea or principle that runs throughout the subtest because it is made up of pictures that you have seen before. Try to remember what the right answer was the first time that you saw the picture and then give that same answer again."

Children's Version—Standard Form. This test is for use with children 5–8 years old or in individuals suspected of being mentally retarded. For this version of the test, the numbered key discs are replaced by colored ones. The sequence 1, 2, 3, 4, changes to Red, Blue, Yellow, Green. Say: "On this screen you will see pictures of different figures and designs.

Each picture will make you think of a color, either red, blue, yellow or green. On this keyboard in front of you, you will notice that the keys are different colors. This one is red, this one is blue, this one is yellow, and this one is green (pointing). Press down on the key that has the same color as the color you think of when you look at the picture. For example, what color does this make you think of?"

Flash on the first picture—red circle. If the subject says "red," ask which key he or she would press. When the subject presses the key, say: "That is the bell which means that you got the right answer. Try another key and see what happens when you get the wrong answer."

After the subject does this, say: "That is the buzzer, which means you got the wrong answer. This way you will know each time whether you are right or wrong, but for each design you may press only one key. If you make a mistake we will go right on to the next one. Let's try some of these."

After the first subtest, say: "That completes the first group of pictures. Now we are going to start the next group. You will have to try to figure out the right reason for picking one key or another. If you are able to figure out the reason why your answers are right or wrong it will help, because the reason stays the same all the way through the group."

Proceed with the second subtest. Any part of the instructions may be repeated at any time, but the subject should never be told the principle. The examiner should be alert to notice what parts of the instructions need repetition. Children frequently need to be reminded to try to figure out the reason for their choices, rather than to make only haphazard guesses. When a subject has difficulty with the test, he or she should be asked to describe stimulus figures before responding, to recall what items had been presented previously, to watch how the pictures change from one to the next, and to try to figure out the reason why one system or another might be correct.

Say: "Now we are going to start the third group. This group may be different from the one you just finished or it may be the same. Let's see if you can figure out the right answers."

Proceed with the fourth subtest using the same type of introductory comments as with the third subtest. Before beginning the fifth subtest, say: *"Now we are going to start the last group. This group will test your memory since it is made up of pictures that you have already seen. Try to remember what the right answer was the first time you saw the picture and give the same answer again."* Do not hesitate to comment favorably at any time during the test when the subject answers correctly.

Booklet Versions (Booklet Category Test, Short Category Test, Children's Category Test). See source. Briefly, the examiner presents a series of cards in sequence. The subject responds by pointing to or verbally identifying one of four colors (for subjects aged 5–8 years) or one of four numerals (for subjects aged 9 years and above) printed on a response card. The examiner says "right" or "wrong" following each response.

Approximate Time for Administration

Standard versions require about 40 minutes, although impaired individuals may take as long as 2 hours. Abbreviated versions take about 20 minutes.

Scoring

Record the total number of errors. Sample scoring sheets for the standard adult, intermediate, and children's versions of the Category Test are provided in Figures 8–1 to 8–3.

Comment

The odd-even split-half method and coefficient alpha have been used to calculate internal consistency values for the standard version of the Category Test. High reliability coefficients were obtained (above .95) for samples of normal and brain-damaged adults (Charter et al., 1987; Moses, 1985; Shaw, 1966). For the booklet versions, SCT and CCT, split-half reliability coefficients are slightly lower (.81 on the SCT; .88 for Level 1 and .86 for Level 2 of the CCT), although still respectable (Boll, 1993; Wetzel & Boll, 1987). Choca et al. (1997)

argue that there is an especially abrupt jump from the difficulty levels of subtest I and II to that of Subtest III.

With intact individuals, test-retest reliability is low ($r = .60$). When severely impaired neurological patients are considered, the Category Test has high retest reliability, $>.90$, even after intervals of 2 years (Matarazzo et al., 1974; Goldstein & Watson, 1989; Russell, 1992). In the case of children and persons with schizophrenia, correlation coefficients are somewhat lower and range from .63 to .72 (Goldstein & Watson, 1989; Wetzel & Boll, 1987). Although coefficients of such magnitude are respectable, one should note that they mean only that subjects were ranked in more or less the same order on both administrations. They do not mean that subjects achieved the same scores on both administrations. In fact, significant changes or practice effects emerge, even in moderately impaired neurological patients (Boll, 1993; Dodrill & Troupin, 1975). Thus, the absence of improvement (practice effects) may be an indicator of abnormality.

Holz and colleagues (1996) administered both booklet and projector versions to a mixed group of brain-injured patients and healthy controls. Individual subtest and total score correlations between the forms were generally large in the brain-damaged sample (total score $r = .88$). The correlations, however, were lower among controls (total score $r = .42$). Mean error scores and variances generated on the projector and booklet formats did not differ significantly. Further, mean administration times for the two forms did not differ in either the brain-injured or control groups. Overall, these data suggest that the two forms can probably be interpreted in the same manner.

The total score shares a high loading with the Performance subtests (Block Design, Object Assembly) of the Wechsler Intelligence Scales (Klonoff, 1971; Lansdell & Donnelly, 1977). Thus, it may not distinguish an ability that is separate from nonverbal intelligence (Lansdell & Donnelly, 1977; but see Donders, 1996, who reported only a modest amount of shared variance, about 13 percent, between WISC-R PIQ and the CCT in children with

Sample Score Sheet
Halstead Category Test (Adult Standard Form)

NAME: ______________________ Date: ______________________
Examiner: ______________________ Score: ______________________

	I	II	III	IV	V	VI	VII	
1.	1	1	1	1	1	1	1	
2.	3	3	3	3	3	3	3	
3.	1	1	1	1	1	1	1	
4.	4	4	4	4	4	4	4	
5.	2	2	2	2	2	2	2	
6.	4	4	4	4	4	4	4	
7.	1	1	1	1	1	1	1	
8.	2	2	2	2	3	2	2	
9.	E–	3	3	3	3	3	3	
10.		2	2	2	2	2	2	
11.		3	3	3	3	3	3	
12.		1	1	1	1	1	1	
13.		4	4	4	4	4	4	
14.		3	3	3	3	3	3	
15.		4	4	4	4	4	4	
16.		2	2	2	2	2	2	
17.		1	1	1	1	1	1	
18.		4	4	4	4	4	4	
19.		1	1	1	1	1	1	
20.		3	3	3	3	3	3	
21.		E–	2	2	2	2	END OF REG. TEST	
22.			1	1	1	1	1	
23.			2	2	2	2	2	EXTRA
24.			4	4	4	4	4	ITEMS
25.			3	3	3	3	3	
26.			2	2	2	2	2	
27.			4	4	4	4		
28.			3	3	3	3		
29.			1	1	1	1		
30.			4	4	4	4		
31.			2	2	2	2		
32.			1	1	1	1		
33.			3	3	3	3		
34.			1	1	1	1		
35.			3	3	3	3		
36.			2	2	2	2		
37.			4	4	4	4		
38.			3	3	3	3		
39.			4	4	4	4		
40.			2	2	2	2		
			E–	E–	E–	E–		

Figure 8—1. Halstead Category Test (Adult Form) sample scoring sheet.

traumatic brain injury). Further, there is a modest association between the Category test and neuropsychological measures of learning and memory (Bertram, Abeles, & Snyder, 1990; Boll, 1993; Fischer & Dean, 1990), providing some evidence of the test's value as a measure of learning ability. It does not, however, assess learning as a pure ability construct.

Despite the fact that the Category Test is composed of several subtests, clinical interpretations and most studies tend to rely (perhaps incorrectly) on a single composite score. There is general agreement that the Category Test is a complex measure, loading on a number of different factors. Recently, Johnstone et al. (1997) investigated the assumption that all seven subtests measure the same reasoning construct using a mixed sample of 308 patients referred for neuropsychological examination. Factor analysis of Category subtests along with other neuropsychological mea-

Sample Score Sheet
Halstead Category Test (Intermediate Form)

Name: _____   Date: _____
Examiner: _____   Score: _____

	I	II	III	IV	V	VI
1.	1	1	1	1	1	1
2.	3	3	3	3	3	3
3.	1	1	1	1	1	1
4.	4	4	4	4	4	4
5.	2	2	2	2	2	2
6.	4	4	4	4	4	4
7.	1	1	1	1	1	1
8.	2	2	2	2	2	2
9.	E=	3	3	3	3	3
10.		2	2	2	2	2
11.		3	3	3	3	3
12.		1	1	1	1	1
13.		4	4	4	4	4
14.		3	3	3	3	3
15.		4	4	4	4	4
16.		2	2	2	2	2
17.		1	1	1	1	1
18.		4	4	4	4	4
19.		1	1	1	1	1
20.		3	3	3	3	3
21.		E=	2	2	2	E=
22.			1	1	1	
23.			2	2	2	
24.			4	4	4	
25.			3	3	3	
26.			2	2	2	
27.			4	4	4	
28.			3	3	3	
29.			1	1	1	
30.			4	4	4	
31.			2	2	2	
32.			1	1	1	
33.			3	3	3	
34.			1	1	1	
35.			3	3	3	
36.			2	2	2	
37.			4	4	4	
38.			3	3	3	
39.			4	4	4	
40.			2	2	2	
			E=	E=	E=	

Figure 8—2. Halstead Category Test (Intermediate Form) sample scoring sheet.

sures (WAIS-R, WMS-R, Trails, TPT) indicated that the Category subtests loaded on three factors distinct from intelligence and other neuropsychological measures, labeled symbol recognition/counting (subtests 1 and 2), spatial position reasoning (subtests 3, 4, and 7), and proportional reasoning (subtests 5 and 6).

The Category Test is sensitive to a variety of brain disturbances (see Choca et al., 1997 for a recent review). One should also note that the Category Test is almost as sensitive as the full Halstead-Reitan battery in determining the presence or absence of neurological damage (Adams & Trenton, 1981). However, impairment on the Category Test shows no consistent relation to specific location or laterality of brain damage (Anderson et al., 1995; Bornstein, 1986; Doehring & Reitan, 1962; Klove, 1974; Hom & Reitan, 1990; Lansdell & Donnelly, 1977; Pendleton & Heaton, 1982; Reitan & Wolfson, 1995), although it was origi-

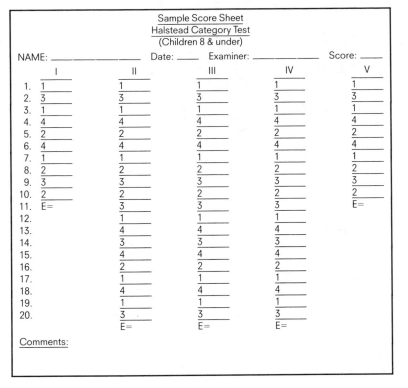

Figure 8—3. Halstead Category Test (Children 8 and Under) sample scoring sheet.

nally designed to detect frontal lobe damage (Halstead, 1947). Diminished performance also occurs in depressed individuals, in the absence of any obvious neurological condition (Savard et al., 1980). Individuals with schizophrenia, particularly of the nondelusional type, also show impairment on this test (Steindl & Boyle, 1995).

A patient's effort may be evaluated on the Category Test. Bolter (personal communication, 1995) has identified 14 items on the HCT that most normal and neurologically impaired individuals pass. These items form the Bolter Validity Index (VI) and include three items in Subtest V (27, 30, 33), five in Subtest VI (4, 18, 21, 24, 30) and three in Subtest VII (6, 10, 13). Approximately 98 percent of normal individuals passed all of these items; only 2 percent failed one item. No normal individual failed more than one item. Among brain-injured individuals, 78 percent passed all 14 items, 16 percent failed one item, 4 percent failed two items, and 2 percent failed four items. In total, 98 percent of the brain-damaged sample

earned a VI score of two or less. Tenhula and Sweet (1996) reported that these infrequently missed items were effective (86 percent hit rate) in discriminating brain-injured individuals from normals instructed to malinger. Trueblood and Schmidt (1993), however, did not find a significant difference between suspected malingerers and brain-injured controls in the number of "rare errors." It may be that this indicator occurs rarely, and therefore its presence would suggest invalidity while its absence would not substantiate a test protocol's validity (Trueblood & Schmidt, 1993). Tenhula and Sweet (1996) suggest that an

Table 8—1. Severity Ranges for the Standard Form of the Adult Halstead Category Test (Errors)

	Perfectly Normal	Normal	Mildly Impaired	Severely Impaired
HCT	0–25	26–45	46–65	65+

Source: Reitan & Wolfson, 1985.

Table 8—2. Category Test (Error Score) Correction for Age and Education

| Age | Years of education ||||||||||||||||| |
	0	1	2	3	4	5	6	7	8	9	10	11	12	13	14	15	16
25	−13.	−11.	−8.	−6.	−3.	−1.	2.	4.	6.	9.	11.	14.	16.	18.	21.	23.	26.
26	−14.	−11.	−9.	−6.	−4.	−2.	1.	3.	6.	8.	11.	13.	15.	18.	20.	23.	25.
27	−14.	−12.	−9.	−7.	−5.	−2.	0.	3.	5.	7.	10.	12.	15.	17.	20.	22.	24.
28	−15.	−13.	−10.	−8.	−5.	−3.	−0.	2.	4.	7.	9.	12.	14.	16.	19.	21.	24.
29	−16.	−13.	−11.	−8.	−6.	−4.	−1.	1.	4.	6.	9.	11.	13.	16.	18.	21.	23.
30	−16.	−14.	−12.	−9.	−7.	−4.	−2.	1.	3.	5.	8.	10.	13.	15.	18.	20.	22.
31	−17.	−15.	−12.	−10.	−7.	−5.	−2.	−0.	2.	5.	7.	10.	12.	14.	17.	19.	22.
32	−18.	−15.	−13.	−10.	−8.	−6.	−3.	−1.	2.	4.	7.	9.	11.	14.	16.	19.	21.
33	−18.	−16.	−14.	−11.	−9.	−6.	−4.	−1.	1.	3.	6.	8.	11.	13.	16.	18.	20.
34	−19.	−17.	−14.	−12.	−9.	−7.	−5.	−2.	0.	3.	5.	8.	10.	12.	15.	17.	20.
35	−20.	−17.	−15.	−12.	−10.	−8.	−5.	−3.	−0.	2.	4.	7.	9.	12.	14.	17.	19.
36	−20.	−18.	−16.	−13.	−11.	−8.	−6.	−3.	−1.	1.	4.	6.	9.	11.	14.	16.	18.
37	−21.	−19.	−16.	−14.	−11.	−9.	−7.	−4.	−2.	1.	3.	6.	8.	10.	13.	15.	18.
38	−22.	−19.	−17.	−14.	−12.	−10.	−7.	−5.	−2.	0.	2.	5.	7.	10.	12.	15.	17.
39	−22.	−20.	−18.	−15.	−13.	−10.	−8.	−5.	−3.	−1.	2.	4.	7.	9.	11.	14.	16.
40	−23.	−21.	−18.	−16.	−13.	−11.	−9.	−6.	−4.	−1.	1.	4.	6.	8.	11.	13.	16.
41	−24.	−21.	−19.	−16.	−14.	−12.	−9.	−7.	−4.	−2.	0.	3.	5.	8.	10.	13.	15.
42	−24.	−22.	−20.	−17.	−15.	−12.	−10.	−7.	−5.	−3.	−0.	2.	5.	7.	9.	12.	14.
43	−25.	−23.	−20.	−18.	−15.	−13.	−11.	−8.	−6.	−3.	−1.	2.	4.	6.	9.	11.	14.
44	−26.	−23.	−21.	−18.	−16.	−14.	−11.	−9.	−6.	−4.	−2.	1.	3.	6.	9.	11.	13.
45	−26.	−24.	−22.	−19.	−17.	−14.	−12.	−9.	−7.	−5.	−2.	0.	3.	5.	8.	10.	12.
46	−27.	−25.	−22.	−20.	−17.	−15.	−13.	−10.	−8.	−5.	−3.	−0.	2.	4.	7.	9.	12.
47	−28.	−25.	−23.	−21.	−18.	−16.	−13.	−11.	−8.	−6.	−4.	−1.	1.	4.	7.	9.	11.
48	−28.	−26.	−24.	−21.	−19.	−16.	−14.	−11.	−9.	−7.	−4.	−2.	1.	3.	6.	8.	11.
49	−29.	−27.	−24.	−22.	−19.	−17.	−15.	−12.	−10.	−7.	−5.	−2.	−0.	2.	5.	7.	10.

50	−30.	−27.	−25.	−23.	−20.	−18.	−15.	−12.	−10.	−8.	−6.	−3.	−1.	2.	4.	7.	9.
51	−30.	−28.	−26.	−23.	−21.	−18.	−16.	−13.	−11.	−9.	−6.	−4.	−1.	1.	3.	6.	8.
52	−31.	−29.	−26.	−24.	−21.	−19.	−17.	−14.	−12.	−9.	−7.	−5.	−2.	0.	3.	5.	8.
53	−32.	−29.	−27.	−25.	−22.	−20.	−17.	−14.	−13.	−10.	−8.	−5.	−3.	−0.	2.	5.	7.
54	−32.	−30.	−28.	−25.	−23.	−20.	−18.	−15.	−14.	−11.	−8.	−6.	−3.	−1.	1.	4.	6.
55	−33.	−31.	−28.	−26.	−23.	−21.	−19.	−16.	−14.	−11.	−9.	−7.	−4.	−2.	1.	3.	6.
56	−34.	−31.	−29.	−27.	−24.	−22.	−19.	−16.	−15.	−12.	−10.	−7.	−5.	−2.	0.	2.	5.
57	−34.	−32.	−30.	−27.	−25.	−22.	−20.	−17.	−16.	−13.	−10.	−8.	−5.	−3.	−1.	2.	4.
58	−35.	−33.	−30.	−28.	−25.	−23.	−21.	−18.	−16.	−13.	−11.	−9.	−6.	−4.	−1.	1.	4.
59	−36.	−33.	−31.	−29.	−26.	−24.	−21.	−18.	−17.	−14.	−12.	−9.	−7.	−4.	−2.	0.	3.
60	−37.	−34.	−32.	−29.	−27.	−24.	−22.	−19.	−18.	−15.	−12.	−10.	−7.	−5.	−3.	−0.	2.
61	−37.	−35.	−32.	−30.	−27.	−25.	−23.	−20.	−18.	−15.	−13.	−11.	−8.	−6.	−3.	−1.	2.
62	−38.	−35.	−33.	−31.	−28.	−26.	−23.	−20.	−19.	−16.	−14.	−11.	−9.	−6.	−4.	−2.	1.
63	−39.	−36.	−34.	−31.	−29.	−26.	−24.	−21.	−20.	−17.	−14.	−12.	−9.	−7.	−5.	−2.	0.
64	−39.	−37.	−34.	−32.	−30.	−27.	−25.	−22.	−21.	−17.	−15.	−13.	−10.	−8.	−5.	−3.	−0.
65	−40.	−37.	−35.	−33.	−30.	−28.	−25.	−22.	−21.	−18.	−16.	−13.	−11.	−8.	−6.	−4.	−1.
66	−41.	−38.	−36.	−33.	−31.	−28.	−26.	−23.	−22.	−19.	−16.	−14.	−11.	−9.	−7.	−4.	−2.
67	−41.	−39.	−36.	−34.	−32.	−29.	−27.	−24.	−23.	−19.	−17.	−15.	−12.	−10.	−7.	−5.	−2.
68	−42.	−39.	−37.	−35.	−32.	−30.	−27.	−24.	−23.	−20.	−18.	−15.	−13.	−10.	−8.	−6.	−3.
69	−43.	−40.	−38.	−35.	−33.	−30.	−28.	−25.	−24.	−21.	−18.	−16.	−14.	−11.	−9.	−6.	−4.
70	−43.	−41.	−38.	−36.	−34.	−31.	−29.	−26.	−25.	−21.	−19.	−17.	−14.	−12.	−9.	−7.	−4.
71	−44.	−41.	−39.	−37.	−34.	−32.	−29.	−26.	−25.	−22.	−20.	−17.	−15.	−12.	−10.	−8.	−5.
72	−45.	−42.	−40.	−37.	−35.	−32.	−30.	−27.	−26.	−23.	−20.	−18.	−16.	−13.	−11.	−8.	−6.
73	−45.	−43.	−40.	−38.	−36.	−33.	−31.	−28.	−27.	−23.	−21.	−19.	−16.	−14.	−11.	−9.	−7.
74	−46.	−43.	−41.	−39.	−36.	−34.	−31.	−28.	−27.	−24.	−22.	−19.	−17.	−14.	−12.	−10.	−7.
75	−47.	−44.	−42.	−39.	−37.	−34.	−32.	−29.	−28.	−25.	−22.	−20.	−18.	−15.	−13.	−10.	−8.
76	−47.	−45.	−42.	−40.	−38.	−35.	−33.	−30.	−28.	−25.	−23.	−21.	−18.	−16.	−13.	−11.	−9.
77	−48.	−46.	−43.	−41.	−38.	−36.	−33.	−31.	−29.	−26.	−24.	−21.	−19.	−16.	−14.	−12.	−9.
78	−49.	−46.	−44.	−41.	−39.	−37.	−34.	−32.	−30.	−27.	−24.	−22.	−20.	−17.	−15.	−12.	−10.

excessive number of errors on Subtests I, II, and VII might also raise the suspicion of malingering.

Both the Category Test and Wisconsin Card Sort Test (WCST) require, in part, the deduction of a classification principle by means of response-contingent feedback, the use of the principle while it remains effective, and the ability to abandon the principle when it is no longer effective. The two tests, however, are not identical (Adams et al., 1995; Donders & Kirsch, 1991; King & Snow, 1981; O'Donnell et al., 1994; Pendleton & Heaton, 1982; Bond & Buchtel, 1984; Gelowitz & Paniak, 1992; Perrine, 1993). Perrine (1993) found that the two tests show only a modest amount of common variance and relate to different facets of concept formation. The WCST is related to attribute identification, which entails discrimination of relevant features, while the CT is more related to rule learning, which assesses the deduction of classification rules. Bond and Buchtel (1984) have pointed out that the perceptual abstraction abilities that are required by the CT are more difficult than those required by the WCST. On the other hand, the WCST requires the subject to realize that the correct matching principle shifts periodically without warning. The CT makes no such demand. The WCST also provides a measure of perseverative tendencies while the CT does not. Recently, Adams et al. (1995) reported that in alcoholic patients, Subtest VII of the HCT correlated with glucose metabolism in cingulate, dorsolateral and orbitomedial regions of the frontal lobe. The summary WCST measure of categories achieved correlated only with glucose metabolism in the cingulate region. On the other hand, Anderson et al. (1995) examined the MRI scans of 68 traumatically brain-injured patients and found that while both CT and WCST performance were altered by brain injury, neither appeared related to volume of focal frontal damage, presence or absence of frontal damage, or to the degree of nonspecific structural (atrophic) changes.

The use of one or both of these tests depends on the diagnostic question. For example, if the examiner wishes to examine for perseverative tendencies, then the WCST should be chosen. On the other hand, if the examiner wishes a more difficult and sensitive measure of abstraction ability, then the CT is the preferred measure. Because of order of administration effects (Brandon & Chavez, 1985; Franzen et al., 1993), the clinician should consider which of the two instruments will provide the best information regarding the referral question and should use only that test for the patient.

Normative Data

Adult Versions. For the 208-item version of the Category Test, Reitan recommends the cutoff error score of 50–51 for adults. Note that this is chance-level performance. Ranges of scores for varying degrees of impairment have been defined for the standard form (Reitan & Wolfson, 1985) (Table 8–1).

Age, education, intellectual level, and ethnicity contribute to performance on the Category Test (Arnold et al., 1994; Boll, 1993; Dodrill, 1987; Ernst, 1987; Heaton, Grant, & Mathews, 1991; Leckliter & Matarazzo, 1989; Prigatano & Parsons, 1976; Seidenberg et al., 1983). Not surprisingly, performance on this measure of complex problem-solving ability is adversely affected by advancing age, lower educational achievement, lower intellectual levels, and non-native status. It is important to note that the norms shown in Table 8–1 for adults are derived from relatively young samples with average intellectual abilities. Use of these scores in subjects above age 40 and in those with lower than average educational achievement or intellectual abilities can result in erroneous diagnostic conclusions. For the standard 208-item version, normative data are available from Heaton, Grant, and Mathews (1991) for use with adults between 20 and 80 years of age. The data are broken down by age (10 levels), education (6 levels) and sex. It is important to note, however, that the total sample size ($n = 486$)—and as a result, the number of subjects within each category—is very small, suggesting that their data may be of limited validity. If their manual is used, raw error scores must be converted initially to scaled scores and then to T-scores. A different method is offered by Alekoubides et al. (1987)

Table 8—3. Corrected and Standard Scores for the Category Test

A	B	A	B	A	B	A	B	A	B
156.	40.	118.	64.	81.	88.	43.	113.	6.	136.
155.	41.	117.	65.	80.	89.	42.	113.	5.	137.
154.	41.	116.	66.	79.	89.	41.	114.	4.	138.
153.	42.	115.	66.	78.	90.	40.	115.	3.	138.
152.	43.	114.	67.	77.	91.	39.	115.	2.	139.
151.	43.	113.	68.	76.	91.	38.	116.	1.	140.
150.	44.	112.	68.	75.	92.	37.	116.	0.	140.
149.	45.	111.	69.	74.	93.	36.	117.	−1.	141.
148.	45.	110.	70.	73.	93.	35.	118.	−2.	141.
147.	46.	109.	70.	72.	94.	34.	118.	−3.	142.
146.	46.	108.	71.	71.	95.	33.	119.	−4.	143.
145.	47.	107.	71.	70.	95.	32.	120.	−5.	143.
144.	48.	106.	72.	69.	96.	31.	120.	−6.	144.
143.	48.	105.	73.	68.	97.	30.	121.	−7.	145.
142.	49.	104.	73.	67.	97.	29.	122.	−8.	145.
141.	50.	103.	74.	66.	98.	28.	122.	−9.	146.
140.	50.	102.	75.	65.	98.	27.	123.	−10.	147.
139.	51.	101.	75.	64.	99.	26.	124.	−11.	147.
138.	52.	100.	76.	63.	100.	25.	124.	−12.	148.
137.	52.	99.	77.	62.	100.	24.	125.	−13.	149.
136.	53.	98.	77.	61.	101.	23.	125.	−14.	149.
135.	54.	97.	78.	60.	102.	22.	126.	−15.	150.
134.	54.	96.	79.	59.	102.	21.	127.	−16.	150.
133.	55.	95.	79.	58.	103.	20.	127.	−17.	151.
132.	55.	94.	80.	57.	104.	19.	128.	−18.	152.
131.	56.	93.	80.	56.	104.	18.	129.	−19.	152.
130.	57.	92.	81.	55.	105.	17.	129.	−20.	153.
129.	57.	91.	82.	54.	106.	16.	130.	−21.	154.
128.	58.	90.	82.	53.	106.	15.	131.	−22.	154.
127.	59.	89.	83.	52.	107.	14.	131.	−23.	155.
126.	59.	88.	84.	51.	107.	13.	132.	−24.	156.
125.	60.	87.	84.	50.	108.	12.	132.	−25.	156.
124.	61.	86.	85.	49.	109.	11.	133.	−26.	157.
123.	61.	85.	86.	48.	109.	10.	134.	−27.	158.
122.	62.	84.	86.	47.	110.	9.	134.	−28.	158.
121.	63.	83.	87.	46.	111.	8.	135.	−29.	159.
120.	63.	82.	88.	45.	111.	7.	136.	−30.	159.
119.	64.			44.	112.			−31.	160.

Note: A = corrected; B = standard.

Source: Alekoumbides et al., 1987.

who prepared a table to correct scores on the standard version for age and education. Table 8–2 contains the numbers to be added or subtracted in order to obtain the corrected score. The corrected score can then be converted to a standard score (mean = 100, SD = 15) by means of Table 8–3. The corrected scores are listed in column A, and the standardized scores are in column B of the table.

For the Short Category Test (Wetzel & Boll, 1987), normative data are based on a relatively small number of healthy individuals ($n = 120$). The manual provides tables broken down by age (45 years and below; 46 years and above). Error raw scores are converted to normalized T-scores and percentile rank equivalents. A cutoff score of 41 is recommended for subjects aged 45 and under while a cutoff score of 46 is suggested for subjects aged 46 and above.

Intermediate Versions. A number of investigators have compiled norms for the standard

Table 8—4. Total Mean Number of Errors for the Intermediate HCT—168 Items

Age	n	M	SD	Range
9	22	59.5	17.7	19–93
10	56	50.0	16.9	15–84
11	50	43.3	18.5	10–79
12	72	36.2	16.5	9–89
13	52	34.6	17.2	7–84
14	43	31.3	11.1	12–53
15	41	30.6	12.3	13–61

Source: Spreen & Gaddes, 1969. Norms are based on a population of normal school children.

Table 8—5. Total Mean Number of Errors for the Children's HCT—80 Items

Age	n	M	SD
2–5	154	38.66	11.10
6	54	22.76	11.16
7	60	18.94	10.80
8	65	13.09	6.39

Source: Klonoff & Low, 1974. Norms are based on a population of normal children referred to pediatricians.

Intermediate version (168 items). Data from Trites (1977) should probably be avoided since they were collected from referrals to a neuropsychology clinic for assessment. Both Knights (1966) and Spreen and Gaddes (1969) give data for the standard Intermediate version for normal schoolchildren. In Knights' (1966) report, the sample sizes at all age levels are very small. The norms provided by Spreen and Gaddes (1969) are more adequate in terms of sample size, and these are shown in Table 8–4. They are, however, somewhat dated.

The manual of the CCT, Level 2 (100 items; Boll, 1993), provides recent normative data for children aged 9–16 derived from a relatively large sample considered representative of the U.S. population. Raw error scores are converted to standard score T-scores and equivalent percentile ranks.

Children's Versions. For the standard format, Knights (1966) provides norms for ages 5–8 years, based on a population of normal schoolchildren. However, the sample sizes at all age levels are very small. The normative data provided by Klonoff and Low (1974) are better since the sample sizes are larger. These data are given in Table 8–5.

Boll (1993) provides more up-to-date norms for the booklet form of the Children's Category Test (CCT), Level 1 (for ages 5 years to 8 years, 11 months) based on a very large sample representative of the U.S. population of children. The new norms establish a higher standard than those reported by Klonoff and Low (1974), in line with the trend for in-

creased average performance of individuals over time (Flynn, 1984). Using tables provided in the manual (Boll, 1993), raw error scores are translated into T-scores and equivalent percentile ranks.

References

Adams, K.M., Gilman, S., Koeppe, R., Klain, K., Junck, L., Lohman, M., Johnson-Greene, D., Berent, S., Dede, D., Kroll, P. (1995). Correlation of neuropsychological function with cerebral metabolic rate in subdivisions of the frontal lobes of older alcoholic patients measured with [18F]Fluorodeoxyglucose and Positron Emission Tomography. *Neuropsychology, 9,* 275–280.

Adams, R.L., & Trenton, S.L. (1981). Development of a paper-and-pen form of the Halstead Category Test. *Journal of Consulting and Clinical Psychology, 49,* 298–299.

Alekoumbides, A., Charter, R.A., Adkins, T.G., & Seacat, G.F. (1987). The diagnosis off brain damage by the WAIS, WMS, and Reitan battery utilizing standardized scores corrected for age and education. *The International Journal of Clinical Neuropsychology, 9,* 11–28.

Anderson, C.V., Bigler, E.D., & Blatter, D.D. (1995). Frontal lobe lesions, diffuse damage, and neuropsychological functioning of traumatic brain-injured patients. *Journal of Clinical and Experimental Neuropsychology, 17,* 900–908.

Arnold, B.R., Montgomery, G.T., Castaneda, I., & Longoria, R. (1994). Acculturation and performance of Hispanics on selected Halstead-Reitan neuropsychological tests. *Assessment, 1,* 239–248.

Bertram, K.W., Abeles, N., & Snyder, P.J. (1990). The role of learning in performance on Halstead's Category Test. *The Clinical Neuropsychologist, 4,* 244–252.

Boll, T. (1993). *Children's Category Test.* San Antonio, TX: The Psychological Corporation.

Bond, J.A., & Buchtel, H.A. (1984). Comparison of the Wisconsin Card Sorting Test and the Halstead Category Test. *Journal of Clinical Psychology, 40,* 1251–1254.

Bornstein, R.A. (1986). Contribution of various neuropsychological measures to detection of frontal lobe impairment. *International Journal of Clinical Neuropsychology, 8,* 18–22.

Boyle, G.L. (1986). Clinical neuropsychological assessment: Abbreviating the Halstead Category Test of brain dysfunction. *Journal of Clinical Psychology, 42,* 615–625.

Brandon, A.D., & Chavez, E.L. (1985). Order and delay effects on neuropsychological test presentation: The Halstead Category and Wisconsin Card Sorting Tests. *International Journal of Clinical Neuropsychology, 7,* 152–153.

Caslyn, D.A., O'Leary, M.R., & Chaney, E.F. (1980). Shortening the Category Test. *Journal of Consulting and Clinical Psychology, 48,* 788–789.

Charter, R.A., Adkins, T.G., Alekoumbides, A., & Seacat, G.F. (1987). Reliability of the WAIS, WMS, and Reitan Battery: Raw scores and standardization scores corrected for age and education. *The International Journal of Clinical Neuropsychology, 9,* 28–32.

Charter, R.A., Swift, K.M., & Blusewicz, M.J. (1997). Age- and education-corrected, standardized short form of the Category Test. *The Clinical Neuropsychologist, 11,* 142–145.

Choca, J., & Morris, J. (1992). Administering the Category Test by computer: Equivalence of results. *The Clinical Neuropsychologist, 6,* 9–15.

Choca, J.P., Laatsch, L., Wetzel, L., & Agresti, A. (1997). The Halstead Category Test: A fifty year perspective. *Neuropsychology Review, 7,* 61–75.

DeFilippis, N.A., & McCampbell, E. (1979, 1991). *Manual for the Booklet Category Test.* Odessa, FL.: Psychological Assessment Resources.

Dodrill, C.B. (1987). What's normal? Paper presented to the Pacific Northwest Neuropsychological Association, Seattle.

Dodrill, C.B., & Troupin, A.S. (1975). Effects of repeated administrations of a comprehensive neuropsychological battery among chronic epileptics. *Journal of Nervous and Mental Disease, 161,* 185–190.

Doehring, D.G., & Reitan, R.M. (1962). Concept attainment of human adults with lateralized cerebral lesions. *Perceptual and Motor Skills, 14,* 27–33.

Donders, J., & Kirsch, N. (1991). Nature and implications on the Booklet Category Test and Wisconsin Card Sorting Test. *The Clinical Neuropsychologist, 5,* 78–82.

Donders, J. (1996). Validity of short forms of Intermediate Halstead Category Test in children with traumatic brain injury. *Archives of Clinical Neuropsychology, 11,* 131–137.

Ernst, J. (1987). Neuropsychological problem-solving skills in the elderly. *Psychology of Aging, 2,* 363–365.

Fischer, W.E., & Dean, R.S. (1990). Factor structure of the Halstead Category Test by age and gender. *International Journal of Clinical Neuropsychology, 12,* 180–183.

Franzen, M.D., Smith, S.S., Paul, D.S., & MacInnes, W.D. (1993). Order effects in the administration of the Booklet Category Test and Wisconsin Card Sorting Test. *Archives of Clinical Neuropsychology, 8,* 105–110.

Flynn, J.R. (1984). The mean IQ of Americans: Massive gains 1932–1978. *Psychological Bulletin, 95,* 29–51.

Gelowitz, D.L., & Paniak, C.E. (1992). Cross-validation of the Short Category Test–Booklet Format. *Neuropsychology, 6,* 287–292.

Gregory, R.J., Paul, J.J., & Morrison, M.W. (1979). A short form of the Category Test for adults. *Journal of Clinical Psychology, 35,* 795–798.

Goldstein, G., & Watson, J.R. (1989). Test–retest reliability of the Halstead-Reitan battery and the WAIS in a neuropsychiatric population. *The Clinical Neuropsychologist, 3,* 265–273.

Halstead, W.C. (1947). *Brain and Intelligence.* Chicago: University of Chicago Press.

Heaton, R.K., Grant, I., & Mathews, C.G. (1991). *Comprehensive Norms for an Expanded Halstead-Reitan Battery.* Odessa, Florida: Psychological Assessment Resources, Inc.

Holz, J.L., Gearhart, L.P., & Watson, C.G. (1996). Comparability of scores on projector- and booklet-administration of the Category Test in brain-impaired veterans and controls. *Neuropsychology, 10,* 194–196.

Hom, J., & Reitan, R.M. (1990). Generalized cognitive function after stroke. *Journal of Clinical and Experimental Neuropsychology, 12,* 644–654.

Johnstone, B., Holland, D., & Hewett, J.E. (1997). The construct validity of the Category Test: Is it a measure of reasoning or intelligence? *Psychological Assessment, 9,* 28–33.

King, M.C., & Snow, W.G. (1981). Problem-solving task performance in brain-damaged subjects. *Journal of Clinical Psychology, 38,* 400–404.

Klonoff, H. (1971). Factor analysis of a neuropsychological battery for children aged 9 to 15. *Perceptual and Motor Skills, 32,* 603–616.

Klonoff, H., & Low, M. (1974). Disordered brain function in young children and early adolescents: Neuropsychological and electroencephalographic correlates. In R. Reitan & L.A. Davidson (Eds.), *Clinical Neuropsychology: Current Status and Applications.* New York: Wiley and Sons.

Klove, H. (1974). Validation studies in adult clinical neuropsychology. In R. Reitan & L. Davison (Eds.), *Clinical Neuropsychology: Current Status and Application.* New York: Wiley and Sons.

Knights, R.M. (1966). Normative data on tests for evaluating brain damage in children from 5 to 14 years of age. *Research Bulletin No. 20,* Department of Psychology, University of Western Ontario, London, Canada.

Labreche, T.M. (1983). *The Victoria Revision of the Halstead Category Test.* Unpublished doctoral dissertation, University of Victoria, Victoria, British Columbia, Canada.

Lansdell, H., & Donnelly, E.F. (1977). Factor analysis of the Wechsler Adult Intelligence Scale and the Halstead-Reitan Category and Tapping tests. *Journal of Consulting and Clinical Psychology, 3,* 412–416.

Leckliter, I.N., & Matarazzo, J.D. (1989). The influence of age, education, IQ, gender, and alcohol abuse on Halstead-Reitan neuropsychological test battery performance. *Journal of Clinical Psychology, 45,* 484–512.

Matarazzo, J.D., Wiens, A.N., Matarazzo, R.G., & Goldstein, S.G. (1974). Psychometric and test–retest reliability of the Halstead impairment index in a sample of healthy, young, normal men. *Journal of Nervous and Mental Disease, 158,* 37–49.

Mercer, W.N., Harrell, E.H., Miller, D.C., Childs, H.W., & Rockers, D.M. (1997). Performance of brain-injured versus healthy adults on three versions of the Category Test. *The Clinical Neuropsychologist, 11,* 174–179.

Moses, J.A. (1985). Internal consistency of standard and short forms of three itemized Halstead-Reitan Neuropsychological Battery Tests. *The International Journal of Clinical Neuropsychology, 3,* 164–166.

O'Donnell, J.P., MacGregor, L.A., Dabrowski, J.J., Oestreicher, J.M., & Romero, J.J. (1994). Construct validity of neuropsychological tests of conceptual and attentional abilities. *Journal of Clinical Psychology, 50,* 596–600.

Pendleton, M.G., & Heaton, R.K. (1982). A comparison of the Wisconsin Card Sorting Test and the Category Test. *Journal of Clinical Psychology, 38,* 392–396.

Perrine, K. (1993). Differential aspects of conceptual processing in the Category Test and Wisconsin Card Sorting Test. *Journal of Clinical and Experimental Neuropsychology, 15,* 461–473.

Prigatano, G.P., & Parsons, O.A. (1976). Relationship of age and education to Halstead test performance in different populations. *Journal of Clinical and Consulting Psychology, 44,* 527–533.

Reed, H.B.C., Reitan, R.M., & Klove, H. (1965). Influence of cerebral lesions on psychological test performances of older children. *Journal of Consulting Psychology, 29,* 247–251.

Reitan, R.M., & Davison, L.A. (1974). *Clinical Neuropsychology: Current status and applications.* Washington: Winston.

Reitan, R.M., & Wolfson, D. (1985). *The Halstead-Reitan Neuropsychological Test Battery: Theory and Clinical Interpretation.* Tucson: Neuropsychology Press.

Reitan, R.M., & Wolfson, D. (1995). Category Test and Trail Making Test as measures of frontal lobe functions. *The Clinical Neuropsychologist, 9,* 50–56.

Russell, E.W., & Levy, M. (1987). Revision of the Halstead Category Test. *Journal of Consulting and Clinical Psychology, 55,* 898–901.

Russell, E.W. (1992). Reliability of the Halstead Impairment Index: A simulation and reanalysis of Matarazzo et al. (1974). *Neuropsychology, 6,* 251–259.

Savard, R.J., Rey, A.C., & Post, R.M. (1980). Halstead-Reitan Category Test in bipolar and unipolar affective disorders: Relationship to age and phase in illness. *Journal of Nervous and Mental Disease, 168,* 297–304.

Seidenberg, M., Giordani, B., Berent, S., & Boll, T.J. (1983). IQ level and performance on the Halstead-Reitan Neuropsychological Test Battery for older children. *Journal of Consulting and Clinical Psychology, 51,* 406–413.

Shaw, D.J. (1966). The reliability and validity of the Halstead Category Test. *Journal of Clinical Psychology, 37,* 847–848.

Spreen, O., & Gaddes, W.H. (1969). Developmental norms for 15 neuropsychological tests age 6 to 15. *Cortex, 5,* 170–191.

Steindl, S.R., & Boyle, G.J. (1995). Use of the Booklet Category Test to assess abstract concept formation in schizophrenic disorders. *Archives of Clinical Neuropsychology, 10,* 205–210.

Tenhula, W.N., & Sweet, J.J. (1996). Double cross-validation of the Booklet Category Test in detecting malingered traumatic brain injury. *The Clinical Neuropsychologist, 10,* 104–116.

Trites, R.L. (1977). *Neuropsychological Test Manual,* Ottawa, Ontario: Royal Ottawa Hospital.

Trueblood, W., & Schmidt, M. (1993). Malingering and other validity considerations in the neuropsychological evaluation of mild head injury. *Journal of Clinical and Experimental Neuropsychology, 15,* 578–590.

Wetzel, L., & Boll, T.J. (1987). *Short Category Test, Booklet Format.* Los Angeles: Western Psychological Services.

COGNITIVE ESTIMATION TEST (CET)

Purpose

This test is used to assess the ability to generate effective problem-solving strategies.

Source

There is no commercial source. Users may refer to the following text in order to design their own material.

Description

Shallice and Evans (1978) focused attention on the ability of brain-damaged patients, particularly those with frontal lobe damage, to produce adequate cognitive estimates. They designed a test that requires subjects to respond to questions that do not have readily apparent answers. For example, answering questions such as "What is the average length of a man's spine?" stresses the abilities of selecting an appropriate plan and of checking the plausibility of the estimate but does not require performing any complex computation. They provided preliminary normative data based on a sample of 25 British neurologically intact individuals. Axelrod and Millis (1994) have recently revised the task. They adapted the task for use with North American populations, eliminated items that required nonnumerative responses, provided a standardized scoring method, and presented some preliminary normative data. The test consists of 10 items, shown in Figure 8–4.

Administration

The examiner provides the sheet containing the test questions and requests that the patient complete the questions with "best guesses" in the spaces provided. There is no time limit.

Approximate Time for Administration

The entire test requires about 5 minutes.

Scoring

Each response is compared with answers provided on the Deviation Scoring sheet (Figure 8–5). The deviation scores for each CET item were developed from percentiles based on the mean performance of a standardization group of 164 employed adults (e.g., deviation score of 0 for responses between 16th to 84th percentiles; deviation score of 1 for responses between 2 to 16 as well as 84th to 98th percentiles; deviation scores of 2 for responses less than the 2nd and greater than the 98th percentiles). The total deviation score is computed by summing item deviation scores for all 10 CET items. Thus, higher deviation scores imply more impaired (bizarre) performance.

Comment

The broad content represented in the CET appears to be multidimensional. Axelrod and Millis (1994) reported that item–total correlations for the American version of the CET ranged from .22 to .57. O'Carroll et al. (1994) found that the internal reliability of the British version CET was .40 (Cronbach's alpha) and .35 (Guttman split-half reliability coefficient). O'Carroll et al. also examined the factor structure of their version of the CET. Principal component analysis followed by varimax rotation resulted in five factors' being extracted from this 10-item scale! Ross et al. (1996) examined reliability in an American college sample ($n = 158$) and reported that internal consistency was low (Cronbach's alpha = .37). Interitem correlations ranged from $r = -.16$ to .31. Forty-four of these individuals were retested following about 37.5 days (SD = 17.5).

Please answer the following questions in the space provided. Although you may not know the exact answer, make a best guess. Be sure to complete all items.

1. How tall is the Empire State Building? _____ feet
2. How fast do race horses gallop? _____ miles per hour
3. How long is the average necktie? _____ feet _____ inches
4. What is the average length of a man's spine? _____ feet _____ inches
5. How tall is the average woman? _____ feet _____ inches
6. How heavy is a full grown elephant? _____ pounds
7. How much does one quart of milk weigh? _____ pound(s)
8. How fast does a commercial jet fly? _____ miles per hour
9. On the average, how many T.V. programs are there on any one channel between the hours of 6 pm and 11 pm? _____
10. What is the average temperature in Anchorage, Alaska on Christmas Day? _____ degrees F.

Total Deviation score = _____

Figure 8—4. Cognitive Estimation Test (Axelrod & Millis, 1994. Reprinted with permission of Psychological Assessment Resources).

Response Empire State Building (ft)	Deviation	Response Elephant Weight (lbs)	Deviation
<78	2	<500	2
78–499	1	500–1000	1
500–3555	0	1001–4999	0
3556–66900	1	5000–20880	1
>66900	2	>20880	2
Race Horse (mph)		Quart of Milk Weight (lbs)	
<5	2	<0.3	2
5–20	1	0.3–0.99	1
21–49	0	1.0–2.2	0
50–100	1	2.3–5.0	1
>100	2	>5.0	2
Necktie Length (inches)		Speed of Commercial Jet (mph)	
<10.5	2	<83	2
10.5–18	1	83–250	1
19–47	0	251–787	0
48–70	1	788–6720	1
>70	2	>6720	2
Spine Length (inches)		Number of TV Shows	
<12	2	<1.3	2
12–24	1	1.3–5.0	1
25–42	0	5.1–9.9	0
43–64	1	10–88	1
>64	2	>88	2
Height of Woman		Temperature in Anchorage (°F)	
<60.5	2	<−37	2
60.5–64.0	1	−37–−10	1
64.1–65.9	0	−9–+32	0
66.0–68.0	1	+33–+59	1
>68	2	>59	2

Figure 8—5. Cognitive Estimation Test deviation scoring sheet. (Axelrod & Millis, 1994. Reprinted with Permission of Psychological Assessment Resources).

The coefficient of stability for the CET was moderate ($r = .57$). On average, slightly better scores were obtained at retest (mean = 4.7, SD = 2.1) than at initial examination (mean = 5.3, SD = 2.3), suggesting a modest practice effect. O'Carroll et al. (1994) reported that the interrater reliability coefficient was high ($r = .91$) for a group of 50 healthy subjects given the British version of the CET in which responses were scored from 0 (good estimate) to 3 (bizarre estimate).

Performance on the CET appears to be relatively unrelated to other executive function tests. Ross et al. (1996) reported that in normal people the CET is significantly correlated with other putative measures of executive functioning (COWAT $r = -.22$, Design Fluency $r = -.19$, Ruff Figural Fluency $r = -.27$, Porteus Mazes $r = .24$, Stroop $r = .22$, Trails B $r = .27$, WCST $r = .19$) with the exception of the Tower of Hanoi ($r = .03$). The magnitude of the associations, however, was low. Further, the CET was moderately related to NAART errors ($r = -.39$), suggesting that level of intelligence contributes to CET performance.

Shallice and Evans (1978) gave their version of the CET to 96 patients with localized cerebral lesions. Patients with anterior lesions performed significantly worse (gave significantly more bizarre answers) than the posterior group on this task. They suggested that the difficulty shown by the patients reflected a deficit in the selection and regulation of cognitive planning. Leng and Parkin (1988) reported that Korsakoff patients performed poorly on the WCST, but normally on the CET, whereas post-encephalitic patients performed adequately on the WCST but poorly on the CET. A single patient with a ruptured anterior communicating artery aneurysm (ACoAA) performed similarly to post-encephalitic amnesics. They suggested that Korsakoff patients have damage to the dorsolateral prefrontal cortex, whereas post-encephalitic (and possibly ACoAA amnesics) have damage to the orbitofrontal cortex. In partial support of Leng and Parkin (1988), Shoqueirat et al. (1990) found that Korsakoff patients were impaired on the CET, WCST, and FAS word fluency, whereas post-encephalitic amnesics were impaired on verbal fluency and the CET, despite performing normally on the WCST. ACoAA amnesics were impaired on both the FAS and the CET, and they scored at a level in between the other amnesic subgroups on the WCST. Further, CET performance was significantly worse in those with lower IQs (FSIQ $r = -.62$), was moderately correlated to verbal fluency ($r = -.34$), but was unrelated to any measure from the WCST. Kopelman (1991) found that both Alzheimer and Korsakoff patients demonstrated poor CET performance. CET scores did not correlate significantly with performance on other putative "frontal" tasks (FAS, Weigl, Nelson version of the WCST, Picture Arrangement errors); however, CET performance was significantly correlated with measures of premorbid (NART $r = -.40$) and current intelligence (Full Scale IQ $r = -.53$), CT scan measures of ventricular-brain ratio ($r = .36$), and measures of retrograde and anterograde memory (.32 to .67). Kopelman (1991) suggested that the CET may be measuring some aspect of access to semantic memory, or alternatively, that it may be sensitive to a different locus of frontal lobe pathology (e.g., in the orbitofrontal region as suggested by Leng & Parkin, 1988) compared with other tests. The fact that Korsakoff patients in the Kopelman (1991) and Shoqueirat et al. (1990) studies performed poorly on the CET, however, means that the latter possibility requires more thorough substantiation. Recently, Taylor and O'Carroll (1995) also reported that patients with Korsakoff syndrome were impaired on the CET. In addition, a subgroup of patients with discrete frontal lesions (confirmed via CT or MRI) was compared with a group with localized nonfrontal lesions. No significant difference in CET performance was observed between the anterior and posterior lesioned groups, calling into question the sensitivity of the CET to anterior brain dysfunction. These authors also noted that CET scores were moderately related to education, IQ (NART errors), and social class in both normal and neurological populations.

Axelrod and Millis (1994) reported that patients with severe head injuries were impaired on the CET relative to a sample of medical outpatients. They suggested that a cutoff ≥7 produced the best differentiation of patients from controls and resulted in an overall correct classification rate of 78 percent. It is worth noting, however, that in this study, patients with TBI had significantly less education than controls, raising the concern that the test may be more sensitive to education than to brain injury.

The evidence suggests that this task is brief, easy to administer, and may capture an important component of executive functioning. The test, however, is relatively new and is in need of further refinement. Future studies should include the development of additional items to increase the scale's internal consistency as well as large-scale studies of normal populations and diverse patient populations, and the subsequent investigation of its temporal stability.

Normative Data

Axelrod and Millis (1994) reported that the average deviation score for a sample of 164 adults (mean age = 39.0, SD = 16.1; mean education = 16.2 years, SD = 2.8; 74 percent female, 26 percent male; 75 percent Caucasian, 23 percent black, 2 percent other) was 4.4 (SD = 2.2). Factually correct responses for each item on the CET result in a total deviation score of 3, which falls within one standard deviation of the sample mean.

Level of education affected performance. In general, deviation scores were lower for in-

Table 8—6. Mean Deviation Score for Cognitive Estimation Performance across Education Groups

Education Level	n	Mean Deviation Score	SD
≤12	16	5.9	2.3
13–15	32	4.8	2.1
16	32	4.2	2.4
17–18	37	3.8	1.9
≥19	25	4.2	2.0

Source: Axelrod and Millis, 1994. Reprinted with permission of Psychological Assessment Resources.

dividuals with more education (see Table 8–6). Age had no effect on performance.

O'Carroll et al. (1994) provide normative data for a 10-item British version of the CET. The data are based on a sample 150 healthy individuals, aged 17–91 years, living in the UK. Mean CET score for the entire sample was 5.3 (SD = 3.6). CET scores were moderately related to general intellectual ability (NART errors r = .30) and gender, with females performing worse than males. Age, education, and social class were not unique predictors of CET performance.

References

Axelrod, B.N., & Millis, S.R. (1994). Preliminary standardization of the Cognitive Estimation Test. *Assessment, 1,* 269–274.

Kopelman, M. (1991). Frontal dysfunction and memory deficits in the alcoholic Korsakoff syndrome and Alzheimer-type dementia. *Brain, 114,* 117–137.

Leng, N.R.C., & Parkin, A.J. (1988). Double dissociation of frontal dysfunction in organic amnesia. *British Journal of Clinical Psychology, 27,* 359–362.

O'Carroll, R., Egan, V., & Mackenzie, D.M. (1994). Assessing cognitive estimation. *British Journal of Clinical Psychology, 33,* 193–197.

Ross, T.P., Hanks, R.A., Kotasek, R.S., & Whitman, R.D. (1996). The reliability and validity of a modified Cognitive Estimation Test. Paper presented to the International Neuropsychological Society, Chicago.

Shallice, T., & Evans, M.E. (1978). The involvement of the frontal lobes in cognitive estimation. *Cortex, 14,* 292–303.

Shoqueirat, M.A., Mayes, A., MacDonald, C., Meudell, P., & Pickering, A. (1990). Performance on tests sensitive to frontal lobe lesions by patients with organic amnesia: Leng and Parkin revisited. *British Journal of Clinical Psychology, 29,* 401–408.

Taylor, R., & O'Carroll, R. (1995). Cognitive estimation in neurological disorders. *British Journal of Clinical Psychology, 34,* 223–228.

DESIGN FLUENCY TEST

Purpose

This test measures the production of novel abstract designs.

Source

No specific material is required.

Description

Design Fluency (Jones-Gotman & Milner, 1977; Jones-Gotman, 1991) was developed as a nonverbal analogue to word-fluency tasks. The task requires the client to generate as many different meaningless designs as possible. The test is composed of a free-response condition, lasting 5 minutes, in which few restrictions are imposed on design generation, and a fixed response condition, lasting 4 minutes, in which the client must produce designs that contain exactly four lines or components.

Administration

The instructions provided in the original article are somewhat vague. More detailed instructions are provided below (from M. Jones-Gotman, personal communication, April 1995).

Use a stopwatch and have the patient comfortably seated before giving the instructions. If more than one page is used per condition, provide new blank paper and place the old one so that the patient can always see what he or she has already drawn. Always use a ballpoint pen to avoid erasures. Use a separate page for examples provided during the instructions, and hide that page after giving the directions. Draw the examples one under the other to illustrate what is expected from the patient.

A. Free Condition (5 minutes). "I want you to do some drawing for me. This test is different from others that you have done, because in this test you must make up the drawings in your head. Do not make drawings that represent something. Do not draw anything you have ever seen before. Do not make drawings that anybody could name; if you draw some- *thing that can be named I won't count it. Instead, what you must do is to make up designs out of your head. For example, you could draw something like this:*

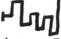

It's nothing, I just made it up. Or you could draw something like this:

It's also nothing and I made it up. But if you were to draw, for example, something like this:

I would call it a star and I would not count it. The only other thing that is not accepted is scribbling. If you draw

and then

each might be slightly different from the other, but they do not require much effort from you and they are too much alike, so they are also not accepted and wouldn't count in your score. All of your drawings must be <u>very different</u> from each other.

Do you have any questions? When I say go, begin drawing. Make as <u>many different</u> drawings as you can in 5 minutes. You can start here, and draw them in columns like I have done. Go."

Remove the examiner's drawings from the patient's view. It is important to watch while the patient draws, so that warnings can be given at the appropriate moment. *One* warning only is given for *each* of the following: Scribbling (*"That is a scribble. Remember scribbling is not allowed."*); Nameable Drawing (*"I can name that. It's a _____. Do not make drawings that represent something."*); Too Similar to a Previous Drawing (*"That is too much like"* . . . indicate which one . . .*"remember, all of your drawings must be very <u>different</u> from each other."*); Too Elaborate (*"Remember, you must make as <u>many</u> different drawings as you can."*) At the end, always question at least one design to probe for nameable drawings (*"What is this?"*).

B. Four-Line Condition (4 minutes). Give the client a separate sheet of paper and write "4 lines" at the top. Use your instruction page to draw examples. Count the lines aloud while drawing the examples in this condition.

"There is a second part to this test. It is like the first one because again you have to make up designs that you invent yourself, but this time each design must be made with exactly four lines. I will show you what I mean by 'a line' for the purposes of this test.

Obviously, a straight line like this

will count as one line. Whenever you draw a sharp angle, such as this

it will make two lines, whether you lift your pen or not. You can also draw a curved line, like this

or like this

or you can even draw a sort of double curve, like this

but avoid making lines that would be difficult to count, such as this

or this

because I must be able to count the lines in your drawing easily. One other thing: a circle

counts as one line, too. So, here is an example of what you could do. You could draw like this, for example

(count components while drawing); *or for another example you could draw this:*

Just like in the first part of the test, you must not make drawings that can be named or that represent anything. Just make up abstract designs, using exactly four lines in each one. Now, when I saw go, make as many different designs as you can in four minutes. Go."

As before, remove the examiner's drawings from the patient's view. Watch the patient so that warnings can be given at the appropriate moment. *One* warning only is given for *each* of

the following: Too Similar to a Previous Drawing (*"That is too much like"* . . . indicate which one . . ."*remember, all of your drawings must be very <u>different</u> from each other.*"); Nameable Drawings (often a letter or a square in this condition); Wrong Number of Lines (count the lines aloud and remind patient to use exactly four lines). Question at least one drawing at the end to probe for nameable designs that you may not recognize as such (*"What is this?"*).

Approximate Time for Administration

The entire test takes about 15 minutes to administer. The time limits are 5 minutes for the free condition and 4 minutes for the fixed condition.

Scoring

There is one basic score for each condition: a *novel output score* which is defined as the total output minus the sum of all perseverative responses, nameable drawings, and drawings with the wrong number of lines.

To score the Design Fluency Test, first determine the perseverative responses. These include rotations or mirror-image versions of previous drawings, variations on a theme, complicated drawings that differ from previous ones by small details, and scribbles. The perseverative responses must be scored harshly and then subtracted from the total number drawn; the remaining drawings should then be all quite different from one another. Occasionally, the patient might reproduce the drawing made by the examiner. This is not counted as a perseverative error.

For nameable drawings, the examiner will have asked "What is this?" for at least one drawing at the end of each condition. Most often patients will deny knowing what the drawing represents, but they sometimes answer with the name of a concrete object or a letter that has been elaborated, etc. The examiner must also use his or her own judgment when something looks obviously nameable.

For each of the two conditions, the final novel output score is the number of drawings remaining after perseverations and rule-breaking items (nameable, wrong number of lines) have been subtracted. This represents the patient's real output of novel designs. The two conditions are not added together. Although the first one may be the more sensitive of the two with regard to frontal lobe dysfunction, Jones-Gotman recommends retaining the two conditions. She found that the fixed condition was particularly sensitive in patients with Binswanger's disease, a group assumed to have primarily frontal-lobe dysfunction (Jones-Gotman, 1995, personal communication).

A perseveration score can also be calculated. Subtract all unacceptable drawings (that is, rule-breaking items) except perseverations from the total output. Then determine the percentage of perseverative responses relative to this subtotal output. For example, if someone has a total output of 22 drawings that contains 10 perseverative responses and 2 nameable items, the 2 nameable items are first subtracted from 22, then 10 (perseverative items) is divided by 20. The perseveration score is .5 or 50 percent.

Comment

When the original scoring criteria (Jones-Gotman & Milner, 1977) are used, there is fair-to-good interrater agreement and rater consistency for the majority of scoring parameters in both conditions (Woodward et al., 1992). They do not, however, produce sufficient reliability for clinical use. Varney et al. (1996) gave the test to 86 patients who suffered closed head injuries and 87 normal controls. Two independent raters agreed 90 percent of the time with respect to the novel design score in the free condition. In a recent study with a college sample, Ross et al. (1996) found good-to-fair interrater reliability with regard to total ($r = .98$) and novel (about .69) responses. Perseverations and other rule violations showed poor interrater agreement (.21 to .48). The supplementary scoring criteria presented above (see Scoring) may enhance overall reliability. Jones-Gotman (1991) assessed scoring reliability in a study of 324 children and 50 adults. Three judges scored all tests independently. Correlation coefficients were above .74.

Ross et al. (1996) retested college students following a one-month interval. The temporal stability ranged from fair to poor (.10 to .70), depending on the measure. Previous exposure to the task resulted in both an increase in design production characterized by more total and novel designs, as well as an increase in test-taking efficiency, marked by a relative decrease in the proportion of perseverative responses.

The cognitive operations underlying the task are not certain. Creating novel designs is a complex task and likely involves several cognitive processes including cognitive flexibility, creativity, and constructional abilities (Bigler et al., 1988), as well as working memory for keeping track of items that have already been produced. Franzen and Petrick (1995) reported a moderate correlation of .55 between the free and fixed conditions in a sample of healthy individuals. They also found positive, but weak, correlations ($r = .12$) between design and verbal fluency (COWAT) measures, suggesting that the two measures are dissociable. The fixed condition correlated modestly with Trails A ($-.39$) and the Stroop color-word interference trial (.36). Similar findings have been reported by Varney et al. (1996) in a sample of 86 patients with closed head injuries. Novel design performance in the free condition showed a modest relation with verbal fluency ($r = .34$). Whereas 47 percent of the patients performed defectively on Design Fluency, only 13 percent performed defectively on the COWAT. Performance on the test was unrelated to WAIS IQ ($r = .14$) and only weakly related to Digit Symbol ($r = .22$), suggesting that task failure was not a reflection of general mental impairment and was only minimally related to problems with concentration or graphomotor speed.

Jones-Gotman and Milner (1977) and Jones-Gotman (1991) showed that patients with right frontal or central damage have difficulty in two different ways: They simply create few new designs and/or tend to make numerous perseverative errors (see also Canavan et al., 1985). Similar deficits in design fluency have been noted in patients diagnosed as suffering from

Table 8—7. Mean Number of Drawings by Children on the Design Fluency Test—Free Condition

Age	n	M	SD
5–6	52	3.2	2.0
7–8	68	6.2	3.2
9–10	68	8.0	3.2
11–14	68	9.4	3.9

Source: Jones-Gotman, 1990, and personal communication, April 1995.

dementia of the Alzheimer's type (AD) (Bigler et al., 1988). The test has also been successful in detecting frontal lobe dementia (Canavan et al., 1985; Neary et al., 1990; Jones-Gotman, personal communication) and is sensitive to even minor closed head injury. Varney et al. (1996) reported that patients with closed head injuries, even of a mild nature, tend to produce fewer novel designs in the free condition than normal controls.

Jones-Gotman (1990) noted that it is normal to produce some drawings that are too similar to others. Furthermore, the greater the total number of drawings produced, the higher the likelihood that some will be repeated. The drawings of an individual may also have a certain resemblance, reflecting the individual's style; however, this is quite different from the pathological repetitiveness or perseveration that is often seen in the productions made by patients with right frontal dysfunction.

Normative Data

Jones-Gotman (1990) tested 324 school children between the ages of 5 and 14 years in the free condition. The mean number of acceptable drawings produced in five minutes for each age group are shown in Table 8–7. Jones-Gotman (personal communication, March 1995) has collected normative data for adults on both the free (5-minute) and fixed or 4-line (4-minute) condition. The data are shown in Table 8–8.

Other researchers have provided data for both children and adults (Daigneault et al., 1992; Franzen & Petrick, 1995; Levin et al., 1991; Varney et al., 1996; Woodward et al., 1992). The values reported are generally higher than those reported here and likely reflect the strictness with which the scoring criteria are applied (Jones-Gotman, personal communication). It is hoped that the more explicit scoring criteria given above (See Scoring) will result in the development of an adequate normative base.

Varney et al. (1996) reported that novel output scores in the free condition are normally distributed, without a "floor effect" in which scores distribute to 0 correct in a significant percentage of cases. They also noted that among 87 normal controls, aged 18–77 years, 95 percent made one or less nameable designs and made three or fewer repeated designs.

The literature suggests improvement in scores during the childhood years and then decreased performance with advancing age (Jones-Gotman, 1990; Levin et al., 1991; Mittenberg et al., 1989). Varney et al. (1996), however, found no significant correlation between number of novel designs and age in adults, aged 18–77. Daigneault, Brun, and Whitaker (1992) found only a higher incidence of perseverative errors in elderly adults (ages 45–65) without any reduction in the number of correct designs. They suggest that fluency and the ability to generate strategies remain intact with advancing age; rather, it is the regulation

Table 8—8. Mean Acceptable Novel Output by Adults on the Design Fluency Test—Free and Fixed Conditions

Age	n	Free Condition			Fixed Condition		
		M	SD	Range	M	SD	Range
14–55	45	15.5	6.1	9.5–21.7	18.9	5.6	13.3–24.5
58–72	10	11.8	4.4	7.4–16.2	12.6	4.3	8.3–16.9

Source: Jones-Gotman, personal communication, June 1996.

of behavior on the basis of preceding responses that is affected.

In adults, education and gender have no effect on the mean number of novel designs (Varney et al., 1996).

References

Bigler, E.D., Schultz, R., Grant, M., Knight, G., Lucas, J., Roman, M., Hall, S., & Sullivan, M. (1988). Design fluency in dementia of the Alzheimer's type: Preliminary findings. *Neuropsychology, 2,* 127–133.

Canavan, S., Janota, I., & Schurr, P.H. (1985). Luria's frontal lobe syndrome: Psychological and anatomical considerations. *Journal of Neurology, Neurosurgery, and Psychiatry, 48,* 1049–1053.

Daigneault, S., Braun, C.M.J., & Whitaker, H.A. (1992). Early effects of normal aging on perseverative and nonperseverative prefrontal measures. *Developmental Neuropsychology, 8,* 99–114.

Franzen, M.D., & Petrick, J.D. (1995). Preliminary norms for Design Fluency. Paper presented to the 103rd meeting of the American Psychological Association, New York.

Jones-Gotman, M. (1990). Presurgical psychological assessment in children: Special tests. *Journal of Epilepsy, 3,* 93–102.

Jones-Gotman, M. (1991). Localization of lesions by neuropsychological testing. *Epilepsia, 32,* S41–S52.

Jones-Gotman, M., & Milner, B. (1977). Design fluency: The invention of nonsense drawings after focal cortical lesions. *Neuropsychologia, 15,* 653–674.

Levin, H.S., Culhane, K.A., Hartmann, J., Harword, H., Ringholtz, G., Ewing-Cobbs, L., & Fletcher, J.M. (1991). Developmental changes in performance on tests of purported frontal lobe functioning. *Developmental Neuropsychology, 7,* 377–395.

Mittenberg, W., Seidenberg, M., O'Leary, D.S., & DiGiulio, D.V. (1989). Changes in cerebral functioning associated with normal aging. *Journal of Clinical and Experimental Neuropsychology, 11,* 918–932.

Neary, D., Snowden, J.S., Mann, D.M.A., Northen, B., Goulding, P.J., & Macdermott, N. (1990). Frontal lobe dementia and motor neuron disease. *Journal of Neurology, Neurosurgery, and Psychiatry, 53,* 23–32.

Ross, T.P., Axelrod, B.N., Hanks, R.A., Kotasek, R.S., & Whitman, R.D. (1996). The interrater and test–retest reliability of the Design Fluency and Ruff Figural Fluency tests. Paper presented to the 24th meeting of the International Neuropsychological Society, Chicago.

Varney, N.R., Roberts, R.J., Struchen, M.A., Hanson, T.V., Franzen, K.M., & Connell, S.K. (1996). Design fluency among normals and patients with closed head injury. *Archives of Clinical Neuropsychology, 11,* 345–353.

Woodward, J.L., Axelrod, B.N., & Henry, R.R. (1992). Interrater reliability of scoring parameters for the Design Fluency Test. *Neuropsychology, 6,* 173–178.

FIVE-POINT TEST

Purpose

This test measures the production of novel designs under time constraints.

Source

Users may make up their own stimuli as described below. Ruff's adaptation is available from PAR, P.O. Box 998, Odessa, Florida 33556, at a cost of $45 US.

Description

Figural fluency tests have been developed as nonverbal analogues to word fluency tasks. Jones-Gotman and Milner's Design Fluency task (1977; see Description earlier in this Chapter) has several problems that restrict its widespread use (Lee et al., 1997). These include adequate normative data, low scoring reliability among different examiners, and difficulty in interpreting the performance of patients with visuoconstructive or motor deficits. In addition, cognitively impaired patients often have difficulty understanding the task demands. In an attempt to overcome some of these limitations, Regard et al. (1982) provided an alternative figural fluency task, the Five-Point Test. This task consists of a sheet of paper (8½ × 11″) with 40 dot matrices arranged in eight rows and five columns. The matrices are identical to the five-dot arrange-

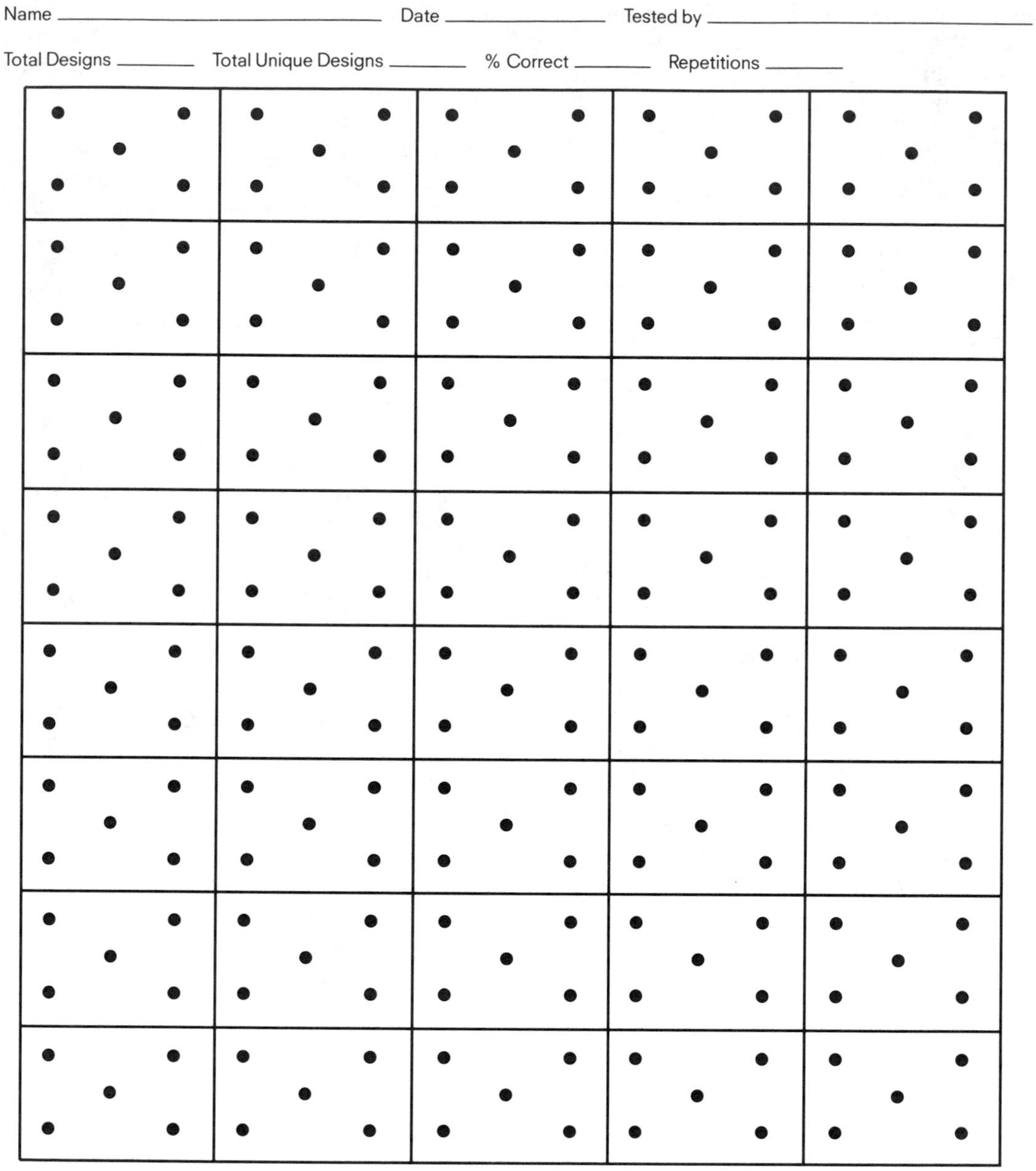

Name _____ Date _____ Tested by _____

Total Designs _____ Total Unique Designs _____ % Correct _____ Repetitions _____

Figure 8—6. Five-Point Test

ment on dice (see Figure 8–6). Patients are asked to produce as many different figures as possible by connecting the dots within each rectangle. Regard et al. (1982) allowed the subjects 5 minutes to perform the task. Others (e.g., Lee et al., 1994) use a three-minute version to make it more comparable to the time limits used for controlled oral word association. We use a 3-minute time limit.

There are a number of adaptations of the Five-Point Test (e.g., Glosser and Goodglass, 1990; Ruff et al., 1987; Ruff, 1988). Ruff, Light and Evan's modification (1987) consists of five different stimuli, each composed of five dots, containing different distractors or variations of the dot matrix, and patients must produce as many design combinations as possible within five separate 60-second time periods. Glosser and Goodglass's (1990) adaptation consists of four different five-dot matrices, and patients are required to draw different patterns by connecting the dots in each matrix using four lines. There are no time limits for this version. We describe here the version used by Regard et al. (1982) with a 3-minute time limit (Lee et al. 1997).

Administration

Place a protocol sheet in front of the patient and indicate that the object is to produce as many different figures or designs as possible in 3 minutes by connecting the dots in each rectangle. The patient is also informed that only straight lines are to be used, that all lines must connect dots, that no figures are to be repeated, and that only single lines are to be used. One warning is given on the first (and only the first) violation of each of these rules. The rules are not repeated on any further infraction.

At the start of the test, two sample solutions are drawn by the examiner. We typically draw the first sample design using all five dots and the second using just two dots in order to demonstrate to the patient that he or she can make either simple or complex designs using some or all of the dots. The patient is permitted to copy the sample designs drawn by the examiner. Most patients do not use more than two test sheets. When a subject exhausts a page, the examiner smoothly and quickly gives the patient a second page while repositioning the first page so that the subject can easily see it.

Patients often ask whether a seemingly trivial variation of a design constitutes a unique production. Reassure the patient that the second design counts. Another frequent question is whether all dots need to be used. Repeat that the patient need not use all dots.

Approximate Time for Administration

The entire test takes about 5–7 minutes to administer. The time limit for the test itself is 3 minutes.

Scoring

A number of scores can be calculated, including the total number of unique designs and the number of repeated designs (perseverations). Because the number of unique designs drawn by patients can influence the number of perseverative errors, the percentage of perseverative errors [(perseverative errors/total unique designs) $\times$ 100] can also be calculated. Patients who are more productive have a greater opportunity to make more perseverative errors, so these scoring variables are not independent.

Comment

Data on reliability are sparse. In a college sample, Ross et al. (1996) found excellent interrater reliability ($r = .80$ to $.98$) for scoring parameters of the Ruff Figural Fluency Test. Ruff (1988) assessed the test–retest reliability of his variant of the Five-Point test following a retest interval of 6 months. He reported a correlation of .76 for the total score. Perseveration scores were less stable (.36). He noted that normal individuals tended to increase the number of unique designs when retested although there was no commensurate increase in perseverations. Similar findings have been reported by Ross et al. (1996) following a retest interval of about 1 month.

Ruff et al. (1994) suggest that the task measures fluid and flexible thinking and the ability to create novel responses without repetitions. The test is moderately correlated with measures of verbal fluency, suggesting that the verbal and nonverbal fluency measures tap similar though not identical functions (Regard et al., 1982; Risser & Andrikopoulos, 1996; but see Ruff et al., 1987). The Five-Point Test and its variants are also moderately correlated with visuospatial and visuoconstructive measures (e.g., Picture Completion, Block Design) and measures of executive control (e.g., Wisconsin Card Sorting Test), but not with measures of motor speed, short-term memory, or aphasia (Glosser & Goodglass, 1990; Regard et al., 1982; Ruff, 1988). Memory for temporal order also appears to be moderately associated with design fluency performance (Parkin et al., 1995).

There is some evidence that the Five-Point Test is sensitive to brain damage generally and to frontal lobe pathology specifically. Lee et al. (1997) gave the test to 196 patients with verified neurologic disease (mostly patients with intractable partial complex seizures) and 62 patients with psychiatric disorder. Psychiatric patients produced significantly more unique designs and a lower percentage of perseverative errors than patients with verified brain damage. Among patients with brain damage, individuals with frontal lobe disease and non–frontal lobe lesions both produced fewer unique designs than controls but did not differ from each other. Patients with frontal lobe disease were, however, distinguished from non–frontal lobe disease neurologic patients and control patients by producing a significantly higher percentage of perseverative errors. There were no significant differences between patients with left and right frontal damage, although there was a trend for patients with right-sided involvement to perform more poorly than their left-sided counterparts. Both Glosser and Goodglass (1990) and Ruff and his colleagues (1994) have reported that poor performance on the variants of the Five Point Test are associated with right hemisphere damage. Ruff et al. (1994) have provided data showing that his variant is sensitive to right anterior damage. There is also some evidence (Lee et al., 1996) that figural fluency is superior to word fluency in detecting frontal lobe disease.

Regard et al. (1982) originally used a 5-minute interval. The 3-minute version, however, appears to accomplish the same discriminatory goals as the 5-minute version and, because of its brevity and high correlation with the 5-minute version, is more attractive (Lee et al., 1997; Risser & Andrikopoulos, 1996). The Ruff Figural Fluency Test stimuli were designed to vary in level of difficulty (e.g., through the use of interference). The research (Ruff, 1988) revealed, however, no significant differences among the five parts of the test, and only the total scores are provided in the manual. Thus, it appears that the use of multiple trials on the Ruff Figural Fluency Test may be redundant and unnecessary (Lee et al., 1997). Finally, Glosser and Goodglass's untimed version of the Five-Point Test may be the most appropriate version to use when time constraints could unduly penalize patients (for example, with patients who have had a stroke or who have Parkinson's disease).

Normative Data

Lee et al. (1997) found that 62 adults with psychiatric disorders (mean age = 35.4, SD = 10.3; mean education = 13.4 years, SD = 3.4; mean FSIQ = 109.1, SD = 11.9) produced about 31.95 acceptable designs (SD = 8.4) in the 3-minute time limit. Few perseverations were made (mean = 1.39, SD = 1.8). The same was true when the percent perseveration score was examined (mean = 4.82, SD = 6.6). The distribution of the percentage of perseverative errors (with percentile ranks) produced by these individuals is shown in Table 8–9.

In adults, IQ appears correlated with the number of unique designs produced (.64) (Lee et al., 1997; see also Ruff et al., 1987; Ruff, 1988, but only for normal, not head-injured patients). Parkin et al. (1995), however, reported that NART IQ was unrelated to performance on Ruff's version in elderly adults. Lee et al. (1997) found that age, education, and gender had no impact on any of the scoring dimensions (see also Glosser and Goodglass, 1990, with regard to age). Ruff et al. (1987), however, noted that both age and education affected performance on his version of the task. Similarly, Parkin et al. (1995) found that elderly individuals (aged 74–95 years) made more perseverative errors out of total responses than did young adults (aged 18–25 years) on Ruff's version.

Regard et al. (1982) provided data (total number of figures, number of rotated figures, number of self-corrections) for the 5-minute version. Their sample consisted of normal children aged 6–13 years. Risser and Andrikopoulos (1996) gave the original 5-minute and a modified 3-minute task to a sample of 30 healthy children, aged 11 years, 9 months to 14 years, 8 months (mean = 13:0 years). Scores on both versions were highly correlated, and the performance of the adolescents was similar to that of the adults (see also Regard et al., 1982). On the 3-minute version, the adolescents produced an average of 29.5 unique designs (SD = 7.77) and made few

Table 8—9. Five-Point Test: Percentile Ranks Associated with the Percentage of Perseverative Errors in Non-Neurologically Impaired Adults

Percent of Perseverations	Cumulative Percentile
0	100
1	56
2	56
3	48
4	39
5	32
6	31
7	27
8	27
9	21
10	21
11	16
12	15
13	11
14	6
15 (cutoff score)	6
16	5
17	0

Source: Lee et al., 1997.

perseverative errors (mean = 1.27, SD = 1.76). On the 5-minute version, the adolescents generated an average of 42.6 unique designs (SD = 11.45) and made few perseverative errors (mean = 2.57, SD = 2.97). No rule-breaking errors were noted on either version.

Regard et al. (1982) found that in children, the task was age-dependent but not sex-dependent. In Risser and Andrikopoulos's small sample of adolescents, however, age and gender had no impact on performance.

References

Glosser, G., & Goodglass, H. (1990). Disorders in executive control functions among aphasic and other brain-damaged patients. *Journal of Clinical and Experimental Neuropsychology, 12,* 485–501.

Jones-Gotman, M., & Milner, B. (1977). Design fluency: The invention of nonsense drawings after focal cortical lesions. *Neuropsychologia, 15,* 653–674.

Lee, G.P., Strauss, E., Loring, D.W., McCloskey, L., & Haworth, J.M. (1997). Sensitivity of figural fluency on the Five-Point Test to focal neurological disease. *The Clinical Neuropsychologist, 11,* 59–68.

Lee, G.P., Loring, D.W., Newell, J., & McCloskey, L. (1994). Figural fluency on the Five-Point Test: Preliminary normative and validity data. *International Neuropsychological Society Program and Abstracts, 1,* 51.

Lee, G., Strauss, E., McCloskey, L., Loring, D., & Drane, D. (1996). Localization of frontal lobe lesions using verbal and nonverbal fluency measures. Paper presented to the International Neuropsychological Society, Chicago.

Parkin, A.J., Walter, B.M., & Hunkin, N.M. (1995). Relationship between normal aging, frontal lobe function, and memory for temporal and spatial information. *Neuropsychology, 9,* 304–312.

Regard, M., Strauss, E., & Knapp, P. (1982). Children's production of verbal and nonverbal fluency tasks. *Perceptual and Motor Skills, 55,* 839–844.

Risser, A.H., & Andrikopoulos, J. (1996). Regard's Five-Point Test: Adolescent Cohort Stability. Paper presented to the International Neuropsychological Society, Chicago.

Ross, T.P., Axelrod, B.N., Hanks, R.A., Kotasek, R.S., & Whitman, R.D. (1996). The interrater and test–retest reliability of the Design Fluency and Ruff Figural Fluency tests. Paper presented to the International Neuropsychological Society, Chicago.

Ruff, R. (1988). *Ruff Figural Fluency Test.* San Diego: Neuropsychological Resources.

Ruff, R.M., Allen, C.C., Farrow, C.E., Niemann, H., & Wylie, T. (1994). Differential impairment in patients with left versus right frontal lobe lesions. *Archives of Clinical Neuropsychology, 9,* 41–55.

Ruff, R.M., Light, R., & Evans, R. (1987). The Ruff Figural Fluency Test: A normative study with adults. *Developmental Neuropsychology, 3,* 37–51.

SELF-ORDERED POINTING TEST (SOPT)

Purpose

This test is used to assess working and strategic memory.

Source

There is no commercial source. Users may refer to the following text and figures in order to design their own material. Alternatively, they may contact Michael Petrides Ph.D., Montreal Neurological Institute, Department of Psychology, 3801 University Street, Montreal, Quebec H3A 2B4.

Description

In the self-ordered pointing test (Petrides & Milner, 1982), the same set of stimulus items is arranged in different layouts on different pages, and subjects are required to point to a different item on each page. Successful performance involves working memory and requires the subjects to organize the stimulus information, maintain a record, and monitor responses.

Petrides and Milner (1982) used four tasks differing in the type of stimulus material: abstract designs, representational drawings, high imagery words, and low imagery words. Usually, however, only one of the tasks need be given. The stimuli used in the longest list (12 items) of Petrides and Milner's abstract designs task are shown in Figure 8–7. Stimuli used in the shortest list (6 items) of a representational drawings task (Courtesy of M. Kates, M.L. Smith, and E. Vriesen) are shown in Figure 8–8. Subjects are presented with a binder containing sheets of paper ($8\frac{1}{2} \times 11$ in.), each one showing an entire set of stimuli (e.g., representational drawings). Each task is divided into four sections, consisting of six, eight, ten and twelve stimulus sheets. Three consecutive trials of each section are administered, the 6-item section is always administered first, followed by the 8-, 10- and 12-item sections, respectively. A different set of stimuli is used for each of the four sections. Within each section, the same stimuli are used, but they are arranged differently on each sheet.

The positions of the stimuli are randomly determined for each sheet of paper, but the layout remains constant (i.e., for 6-item: 2×3, for 8-item: 2×4). For example, the six-item section contains six pages displaying the same six drawings in a different random order on each sheet. The eight-item section displays a new set of eight drawings on eight separate sheets, and so on. After the first six sheets, there is a blank sheet indicating completion of the first block. Similarly, a blank sheet after the 8th, 10th and 12th sheets indicates completion of the second, third and fourth sections, respectively. On each trial, subjects are instructed to point to one of the drawings with the restriction that they should point to a different one on each trial. The demand on working memory is increased by having the subjects perform each section three times before moving on to the next section.

Administration

Instruct the patient as follows: "*Look, here are six pictures. I have pages with the same pictures but they are in different places each time. See, the orange is up here* (point to orange on first page), *but now it is down here* (point to orange on second page). *I want you to point to one picture on each page. I want you to point to a different picture each time. Once you point to a picture, you can't choose it again. Do you understand? Point to a picture on this page.*"

The examiner turns the sheets in order to maintain a comfortable pace. Testing begins only after it is clear that the patient understands the task. When the patient encounters the first blank sheet (indicating completion of that trial), the patient is instructed to start all over again. Say, "Now we are going to do it again beginning with a different one than last time." Again, emphasize that the patient is not to touch any stimulus more than once, but can touch the stimuli in any order.

The patient is not allowed to respond consistently to the same location on any given trial, because by adopting such a strategy the patient merely has to recognize the recurrence

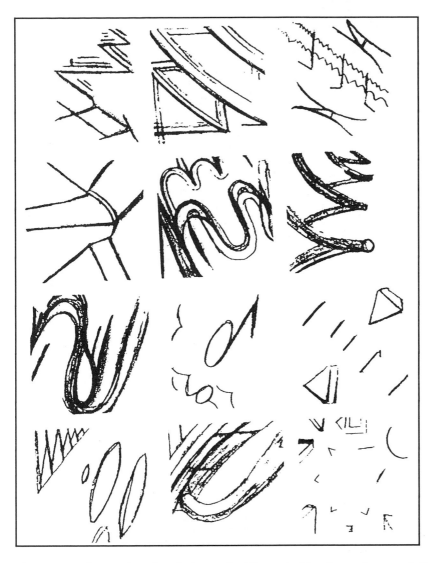

Figure 8—7. The stimuli used in the longest list (12 items) of the abstract-designs task (Petrides and Milner, 1982).

of a given item in that location rather than plan a sequence of responses. The patients are also not allowed to verbalize items as they point. There is no time limit.

Approximate Time for Administration

About 20 minutes are required for the representational drawings task consisting of 6-, 8-, 10-, and 12-item sections.

Scoring

The examiner numbers the order in which the stimuli are touched on the record sheet (see Fig. 8–9). An error is recorded each time the subject selects a picture chosen previously in that trial. The number of errors is readily evident since there will be two or more numbers associated with a particular item. The total number of errors summed across the four sections (6- to 12-item sets) is recorded.

Comment

Information on test reliability is currently not available. In terms of validity, Daigneault et al. (1992) reported that in normal individuals, the SOPT (abstract designs condition) correlated with the WCST ($r = .33$), the Porteus Mazes ($r = .38$), and the Stroop test ($r = .36$).

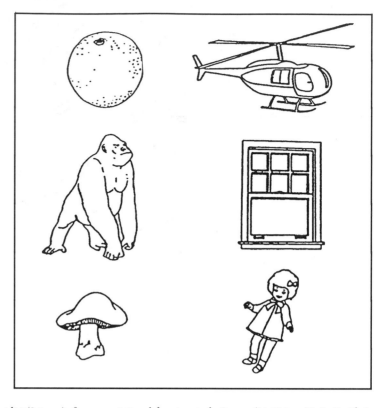

Figure 8—8. Stimuli used in shortest list (6 items) of representational drawings task. *Source* (M. Kates, M. L. Smith & E. Vriesen, April 1997).

The task may be distinguished from other tasks that require the patient to execute a particular response sequence, such as the Visual Memory Span subtest of the Wechsler Memory Scale-Revised, in that the SOPT requires patients to plan, sequence, initiate, and monitor their own pointing responses, rather than follow a sequence dictated by the examiner (Rich et al., 1996). Patients with frontal-lobe lesions are impaired on this task, whereas patients with temporal lobe lesions not extending beyond the pes of the hippocampus (i.e., involving only the anterior temporal neocortex, the amygdala, and/or the pes hippocampus) perform normally (Petrides & Milner, 1982). However, patients with extensive temporal-lobe excisions (that is, those with radical hippocampectomies) exhibit material-specific deficits on the SOPT that correspond to the side of the lesion. Thus, the ability to carry out the general task demands of the SOPT requires intact frontal-lobe functioning, whereas success on material-specific

SOPT tasks requires intact left or right hippocampal functioning for verbal or nonverbal material, respectively. Petrides and his colleagues (1993a, 1993b) have also observed PET rCBF activation of mid-dorsolateral frontal cortex when normal individuals must monitor a series of responses within working memory. This is consistent with data from non-human primates showing that lesions limited to the mid-dorsolateral frontal cortex (areas 46 and 9) give rise to severe impairment on analogous tasks (Petrides, 1991, 1995).

In line with findings of age-related changes in the frontal lobes, Shimamura and Jurica (1994) and Daigneault and colleagues (1992, 1993) have demonstrated an impairment, in the form of more errors and an increase in perseveration, on versions of the SOPT in adults, aged 45 years and older. Daigneault and Braun (1993) suggest that, with advancing age, there is significantly less effective exploitation of top-down clustering strategy. That is, young adults seem to benefit significantly

6-Item Set
doll   _____   _____   _____
gorilla   _____   _____   _____
helicopter _____   _____   _____
mushroom   _____   _____   _____
orange   _____   _____   _____
window   _____   _____   _____
                                                        errors_____

8-Item Set
ball   _____   _____
basket   _____   _____
belt   _____   _____   _____
bowl   _____   _____   _____
flag   _____   _____   _____
kettle   _____   _____   _____
tiger   _____   _____   _____
wagon   _____   _____   _____
                                                        errors_____

10-Item Set
banana   _____   _____   _____
couch   _____   _____   _____
ear   _____   _____   _____
envelope   _____   _____   _____
giraffe   _____   _____   _____
guitar   _____   _____   _____
motorcycle _____   _____   _____
mountain   _____   _____   _____
pot   _____   _____   _____
sandwich   _____   _____   _____
                                                        errors_____

12-Item Set
bottle   _____   _____   _____
bow   _____   _____   _____
brush   _____   _____   _____
candle   _____   _____   _____
fence   _____   _____   _____
finger   _____   _____   _____
hanger   _____   _____   _____
moon   _____   _____   _____
purse   _____   _____   _____
squirrel   _____   _____   _____
strawberry _____   _____   _____
toaster   _____   _____   _____
                                                        errors_____
                                                        total errors_____

Figure 8—9. Sample score sheet for SOPT (*Source:* Mary Lou Smith, April 1997)

from the use of strategy, whereas older individuals do not.

Some investigators have proposed that frontal lobe dysfunction may serve as a conceptual model for Attention Deficit Hyperactivity Disorder (ADHD). In support of this hypothesis, Shue and Douglas (1992) reported that ADHD children differed significantly from normal controls on measures such as the WCST and the SOPT, but not on tests of temporal lobe function (e.g., Wechsler Memory Scale).

Given the integral connections between prefrontal cortex and the striatum, one might expect compromised functioning in patients with primary pathology in the basal ganglia. Gabrielli et al. (1996) gave a version of the SOPT (10-, 12- and 14-word tests) to untreated patients with Parkinson's Disease (PD) and to normal controls. PD patients made more errors than controls on strategic tests of self-ordered pointing, temporal ordering, and free recall but were not impaired on tests of recognition memory and semantic memory. Rich et al. (1996) found that patients with Huntington's disease (HD) made more SOPT errors than controls. Further, performance on the task showed a moderate correlation with activities of daily living. Patients with greater impairment in everyday life made proportionately more errors.

The evidence so far suggests that this task may capture an important component of executive functioning. The test, however, is relatively new and is in need of further refinement (e.g., studies of temporal stability, divergent validity). In addition, research is needed to determine if the SOPT variants are measuring similar cognitive processes. Finally, the test is somewhat lengthy to administer and research into short forms may be useful.

Normative Data

On the representational designs task, Archibald (1997) reported that 89 healthy children, aged 6 to 12 years, made about 14.09 (SD = 5.29) errors. Age had a significant effect on performance (age 6–8: n = 27, mean errors = 17.33, SD = 6.57; age 9–10: n = 38, mean errors = 13.13, SD = 4.15; age 11–12: n = 24, mean errors = 11.96, SD = 3.46). IQ, but not gender, also affected scores. Somewhat better performance was found by Shue and Douglas (1992), although the sample was smaller. Shue and Douglas (1992) reported that 24 normal children (mean age = 10.3, SD = 1.54, Mean Wechsler IQ = 96.88, SD = 11.57) made an average of 9.31 errors (SD = 4.55). They made an average of 24.15 errors (SD = 25.15) when abstract drawings were used as stimuli.

Twenty-two adults, aged 19–35 years (mean = 24.1), of average IQ (mean = 102) made 4.68 (SD = 2.53) errors on the representational drawings task (Smith et al., 1996). Normative data for the abstract designs condition have been provided by Daigneault et al. (1992). A group of 70 healthy young adults aged 20–35 (mean education = 12.36 years, SD = 2.09) made on average 15.2 errors (SD = 6.22). A group of 58 healthy older adults, aged 45–65 years, made about 21.67 (SD = 5.58) errors.

In adults, performance declines with advancing age (Daigneault et al., 1992; Daigneault & Braun, 1993; Shimamura & Jurica, 1994). Daigneault and Braun (1993) report that sex had no effect on SOPT performance in their sample of adults.

References

Archibald, S. (1997). Personal communication.

Daigneault, S., Braun, C.M., & Whitaker, H.A. (1992). Early effects of normal aging on perseverative and non-perseverative prefrontal measures. *Developmental Neuropsychology, 8*, 99–114.

Daigneault, S., & Braun, C.M. (1993). Working memory and the Self-Ordered Pointing Task: Further evidence of early prefrontal decline in normal aging. *Journal of Clinical and Experimental Neuropsychology, 15*, 881–895.

Gabrieli, J.D.E., Singh, J., Stebbins, G.T., & Goetz, C.G. (1996). Reduced working memory span in Parkinson's disease: Evidence for the role of a frontostriatal system in working and strategic memory. *Neuropsychology, 10*, 322–332.

Petrides, M. (1991). Monitoring of selections of visual stimuli and the primate frontal cortex. *Proceedings of the Royal Society of London* (Biol) *246*, 293–298.

Petrides, M. (1995). Impairments on nonspatial self-ordered and externally ordered working memory tasks after lesions of the mid-dorsal part of the lateral frontal cortex in the monkey. *Journal of Neuroscience, 15*, 359–375.

Petrides, M., Alivisatos, B., Meyer, E., & Evans, A. (1993a). Functional activation of the human frontal cortex during the performance of verbal working memory tasks. *Neurobiology, 90*, 878–882.

Petrides, M., Alivisatos, B., Evans, A., & Meyer, E. (1993b). Dissociation of human mid-dorsolateral from posterior dorsolateral frontal cortex in memory processing. *Society for Neuroscience Abstracts, 90*, 873–877.

Petrides, M., & Milner, B. (1982). Deficits on subject-ordered tasks after frontal- and temporal-lobe lesions in man. *Neuropsychologia 20*, 249–262.

Rich, J.B., Blysma, F.W., & Brandt, J. (1996). Self-ordered pointing performance in Huntington's disease patients. *Neuropsychiatry, Neuropsychology and Behavioral Neurology, 9*, 99–106.

Shimamura, A.P., & Jurica, P.J. (1994). Memory interference effects and aging: Findings from a test of frontal lobe function. *Neuropsychology, 8*, 408–412.

Shue, K.L., & Douglas, V.I. (1992). Attention deficit hyperactivity disorders and the frontal lobe syndrome. *Brain and Cognition, 20*, 104–124.

Smith, M.L., Klim, P., Mallozzi, E., & Hanley, W. (1996). A test of the frontal specificity hypothesis in the cognitive performance of young adults with phenylketonuria. *Developmental Neuropsychology, 12*, 327–341.

STROOP TEST

Purpose

This test measures the ease with which a person can shift his or her perceptual set to conform to changing demands and suppress a habitual response in favor of an unusual one.

Source

There are a number of versions of the Stroop test. One version, developed by Golden (1978), can be ordered from Stoelting Company, 620 Wheat Lane, Wood Dale, Illinois, 60191, at a cost of $75 US. A Spanish edition is also available from this company. Sachs et al., (1991) have developed five equivalent forms of the Dodrill version. The alternate forms are available in packs of 50 from Dr. T.L. Sacks, Hillcrest Hospital, P.O. Box 233, Greenacres SA 5087 Australia. Another variation, by Trenarry, Crosson, DeBoe and Leber (1989), is available from Psychological Assessment Resources, Inc., P.O. Box 998, Odessa, Florida 33556, at a cost of $62 US. The Victoria version of the test can be ordered from the Neuropsychology Laboratory, University of Victoria, P.O. Box 1700, Victoria, B.C., for approximately $40 US. Alternatively, users may make their own cards as described below.

Description

This measure of selective attention and cognitive flexibility was originally developed by Stroop (1935). His version consisted of three white cards, each containing 10 rows of five items. There are four parts to the test. In Part 1, the subject reads randomized color names (blue, green, red, brown, purple) printed in black type. In Part 2, the subject reads the color names (blue, green, red, brown, purple) printed in colored ink (blue, green, red, yellow), ignoring the color of the print (the print color never corresponds to the color name). In part 3, the subject has to name the color of squares (blue, green, red, brown, purple). In Part 4, the subject is given the card used in Part 2. This time, however, he or she must name the color in which the color names are printed and disregard their verbal content. Of major interest is the subject's behavior when presented with colored words printed in nonmatching colored inks. Stroop reported that normal people can read color words printed in colored ink as fast as when the words are presented in black ink (Part 2 versus Part 1). However, the time to complete the task increases significantly when the subject is asked to name the color of the ink rather than read the word (Part 4 versus Part 3). This decrease in color-naming speed is called the "color-word interference effect."

A number of versions of the Stroop Test have been developed (e.g., Dodrill, 1978; Golden, 1976, 1978; Graf, Uttl, & Tuokko, 1995; Trenerry et al., 1989). Tests differ in the number of cards used. For example, sometimes the card containing color-words printed in black ink is omitted (e.g., Trenerry et al., 1989), and sometimes a congruent color card is included in which the color words are printed in their congruent ink colors (e.g., Graf et al., 1995). Tests also differ in the use of colored dots (e.g., Victoria version) or colored XXXs (Golden, 1976; Graf et al., 1995), the number of items on each test card (e.g., 24 per card on the Victoria version versus 100 items on the Golden version), and the number of colors used (e.g., three in the version by Graf et al., four in the Victoria and Golden versions, and five in the original form used by Stroop).

The Victoria version (Regard, 1981) is similar to that devised by Perret (1974). We use this version in part because of its short administration time and sensitivity to frontal lobe disorders. Further, baseline (neutral) conditions are included in order to tease apart general performance (e.g., general slowness) and

interference effects. It consists of three 21.5 ×
14 cm cards, each containing six rows of four
items (Helvetica, 28 point). The rows are
spaced 1 cm apart. In Part D, the subject must
name as quickly as possible the color of 24 dots
printed in blue, green, red, or yellow. Each
color is used six times, and the four colors are
arranged in a pseudo-random order within the
array, each color appearing once in each row.
Unlike the original Stroop Test, Part W is similar to Part D, except that the dots are replaced by common words (when, hard, and
over), printed in lower-case letters. The subject is required to name the colors in which
the stimuli are printed, and to disregard their
verbal content. Part C is similar to Parts D and
W, but here the colored stimuli are the color
names "blue, green, red, and yellow" printed
in lower case so that the print color never corresponds to the color name.

Administration

In the Victoria version, the three cards are always presented in the same sequence: D, W,
C. The subject is instructed to read or call out
the color name as quickly as possible. Start the
timer immediately after providing instruction. Instruct as follows:

Part D. "*Name the colors of the dots as quickly as you can. Begin here and go across the
rows from left to right.*" Direct the patient's
eyes across the rows from left to right.

Part W. "*This time, name the colors of the
words as quickly as you can. Begin here and
go across the rows from left to right.*" Clarify,
if necessary: "*Name the colors in which the
words are printed.*"

Part C. "*Again, name the colors in which the
words are printed as quickly as you can.*"
Clarify if necessary: "*Don't read the word, tell
me the color in which the word is printed.*'

The errors in color naming on each part are
corrected immediately, if not spontaneously
corrected by the patient. The subject is then
instructed to go on as rapidly as possible.

Approximate Time for Administration

The approximate time required is 5 minutes.

Scoring

For each part, record both the time to complete and the number of errors. Score spontaneous corrections as correct. For sample scoring sheet, see Figure 8-10. Researchers have
typically relied on a difference score, defined
as the difference in the amount of time required for the interference card (e.g., Part C)
versus the color card (e.g., Part D) (McLeod,
1991). Graf et al. (1995) contend that a difference score is insensitive to age-related slowing and recommend the use of a ratio index of
interference (e.g., Card C/Part D).

Comment

Uttl and Graf (in press) gave healthy individuals a Stroop test which had three trials in each
condition. Trial-to-trial reliabilities and the
estimated reliabilities for the average of three
trials were respectable, above .75. We have
looked at test–retest reliability, using a one-
month interval between test sessions. We
found reliability coefficients of .90, .83, and
.91 for the three parts of the test. However,
experience with the test does affect performance. Normal college students showed significant practice effects (p < .001). On the
second administration, performance improved by about 2 seconds on parts D and W,
and by about 5 seconds on part C. Similar results have been reported for other versions of
the test (Connor, Franzen, & Sharp, 1988;
Feinstein et al., 1994; Graf et al., 1995; Sachs
et al., 1991; Stroop, 1935; Trenerry et al.,
1989). These increases may not affect interpretation of the results if interpretation is
based on pattern and not level because all
scores increase consistently (Connor et al.,
1988; but see Feinstein et al., 1994, who found
marked practice effects on the color-naming
and interference trials but not on the color-
reading trial). The reason for the improvement in performance is not certain but may
reflect an active learning process that sup-
presses distraction and/or a habituation of
competing responses (Reisberg et al., 1980).

```
┌─────────────────────────────────────────────────────────────────┐
│                      Sample Score Sheet                            │
│                        Stroop Test                                 │
│  NAME _____    DATE _____    │
│  AGE _____                                                    │
│  DOTS:    G  B  Y  R          WORDS:    G  B  Y  R                 │
│           Y  R  G  B                    Y  R  G  B                 │
│           B  G  Y  R                    B  G  Y  R                 │
│           B  Y  R  G                    B  Y  R  G                 │
│           R  G  B  Y                    R  G  B  Y                 │
│           Y  G  B  R                    Y  G  B  R                 │
│                                                                    │
│  COLORS:  G  B  Y  R                                               │
│           Y  R  G  B          ┌──────┬──────────┬──────────┐      │
│           B  G  Y  R          │      │  Time    │  Errors  │      │
│           B  Y  R  G          │  I   │          │          │      │
│           R  G  B  Y          │  II  │          │          │      │
│           Y  G  B  R          │  III │          │          │      │
│                               └──────┴──────────┴──────────┘      │
└─────────────────────────────────────────────────────────────────┘
```

Figure 8—10. Stroop Test sample scoring sheet.

Although Stroop (1935) made an equivalent form of the test by printing the cards in reverse order, most examiners have generally retested subjects with the same set of cards. Sachs et al., (1991) have developed five equivalent forms of the Dodrill version (see source). Due to the presence of significant practice effects, examiners interested in documenting change by repeated measurement on the same or alternate forms should ensure that patients have sufficient practice with the test, at least more than one practice trial (Franzen et al., 1987; Sachs et al., 1991).

Factor analytic studies (Graf et al., 1995) suggest that speed of processing and conceptual abilities (Block Design, Digit Symbol, Similarities, Digit Span) contribute to performance on Stroop tasks involving color naming. Similarly, Sherman and colleagues (1995) found that rapid response on the interference trial of the Stroop was moderately related to the Perceptual Organization ($r = .37$) and Freedom from Distractability ($r = .29$) factors of the WAIS-R. It was unrelated to the Verbal Comprehension factor ($r = .17$). Shum et al. (1990) reported that the Stroop test (interference score) loaded on the same factor as serial subtraction tasks (time to finish serial 7s and 13s) and reflects the ability to sustain mental processes and select appropriate features. MacLeod and Prior (1996) reported that in adolescents with and without ADHD, the interference score was not correlated with Slosson IQ, but showed a moderate relation with the PASAT, a task thought to require speeded processing and the ability to divide attention. Consistent with the notion that the task measures some aspects involved in planning and organization of behavior, Hanes et al. (1996) found that the Stroop (interference score) showed strong relations with performance on a semantic (Category) fluency task ($r = .58$) and a version of the Tower of London ($r = .65$), but only modest or little relations with other tasks, such as delayed recall of the Rey figure ($r = .31$) and peg placement on the Purdue Pegboard ($r = .12$).

The Stroop test has been studied in psychiatric and brain-damaged patients. The test is fairly effective in distinguishing between normal controls and brain-damaged patients, and between psychiatric and brain-damaged samples (Golden, 1976; Hanes et al., 1996; Trenerry et al., 1989). For example, Hanes et al. (1996) found impaired Stroop performance (as reflected in increased time taken to name colors subtracted from the time to read words) in patients with schizophrenia, Parkinson's disease, and Huntington's disease. Head-injured patients are typically slower to respond on all subtasks, although they do not consistently demonstrate disproportionate difficulty on the interference condition (Batchelor et al., 1995; McLean et al., 1983; Ponsford & Kinsella, 1992). The interference effect can be elicited more readily in mildly head-injured patients with a more challenging version of the Stroop test (Batchelor et al., 1995; Bohnen et al., 1992). The modification (Bohnen et al., 1992) consists of drawing rectangular lines around a random selection of one-fifth of the items comprising the color-word subtest. On the boxed items, subjects are required to read the word rather than name the color of the print. Thus, task complexity is increased by requiring flexibility in directing attention to the naming and reading of the different items. Aloia et al. (1997) suggest, however, that a more drastic modification may be necessary to elicit interference.

The Stroop test also appears to be sensitive to severity of dementia (Koss et al., 1984). There is evidence that impairment on our version of the Stroop is related to the location of the cerebral lesion. Both Perret (1974) and Regard (1981) reported that the interference effect of Part C (relative to Part W) was greater for patients with left frontal lobe damage than for other patient or control groups.

Diminished performance on the Stroop test has also been documented in depressed (Raskin et al., 1982) and anxious patients (Batchelor et al., 1995; but see Vingerhoets et al., 1995, who found no relation between psychological distress and cognitive performance in patients before or after open-heart surgery). The implication is that the clinician should not necessarily conclude that poor performance on the task is indicative of neurological dysfunction.

It is important to note that Stroop (1935) employed neutral and incongruent conditions in order to measure interference. If no baseline (neutral) condition is employed, discussion of the data as measuring interference is not warranted (Henik, 1996). The incongruent condition measures general performance (e.g., general slowness) and also interference; if only one condition is given, it is impossible to tease them apart. Sometimes, patients are given the card used for the incongruent condition and are asked once to read the word and ignore the color and as a second condition, they are asked to name the color and ignore the word (e.g., Dodrill, 1978; Trenerry et al., 1989). This comparison is also problematic since it confounds differences between tasks and interference (Henik, 1996).

For example, this difference between color naming and word reading could reflect interference of color on word or word on color.

As Lezak (1995) points out, visual competence is important. Color-blindness precludes use of this test. Similarly, patients with visual disturbances may find the word degraded and therefore have an advantage on the color-word interference trial since the interference will be diminished as a result of the decreased clarity of the word. The amount of interference also depends on the subject's familiarity with the stimuli and the semantic relatedness of the material (e.g., pictures versus words) (Graf et al., 1995). The degree of automaticity of the reading response is also a critical factor. Cox et al. (1997) recommend that interpretation of the interference score as a measure of response inhibition be restricted to those whose single word readings are at least equal to their Full Scale IQs.

Normative Data

Bullock, Brulot, and Strauss (unpublished data) have collected normative data for the Victoria version (See Table 8–10). The values are derived from a sample of 188 healthy adults with above-average educational achievement (mean = 14.28 years, SD = 2.29).

Both age and intellectual level are predictors of performance on the Stroop test (Bullock et al., 1996; Comalli, 1965; Comalli et al., 1962; Das, 1970; Ivnik et al., 1996; Klein et al., 1997; Regard, 1981; Sherman et al., 1995; Trenerry et al., 1989). In adults, aging appears to be linked with a slowing in color naming and an increase in the Stroop interference effect, expressed as difference (e.g., C-D), ratio (e.g., C/D) or error scores. Graf et al. (1995) found no effect of age on the ratio index of interference in adults aged 65 or older, but they only examined older adults. Using a broader sample, aged 12–83 years, Uttl and Graf (in press) found a small influence of age in the incongruent condition. They have interpreted the age effects in Stroop interference as due to age-related decline in processing speed (indexed also by color naming and by word reading), and not as evidence of a selective age-related decline in specific cognitive functions, such as cognitive flexibility and control. Klein

Table 8—10. Modified Stroop Test: Mean Reading Time (Seconds) and Errors
for the 24 Item/Card Form

	Age (years)						
	17–29 (n = 40)	30–39 (n = 26)	40–49 (n = 18)	50–59 (n = 36)	60–69 (n = 26)	70–79 (n = 24)	80+ (n = 13)
Name Color of Dots "D"							
Sec	11.79	11.14	12.16	12.84	12.56	14.98	19.31
SD	2.79	1.68	1.96	2.43	1.89	5.10	4.91
Errors	.19	.12	.06	.00	.00	.08	.15
SD	.40	.33	.24	.00	.00	.28	.55
Name Color Print of Non-Color Words "W"							
Sec	13.46	13.81	14.82	15.96	16.16	19.11	23.91
SD	3.11	2.66	2.46	2.93	3.46	5.13	5.30
Errors	.09	.08	.06	.00	.00	.00	.15
SD	.29	.27	.24	.00	.00	.00	.38
Name Color Print of Color Words "C"							
Sec	21.28	25.08	27.20	28.48	31.32	39.56	56.98
SD	5.37	9.52	8.15	8.07	8.22	13.26	23.70
Errors	.68	.80	.78	.64	.31	.75	2.54
SD	.96	1.04	.88	.96	.62	1.15	2.03
C/D	1.85	2.25	2.28	2.28	2.55	2.81	2.95
SD	.44	.75	.73	.70	.75	1.12	.93

Source: Bullock, Brulot & Strauss (1996). Unpublished data.

et al. (1997), however, reported that test duration differentially affects the performance of young and old subjects. Young individuals (aged 25–35 years) were relatively fast on the first part of their interference test but slower on the second part. Older subjects (aged 70–80 years) were relatively slower on the first part but speeded up on the second part. They attributed the slow-starting phenomenon to the possibility that elderly subjects are less adept at developing new automatic processes or at adapting existing processes.

Although women tend to have superior color naming skills (Stroop, 1935), sex differences on the color-word interference card are not always present (Bullock et al., 1996; Golden, 1978; Ivnik et al., 1996). Education shows a small relation with the Stroop interference score (Bullock et al., 1996; Ivnik et al., 1996).

References

Aloia, M.S., Weed, N.C., & Marx, B. (1997). Some construct network effects of modifying the Stroop Color and Word Test. *The Clinical Neuropsychologist, 11,* 54–58.

Batchelor, J., Harvery, A.G., & Bryant, R.A. (1995). Stroop Color Word Test as a measure of attentional deficit following mild head injury. *The Clinical Neuropsychologist, 9,* 180–186.

Bohnen, N., Jolles, J., & Twijnstra, A. (1992). Modification of the Stroop Color Word Test improves differentiation between patients with mild head injury and matched controls. *The Clinical Neuropsychologist, 6,* 178–188.

Bullock, L., Brulot, M., & Strauss, E. (1996). Unpublished data.

Comalli, P.E. (1965). Cognitive functioning in a group of 80–90 year-old men. *Journal of Gerontology, 20,* 14–17.

Comalli, P.E., Jr., Wapner, S., & Werner, H. (1962). Interference effects of Stroop color-word test in childhood, adulthood and aging. *Journal of Genetic Psychology, 100,* 47–53.

Connor, A., Franzen, M., & Sharp, B. (1988). Effects of practice and differential instructions on Stroop performance. *International Journal of Clinical Neuropsychology, 10,* 1–4.

Cox, C.S., Chee, E., Chase, G.A., Baumgardner, T.L., Schuerholz, L.J., Reader, M.J., Mohr, J., & Denkla, M.B. (1997). Reading proficiency affects the construct validity of the Stroop Test Interference Score. *The Clinical Neuropsychologist, 11,* 105–110.

Das, J.P. (1970). Changes in Stroop-test responses

as a function of mental age. *British Journal of Clinical and Social Psychology, 9*, 68–73.

Dodrill, C.B. (1978). A neuropsychological battery for epilepsy. *Epilepsia, 19*, 611–623.

Feinstein, A., Brown, R., & Ron, M. (1994). Effects of practice on serial tests of attention in healthy subjects. *Journal of Clinical and Experimental Neuropsychology, 16*, 436–447.

Franzen, M.D., Tishelman, A.C., Sharp, B.H., & Friedman, A.G. (1987). An investigation of the test–retest reliability of the Stroop Color-Word Test across two intervals. *Archives of Clinical Neuropsychology, 2*, 265–272.

Golden, J.C. (1976). Identification of brain disorders by the Stroop color and word test. *Journal of Clinical Psychology, 32*, 654–658.

Golden, J.C. (1978). *Stroop Color and Word Test.* Stoelting Co., Chicago, IL.

Graf, P., Uttl, B., & Tuokko, H. (1995). Color- and picture-word Stroop tests: Performance changes in old age. *Journal of Clinical and Experimental Neuropsychology, 17*, 390–415.

Hanes, K.R., Andrewes, D.G., Smith, D.J., & Pantelis, C. (1996). A brief assessment of executive control dysfunction: Discriminant validity and homogeneity of planning, set shift, and fluency measures. *Archives of Clinical Neuropsychology, 11*, 185–191.

Henik, A. (1996). Paying attention to the Stroop effect. *Journal of the International Neuropsychological Society, 2*, 467–470.

Ivnik, R.J., Malec, J.F., Smith, G.E., & Tangalos, E.G. (1996). Neuropsychological test norms above age 55: COWAT, BNT, MAE Token, WRAT-R Reading, AMNART, Stroop, TMT, and JLO. *The Clinical Neuropsychologist, 10*, 262–278.

Klein, M., Ponds, R.W.H.M., Houx, P.J., & Jolles, J. (1997). Effect of test duration on age-related differences in Stroop interference. *Journal of Clinical and Experimental Neuropsychology, 19*, 77–82.

Koss, E., Ober, B.A., Delis, D.C., & Friedland, R.P. (1984). The Stroop Color-Word Test: Indicator of dementia severity. *International Journal of Neuroscience, 24*, 53–61.

Lezak, M.D. (1995). *Neuropsychological Assessment* (3rd ed.). New York: Oxford University Press.

MacLeod, C.M. (1991). Half a century of research on the Stroop effect: An integrative review. *Psychological Bulletin, 109*, 163–203.

MacLeod, D., & Prior, M. (1996). Attention deficits in adolescents with ADHD and other clinical groups. *Child Neuropsychiatry, 2*, 1–10.

McLean, A., Temkin, N.R., Dikmen, S., & Wyler, A.R. (1983). The behavioral sequelae of head injury. *Journal of Clinical Neuropsychology, 5*, 361–376.

Perret, E. (1974). The left frontal lobe of man and the suppression of habitual responses in verbal categorical behavior. *Neuropsychologia, 12*, 323–330.

Ponsford, J., & Kinsella, G. (1992). Attentional deficits following closed head injury. *Journal of Clinical and Experimental Neuropsychology, 14*, 822–828.

Raskin, A., Friedman, A.S., & DiMascio, A. (1982). Cognitive and performance deficits in depression. *Psychopharmacology Bulletin, 18*, 196–202.

Regard, M. (1981). *Cognitive rigidity and flexibility: A neuropsychological study.* Unpublished Ph.D. dissertation, University of Victoria.

Reisberg, D., Baron, J., & Kemler, D.G. (1980). Overcoming Stroop interference: Effects of practice on distractor potency. *Journal of Experimental Psychology: Human Perception and Performance, 6*, 14–150.

Sachs, T.L., Clark, C.R., Pols, R.G., & Geffen, L.B. (1991). Comparability and stability of performance of six alternate forms of the Dodrill-Stroop Color-Word Test. *The Clinical Neuropsychologist, 5*, 220–225.

Sherman, E.M.S., Strauss, E., Spellacy, F., & Hunter, M. (1995). Construct validity of WAIS-R factors: Neuropsychological test correlates in adults referred for possible head injury. *Psychological Assessment, 7*, 440–444.

Shum, D.H.K., McFarland, K.A., & Bain, J.D. (1990). Construct validity of eight tests of attention: Comparison of normal and closed head injured samples. *The Clinical Neuropsychologist, 4*, 141–162.

Stroop, J.R. (1935). Studies of interference in serial verbal reaction. *Journal of Experimental Psychology, 18*, 643–662.

Trenerry, M.R., Crosson, B., DeBoe, J., and Leber, W.R. (1989). *Stroop Neurological Screening Test.* Florida: Psychological Assessment Resources.

Vingerhoets, G., De Soete, G., and Jannes, C. (1995). Relationship between emotional variables and cognitive test performance before and after open-heart surgery. *The Clinical Neuropsychologist, 9*, 198–202.

Uttl, B., & Graf, P. (in press). Color Word Stroop Test performance across the adult life span. *Journal of Clinical and Experimental Neuropsychology.*

WISCONSIN CARD SORTING TEST (WCST)

Purpose

The purpose of this test is to assess the ability to form abstract concepts, to shift and maintain set, and utilize feedback.

Source

The test, including the WCST Manual—Revised and Expanded by Heaton, Chelune, Talley, Kay and Curtiss (1993), can be obtained from Psychological Assessment Resources, Inc., P.O. Box 98, Odessa FL, 33556-0998, for about $185 US or from the Institute of Psychological Research, Inc., 34 Fleury St. W., Montreal PQ, H3L 1S9, for approximately $245 Cdn. A scoring program ($299 US) as well as a computer version (2nd research edition) ($545 US or $665 Cdn) are also available from these companies.

Description

This test was developed by Berg and Grant (Berg, 1948; Grant and Berg, 1948) to assess abstraction ability and the ability to shift cognitive strategies in response to changing environmental contingencies. The test is considered a measure of executive function (Heaton et al., 1993) in that it requires strategic planning, organized searching, the ability to use environmental feedback to shift cognitive sets, goal-oriented behavior, and the ability to modulate impulsive responding. Heaton and his colleagues (1981, 1993) point out that there has been increasing interest in the test, in part because it provides information on several aspects of problem-solving behavior beyond such basic indices as task success or failure. Examples of such indices include the number of perseverative errors, the failure to maintain set, and the number of categories achieved. Heaton (1981) standardized the test instructions and scoring procedures and formally published it as a clinical instrument. In the updated manual (Heaton et al., 1993), scoring rules were refined, the recording form was revised, and normative data were provided for individuals, aged 6 years 5 months to 89 years.

The test consists of four stimulus cards, placed in front of the subject, the first with a red triangle, the second with two green stars, the third with three yellow crosses, the fourth with four blue circles on them. The subject is then given two packs each containing 64 response cards, which have designs similar to those on the stimulus cards, varying in color, geometric form, and number. The subject is told to match each of the cards in the decks to one of the four key cards and is given feedback each time whether he or she is right or wrong. There is no time limit to this test.

While there are other versions of the test (e.g., Modified Card Sorting Test, by Nelson, 1976; Milwaukee Card Sorting Test by Osmon and Suchy, 1996), we use Heaton's procedure. Nelson (1976) removed the response cards which shared more than one attribute with the stimulus card, thus eliminating ambiguity. In addition, subjects were told when the target category was changed. Nelson's version, however, changes the quality of the test. The literature suggests that the Modified Card Sorting Test and WCST are not equivalent and should be regarded as separate tests (de Zubicaray and Ashton, 1996). The Milwaukee Card Sorting Test (Osmon & Suchy, 1996) requires that patients verbalize prior to sorting and provides additional scores that may be useful in characterizing a patient's difficulty in forming, maintaining, and switching mental set. Further research is needed, however, to evaluate the reliability and validity of this version. Normative data are also required. An abbreviated form of the WCST has been suggested (Axelrod et al., 1992b) which involves giving only the first deck of 64 cards. Although the use of a short form reduces reliability, the WCST-64 correlates highly with the long form. Some normative data are available for this version (Axelrod et al., 1993). The use of the WCST manual's norms for 128 cards to estimate normative data from the WCST-64 is not recommended since there is poor consistency across versions (Axelrod et al., 1997). Studies of the WCST-64 performance in patients with focal frontal lobe dysfunction and other disorders compromising executive function are also needed. There is some recent evidence that this short form is sensitive to deficits in AD and PD (Paolo et al., 1996b).

Administration

See source. Clients should have normal or corrected vision and hearing sufficient to adequately comprehend the test instructions and to discriminate visually the stimulus parameters of color, form, and number. The two packs of cards are placed in front of the subject. The examiner instructs the subject to place each response card in piles below one of the four stimulus (key) cards, wherever he or she thinks it should go, and is told that the experimenter will then inform him or her whether the choice is "right" or "wrong." The subject is directed to make use of this information and to try to get as many cards "right" as possible. While it is permissible to clarify the meaning of the stimulus (key) cards and the manner in which the client is to respond, the examiner must never violate the integrity of the WCST by giving any indication of the sorting principles or the nature of the shift from one category to the next.

The subject is required to sort first to *color*, all other responses being called "wrong"; then, once 10 consecutive correct responses to color have been achieved, the required sorting principle shifts, without warning, to *form;* color responses are now "wrong." After 10 consecutive correct responses to form, the principle shifts to *number*, and then back to color once more. This procedure continues until the subject has successfully completed six sorting categories (color, form, number, color, form number), or until all 128 cards have been placed.

Computer implementation of the WCST is available (see Source). Fortuny and Heaton (1996) report that the computerized (PAR) and standard versions yield fairly similar results in normal individuals. Hellman et al. (1992) found no significant differences between computerized (Loong, 1990) and standard versions in a small and heterogeneous group of psychiatric patients. The computerized and standard formats, however, may not be equivalent in all clinical populations. Ozonoff (1995) reported that autistic children make fewer errors on the computer version (Loong, 1990). Accordingly, norms collected under standard administration conditions and impairment thresholds may not apply to all patient populations.

Approximate Time for Administration

The time required is about 15–30 minutes.

Scoring

The WCST Record Booklet consists of four pages designed for recording information about the client, recording the client's responses to the WCST items, and calculating and recording WCST scores.

Scoring rules of the WCST, originally delineated by Heaton (1981), caused some confusion (Flashman, Horner, & Freides, 1991). The revised manual (Heaton et al., 1993) provides detailed scoring criteria and clarifies common sources of difficulty. Performance is scored in a number of different ways. *Categories Completed* refers to the number of categories (i.e., each sequence of 10 consecutive correct matches to the criterion sorting category) completed during the test. Scores can range from 0 for the subject who never gets the idea at all to 6, at which point the test is normally discontinued. The total number of *Trials to Complete First Category* gives an indication of initial conceptualization before a shift of set is required. When a client persists in responding to a stimulus characteristic that is incorrect, the response is said to match the "perseverated-to" principle and is scored as perseverative ("p"). *Percent Perseverative Errors* reflects the concentration of perseverative errors in relation to overall test performance. Heaton et al. (1993) describe the situations that define the perseverated-to principle, and the reader should refer to their updated manual. Berry (1996) summarizes the relevant rules for scoring perseveration in a diagrammatic format that can also be used as an aid to scoring. The perseverative response may reveal an inability to relinquish the old category for the new one, or the inability to see a new possibility.

There are a number of other measures that can be derived from the test. The score for *Failure to Maintain Set* is the number of times the subject makes 5 or more correct responses in a row and then makes an error before successfully achieving a category. It indicates the inability to continue using a strategy that has been successful. *Percent Conceptual Level Responses* is defined as consecutive correct responses occurring in runs of three or more. It is thought to reflect some insight into correct sorting principles. A final score, *Learning to Learn*, reflects the subject's average change in conceptual efficiency across the successive stages (categories) of the WCST.

Percent Errors, Percent Perseverative Responses, and Percent Nonperseverative Errors can also be calculated to assist in research investigations. Use of these scores is not recommended for clinical interpretation, in part because reliabilities of these "percent" scores are lower than those of their respective basic scores.

Recording a performance, particularly if the patient works rapidly, can be difficult. Briefly, the recording form has 128 response items, each one "CFNO" (C = color, F = form, N = number, O = other). The examiner records the patient's response by making a slash through those dimensions that are the same on the response and stimulus cards. To assist in later scoring, the examiner consecutively numbers continuous correct responses, up to 10, in the space provided in the record booklet to the left of each item. Any time a client interrupts a sequence of correct responses by making an error, the examiner begins renumbering the next series with the number 1. In addition, a line is drawn under the last item when the criterion of 10 consecutive correct responses has been reached, and to indicate the new correct sorting category below that line.

Scoring errors are common, even among experienced clinicians (Greve, 1993; Paolo et al., 1994). Errors are likely to occur when response cards match a stimulus card on two attributes (Paolo et al., 1994). Clinicians might consider purchasing computer scoring software in order to eliminate recording and scoring errors.

Comment

See the Comment sections of the California Sorting Test and the Category Test for discussions of the similarities and differences between these tasks. Interscorer and intrascorer reliability were excellent in some studies (Interclass correlations above .83) (Axelrod et al., 1992a; Greve, 1993), whereas another study (Flashman et al., 1991) indicated that interscorer reliability on indices of perseveration was quite low (correlations not reported). The detailed criteria provided in the newly revised manual (Heaton et al., 1993) and/or the use of computer software may increase reliability.

A group of 46 healthy children and adolescents were given the WCST on two occasions, spaced about one month apart (Heaton et al., 1993). The investigators report generalizability coefficients (i.e., how well the instrument measures subjects' true scores) that appear to be only moderate in value, ranging from .37 (percent perseverative errors) to .72 (nonperseverative errors). It is also worth noting that the standard errors of measurement for WCST standard scores in normal children are quite large (e.g., 10.28 for perseverative responses, see Source). Thus, retesting may well yield different results and WCST scores should be interpreted with considerable caution. In line with this notion are the recent findings of Paolo et al. (1996a). They retested 87 normal elderly following an interval of about 1 year. To ensure that each participant displayed normal cognitive functions at both assessment probes, each participant had to have an initial DRS score greater than 130 and display no evidence of significant decline (i.e., a drop of 10 points or more). Stability coefficients ranged from .12 on the Learning to Learn scale to .66 for the Total number of Errors scale. The majority of individuals improved on retest with five WCST scores demonstrating significant average retest gains of 5 to 7 standard score points. They calculated standard error of prediction, standard error of difference, and abnormal test-retest discrepancy scores to assist in detecting possible meaningful changes in WCST scores on retest. Table 8–11 presents the 90% cutoff scores for WCST Standard scores with 5% of the cases falling in the positive direction (gain) and 5% falling in the negative direction (loss). To use the cutoff scores, first convert the raw scores to normalized age- and education-corrected standard scores according to the WCST manual (Heaton et al., 1993). Next, subtract the initial score from the score ob-

Table 8—11. Cutoff Scores at the 90% Level of Abnormality for the Detection of Change on Retest

Scale	Abnormal Cutoff	
	Loss	Gain
Total number of errors	18	35
Perseverative responses	12	20
Perseverative errors	15	35
Nonperseverative errors	29	40
Percent conceptual level response	24	35

Source: Paolo et al., 1996. Reprinted with permission of Psychological Assessment Resources.

tained on retest. If the difference score is negative, it reflects a loss on retest; if it is positive, it represents a retest gain. Next, compare the difference score to the cutoff values provided in Table 8–11. If the difference score equals or exceeds the tabled values, then the test-retest change is considered unusual, because it occurred in 5% or less of the normal sample. Note that the magnitude of the difference required for an unusual change on retest is quite large, typically more than one standard deviation.

It has been argued that once a person with reasonably intact memory has figured out the category sorts and shift principle, the WCST no longer measures problem-solving ability (Lezak, 1995). This suggests that the low stability of the WCST for normal people may reflect that, on retesting, it is no longer measuring problem-solving abilities in the same manner (Paolo et al., 1996a). In clinical samples, however, reliability estimates may be considerably higher. In line with this notion, Ozonoff (1995) retested autistic and learning-disabled children over a two and a half year-interval and reported test-retest generalizeability coefficients greater than .90.

Measures of concept achievement and perseveration on the WCST are not independent (Beatty & Monson, 1996). There is evidence, however, that the WCST is multidimensional and that some WCST scores may provide unique information regarding an individual's ability to solve problems. Goldman et al. (1996), making use of the WCST standardization sample, found that, in normal individu-

als, the WCST is best described by a unitary factor. In contrast, in neurological patients with either focal or diffuse impairment, performance is primarily explained on the basis of two factors: "problem solving/perseveration" and "loss of set." The inclusion of nonperseverative errors on this second factor was more obvious in neurological patients with focal lesions. Paolo et al. (1995) factor-analyzed the WCST in a sample of normal elderly subjects and individuals with Parkinson's disease (PD). Three factors emerged in the normal sample. The first factor, reflecting "overall conceptualization/problem-solving," consisted of number of categories completed, number of errors, perseverative responses and errors, nonperseverative errors, and conceptual level response. The second factor consisted of only the "failure to maintain set" score. The third factor was labeled "learning" and included the number of trials to complete the first category and learning to learn. The factor structure for the PD group was similar, though not completely identical (e.g., perseverative and nonperseverative errors were related for the normal, but not the PD group), again suggesting that the factor structure of the WCST and what the scores represent may vary according to sample used and type of neurological impairment.

Other investigators (Greve et al., 1993; Salthouse et al., 1996; Sullivan et al., 1993), using a variety of populations (e.g., mixed psychiatric or neurologic patients and normals; normal elderly) have also found evidence in favor of a 3- or 2-factor solution, where the first factor appears to reflect problem-solving (on which measures of perseveration load highly) and the second measures some aspect of attentional processes (reflected in failure to maintain set). Some support for the suggestion that Factor 2 reflects attentional dysfunction derives from studies of WCST performance in which color overlays (blue versus red) are used to manipulate visual attention (Greve et al., 1996; Williams et al., 1994). The underlying rationale is that the wavelength (color) of a stimulus affects processing in the dorsal neural stream which is believed to mediate key attentional operations.

The variability in findings from factor analytic studies is due in part to the use of different populations, as well as variable redundancy in the factor analyses (e.g., perseverative errors and perseverative responses) (Goldman et al., 1996). Based on the available data, it is premature to abandon individual scores and derive factor scores. Rather, one might consider problem-solving (as reflected in a number of categories, total errors, or perseverative responses) and failure to maintain set as measures that may potentially tap unique cognitive processes in performance on the WCST.

Based on a computational analysis, Dehaene and Changeux (1991) suggested that the task requires the ability to change the current rule rapidly subsequent to a negative reward (rule selection), the ability to memorize previously tested rules and to avoid testing them twice (episodic memory), and the ability to reject some rules *a priori* by reasoning on the possible outcomes of using one rule or the other (reasoning). In a study of patients with closed head injury (Sherman et al., 1995), both the number of categories achieved and the number of perseverative responses were associated with the Verbal Comprehension and Perceptual Organization factors of the WAIS-R ($r = -.28$ to .32). Both WCST measures were unrelated to the Freedom From Distractability factor. Paolo et al. (1995) factor analyzed the WCST scores along with measures of attention and memory. In neither normal elderly nor patients with Parkinson's disease did WCST scores load with the memory and attention measures. The implication from these studies is that the WCST measures some general reasoning ability that is relatively independent of memory and attention. On the other hand, some investigators (e.g., O'Donnell et al., 1994; Vanderploeg et al., 1994) have reported that the number of perseverative responses or errors on the WCST show modest correlations (.28 to .38) with Part B of the Trail Making Test and various measures of the CVLT. Moreover, there is evidence (see above) that response maintenance (in the form of FMS) is affected by experimental manipulations (e.g., color overlays) that influence neural systems linked to attention (Greve et al., 1996). Fristoe et al. (1997) gave the WCST as

well as measures of working memory and processing speed to both young and older adults. Their study suggested that WCST performance is related to both working memory and effective processing of feedback information, and both of these components are mediated by a speed of processing measure.

The WCST appears to measure a dimension of conceptual processing similar, but not identical, to that of the Category Test (e.g., Pendleton & Heaton, 1982; Perrine, 1993; O'Donnell et al., 1994). Shute and Huertas (1990) found that the perseverative error score loaded on a factor defined by a measure of Piagetian formal operations. Perrine (1993) reported that the WCST was associated with attribute identification, which entails discrimination of relevant features. Welsh et al. (1991) found that in normal individuals aged 8 years and older, the number of perseverative responses loaded on the same factor as the number of errors made on the Matching Familiar Figures Test, a task thought to measure impulse control. Measures reflecting speeded responding (e.g., Verbal Fluency, Visual Search) and planning (Tower of Hanoi) loaded on separate factors. Finally, Ozonoff (1995) suggested that adequate performance on the WCST also requires a certain level of social awareness and motivation to attend to verbal feedback.

In her classic study with the WCST, Milner (1963) found clear differences between patients with dorsolateral frontal excisions and those with orbitofrontal and posterior lesions. Patients with dorsolateral lesions showed an inability "to shift from one sorting principle to another, apparently due to perseverative interference from previous modes of response" (p. 99). Some subsequent studies, using patients, and functional (PET or SPECT) and MRI imaging, have supported the notion that the WCST is sensitive to frontal lobe function (Arnett et al., 1994; Heaton et al., 1993; Rezai et al., 1993; Weinberger et al., 1988), although others have found that patients with frontal damage do not differ from controls subjects on this measure (Cantor-Graae et al., 1993; Stuss et al., 1983). It is important to note that patients with diffuse cerebral lesions as well as patients with disturbances outside the frontal lobes may perform about the same as focal frontal patients on the WCST (Anderson et al., 1991; Axelrod et al., 1996; Grafman et al., 1990; Heaton et al., 1993; Hermann et al., 1988; Huber et al., 1992; Robinson et al., 1980; Strauss et al., 1993). For example, Axelrod et al. (1996), used the normal and four neurological groups (focal frontal lesions, focal lesions in both frontal and nonfrontal areas, nonfrontal lobe lesions, and diffuse lesions) from the standardization sample. They found that the WCST indices could differentiate normals from patients, with classification rates falling at about 71% accuracy, regardless of the WCST variable used. However, patient groups were not consistently discriminable from each other. S.W. Anderson et al. (1991) examined the CT/MRI scans of 91 patients with focal brain lesions (e.g., CVA, tumor, or seizures) and found no significant differences in WCST performance between subjects with frontal vs. nonfrontal damage. Similarly, C.V. Anderson et al. (1995) examined MRI scans of 68 TBI patients and found that while WCST performance was impaired by brain injury, it was not related to volume of focal frontal damage, presence or absence of frontal damage, or to the degree of nonspecific structural (atrophic) changes. Based on their findings, they suggested that the important variable in WCST performance in TBI patients is the injury itself, regardless of the location or amount of structural damage. The WCST did not add anything unique about frontal lobe integrity in TBI patients. Hermann and Seidenberg (1995) have found that deficits on the WCST that occur in temporal lobe epilepsy do not appear to be directly attributable to temporal lobe/hippocampal compromise, but rather are due to the influence of nociferous cortex on extratemporal systems. While suspicion may be focused on the frontal regions as the extratemporal mediator, there are no data in support of this notion. Indeed, Horner et al. (1996) reported that performance of patients with temporal lobe foci was more impaired than that of patients with frontal lobe foci. Overall, the WCST cannot be used by itself to predict a focal frontal lesion (Anderson et al., 1995; Heaton et al., 1993; Mountain & Snow, 1993). Rather, it may be more plausible

to conceive of the WCST as a complex measure of executive functioning that is not linked to a single neuroanatomical region, but to the integration of multiple brain regions, of which the frontal lobes are important constituents (Axelrod et al., 1996).

There also appears to be little consistency in the literature with regard to laterality of dysfunction. Both Milner (1963) and Taylor (1979) suggested that the test is sensitive to function in the dorsolateral areas of both frontal lobes, but more to the left than to the right side, although some have reported excessive impairment (typically in the form of more perseveration) in patients with right as compared to left-sided damage (Bornstein, 1986; Drewe, 1974; Hermann et al., 1988; Robinson et al., 1980). Horner et al. (1996) found no differences in performance between patients with language dominant and non-dominant temporal foci. The reason for the left-right inconsistency may relate to the developmental state of the group of cells at the time of insult. Strauss, Hunter and Wada (1993) found that excessive perseveration tends to occur with left temporal-lobe dysfunction, but only when the damage occurs very early in life. Left temporal-lobe dysfunction after one year of age leaves sorting behavior relatively intact. Perseveration may also occur in the context of right temporal-lobe dysfunction, regardless of the age of onset of the damage, although the deficit tends to be less marked.

Impaired performance has been documented in a number of neurologic conditions including alcoholism, autism, multiple sclerosis, Parkinson's disease, Korsakoff's Syndrome, and chronic cocaine and polydrug use (for a recent review see Adams et al., 1995; Arnett et al., 1994; Beatty and Monson, 1996; Heaton et al., 1993; Lezak, 1995; Ozonoff, 1995; Paolo et al., 1995; Rosselli & Ardilla, 1996; van Spaendonck et al., 1995). In traumatically brain-injured patients, injury severity as measured by Glascow Coma Scale scores has been found to correlate moderately with both perseverative errors ($r = .49$) and number of categories ($r = .33$) (Anderson et al., 1995). There is also evidence that patients with schizophrenia demonstrate impaired levels of performance on the WCST (for recent reviews, see Beatty et al., 1994; Van der Does & Van den Bosch, 1992). In addition, the literature suggests (Heinrichs, 1990; Martin, Oren, & Boone, 1991) that depression may affect performance on the WCST, particularly as reflected in increased perseveration, failure to maintain set, and decreased percent conceptual level response. Depression is related to diminished problem-solving ability, and performance worsens as symptom severity increases. An obvious implication is that neuropsychological test batteries should include an assessment for depression. If depressive symptoms emerge, the clinician should not conclude that abnormal WCST test findings are indicative of organic dysfunction since poor performance appears to be characteristic of depressive cognitive function in the absence of any obvious neurological condition. There is also some evidence that the WCST may have value as a predictor of the capacity to manage independently outside of a hospital setting (Heinrichs, 1990).

Performance on the WCST may also be useful in detecting malingering. Bernard et al. (1996) have reported that people simulating malingering do more poorly on obvious versus subtle tasks compared to people with verified brain damage. Thus, they present with poorer performance ratios on categories (suppression on the obvious measure) compared to perseverative errors (the more subtle measure). Compared to individuals with mild-to-moderate closed head injuries, people instructed to malinger had only about twice the number of perseverative errors, while on the obvious task, malingerers completed only one-seventh as many categories as the closed head injury group. That is, if one obtains a low Category score, one must also obtain an elevated perseverative error score in order to be considered a nonmalingering individual. Bernard et al. provide classification function coefficients to detect malingering on the WCST. Note, however, that these findings are based on subjects simulating malingering, not "real" malingerers. The discriminant functions should be considered as helpful in recognizing malingering but should not be used as the sole basis for such decisions.

Finally, most of the work has been done with the WCST on adult populations. There is some evidence (Chelune & Thompson, 1987; Heaton et al., 1993; Levin et al., 1991) that the test may also be useful in identifying differences in developmental skill acquisition in various diagnostic groups of children and adolescents (e.g., traumatic brain injury, seizure disorders, attention deficit disorder). Preliminary findings (Heaton et al., 1993) on children and adolescents who have structural cerebral lesions suggest that the test is sensitive (but not necessarily specific) to frontal lobe dysfunction in this age group.

Normative Data

For the standard version, Heaton et al. (1993) provide norms for individuals aged 6 years, 5 months to 89 years of age. The data were derived from a total group of 899 normal subjects aggregated from six samples. The educational level of the adult sample was somewhat higher than that of the U.S. population in 1987. Tables are provided (see source) based on the client's age or combination of age and years of education (for adults 20 years and older). Raw scores are converted to percentile scores. For some scores, corresponding standard scores (mean = 100, SD = 15) and T-scores (mean = 50, SD = 10) can also be recorded. Because both age and education influence performance, demographically corrected normative data are recommended (see Appendix D in source), particularly for diagnostic purposes. When making inferences about the adequacy of a client's capacity for everyday functioning (e.g., job placement), U.S. census-based data may be preferred (Appendix C in source). To assist in interpretation of the WCST performance, "base rate" information is also provided separately for adults, adolescents, and children (Appendix E in source).

The WCST manual includes norms for 250 normal children, ages 9–14 years. Paniak et al. (1996) have recently provided data on 685 healthy Canadian children in this age range. The mean WISC-III Vocabulary scaled score was 10.3 (SD = 2.69). The children showed general improvement with increasing age, but did not reach adult levels of performance. The data reported by Paniak et al. (1996) are pre-

Table 8—12. Test Scores for Children on the WCST

	9 (n = 80)	10 (n = 140)	11 (n = 131)	12 (n = 123)	13 (n = 96)	14 (n = 115)
			Age, in years			
ERR						
M	43.79	41.44	38.25	30.12	27.95	24.13
Mdn	42	42	34	24	23	18
SD	18.04	19.25	19.53	17.50	15.96	15.41
PERRES						
M	26.76	24.66	20.64	17.61	15.70	12.89
Mdn	23	22	17	13	11	9
SD	16.25	14.64	12.39	12.69	10.66	8.96
NONPER						
M	20.34	19.31	19.15	14.30	13.66	12.33
Mdn	17	18	15	11	11	9
SD	10.92	10.55	12.41	9.37	8.45	9.40
PERERR						
M	23.45	21.94	18.78	15.81	14.29	11.80
Mdn	21	20	16	12	10	9
SD	13.08	11.90	10.49	10.52	9.15	7.41

Note: ERR = Errors, PERRES = Perseverative Responses, NONPER = Nonperseverative Errors, PERERR = Perseverative Errors.

Source: Paniak et al., 1996. Reprinted with permission.

ferred over those by Heaton et al. (1993), Chelune and Baer (1986) (n = 105), and Roselli and Ardilla (1993) (n = 233) because their sample is larger and appears representative of the North American population with regard to verbal intelligence. The data are shown in Tables 8–12 and 8–13.

For children, aged 5 to 8 years, the data collected in Bogota, Colombia by Rosselli and Ardilla (1993) are given in Table 8–14. No differences between socioeconomic groups were observed. The normative scores are somewhat higher than those reported by Chelune and Baer (1986) for a small American sample. For Categories achieved, Chelune and Baer reported means of 2.73 (SD = 2.10) for 6 year-olds (n = 11), 4.07 (SD = 1.94) for 7 year-olds (n = 14) and 4.05 (SD = 2.01) for 8 year-olds (n = 22). By the same token, perseverative errors were higher in their sample (6 year olds: mean = 40.64, SD = 28.03; 7 year olds: mean = 25.07, SD = 18.43; 8 year olds: mean = 23.18, SD = 13.23).

Age has the strongest relationship to WCST performance (Heaton et al., 1993). Performance increases from 5 years through 19 years of age and remains fairly stable between the 20- to 50-year age decades. Declines in some aspects of performance become apparent after age 60. Similar findings have been reported by others (Axelrod & Henry, 1992; Axelrod et al., 1993; Beatty, 1993; Boone et al., 1993; Chelune & Baer, 1986; Daigneault et al., 1992; Haaland et al., 1987; Heaton, 1981; Heaton et al., 1993; Heinrichs, 1990; Levin et al., 1991; Levine et al., 1995; Parkin et al., 1995; Rosselli & Ardila, 1993; Welsh et al., 1988, 1991). Fristoe et al. (1997) propose that although use of feedback information and working memory are important determinants of WCST age-related differences, these age-related differences are largely predictable from more basic speed-of-processing factors.

Educational level shows modest correlations with some WCST scores (Boone et al., 1993; Heaton et al., 1993; Heinrichs, 1990).

Table 8—13. Test Scores for Skewed Variables

		WCST Variables		
	Percentiles	CATS	TTF	FMS
Age 9	>16	4–6	10–17	0–2
	11–16	2–3	18–22	3
	6–10	2	23–25	3–4
	2–5	1–2	26–78	4–5
	<1	0–1	79–128	6–21
Age 10	>16	4–6	10–17	0–2
	11–16	2–3	18–21	2–3
	6–10	2	22–37	3
	2–5	2	38–51	4
	<1	0–1	52–128	5–21
Age 11	>16	4–6	10–14	0–1
	11–16	3	15–19	2–3
	6–10	2–3	20–25	3
	2–5	1–2	32–63	3–4
	<1	0–1	64–128	5–21
Age 12	>16	5–6	10–12	0–1
	11–16	4	13–16	2
	6–10	2–4	17–19	2–3
	2–5	2	20–38	3
	<1	0–1	39–128	4–21
Age 13	>16	5–6	10–12	0–1
	11–16	4	13–15	2–3
	6–10	4	16–22	3
	2–5	3–4	23–31	3–5
	<1	0–2	32–128	6–21
Age 14	>16	6	10–15	0–1
	11–16	4–5	16–18	1–2
	6–10	4	19–21	2
	2–5	3–4	22–39	3–4
	<1	0–3	40–128	4–21

Note: CATS = Categories Achieved, TTF = Trials to Complete First Category, FMS = Failure to Maintain Set.

Source: Paniak et al. (1996). Reprinted with permission.

For adults, there is a gradual increase in proficiency in WCST performance from lower to higher levels of education.

The influence of gender is controversial. Heaton et al. (1993), Paniak et al. (1996) and Rosselli and Ardilla (1993) report that gender is not significantly related to WCST performance. By contrast, Boone et al. (1993) found that women tend to outperform men on the WCST.

IQ appears related to performance. Chelune and Baer (1986), Heaton (1981), Heinrichs (1990), Paniak et al. (1996), and Parkin et al. (1995) documented a modest relation between IQ and WCST scores, although Boone et al. (1993) reported that IQ did not affect WCST performance.

References

Adams, K.M., Gilman, S., Koeppe, R., Klain, K., Junck, L., Lohman, M., Johnson-Greene, D., Berent, S., Dede, D., Kroll, P. (1995). Correlation of neuropsychological function with cerebral metabolic rate in subdivisions of the frontal lobes of older alcoholic patients measured with [18F] Fluorodeoxyglucose and Positron Emission Tomography. *Neuropsychology, 9,* 275–280.

Anderson, C.V., Bigler, E.D., & Blatter, D.D. (1995). Frontal lobe lesions, diffuse damage, and neuropsychological functioning in traumatic brain-injured patients. *Journal of Clinical and Experimental Neuropsychology, 17,* 900–908.

Anderson, S.W., Damasio, H., Jones, R.D., & Tranel, D. (1991). Wisconsin Card Sorting Test performance as a measure of frontal lobe dam-

Table 8—14. WCST Scores for Children Aged 5 to 8 Years Grouped by Age and Socioeconomic Level

	Age 5–6 years (*n* = 49)				Age 7–8 years (*n* = 63)			
	High socioeconomic level		Low socioeconomic level		High socioeconomic level		Low socioeconomic level	
Variable	Score	SD	Score	SD	Score	SD	Score	SD
Categories achieved	4.2	1.8	4.2	2.2	4.9	1.7	4.4	1.9
Correct responses	66.9	15.1	67.0	17.8	67.8	11.6	70.5	14.4
Errors	46.1	23.0	51.6	24.7	48.4	20.9	48.4	23.0
Perseverative responses	21.7	11.3	29.5	21.7	19.1	8.7	24.4	18.2
Perseverative errors	21.3	15.7	25.3	10.6	17.9	8.1	20.9	10.5
Nonperseverative errors	24.6	17.6	25.9	12.0	30.5	16.3	27.2	17.1
Failure to maintain set	0.8	0.6	0.0	0.0	0.8	0.7	0.4	0.6

Source: Rosselli and Ardilla, 1993. Reprinted with permission of Swets and Zeitlinger.

age. *Journal of Clinical and Experimental Neuropsychology, 13,* 909–922.

Arnett, P.A., Rao, S.M., Bernardin, L., Grafman, J., Yetkin, F.Z., & Lobeck, L. (1994). Relationship between frontal lobe lesions and Wisconsin Card Sorting Test performance in patients with multiple sclerosis. *Neurology, 44,* 420–425.

Axelrod, B.N., & Henry, R.R. (1992). Age-related performance on the Wisconsin Card Sorting, Similarities, and Controlled Oral Word Association Tests. *The Clinical Neuropsychologist, 6,* 16–26.

Axelrod, B.N., Goldman, R.S., & Woodard, J.L. (1992a). Interrater reliability in scoring the Wisconsin Card Sorting Test. *The Clinical Neuropsychologist, 6,* 143–155.

Axelrod, B.N., Woodard, J.L., & Henry, R.R. (1992b). Analysis of an abbreviated form of the Wisconsin Card Sorting Test. *The Clinical Neuropsychologist, 6,* 27–31.

Axelrod, B.N., Jiron, C.C., & Henry, R.R. (1993). Performance of adults ages 20 to 90 on the abbreviated Wisconsin Card Sorting Test. *The Clinical Neuropsychologist, 7,* 205–209.

Axelrod, B.N., Goldman, R.S., Heaton, R.K., Lawless, G., Thompson, L.L., Chelune, G.J., Kay, G.G. (1996). Discriminability of the Wisconsin Card Sorting Test using the standardization sample. *Journal of Clinical and Experimental Neuropsychology, 18,* 338–342.

Axelrod, B.N., Paolo, A.M., & Abraham, E. (1997). Do normative data from the full WCST extend to the abbreviated WCST? *Assessment, 4,* 41—46.

Beatty, W.W. (1993). Age differences on the California Card Sorting Test: Implications for the assessment of problem solving by the elderly. *Bulletin of the Psychonomic Society, 31,* 511–514.

Beatty, W.B., Jocic, Z., Monson, N., & Katzung, V.M. (1994). Problem solving by schizophrenic and schizoaffective patients on the Wisconsin and California Card Sorting Tests. *Neuropsychology, 8,* 49–54.

Beatty, W.W., & Monson, N. (1996). Problem solving by patients with multiple sclerosis: Comparison of performance on the Wisconsin and California Card Sorting Tests. *Journal of the International Neuropsychological Society, 2,* 134–140.

Berg, E.A. (1948). A simple objective technique for measuring flexibility in thinking. *Journal of General Psychology, 39,* 15–22.

Bernard, L.C., McGrath, M.J., & Houston, W. (1996). The differential effects of simulating malingering, closed head injury, and other CNS pathology on the Wisconsin Card Sorting Test: Support for the "pattern of performance" hypothesis. *Archives of Clinical Neuropsychology, 11,* 231–245.

Berry, S. (1996). Diagrammatic procedure for scoring the Wisconsin Card Sorting Test. *The Clinical Neuropsychologist, 10,* 117–121.

Boone, K.B., Gharffarian, S., Lesser, I.M., Hill-Gutierrez, E., & Berman, N.G. (1993). Wisconsin Card Sorting Test performance in healthy, older adults: Relationship to age, sex, education, and IQ. *Journal of Clinical Psychology, 49,* 54–60.

Bornstein, R.A. (1986). Contribution of various neuropsychological measures to detection of frontal lobe impairment. *International Journal of Clinical Neuropsychology, 8,* 18–22.

Cantor-Graae, E., Warkentin, S., Franzen, G., & Risberg, J. (1993). Frontal lobe challenge: A comparison of activation procedures during rCBF measurements in normal subjects. *Neuropsychiatry, Neuropsychology, and Behavioral Neurology, 6,* 83–92.

Chelune, G.J., & Baer, R.A. (1986). Developmental norms for the Wisconsin Card Sorting Test. *Journal of Clinical and Experimental Neuropsychology, 8,* 219–228.

Chelune, G.J., & Thompson, L.T. (1987). Evaluation of the general sensitivity of the Wisconsin Card Sorting Test among younger and older children. *Developmental Neuropsychology, 3,* 81–89.

Daigneault, S., Braun, C.M.J., & Whitaker, H.A. (1992). Early effects of normal aging on perseverative and non-perseverative prefrontal measures. *Developmental Neuropsychology, 8,* 99–114.

Dehaene, S., & Changeux, J.P. (1991). The Wisconsin Card Sorting Test: Theoretical analysis and modeling in a neuronal network. *Cerebral Cortex, 1,* 62–79.

de Zubicaray, G., & Ashton, R. (1996). Nelson's Modified Card Sorting Test: A review. *The Clinical Neuropsychologist, 10,* 245–254.

Drewe, E.A. (1974). The effect of type and area of brain lesion on Wisconsin Cart Sorting Test performance. *Cortex, 10,* 159–170.

Flashman, L.A., Horner, M.D., & Freides, D. (1991). Note on scoring perseveration on the Wisconsin Card Sorting Test. *The Clinical Neuropsychologist, 5,* 190–194.

Fortuny, L.A., & Heaton, R.K. (1996). Standard versus computerized administration of the Wisconsin Card Sorting Test. *The Clinical Neuropsychologist, 10,* 419–424.

Fristoe, N.M., Salthouse, T.A., & Woodard, J.L. (1997). Examination of age-related deficits on the Wisconsin Card Sorting Test. *Neuropsychology, 11*, 428–436.

Goldman, R.S., Axelrod, B.N., Heaton, R.K., Chelune, G.J., Curtiss, G., Kay, G.G., & Thompson, L.L. (1996). Latent structure of the WCST with the standardization samples. *Assessment, 3*, 73–78.

Grafman, J., Jones, B., & Salazar, A. (1990). Wisconsin Card Sorting Test performance based on location and size of neuroanatomical lesion in Vietnam veterans with penetrating head injury. *Perceptual and Motor Skills, 71*, 1120–1122.

Grant, D.A., & Berg, E.A. (1948). A behavioral analysis of degree of impairment and ease of shifting to new responses in a Weigl-type card sorting problem. *Journal of Experimental Psychology, 39*, 404–411.

Greve, K.W. (1993). Can perseverative responses on the Wisconsin Card Sorting Test be scored accurately? *Archives of Clinical Neuropsychology, 8*, 511–517.

Greve, K.W., Brooks, J., Crouch, J., Rice, W.J., Cicerone, K., & Rowland, L. (1993). Factorial structure of the Wisconsin Card Sorting Test. *The Clinical Neuropsychologist, 7*, 350–351.

Greve, K.W., Williams, M.C., Haas, W.G., Lettell, R.R., & Reinoso, C. (1996). The role of attention in Wisconsin Card Sorting Test performance. *Archives of Clinical Neuropsychology, 11*, 215–222.

Haaland, K., Vranes, L.F., Goodwin, J.S., & Garry, J.P. (1987). Wisconsin Cart Sorting Test performance in a healthy elderly population. *Journal of Gerontology, 42*, 345–346.

Heaton, R.K. (1981). *Wisconsin Card Sorting Test Manual*. Odessa, Fl: Psychological Assessment Resources, Inc.

Heaton, R.K., Chelune, G.J., Talley, J.L., Kay, G.G., & Curtis, G. (1993). *Wisconsin Card Sorting Test (WCST) Manual Revised and Expanded*. Odessa, Fl: Psychological Assessment Resources.

Heinrichs, R.W. (1990). Variables associated with Wisconsin Card Sorting Test performance in neuropsychiatric patients referred for assessment. *Neuropsychiatry, Neuropsychology and Behavioral Neurology, 3*, 107–112.

Hellman, S.G., Green, M.F., Kern, R.S., & Christenson, C.D. (1992). Comparison of card and computer versions of the Wisconsin Card Sorting Test for psychotic patients. *International Journal of Methods in Psychiatric Research, 2*, 151–155.

Hermann, B.P., Wyler, A.R., & Richey, E.T. (1988). Wisconsin Card Sorting Test performance in patients with complex partial seizure of temporal lobe origin. *Journal of Clinical and Experimental Psychology, 10*, 467–476.

Hermann, B., & Seidenberg, M. (1995). Executive system dysfunction in temporal lobe epilepsy: Effects of nociferous cortex versus hippocampal pathology. *Journal of Clinical and Experimental Neuropsychology, 17*, 809–819.

Horner, M.D., Flashman, L.A., Freides, D., Epstein, C.M., & Bakay, R.A.E. (1996). Temporal lobe epilepsy and performance on the Wisconsin Card Sorting Test. *Journal of Clinical and Experimental Neuropsychology, 18*, 310–313.

Huber, S.J., Bornstein, R.A., Rammohan, K.W. et al. (1992). Magnetic resonance imaging correlates of executive function impairments in multiple sclerosis. *Neuropsychiatry, Neuropsychology, and Behavioral Neurology, 5*, 33–36.

Levin, H.S., Culhane, K.A., Hartmann, J., Evankovitch, K., Mattson, A.J., Harward, H., Ringholz, G., Ewing-Cobbs, L., & Fletcher, J.M. (1991). Developmental changes in performance on tests of purported frontal lobe functioning. *Developmental Neuropsychology, 7*, 377–395.

Levine, B., Stuss, D.T., & Milberg, W.P. (1995). Concept generation: Validation of a test of executive functioning in a normal aging population. *Journal of Clinical and Experimental Neuropsychology, 17*, 740–758.

Lezak, M.D. (1995). *Neuropsychological Assessment* (3rd ed.). New York: Oxford University Press.

Loong, J.W.K. (1990). *The Wisconsin Card Sorting Test* (IBM version). San Luis Obispo, CA: Wang Neuropsychological Laboratory.

Martin, D.J., Oren, Z., & Boone, K. (1991). Major depressives' and dysthymics' performance on the Wisconsin Card Sorting Test. *Journal of Clinical Psychology, 47*, 685–690.

Milner, B. (1963). Effects of different brain lesions on card sorting. *Archives of Neurology, 9*, 90–100.

Mountain, M.A., & Snow, G. (1993). Wisconsin Card Sorting Test as a measure of frontal pathology: A review. *The Clinical Neuropsychologist, 7*, 108–118.

Nelson, H.E. (1976). A modified card sorting test sensitive to frontal lobe defects. *Cortex, 12*, 313–324.

O'Donnell, J.P., MacGregor, L.A., Dabrowski, J.J., Oestreicher, J.M., & Romero, J.J. (1994). Construct validity of neuropsychological tests of conceptual and attentional abilities. *Journal of Clinical Psychology, 50*, 596–600.

Osmon, D.C., & Suchy, Y. (1996). Fractionating frontal lobe functions: Factors of the Milwaukee Card Sorting Test. *Archives of Clinical Neuropsychology, 11*, 451–552.

Ozonoff, S. (1995). Reliability and validity of the Wisconsin Card Sorting Test in studies of autism. *Neuropsychology, 9*, 491–500.

Paniak, C., Miller, H.B., Murphy, D., Patterson, L., & Keizer, J. (1996). Canadian developmental norms for 9- to 14-year-olds on the Wisconsin Card Sorting Test. *Canadian Journal of Rehabilitation, 9*, 233–237.

Paolo, A.M., Axelrod, B.N., Ryan, J.J., & Goldman, R.S. (1994). Administration accuracy of the Wisconsin Card Sorting Test. *The Clinical Neuropsychologist, 8*, 112–116.

Paolo, A.M., Troster, A.I., Axelrod, B.N., & Koller, W.C. (1995). Construct validity of the WCST in normal elderly and persons with Parkinson's disease. *Archives of Clinical Neuropsychology, 10*, 463–473.

Paolo, A.M., Axelrod, B.N., & Troster, A.I. (1996a). Test-retest stability of the Wisconsin Card Sorting Test. *Assessment, 3*, 137–143.

Paolo, A.M., Axelrod, B.N., Troster, A.I., Blackwell, K.T., & Koller, W.C. (1996b). Utility of a Wisconsin Card Sorting Test short form in persons with Alzheimer's and Parkinson's Disease. *Journal of Clinical and Experimental Neuropsychology, 18*, 892–897.

Parkin, A.J., Walter, B.M., & Hunkin, N.M. (1995). Relationships between normal aging, frontal lobe function, and memory for temporal and spatial information. *Neuropsychology, 9*, 304–312.

Pendleton, M.G., & Heaton, R.K. (1982). A comparison of the Wisconsin Card Sorting Test and the Category Test. *Journal of Clinical Psychology, 38*, 392–396.

Perrine, K. (1993). Differential aspects of conceptual processing in the Category Test and Wisconsin Card Sorting Test. *Journal of Clinical and Experimental Neuropsychology, 15*, 461–473.

Rezai, K., Andreasen, N.C., Alliger, R., Cohen, G., Swayze II, V., & O'Leary, D.S. (1993). The neuropsychology of the prefrontal cortex. *Archives of Neurology, 59*, 636–642.

Robinson, A.L., Heaton, R.K., Lehman, R.A.W., & Stilson, D.W. (1980). The utility of the Wisconsin Card Sorting Test in detecting and localizing frontal lobe lesions. *Journal of Consulting and Clinical Psychology, 48*, 605–614.

Rosselli, M., & Ardila, A. (1993). Developmental norms for the Wisconsin Card Sorting Test in 5- to 12-year-old children. *The Clinical Neuropsychologist, 7*, 145–154.

Rosselli, M., & Ardila, A. (1996). Cognitive effects of cocaine and polydrug abuse. *Journal of Clinical and Experimental Neuropsychology, 18*, 122–135.

Salthouse, T.A., Fristoe, N., & Rhee, S.H. (1996). How localized are age-related effects on neuropsychological measures? *Neuropsychology, 10*, 272–285.

Sherman, E.M., Strauss, E., Spellacy, F., & Hunter, M. (1995). Construct validity of WAIS-R factors: Neuropsychological correlates in adults referred for possible head injury. *Psychological Assessment, 7*, 440–444.

Shute, G.E., & Huertas, V. (1990). Developmental variability in frontal lobe function. *Developmental Neuropsychology, 6*, 1–11.

Strauss, E., Hunter, M., & Wada, J. (1993). Wisconsin Card Sort performance: Effects of age of onset and laterality of dysfunction. *Journal of Clinical and Experimental Neuropsychology, 15*, 896–902.

Stuss, D.T., Benson, D.F., Kaplan, E.F., et al. (1983). The involvement of orbitofrontal cerebrum in cognitive tasks. *Neuropsychologia, 21*, 235–248.

Sullivan, E.V., Mathalon, D.H., Zipursky, R.B., Kersteen-Tucker, Z., Knight, R.T., & Pfefferbaum, A. (1993). Factors of the Wisconsin Card Sorting Test as measures of frontal-lobe function in schizophrenia and in chronic alcoholism. *Psychiatry Research, 46*, 175–199.

Taylor, L.B. (1979). Psychological assessment of neurological patients. In T. Rasmussen and R. Marino (Eds.), *Functional Neurosurgery*. New York: Raven Press.

Van der Does, A.J.W., & Van den Bosch, R.J. (1992). What determines Wisconsin Card Sorting performance in schizophrenia? *Clinical Psychology Review, 12*, 567–583.

Vanderploeg, R.D., Schinka, J.A., & Retzlaff, P. (1994). Relationships between measures of auditory verbal learning and executive functioning. *Journal of Clinical and Experimental Neuropsychology, 16*, 243–252.

van Spaendonck, K.P.M., Berger, H.J.C., Horstink, M.W.I.M., Borm, G.F., & Cools, A.R. (1995). Card sorting performance in Parkinson's Disease: A comparison between acquisition and shifting performance. *Journal of Clinical and Experimental Neuropsychology, 17*, 918–925.

Weinberger, D.R., Berman, K.F., & Zec, R.F.

(1988). Physiological dysfunction of dorsolateral prefrontal cortex in schizophrenia; I: Regional cerebral blood flow (rCBF) evidence. *Archives of General Psychiatry, 45,* 609–615.

Welsh, M.C., Groisser, D., & Pennington, B.F. (1988). A normative-developmental study of performance on measures hypothesized to tap prefrontal functions. Paper presented to the International Neuropsychological Society, New Orleans.

Welsh, M.C., Pennington, B.F., & Grossier, D.B. (1991). A normative-developmental study of executive function: A window on prefrontal function in children. *Developmental Neuropsychology, 7,* 131–149.

Williams, M.C., Littell, R.R., Reinoso, C., & Greve, K.W. (1994). The effect of wavelength on the performance of attention-disordered and normal children on the Wisconsin Card Sorting Test. *Neuropsychology, 8,* 187–193.

9

Attention

Attentional processes play a major role in the daily behavior of patients with neuropsychological disorders. They may affect learning and memory as well as other aspects of cognition. Several models of attention have been proposed (e.g., Mirsky, 1987; Posner & Peterson, 1990; Schum et al., 1990; Schmidt et al., 1994; Sohlberg & Mateer, 1989). In an effort to integrate different models, Mateer and Mapou (1996) proposed an assessment model that separates attention into two major areas: deployment and encoding. Deployment refers to how well an individual can channel and focus attentional resources and includes arousal, focused, and sustained attention. Arousal is usually evaluated by direct observation. Focused attention requires the individual to reject irrelevant information while attending to relevant input. It can be assessed by tasks that require rapid scanning and identification of targets such as the Digit Symbol (from Wechsler Intelligence Scale), Symbol Digit Modalities, Trail Making, Stroop, d2, and VSAT tests. Sustained attention can be assessed by continuous performance tests. The second area, capacity/encoding, refers to how well an individual can hold information in mind and then process it, even if distracted or required to divide attention (allocate attentional resources) among tasks. It includes span of attention (e.g., Digit Span Forward, Trial 1 of the CVLT or RAVLT, Sentence Repetition, Visual Span Forward), resistance to interference (e.g., Consonant Trigrams, comparison of List B to List A on the CVLT or RAVLT),

and mental manipulation (Digit Span Backwards, Arithmetic, PASAT, Brief Test of Attention). It is important to bear in mind, however, that most measures of attention are multifaceted and cannot easily be fit into distinct components. Many can also be considered measures of working memory.

Attention deficits may be related to slowed processing speed which can be evaluated by measures of reaction time (see Reaction Time in the chapter on Visual, Visuomotor, and Auditory tests; MicroCog in General Intellectual Ability) and information processing speed (e.g., MicroCog in General Intellectual Ability).

Clinicians may also refer to the recently published Test of Everyday Attention (TEA, distributed by Northern Speech Services, 117 N. Elm, P.O. Box 1247, Gaylord, MI 49735 or from Thames Valley Test Company, 7–9 The Green, Flempton, Bury St. Edmunds, Suffolk IP28 6EI, UK), but not yet available to us. According to Robertson et al. (1996), the TEA consists of a series of eight tests of attention, which are based on ecologically plausible activities such as searching maps, looking through telephone directories, and listening to lottery-number broadcasts. The TEA has three parallel forms, has good test-retest reliability and appears to correlate with existing measures of attention (e.g., d2, PASAT, Trails B). Robertson et al. report that the TEA is applicable to a wide variety of clinical conditions and appears to correlate with functional status. Further, the tasks show little relation to

NART-measured verbal intelligence. An age-, sex- and IQ-stratified sample of 154 normal participants was given these tasks, along with a number of other measures of attention. The factor structure of this data set included factors for sustained attention, selective attention, attentional switching, and auditory-verbal working memory. A children's version of the TEA is currently being developed.

References

Mateer, C.A., & Mapou, R. (1996). Understanding, evaluating and managing attention disorders following traumatic brain injury. *Journal of Head Trauma Rehabilitation, 11*, 1–16.

Mirsky, A.F. (1987). Behavioral and psychophysiological markers of disordered attention. *Environmental Health Perspectives, 74*, 191–199.

Posner, M.I., & Peterson, S.E. (1990). The attention system of the human brain. *Annual Review of Neuroscience, 13*, 25–42.

Robertson, I.H., Ward, T., Ridgeway, V., & Nimmo-Smith, I. (1996). The structure of normal human attention: The Test of Everyday Attention. *Journal of the International Neuropsychological Society, 2*, 525–534.

Schmidt, M., Trueblood, W., & Merwin, M. (1994). How much do "Attention" tests tell us? *Archives of Clinical Neuropsychology, 9*, 383–394.

Shum, D.H.K., McFarland, K.A., & Bain, J.D. (1990). Construct validity of eight tests of attention: Comparison of normal and closed head injured subjects. *Clinical Neuropsychologist, 4*, 151–162.

Sohlberg, M.M., & Mateer, C.A. (1989). *Introduction to Cognitive Rehabilitation: Theory and Practice.* New York: Guilford Press.

BRIEF TEST OF ATTENTION (BTA)

Purpose

This test is used to assess the ability to divide auditory attention.

Source

The tape (including instructions and sample scoring sheet) can be ordered from David Schretlen, Johns Hopkins Hospital, 600 N. Wolfe St., Meyer 218, Baltimore, MD 21287-7218.

Description

This test was devised by Schretlen and colleagues (Schretlen, Bobholz, & Brandt, 1996a; Schretlen, Brandt, & Bobholz, 1996b) and consists of two parallel forms that are presented via audiocassette. Subjects are administered both forms; each requires 4 minutes to administer and score. Form N consists of ten lists of letters and numbers (e.g., "M-6-3-R-2") that increase in length from 4 to 18 items. The subject's task is to disregard the letters and count how many *numbers* are read aloud. Each list is followed by five seconds of silence, during which the subject reports how many numbers were recited. The *same* ten lists are presented as Form L, in which the subject's task is to disregard the numbers and count how many *letters* are read aloud. Unlike digit span tests, this test does not require the subject to recall which numbers (or letters) are presented.

Administration

The examiner may begin with Form N or L, but both forms should be administered. If a subject finds the test particularly frustrating, it is better to interpose some other task between forms than to eliminate one form entirely. This is because the reliability of each form alone is considerably lower than for both together.

Instructions for administering the BTA appear at the top of each answer sheet. Test instructions should be read to the subject. The instructions for Form N are as follows:

"This is a brief test of attention. A voice on the tape recorder will read a list of letters and numbers. You are to keep track only of how many numbers you hear. Then, tell me how many NUMBERS were on the list. While the list is being read, please make your hands into fists and put them on the table. We will begin with two examples to make sure that you have

the idea, Remember, tell me HOW MANY NUMBERS *are on each list."*

Subjects are instructed to make their hands into fists and place them on the table in order to prevent them from counting test stimuli on their fingers. The examiner then reads the first of two sample items from the answer sheet. After each sample, the examiner asks, *"How many numbers were on the list?"* Give up to two additional trials of each sample item. If the subject fails all three trials of both samples, discontinue the test. Otherwise, the examiner should continue reading the directions from the answer sheet and start the tape recorder.

"Now I will start the tape. After each trial, tell me how many numbers you heard. If you are not sure, guess!"

Subjects should be urged to indicate if the volume is too high or low. Also, the examiner should emphasize the importance of guessing, even if the subject is unsure of the correct answer. However, the tape *should not* be stopped between trials.

The tape begins with the following introduction, *"Brief test of attention—Part A."* It is introduced in this way so that the examiner may select which form to administer first. Each trial is announced by number (e.g., *"Trial number one . . . ready! . . ."*), and is followed by a 5-second pause during which the subject is to give the answer. Subjects may be prompted by the examiner with such questions as, *"How many numbers were on the list?"* After each trial, the examiner notes the subject's response in the space provided on the answer sheet. At the conclusion of trial number 10, the examiner stops the tape. The examiner then repeats the instructions and procedures outlined above for the alternate form of the test, using the appropriate answer sheet. When the tape is restarted, the alternate form will begin with the following recorded introduction, *"Brief test of attention—Part B."* Because the entire BTA (Parts A and B) is recorded on both sides of the tape, it is not necessary to rewind the tape after each use. Simply fast-forward to the end of whichever side is being used, and reverse the tape for the next administration. Repeat instructions for the second part.

Approximate Time for Administration

About 10 minutes are required for the entire test.

Scoring

Each response is compared with the correct answer (provided on the answer sheet), and the total number of correctly monitored lists is recorded. Thus, for each form, scores range from 0 to 10, and total scores range from 0 to 20.

Comment

Schretlen et al. (1996a) report that internal consistency is high (above .8) for both normal adults and children and a mixed clinical sample. In normal people, the Pearson correlation between Form N and Form L was 0.69 but increased to .81 for the combined (n = 926) normal and clinical samples. Neither practice nor interference effects were found to influence performance from the first to the second form administered. Over 97 percent of normal subjects and 93 percent of patients produced scores that differed by ≤3 points between Forms L and N.

Regarding test–retest data, Schretlen and his colleagues (personal communication, September 1995) collected data on 60 adults (range: 30–78 years, mean = 66.2, SD = 4.8) who took the test twice, about 8.7 months apart (range: 6.7–12.6), as part of a study of behavior/dietary control of mild hypertension. When their initial scores were subtracted from their follow-up scores, the mean difference was 0.6 points (SD = 2.5, range: −3 to +8). On follow-up testing, 56 out of 60 (93 percent) of the subjects scored between −3 and +4 points of their initial score. The test–retest correlation (Pearson *r*) was .70 for BTA total scores.

Correlation analyses and principal components analyses (Schretlen et al., 1996a,b) showed that the BTA correlated more strongly with the complex (e.g., Trails B, Digit Span backward, Stroop) than with the simple tests of attention (e.g., Trails A, Digit Span forward) and correlated more strongly with measures of attention than with other cognitive tasks (e.g., Rey-Osterrieth, Boston Naming Test, WMS-R Logical Memory, General Memory, and Delayed Memory Indices). Like most neuropsychological tests, however, the BTA also shows moderate relations with measures of general mental ability. Tagami and Strauss (1996) found in a sample of 33 university students, aged 18–44 years (mean = 22.12, SD = 6.33), that scores on the BTA correlated significantly with scores on the first trial of the PASAT ($r = .55$). Whereas the PASAT showed a moderate relation with performance on the Wonderlic ($r = .33$), the BTA was unrelated to this brief measure of intellectual functioning ($r = .05$).

Schretlen and colleagues (1996b) reported that patients with impaired attention (that is, nondemented patients with Huntington's disease) performed poorly on the BTA. Amnesic patients, however, were not impaired, suggesting that the BTA does not require intact memory for successful performance. No other studies of patients with neurological disorders are available yet.

Normative Data

Schretlen and colleagues (1996a) report that in normal children, BTA scores are influenced by age and sex, with boys producing significantly lower scores than females. In normal adults, only age accounted for significant variance in BTA performance. There is a decline in performance with advancing age, after about age 60. Sex, race, and education did not have unique contributions in adults. In a heterogeneous clinical sample, however, the effect of race was significant, with black patients scoring 1.5–2.0 points lower than white patients in higher education subgroups. Race-related differences were not found among patients with less than 9 years of education.

Cumulative frequency data for the BTA are shown in Table 9–1. The authors report that when adult patients score <4/10 or >7/10 on the first form given, the second form may be omitted without compromising the reliability of clinical judgments regarding the presence or absence of impaired attention.

Table 9—1. Percent Cumulative Frequency of BTA Scores for Normal Subjects by Age

Score	Age 6–8 (n = 24)	Age 9–11 (n = 25)	Age 12–14 (n = 25)	Age 17–19 (n = 24)	Age 20–39 (n = 89)	Age 40–59 (n = 54)	Age 60–69 (n = 68)	Age 70–81 (n = 40)
20			100	100	100	100	100	100
19				96	67	75	82	82	93
18			100	84	50	55	67	68	78
17			96	84	46	40	44	60	65
16			88	72	29	23	35	47	55
15			76	68	17	15	26	38	40
14	100	72	36	4	9	17	24	35
13	96	52	24		3	13	16	30
12	88	44	20			9	9	23
11	75	36	12			4	4	15
10	63	28	8			2	3	15
9	58	12	8				3	10
8	50	8	4				2	5
7	33	8						3
6	21							
5	13							
4	8							
3	4							
2	4							
1	4							
0	4							

Source: Schretlen et al., 1996a. Reprinted with permission.

References

Schretlen, D., Bobholz, J.H., & Brandt, J. (1996a). Development and psychometric properties of the Brief Test of Attention. *The Clinical Neuropsychologist*, *10*, 80–89.

Schretlen, D., Brandt, J., & Bobholz, J.H. (1996b). Validation of the Brief Test of Attention in patients with Huntington's Disease and amnesia. *The Clinical Neuropsychologist*, *10*, 90–95.

Tagami, Y., & Strauss, E. (1996). The Brief Test of Attention: Relationship to the PASAT and to IQ. B.A. Honors Thesis. University of Victoria.

CONTINUOUS PERFORMANCE TEST (CPT)

Purpose

This test is used to assess lapses in attention or vigilance and impulsivity.

Source

The Conners' Continuous Performance Test (including manual and computer disk for unlimited use) can be ordered from Multi-Health Systems, Inc. (MHS), 65 Overlea Blvd., Suite 210, Toronto, Ontario, M4H 1P1, at a cost of $495 Cdn.

Description

The continuous performance test (CPT) was initially introduced by Rosvold et al. (1956) to detect lapses of attention in patients with petit mal epilepsy. In their version, subjects pressed a key when a target letter appeared (e.g., X), or when the target letter was preceded by another letter (e.g., A–X). Subsequent CPTs have been modeled after Rosvold et al.'s task although they vary with regard to modality (i.e., visual or auditory), the type of stimuli (e.g., letters, numbers, colors, or geometric figures), the nature of the task (e.g., respond to a single stimulus such as X; respond to a designated sequence of stimuli, such as A followed by X; respond to every stimulus other than a designated one), and the type of data that are evaluated (omissions; commissions; interstimulus interval; measures of sensitivity—d′, and response criterion—β). It is likely that these different tasks and approaches generate data with diverse meanings (Halperin, 1991; Seidel & Joschko, 1990).

Several CPT versions are available commercially (e.g., Gordon, 1983). We use the Connors' CPT (1995) because of the wide range of subject-response parameters that are evaluated and the flexibility of the program.

The Standard CPT in Conners' program (1995) requires the subject to press the appropriate key for any letter *except* the letter X. There are six blocks, each with three 20-trial sub-blocks (letters presented, whether targets or not). For each block, the sub-blocks have different interstimulus intervals (ISIs): 1, 2, or 4 seconds. The order of the ISIs varies between blocks. Each letter is displayed for 250 milliseconds. This paradigm is the default program although the Conners' CPT computer program allows the examiner to create customized paradigms (including X and A–X paradigms), to select the number of trials (or blocks), and to select most of the other parameters (e.g., interstimulus interval, display time). After the test session, the program generates a report that includes the total number of stimuli, the number correct, omission errors, commission errors, and various reaction times.

Administration

Test presentation is controlled by the computer program. The program allows the examiner to administer one or more practice tests to patients.

Approximate Time for Administration

The standard form takes about 14 minutes.

Scoring

The information is presented in several forms: raw scores, T-scores (mean = 50, SD = 10), percentiles, and guidelines (e.g., within average range, mildly or markedly atypical) that are based on comparisons to groups of the same age and gender. The program provides an overall summary of the data and an interpretive (narrative) guide. For example, summary may indicate that the subject gave slower responses at the end of the test than at the beginning, indicating an inability to sustain attention.

High T-scores (above 60) and percentiles indicate a problem for all measures, although both high and low T-scores or percentiles can be associated with attention problems for hit reaction times and β. The patient's report is broken down into several categories:

Hits: The number of targets the person responded to correctly (and the percentage correct out of the total number of targets).

Omissions: The number of targets the person did not respond to (and the percentage of omissions out of the total number of targets).

Commissions: The number of times the person responded to a non-target ("X"). The percentage is the number of commissions out of all non-targets presented.

Hit RT: The mean response time (in milliseconds).

Hit RT Standard Error: The consistency of response times to targets.

Variability of SEs: A different method for calculating response consistency; the standard deviation of the 18 standard error values is calculated for each sub-block.

Attentiveness (d'): A measure of how well the individual discriminates between targets and non-targets.

Risk Taking (β): An individual's response tendency. Individuals who are cautious and tend not to respond very often obtain high β T-scores. Those who are more risk-taking or impulsive and respond more frequently obtain low β T-scores.

Hit RT Block Change: The slope of change in reaction times over the six time blocks. A positive slope indicates a slowing in reaction time, while a negative slope indicates quicker reaction times as the test progressed.

Hit SE Block Change: The slope of change in reaction time standard errors over the six time blocks. A positive slope indicates that reaction times became less consistent as the test progressed. Negative slopes imply reaction times became more consistent as the test progressed.

Hit RT ISI Change: The slope of change in reaction times over the three ISIs (1, 2, and 4 sec). A positive slope indicates a slowing of reaction times as the time between targets increased, while a negative slope indicates faster reaction times as the time between targets increased.

Hit SE ISI Change: The slope of change in reaction time standard errors over the three ISIs. A positive slope means the person's reaction times became more erratic as the time between targets increased. A negative slope indicates increased consistency as the time between targets increased.

Overall Index: A weighted sum of the measures.

Comment

Connors and colleagues (1995) report that there is little practice effect. Rather, a slight negative practice effect occurs because of repeating an essentially repetitive and boring task. They suggest, therefore, that any improvement on repeat testing reflects real change, not just task familiarity. Unfortunately, the data supporting these assertions are not provided in the manual. Inattention and impulsivity measures derived from AX versions of the CPT appear to have adequate split-half reliabilities, test–retest reliability, and stability over time (Gordon, 1983; Halperin et al., 1991b; Rosvold et al., 1956; Seidel & Joschko, 1991).

The cognitive processes assessed by the CPT are unclear. Most investigators agree that omission errors reflect deficits in sustained attention or vigilance (Halperin et al., 1991a). Commission errors appear to reflect a mixture of different underlying processes, including impulsivity and inattention/memory deficit (Halperin et al., 1991a).

Low-to-moderate correlations have been reported between various versions of the continuous-performance test and measures of attention, such as behavioral ratings/checklists, the Wechsler Freedom From Distractibility Factor (FFD), the Stroop, the

PASAT, and cancellation tests (Burg et al., 1995; Campbell et al., 1991; DuPaul et al., 1992; Halperin, 1991; Halperin et al., 1991a; Halperin et al., 1991b; Lassiter et al., 1994; Newcorn et al., 1989; Rasile et al., 1995; Seidel & Joschko, 1991; Thompson & Nichols, 1992). There are several reasons that the relationships between scores generated by various measures of attention such as rating scales, FFD, and CPTs are not very robust (Halperin, 1991; Halperin et al., 1991b; Thompson & Nichols, 1992). One possibility relates to the multidimensional nature of attention problems and the fact that the measures tap different aspects of attention. Another possibility is that, in addition to measuring attention, each measure assesses a wide range of other cognitive functions, which distinguishes it from the other measures. Thus, the common variance accounted for by attention may only amount to a small proportion of the total variance of these measures. A final possibility relates to differences in task and environmental demands. For example, rating scales are typically based on observations across extended time periods (e.g., several weeks), whereas CPTs usually take less than 15 minutes to complete. Thus, repeated testing procedures may be necessary to obtain a sample of behavior equivalent to that of other assessment measures.

Factors affecting vigilance performance include specific parameters of the task itself (e.g., subject expectancies, modality, interstimulus interval, signal to noise ratio), environmental or situational conditions during task performance (e.g., noise, presence of observers) and subject characteristics (Ballard, 1997a, 1997b).

Early studies suggested that performance on vigilance tasks was unrelated to IQ. Rosvold et al. (1956) reported that brain-damaged patients, whether retarded or with a relatively normal IQ, performed more poorly than retarded or normal-IQ individuals who were not brain-damaged, suggesting that the CPT was more directly associated with neurologic impairment than with low IQ. More recent studies suggest a consistent relation between better CPT performance and higher IQ scores (see Ballard, 1997a), raising the concern that the CPT is merely a crude measure of cognitive ability. CPT scores have also been linked with academic achievement (See Ballard, 1997a for review). Anxiety also affects CPT scores, particularly omissions (Ballard, 1997b).

Various versions of the CPT have been shown to distinguish between normal controls and certain patient groups including adults with head injuries (Burg et al., 1995), children with attention-deficit disorder, conduct disorder, learning disabilities, and those at high risk for schizophrenia (see Ballard, 1997a; Cornblatt and Keilp, 1994; Halperin et al., 1991a; Seidel & Joschko, 1990; for a review). Children with severe closed-head injuries have also been shown to demonstrate significantly poorer CPT scores than do mildly or moderately injured individuals six months after injury (Kauffman et al., 1993). In this study, the CPT revealed impaired attention that was not evident on the WISC-R Digit Span subtest. The Conners' CPT has been given to 670 clinical cases (children and adults) diagnosed with ADD/ADHD, comorbid cases (including ADD/ADHD as one of the diagnoses), and other diagnoses (e.g., oppositional defiant disorder, anxiety disorder) (Conners et al., 1995). The ADD/ADHD group scored most poorly, the comorbid group next, and the "other" group performed best. The ADD/ADHD group, however, was significantly different from the comorbid group on only one of the scores. An overall summary index derived from CPT measures misclassified 18 out of 200 clinical cases (9 percent false negative rate) and 35 out of 452 individuals in the general population (7.7 percent false positive). Sixty-eight out of a total of 720 clinical and general population cases over the age of 6 years (9.4 percent) were considered unclear cases, warranting further investigation. Cross-validation with different clinical data yielded false positive and negative rates of about 29 percent each.

There is some evidence that the task is sensitive to medication effects (Ritalin treatment) in attention deficit with hyperactivity. Kirby, Vandenberg, and Sullins (1993, cited in Conners et al., 1995) found that in children diagnosed as ADHD, reaction times were faster on medication than off medication; standard errors were significantly smaller; and percentage of hits was significantly higher.

Rezai et al. (1993) used single-photon-emission-computed tomography with the xenon-inhalation technique to compare activation of regional cerebral blood flow in frontal brain regions during the performance of four tests including the CPT (AX paradigm). In normal individuals, the CPT produced activation in the mesial frontal lobes bilaterally with somewhat greater activity on the left side.

The Conners' CPT has a number of advantages. First, it allows for considerable data to be gathered on a number of important measures. Second, detailed analyses of the various measures may be useful in describing the nature of the deficit and in distinguishing among different disorders. Third, the computerized nature of the task may appeal to some patients, particularly children. On the other hand, research on the validity and reliability of this version is somewhat limited. Further, the Connors' CPT and CPTs in general have not been shown to consistently discriminate between patient groups, and no diagnostic group has been shown to uniformly perform poorly on the CPT (DuPaul et al., 1992; Halperin et al., 1991b; Trommer et al., 1988). Therefore, while the inclusion of data from the CPT is an important component, diagnosis (for example, of hyperactivity) should not depend solely on this instrument.

Normative Data

Data for the Connors' CPT are based on 520 normal individuals, aged 4–70, and on 670 patients with a variety of attentional problems, aged 4–61 years. Demographic data provided on these samples are, however, sparse. Conners et al. (1995) report that 51.2 percent of the general population were male. Note that only 74 subjects were tested who were 18 years and older and that a high proportion of the adult sample (61 of 74, or 82.4 percent) was between the ages of 18 and 34 years. Until data for older adults become available, the CPT may be most useful for individuals between 6 and 30 years. For the clin-ical sample, 75.4 percent were male. The mean age of the patient sample was not reported.

Conners et al. (1995) reported that both age and sex affected many CPT measures. For example, as age increases, reaction times get faster, responses increase in consistency (SEs get lower), and commission and omission errors decrease. Therefore, the CPT scores should be evaluated relative to scores obtained by same-age and same-sex peers in the general population. Although data based on an ADHD group are provided, it is recommended that the general population norms be used as a basis for interpreting CPT results (Conners et al., 1995).

According to Conners et al. (1995), high omission-error rates indicate that an individual is not orienting or responding to stimuli, or that he or she has a very slow response. Reaction times averaging over 900 msec are considered sluggish responses. Normal adults and children tend to make most of their errors early on, learning to inhibit appropriately as the test continues. Further, by the end of the test, they tend to modulate their response tempos to conform to the amount of time given to respond (i.e., 1, 2, and 4 seconds). This can be determined by examining mean reaction times and standard errors over the six time blocks. Small standard errors indicate that the individual is adjusting his or her tempo. Thus, the inability to modulate responses, a slowing of response latency over time, or very fast responses in conjunction with a high error rate may indicate impulsive or inattentive behavior.

References

Ballard, J.C. (1997a). Computerized assessment of sustained attention: A review of factors affecting vigilance performance. *Journal of Clinical and Experimental Neuropsychology, 18,* 843–863.

Ballard, J.C. (1997b). Computerized assessment of sustained attention: Interactive effects of task demand, noise, and anxiety. *Journal of Clinical and Experimental Neuropsychology, 18,* 864–882.

Burg, J.S., Burright, R.G., & Donovick, P.J. (1995). Performance data for traumatic brain-injured subjects on the Gordon Diagnostic System (GDS) tests of attention. *Brain Injury, 9,* 395–403.

Campbell, J., D'Amato, R.C., Raggio, D.J., & Stephens, K.D. (1991). Construct validity of the computerized continous performance test with measures of intelligence, achievement, and behavior. *Journal of School Psychology, 29,* 143–150.

Conners, C.K., & Multi-Health Systems Staff. (1995). *Conners' Continuous Performance Test.* Toronto: MHS.

Cornblatt, B.A., & Keilp, J.G. (1994). Impaired attention, genetics, and the pathophysiology of schizophrenia. *Schizophrenia Bulletin, 20,* 31–46.

DuPaul, G.J., Anastopoulos, A.D., Shelton, T.L., Guevremont, D.C., & Metvia, L. (1992). Multimethod assessment of attention-deficit hyperactivity disorder: The utility of clinic-based tests. *Journal of Clinical Child Psychology, 21,* 394–402.

Gordon, M. (1983). *The Gordon Diagnostic System.* DeWitt, NY: Gordon Systems.

Halperin, J.M. (1991). The clinical assessment of attention. *International Journal of Neuroscience, 58,* 171–182.

Halperin, J.M., Wolf, I., Greenblatt, E.R., & Young, G. (1991a). Subtype analysis of commission errors on the continuous performance test in children. *Developmental Neuropsychology, 7,* 207–212.

Halperin, J.M., Sharma, V., Greenblatt, E., & Schwartz, S.T. (1991b). Assessment of the Continuous Performance Test: Reliability and validity in a nonreferred sample. *Psychological Assessment, 3,* 603–608.

Kaufmann, P.M., Fletcher, J.M., Levin, H.S., Miner, M.E., et al. (1993). Attentional disturbance after pediatric closed head injury. *Journal of Child Neurology, 8,* 348–353.

Lassiter, K.S., D'Amato, R.C., Raggio, J., Whitten, J.C., et al. (1994). The construct specificity of the Continuous Performance Test: Does inattention relate to behavior and achievement? *Development Neuropsychology, 10,* 179–188.

Newcorn, J.H., Halperin, J.M., Healey, J.M., et al. (1989). Are ADDH and ADHD the same or different? *Journal of the Academy of Child and Adolescence Psychiatry, 285,* 734–738.

Rasile, D.A., Burg, J.S., Burright, R.G., & Donovick, R.J. (1995). The relationship between performance on the Gordon Diagnostic System and other measures of attention. *International Journal of Psychology, 30,* 35–45.

Rezai, K., Andreasen, N.C., Alliger, R., Cohen, G., Swayze, V., & O'Leary, S. (1993). The neuropsychology of the prefrontal cortex. *Archives of Neurology, 50,* 636–642.

Rosvold, H.E., Mirsky, A.F., Sarason, I., Bransome, E.D. Jr., & Beck, L.H. (1956). A continuous performance test of brain damage. *Journal of Consulting Psychology, 20,* 343–350.

Seidel, W.T., & Joshko, M. (1990). Evidence of difficulties in sustained attention in children with ADDH. *Journal of Abnormal Child Psychology, 18,* 217–229.

Seidel, W.T., & Joschko, M. (1991). Assessment of attention in children. *The Clinical Neuropsychologist, 5,* 53–66.

Thompson, R.W., & Nichols, G.T. (1992). Correlations between scores on a continuous performance test and parents' ratings of attention problems and impulsivity in children. *Psychological Reports, 70,* 739–742.

Trommer, B.A., Hoeppner, J.B., Lorber, R., & Armstrong, K. (1988). Pitfalls in the use of a continuous performance test as a diagnostic tool in attention deficit disorder. *Developmental and Behavioral Pediatrics, 9,* 339–345.

d2 TEST: CONCENTRATION ENDURANCE TEST

Purpose

The purpose of this test is to assess sustained attention and visual scanning ability.

Source

The manual (7th ed. in German), recording sheets, and scoring key can be obtained from Hogrefe & Huber Publishers, P.O. Box 2487, Kirkland, WA 98083-2487, or 12–14 Bruce-park Avenue, Toronto, Ontario M4P 2S3, at a cost of about $28 US or $35 Cdn.

Description

This paper-and-pencil test was developed by Brickenkamp (1981) and modeled after other cancellation tasks (Bourdon, cited in Brickenkamp, 1981). It can be given individually or as a group measure. The test is composed of 14 lines with 47 letters each (see Figure 9–1).

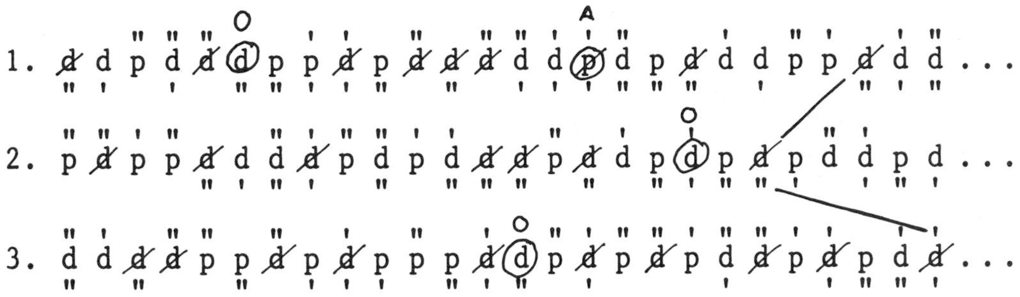

Figure 9–1. d2 Test sample.

The target is the letter "d" with two quotation marks (") either above, below, or separated, one mark (') above and one mark below. Distractors are the letter "p" with one to four marks and the letter "d" with one, three, or four marks. The subject's task is to mark as many targets per line as possible. The time limit is 20 seconds per line.

Administration

The instructions (translated by H. Niemann) are as follows: Place the front page in front of the subject. *"Now I want to see how well you can concentrate on a task. Look down here* (Point to the three "d's"). *You see three "d's" like in the word "dash". Each one has two dots. The first one has two dots above, the second two dots below, and the last one has one dot above and one dot below, so that makes two dots again for this letter. You should cross out all "d's" that have two dots. Now I want you to cross out these three "d's" in the example. Afterwards, go down to the practice row below and cross out every "d" with two dots. You should not cross out "d's" with less or more than two dots, and you should not cross out "p's", like in "Paul" regardless of the number of dots. Use only one slash for crossing out the correct letters. If you realize that you crossed out a wrong letter, put a second slash through it."* Demonstrate on the first four letters of the practice trial.

"Now let us see how well you did on this practice trial." Be sure that the subject has understood the instructions before continuing the test. Before turning the page over, say: *"On the back page you will find 14 rows like the practice row. On every row you will be asked to go from left to right crossing out every "d" with two dots. After 20 seconds, I will say, "Next line!". Then you have to stop crossing out on that line and start immediately at the beginning of the next line. Work as quickly as you can, but try to be as accurate as you can. Don't make mistakes!"* Turn the page over and point to the beginning of the first line and say: *"Ready, go!"*

Approximate Time for Administration

The time required is about 10 minutes.

Abbreviations

Abbreviations used in the manual are PR = Percentile Rank; SW = Standard Score; GZ = Total Score; GZ − F = Total Score − Errors; F% = Error Percentage; SB = Fluctuations; Erw = Adults; Vo = Volksschule (elementary school); Be = Berufsschule (occupational school); and Ob = Oberschule (high school).

Scoring

Several scores can be computed to evaluate the patient's speed, accuracy, persistence, and learning (see source). Briefly, the scoring is as follows:

Total Raw Score (TS or GZ in the Manual) refers to the number of letters the subject has considered regardless of errors. The number of letters per line must be added together in order to derive the Total Raw Score. Counting is facilitated by the use of an overlay.

Errors: Two types of errors are recorded:

1. *Omissions* refer to the number of "d's" with two dots that have been missed up to the last letter in every line that has been crossed out.

2. *Additions* refer to every "d" with less or more than two dots and every "p" that have been crossed out. The sum of Omissions and Additions equals the total number of errors (F) across all rows.

Percentage of Errors (F% in the Manual) is derived from the formula $F\% = 100 \times F/TS$.

Distribution of Errors:

1. Sum the number of errors for the first four rows.

2. Sum the number of errors for the last four rows.

Large differences between the first and last four rows may be due to shifts in test-taking attitude, practice effects, or fatigue.

Total Score Minus Errors (TS−F): This score is derived by subtracting the total number of errors (F) from the Total Score (TS) and represents the number of correctly crossed-out letters across all rows.

Fluctuation (FL) refers to *Schwankungsbreite* (SB) in the Manual. This measure is derived by subtracting the score for the row with the lowest rate of production (TS) from the row with the highest rate.

Comment

Internal consistency is reported to be high, above .8 (see source). Test-retest reliabilities are high, ranging from .89 to .92 for the total score after a 5-hour interval, and .92 for the total score minus errors after a 12-month interval (Brickenkamp, 1981). With normal people, practice effects of about 25 percent can be expected on retesting. However, Sturm et al. (1983) did not find any practice effects after retesting a group of brain-damaged subjects following a 4-week interval.

Brickenkamp (1981) reported that the Digit Symbol subtest of the WAIS was the only subtest that correlated significantly with the d2

Test ($r = .45$), suggesting that it is relatively independent of factors evaluated by standardized tests of intelligence. This is also confirmed by Jager (1973), although Wiese and Kroj (1972) reported higher correlations with the German WAIS in young adults (18–48 years). Correlations with other tests of attention and concentration ranged from .31 to .72, depending on the sample, the comparison measure, and the score used for the statistical analysis (Niemann, 1989). Factor analytic studies with normal people consistently report high loadings on an attentional factor, but not on factors of motor speed, motor coordination, or visual discrimination (Brickenkamp, 1981). Sherman and colleagues (1995) compared the WAIS-R factor scores of head-injured adults to various neuropsychological tests. Contrary to expectation, the d2 total score showed little relation with the Freedom From Distractibility factor ($r = .14$). It showed a moderate relation to the Perceptual Organization factor of the WAIS-R ($r = .32$).

Cancellation tasks assess many functions (Lezak, 1983), not the least of which is the capacity for sustained attention. In addition, accurate visual scanning and activation and inhibition of rapid responses are required. Lowered scores on cancellation tasks may reflect inattentiveness, general response slowing, problems with shifting of responses, or problems with unilateral spatial neglect.

Normative Data

Normative data given in the test manual are derived from rather large samples ($n = 3,132$) of normal students and adults, ages 9–60 years. Tables are provided for transforming the scores into percentiles, standard scores, stanines, and scaled scores. In the German school system, children are separated at age 11 into groups of average ability and higher academic potential. In the tables, "Vo" is like middle school and junior secondary school. The "Be" group are in vocational training settings, and the "Ob" group consists of students who are preparing for college. Consequently, when these tables are used for North American students, one should check the norms for the appropriate age at both kinds of schools.

Table 9—2. Total Raw Score and Errors for
Adults, Ages 50 to 85

Age	Sex	*n*	Total raw score		Errors	
			M	SD	M	SD
50–59	M	5	470.8	79.4	26.6	35.2
	F	14	403.0	87.7	11.4	6.5
60–69	M	4	420.3	53.6	44.0	27.6
	F	23	432.0	87.7	17.9	18.1
70–79	M	9	383.6	47.9	16.1	8.1
	F	14	360.2	76.0	27.9	36.1
80+	M	5	289.2	75.3	39.0	20.9
	F	6	360.0	70.3	63.5	56.3

Source: Our data, collected in 1989, are derived from a
sample of healthy, well-educated elderly volunteers.

We have collected normative data on a small
group of healthy well-educated (about 13
years) adults, ages 50–85. Table 9–2 shows the
data for two variables, Total Raw Score and
Errors, broken down by age and sex.

Sex, age, and intellectual level contribute
to performance on the d2 Test. In general, females perform better than males. Scores increase with age from TS-F = 240 at age 10 to
approximately 340–440 at age 17. Adult levels
are reached at about age 17. There is little decrement in scores until about age 40.

References

Brickenkamp, R. (1981). *Test d2:/Aufmerksam-
keits-Belastungs-Test* (Handanweisung, 7th ed.)
[Test d2: Concentration-Endurance-Test: Manual, 7th ed.]. Gottingen, Toronto, Zurich: Verlag
für Psychologie, C.J. Hogrefe.

Jager, R. (1973). Remarks on W. Wiese and G.
Kroj's article "Investigation on the relationship
between intelligence (Wechsler) and the ability
to concentrate (test d2) by R. Brickenkamp."
*Zeitschrift für Experimentelle und Angewandte
Psychologie, 20,* 572–574.

Lezak, M.D. (1983). *Neuropsychological Assessment* (2nd ed.). New York: Oxford University
Press.

Niemann, H. (1989). Computer-assisted retraining
of head-injured patients. Unpublished Ph.D.
dissertation. University of Victoria.

Sherman, E.M.S., Strauss, E., Spellacy, F., &
Hunter, M. (1995). Construct validity of WAIS-R
factors: Neuropsychological test correlates in
adults referred for possible head injury. *Psychological Assessment, 7,* 440–444.

Sturm, W., Dahmen, W., Hartje, W., & Wilmes,
K. (1983). Ergebnisse eines Trainingsprogramms
zur Verbesserung der visuellen Auffassungs-
schnelligkeit und Konzentrationsfähigkeit bei
Hirngeschädigten [Results of a program for the
training of perceptual speed and concentration
in brain-damaged patients]. *Archiv für Psychiatrie und Nervenkrankheiten, 233,* 9–22.

Wiese, W., & Kroj, G. (1972). Investigation on the
relationship between intelligence (Wechsler)
and ability to concentrate (test d2, Brickenkamp). *Zeitschrift für Experimentelle und Angewandte Psychologie, 19,* 690–699.

PACED AUDITORY SERIAL ADDITION TEST (PASAT)

Purpose

This test is a serial-addition task used to assess
capacity and rate of information processing
and sustained and divided attention.

Source

The tape (including instructions and sample
scoring sheet) can be ordered from the Neuropsychology Laboratory, University of Victoria, P.O. Box 1700, Victoria, BC V8W 2Y2,
Canada at a cost of $50 US. The Psychological
Corporation (555 Academic Court, San Antonio, TX 78204-2498 or 55 Horner Avenue,
Toronto, Ontario M8Z 4X6) offers a computerized version (IBM compatible) of the test
(disks) for $716.50 US or $1,255 Cdn. A
soundboard, microphone, and two speakers
are needed for this version. For children, the
CHIPASAT can be obtained from D. Johnson,
Department of Neuropsychology, Atkinson
Morley's Hospital, Copse Hill, London SW 20
0NE, U.K., at a cost of $50.

Description

This test was devised by Gronwall and colleagues (Gronwall & Sampson, 1974; Gron-

wall & Wrightson, 1974; Gronwall, 1977) to provide an estimate of the subject's rate of information processing (or the amount of information that can be handled at one time). The subject is required to comprehend the auditory input, respond verbally, inhibit encoding of his or her own response while attending to the next stimulus in a series, and perform at an externally determined pace. A prerecorded tape delivers a random series of 61 numbers from 1 to 9. The subject is instructed to add pairs of numbers such that each number is added to the one that immediately precedes it: the second is added to the first, the third to the second, the fourth to the third, and so on. For example, after the numbers "1,9" the answer is "10"; if the next number is "4", this is added to the previous "9" to give the answer "13"; and so on. The same 61 numbers, given in the same sequence, are presented in four different trials, each trial differing in its rate of digit presentation (2.4, 2.0, 1.6, 1.2 sec). The PASAT thus increases processing demands by increasing the speed of stimulus input. Duration of each spoken digit is about 0.4 seconds.

There are different versions of the test. For example, in the adaptation by Levin et al. (1987), 50 single digits are used in different random sequences for each of the four trials. A version of the PASAT has been developed for use with children (CHIPASAT) (Dyche & Johnson, 1991a, 1991b; Johnson et al., 1988). The CHIPASAT consists of tape-recorded single-digit numbers presented in five trials of differing speeds; 61 digits per trial, presented at speeds of one digit every 2.8, 2.4, 2.0, 1.6, 1.2 seconds. The sum of any number pair never exceeds 10 on this version.

Administration

Instructions are on the tape. For some very impaired subjects, the instructions may need to be expanded as follows:

Oral and Written Demonstration. "I am going to ask you to add together pairs of single-digit numbers. You will hear a tape-recorded list of numbers read one after the other. I will ask you to add the numbers in pairs and give your answers out loud. Al-

though this is really a concentration task, and not a test to see how well you can add, it might help to do a little adding before I explain the task in more detail. Please add the following pairs of numbers together as fast as you can and give your answers out loud: 3,8 (11); 4,9 (13); 7,8 (15); 8,6 (14); 8,9 (17); 5,7 (12); 6,5 (11); 6,9 (15); 4,7 (11); 7,6 (13). Good.

The task that I want you to do involves adding together pairs of numbers, just like you have done, except that the numbers will be read as a list, one after the other. Let me give you an example with a short, easy list. Suppose I gave you the following: 1,2,3,4. Here is what you would do. After hearing the first two numbers on the list, which were 1,2, you would add these together and give your answer, 1 + 2 = 3. The next number on the list is 3, so when you heard it, you would add this number to the number right before it on the list, which was 2, and give your answer, 2 + 3 = 5. Are you following so far? The last number you heard is 4 (Remember the list is 1,2,3,4), so you would add 4 to the number right before it, which was 3, and give your answer, 3 + 4 = 7. The important thing to remember is that you must add each number on the list to the number right before it on the list, and not to the answer you have just given. You can forget your answers as soon as you have said them. All you have to remember is the last digit that you have heard and add it to the next digit that you hear. O.K.? Let's try that short list again, only this time you say the answers. Ready? 1,2, (3), 3, (5), 4, (7). Now let's try another, longer practice list of numbers. This time the numbers on the list won't be in any particular order. Ready? 4,6, (10), 1, (7), 8, (9), 8, (16), 4, (12), 3, (7), 8, (11), 2, (10), 7, (9). Good."

If the subject has difficulty understanding the oral instruction, then provide a written demonstration. Say: *"That sounds complicated. Let me show you what I mean."* Write down a list of five numbers: 5, 3, 7, 4, 2 *"You see, you add the 5 and the 3 together, and say 8, then you have to forget the 8 and remember the 3. When the 7 comes along you add it to the 3, and say 10, and you have to remember the 7. All right, what do you say after 4?"* Continue until the subject understands what he or she is to do. Say: *"It's very easy when all the numbers are written down for you. Try it with me saying some numbers to you.* See above list. Discontinue if the subject is unable to get at least the first three answers from the unpaced practice list correct, after two trials.

Paced Practice. "Remember, I said the numbers would be tape-recorded? The task is not easy and no one is expected to get all of the answers right. The hard part is keeping up with the speed of the recording. However, if you can't answer in time, don't worry; just wait until you hear two more numbers, add them together and go on from there. O.K.? Any questions? I'll play a practice list of numbers and get you to give the answers." Play to the end of the first practice list.

Test Trials. "You see what I meant about the task measuring how well you can concentrate. It doesn't have anything to do with how smart you are. Now we'll try the first real trial. This trial is just the same as the practice trial you've just done, except that it is six times as long, so it goes on for almost two and a half minutes. Don't worry if you make adding mistakes or miss some answers. This is a difficult task. I want to see not only how long you can keep going without stopping, but also how quickly you can pick up again if you do stop. No one is expected to get all the answers. After this trial, we will take a break and then do another trial at a faster speed."

Play the first trial (at the rate of 2.4 seconds). Allow at least 60 seconds before playing the next trial. Warn the subject before each trial that it will be faster than the previous one.

Many patients find even the slow presentation trials (2.4, 2.0) difficult. Consequently, the two faster rates (1.6, 1.2) are given only if subjects perform adequately at the slower rates (above 20 at the pacing rate of 2.0) unless the subject scored more than 40 on the first trial (2.4 second pacing). Loudness should be well above threshold and adjusted to a comfortable listening level for each subject.

Follow-up Administrations (Retests). Do not repeat instructions, written demonstration,

or unpaced practice trial unless the subject demonstrates on the paced practice trial that he or she has forgotten what to do. Record this information.

Approximate Time for Administration

About 15–20 minutes are required if all four trials are given.

Scoring

See sample sheet (Figure 9–2). Record the number of correct and incorrect responses per trial (i.e., at the four pacing rates). To be correct, a response must be made before presentation of the next stimulus. The maximum score per trial is 60.

For subjects below the age of 40, convert the total correct scores to time per correct response using Table 9–3. There should be no more than a 0.6-second difference between the time scores if all four trials were given. If one trial differs by more than this, discard the data from that trial. If more than one trial differs by more than 0.6 seconds from all other trials, data from the whole session may be difficult to interpret.

The examiner should also compute the proportion of responses that were errors (sum across all trials). This proportion should be less than 10 percent. If the proportion exceeds 20 percent, the interpretation of results as a measure of attention is difficult. One can also compute the mean time score by averaging time scores for the four (or three, if one was discarded) trials.

Comment

The PASAT's split-half reliability is about .9, implying high internal consistency (Egan, 1988; Johnson et al., 1988). Cronbach's alpha from scores on the four PASAT trials is reported to be .90 (Crawford et al., in press). Performance measures across the different pacings are highly correlated (*r*'s between .76 and .95) (MacLeod & Prior, 1996). Test–retest correlations, following short re-test intervals (7 to 10 days) are high (>.9) (McCaffrey et al., 1995). There are, however, significant practice ef-

PASAT

Name _____ Date _____ Tested by _____

	2.4″	2.0″	1.6″	1.2″		2.4″	2.0″	1.6″	1.2″		2.4″	2.0″	1.6″	1.2″
7 (9)					8 (12)					5 (13)				
5 (12)					7 (15)					4 (9)				
1 (6)					1 (8)					8 (12)				
4 (5)					6 (7)					2 (10)				
9 (13)					3 (9)					1 (3)				
6 (15)					5 (8)					7 (8)				
5 (11)					9 (14)					5 (12)				
3 (8)					2 (11)					9 (14)				
8 (11)					7 (9)					1 (10)				
4 (12)					5 (12)					3 (4)				
3 (7)					3 (8)					6 (9)				
2 (5)					4 (7)					2 (8)				
6 (8)					7 (11)					9 (11)				
9 (15)					1 (8)					7 (16)				
3 (12)					5 (6)					8 (15)				
4 (7)					8 (13)					2 (10)				
5 (9)					3 (11)					4 (6)				
8 (13)					4 (7)					7 (11)				
6 (14)					6 (10)					6 (13)				
4 (10)					8 (14)					3 (9)				

	Total Correct	z	%ile	Time/Resp.	z	%ile
2.4″ pacing	_____	_____	_____	_____	_____	_____
2.0″ pacing	_____	_____	_____	_____	_____	_____
1.6″ pacing	_____	_____	_____	_____	_____	_____
1.2″ pacing	_____	_____	_____	_____	_____	_____

Figure 9—2. Paced Auditory Serial Addition Test sample scoring sheet.

fects (Gronwall, 1977). Normal subjects who are given the PASAT on two occasions, spaced one week apart, perform about six points higher on the second visit (Stuss et al., 1987). Similar practice effects have been reported in adults with traumatic brain injury (Stuss et al., 1989), HIV infection (McCaffrey et al., 1995), and in children (Dyche & Johnson, 1991a). Gronwall (1977) reports that after the second presentation, practice effects tend to be minimal. Feinstein et al. (1994), however, noted linear improvement over multiple sessions. Younger subjects (aged 25 to 30 years) improved over a longer period compared to their older counterparts (41 to 57 years) who plateaued after six sessions spaced 2 to 4 weeks apart.

The PASAT is thought to measure some central information-processing capacity simi-lar to that seen on reaction-time and divided-attention tasks (Gronwall & Sampson, 1974; Ponsford & Kinsella, 1992). Gronwall (1977) likens the deficit on this task to what a 65-year old man would have if suddenly confronted with the work schedule he had coped with at age 25. There is some corroborative evidence for construct validity. The test is moderately correlated to other measures of attention, such as Digit Span, Brown-Peterson Trigrams, d2 Test, Trail Making Test, Visual Search and Attention Test (VSAT), and Stroop test (Gronwall & Wrightson, 1981; Dyche & Johnson, 1991a; McLeod & Prior, 1996; O'Donnell et al. 1994; Sherman et al. 1997). Based on a factor analysis of test scores (WAIS-R, PASAT, RAVLT) of diabetics, Deary and colleagues (1991) argue that the PASAT loads highest on the third WAIS-R factor, Freedom From Distractibility

Table 9—3. PASAT Total Correct per Trial Converted to Time per Correct Response

n*	2.4"	2.0"	1.6"	1.2"	n*	2.4"	2.0"	1.6"	1.2"
1	144	120	96	72	31	4.7	3.9	3.1	2.3
2	72	60	48	36	32	4.5	3.8	3.0	2.3
3	48	40	32	24	33	4.4	3.6	2.9	2.2
4	36	30	24	18	34	4.2	3.5	2.8	2.1
5	28.8	24	19.2	14.4	35	4.1	3.4	2.7	2.1
6	24	20	16	12	36	4.0	3.3	2.7	2.0
7	10.6	17.1	13.7	10.3	37	3.9	3.2	2.6	2.0
8	18	15	12	9	38	3.8	3.2	2.5	1.9
9	16	13.3	10.7	8	39	3.7	3.1	2.4	1.9
10	14.4	12	9.6	7.2	40	3.6	3.0	2.4	1.8
11	13.1	10.9	8.7	6.6	41	3.5	2.9	2.3	1.8
12	12	10	8.0	6.0	42	3.4	2.9	2.3	1.7
13	11.1	9.2	7.4	5.5	43	3.3	2.8	2.2	1.7
14	10.3	8.6	6.9	5.1	44	3.3	2.7	2.2	1.6
15	9.6	8.0	6.4	4.8	45	3.2	2.7	2.1	1.6
16	9.0	7.5	6.0	4.5	46	3.1	2.6	2.1	1.6
17	8.5	7.1	5.7	4.2	47	3.1	2.6	2.0	1.5
18	8.0	6.7	5.3	4.0	48	3.0	2.5	2.0	1.5
19	7.6	6.3	5.1	3.8	49	3.0	2.5	2.0	1.5
20	7.2	6.0	4.8	3.6	50	2.9	2.4	1.9	1.4
21	6.9	5.7	4.6	3.4	51	2.8	2.4	1.9	1.4
22	6.5	5.5	4.4	3.3	52	2.8	2.3	1.9	1.4
23	6.3	5.2	4.2	3.1	53	2.7	2.3	1.8	1.4
24	6.0	5.0	4.0	3.0	54	2.7	2.2	1.8	1.3
25	5.8	4.8	3.8	2.9	55	2.6	2.1	1.7	1.3
26	5.5	4.6	3.7	2.8	56	2.6	2.1	1.7	1.3
27	5.3	4.4	3.6	2.7	57	2.5	2.1	1.7	1.3
28	5.1	4.3	3.4	2.6	58	2.5	2.1	1.7	1.2
29	5.0	4.1	3.3	2.5	59	2.4	2.0	1.6	1.2
30	4.8	4.0	3.2	2.4	60	2.4	2.0	1.6	1.2

*Number correct per trial.

Interpretation of Time Scores
N.B. Applies ONLY to ages between 14 and 40 years.
First Test: Control mean time score = 3.2 (SD = .25) on each trial
Subsequent Retests: Control mean time score = 2.6 (SD = .25) on each trial

Source: D. Gronwall. Reprinted with permission.

(FFD). Similar results have recently been reported by Crawford et al. (in press). Sherman and colleagues (1995) compared the PASAT to the WAIS-R factor scores of head-injured adults. They reported a correlation of .30 with the verbal comprehension factor, .23 with the perceptual organization factor, and .46 with the Freedom From Distractibility factor. Larrabee and Curtiss (1995) evaluated the factor structure of various tests of memory and information-processing ability in a group of outpatients. The PASAT loaded on the same factor as the WMS Mental Control and WAIS-R Digit Span subtests. Haslam et al. (1995) analyzed the performance of severely head-injured patients on the PASAT, Symbol Digit Modalities Test, Rey Auditory Verbal Learning Test, and Vocabulary subtest of the WAIS-R. The PASAT loaded on the same factor as the Symbol Digit Modalities Test. These findings provide additional support for the construct validity of the PASAT.

There is also some evidence that different PASAT speeds may index different processing stages. Deary et al. (1991) found that slower rates of presentation also correlated moderately with scores from the RAVLT, whereas a faster rate showed little correlation with memory measures. On the other hand, Sherman et al. (1997) found that in patients with mild-to-moderate head injury, the different PASAT trials were not consistently related to memory measures.

Gronwall claims that, although it is a cognitive task, the PASAT is only weakly correlated with arithmetic ability (.28) and general intelligence (.28) (Gronwall & Sampson, 1974; Gronwall & Wrightson, 1981; see also Dyche & Johnson, 1991a; Johnson et al., 1988; Roman et al., 1991). Egan (1988), Crawford et al. (in press), Deary et al. (1991), MacLeod & Prior, (1996) and Sherman et al. (1997), however, found that the PASAT shows a modest correlation with general intelligence and numerical ability (.41 to .68). Crawford et al. (in press) gave the PASAT and WAIS-R to a sample of 152 healthy individuals. Principal components analysis revealed that the PASAT's loading on general intelligence was substantial and exceeded that of many WAIS-R subtests. Sherman et al., (1997) have found that in head-injured patients, math-related tests (WAIS-R Arithmetic, WRAT-3 Mathematics) are the strongest unique predictors of PASAT performance suggesting that the test is possibly as much a test of mathematical ability as it is of attention. Verbal achievement (WRAT3 Reading) and complex motor skills (Purdue Pegs Assembly) emerged as lesser unique predictors, implying that adequate performance on the PASAT also requires adequate general cognitive ability and speed of processing. Thus, low PASAT performance should only be interpreted as an indicator of impaired information-processing capacity in the absence of poor performance on measures of mathematics, verbal ability/achievement, and complex motor skills. The implication is that the PASAT may only be suitable for high-functioning patients.

The PASAT can be quite a demanding and frustrating test, and the clinical impression is that it may also not be appropriate for excessively anxious individuals (Roman et al., 1991; Weber, 1986).

Some have suggested that the PASAT is sensitive to mild concussions (Gronwall & Sampson, 1974; Gronwall & Wrightson, 1974), is related to the patient's experience of symptoms (Gronwall, 1976), is related to a close associate's perception of change in the patient's personality (O'Shaughnessy et al., 1984), and is an indication of readiness to return to work (Gronwall, 1977). It also appears to be a more sensitive indicator of information-processing capacity in head-injured patients than other measures such as the Attention/Concentration Index of the Wechsler Memory Scale—Revised (Crossen & Wiens, 1988). Although it is a better predictor of subsequent memory difficulties than post-traumatic amnesia (PTA) (Gronwall, 1981), the PASAT is not primarily a memory task itself (Gronwall & Wrightson, 1981).

Not all studies are consistent with the view that the PASAT is sensitive to information-processing deficits in head-injured patients. A number of investigators (e.g., Levin et al., 1982; O'Shaughnessy et al., 1984; Sherman et al., 1997; Stuss et al., 1989) found no relation between the PASAT and measures of head-injury severity, such as PTA or loss of consciousness (LOC). For example, Stuss et al. (1989) found that in comparison to the PASAT and Trail Making Test, only the auditory Consonant Trigrams Task explained more than 30 percent of the shared variance in PTA and coma duration (43 percent and 30 percent, respectively) in a group with severe head injuries. In a mild-concussion group, indices of head-injury severity were not correlated with the PASAT, and only the Consonant Trigrams task distinguished patients from controls.

The PASAT's sensitivity to head injury may relate, at least in part, to the type of injury sustained. Roman et al. (1991) suggested that the PASAT's ability to detect head injury is best in samples where injury is secondary to marked acceleration/deceleration forces and concomitant subcortical involvement, such as that following motor vehicle accidents. Head injuries secondary to assault, therefore, where acceleration/deceleration forces are less marked, and associated subcortical or white matter damage is less extensive, are less likely to be associated with measurable impairments on the PASAT. Such an explanation, however, is unlikely to account for the findings of Sherman et al. (1997). Individuals involved in motor vehicle accidents comprised the majority

Table 9—4. Mean Number of Correct Responses at Each Age Range

| Presentation rate (in sec) | Age in years | | | | | |
| | 16–29 (n = 30) | | 30–49 (n = 30) | | 50–69 (n = 30) | |
	M	SD	M	SD	M	SD
2.4	47.4	10.1	43.4	10.2	43.5	13.6
2.0	42.0	12.5	41.9	10.2	35.6	14.6
1.6	36.0	13.0	33.1	12.2	30.8	15.9
1.2	27.4	9.9	24.6	10.6	21.2	14.4

Source: Stuss et al. (1988) provide normative data derived from a sample of healthy, relatively well-educated adults, ages 16–69 years.

of their sample. Nonetheless, in that study, PASAT scores were unrelated to PTA or LOC.

The PASAT is sensitive to dissimulation (Strauss et al., 1994). Persons attempting to feign the effects of brain injury perform more poorly than non-malingerers on the PASAT.

Overall, the PASAT appears to be an interesting measure, assessing some processes not tapped by other measures of attention. However, numerous weaknesses are also associated with the PASAT. One problem is its heavy demand on fast speech responses, a feature that prevents its use with dysarthric or other speech-impaired patients (Weber, 1986). Further, it may be a sensitive test of deficit in high functioning, mildly brain-injured patients, particularly those with acceleration/deceleration-type injuries, but it is not appropriate cognitively for low-functioning patients (Sherman et al., 1997; Weber, 1986), for those with mathematical deficits (Sherman et al.,

1997), or for excessively anxious ones (Roman et al., 1991).

Normative Data

Table 9–4 shows the mean number correct at different age ranges. The normative data are based on samples of healthy adults. The data shown for young adults are similar to those reported by others (e.g., Gronwall, 1977; Weber, 1986) but somewhat lower than those provided by Crawford et al. (in press) for a sample considered representative of the United Kingdom (ages 16–29, N = 38, mean Total PASAT = 169.2, SD = 30.12; ages 30–49, n = 78, mean Total PASAT = 149.8, SD = 40.29; ages 50–74, n = 36, mean Total PASAT = 136.9, SD = 43.79). Examination of Table 9–4 reveals that the faster the rate of presentation, the worse the performance, regardless of age. Although the table suggests that perfor-

Table 9—5. Regression Equations to Predict PASAT Scores from NART Plus Age and WAIS-R FSIQ Plus Age

| Predictors | Equations | Multiple R | SEest | Discrepancy required for one-tailed significance | | |
				.15	.10	.05
NART errors and Age	$215.74 - (1.85 \times NART) - (.77 \times Age)$	.52	34.87	35.9	44.6	57.2
WAIS-R FSIQ and Age	$12.87 + (1.65 \times FSIQ) - (.87 \times Age)$	.66	30.66	31.6	39.3	50.3

Source: Crawford et al. (in press).

Table 9—6. Children's Paced Auditory Serial Addition Task (CHIPASAT)

Age	CHIPASAT 2.4 Correct responses M	SD	%	Average speed of response in sec.	CHIPASAT 2.0 Correct responses M	SD	%	Average speed of response in sec.	CHIPASAT 1.6 Correct responses M	SD	%	Average speed of responses in sec.	CHIPASAT 1.2 Correct responses M	SD	%	Average speed of responses in sec.	CHIPASAT OVERALL Correct responses M	SD	%	Average speed of response in sec. M	SD
8–9 n = 51	22.5	5.5	37.5	6.8	19.4	6.5	32.4	7.0	16.4	6.4	27.4	7.0	9.9	5.2	16.5	11.6	17.1	5.5	28.5	8.1	5.0
9–10 yrs n = 58	27.1	7.1	45.2	5.7	23.0	6.6	38.3	5.9	19.8	6.5	33.0	5.7	13.1	5.9	21.8	7.9	20.7	5.8	34.6	6.3	3.1
10–11 yrs n = 60	30.5	8.3	50.9	5.1	26.2	7.1	43.7	5.0	20.8	6.3	34.6	5.3	14.9	5.9	24.8	5.9	23.1	6.2	38.5	5.3	1.9
11–12 yrs n = 51	33.8	8.5	56.3	4.6	28.3	7.2	47.2	4.5	23.1	6.2	38.4	4.5	16.6	5.4	27.7	5.0	25.5	6.2	42.4	4.6	1.4
12–13 yrs n = 36	32.3	9.1	53.8	5.1	29.6	7.9	49.4	4.9	24.4	7.4	40.6	5.3	16.1	6.8	26.8	4.7	25.6	7.0	42.7	4.4	1.2
13–14 yrs n = 51	37.4	9.4	62.4	4.2	33.4	10.1	55.7	4.1	27.7	9.1	46.1	3.9	19.3	7.4	32.2	4.7	29.4	8.4	49.1	4.2	1.8
14–15 yrs n = 8	41.1	9.9	68.5	3.7	38.3	8.0	63.8	3.3	31.5	6.8	52.5	3.2	20.6	5.7	34.4	3.8	32.9	6.9	54.8	3.5	0.9

Source: Johnson et al., 1988. Reprinted with permission from Elsevier Science Ltd.

mance declines with age, the correlation between age and performance on the PASAT is not significant (Stuss et al., 1987; see also Macleod & Prior, 1996; but see Crawford et al., in press). Performance is, however, correlated with education; the higher the educational level, the better the performance (Stuss et al., 1987; Stuss et al., 1989). Similarly, performance is related to mathematical ability (Sherman et al., 1997) and to IQ (Crawford et al., in press; Sherman et al., 1997).

Given the strength of the relation between PASAT and IQ, a low PASAT does not necessarily mean that the individual has a specific acquired deficit when the person has only a modest cognitive capacity. Conversely, an "average" score in a patient of above-average premorbid ability does not necessarily imply adequate attentional capacity. To assist with interpretation, Crawford et al. (in press) have developed regression equations that allow the clinician to compare PASAT performance with *current* general level of intellectual functioning and with NART estimated *premorbid* performance. The equations are provided in Table 9–5.

Brittain et al. (1991) provide data (total correct responses per trial as well as seconds per correct response) broken down by age and IQ, compiled from 526 normal healthy American adults, ages 17–88, on the Levin modification (Levin et al., 1987) of the PASAT. In contrast to the findings of Stuss et al. (1987), Brittain et al. report that education and race have little effect on performance; gender exerts minimal statistical significance (males perform slightly better than females), but the effect is not considered clinically meaningful; age and IQ have significant effects on PASAT performance. Younger subjects performed better than older subjects, particularly those aged 55 and above, and good Shipley performance was associated with good PASAT performance. Roman et al. (1991) gave the Levin version to a smaller group ($n = 143$) of normal subjects, ages 18–75 years. The norms were higher than those of Brittain et al.'s (1991) sample, perhaps reflecting education differences between the samples. Other findings were relatively similar to those reported by Brittain et al. (1991); namely, Roman and colleagues

noted no significant effect of gender. There was an age-related decline in performance, particularly after age 50. Modest correlations (.26–.38) were found between PASAT performance and IQ estimated from the Vocabulary and Block Design subtests of the WAIS-R.

Data for children, aged 8–14:6 years, on the CHIPASAT are provided by Johnson et al. (1988) and are shown in Table 9–6. Age, and to a lesser extent arithmetic ability, affected information-processing capacity. Older children achieve a greater number of correct responses in a given time than younger ones. Similarly, information-processing rate, as reflected in the average speed of response, improves with age, the greatest changes occurring in children under 10 years. Because young children may be less fluent in arithmetic, caution is needed in interpreting CHIPASAT performances of young children, especially those under 9 years, 6 months.

References

Brittain, J.L., La Marche, J.A., Reeder, K.P., Roth, D.L., & Boll, T.J. (1991). Effects of age and IQ on Paced Auditory Serial Addition Task (PASAT) performance. *The Clinical Neuropsychologist, 5*, 163–175.

Crawford, J.R., Obansawin, M.C., & Allan, K.M. (in press). PASAT and components of WAIS-R performance: Convergent and discriminant validity. *Neuropsychological Rehabilitation.*

Crossen, J.R., & Wiens, A.N. (1988). Residual neuropsychological deficits following head-injury on the Wechsler Memory Scale-Revised. *The Clinical Neuropsychologist, 2*, 393–399.

Deary, I.J., Langan, S.J., Hepburn, D.A., & Frier, B.M. (1991). Which abilities does the PASAT test? *Personality and Individual Differences, 12*, 983–987.

Dyche, G.E., & Johnson, D.A. (1991a). Development and evaluation of CHIPASAT, an attention test for children: II. Test-retest reliability and practice effect for a normal sample. *Perceptual and Motor Skills, 72*, 563–572.

Dyche, G.M., & Johnson, D.A. (1991b). Information-processing rates derived from CHIPASAT. *Perceptual and Motor Skills, 73*, 720–722.

Egan, V. (1988). PASAT: Observed correlations with IQ. *Personality and Individual Differences, 9*, 179–180.

Feinstein, A., Brown, R., & Ron, M. (1994). Effects

of practice of serial tests of attention in healthy adults. *Journal of Clinical and Experimental Neuropsychology, 16,* 436–447.

Gronwall, D. (1976). Performance changes during recovery from closed head injury. *Proceedings of the Australian Association of Neurologists, 5,* 72–78.

Gronwall, D.M.A. (1977). Paced auditory serial-addition task: A measure of recovery from concussion. *Perceptual and Motor Skills, 44,* 367–373.

Gronwall, D. (1981). Information processing capacity and memory after closed head injury. *International Journal of Neuroscience, 12,* 171.

Gronwall, D.M.A., & Sampson, H. (1974). *The Psychological Effects of Concussion.* New Zealand: Auckland University Press.

Gronwall, D., & Wrightson, P. (1974). Delayed recovery of intellectual function after minor head injury. *The Lancet, 2,* 605–609.

Gronwall, D., & Wrightson, P. (1981). Memory and information processing capacity after closed head injury. *Journal of Neurology, Neurosurgery, and Psychiatry, 44,* 889–895.

Haslam, C., Batchelor, J., Fearnside, M.R., Haslam, A.S., & Hawkins, S. (1995). Further examination of post-traumatic amnesia and post-coma disturbance as non-linear predictors of outcome after head injury. *Neuropsychology, 9,* 599–605.

Johnson, D.A., Roethig-Johnson, K., & Middleton, J. (1988). Development and evaluation of an attentional test for head-injured children: 1. Information processing capacity in a normal sample. *Journal of Child Psychology and Psychiatry, 2,* 199–208.

Larrabee, G.J., & Curtiss, G. (1995). Construct validity of various verbal and visual memory tests. *Journal of Clinical and Experimental Neuropsychology, 17,* 536–547.

Levin, H.S., Benton, A.L., & Grossman, R.G. (1982). *Neurobehavioral Consequences of Closed Head Injury.* New York: Oxford University Press.

Levin, H.S., Mattis, S., Ruff, R.M., Eisenberg, H.M., et al. (1987). Neurobehavioral outcome following minor head injury: A three-center study. *Journal of Neurosurgery 66,* 234–243.

MacLeod, D., & Prior, M. (1996). Attention deficits in adolescents with ADHD and other clinical groups. *Child Neuropsychology, 2,* 1–10.

McCaffrey, R.J., Cousins, J.P., Westervelt, H.J., Martnowicz, M., Remick, S.C., Szebenyi, S.,

Wagle, W.A., Bottomley, P.A., Hardy, C.J., & Haase, R.F. (1995). Practice effect with the NIMH AIDS abbreviated neuropsychological battery. *Archives of Clinical Neuropsychology, 10,* 241–250.

O'Donnell, J.P., MacGregor, L.A., Dabrowski, J.J., Oestreicher, J.M., & Romero, J.J. (1994). Construct validity of neuropsychological tests of conceptual and attentional abilities. *Journal of Clinical Psychology, 50,* 596–600.

O'Shaughnessy, E.J., Fowler, R.S., & Reid, V. (1984). Sequelae of mild closed head injuries. *The Journal of Family Practice, 18,* 391–394.

Ponsford, J., and Kinsella, G. (1992). Attentional deficits following closed-head injury. *Journal of Clinical and Experimental Neuropsychology, 14,* 822–838.

Roman, D.D., Edwall, G.E., Buchanan, R.J., & Patton, J.H. (1991). Extended norms for the Paced Auditory Serial Addition Task. *The Clinical Neuropsychologist, 5,* 33–40.

Sherman, E.M.S., Strauss, E., Spellacy, F., & Hunter, M. (1995). Construct validity of WAIS-R factors: Neuropsychological correlates in adults referred for possible head injury. *Psychological Assessment, 7,* 440–444.

Sherman, E.M.S., Strauss, E., & Spellacy, F. (1997). Testing the validity of the Paced Auditory Serial Addition Test (PASAT) in adults with head injury. *The Clinical Neuropsychologist, 11,* 34–45.

Strauss, E., Spellacy, F., Hunter, M., & Berry, T. (1994). Assessing believable deficits on measures of attention and information processing capacity. *Archives of Clinical Neuropsychology, 9,* 483–490.

Stuss, D.T., Stethem, L.L., & Poirier, C.A. (1987). Comparison of three tests of attention and rapid information processing across six age groups. *The Clinical Neuropsychologist, 1,* 139–152.

Stuss, D.T., Stethem, L.L., & Pelchat, G. (1988). Three tests of attention and rapid information processing: An extension. *The Clinical Neuropsychologist, 2,* 246–250.

Stuss, D.T., Stethem, L.L., Hugenholtz, H., & Richard, M.T. (1989). Traumatic brain injury: A comparison of three clinical tests and analysis of recovery. *The Clinical Neuropsychologist, 3,* 145–156.

Weber, M.A. (1986). Measuring attentional capacity. Unpublished Ph.D. Thesis. University of Victoria.

SYMBOL DIGIT MODALITIES TEST (SDMT)

Purpose

This test is used to assess visual scanning, tracking, and motoric speed and allows comparison between oral and written responses.

Source

The kit (including manual and 25 test forms) can be ordered from Western Psychological Services, 12031 Wilshire Blvd., Los Angeles, CA 90025-1251, at a cost of $60 US.

Description

This test, originally published in 1973 and revised in 1982, was developed by Aaron Smith as a measure for screening for cerebral dysfunction in children and adults. The test is similar to the Digit Symbol subtest of the Wechsler Intelligence Scale in requiring substitution under time constraints, but it alters the format by requiring that the patient examine a series of nine meaningless geometric designs and for each symbol in the sequence, search a key for that symbol and substitute a number, either orally or in writing, for the symbols. Group administration of the written form is possible.

Administration

The test form is placed before the patient, and the examiner reads the instructions that are provided in the SDMT manual. As in the Wechsler Digit Symbol subtest, 90 seconds are allowed to complete the trial. In the written version, the patient places the numbers in boxes below the marks according to the key provided at the top of the page. In the oral version, the examiner records the numbers spoken by the patient. When administering both forms of the test, the recommended procedure is to give the written version first.

Uchiyama et al. (1994) vary the procedure by giving an incidental recall task immediately following the written portion of the test. Clients are given a new sheet composed of a line of 15 symbols in which all nine original symbols are included at least once. The clients are asked to fill in the number associated with the symbol. In those cases where a symbol is presented more than once, and the client correctly identifies the number on one occasion and incorrectly on another, the client is given credit for the correct identification.

Approximate Time for Administration

About 5 minutes are required for the entire test.

Scoring

The score in both written and oral administrations of the test is the number of correct substitutions in each 90-second interval. The maximum score is 110 on each form.

Comment

Smith (1991) reports that 80 normal adults were given two administrations of the written and oral forms with an average retest interval of 29 days. The test-retest correlations were .80 for the written SDMT and .76 for the oral version. Gains of about four points were noted on retest for either version. Feinstein et al. (1994) gave a computerized version of the test to healthy volunteers who were tested at 2- to 4-week intervals over eight test sessions. Subjects showed a trend toward improvement in their performances over time. Uchiyama et al. (1994), however, noted no significant practice effects when the written version was given at yearly intervals over a 2-year period, suggesting relative stability over longer time intervals. Moderately large ($>.72$) correlations are reported.

In normal adults, the correlations between written and oral forms is above .78 (see source), suggesting that the two forms are fairly equivalent (see source). Ponsford and Kinsella (1992) reported that performance on the written version correlated .88 with performance on the oral version in head-injured patients. When the oral version was given to healthy children after the written version, a general tendency to produce higher oral scores was found for all age groups, with the largest score gains evident in the earlier years (source). These results must be viewed with caution, however, since written scores were obtained from group-administered tests, whereas oral scores were obtained from these same children using individual administration. Therefore, differences in performance might be attributable to differences in methods of testing (see source). Yeudall et al. (1986) gave both versions of the test to 225 healthy volunteers, aged 15–40 years. Oral scores were higher (about 11 points) than written ones, but order of test administration was not reported.

In addition to the standard versions (see source), other forms have been used (e.g., Feinstein et al., 1994; Hinton-Bayre et al., 1997; Royer et al., 1981; Uchiyama et al., 1994). Hinton-Bayre et al. (1997) have developed three new written forms that appear to be equivalent to the original. Feinstein et al. (1994) used a computerized version, while Royer et al. (1981) developed written versions that vary in difficulty (none were identical to the standard form). The version described by Uchiyama et al. (1994) consists of the same symbols as the standard version. Although the symbols are paired with different numbers in the test key, the order in which the symbols are presented in the alternate version is the same as in the standard version. Adult subjects were administered the test according to standard procedures. Total scores were significantly higher for the standard form (standard: 54.91, SD = 9.54; alternate: 52.82, SD = 10.33), whereas incidental recall scores were significantly higher for the alternate form (standard: 5.85, SD = 2.46; alternate: 6.39, SD = 2.51). Discrepancies were also noted between these two versions when they were examined longitudinally over the course of 2 years. Uchiyama et al. suggest that although the two versions differed on both initial and longitudinal testing, they may be of clinical and research utility when used with the appropriate normative data.

The SDMT is similar to the Wechsler Digit Symbol (DSym) subtest. For example, Lewandowski (1984) found a correlation of .62 between the SDMT and the Coding subtest of the WISC-R. Bowler et al. (1992) gave the WAIS-R DSym subtest and the written form of the SDMT to former microelectronics workers with organic solvent exposure and to unexposed comparison subjects. Scores between the tests correlated highly for the former workers ($r = .78$) and the comparison subjects ($r = .73$). Morgan and Wheelock (1992) gave both the SDMT and the DSym subtest of the WAIS to 45 individuals referred for neuropsychological examination. The written form of the SDMT and DSym scores correlated highly ($r = .91$). However, the SDMT yielded lower scores than the Dsym subtest, likely the result of different normative bases. Note that the DSym subtest may also be somewhat easier than the SDMT (Glosser et al., 1977). On DSym, cues to spatial location are contained in the key since stimulus items (digits) are arranged in arithmetic progression across the page. In the case of the SDMT, the sequence of symbols is random, with no cues to spatial location contained within the key (Glosser et al., 1977; Stones & Kozma, 1989).

The SDMT primarily assesses the scanning and tracking aspect of attention, tapping aspects of performance similar to those of Letter Cancellation, Trail Making, Digit Symbol, and choice reaction-time tests (McCaffrey et al., 1988; Ponsford & Kinsella, 1992; Shum et al., 1990). Motor speed and agility are also related to SDMT performance (Polubinski & Melamed, 1986).

The test is sensitive to brain insult in adults as well as children (see source; Lewandowski, 1984). Impaired performance has been associated with a number of conditions including long-standing epilepsy (Campbell et al., 1981); stroke (see source); organic solvent exposure (Bowler et al., 1992); Parkinson's disease (Starkstein et al., 1989); lack of excercise in older adults (Stones & Kozma, 1989); aging, general fitness, and the P3 component of event-related brain potentials (Emmerson et al., 1990); substance abuse (McCaffrey et al., 1988; O'Malley et al., 1992); and closed-head injury (Hinton-Bayre et al., 1997; Ponsford & Kinsella, 1992). No systematic differences between right- versus left-hemisphere-damaged groups have been observed (see source). Tsolaki et al. (1994) reported, however, that in patients diagnosed with multiple sclerosis, lesions in the internal capsule (as visualized on MRI) were related to SDMT performance.

Smith (see source) claimed that the SDMT was the most sensitive measure of cerebral integrity. In line with his view, Ponsford and Kinsella (1992) found that reaction-time tasks, the Stroop, and the PASAT were good discriminators of information-processing deficits in head-injured patients; however, the oral version of the SDMT was the single best measure of their reduced speed of processing. Pfeffer et al. (1981) found the SDMT to be the best discriminator among all tests (including a Mini-Mental State Test and the Raven Colored Progressive Matrices) used to discriminate between groups considered demented versus cognitively intact (that is, normal or depressed).

Performance on the SDMT also appears to be related to real-world functioning. Stenager et al. (1994) reported a significant correlation between the SDMT and the ability to read TV subtitles in patients with multiple sclerosis. No correlations were found with other measures such as the RAVLT, Trails, and Recurring Figures Test.

Although the SDMT appears to be sensitive to brain damage, performance can be depressed by other factors. For example, the medical-legal context may affect performance on the SDMT. Lees-Hayley (1990) gave the test to 20 personal injury litigants with no history of brain injury and no claim for brain injury. One half of the subjects scored in the potentially impaired range (that is, at or below −1.5 SD from the mean). Accordingly, caution is advised in the interpretation of SDMT scores of litigating clients.

Normative Data

Smith (Table 1 in source) provides data, by sex and age, based on a sample of 3,680 normal children, aged 8–17 years. The children were in the Omaha, Nebraska, school system. While the sample might be considered representative of urban Omaha, the scores may not be applicable to other populations. Note, too, that the mean scores for the written SDMT were obtained when this version was the initial or only test given. All written scores were derived from group administration of the test. The mean scores for the oral SDMT were obtained when this version was the only test given. Smith reported that both age and sex affected performance. Scores tend to improve with increasing age, and girls tend to outperform boys. In general, both boys and girls show consistently higher oral than written scores for ages 8–13 years. However, the difference between written and oral scores diminishes as age increases, particularly from ages 14–17 years.

Smith (see source) also provides data based on a sample of 1,307 normal adults, aged 18–78 years. Note that the data for the oral form are based on the "retest" version, given shortly after the written form. The SDMT manual (Table 2 in source) presents the means and standard deviations by age and educational level. The influence of gender was judged not to be of sufficient magnitude (that is, less than one-third of a standard deviation difference between sexes) to justify separate male and female norms.

Smith (see source) suggests that SDMT scores 1–1.5 SD below the mean age norms should be considered suggestive of cerebral dysfunction. A table is provided in the SDMT manual (Table 3 in source) that shows the raw scores at each of several points in the distribution of scores for each subgroup, ranging from −3.0 SD below the mean to +3.0 SD above the mean.

Richardson and Marottoli (1996) provide normative information on the written version for individuals beyond age 75 years. The data derive from a sample of urban drivers (mean age = 81.47, SD = 3.3; mean education = 11.02, SD = 3.68) and are shown in Table 9–7.

Yeudall et al. (1986) provide data for both written and oral administrations based on a sample of healthy, well-educated volunteers of above average IQ, aged 15–40 years. The data are stratified by age and sex. The data for the written form are similar to those reported by Smith (see source) and Uchiyama et al. (1994). The oral scores are somewhat higher than those reported by Smith, perhaps reflecting differences in intellectual status between the samples.

Table 9—7. SDMT Means and Standard
Deviations for Elderly Individuals

	Age 76–80		Age 81–91	
Education	<12	>12	<12	>12
n	26	24	18	33
Mean	20.08	32.75	21.25	28.84
SD	9.08	10.16	9.48	8.93

Source: Richardson & Marottoli, 1996. Reprinted with
permission.

Nielsen et al. (1989) give data on the written
version based on a sample of 101 Danish individuals, most of whom were undergoing minor surgery (mean WAIS-R IQ = 98.61, SD =
12.21). The scores are somewhat lower than
those reported by Smith, possibly the result of
differences in cultural and general intellectual
factors. The possible influence of psychological distress should also be kept in mind.

In adults, age, IQ, education, and ethnicity
affect performance. Scores decline with advancing age on both written and oral forms
(see source; Bowler et al., 1992; Emmerson et
al., 1990; Feinstein et al., 1994; Gilmore et
al., 1983; Richardson & Marottoli, 1996;
Selnes et al., 1991; Stones & Kozma, 1989;
Uchiyama et al., 1994; Yeudall et al., 1986),
perhaps reflecting changes in speed of motor
components and speed of two information-
processing operations: symbol encoding and
visual search (Gilmore et al., 1983). Scores improve with increasing IQ (Nielsen et al., 1989;
Uchiyama et al., 1994; Waldmann et al., 1992;
Yeudall et al., 1986), underscoring the need to
consider intellectual level, particularly when
dealing with low-ability individuals (that is,
IQs less than 80). Further, better-educated
subjects (13 years of school or more) have
higher scores than less-educated individuals
(12 years of school or less) (see source; Richardson & Marottoli, 1996; Selnes et al., 1991;
Uchiyama et al., 1994; Yeudall et al., 1986).
Although some have not found gender differences (Gilmore et al., 1993; Waldmann et al.,
1992), others have reported that females outperform males (see source; Polubinski &
Melamed, 1986; Yeudall et al., 1986). Aspects
of motor ability may be involved in the sex-
related difference in performance (Polubinski

& Melamed, 1986). Hand preference may
moderate performance, but it has no direct
impact on oral test scores (Polubinski &
Melamed, 1986).

References

Bowler, R., Sudia, S., Mergler, D., Harrison, R.,
& Cone, J. (1992). Comparison of Digit Symbol
and Symbol Digit Modalities Tests for assessing
neurotoxic exposure. *The Clinical Neuropsychologist, 6,* 103–104.

Campbell, A.L. Jr., Bogen, J.E., & Smith, A.
(1981). Disorganization and reorganization of
cognitive and sensorimotor functions in cerebral
commissurotomy. *Brain, 104,* 493–511.

Emmerson, R.Y., Dustman, R.E., Shearer, D.E.,
& Turner, C.W. (1990). P3 latency and Symbol
Digit performance correlations in aging. *Experi-
mental Aging Research, 15,* 151–159.

Feinstein, A., Brown, R., & Ron, M. (1994). Effects
of practice on serial tests of attention in healthy
subjects. *Journal of Clinical and Experimental
Neuropsychology, 16,* 436–447.

Gilmore, G.C., Royer, F.L., & Gruhn, J.J. (1983).
Age differences in symbol-digit substitution task
performance. *Journal of Clinical Psychology, 39,*
114–124.

Glosser, G., Butters, N., & Kaplan, E. (1977).
Visuoperceptual processes in brain-damaged patients on the Digit Symbol Substitution task. *International Journal of Neuroscience, 7,* 59–66.

Hinton-Bayre, A.D., Geffen, G., & McFarland, K.
(1997). Mild head injury and speed of information processing: A prospective study of professional rugby league players. *Journal of Clinical
and Experimental Neuropsychology, 19,* 275–
289.

Lees-Haley, P.R. (1990). Contamination of neuropsychological testing by litigation. *Forensic Reports, 3,* 421–426.

Lewandowski, L.J. (1984). The Symbol Digit Modalities Test: A screening instrument for brain-
damaged children. *Perceptual and Motor Skills,
59,* 615–618.

McCaffrey, R.J., Krahula, M.M., Heimberg, R.G.,
Keller, K.E., & Purcell, M.J. (1988). A comparison of the Trail Making Test, Symbol Digit Modalities Test, and the Hooper Visual Organization Test in an inpatient substance abuse
population. *Archives of Clinical Neuropsychology, 3,* 181–187.

Morgan, S.F., & Wheelock, J. (1992). Digit Symbol and Symbol Digit Modalities Tests: Are they

directly interchangeable? *Neuropsychology, 6*, 327–330.

O'Malley, S., Adams, M., Heaton, R.K., & Gawin, F. (1992). Neuropsychological impairment in chronic cocaine abusers. *American Journal of Drug and Alcohol Abuse, 18*, 131–144.

Nielsen, H., Knidsen, L., & Daugbjerg, O. (1989). Normative data for eight neuropsychological tests based on a Danish sample. *Scandinavian Journal of Psychology, 30*, 37–45.

Pfeffer, R.I., Kuroskai, T.T., Harrah, C.H., Jr., Chance, J.M., et al. (1981). A survey diagnostic tool for senile dementia. *American Journal of Epidemiology, 114*, 515–527.

Polubinski, J.P., & Melamed, L.E. (1986). Examination of the sex difference on a symbol digit substitution task. *Perceptual and Motor Skills, 62*, 975–982.

Ponsford, J., & Kinsella, G. (1992). Attentional deficits following closed head injury. *Journal of Clinical and Experimental Neuropsychology, 14*, 822–838.

Richardson, E.D., & Marottoli, R.A. (1996). Education-specific normative data on common neuropsychological indices for individuals older than 75 years. *The Clinical Neuropsychologist, 10*, 375–381.

Royer, F.L., Gilmore, G.C., & Gruhn, J.J. (1981). Normative data for the symbol substitution task. *Journal of Clinical Psychology, 37*, 608–614.

Selnes, O.A., Jacobson, L., Machado, A.M., Becker, J.T., Wesch, J., Miller, E.N., Visscher, B., & McArthur, J.C. (1991). Normative data for a brief neuropsychological screening battery. *Perceptual and Motor Skills, 73*, 539–550.

Shum, D.H.K., McFarland, K.A., & Bain, J.D. (1990). Construct validity of eight tests of attention: Comparison of normal and closed head injured samples. *The Clinical Neuropsychologist, 4*, 151–162.

Smith, A. (1991). *Symbol Digit Modalities Test*. Los Angeles: Western Psychological Services.

Starkstein, S.E., Bolduc, P.L., Presiosi, T.J., & Robinson, R.G. (1989). Cognitive impairments in different stages of Parkinson's disease. *Journal of Neuropsychiatry and Clinical Neurosciences, 1*, 243–248.

Stenager, E., Knudsen, L., & Jensen, K. (1994). Multiple sclerosis: Methodological aspects of cognitive functioning. *Acta Neurologica Belgica, 94*, 53–56.

Stones, M.J., & Kozma, A. (1989). Age, exercise, and coding performance. *Psychology and Aging, 4*, 190–194.

Tsolaki, M., Drevelegas, A., Karachristianou, S., Kapinas, K., Divanoglou, D., & Roustonis, K. (1994). Correlation of dementia, neuropsychological and MRI findings in multiple sclerosis. *Dementia, 5*, 48–52.

Uchiyama, C.L., D'Elia, L.F., Dellinger, A.M., Selnes, O.A., Becker, J.T., Wesch, J.E., Chen, B.B., Satz, P., Van Gorp, W., & Miller, E.N. (1994). Longitudinal comparison of alternate versions of the Symbol Digit Modalities Test: Issues of form comparability and moderating demographic variables. *The Clinical Neuropsychologist, 8*, 209–218.

Waldmann, B.W., Dickson, A.L., Monahan, M.C., & Kazelskis, R. (1992). The relationship between intellectual ability and adult performance on the Trail Making Test and the Symbol Digit Modalities Test. *Journal of Clinical Psychology, 48*, 360–363.

Yeudall, L.T., Fromm, D., Reddon, J.R., & Stefanyk, W.O. (1986). Normative data stratified by age and sex for 12 neuropsychological tests. *Journal of Clinical Psychology, 42*, 918–946.

VISUAL SEARCH AND ATTENTION TEST (VSAT)

Purpose

This test is used to assess visual scanning and sustained attention in adults.

Source

The test (including manual and 25 test booklets) can be ordered from Psychological Assessment Resources, P.O. Box 998, Odessa, Florida 33556, at a cost of $58 US.

Description

This test was developed by Trenerry, Crosson, DeBose, and Leber (1990) and consists of four different cancellation tasks. The first two tasks (1 and 2) serve as practice trials and require that the patient cross out a letter or symbol that matches the target. Tasks 3 and 4 require the patient to cancel blue Hs and blue slashes from an array of letters or symbols printed in blue, green, or red ink. Each task consists of

10 rows, each containing 40 stimuli. There are 10 randomly placed targets in each row. The tasks are oriented horizontally, one task per page, on $11 \times 8\frac{1}{2}$ inch paper. The target is centrally located at the top of each page. Each task is timed and allows 60 seconds for the patient to respond.

Although only Tasks 3 and 4 are scored, Tasks 1 and 2 should be given since the normative data were collected under the condition that all four tasks were administered in order. The VSAT provides an overall attention score and also provides separate scores for left- and right-side performance that may be useful in assessing visual field defects and spatial neglect syndromes.

Administration

The examiner places the Test Booklet in front of the respondent, checks color discrimination (using a color strip located on the front of the booklet), and directs the patient's attention to the relevant task targets. Instructions for administration and timing are provided in the VSAT manual. The authors warn that the VSAT should not be given to patients who have physical disabilities that would adversely affect performance (e.g., patients who cannot distinguish colors; hemiparesis of the dominant hand).

Approximate Time for Administration

The test takes about 6 minutes to administer.

Scoring

For Tasks 3 and 4, the examiner draws a vertical line from the centrally placed target to just below the last row of stimuli, dividing each row of the task stimuli in half. The examiner records for each task the number of targets correctly canceled on each side, within the time limit. The sum of the left-side raw scores (L3 and L4), the sum of the right-side raw scores (R3 and R4), and the total raw score (Left and Right) are recorded on the face sheet of the Test Booklet. Percentile scores are used to interpret a patient's performance on the VSAT.

Comment

Trenerry et al. (1990) gave the VSAT to 28 normal individuals on two separate occasions, with an average retest interval of about 2 months. Test-retest reliability was .95. Practice, however, had a significant impact on performance, with gains of about 15 points recorded for total scores.

Trenerry et al. (1990) administered the WAIS-R and Category Test to a sample of brain-damaged individuals (sample sizes varied from 41 to 75 depending on the measure). Moderate correlations were noted between the VSAT and the Category Test errors ($-.52$), Block Design (.54), Digit Symbol (.65), Vocabulary (.30), and Digit Span (.24) subtests. O'Donnell et al. (1994) administered the VSAT along with the Category Test, WCST, PASAT, and Trail Making Test (part B) to 117 adults, aged 18–61 years, referred for neuropsychological examination. Modest correlations (.20–.30) were reported between the VSAT and the other tasks. Principal components analysis showed that the VSAT, PASAT, and Trails-B defined an attention factor, whereas the Category Test and WCST loaded on a conceptual factor. Thus, the VSAT appears to be measuring a component similar to that of other measures of attention, but the tests are not interchangeable.

According to Trenerry et al. (1990), Tasks 3 and 4 provided good discrimination between 272 normal and 100 brain-damaged individuals (overall hit rates above .84). Meaningful differences between Left and Right raw scores occurred infrequently in this sample and were unrelated to side of lesion or type of brain damage. Accordingly, the authors caution that performance on the VSAT should not be the sole measure of determining whether a specific syndrome (e.g., unilateral neglect) exists. As yet, no other studies with neurological populations are available.

Normative Data

Trenerry et al. (1990) report that in normal adults, VSAT scores are influenced by age. There is a decline in performance with advancing age. Sex and education did not have unique contributions. Normative data are based on a sample of 272 healthy adults (89 males and 183 females) ranging in age from 18 through 85 years. Percentile scores for six separate age groups (18–19, 20–29, 30–39, 40–19, 50–59, 60+) are provided in the VSAT manual. Normative data are provided for the total score as well as for the Left and Right scores. The patient's Left and Right scores can be compared to those of the normative sample by examining Left and Right percentile scores. Similarly, the Left and Right raw scores can be compared to each other. Trenerry et al. (1990) reported that the mean difference between Left and Right raw scores in the normative sample was approximately 4 (SD = 3). Young adults (age 20–30) typically obtain a total score of about 166/200 with 84/100 correct on the Left side and 82/100 on the right side. In elderly individuals, the average total score is lower (about 100/200), and the mean difference is about 5 points between left- and right-side scores.

References

O'Donnell, J.P., MacGregor, L.A., Dabrowski, J.J., Oestreicher, J.M., & Romero, J.J. (1994). Construct validity of neuropsychological tests of conceptual and attentional abilities. *Journal of Clinical Psychology, 50*, 596–600.

Trenerry, M.R., Crosson, B., DeBoe, J., & Leber, W.R. (1990). *Visual Search and Attention Test.* Odessa, FL.: Psychological Assessment Resources.

10

Memory

Memory is a complex process by which the individual registers, retains, and retrieves information. The literature suggests that short-term (or working) memory has a structural basis different from that of long-term memory. Moreover, retrieval processes are supported by multiple systems including explicit or declarative memory and implicit or procedural memory (Kolb & Whishaw, 1995; Schacter & Tulving, 1994). Explicit memory entails intentional or conscious recollection of previous experiences. In a typical explicit memory task, the patient is shown a series of words, pictures, or some other set of to-be-remembered material and is later given a recall or recognition test that requires the patient to think back to the study episode in order to produce or select a correct response (Schacter et al., 1993). Implicit memory, by contrast, refers to a heterogeneous collection of abilities (e.g., skill learning, habit formation, priming) involving a facilitation or change in test performance that is attributable to information or skills acquired during a prior study episode, even though the patient is not required to, and may even be unable to recollect the study phase. Implicit memory is assessed by examining the impact of study episodes on subsequent performance of tasks that do not require recollection of those episodes, such as completing a word fragment, choosing which of two stimuli the patient prefers, or reading inverted text (Schacter et al., 1993). Damage to the temporal-limbic system is thought to disrupt the formation/retrieval of new explicit memories but spare old and implicit memories. Implicit memory functions are considered to be independent of the hippocampal system. Unfortunately, most of the standard neuropsychological tests evaluate declarative as opposed to implicit memory.

In order to test different diagnostic hypotheses and facilitate efforts of rehabilitation, the memory examination should cover immediate or short-term retention, rate and pattern of acquisition of new information, efficiency of encoding under both explicit and incidental conditions, efficiency of retrieval of both recently learned and remote information, retrieval under both explicit and implicit conditions, rate of decay of information, and proactive and retroactive interference. Further, these component processes should be evaluated for both verbal and nonverbal domains, using both recall and recognition techniques since inferences about the relative integrity of encoding and retrieval processes are usually made by contrasting free recall and recognition performance.

Clinicians often turn to an assortment of materials and procedures to evaluate meaningful components of memory. When *batteries* are considered, the Wechsler Memory Scale (WMS, Wechsler, 1945) or the Wechsler Memory Scale—Revised (WMS-R; Wechsler, 1987) may offer a first step in the assessment of explicit memory. The WMS-R is an improvement over its predecessor in terms of task content, adequacy of scoring criteria and normative data. However, a wealth of data has accumulated with the WMS, and clinicians frequently rely on the original version. Accordingly, we present both versions. For children, the Wide Range Assessment of Memory and Learning (Adams & Sheslow, 1990) can be used. The Rivermead Behavioral Memory Test (Wilson, Cockburn, & Baddeley, 1985) is useful for detecting impairment in everyday memory functioning in both adults and children, even in the presence of other difficulties (e.g., language or perceptual problems). The inclusion of prospective memory tasks is also particularly appealing. The Colorado Neuropsychology Tests (Davis et al., 1995), while technically not a battery, are a computerized collection of tests that assess explicit as well as implicit memory. In addition to standard measures of recall and recognition, the battery includes Towers of Hanoi, Toronto, and London, a test of mirror-reading as well as a measure of priming.

As Lezak (1995) notes, an advantage of some batteries is that they review a number of different components of memory and, at the same time, allow for intersubtest comparisons. On the other hand, they can be time-consuming to give, and all subtests may not be relevant to a patient's problems. Further, they do not tap all critical aspects of memory and may therefore miss the crucial features relevant for a particular patient. The availability of a host of new and sophisticated *individual tests* allows the knowledgeable examiner the flexibility to tailor the examination in an efficient manner, sampling particular domains and selecting those tasks most appropriate for a specific patient.

Verbal memory tests, such as the Consonant Trigrams (Brown, 1958; Peterson & Peterson, 1959), Sentence Repetition (Spreen & Benton, 1977), the Selective Reminding Test (SRT; Bushke, 1973; Bushke & Fuld, 1974), the California Verbal Learning Test (CVLT; Delis et al., 1987; Delis et al., 1994), and the Rey Auditory Verbal Learning Test (RAVLT; Rey, 1964) can be used to delineate the specific component processes that are affected. The Consonant Trigrams and Sentence Repetition tests assess attention/short-term memo-

ry, whereas the other tests are supra-span word-list learning tasks that include measures of immediate and long-term recall and recognition, increased vulnerability to proactive and retroactive interference, and also reveal learning ability. Although the CVLT yields more information about multiple aspects of learning/memory, the RAVLT or SRT have more adequate normative data as well as alternate forms.

Clinical assessment of visuospatial memory typically relies on the brief presentation of visual designs followed by recall or recognition at varying length of delay. Commonly used measures are the Benton Visual Retention Test (BVRT; Sivan, 1992) and the Recognition Memory Test (Warrington, 1984). The Brief Visuospatial Memory Test—Revised (BVMT-R; Benedict, 1997) is a new nonverbal analog to the widely used supra-span word-list learning technique. Some of the tests of visuospatial memory confound the effects of visuoperceptual and constructional impairments with possible disorders in memory. The inclusion of both multiple-choice (e.g., BVRT, BVMT-R) and copy (BVRT) administrations may help the examiner to discriminate among perceptual, constructional, and memory disorders.

The verbal and nonverbal tests considered above assess learning/memory under explicit encoding conditions. However, much of learning occurs incidentally, without directed effort. The Rey-Osterrieth Complex Figure (Rey, 1941; Osterrieth, 1944) is a test of incidental learning. Measures such as the Wechsler Digit Symbol subtest (Collaer & Evans, 1982; Hultsch et al., 1997; Kaplan et al., 1991) and the Symbol Digit Modalities Test (Uchiyama et al., 1994) have also been adapted to provide not only the standard scores but also measures of incidental learning.

The tests discussed above relate to anterograde memory, that is, the ability to retain information beginning with the onset of the disorder. Neuropsychological assessment of remote or retrograde memory (that is, the ability to retrieve information that was acquired prior to the onset of the insult) can be approached in a number of ways. The Crovitz and Schiffman technique (1974) requires the patient to describe past incidents in response to cue words provided by the examiner. The patient's recollections are evaluated for their vividness, as well as their temporal and locational specificity. A limitation of this technique (Brandt & Benedict, 1993; Kopelman et al., 1989) is the fact that there is no way to determine whether a subject's remote memory is temporally graded because time periods are not sampled systematically. Remote memory tests that use public events (e.g., Albert et al., 1979; Brandt & Benedict, 1993) avoid this difficulty but may become out of date and require frequent restandardization. We describe here another technique for examining personal remote memory, the Autobiographical Memory Interview (AMI) (Kopelman et al., 1990). It is a semistructured interview that allows quantification of both the patient's personal semantic memory (e.g., names of schools) and episodic memory (e.g., specific incidents that occurred while in high school) from childhood (ages 2–18 years), early adulthood (ages 19–39), and recent years (last 5 years).

References

Adams, W., & Sheslow, D. (1990). *WRAML Manual*. Wilmington, DE: Jastak Associates.

Albert, M.S., Butters, N., & Levin, J.A. (1979). Temporal gradients in the retrograde amnesia of patients with alcoholic Korsakoff's disease. *Archives of Neurology, 36*, 211–216.

Benedict, R.H.B. (in press). Brief Visuospatial Memory Test—Revised. Odessa, FL: Psychological Assessment Resources.

Brandt, J., & Benedict, R.H.B. (1993). Assessment of retrograde amnesia: Findings with a new public events procedure. *Neuropsychology, 7*, 217–227.

Brown, J. (1958). Some tests of the decay of immediate memory. *Quarterly Journal of Experimental Psychology, 10*, 12–21.

Bushke, H. (1973). Selective reminding for analysis of memory and learning. *Journal of Verbal Learning and Verbal Behavior, 12*, 543–550.

Bushke, H., & Fuld, P. (1974). Evaluating storage, retention, and retrieval in disordered memory and learning. *Neurology, 24*, 1019–1025.

Collaer, M.L., & Evans, J.R. (1982). A measure of short-term visual memory based on the WISC-R Coding subtest. *Journal of Clinical Psychology, 38*, 641–644.

Crovitz, H.F., & Schiffman, H. (1974). Frequency of episodic memories as a function of their age. *Bulletin of the Psychonomic Society, 4*, 517–518.

Davis, H.P., Bajszar, G.M., & Squire, L.R. (1995). *Colorado Neuropsychology Tests*. Colorado Springs, CO: Colorado Neuropsychology Company.

Delis, D.C., Kramer, J.H., Kaplan, E., & Ober, B.A. (1987). *California Verbal Learning Test: Adult Version Manual*. San Antonio, TX: The Psychological Corporation.

Delis, D.C., Kramer, J.H., Kaplan, E., & Ober, B.A. (1994). *CVLT-C: California Verbal Learning Test—Children's Version*. San Antonio, TX: The Psychological Corporation.

Hultsch, D., Dixon, R., & Hertzog, C. (1997). Unpublished data.

Kaplan, E., Fein, D., Morris, R., & Delis, D.C. (1991). *WAIS-R NI Manual*. San Antonio, TX: The Psychological Corporation.

Kolb, B., & Whishaw, I.Q. (1995). *Fundamentals of Human Neuropsychology* (4th ed.). New York: W.H. Freeman.

Kopelman, M.D., Wilson, B.A., & Baddeley, A.D. (1989). The Autobiographical Memory Interview: A new assessment of autobiographical and personal semantic memory in amnesic patients. *Journal of Clinical and Experimental Neuropsychology, 11*, 724–744.

Kopelman, M., Wilson, B., & Baddeley, A. (1990). *The Autobiographical Memory Interview*. Bury St. Edmunds, England: Thames Valley Test Company.

Lezak, M.D. (1995). *Neuropsychological Assessment* (3rd ed.). New York: Oxford University Press.

Osterrieth, P.A. (1944). Le test de copie d'une figure complex: Contribution à l'étude de la perception et de la mémoire. *Archives de Psychologie, 30*, 286–356.

Peterson, L.R., & Peterson, M.J. (1959). Short-term retention of individual verbal items. *Journal of Experimental Psychology, 58*, 193–198.

Rey, A. (1964). *L'examen clinique en psychologie*. Paris: Press Universitaire de France.

Rey, A. (1941). L'examen psychologique dans les cas d'encephalopathie traumatique. *Archives de Psychologie, 28*, 286–340.

Schacter, D.L., & Tulving, E. (1994). *Memory Systems*. Cambridge, MA: MIT Press.

Schacter, D.L., Chiu, C-Y-P., & Ochsner, K.N. (1993). Implicit memory: A selective review. *Annual Review of Neuroscience, 16*, 159–182.

Sivan, A.B. (1992). *Revised Visual Retention Test*

(5th ed.). New York: The Psychological Corporation.

Spreen, O., & Benton, A.L. (1977). *Neurosensory Center Comprehensive Examination for Aphasia*. Victoria, BC: University of Victoria, Psychology Laboratory.

Uchiyama, C.L., D'Elia, L.F., Dellinger, A.M., Selnes, O.A., Becker, J.T., Wesch, J.E., Chen, B.B., Satz, P., Van Gorp, W., & Miller, E.N. (1994). Longitudinal comparison of alternate versions of the Symbol Digit Modalities Test: Issues of form comparability and moderating demographic variables. *The Clinical Neuropsychologist, 8*, 209–218.

Warrington, E.K. (1984). *Recognition Memory Test Manual*. Windsor, Berkshire: NFER-Nelson.

Wechsler, D. (1945). A standardized memory scale for clinical use. *Journal of Psychology, 19*, 87–95.

Wechsler, D. (1987). *Wechsler Memory Scale—Revised*. San Antonio, TX: The Psychological Corporation.

Wilson, B., Cockburn, J., & Baddeley, A. (1985). *The Rivermead Behavioral Memory Test*. Bury St. Edmunds, England: Thames Valley Test Company.

AUDITORY CONSONANT TRIGRAMS (CCC)

Other Test Name

The task is also known as the Brown-Peterson procedure.

Purpose

The purpose of this test is to assess short-term memory, divided attention, and information-processing capacity in adults.

Source

There is no commercial source for this test.

Description

The Brown-Peterson test of memory (Brown, 1958; Peterson & Peterson, 1959), although frequently used as a measure of decay of short-term memory, also measures divided attention and information-processing capacity (Stuss et al., 1987, 1989). A consonant trigram (CCC) is delivered to the subject verbally at a rate of one letter per second followed immediately by a three-digit random number. The subject is asked to count out loud backwards from a number by threes for interval delays of 9, 18, and 36 seconds used at random. The subject is then asked to recall the trigram. Five trials are given for each delay period with intertrial delays of 2–5 seconds. The delays of 9, 18, and 36 seconds are chosen in order to minimize any ceiling effect. Dependent measures are the total number of letters correctly recalled at each of the three delay intervals.

Recently, Paniak et al. (1997) developed a version of the task that is appropriate for children aged 9–15 years. Delays of 3, 9, and 18 seconds are used. Having the children count backward by threes proved too difficult for them. Accordingly, the children count backwards by ones instead.

Administration

The instructions provided here are adapted from Stuss (personal communication, May 1994). For adults, three consonants are presented, as shown in Figure 10–1. The subject must remember these consonants after intervals of 0, 9, 18, and 36 seconds. During the intervals of 9, 18, and 36 seconds, the subject is required to count backwards aloud by threes from different numbers; e.g., 100–97–94. If this is too difficult, variations may be used, e.g., backwards by ones.

The consonants are read by the examiner at the speed of one consonant per second. The subject is not allowed to repeat the consonants aloud at any time. After the presentation of the third consonant, the examiner immediately initiates the counting backwards by counting aloud himself or herself, urging the subject to do likewise. The examiner then stops counting. If the subject stops counting before the prescribed delay interval, the examiner again counts out loud with the subject. It is important that interference be sustained throughout the delay interval by the subject himself or herself.

Stimulus	Starting Number	Delay (sec)	Response	Number Correct
QLX	—	0		
SZB	—	0		
HJT	—	0		
GPW	—	0		
DLH	—	0		
XCP	75	18		
NDJ	28	9		
FXB	194	36		
JCN	20	9		
BGQ	167	18		
KMC	180	36		
RXT	82	18		
KFN	47	9		
MBW	188	36		
TDH	51	9		
LRP	117	36		
ZWS	141	18		
PHQ	89	9		
XGD	91	18		
CZQ	158	36		

Number Correct
0″ delay _____
9″ delay _____
18″ delay _____
36″ delay _____

Figure 10—1. Auditory Consonant Trigrams sample score sheet—Adults. Adapted from D. Stuss (May 1994).

All intervals are timed, the timing beginning after presentation of the last consonant. The examiner signals when the consonants are to be recalled by some prescribed movement or sign (e.g., a knock on the table).

Instruct as follows: *"I'm going to say three letters of the alphabet, which I want you to remember. When I signal you, like this* (give sign), *you tell me what the letters were. Sometimes, after I say the letters, you must count backwards from a number by threes, like this: 100–97–94. Count out loud, and continue until I give you the signal to tell me the letters. I'll tell you each time what the number is from which you should count backward."*

"Let's try one for practice. F–D–B–98–95– . . . ." (The examiner immediately starts counting, and urges that the subject also do so. After the defined delay interval, the examiner signals the subject to say the letter). *"That's right. You start counting with me, and keep on counting out loud until I knock. Then try to remember the three letters."* The subject is not instructed to repeat them in the exact order.

For children, three consonants are also presented, as shown in Figure 10–2. Say to the child: *"I am going to say three letters and when I am through, I am going to knock like this. When I do, I want you to say the letters back."* Present the first five (0 delay) trials. Then say: *"This time, I am going to say three letters followed immediately by a number. As soon as you get the number, I want you to start counting backward by ones out loud, like this: 29–28–27. Continue counting out loud until I knock as before."* Demonstrate knocking on the desk. *"When I knock, I want you to recall the three letters. Do you have any questions?"*

Approximate Time for Administration

The time required is about 10 minutes.

Scoring

Record the responses verbatim. The number of letters correctly remembered is tallied for

Stimulus	Starting Number	Delay (sec)	Response	Number Correct
XTN	—	0		
TQJ	—	0		
LNP	—	0		
SJH	—	0		
KPW	—	0		
NKR	94	18		
FBM	69	9		
KXQ	53	3		
GQS	46	9		
DLX	47	18		
BFM	48	3		
ZGK	55	18		
WGP	62	9		
ZDL	38	3		
RLB	22	3		
QDH	35	3		
GWB	47	18		
CSJ	39	9		
FMH	77	18		
HFZ	49	3		

Number Correct
0″ delay _____
3″ delay _____
9″ delay _____
18″ delay _____
Total _____

Figure 10—2. Auditory Constant Trigrams sample score sheet—Children. From Paniak et al. (1997).

each category of delay interval. The order in which the consonants are recalled does not matter for scoring purposes. The maximum score at each delay interval is 15. To calculate the total score, sum the number of consonants recalled correctly on each trial, including those from the 0-second delay trials. The maximum score obtainable is 60.

Comment

Stuss and his colleagues (1987, 1989) gave the test to both normal and head-injured individuals on two separate occasions with an inter-session duration of one week. Both healthy and neurologically impaired subjects scored significantly higher on their second visit than they did on their first (see Table 10–1).

The Brown-Peterson task captures an everyday experience; namely, momentary distraction and the subsequent loss of very recent information (Crowder, 1982). Forgetting is influenced by both proactive and retroactive interference as well as the success with which the distractor task blocks rehearsal (Morris, 1986). It has been proposed that retention of the to-be-remembered material on the Brown-Peterson task involves mainly maintenance rehearsal, making significant demands on central-processing resources (cf. Valler & Baddeley, 1984). Thus, one reason the distractor task causes forgetting is that it uses up central-processing resources that would otherwise be devoted to rehearsing the to-be-remembered items (Morris, 1986).

Impaired performance on the Brown-Peterson task is observed in a variety of conditions, including those induced by Alzheimer's disease, herpes encephalitis, Korsakoff's syndrome, Anterior Communicating Artery aneurysms (ACoA), and frontal leucotomy (Cermak & Butters, 1972; Corkin, 1982; Dannenbaum et al., 1988; Kopelman & Stanhope, 1997; Morris, 1986; Parkin et al., 1988; Stuss et al., 1988). A number of researchers (Parkin et al., 1988; Stuss et al., 1982) have suggested that the test is particularly sensitive to frontal lobe or frontal/brainstem system deficits. Correlation with regard to frontal-lobe disturbance, however, has not been perfect. For example, Winocur and colleagues (1984) examined a patient whose lesion was restricted to the thalamus and who showed impairment on the Brown-Peterson task. Second, Parkin (1984) noted that postencephalitic amnesics often have frontal involvement but, in general, show normal performance on the task. Third, performance on the task has been found to be impaired in some ACoA patients and not others (for recent review, see DeLuca & Diamond, 1995). Finally, Kopelman and Stanhope (1997) reported that in patients with diencephalic, frontal, or temporal damage, scores on a word version of the task correlated moderately with age ($r = -.24$), IQ ($r = .50$) and with modified card-sorting percent perseverations ($r = -.38$), but correlations with other frontal-lobe measures (card-sorting categories, FAS, Cognitive Estimation) were non-significant. In short, the exact interpretation of task impairment remains to be determined. Kopelman and Stanhope (1997) suggest that impairment on the task is related to generalized deficits in information processing rather than to specifically frontal functions.

Stuss and colleagues (1989) have found that the test does distinguish normal individuals from patients who have suffered a traumatic brain injury. The longer the duration of post-traumatic amnesia or coma, the worse the performance on the auditory consonant trigrams test. In comparison to the PASAT and the Trail Making Test, only the CCC was sufficiently sensitive to differentiate mildly concussed patients from their control group.

In short, the CCC is a relatively brief measure of short-term or working memory. Stuss et al. (1989) suggested that it is less affected by moderator variables such as age and education, and it is perhaps less stressful than the PASAT. They warn, however, that the CCC is difficult to administer in a rigid standardized manner that would make results equivalent across laboratories.

Normative Data

Age-based normative data for adults are provided by Stuss and colleagues (1987, 1988) and are shown in Table 10–1. With this technique, normal subjects have essentially perfect recall with no distraction delay. In gener-

Table 10—1. Performance on the Consonant Trigrams Test on Two Separate Occasions (One Week Apart) by Age (SD in Parentheses)

Condition	16–29 years ($n = 30$)		30–49 years ($n = 30$)		50–69 years ($n = 30$)	
	1st visit	2nd visit	1st visit	2nd visit	1st visit	2nd visit
9-sec delay	12.03 (2.24)	12.57 (2.03)	12.00 (2.52)	12.10 (2.85)	11.47 (2.33)	11.70 (2.28)
18-sec delay	11.37 (2.82)	12.27 (2.41)	10.50 (3.11)	12.00 (2.59)	10.23 (2.46)	10.67 (2.92)
36-sec delay	9.43 (2.71)	10.93 (2.88)	9.90 (3.04)	11.10 (2.37)	8.67 (2.85)	8.57 (3.54)

Source: Stuss et al. (1988). Reprinted with permission of Swets & Zeitlinger.

Table 10—2. CTT Scores for Children

Delay (in sec)	Age													
	9 ($n = 82$)		10 ($n = 140$)		11 ($n = 32$)		12 ($n = 122$)		13 ($n = 96$)		14 ($n = 115$)		15 ($n = 28$)	
	M	SD	M	SD	M	SD	M	SD	M	SD	M	SD	M	SD
0	15.0	0.2	14.9	0.3	14.9	0.4	14.9	0.4	14.9	0.4	15.0	0.1	14.9	0.3
3	9.9	2.7	10.5	2.6	10.9	2.3	11.5	2.5	12.2	2.0	12.1	2.0	12.1	1.9
9	6.6	2.6	6.9	2.7	7.8	2.4	8.6	2.6	9.9	2.8	10.1	2.6	10.9	2.2
18	5.7	2.5	6.0	2.1	6.7	2.4	7.8	2.6	8.7	2.9	9.3	2.6	9.5	2.8
Total score	37.1	6.2	38.2	6.0	40.3	6.0	42.8	6.2	45.8	6.5	46.4	5.6	47.4	5.5

Source: Paniak et al. (1997). Reprinted with permission of Swets & Zeitlinger.

al, the greater the delay, the worse the performance. Stuss et al. (1987, 1989) reported that in normal individuals, age and education showed little relation with scores on the test. In head-injured patients, education correlated significantly with the results from the 9- and 18-second-delay trials.

Paniak et al. (1997) provided normative data based on 715 students (326 males, 389 females), ages 9–15 who attended Edmonton schools. Estimated verbal intelligence (based on the WISC-R Vocabulary subtest) was near the WISCIII normative sample's mean. The data are shown in Table 10–2. Scores improved with age but were not influenced by gender. Note that even though the test was simpler than the adult version, scores appear not to have reached adult levels by age 15 years.

References

Brown, J. (1958). Some tests of the decay of immediate memory. *Quarterly Journal of Experimental Psychology, 10*, 12–21.

Cermak, L.S., & Butters, N. (1972). The role of interference and encoding in the short-term memory of Korsakoff patients. *Neuropsychologia, 10*, 89–95.

Corkin, S. (1982). Some relationships between global amnesias and the memory impairments in Alzheimer's disease. In S. Corkin, K.L. Davis, J.H. Groudin, E. Usdin, & R.J. Wurtman (Eds.), *Alzheimer's Disease: A Report of Progress in Research.* Hillsdale, NJ: Lawrence Erlbaum Associates, Inc.

Crowder, R.G. (1982). The demise of short-term memory. *Acta Psychologia, 50*, 291–323.

Dannenbaum, S.E., Parkinson, S.R., & Inman, V.W. (1988). Short-term forgetting: Comparisons between patients with dementia of the Alzheimer type, depressed, and normal elderly. *Cognitive Neuropsychology, 5*, 213–234.

DeLuca, J., & Diamond, B.J. (1995). Aneurysm of the anterior communicating artery: A review of neuroanatomical and neuropsychological sequelae. *Journal of Clinical and Experimental Neuropsychology, 17*, 100–121.

Kopelman, M.D., & Stanhope, N. (1997). Rates of forgetting in organic amnesia following temporal lobe, diencephalic, or frontal lobe lesions. *Neuropsychology, 11*, 343–356.

Morris, R.G. (1986). Short-term forgetting in senile dementia of the Alzheimer's type. *Cognitive Neuropsychology, 3*, 77–97.

Paniak, C.E., Millar, H.B., Murphy, D., & Keizer, J. (1997). A Consonant Trigrams test for children: Development and norms. *The Clinical Neuropsychologist, 11*, 198–200.

Parkin, A.J. (1984). Amnesic syndrome: A lesion specific disorder? *Cortex, 20*, 478–508.

Parkin, A.J., Leng, N.R., Stanhope, N., & Smith, A.P. (1988). Memory impairment following ruptured aneurysm of the anterior communicating artery. *Brain and Cognition, 7*, 231–243.

Peterson, L.R., & Peterson, M.J. (1959). Short-term retention of individual verbal items. *Journal of Experimental Psychology, 58*, 193–198.

Stuss, D.T., Kaplan, E.F., Benson, D.F., Weir, W.S., Chuilli, S., & Sarazin, F. (1982). Evidence for the involvement of orbitofrontal cortex in memory functions: An interference effect. *Journal of Comparative and Physiological Psychology, 5*, 913–925.

Stuss, D.T., Stethem, L.L., Hugenholtz, H., & Richard, M.T. (1989). Traumatic brain injury: A comparison of three clinical tests, and analysis of recovery. *The Clinical Neuropsychologist, 3*, 145–156.

Stuss, D.T., Stethem, L.L., & Pelchat, G. (1988). Three tests of attention and rapid information processing: An extension. *The Clinical Neuropsychologist, 2*, 246–250.

Stuss, D.T., Stethem, L.L., & Poirier, C.A. (1987). Comparison of three tests of attention and rapid information processing across six age groups. *The Clinical Neuropsychologist, 1*, 139–152.

Vallar, G., & Baddeley, A.D. (1984). Fractionation of working memory: Neuropsychological evidence for a phonological short-term store. *Journal of Verbal Learning and Verbal Behavior, 23*, 151–161.

Winocur, G., Oxbury, S., Roberts, R., Agnetti, V., & Davis, C. (1984). Amnesia in a patient with bilateral lesions to the thalamus. *Neuropsychologia, 22*, 123–144.

AUTOBIOGRAPHICAL MEMORY INTERVIEW (AMI)

Purpose

This test is used to assess retrograde amnesia, the inability to remember events and facts preceding injury or illness.

Source

The test (including manual and 25 scoring sheets) can be ordered from Western Psychological Services, 12031 Wilshire Boulevard, Los Angeles, CA 90025-1251, at a cost of $140 US.

Description

This test was devised by Kopelman and colleagues (Kopelman, Wilson, & Baddely, 1990) to assess the intactness of a client's remote memory, including the pattern of any deficit and its temporal gradient (e.g., relative sparing of early compared with more recent memories). The AMI consists of a semi-structured interview schedule, encompassing two components. The first, called the "personal semantic" schedule, assesses patients' recall of *facts* from their own past life, relating to childhood (e.g., names of schools or teachers), early adult life (e.g., name of first employer, date uand place of wedding), and more recent facts (e.g., holidays, journeys, previous hospitalizations). The second component, called the "autobiographical incidents" schedule, assesses patients' recall of specific *events or incidents* in the same three time periods: three from childhood, three from early adult life, and three recent events. (For example, recall an incident while at primary school; recall an incident from college or the first job; and recall an incident that took place while on holiday in the last 5 years). The test constrains subjects to produce memories from these three specific time periods and is appropriate across the adult age range from 18 years to old age.

Administration

The examiner asks questions and records responses on the scoring sheet as close to verbatim as possible. Instructions for administering the AMI appear in the manual. Where a client fails to produce any memory, some specific prompts may be used, and these are provided on the answer sheet (see AMI scoring sheet). It is permissible, but not obligatory, to tape-record the interview.

Approximate Time for Administration

About 20–30 minutes are required for the test.

Scoring

Items in the personal semantic schedule are scored from one to three points. Each of these subsections (childhood, early adult life, recent life) is scored out of 21 points for a maximum total of 63 points. Partial credit can be given for many of the items.

On the autobiographical incident schedule, three points are given for an episodic memory, specific in time and place; two points for a specific memory, in which time and place are not recalled, or for a less specific event in which time and place are recalled; one point for a vague personal memory; and no points in the absence of a response or for a response based purely on general knowledge (semantic memory). Examples are provided in the appendix of the AMI manual. Scores for each subsection range from 0 to 9, and the maximum total score is 27.

Comment

Kopelman et al. (1990) reported that interrater reliability is high. Three raters independently scored written descriptions of memories recalled. The correlations between pairs of testers varied between .83 and .86. Information on test–retest reliability is currently not available.

The AMI discriminates amnesics from healthy controls. Kopelman, Wilson, and Baddeley (1989) found that patients with memory deficits, although matched in estimated premorbid intelligence (NART) and age with controls, showed reduced capacity for new learning, and showed impaired remote memory when assessed on the AMI as well as other existing tests, such as the Logical Memory (WMS), the Recognition Memory Test, the Rivermead Behavioral Memory Test, the Prices test (in which subjects have to estimate the prices of common objects), and the Crovitz Test of Autobiographical Memory.

In a group of amnesic patients ($n = 62$), the personal semantic score correlated about .60 with the autobiographical incidents score (Kopelman et al., 1990). Both the personal semantic and autobiographical incidents scores showed weak-to-moderate correlations with other measures of remote memory. When normal and memory-impaired groups were merged, increasing the variability in performance, the two components of the AMI correlated highly (.77), casting some doubt on the usefulness of a simple episodic/semantic distinction in characterizing the effects of organic amnesia (but see Paul et al. 1997, who found that MS patients were significantly impaired on recall of semantic, but not episodic memories on the AMI). Further, all the remote memory tests correlated moderately with one another (.28–.64), suggesting that the AMI and other retrograde memory tests are measuring similar but not identical components of memory (see also Brandt & Benedict, 1993). Correlations between the AMI and the WMS MQ, as an index of anterograde impairment, ranged from .32 to .35 in Korsakoff patients and from .52 to .65 in Alzheimer's patients (Kopelman, 1989). This finding is consistent with the observation that in some cases of head injury, anterograde amnesia can occur in the presence of little or no retrograde loss.

There is also evidence that the test is sensitive to temporal gradients, with certain amnesic patients showing relative sparing of the most remote memories. Kopelman (1989) found, for both components of the AMI, that healthy subjects showed a gentle recency effect whereas amnesic patients with damage to the hippocampal circuit were most severely impaired in the recall of recent facts and events. Patients with Korsakoff's disease showed gradients that were steeper than those found in patients with Alzheimer's, while the latter showed gentler temporal gradients. Kopelman suggested that there might be relative sparing of early memories in both the Korsakoff and Alzheimer groups because these memories are particularly salient and well-rehearsed, and are thereby protected from any retrieval deficit. The steeper gradient in the Korsakoff patients might result from an additional, progressive anterograde impairment arising from their period of heavy drinking.

Graham and Hodges (1997) reported that amnesic AD patients showed a clear temporal gradient on the AMI, with preserved older memories and impaired recent memories, consistent with other studies (Kopelman, 1989). Patients with semantic dementia (that is, with primary progressive aphasia) whose lesions involve the left temporal neocortex with sparing of the hippocampal region, showed the reverse pattern for both personal semantic and autobiographical events. The patients were able to produce more detailed information from the recent past than from their childhood or early adulthood. This double dissociation in performance on autobiographical components of the AMI provides evidence that the hippocampal structures and the neocortex play temporally distinct roles in long-term storage.

Pathology in the frontal lobes has also been proposed as important for producing an extensive retrograde loss (Kopelman, 1993). In Korsakoff and Alzheimer's patients, performance on "frontal-lobe" tests (e.g., verbal fluency, card sorting, cognitive estimation) is correlated with recall of autobiographical memories.

Kopelman and his colleagues (1989, 1990) have checked patients' recall against a number of corroborative sources. They report that while some inaccuracy and confabulation occurs, the amount is small. They suggest that detailed checking of responses with relatives is probably not necessary for routine assessments, except in the case of patients who are clearly confabulating. Paul et al. (1997) also found that MS patients and healthy controls rarely confabulate on the AMI.

The AMI has several advantages. First, it assesses information that any person is likely to possess and is not dependent on an individual's interest in current affairs and inclination to read the newspaper or watch television. Second, the test does not quickly become out of date and require restandardization. On the other hand, it does not assess remote memory on a year-by-year basis, and as a result some deficits may go undetected.

Normative Data

Kopelman and colleagues (1990) provide cut-off points based on a small sample ($n = 34$) of healthy adults. The authors report that neither age nor IQ (estimated by the NART) affect performance. The influence of gender and education is not reported.

References

Brandt, J., & Benedict, R.H.B. (1993). Assessment of retrograde amnesia: Findings with a new public events procedure. *Neuropsychology, 7,* 217–227.

Graham, K.S., & Hodges, J.R. (1997). Differentiating the roles of the hippocampal complex and the neocortex in long-term memory storage: Evidence from the study of Semantic Dementia and Alzheimer's disease. *Neuropsychology, 11,* 77–89.

Kopelman, M.D. (1989). Remote and autobiographical memory, temporal context memory, and frontal atrophy in Korsakoff and Alzheimer patients. *Neuropsychologia, 27,* 437–460.

Kopelman, M.D., Wilson, B.A., & Baddeley, A.D. (1989). The Autobiographical Memory Interview: A new assessment of autobiographical and personal semantic memory in amnesic patients. *Journal of Clinical and Experimental Neuropsychology, 11,* 724–744.

Kopelman, M., Wilson, B., & Baddely, A. (1990). *The Autobiographical Memory Interview.* Bury St. Edmunds U.K.: Thames Valley Test Company.

Kopelman, M.D. (1993). The neuropsychology of memory. In F. Boller & J. Grafman (Eds.), *Handbook of Neuropsychology,* Vol. 8. Amsterdam: Elsevier.

Paul, R.H., Blanco, C.R., Hames, K.A., & Beatty, W.W. (1997). Autobiographical memory in multiple sclerosis. *Journal of International Neuropsychological Society, 3,* 246–251.

BENTON VISUAL RETENTION TEST—REVISED (BVRT-R)

Other Test Names

Other test names are Visual Retention Test—Revised (VRT-R) and Benton-Test.

Purpose

The purpose of this test is to assess visual memory, visual perception, and visuoconstructive abilities.

Source

The manual (5th edition; Sivan, 1992) for the drawing administrations, design cards (forms C, D, and E bound together, with easel support), and record forms can be obtained from the Psychological Corporation, P.O. Box 9954, San Antonio, TX 78204-0954, at a cost of $118 US, or from the Institute of Psychological Research, Inc., 34 Fleury St. West, Montreal, Quebec H3L 1S9, for $100 Cdn. The German version (Der Benton-Test; Sivan & Spreen, 1996) includes the multiple-choice version; stimulus booklets and answer sheets can be obtained from Hogrefe and Huber Publishers, P.O. Box 2487, Kirkland, WA 98083-2487, or Brucepark Avenue, Toronto, Ontario M4P 2S3, at a cost of about $100 Cdn.

Description

The drawing administrations of the Benton Visual Retention Test (BVRT) have three alternate forms (C, D, and E) that are roughly of equivalent difficulty. Each form is composed of 10 designs; the first two designs consist of one major geometric figure, and the other eight designs consist of two major figures and a smaller peripheral figure. Under Administration A, the standard procedure, each design is displayed for 10 seconds and then withdrawn. Immediately after this, the subject is required to reproduce the design from memory at his or her own pace on a blank piece of paper. Administration B is similar to A except that each design is exposed for only 5 seconds. Administration C (copying) requires the subject to copy each of the designs without removing the stimulus card from sight. In Administration D, each design is exposed for 10 seconds and the subject must reproduce the design after a 15-second delay. Two additional multiple-choice forms (F and G) are available only in the German edition of the test and measure the subject's recognition, rather than reproduction, ability (Administration M). The multiple-choice administration can be used for people with motor handicaps or for people without motor handicaps, in order to determine whether the person's disability lies in the area of memory, perception, or drawing ability.

Administration

See manual. Briefly, for Administrations A to D, the subject is given 10 blank, white 21.5- × 14-cm pieces of paper. The subject either reproduces each design from memory (Administrations A, B, D) or copies each design (Administration C). Benton (1972) suggested that form C can be abbreviated to only the first eight designs because the eight-design score correlated .97 with the 10-design score. Drawings should be numbered in the right-hand corner by the examiner after completion of the drawing in order to identify the spatial orientation of the drawing, as well as the specific design that was drawn (Wellman, 1985). For Administration M, each of the 15 stimulus cards, consisting of one to three geometric figures, is exposed for 10 seconds. Immediately after each exposure, the subject is shown a multiple-choice card with four similar stimuli labeled A, B, C, D; he or she must choose (point to or name by letter) the one that is identical to the stimulus card.

Approximate Time for Administration

The time required for each administration is about 5–10 minutes.

Scoring

Scoring is accomplished according to explicit criteria that are detailed in the manual (see source). Briefly, two scoring systems (the number of correct reproductions and the error score) are available for the evaluation of a subject's performance on the drawing forms (Administrations A to D). The number correct score has a range of 0–10 as each of the 10 designs is scored on an all-or-none basis and given a credit of 1 or 0. Principles underlying the scoring of the designs, together with specific scoring samples illustrating correct and incorrect reproductions, are located in the manual. The scoring of errors allows for both a quantitative and qualitative analysis of a subject's performance. Six major types of errors are noted: (1) omissions, (2) distortions, (3) perseverations, (4) rotations, (5) misplacements, and (6) size errors. Each major category contains a variety of specific error subtypes. Provision is also made for noting right- and left-sided errors. Scoring is recorded and summarized on the record form. This form allows the examiner to indicate the correct designs as well as to summarize the types of errors made on each design.

Comment

This popular test has been in use since 1946 (Benton, 1946) and has stimulated numerous psychometric and clinical studies, partially summarized by Sivan (1992). For the drawing administrations of the BVRT, interscorer agreement for number correct and the total error score is high (above .95, Swan et al., 1990; Wahler, 1956). Similarly, interrater agreement of some qualitative aspects of the scoring system is good (omissions .96, perseverations .88, rotations .88), but less acceptable for scoring of misplacement and size errors (Swan et al., 1990). This may improve because of the introduction of augmented scoring rules and examples in the current edition. Alternate form reliability is good. Sivan (1992) reports correlation coefficients ranging from .79 to .84 between the three forms (C, D, and E) of the test. There is some evidence (Breidt, 1970) that Form D is slightly more difficult than Form C for the memory, but not the copying task, with Form E occupying an intermediate position, although other studies have found virtually no difference among forms (Brown & Rice, 1967; Weiss, 1974). There is a modest relation (.41–.52) between

performance levels on the copying (Administration C) and memory (Administration B) tasks (Benton, 1974). Positive correlations, ranging from .40 to .83, have also been reported between immediate (Administration A) and delayed (Administration D) reproduction versions (Benton, 1974). Retest reliability for Administration A is high (.85; Benton, 1974), but Cronbach internal consistency coefficients were reported to be .76 for Form C, .79 for Form D, and .79 for Form E (number correct, Steck et al., 1990). For number of errors, the corresponding values were .71, .82, and .80. Steck also noted that internal consistency rises to .911 when all 30 items (Form C + D + E) are administered.

Practice effects of retesting are in dispute: Botwinick et al. (1986) found virtually no change in scores for 64- to 81-year olds tested four times at 1½-year intervals, but Larrabee et al. (1986) found an improvement of more than one point on retest of 60- to 90-year olds after 10–13 months.

For the multiple-choice administration (M), alternate-form reliability (Forms F and G) is good (.80, Sivan & Spreen, 1996). Split-half reliability of the multiple-choice forms is .76. The correlation between the multiple-choice and reproduction forms is, however, considerably lower, (.55, Sivan & Spreen, 1996). Based on the analysis of the performance of 52 10-year-old school counseling clients, Wagner (1992) argued that the item difficulty range for this age was unsatisfactory.

Although performance is intended to measure nonverbal memory, some of the geometric figures can be verbalized (Arenberg, 1978). Further, the reproduction administrations are more closely associated with visual-perceptual-motor ability than with visual memory. Factor analyses revealed that the BVRT (Administration A) loads primarily on a visual-perceptual-motor factor, and only secondarily on a memory-concentration-attention factor (Larabee et al., 1985; Crook and Larrabee, 1988). A second factor analytic study (Larrabee & Crook, 1989) found that the test loaded on two factors, "vigilance" and "psychomotor speed," when analyzed in the context of other memory tests and measures of everyday memory performance. Moses (1986), however, showed that Administration A and the multiple-choice administration both loaded on a first factor representing primarily memory skills, and on a second factor, described as attention span and perceptual-analytic ability. The copying form (Form C) loaded primarily on the second factor. A replication study with 162 neuropsychiatric patients (Moses, 1989) confirmed that the BVRT copy and memory scores form separable factorial components. In both analyses, number correct and error scores were considered redundant.

Finally, some of the items on the multiple-choice version of the BVRT can be correctly completed without viewing the target stimuli, merely by solving the task as an oddity problem (Blanton & Gouvier, 1985). Thus, the validity of the test may be compromised in subjects who respond strategically rather than by relying on their visual memory. The examiner should interview the subject after the test to determine the type of strategy that was used (Franzen, 1989).

A number of studies have examined the ability of the BVRT to detect brain injury (Heaton et al., 1978; Marsh & Hirsch, 1982; Schwerd & Salgueiro-Feik, 1980; Tamkin & Kunce, 1985; Zonderman et al., 1995). Overall, these studies show that the test is sensitive to the presence of brain damage, although its predictive ability is not high. Steck et al. (1990) reported that even a 30-item version did not show significant score or type-of-error differences among small groups of depressives, schizophrenics, alcoholics, and brain-damaged patients, although all groups showed error scores well below those of 145 healthy control subjects. A similar result for chronic and subchronic schizophrenics was reported by Milech et al. (1990). Crockett et al. (1990) found that patients with anterior or posterior brain dysfunction showed more impairment than a psychiatric group, but the difference was not significant. Levin et al. (1990) found that head-trauma patients made an average of five errors (SD = 5.0) compared to only two errors (SD = 4.0) in matched controls, and Davidson et al. (1987) found that omissions, but not number correct or error scores, correlated with length of posttraumatic amnesia.

Davidson also found that the test did not correlate significantly with the Otago computerized neuropsychological test battery in 16 head-injured patients. The clinical impression is that patients with right posterior lesions tend to be most impaired on the reproduction administrations of the BVRT, but the evidence is inconsistent (Sivan, 1992). Both DeRenzi et al. (1977) and Vakil et al. (1989) found that patients with right- and left-hemisphere lesions did not differ on Administration A, although their performance was significantly below that of a control group; with a 15-second delay administration (Administration D), however, right-hemisphere patients showed more impairment than left-hemisphere patients on the number correct, but not the error score. Vakil et al. argue that this justifies the use of both scores. Mann et al. (1989) found a relationship between MRI lesion volume in multiple sclerosis (MS) and impairment of BVRT performance. Patients with lesions in both hemispheres showed impairment, but there was a trend for more impairment to be related to left parietal lobe lesions. The copying (Administration C) and multiple-choice (Administration M) versions of the BVRT do not distinguish between hemispheric side of lesion (Arena & Gainotti, 1978). Some types of errors may, however, be of localizing significance. For example, patients with unilateral neglect may consistently omit peripheral figures appearing on one side. Ryan et al. (1996) found impaired performance on the BVRT (Administration A) to be related to lesions in the corpus callosum, especially in the genu, in MS patients. A study of patients with infarct of the thalamus indicated that, after 1 year, six out of 19 patients showed impairment on the BVRT, two with left-sided and four with right-sided lesions (Buttner et al., 1991); all patients had additional older infarcts outside the area of the thalamus. P2 and N2 latencies of evoked potentials in tumor and trauma patients correlated significantly (.67 and −.49) with BVRT scores (Olbrich et al., 1986); Pelosi et al. (1992) found similar results in studies of evoked potentials with healthy adults and interpreted them as indicators of objective and subjective task difficulty. BVRT results corresponded well to depth of coma in patients with craniocephalic damage (Buzon-Reyes et al., 1992).

The test has been used with Alzheimer's disease patients: Robinson-Whelen (1992) reported significant differences between normal controls and patients with very mild and moderate dementia for both Administration A and C. Omission errors were significantly higher on both administrations, although other error types also showed significant differences. Storandt et al. (1986) also reported that patients with mild Alzheimer's dementia showed significantly more errors on Administration C (mean = 3.3 ± 5.1) than age-matched controls; further, 2½ years later the error score had climbed rapidly (mean = 13.5 ± 11.7), while the controls showed virtually no change. In the Baltimore Longitudinal Study, Zonderman et al. (1995) found the test to be a strong predictor of Alzheimer's disease as early as 6 years prior to the diagnosed onset of the disease, and Swan, Carmelli, and Larue (1996) found the test to be a significant predictor of mortality in a follow-up of older adults, even in the context of a regression analysis including health factors such as cancer, cardiovascular disease, systolic blood pressure, and cholesterol level. Baum et al. (1996) conducted a canonical analysis of a variety of measures of activities of daily living and a set of neuropsychological tests. The BVRT had a loading of .85 (memory) and .69 (copying) on the first canonical variate, indicating good ecological validity in this AD population. Pakesch et al. (1992a, b) found significant differences between HIV-infected drug addicts and healthy homosexual controls, but a group off seronegative drug addicts showed similar impairment, suggesting that drug effects rather than cognitive HIV impairment were responsible.

The test has also been used in case study designs to estimate the effect of memory training in patients with brain trauma (Kaschel, 1994), in alcoholics (Unterholzner et al., 1992), and of cognitive/communicative training in schizophrenics (Roder et al., 1987). In a group design ($n = 168$), John et al. (1991) found that significant improvement compared to controls during an alcohol detoxification program oc-

curred mainly during the first week, whereas subsequent weeks did not show further improvement. Bach et al. (1993) found improvement of BVRT scores in a group of 22 geriatric patients undergoing 24 weeks of activation therapy as compared to a matched group without therapy.

Studies with children showed that the standard administration of the test discriminates well between reading-retarded and normal 5th graders (Arnkelsson, 1993).

The BVRT has a number of advantages (Wellman, 1985) that are worth noting. These include short administration time, precise scoring criteria, and many alternate forms. Further, because of its multiple-choice, drawing from memory, and copying administrations, the examiner may be able to discriminate among perceptual, motor, and memory deficits. Finally, the BVRT is one of the neuropsychological tests for which patterns of dissimulation are known (Franzen, 1989). Simulators produce more errors than brain-damaged subjects; they produce more distortions, fewer perseverations, and fewer errors than brain-damaged patients (Benton & Spreen, 1961).

Normative Data

Performance on the BVRT shows a moderate correlation with intelligence (about .7, Benton, 1974) and age (Arenberg, 1978; Benton, 1974; Benton et al., 1981; Poitrenaud & Clement, 1965). Consequently, normative data presented in the manuals (Sivan, 1992; Sivan & Spreen, 1996) are provided within the context of age and presumed premorbid IQ. The data were derived from relatively large samples of individuals with no history or evidence of brain damage. It should be noted that Dartigues et al. (1992) found that in 2,720 healthy elderly community residents BVRT results corresponded strongly with life-time occupation regardless of education level; in particular, farmers, domestic service employees, and blue-collar workers showed poor memory two to three times more often than people with professional/management occupations. In elderly subjects, distortion errors were most frequent (45 percent), followed by rotations

(18 percent) and omissions (14 percent) (Eslinger et al., 1988; LaRue et al., 1986). Similarly, Steck et al. (1990) found that in healthy subjects distortions were most frequent (42 percent), followed by rotations (19.5 percent), misplacements (19 percent), and perseverations (14 percent), while omissions (5 percent) and size errors (0.5 percent) were rare.

For Administration A (10-second exposure, immediate reproduction), rounded normative scores broken down by IQ level and age are provided in the manual for adult subjects aged 18–69 years (Benton, 1963). Whereas this facilitates direct comparison with a given subject's expected score, the lack of precise means and SDs does not allow calculation of z-scores or similar statistics. However, the new manual (1992) provides more detailed norms with SD (age <30 to 80+) from three studies (Arenberg, 1978; Benton et al., 1981; Poitrenaud & Clement, 1965) in a section on "Performance in Old Age." Very similar results, shown in Table 10–3, were obtained in a recent study of over 1,000 subjects by Youngjohn et al. (1993). They correspond very closely to results by Steck et al. (1990), even though his data were based on the administration of

30 (Form C + D + E) rather than the 10 items required under administration A. Youngjohn et al. also calculated regression equations that may be useful for the practitioner:

Predicted BVRT # correct (± 1.57) = 7.87 − .045 (age) + .098 (years of education)

Predicted BVRT # of errors (± 2.88) = 1.73 + .088 (age) − .126 (years of education)

The ± value indicates the standard error of measurement.

A study by Randall et al. (1988) suggests that both number correct and error scores suggested in the manual for the borderline and mentally retarded range may be too conservative. As Table 10–4 shows, performance level dropped dramatically in this range.

In children, performance on Administration A shows a progressive rise from age 8 years until a plateau is reached at the age of 14–15. This plateau is maintained into the 30s, and a progressive decline in performance occurs from the 40s onwards. Recent studies indicate that there is a marked decline in performance, particularly after age 70 (Robertson-Tchabo & Arenberg, 1989; Benton et al.,

Table 10—3. Mean Number of Correct Responses and Errors by Age and Education Level for Administration A

Age	Education								
	12–14 years			15–17 years			18+ years		
	n	M	SD	n	M	SD	n	M	SD
Number Correct									
18–39	29	7.59	1.52	27	8.04	1.19	18	8.11	1.28
40–49	18	7.11	1.53	23	7.78	1.54	19	7.42	1.22
50–59	130	6.66	1.47	146	7.08	1.70	133	7.55	1.53
60–69	129	6.18	1.67	159	6.70	1.47	134	6.80	1.55
70+	53	5.62	1.73	54	6.06	1.84	49	6.22	1.57
Number of Errors									
18–39	29	3.38	2.37	27	2.52	1.70	18	2.67	1.78
40–49	18	4.22	2.62	23	3.48	2.78	19	3.74	2.47
50–59	130	4.90	2.42	146	4.21	2.85	133	3.64	2.76
60–69	129	5.55	2.74	159	4.99	2.78	134	4.93	2.87
70+	53	7.28	3.55	54	7.74	4.34	49	6.33	3.63

Source: Youngjohn et al. (1993). With permission of Swets & Zeitlinger. Data are derived from 1,128 well-educated volunteers aged 17–84.

Table 10—4. Number Correct and Number of Errors
under Administration D and A

IQ Group	Administration D		Administration A	
	M	SD	M	SD
Number Correct				
60–69 (mentally retarded)	1.80	1.32	2.50	1.64
70–79 (borderline)	4.50	2.21	4.30	1.26
80–89 (low average)	6.50	2.01	6.50	1.90
90–109 (average)	8.75	.85	8.30	1.34
110–119 (high average)	8.50	1.10	8.05	1.19
120+ (superior)	8.40	.94	8.25	.79
Number of Errors				
60–69	19.10	6.62	15.50	5.05
70–79	9.30	6.15	10.15	2.00
80–89	4.80	3.16	5.40	2.99
90–109	1.35	.93	2.10	1.83
110–119	1.60	1.31	2.50	1.79
120+	1.90	1.21	2.00	1.07

Source: Randall et al., 1988. Administration D (15-seconds delayed recall of Form D)
and Administration A (Form C) in college-student volunteers between 18 and 30 years
of age. Based on 120 subjects with approximately equal *n* in each group. IQ estimates
based on a Satz-Mogul abbreviated WAIS-R score.

1981). One study with 12- to 13-year-old adolescents (Knuckle & Asbury, 1986) suggested effects of both ethnicity and gender. This group of black average-learning students scored lower than expected on the basis of norms, and boys did more poorly than girls. However, since no other gender effects have been reported in the literature and this is the only study of black children, without a comparison group, further replication is warranted.

For Administration B (5-second exposure, immediate reproduction), the manual (Sivan, 1992) suggests that one point should be subtracted from the expected Number Correct score for Administration A.

Normative data for Administration C (copying) are also provided in the manual. For adults, only rounded error scores without SD are provided. In general, adults make two or fewer errors on this form of the test. Robinson-Whelen (1992) reported means of 9.38 (correct) and 0.65 (errors) for a group of 122 healthy community volunteers with an average of 12.8 years of education (mean age 72

years). This suggests that less than one error is made, even in elderly subjects. For children aged 7–13 years, exact number correct and error scores with SDs are given. Additional data gathered by Brasfield (1971) and Beames and Russell (1970) for young children, aged 5–6 years, are also summarized in the manual (Sivan, 1992). There is a rapid rise in performance between the ages of 5 and 10, and a much slower rise between ages 10 and 13. The performance of 13-year-old children is very close to the adult level.

The manual (Sivan, 1992) indicates that normal adults obtain Number Correct scores of about .4 points less under Administration D (10-second exposure, 15-second delay) as compared with Administration A. Randall et al. (1988) present actual score distributions, shown in Table 10–4. The lack of variance in the average-to-superior IQ groups suggests a possible ceiling effect.

For Administration M (10-second exposure, immediate multiple-choice), Sivan (1992) provides normative data for children aged 7–

Table 10—5. Performance by Elderly Subjects on the BVRT—Multiple-Choice Administration

Score	Percentile
6	2.4
7	4.7
8	12.9
9	24.7
10	42.4
11	55.3
12	82.4
13	95.3
14	100.0

Source: Montgomery and Costa, 1983. Note that their administration differed from the standard administration in that stimulus exposure was 5, not 10, seconds. Data are based on 85 healthy, well-educated elderly volunteers, aged 65–89, with a mean age of 74.04. Reprinted with permission.

13 years, and adolescents through adults aged 14–55 years. Adult levels are obtained by about age 12. In general, adults tend to make two or fewer errors. Caplan and Caffery (1997) used a 16-item multiple-choice version, but reported similar means of 12.6 (SD = 1.9) for 51 adult control subjects (aged 29–71 years, mean age = 36.6). They found that this form of the test correlated significantly with age ($r = -.43$), with education ($r = .33$), and with age-corrected WAIS-R Vocabulary (.35). Montgomery and Costa (1983) gave the test to a sample of healthy elderly subjects aged 65–89 (mean = 74.04) years. Their administration differed from the standard administration in that they used a 5-second, rather than a 10-second, exposure. The data are given in Table

Table 10—6. Normative Data for the Multiple-Choice Form for Adults Aged 65–90 Years

Age	Male, Education (in years)			Female, Education (in years)		
	7	11	16	7	11	16
65	12.8	13.7	14.5	12.8	13.7	14.6
70	12.4	13.1	14.1	12.3	13.2	13.9
75	11.9	12.4	13.4	11.8	12.4	13.5
80	11.7	11.8	12.2	11.4	11.9	12.8
85	10.4	11.4	12.3	10.5	11.5	12.3
90	10.1	10.8	11.8	10.2	10.8	11.7

Source: Extrapolated from Tuokko & Woodward, 1996.

10–5. In contrast to Caplan and Caffery's findings, performance did not decline significantly with age. Their findings suggest that in the elderly, graphomotor or visuoconstructional impairments, not memory deficits, contribute to reduced performance on the reproduction form. The Canadian Study of Health and Aging (Tuokko & Woodward, 1996) investigated a representative Canadian sample of 265 normal community-dwelling adults, aged 65–90 years (mean = 78.4 years, average education 11.3 years) with distinct age effects. Table 10–6 presents the extrapolated normative data. Steenhuis and Ostbye (1995) report somewhat higher values (mean = 11.85) for a sample of 591 subjects from the same study. The average SD was 2.13. As seen in Table 10–6, gender differences are minimal even at this age. Tuokko & Woodward (1995) list the sensitivity of the test as 75 and 77 percent (with 1 or 2 SD) for correct negative diagnosis, and as 82 and 84 percent for correct positive diagnosis when compared to a dementia group.

Some of the normative data provided in the manual were compiled over 30 years ago and interpreted with reference to IQ levels. Most have been updated by more recent studies (Benton, Eslinger & Damasio, 1981; Brook, 1975; Robertson-Tchabo & Arenberg, 1989) and appear not to be significantly different from those presented in the earlier studies.

References

Arena, R., & Gainotti, G. (1978). Constructional apraxia and visuoperceptive disabilities in relation to laterality of lesions. *Cortex, 14,* 463–473.

Arenberg, D. (1978). Differences and changes with age in the Benton Visual Retention Test. *Journal of Gerontology, 33,* 534–540.

Arnkelsson, G. B. (1993). Reading-retarded Icelandic children: The discriminant validity of psychological tests. *Scandinavian Journal of Educational Research, 37,* 163–174.

Bach, D., Boehmer, F., Frühwald, F., & Grilc, B. (1993). Aktivierende Ergotherapie—Eine Methode zur Steigerung der kognitiven Leistungsfähigkeit bei geriatrischen Patienten. *Zeitschrift für Gerontologie, 26,* 476–481.

Baum, C., Edwards, D., Yonan, C., & Storandt, M. (1996). The relation of neuropsychological test performance to performance on functional tasks in dementia of the Alzheimer type. *Archives of Clinical Neuropsychology, 11*, 69–75.

Beames, T.B., & Russell, R.L. (1970). Normative data by age and sex for five preschool tests. Report. Neuropsychology Laboratory, University of Victoria.

Benton, A.L. (1946). *A Visual Retention Test for Clinical Use.* New York: Psychological Corporation.

Benton, A.L. (1963). *Revised Visual Retention Test: Clinical and Experimental Applications* (3rd ed.). New York: Psychological Corporation.

Benton, A.L. (1972). Abbreviated versions of the Visual Retention Test. *Journal of Psychology, 80*, 189–192.

Benton, A.L. (1974). *Revised Visual Retention Test* (4th ed.). New York: The Psychological Corporation.

Benton, A.L., Eslinger, P.J., & Damasio, A.R. (1981). Normative observations on neuropsychological test performances in old age. *Journal of Clinical Psychology, 3*, 33–42.

Benton, A.L., & Spreen, O. (1961). Visual Memory Test: The simulation of mental incompetence. *Archives of General Psychiatry, 4*, 79–83.

Blanton, P.D., & Gouvier, W.D. (1985). A systematic solution to the Benton Visual Retention Test: A caveat to examiners. *International Journal of Clinical Neuropsychology, 7*, 95–96.

Botwinick, J., Storandt, M., & Berg, L. (1986). A longitudinal, behavioral study of senile dementia of the Alzheimer type. *Archives of Neurology, 43*, 1124–1127.

Brasfield, D.M. (1971). An investigation of the use of the Benton Visual Retention Test with preschool children. M.A. Thesis, University of Victoria.

Breidt, R. (1970). Möglichkeiten des Benton-Tests in der Untersuchung psychoorganischer Störungen nach Hirnverletzungen. *Archiv für Psychologie, 122*, 314–326.

Brook, R.M. (1975). Visual retention test: Local norms and impact of short-term memory. *Perceptual and Motor Skills, 40*, 967–970.

Brown, L.F., & Rice, J.A. (1967). Form equivalence analysis of the Benton Visual Retention Test in children with low IQ. *Perceptual and Motor Skills, 24*, 737–738.

Buttner, T., Schilling, G., Hornig, C.R., & Dorndorf, W. (1991). Thalamusinfarkte-Klinik, neuropsychologische Befunde, Prognose. *Fortschritte der Neurologie und Psychiatrie, 59*, 479–487.

Buzon-Reyes, J.M., Leon-Carrion, J., Murillo, F., & Forastero, P. (1992). Deficits visuoconstructivos y profundidad del coma. *Archivos de Neurobiologia, 55*, 156–161.

Caplan, B., & Caffery, D. (1997). Visual form discrimination as a multiple-choice visual memory test: Preliminary normative data. *The Clinical Neuropsychologist, 10*, 152–158.

Crockett, D.J., Hurwitz, T., & Vernon-Wilkinson, R. (1990). Differences in neuropsychological performance in psychiatric, anterior- and posterior-cerebral dysfunctioning groups. *International Journal of Neuroscience, 52*, 45–57.

Crook, T.H., & Larrabee, G.J. (1988). Interrelationship among everyday memory tests: Stability of factor structure with age. *Neuropsychology, 2*, 1–12.

Dartigues, J.F., Gagnon, M., Mazaux, J.M., & Barberger-Gateau, P. (1992). Occupation during life and memory performance in nondemented French elderly community residents. *Neurology, 42*, 1697–1701.

Davidson, O.R., Stevens, D.E., Goddard, G.V., Bilkey, D.K., & Bishara, S.N. (1987). The performance of a sample of traumatic head-injured patients on some novel computer-assisted neuropsychological tests. *Applied Psychology and International Review, 36*, 329–342.

DeRenzi, E., Faglioni, P., & Previdi, P. (1977). Spatial memory and hemispheric locus of lesion. *Cortex, 13*, 424–433.

Eslinger, P.J., Pepin, L., & Benton, A.L. (1988). Different patterns of visual memory errors occur with aging and dementia. *Journal of Clinical and Experimental Psychology, 10*, 60–61 (abstract).

Franzen, M.D. (1989). *Reliability and Validity in Neuropsychological Assessment.* New York: Plenum Press.

Heaton, R., Baade, L.E., & Johnson, K.L. (1978). Neuropsychological test results associated with psychiatric disorders in adults. *Psychological Bulletin, 85*, 141–162.

John, U., Veltrup, C., Schnofl, A., Wetterling, T., Kanitz, W.D., & Dilling, H. (1991). Gedächtnisdefizite Alkoholabhängiger in der ersten Woche der Abstinenz. *Zeitschrift für klinische Psychologie, Psychopathologie und Psychotherapie, 39*, 348–356.

Kaschel, R. (1994). *Neuropsychologische Rehabilitation von Gedächtnisleistungen.* Weinheim, Germany: Beltz Psychologie Verlags Union.

Knuckle, E.P., & Asbury, C.A. (1986). Benton Revised Visual Retention Test performance of black adolescents according to age, sex, and ethnic identity. *Perceptual and Motor Skills, 63*, 319–327.

Larrabee, G.J., Kane, R.L., Schuck, J.R., & Francis, D.J. (1985). Construct validity of various memory testing procedures. *Journal of Clinical and Experimental Neuropsychology, 7*, 239–250.

Larrabee, G.J., & Crook, T.H. (1989). Dimensions of everyday memory in age-associated memory impairment. *Psychological Assessment, 1*, 92–97.

Larrabee, G.J., Levin, H.S., & High, W.M. (1986). Senescent forgetfulness: A quantitative study. *Developmental Neuropsychology, 2*, 373–385.

LaRue, A., D'Elia, L.F., & Clarke, E.O. (1986). Patterns of performance on the Fuld Object Memory Evaluation in elderly inpatients with depression or dementia. *Journal of Clinical and Experimental Neuropsychology, 11*, 409–422.

Levin, H.S., Gary, H.E., & Eisenberg, H.M. (1990). Neurobehavioral outcome 1 year after severe head injury: Experience of the Traumatic Coma Data Bank. *Journal of Neurosurgery, 73*, 699–709.

Mann, U., Staedt, D., Kappos, L., Wense, A.V.D., & Haubitz, I. (1989). Correlation of MRI findings and neuropsychological results in patients with multiple sclerosis. *Psychiatry Research, 29*, 293–294.

Marsh, G.G., & Hirsch, S.H. (1982). Effectiveness of two tests of visual retention. *Journal of Clinical Psychology, 38*, 115–118.

Milech, U., Boening, J., & Classen, W. (1990). Leistungspsychologische Querschnittsuntersuchug bei jungen Schizophrenen mit subchronischem und chronischem Krankheitsverlauf. *Psychiatrie, Neurologie, und medizinische Psychologie, 42*, 385–393.

Montgomery, C., & Costa, L. (1983). Paper presented to the International Neuropsychological Society, Mexico City.

Moses, J.A. (1986). Factor structure of Benton's tests of visual retention, visual construction, and visual form discrimination. *Archives of Clinical Neuropsychology, 1*, 147–156.

Moses, J.A. (1989). Replicated factor structure of Benton's tests of visual retention, visual construction, and visual form discrimination. *International Journal of Clinical Neuropsychology, 11*, 30–37.

Olbrich, H.M., Lanczos, L., Lodemann, E., Zerbin, D., Engelmeier, M.P., Nau, H.E., & Schmitt-Neuerburg, K.P. (1986). Ereigniskorrelierte Hirnpotentiale und intellektuelle Beeinträchtigung—Eine Untersuchung bei Patienten mit Hirntumor und Schädelhirntrauma. *Fortschritte der Neurologie und Psychiatrie, 54*, 182–188.

Pakesch, G., Pfersmann, D., Loimer, N., Gruenberger, J., Linzmayer, L., & Mayerhofer, S. (1992a). Noopsychische Veränderungen und psychopathologische Auffälligkeiten bei HIV-1 Patienten unterschiedlicher Risikogruppen. *Fortschritte der Neurologie und Psychiatrie, 60*, 17–27.

Pakesch, G., Loimer, N., Gruenberger, J., Pfersmann, D., Linzmayer, L., & Mayerhofer, S. (1992b). Neuropsychological findings and psychiatric symptoms in HIV-1 infected and noninfected drug users. *Psychiatry Research, 41*, 163–177.

Pelosi, L., Holly, M., Slade, T., & Hayward, M. (1992). Wave form variations in auditory event-related potentials evoked by a memory-scanning task and their relationship with tests of intellectual function. *Electroencephalography and Clinical Neurophysiology Evoked Potentials, 84*, 344–352.

Poitrenaud, J., & Clement, F. (1965). La déterioration physiologique dans le Test de Retention Visuelle de Benton: Résultats obtenue par 500 sujets normaux. *Psychologie Française, 10*, 359–368.

Randall, C.M., Dickson, A.L., & Plasay, M.T. (1988). The relationship between intellectual function and adult performance on the Benton Visual Retention Test. *Cortex, 24*, 277–289.

Robertson-Tchabo, E.A., & Arenberg, D. (1989). Assessment of memory in older adults. In T. Huntert & C. Lindley (Eds.) *Testing Older Adults*. Austin, TX: Pro-Ed.

Robinson-Whelen, S. (1992). Benton Visual Retention Test performance among normal and demented older adults. *Neuropsychology, 6*, 261–269.

Roder, V., Studer, K., & Brenner, H. (1987). Erfahrungen mit einem integrierten psychologischen Therapieprogramm zum Training kommunikativer und kognitiver Fähigkeiten in der Rehabilitation schwer chronisch schizophrener Patienten. *Schweizer Archiv für Neurologie und Psychiatrie, 138*, 31–44.

Ryan, L., Clark, C.M., Klonoff, H., et al. (1996). Patterns of cognitive impairment in relapsing-remitting multiple sclerosis and their relationship to neuropathology on magnetic resonance images. *Neuropsychology. 10*, 176–193.

Schwerd, A., & Salgueiro-Feik, M. (1980). Untersuchung zur Diagnostischen Validität des

Benton-Test bei Kindern und Jugendlichen. *Zeitschrift für Kinder und Jugendpsychiatrie, 8,* 300–313.

Sivan, A.B. (1992). *Benton Visual Retention Test* (5th ed.). San Antonio, TX: The Psychological Corporation.

Sivan, A.B., & Spreen, O. (1906). *Der Benton-Test* (7th ed.). Berne, Switzerland: Verlag Hans Huber.

Steck, P., Beer, U., Frey, A., Frühschütz, H.G., & Körner, A. (1990). Testkritische Überprüfung einer 30-Item Version des Visual Retention Tests nach A. L. Benton. *Diagnostica, 36,* 38–49.

Steenhuis, R. E., & Ostbye, T. (1995). Neuropsychological test performance of specific groups in the Canadian Study of Health and Aging (CSHA). *Journal of Clinical and Experimental Neuropsychology, 17,* 773–785.

Storandt, M., Botwinick, J., & Danzinger, W.L. (1986). Longitudinal changes: Patients with mild SDAT and matched healthy controls. In L. W. Poon (ed.), *Handbook for Clinical Memory Assessment of Older Adults.* Washington, DC: American Psychological Association.

Swan, G.E., Morrison, E., & Eslinger, P.J. (1990). Interrater agreement on the Benton Visual Retention Test. *The Clinical Neuropsychologist, 4,* 37–44.

Swan, G.E., Carmelli, D., & Larue, A. (1996). Psychomotor speed and visual memory as predictors of 7-year all-cause mortality in older adults. Paper presented at the meeting of the International Neuropsychological Society, Chicago.

Tamkin, A.S., & Kunce, J.T. (1985). A comparison of three neuropsychological tests: The Weigl, Hooper, and Benton. *Journal of Clinical Psychology, 41,* 660–664.

Tuokko, H., & Woodward, T.S. (1995). Development and validation of the demographic correc-

tion system for neuropsychological measures used in the Canadian Study of Health and Aging. *Journal of Clinical and Experimental Neuropsychology, 18,* 479–616.

Unterholzner, G., Sagstetter, E., & Bauer, M.G. (1992). Mehrstufiges Trainingsprogramm (MKT) zur Verbesserung kognitiver Funktionen bei chronischen Alkoholikern. *Zeitschrift für klinische Psychologie, Psychopathologie und Psychotherapie, 40,* 378–395.

Vakil, E., Blachstein, H., Sheleff, P., & Grossman, S. (1989). BVRT-Scoring system and time delay in the differentiation of lateralized hemispheric damage. *International Journal of Clinical Neuropsychology, 11,* 125–128.

Wagner, H. (1992). The Benton test in school counselling diagnostics. *Acta Paedopsychiatrica, 55,* 179–181.

Wahler, H.J. (1956). A comparison of reproduction errors made by brain-damaged and control patients on a memory-for-designs test. *Journal of Abnormal and Social Psychology, 52,* 251–255.

Weiss, A.A. (1974). Equivalence of three alternate forms of Benton's Visual Retention Test. *Perceptual and Motor Skills, 38,* 623–635.

Wellman, M.M. (1985). Benton Revised Visual Retention Test. In D.J. Keyser & R.C. Sweetland (Eds.), *Test Critiques.* Kansas City, MO: Test Corporation of America.

Youngjohn, J.R., Larrabee, G.J., & Crook, T.H. (1993). New adult- and education-correction norms for the Benton Visual Retention Test. *The Clinical Neuropsychologist, 7,* 155–160.

Zonderman, A.B., Giamba, L.M., Arenberg, D., Resnick, S.M., & Costa, P.T. (1995). Changes in immediate visual memory predict cognitive impairment. *Archives of Clinical Neuropsychology, 10,* 111–123.

BRIEF VISUOSPATIAL MEMORY TEST—REVISED (BVMT-R)

Purpose

This test is used to assess visual memory.

Source

The test (including manual, stimuli, and scoring sheets) can be ordered from Psychological Assessment Resources, Inc., P.O. Box 998, Odessa, FL 33556, at a cost of $119.00 U.S.

Description

This test was devised by Benedict and colleagues (Benedict & Groninger, 1995; Benedict et al., 1996; Benedict, 1997) and modeled after the Visual Reproduction subtest of the Wechsler Memory Scale (Russell Revision). It consists of six alternate forms that yield measures of immediate recall, rate of acquisition, delayed recall, and recognition. The subject is shown the same 8- × 11-inch plate containing six simple geometric visual designs in a 2 × 3 matrix. The matrix is presented for 10 seconds, after which time the patient is asked to reproduce (on a blank sheet of paper) as many of the designs as possible, in the same location as they appeared on the display. There is no time limit for recall. The patient is then asked to complete two additional learning trials using the same plate and encouraged to improve his or her performance. After 25 minutes of distracting tasks, the patient is asked to reproduce the designs again. This delayed recall trial is followed by a recognition trial in which the patient is shown 12 designs (each printed on a 3- × 5-inch card) one at a time. The patient is asked to respond "yes" to those designs included in the original matrix and to respond "no" to foils. This yes/no delayed recognition task includes six targets and six nontargets.

Administration

The instructions for administering the BVMT-R are provided in the test manual. Briefly, the examiner presents the displays and reads the instructions. Recall performance is recorded on a scoring sheet for each of the immediate recall trials (1 to 3), and for the delayed recall and recognition trials.

Approximate Time for Administration

About 15 minutes are required for the test, excluding the delay interval.

Scoring

Each response is evaluated in terms of two dimensions: accuracy and location. Two points are awarded for each reproduction that is correct with regard to accuracy and location. One point is given if the reproduction is correct with regard to accuracy but incorrectly placed or incorrect but recognizable as the target and correctly placed. If the drawing is incorrect (not present or present but not recognizable), 0 points are given. Scoring examples for each design are provided in the manual. The maximum total for each recall trial is 12.

The recall scores are combined to form three additional measures of learning and memory. The total immediate recall score is the sum of Trials 1 to 3. The learning score is the best of Trials 2 and 3 minus the trial 1 score. The percent retained after the delay is also calculated as Trial 4 recall divided by the best of Trials 2 and 3. Finally, measures of target discriminability and response bias are calculated from the total number of true- and false-positives obtained from the delayed recognition trial. The discrimination index is the number of true-positives minus the number of false positives. The response bias measure ranges from 0 to 1, with higher scores reflecting a liberal, as opposed to conservative response bias. Raw scores on Trials 1–3, total recall, learning, and delayed recall are converted to T-scores and percentile equivalents. Scores on percent retained, recognition hits, false alarms, discrimination index, and response bias all had highly skewed distributions, and only percentile ranks were calculated (e.g., 6–10th percentile).

Comment

Interrater reliability is reported to be high, above .90 (Benedict, 1997). Seventy-one subjects completed the same form after an interval of about 2 months. Reliability coefficients are above .4. When the sample is combined across the six test forms, the reliability coefficients range from .60 for Trial 1 to .84 for Trial 3 (Benedict, 1997). Benedict et al. (1996) report that the six different test forms were randomly assigned to a large sample of healthy individuals ($n = 457$). In addition, a sample of 18 college students completed all six forms at weekly intervals. Both between-groups and within-subjects analyses revealed equivalence of the alternate forms. There are, however, subtle practice effects despite the use of alternate forms. Healthy college students, administered alternate forms at six weekly intervals, improved their BVMT-R total recall scores from 28.9 (SD = 3.1) on session one to 30.8 (SD = 1.8) by session six.

With regard to construct validity, Benedict et al. (1996) found that in patients with either nonlateralized cerebral pathology or psychiatric disease, indices of learning and delayed recall correlated most strongly with other tests of explicit memory, such as the Hopkins Verbal Learning Test, the Visual Reproduction subtest of the WMS-R, and Rey Figure recall (.65–.80), less strongly with a measure of visuospatial construction, the copy portion of the Rey figure (.65 to .66), and most weakly with measures of expressive language, FAS word fluency, and the Boston Naming Test (.24–.54). The implication is that the BVMT-R involves both verbal and nonverbal memory processes. On the other hand, in a factor analysis that also included the Trail Making Test, Controlled Oral Word Association Test, VMI, and Hopkins Verbal Learning Test, the BVMT-R loaded on a separate factor, suggesting that it does indeed measure visuospatial learning and memory with a reasonable degree of specificity (Benedict et al., 1996).

Further, the test seems sensitive to brain integrity. Impaired performance has been noted in patients with HIV infection, dementia of the Alzheimer type (AD) and/or vascular dementia (VaD) (Benedict et al., 1996). None of the BVMT-R measures, however, discriminated between the AD and VaD patients. Information regarding the performance of patients with lateralized dysfunction is not yet available.

In summary, the test has a number of advantages including brevity, the availability of six equivalent forms, and the inclusion of learning, delayed recall, and recognition components. On the other hand, at this stage, the test is still under development, and the ability of the task to characterize the unique learning and memory deficits associated with various disorders is not known. In addition, the distribution of scores on some of the measures is skewed, rendering interpretation of some scores (e.g., the discrimination index) difficult.

Normative Data

The standardization sample included 588 healthy volunteers (210 males, 378 females) with an average age of 38.6 years (SD = 18.0, range 18–88) and an average level of education of 13.4 years (SD = 1.8). Normative data, subdivided according to age, are provided in the manual (Benedict, 1997). Normative tables were constructed using the method of overlapping midpoint age cells. Normative data are also given for a U.S. census aged-matched sample. Base-rate data are also provided that show the proportion of normals and patients with neurological disorders who fall within the various score ranges.

Benedict et al. (1996) reported that age was moderately correlated with single trial recall scores (−.44−−.50). Correlations between age and recognition performance were not significant. Correlations with education were weak (<.20). Gender did not influence most aspects of recall and recognition performance. In a mixed sample of patients, IQ showed a moderate relation with most of the BVMT measures (Benedict, personal communication, September 1996). Accordingly, data need to be provided, broken down by both age and intellectual level.

References

Benedict, R.H.B. (1997). *Brief Visuospatial Memory Test—Revised*. Odessa: FL: Psychological Assessment Resources, Inc.

Benedict, R.H.B., & Groninger, L. (1995). Preliminary standardization of a new visuospatial memory test with six alternate forms. *The Clinical Neuropsychologist*, 9, 11–16.

Benedict, R.H.B., Schretlen, D., Groninger, L., Dobraski, M., & Shpritz, B. (1996). Revision of the Brief Visuospatial Memory Test: Studies of normal performance, reliability, and validity. *Psychological Assessment*, 8, 145–153.

BUSCHKE SELECTIVE REMINDING TEST (SRT)

Other Test Name

Another test name is the Selective Reminding Test (SRT).

Purpose

The purpose of the test is to measure verbal learning and memory during a multiple-trial list-learning task.

Source

There is no commercial source. Users may refer to the following text in order to design their own material.

Description

The SRT materials include a list of words, index cards containing the first two to three letters of each list word, and index cards containing the multiple-choice recognition items. The procedure (Buschke, 1973; Buschke & Fuld, 1974) involves reading to the subject a list of words and then having the subject recall as many of these words as possible. Each subsequent learning trial involves the selective presentation of only those items that were not recalled on the immediately preceding trial. The SRT distinguishes between short-term and long-term components of memory by measuring recall of items that were not presented on a given trial. The rate at which subjects learn can also be evaluated.

A number of different versions of the test exist. For adults, our version is the same as that developed by Hannay and Levin (1985; Hannay, 1986). Briefly, the test consists of a series of 12 unrelated words presented over 12 selective reminding (SR) trials, or until the subject is able to recall the entire list on three consecutive trials. Several trials are added to help identify the conditions that promote otherwise impaired memory (e.g., cueing, multiple-choice recognition), or disclose forgetting (e.g., delayed recall) (Hannay & Levin, 1985). A cued-recall trial is presented after the 12th or last selective-reminding trial. The first two or three letters of each word are presented on

an index card, and the subject is asked to recall the corresponding list word. Following the cued-recall trial, the examiner presents a multiple-choice recognition trial. Here the examiner presents a series of 12 index cards, each card consisting of a list word, a synonym, a homonym, and an unrelated distractor word. Finally, a delayed-recall trial is given without forewarning 30 minutes after the multiple-choice recognition trial. Four different forms of the test are available. Figure 10–3 provides the word lists, and Figure 10–4 gives the multiple-choice and cued-recall items for the versions of the test used with adults. For adolescents, ages 13–15, the test can be modified by reducing the number of learning trials to eight (Miller et al., personal communication, September 1996).

Similar selective reminding (SR) procedures have been developed for use with children. Clodfelter et al. (1987) developed two alternate forms for children aged 9–12 years, and these are shown in Figure 10–5. A list of 12 words is presented for eight trials or until the child recalls all 12 words on two consecutive trials. Morgan (1982) developed alternate forms for children aged 5–8 years, and these are shown in Figure 10–6. The examiner presents a list of eight words that the subject must recall, in any order. The test continues for six

Form 1	Form 2	Form 3	Form 4
bowl	shine	throw	egg
passion	dis-agree	lily	runway
dawn	fat	film	fort
judge-ment	wealthy	dis-creet	tooth-ache
grant	drunk	loft	drown
bee	pin	beef	baby
plane	grass	street	lava
county	moon	helmet	damp
choice	prepare	snake	pure
seed	prize	dug	vote
wool	duck	pack	strip
meal	leaf	tin	truth

Figure 10—3. Word list for Forms 1–4 for Adult Version of SRT. Source: Hannay and Levin (1985).

Form 1

1.	bowl	dish	bell	view
2.	love	poison	conform	passion
3.	dawn	sunrise	bet	down
4.	pasteboard	verdict	judgement	fudge
5.	grand	grant	give	jazz
6.	see	sting	fold	bee
7.	pain	plane	pulled	jet
8.	county	state	tasted	counter
9.	voice	select	choice	cheese
10.	flower	seed	herd	seek
11.	date	sheep	wool	would
12.	mill	queen	food	meal

Form 2

1.	shine	glow	chime	cast
2.	dispute	disappear	contour	disagree
3.	fat	oil	trail	fit
4.	stopwatch	affluent	wealthy	worthy
5.	trunk	drunk	stoned	blunt
6.	fin	peg	wake	pin
7.	glass	grass	plan	lawn
8.	moon	beam	spark	noon
9.	propose	ready	prepare	husband
10.	award	prize	pot	size
11.	bark	bird	duck	luck
12.	leap	ranch	blade	leaf

Form 3

1.	throw	toss	through	plate
2.	flower	lilt	intent	lily
3.	film	movie	slave	kiln
4.	waver	cautious	discreet	distinct
5.	soft	loft	attic	tack
6.	beet	meat	clue	beef
7.	stream	street	speed	road
8.	helmet	armor	bacon	velvet
9.	smoke	serpent	snake	pool
10.	hoed	dug	hay	dog
11.	blank	bundle	pack	puck
12.	ton	shirt	foil	tin

Form 4

1.	egg	shell	beg	source
2.	airline	runner	darling	runway
3.	fort	castle	sink	fork
4.	boldness	dentist	toothache	headache
5.	blown	drown	float	rib
6.	body	infant	middle	baby
7.	larva	lava	echo	rock
8.	damp	moist	hook	stamp
9.	purse	clean	pure	bare
10.	ballot	vote	dish	note
11.	chain	peal	strip	slip
12.	trust	rise	fact	truth

Cued Recall Words

Form 1		Form 2		Form 3		Form 4	
BO	PL	SH	GR	TH	ST	—	LA
PA	COU	DI	MO	LI	HE	RU	DA
DA	CH	FA	PRE	FI	SN	FO	PU
JUD	SE	WEA	PR	DI	DU	TO	VO
GR	WO	DR	DU	LO	PA	DR	ST
—	ME	—	LE	BE	—	BA	TR

Figure 10—4. Multiple-choice and cued-recall items for Forms 1–4 of SRT. Source: Hannay (1986) and Hannay & Levin (1985).

List 1	List 2
garden	market
doctor	palace
metal	flower
city	picture
money	dollar
cattle	river
prison	cotton
clothing	sugar
water	college
cabin	baby
tower	temple
bottle	butter

Figure 10—5. Alternate forms of SRT for children, aged 9 to 12. Source: Clodfelter et al. (1987).

SR trials or until the subject is able to recall correctly the entire list in two consecutive trials.

Administration

Say to the subject: *"This test is to see how quickly you can learn a list of words. I am going to read you a list of 12* (for young children, eight) *words. I want you to listen carefully because when I stop, I want you to tell me as many of the words as you can recall. The words do not have to be in any particular order. When you have given me all the words that you can recall, I will tell you the words that you didn't give me from the list; then I want you to give me the entire list all over again. We do this 12* (for older children, eight; for younger children, six) *times, and each time I want you to try to give me all 12* (for younger children, eight) *words."*

Read the list of words at a rate of one word per 2 seconds and always present the words in order, beginning with the top of the list and

List 1	List 2	List 3
dog	balloon	apple
horse	crayons	meat
turtle	doll	egg
lion	bicycle	candy
squirrel	paints	carrot
bear	baseball	cereal
elephant	clay	bread
rabbit	book	banana

Figure 10—6. Word lists for three forms of SRT for children, aged 5 to 8. Source: Morgan (1982).

working to the bottom. The presentation of words will, of course, skip over the words that were recalled correctly on the preceding trial. If the subject is able to recall correctly all 12 (for younger children, eight) words on three (for children, two) consecutive trials, discontinue, but score as if all trials had been given. If the subject recalls words not on the list, inform the subject, and note the extra words. The total number of words on the list is not disclosed.

For the cued-recall trial, the first two to three letters of each list word are presented on an index card and the subject is asked to say the word from the list that would begin with the first two letters on the card (see Figure 10–4). The cue cards are presented one at a time in the same order as the words on the list. There is no time limit, and the subject is allowed to return to a previous card if he or she wishes. Since one word on Form 1 (bee) can be clearly identified by the first two letters, it is omitted from cued recall as well as pin, tin, and egg on Forms 2, 3, and 4, respectively. Cues that fail initially to evoke the list word are presented a second time after each cue has been given once. For the multiple-choice recognition trial, the subject is shown each of the 12 index cards and is asked to identify the list word. Give the cued-recall and multiple-choice trials even if the subject has recalled the entire list on the SR trials. After a 30-minute delay, ask the subject to recall all 12 words. During the 30-minute delay, the subject should be given nonverbal tasks to perform.

Approximate Time for Administration

The adult version requires 30 minutes; the children's version takes 10 minutes.

Scoring

See samples shown in Figures 10–7 through 10–9. A number of different scores are calculated (Buschke, 1973; Buschke & Fuld, 1974; Hannay & Levin, 1985). If a word is recalled on two consecutive trials, it is assumed to have entered long-term storage (LTS) on the first of these trials. Once a word enters LTS, it is considered to be in permanent storage, and it is

Sample SRT Score Sheet—Form 1 (Adult)

Name _____ Date _____ Examiner _____

	1	2	3	4	5	6	7	8	9	10	11	12	CR	MC	30 min
bowl															
passion															
dawn															
judgement															
grant															
bee															
plane															
county															
choice															
seed															
wool															
meal															
Total Recall															
LTR															
STR															
LTS															
CLTR															
RLTR															
Reminders															
Intrusions															

Trial 1   ____
Total Recall   ____ (Number recalled over 12 trials)
LTS   ____ (Words recalled twice in a row, assumed to be in LTS from that point on. Mark with red underliner, counting blanks. Compute sum over the 12 trials.)
STR   ____ (Words that are not underlined. Compute sum over the 12 trials.)
CLTR   ____ (Words that are continuously recalled. Mark with highlighter. Compute sum across 12 trials.)
RLTR   ____ (Words that are underlined but NOT CLTR. Do not count blanks. Compute sum across 12 trials.)
Reminders   ____ (Compute sum over 12 trials. Maximum = 144)
Intrusions   ____ (Compute sum over 12 trials.)
Cued Recall   ____ (Maximum = 11)
Mult. Choice   ____ (Maximum = 12)
30-Min Recall   ____ (Maximum = 12)

Figure 10—7. Selective Reminding Test sample scoring sheet.

scored as LTS on all following trials, regardless of the subject's subsequent recall. When a subject recalls a word that has entered LTS, it is scored as long-term retrieval (LTR). When a subject begins to recall a word in LTS consistently on all subsequent trials, it is also scored as consistent long-term retrieval (CLTR) or list-learning, beginning on the first of the uninterrupted successful recall trials. Inconsistent LTR refers to recall of a word in LTS followed by subsequent failure to recall the word. It is scored as random long-term retrieval (RLTR) until it is recalled consistently. Short-term recall (STR) refers to recall of a word that has not entered LTS. The total recall (Sum Recall) on each trial is the sum of STR and LTR. The number of reminders given by the examiner before the next recall attempt is equal to 12 − Sum Recall (for young children, 8 − Sum Recall) of the previous trial. Record by number the order of the subject's recall on each trial. Intrusions of extra-list words are also recorded on each trial.

Comment

It has been difficult to develop lists of equal difficulty and reliability for repeated testing of

Sample SRT Score Sheet–Form 1 (Children 9–12 years)

Name _____ Date _____ Examiner _____

	1	2	3	4	5	6	7	8
garden								
doctor								
metal								
city								
money								
cattle								
prison								
clothing								
water								
cabin								
tower								
bottle								

Total Recall

LTR _____

STR _____

LTS _____

CLTR _____

RLTR _____

Reminders _____

Intrusions _____

_____

_____

_____

_____

Total Recall _____ (Number recalled over 8 trials)

LTS _____ (Words recalled twice in a row, assumed to be in LTS from that point on. Mark with red underliner, counting blanks. Compute sum over the 8 trials.)

STR _____ (Words that are not underlined. Compute sum over the 8 trials.)

CLTR _____ (Words that are continuously recalled. Mark with highlighter. Compute sum across 8 trials.)

RLTR _____ (Words that are underlined but NOT CLTR. Do not count blanks. Compute sum across 8 trials.)

Reminders _____ (Compute sum over 8 trials. Maximum = 96)

Intrusions _____ (Compute sum over 8 trials.)

Figure 10—8. Selective Reminding Test sample score sheet for children ages 9–12.

individuals (Hannay & Levin, 1985; Kraemer et al., 1983; Loring & Papanicolaou, 1987; Said et al., 1990). The separate forms for the children's version are roughly of equivalent difficulty (Clodfelter et al., 1987; Morgan, 1982). For adults, we use the forms developed by Hannay and Levin (1985; Hannay, 1986) although other forms are available (e.g., Coen et al., 1990; Deptula et al., 1990). For college students, Forms 2 to 4 are of equivalent difficulty, whereas Form 1 is about 10 percent harder than Forms 3, 4, and 5 (Hannay & Levin, 1985). The four forms, however, appear to be of equivalent difficulty for elderly subjects

(Masur et al., 1989) and patients with clinical memory disorders, at least for those with medically refractory epilepsy (Sass et al., in press; Westerveld et al., 1994).

There was no significant practice effect when patients with seizures underwent multiple administrations of alternate forms on four consecutive days (Sass et al., in press; Westerveld et al., 1994). With normal individuals, however, there appears to be a nonspecific practice effect with repeated administration of alternate forms (Clodfelter et al., 1987; Hannay & Levin, 1985; Loring & Papanicolaou, 1987). Thus, the ability to learn how to per-

Sample SRT Score Sheet—Form 1 (Children 5–8 years)

Name _____ Date _____ Examiner _____

	1	2	3	4	5	6
dog						
horse						
turtle						
lion						
squirrel						
bear						
elephant						
rabbit						

Total Recall _____
LTR _____
STR _____
LTS _____
CLTR _____
RLTR _____
Reminders _____
Intrusions _____
_____
_____
_____
_____

Total Recall	_____ (Number recalled over 6 trials)
LTS	_____ (Words recalled twice in a row, assumed to be in LTS from that point on. Mark with red underliner, counting blanks. Compute sum over the 6 trials.)
STR	_____ (Words that are not underlined. Compute sum over the 6 trials.)
CLTR	_____ (Words that are continuously recalled. Mark with highlighter. Compute sum across 6 trials.)
RLTR	_____ (Words that are underlined but NOT CLTR. Do not count blanks. Compute sum across 6 trials.)
Reminders	_____ (Compute sum over 6 trials. Maximum = 48)
Intrusions	_____ (Compute sum over 6 trials.)

Figure 10—9. Selective Reminding Test sample score sheet for children ages 5–8.

form a complex task, as well as the ability to form associations between stimuli, may be accounting for group differences in research involving some populations (Loring & Papanicolaou, 1987; Sass et al., in press).

Alternate form reliability coefficients, while significant, tend to be moderate in magnitude for both normal and neurological samples (Clodfelter et al., 1987; Hannay & Levin, 1985; Morgan, 1982; Ruff et al., 1988; Sass et al., in press; Westerveld et al., 1994), although high values (.92 for consistent retrieval) have been reported for patients suffering from Alzheimer's disease (Masur et al., 1989). Total Recall scores are the most stable, and STM scores are the least stable (Sass et al., in press). Variance in performance on alternate

forms can be extreme, particularly for the measure of CLTR (Sass et al., in press; Westerveld et al., 1994). Sass et al. (in press) reported that 6 of 24 patients with epilepsy achieved CLTR scores that varied by 50 points or more. Westerveld and colleagues suggest that use of the mean or the better of two baseline assessments minimizes error variance, thereby enhancing interpretation of change. Alternatively, given that Total Recall scores generally are less variable and that SRT scores appear to measure a single construct, examiners may choose to rely on Total Recall scores (Sass et al., in press).

Smith et al. (1995) point out that there is no theoretical rationale for choosing 12 as the requisite number of trials. They found that as

Table 10—7. Norms for Verbal Selective Reminding Test

Variables[a]	Age Groups						
	18–29	30–39	40–49	50–59	60–69	70–79	80–91
Age							
Mean	22.55	34.62	43.71	54.17	66.0	74.49	83.48
SD	3.30	2.69	2.91	2.74	2.47	2.92	3.10
Education							
Mean	12.88	14.90	14.71	12.92	13.40	13.46	13.22
SD	1.73	2.47	2.72	1.98	3.57	3.78	3.76
n							
Total n	51	29	31	24	50	59	27
Female/male	23/28	15/14	19/12	22/2	33/17	38/21	23/4
Total							
Mean	128.18	124.59	125.03	121.62	114.82	105.27	97.96
SD	9.16	13.40	12.00	10.46	15.77	16.67	17.49
LTR							
Mean	122.16	118.14	118.55	112.71	101.52	89.95	77.22
SD	13.12	20.64	17.96	16.10	24.68	29.23	26.26
STR							
Mean	6.14	6.72	6.48	8.96	13.52	17.47	20.74
SD	4.82	7.59	6.72	6.40	9.52	10.41	9.62
LTS							
Mean	124.00	121.62	122.45	116.67	107.00	95.54	87.48
SD	10.47	18.36	15.64	14.52	21.79	24.86	25.26
CLTR							
Mean	115.12	107.93	107.10	101.50	88.92	69.68	54.96
SD	19.67	27.62	26.62	22.39	35.85	35.96	29.04

few as six trials provide information highly consistent with that provided by 12 trials. The only score with consistently lower correlations with 12-trial scores is RLTR, a not surprising finding since it is a measure of random long-term recall and is not expected to be consistent across trials. A 6- or 8-trial SRT would significantly reduce administration time and patient fatigue. Normative data are available for a 6-trial, 10-item form, but only for elderly individuals (Wiederholt et al., 1993).

The SRT is popular because it purports to parcel verbal memory into distinct component processes (e.g., LTS, LTR, CLTR, STR). In support of this notion, Beatty et al. (1996a) reported that in MS patients and controls, the probability of recall or recognition varied in a consistent manner as a function of the status of the words (CLTR, RLTR, or STR) in the subject's memory at the conclusion of training. Thus, words that were being retrieved from CLTR at the end of acquisition were more likely to be recalled after delay than were words that were not being consistently retrieved from LTS. Words that were being retrieved from STR were the least likely to be recalled after delay. On the other hand, there is evidence that the numerous scores that can be derived from the test tend to be highly intercorrelated, suggesting that these measures are assessing similar constructs (Kenisten, cited in Kraemer et al., 1983; Larrabee et al., 1988; Loring & Papanicolaou, 1987; Paniak et al., 1989; Sass et al., in press; Smith et al., 1995; Westerveld et al., 1994). Further, although the SR procedure offers information

Table 10—7. *(Continued)*

Variables[a]	Age Groups						
	18–29	30–39	40–49	50–59	60–69	70–79	80–91
RLTR							
Mean	8.12	10.12	11.19	10.79	14.66	20.71	22.19
SD	9.42	9.73	11.34	9.25	11.83	14.37	10.70
Reminders							
Mean	16.0	18.10	19.03	22.25	28.12	36.95	43.96
SD	8.42	13.12	11.26	10.06	15.16	15.17	15.77
Intrusions							
Mean	.84	.97	1.81	1.17	3.90	4.22	3.30
SD	1.29	1.43	3.10	1.49	7.29	5.76	5.09
Cued Recall							
Mean	—	—	—	—	9.58[b]	8.95[c]	8.16[d]
SD					1.93	2.12	2.22
Multiple Choice							
Mean	12.0	12.0	12.0	12.0	11.96	11.85	11.93
SD	0.0	0.0	0.0	0.0	0.20	0.58	0.27
Delayed Recall							
Mean	11.53	10.66	11.03	10.83	9.58	9.05	8.37
SD	.83	1.97	1.43	1.40	2.46	2.62	2.45

[a]Correction values for raw scores of males (calculate before entering normative tables). Total = +5; LTR = +9; STR = −4; LTS = +7; CLTR = +13; RLTR = −5; Reminders = −5; Intrusions = 0; Cued Recall = 0; Multiple Choice = 0; Delayed Recall = +1. Caution: Do not correct LTS or CLTR if raw score is 0. See text for definitions of Total, LTR, STR, LTS, CLTR, RLTR, Reminders by Examiner, Intrusions, Cued Recall, Multiple Choice, Delayed Recall.

[b]$n = 31$.

[c]$n = 38$.

[d]$n = 19$.

Source: Larabee et al., 1988. Reprinted with permission.

regarding short- and long-term memory, the operational distinction between long-term storage and retrieval is problematic (Loring & Papanicolaou, 1987). According to Bushke's definition, a word has entered LTS if it has been successfully recalled on two successive trials. By definition, failure to recall is due to a retrieval difficulty. However, the item may have been stored in a weak or degraded form and through the process of additional repetition by the examiner, the word is encoded more deeply and efficiently (Loring & Papanicolaou, 1987). Therefore, operationally defined retrieval may have little to do with retrieval itself.

A single index from among those obtained using standard scoring methods may adequately convey the SRT result, given the redundancy of the scores. The total number of words recalled on all trials throughout the test, a fairly reliable measure, is recommended by Westerveld et al. (1994) and Sass et al. (in press) as a measure of learning. To measure forgetting, Trahan and Larrabee (1993) recommend computing a score based on the number of words in long-term storage on the final learning trial (Trial 12 LTS) minus the 30-minute delayed recall score.

Modest correlations have been demonstrated among the SRT and other tests (e.g.,

Table 10—8. Normative Data for Selective Reminding Test, Ages 13–15

	Females											
	Age 13 ($n = 48$)				Age 14 ($n = 58$)				Age 15 ($n = 22$)			
	Low IQ		High IQ		Low IQ		High IQ		Low IQ		High IQ	
	M	SD	M	SD	M	SD	M	SD	M	SD	M	SD
CLTR	60.56	(14.03)	65.91	(16.88)	60.50	(17.15)	69.66	(16.25)	61.56	(14.99)	68.75	(11.44)
STR	5.44	(3.15)	5.61	(4.32)	6.12	(3.44)	4.87	(4.83)	4.78	(3.78)	2.75	(1.26)
LTS	76.36	(7.50)	76.74	(10.12)	74.42	(7.20)	78.13	(10.57)	77.33	(8.77)	81.25	(7.36)
30″ DEL	10.24	(1.36)	10.48	(1.59)	10.35	(1.20)	10.75	(1.44)	10.61	(1.54)	11.25	(0.96)
RECG	11.12	(1.17)	11.22	(1.09)	10.36	(1.48)	11.53	(0.80)	10.94	(1.30)	12.75	(0.50)
SAV	92.36	(10.28)	93.25	(9.67)	95.47	(11.92)	93.47	(10.52)	96.85	(11.62)	95.65	(5.03)

Source: Miller et al., 1996. Reprinted with permission.

CVLT, RAVLT, WMS) of verbal learning and memory (McCartney-Filgate & Vriezen, 1988; Shear & Craft, 1989). Larrabee and Curtiss (1995) evaluated the factor structure of several tests of memory and information-processing ability and found that the SRT loaded on a general verbal visual memory factor (along with the Expanded Paired Associates Test, Continuous Recognition Memory Test, and Continuous Visual Memory Test).

The SRT has become one of the more widely used procedures for assessing memory functioning following head injury (e.g., Levin & Grossman, 1976; Paniak et al., 1989). SRT performance is impaired following severe closed-head injury. Further, the severity of the injury (e.g., determined by length of unconsciousness) is related to the level of memory performance. Levin et al. (1979) have reported that the degree of long-term memory impairment 1 year after severe head injury corresponds to the overall level of disability in survivors. Patients who attained good recovery (i.e., resumption of work and normal social functioning) consistently recalled words without further reminding at a level comparable to that of normal adults. In contrast, consistent recall was grossly impaired in patients who were moderately or severely disabled at the time of the study.

The SRT has also proved useful in differentiating normal children from those at risk for memory disorders: learning disabled and those with seizures of left-hemisphere origin (Snow et al., 1992). In patients with MS, the SRT has served to emphasize the heterogeneity of the memory disturbances. Beatty et al. (1996b) found evidence of three distinct patterns of SRT performance in these patients: unimpaired, mildly impaired with mainly retrieval problems, and more severely impaired with encoding as well as retrieval difficulties. In addition, the test is useful in distinguishing normal adults from demented elderly persons (Larrabee, Largen, & Levin, 1985; Masur et al., 1989; Sabe et al., 1995). The measures LTR and CLTR were most valuable in distinguishing mild dementia from normal aging (Masur et al., 1989). Scores from the SRT may also be useful as preclinical indicators of the development of dementia. Masur and colleagues (1990), using a modified SRT procedure (six trials, delayed recall and recognition after a 5-minute period of distraction), reported that the sum of recall and delayed recall were the measures best able to predict dementia, with sensitivities of 47 percent and 44 percent, respectively. The predictive values were 37 percent and 40 percent, respectively, or better than 2.5 times the base rate.

Further, there is an association between impairment of verbal learning and memory, as measured by the SRT, and left temporal-lobe abnormality (Lee et al., 1989; Lee et al., 1990; Lencz et al., 1992; Levin et al., 1982; Martin et al., 1988; Snow et al., 1992). For example, Sass and colleagues (1990) showed that SRT scores correlated significantly with hippocampal pyramidal cell density obtained from pathologic analysis of excised tissue from the

	Males											
	Age 13 ($n = 33$)				Age 14 ($n = 42$)				Age 15 ($n = 24$)			
	Low IQ		High IQ		Low IQ		High IQ		Low IQ		High IQ	
	M	SD	M	SD	M	SD	M	SD	M	SD	M	SD
CLTR	42.08	(13.20)	59.14	(15.05)	59.75	(16.80)	68.35	(15.96)	36.00	(16.51)	63.67	(14.61)
STR	10.08	(4.63)	7.14	(6.14)	7.65	(5.39)	5.27	(4.53)	8.11	(4.60)	4.67	(3.85)
LTS	64.67	(8.96)	73.67	(12.29)	72.60	(13.09)	77.77	(10.06)	70.39	(9.60)	81.00	(6.90)
30″ DEL	8.08	(1.76)	10.00	(2.43)	10.50	(1.85)	10.77	(1.19)	10.11	(2.25)	30.83	(1.83)
RECG	10.08	(1.20)	10.86	(1.24)	11.15	(1.18)	11.73	(0.70)	10.72	(1.23)	11.67	(0.82)
SAV	79.73	(17.92)	92.65	(22.87)	94.28	(13.75)	92.04	(10.09)	93.82	(17.22)	92.50	(11.73)

left, but not the right hippocampus, of left-speech dominant adults. Further, left-speech dominant patients with severe hippocampal neuron loss experience no significant decrement in SRT performance following total excision of the left hippocampus (Sass et al., in press). However, those with mild or moderate neuron loss decline significantly. It is important to note, however, that patients with diffuse cerebral lesions perform about the same as patients with focal involvement of the left temporal lobe on the SRT (Levin et al., 1982). There is also evidence that individuals with emotional disorders (e.g., combat-related post-traumatic stress disorder, schizophrenia, depression) perform poorly on the SRT (Bremner et al., 1993; Goldberg et al., 1989; Sabe et al., 1995; but see Gass, 1996). Therefore, the SRT should not be used by itself to predict left temporal lobe abnormality.

In short, the SRT has a number of advantages. The examiner has available four equivalent forms that are sensitive, but not specific, to side of seizure onset and degree of hippocampal neuron loss. Further, the literature suggests an absence of practice effects in neurological patients, even when test sessions are on successive days. Therefore, the SRT has special merit when changes in memory function need to be evaluated (e.g., pre- and post-temporal lobectomy). On the other hand, extreme variance can occur in some SRT indices. Emotional distress and intellectual level may also affect performance on the test.

Normative Data

Both age and sex affect performance, with age being the most salient of these two subject variables. In general, females perform better than males (Bishop et al., 1990; Miller et al., 1996; Trahan & Quintana, 1990; Wiederholt et al., 1993). Further, with increasing age, the performance of men declines more rapidly than that of women (Wiederholt et al., 1993). Psychometric intelligence is moderately related to SRT performance. Sherman and colleagues (1995) found that the Verbal Comprehension factor of the WAIS-R correlated moderately ($r = .33$) with the LTR score of the SRT. Similarly, Bishop et al. (1990) found that scores of college students in the low-average range fell approximately 1 SD below comparable SRT data. Miller et al. (1996) reported that in adolescents, scores improved with increasing IQ. Goldberg et al. (1989) noted that scores on the Mini Mental State Examination correlated significantly with total recall scores on the SRT. Thus, use of SRT normative data that does not consider intellectual level may put clinicians at risk of overestimating memory deficits in individuals with low-average IQs (Bishop et al., 1990). The influence of education is inconsistent, with some studies finding it to be relatively unimportant (Goldberg et al., 1989; Larrabee et al., 1988; Petersen et al., 1992; Ruff et al., 1989; Trahan & Quintana, 1990), whereas others (Wiederholt et al., 1993) note significantly better perfor-

Table 10—9. Normative Data for Selective Reminding Test, Ages 9–12

	Age 9 (n = 77; m = 32, f = 45)				Age 10 (n = 126; m = 59, f = 67)				Age 11 (n = 110; m = 49, f = 61)				Age 12 (n = 98; m = 50, f = 48)			
	Low IQ		High IQ		Low IQ		High IQ		Low IQ		High IQ		Low IQ		High IQ	
	M	SD	M	SD	M	SD	M	SD	M	SD	M	SD	M	SD	M	SD
CLTR	49.88	(18.69)	53.56	(17.91)	56.00	(18.22)	61.96	(16.41)	51.69	(18.14)	55.16	(17.25)	57.64	(16.98)	66.15	(17.21)
STR	6.50	(3.92)	5.42	(3.74)	6.05	(4.17)	5.84	(4.30)	7.06	(5.45)	6.36	(4.86)	3.36	(4.46)	5.13	(4.40)
LTS(M)	66.94	(12.36)	71.90	(10.15)	71.36	(9.84)	76.25	(6.63)	58.70	(10.73)	70.54	(11.97)	76.59	(10.45)	76.28	(11.05)
LTS(F)	72.31	(10.18)	76.62	(8.30)	73.34	(10.13)	74.26	(11.38)	74.61	(13.75)	74.46	(10.70)	74.82	(10.96)	80.00	(8.64)
30" DEL	9.66	(2.24)	10.09	(1.58)	10.07	(1.67)	10.49	(1.42)	10.82	(1.97)	10.31	(1.43)	10.62	(1.52)	10.79	(1.34)
RECG	10.34	(1.78)	10.64	(1.48)	11.00	(1.31)	11.18	(1.27)	10.76	(1.22)	10.77	(1.36)	10.98	(1.12)	11.40	(0.87)
SAV	93.28	(19.53)	95.66	(15.86)	91.69	(11.90)	93.72	(10.52)	93.41	(17.56)	96.40	(13.05)	96.90	(11.30)	94.79	(11.79)

Source: Miller et al., 1996, personal communication.

Table 10—10. Mean Scores of Children,
Aged 5–8, on SRT

	Age 5–6 (n = 16)		Age 7–8 (n = 14)	
	M	SD	M	SD
Recall/trial	5.3	1.2	6.1	1.1
LTS	28.6	10.1	35.7	9.1
LTR	25.7	9.9	33.4	10.2
CLTR	18.9	11.3	27.7	13.2

Source: Morgan, 1982. Scores are derived from a small group of healthy schoolchildren, of average intelligence.

mance for those with some college education on all indices except the short-term memory index. The finding that some measures are relatively unaffected by intelligence makes the SRT a valuable clinical tool, particularly for the examination of those with less than a high school education.

Larrabee et al. (1988) provided norms for the adult version (Form I) of the SRT, organized by age and sex, shown in Table 10–7. The reader should note that corrections need to be made for gender (see Note *a* on Table 10–7). In addition, note that the mean values for LTR and STR do not sum to the exact value of the total correct score. The same is true for the relationship of the mean values for CLTR and RLTR to LTR. These small discrepancies appeared because different gender corrections were used for these respective scores. Note too that various indices of acquisition (LTS, CLTR) decline with age, particularly after age 50. There are also age-related differences in rate of forgetting, but the effects tend to be quite modest and dependent upon the particular index used to measure what was stored in acquisition (Petersen et al., 1992; Trahan & Larrabee, 1993). To measure forgetting, Trahan and Larrabee (1993) recommend the use of the acquisition score (defined as Trial 12 LTS) minus the Delay score.

Similar data have been reported for middle-aged adults by Ruff et al. (1989). Masur et al. (1989) also provide normative data for a large sample of elderly subjects. Their sample, however, contains a large number of non–native English speakers. This may account for the fact that their scores are somewhat lower

than those reported here. Wiederholt and colleagues (1993) also give data for a large sample of community-dwelling elderly individuals. The data, however, are based on a somewhat different version of the SRT than that presented here, one in which 10 (not 12) items are presented for 6 (not 12) trials.

Levin has also used Form I of the SRT with adolescents, aged 13–18 (Levin & Grossman, 1976; Levin, Benton, & Grossman, 1982), and gives data based on small samples of males (*n* = 23) and females (*n* = 27) for Form I for two measures, LTS and CLTR. Levin reports that there were no significant effects of age on performance between the ages of 13 and 18. Girls, however, performed at a superior level compared to boys. Miller et al. (1996) modified the adult form by reducing the number of learning trials to eight. Sex, age, and verbal IQ level (low = 110 or less and high = 111 and above) affected test scores among adolescents. Table 10–8 provides data for 227 students, aged 13–15 years, stratified on the basis of sex, age, and verbal IQ. The savings score is calculated as a ratio of the number of words recalled on delay divided by the number recalled on the eighth and last learning trial.

Clodfelter et al. (1987) provide normative data, based on 58 children, for alternate forms of the SRT for children, aged 9–12 years. Clodfelter et al., however, provided data on only a few variables and did not address retention following delay. Miller et al. (1986) give more extensive norms, based on 417 schoolchildren (Table 10–9). Both age and verbal IQ affected results. Normative data for parallel forms of the SRT for children, aged 5–8, have been provided by Morgan (1982). Table 10–10 presents the means and standard deviations by age for four SRT variables (recall per trial, LTS, LTR, CLTR). The tables show that children's performance increases substantially with age. It should be noted that the data presented are of limited value since the sample sizes are quite small.

References

Beatty, W.W., Krull, K.R., Wilbanks, S.L., Blanco, C.R., Hames, K.A., & Paul, R.H. (1996a). Further validation of constructs from the Selective Reminding Test. *Journal of Clinical and Experimental Neuropsychology, 18*, 52–55.

Beatty, W.W., Krull, K.R., Wilbanks, S.L., Blanco, C.R., Hames, K.A., Tivis, R., & Paul, R.H. (1996b). Memory disturbance in multiple sclerosis: Reconsideration of patterns of performance on the Selective Reminding Test. *Journal of Clinical and Experimental Neuropsychology, 18*, 56–62.

Bishop, E.G., Dickson, A.L., & Allen, M.T. (1990). Psychometric intelligence and performance on Selective Reminding. *The Clinical Neuropsychologist, 4*, 141–150.

Bremner, J.D., Scott, T.M., Delaney, R.C., et al. (1993). Deficits in short-term memory in posttraumatic stress disorder. *American Journal of Psychiatry, 150*, 1015–1019.

Buschke, H. (1973). Selective reminding for analysis of memory and learning. *Journal of Verbal Learning and Verbal Behavior, 12*, 543–550.

Buschke, H., & Fuld, P.A. (1974). Evaluating storage, retention, and retrieval in disordered memory and learning. *Neurology, 24*, 1019–1025.

Coen, R.F., Kinsella, A., Lambe, R., et al. (1990). Creating equivalent word lists for the Buschke Selective Reminding Test. *Human Psychopharmacology; Clinical and Experimental, 5*, 47–51.

Clodfelter, C.J., Dickson, A.L., Newton Wilkes, C., & Johnson, R.B. (1987). Alternate forms of selective reminding for children. *The Clinical Neuropsychologist, 1*, 243–249.

Deptula, D., Singh, R., Goldsmith, S., et al. (1990). Equivalence of five forms of the Selective Reminding Test in young and elderly subjects. *Psychological Reports, 3*, 1287–1295.

Gass, C.S. (1996). MMPI-2 variables in attention and memory test performance. *Psychological Assessment, 8*, 135–138.

Goldberg, T.E., Weinberger, D.R., Pliskin, N.H., Berman, K.F., & Podd, M.H. (1989). Recall memory deficit in schizophrenia. *Schizophrenia Research, 2*, 251–257.

Hannay, H.J. (1986). *Experimental Techniques in Human Neuropsychology.* New York: Oxford.

Hannay, J.H., & Levin, H.S. (1985). Selective reminding test: An examination of the equivalence of four forms. *Journal of Clinical and Experimental Neuropsychology, 7*, 251–263.

Kraemer, H.C., Peabody, C.A., Tinklenberg, J.R., & Yesavage, J.A. (1983). Mathematical and empirical development of a test of memory for clinical and research use. *Psychological Bulletin, 94*, 367–380.

Larrabee, G.J., Largen, J.W., & Levin, H.S. (1985). Sensitivity of age-decline resistant

("Hold") WAIS subtests to Alzheimer's disease. *Journal of Clinical and Experimental Neuropsychology, 7*, 497–504.

Larrabee, G.L., Trahan, D.E., Curtiss, G., & Levin, H.S. (1988). Normative data for the verbal selective reminding test. *Neuropsychology, 2*, 173–182.

Larrabee, G.J., and Curtiss, G. (1995). Construct validity of various verbal and visual memory tests. *Journal of Clinical and Experimental Neuropsychology, 17*, 536–547.

Lee, G.P., Loring, D.W., & Thompson, J.L. (1989). Construct validity of material-specific memory measures following unilateral temporal lobe ablations. *Psychological Assessment, 1*, 192–197.

Lee, G.P., Meador, K.J., Loring, D.W., et al. (1990). Behavioral activation of human hippocampal EEG: Relationship to recent memory. *Journal of Epilepsy, 3*, 137–142.

Lencz, T., McCarthy, G., Bronen, R.A., et al. (1992). Quantitative magnetic resonance imaging in temporal lobe epilepsy: Relationship to neuropathology and neuropsychological function. *Annals of Neurology, 31*, 629–637.

Levin, H.S., Benton, A.L., & Grossman, R.G. (1982). *Neurobehavioral Consequences of Closed Head Injury.* New York: Oxford University Press.

Levin, H.S., & Grossman, R.G. (1976). Storage and retrieval. *Journal of Pediatric Psychology, 1*, 38–42.

Levin, H.S., Grossman, R.G., Rose, J.E., & Teasdale, G. (1979). Long-term neuropsychological outcome of closed head injury. *Journal of Neurosurgery, 50*, 412–422.

Loring, D.W., & Papanicolaou, A.C. (1987). Memory assessment in neuropsychology: Theoretical considerations and practical utility. *Journal of Clinical and Experimental Neuropsychology, 9*, 340–358.

Macartney-Filgate, M.S., & Vriezen, E.R. (1988). Intercorrelation of clinical tests of verbal memory. *Archives of Clinical Neuropsychology, 3*, 121–126.

Martin, R.C., Loring, D.W., Meador, K.J., & Lee, G.P. (1988). Differential forgetting in patients with temporal lobe dysfunction. *Archives of Clinical Neuropsychology, 3*, 351–358.

Masur, D.M., Fuld, P.A., Blau, A.D., Thal, L.J., Levin, H.S., & Aronson, M.K. (1989). Distinguishing normal and demented elderly with the Selective Reminding Test. *Journal of Clinical and Experimental Neuropsychology, 11*, 615–630.

Masur, D.A., Fuld, P.A., Blau, A.D., Crystal, H., & Aronson, M.K. (1990). Predicting development of dementia in the elderly with the Selective Reminding Test. *Journal of Clinical and Experimental Neuropsychology, 12,* 529–538.

Miller, H.B., Murphy, D., Paniak, C., & Spackman, L., & LaBonte, M. (1996). Selective Reminding Test: Norms for children ages 9 to 15. Personal communication.

Morgan, S.F. (1982). Measuring long-term memory, storage and retrieval in children. *Journal of Clinical Psychology, 4,* 77–85.

Paniak, C.E., Shore, D.L., & Rourke, B.P. (1989). Recovery of memory after severe closed head injury: Dissociations in recovery of memory parameters and predictors of outcome. *Journal of Clinical and Experimental Neuropsychology, 11,* 631–644.

Petersen, R.C., Smith, G., Kokmen, E., et al., (1992). Memory function in normal aging. *Neurology, 42,* 396–401.

Ruff, R.M., Quayhagen, M., & Light, R.H. (1989). Selective reminding tests: A normative study of verbal learning in adults. *Journal of Clinical and Experimental Neuropsychology, 11,* 539–550.

Sabe, L., Jason, L., Juejati, M., Leiguarda, R., & Strakstein, S.E. (1995). Dissociation between declarative and procedural learning in dementia and depression. *Journal of Clinical and Experimental Neuropsychology, 17,* 841–848.

Said, J.A., Shores, A., Batchelor, J., Thomas, D., et al. (1990). The children's Auditory-Verbal Selective Reminding Test: Equivalence and test–retest reliability of two forms with boys and girls. *Developmental Neuropsychology, 6,* 225–230.

Sass, K.J., Spencer, D.D., Kim, J.H., Westerveld, M., Novelly, R.A., & Lencz, T. (1990). Verbal memory impairment correlates with hippocampal pyramidal cell density. *Neurology, 40,* 1694–1697.

Sass, K.J., Westerveld, M., Spencer, S.S., Kim, J.H., & Spencer, D.D. (in press). Degree of hippocampal neuron loss mediates verbal memory decline following left anteromedial temporal lobectomy. *Epilepsia.*

Sass, K.J., Dorfinger, J., Henry, H., Buchanan, C.P., & Westerveld, M. (in press). Examining the verbal memory of adults with epilepsy: A replication of Verbal Selective Reminding Test reliability and alternate forms equivalence. *Journal of Epilepsy.*

Shear, J.M., & Craft, R.B. (1989). Examination of the concurrent validity of the California Verbal Learning Test. *The Clinical Neuropsychologist, 3,* 162–168.

Sherman, E.M.S., Strauss, E., Spellacy, F., & Hunter, M. (1995). Construct validity of WAIS-R factors: Neuropsychological test correlates in adults referred for possible head injury. *Psychological Assessment, 7,* 440–444.

Smith, R.L., Goode, K.T., la Marche, J.A., & Boll, T.J. (1995). Selective reminding test short form administration: A comparison of two through twelve trials. *Psychological Assessment, 7,* 177–182.

Snow, J.H., English, R., & Lange, B. (1992). Clinical utility of the Selective Reminding Test—children's version. *Journal of Psychoeducational Assessment, 10,* 153–160.

Trahan, D.E., & Quintana, J.W. (1990). Analysis of gender effects upon verbal and visual memory performance in adults. *Archives of Clinical Neuropsychology, 5,* 325–334.

Trahan, D.E., & Larrabee, G.J. (1993). Clinical and methodological issues in measuring rate of forgetting with the Verbal Selective Reminding Test. *Psychological Assessment, 5,* 67–71.

Westerveld, M., Sass, K.J., Sass, A., & Henry, H.G. (1994). Assessment of verbal memory in temporal lobe epilepsy using the Selective Reminding Test: Equivalence and reliability of alternate forms. *Journal of Epilepsy, 7,* 57–63.

Wiederholt, W.C., Cahn, D., Butters, N.M., Salmon, D.P., Kritz-Silverstein, D., & Barrett-Connor, E. (1993). Effects of age, gender, and education on selected neuropsychological tests in an elderly community cohort. *Journal of the American Geriatrics Society, 41,* 639–647.

CALIFORNIA VERBAL LEARNING TEST (CVLT)

Purpose

The purpose of this test is to provide an assessment of the strategies and processes involved in learning and remembering verbal material.

Source

The kit (includes manual and 25 record forms) can be ordered from The Psychological Corporation, 555 Academic Court, San Antonio, TX 78204-2498, or 55 Horner Avenue, Toronto, Ontario M8Z 4X6, at a cost of $121 US or $185 Cdn. CVLT Computer scoring software (for IBM) is available for an unlimited number of scorings at an additional cost of $270 US or $405 Cdn. The children's version of the test, CVLT-C (including the manual, 25 record forms, and software), costs $315.50 US or $475 Cdn.

Description

This test (Delis et al., 1987) has become increasingly popular because it assesses multiple aspects of how verbal learning occurs as well as the amount of verbal material learned. It uses items that make up two shopping lists, presented to the patient as the "Monday" and "Tuesday" lists. The CVLT measures both recall and recognition of the word lists over a number of trials. Administration begins by evaluating an individual's ability to recall a list (List A) of 16 words (four words from each of four semantic categories) over five trials. An interference list (List B) of 16 words (four words from each of four semantic categories) is then presented for one trial. Two of the semantic categories on List B are the same as categories on List A ("shared" categories), while the other two categories are different ("nonshared" categories). The interference List B is immediately followed by free and category-cued recall of the first list (List A). After a 20-minute delay during which nonverbal testing (e.g., block construction or finger tapping) occurs, free recall, cued recall, and recognition of the first list (using a yes/no paradigm) are assessed. From this procedure, the CVLT quantifies the following parameters:

• levels of total recall and recognition on all trials
• semantic and serial learning strategies
• serial position effects
• learning rate across trials
• recall consistency across trials
• degree of vulnerability to proactive and retroactive interference
• retention of information over short and longer delays
• enhancement of recall performance by category cuing and recognition testing
• indices of recognition performance (discriminability and response bias) derived from signal detection theory
• perseverations and intrusions in recall
• false positives in recognition.

The adult version is appropriate for individuals aged 17–80 years. An alternate form has been developed for research purposes (Delis et al., 1991) and is available by writing to Dr. Delis directly (Psychology Service 116B, V.A. Medical Center, 3350 La Jolla Village Drive, San Diego, CA 92161). A short nine-word form has recently been developed, particularly for use with older individuals who are already cognitively impaired (Libon et al., 1996). The test is reproduced in Figure 10–10. The A 'shopping list' is composed of three items, from each of three categories (fruits, vegetables and clothing). It is presented over five immediate free recall trials. A second nine-word 'shopping list,' List B, is also drawn from three categories (fruits, tools, and baked goods). After a 20-minute filled delay, free recall, category-cued recall, and recognition are assessed for List A. The recognition test contains 33 words; nine from List A, six from List B, and 18 distractor items including nine unrelated words, six prototypical or high probability distractor items, and three phonemic distractor items related to words from List A.

A children's version, the CVLT-C, can be given to individuals aged 5–16 (Delis et al., 1994). It is similar in format to the adult version except that the child is asked to learn and recall 15 words (five words from each of three semantic categories).

Trial 1: Let's suppose you were going shopping on Monday. I am going to read a list of things for you to buy. Listen carefully, because when I am through I want you to tell me as many of these things as you can.

Trial 2: I am going to read the Monday shopping list again, tell me as many of the things as you can in any order you wish.

Trial 3-5: I am going to read the Monday shopping list again. Like before, tell as many of the things as you can.

List A - Test Items Sequence	Trial 1	Trial 2	Trial 3	Trial 4	Trial 5
cherries					
sweater					
lettuce					
jacket					
cabbage					
plums					
shorts					
grapes					
spinach					

total trials 1-5
correct -
intrusions -
persev. -
clusters -

correct _____ _____ _____ _____ _____
intrusions _____ _____ _____ _____ _____
perseverations _____ _____ _____ _____ _____
clusters _____ _____ _____ _____ _____

Interference - List B (trial 6p): Now let's suppose you were going shopping again, this time on Tuesday. I am going to read a new list of things for you to buy. When I am through, I want you to tell me as many of these things from this new list as you can. You can say them in any order.

Short Delay Free Recall (trial 7r): Now I want you to tell me all the things you can from the Monday shopping list. The Monday list was the first list, the one I read you five times. Don't tell me the things that were on the Tuesday list. Only tell me the things that were on the Monday list.

Short Delay Cued Recall (trial 8): Tell me the things from the Monday list that were clothing . . . vegetables . . . fruits.

List B - Test Items sequence	Interference (trial 6p)	Short Delay Free Recall (trial 7r)	Short Delay Cued Recall (trial 8) Clothing	Vegetables	Fruit
cookies					
peaches					
drill					
bananas					
wrench					
cupcakes					
pliers					
brownies					
strawberries					

proactive interference
tr1 minus tr6p

retroactive interference
tr5 minus tr7r

correct _____
intrusions _____
perseverations _____
clusters _____

Recognition: Now I am going to read a bunch of things that people can buy. After I read each one, say "yes" if it was on the Monday list, and say "no" if it was not on the Monday list.

Long Delay Free Recall (trial 9d): I read two shopping lists to you before, the Monday list and the Tuesday list. I want you to tell me all the things you can remember from the Monday list . . . that's the Monday list.

Long Delay Cued Recall (trial 10): Tell me all the things from the Monday shopping list that are clothing . . . vegetables . . . fruit.

Long Delay Cued Recall (trial 10)

Long Delay Free Recall (trial 9d)	Clothing	Vegetables	Fruit

cor. _____
intru _____
per. _____
cl. _____

Recognition

Item	M	TS	TO	TU	NP	NU	PS
shorts		X	X	X	X	X	X
glasses	X	X	X	X	X		X
soap	X	X	X	X	X		X
drill	X	X	X		X	X	X
pants	X	X	X	X		X	X
mop	X	X	X	X	X		X
cherries		X	X	X		X	X
lettuce		X	X	X	X	X	X
brownies	X	X		X	X	X	X
apples	X	X	X	X		X	X
racquet	X	X	X	X	X	X	X
keys	X	X	X	X	X		X
grapes		X	X	X	X	X	X
corn	X	X	X	X		X	X
rug	X	X	X	X	X		X
spinach		X	X	X	X	X	X
oranges	X	X	X	X		X	X
sweater		X	X	X	X	X	X
radio	X	X	X		X		X
cookies	X	X	X	X	X		X
strawberries	X		X	X	X	X	X
jacket		X		X	X	X	X
peaches	X		X	X	X	X	X
socks	X	X	X	X		X	X
roses	X	X	X	X	X		X
plums		X	X	X	X	X	X
drapes	X	X	X	X	X	X	
cabbage		X	X		X	X	X
wrench	X	X	X	X	X	X	
pencil	X	X	X	X			X
wallet	X	X	X	X	X		X
carrots	X	X	X	X		X	X
baggage	X	X	X	X		X	X
Correct			X	X	X	X	
TO	X	X	X	X	X	X	X
TS	X	X	X	X	X	X	X
TU	X	X	X	X	X	X	X
NP	X	X	X	X	X	X	X
NU	X	X	X	X	X	X	X
PS	X		X	X	X	X	X

Figure 10—10. California Verbal Learning Test (nine-word version). Source: D. Libon, personal communication. M = Monday, TS = Tuesday items from shared semantic category, TO = Tuesday items from a related but different semantic category, TU = Tuesday items from an unrelated semantic category, NP = semantic prototypical foils, NU = non-prototypical foils unrelated to any semantic category in list A or B, PS = foils that are phonemically related to list A words.

Administration

Instructions for administration are given in the CVLT/CVLT-C manual. Briefly, the CVLT can be given using either the paper-and-pencil Record Form, or the CVLT Administration and Scoring Software. The computer does not replace the examiner but rather facilitates administration and response recording, and automatically performs data analysis. Administration is the same for both formats.

In the pencil-and-paper format, the examiner reads aloud the instructions, stimulus words, and then records and summarizes the patient's oral responses. Instructions for each part of the test are printed on the Record Form.

In the computer-assisted format, the examiner enters the patient's responses directly into the computer during administration by using designated single-key input or light pen touching of the target words displayed on the monitor. Error types (i.e., perseverations and intrusions) are also entered directly into the computer during administration.

The nine-word CVLT should be reserved for those with obvious memory impairment (e.g., frank dementia) (see Libon et al., 1996). If patients appear to be relatively intact or there is suspicion of very mild or subtle impairment, the 16-word CVLT should be given.

Approximate Time for Administration

The test can be given in about 35 minutes.

Scoring

Scoring can be done manually or automatically using the CVLT/CVLT-C software. Computer-assisted scoring can be used regardless of the administration format (i.e., computer-assisted or paper-and-pencil) and is recommended since it is cost-effective and efficient in tabulating the results of the numerous analyses that provide summary measures. Detailed scoring guidelines and computational formulae are also found in the CVLT manual.

Comment

Reliability. For the adult standard version, measures of internal consistency (split-half,

coefficient alpha) fall in the moderate-to-high range (see source). Unfortunately, standard errors of measurement and confidence intervals are not provided in the manual.

The authors report that 21 normal adults were retested on the same form of the CVLT after 1 year. Correlation coefficients for various scores ranged from poor to moderate (.12–.79). The average improvement on the second testing in the total immediate recall of List A across five trials was about two words. The average improvement on Short- and Long-Delay Recall Trials and on Recognition hits was about one word. Over shorter intervals (7–10 days), practice effects are very pronounced, with an average increase of 12–15 words (overall score for trials 1–5) on the second test administration (McCaffrey et al., 1995). Delis et al. (1991) report preliminary data showing that the two forms of the CVLT yielded equivalent mean scores for the various learning and memory measures. Practice effects were not found regardless of the order in which the forms were administered. Alternate form reliability coefficients for the traditional recall measures of the CVLT were robust (e.g., List A Total Trials 1–5 index $r = .84$), although some of the correlations for variables derived from cognitive science (e.g., semantic clustering and recognition discriminability) were not (Delis et al., 1991).

For the CVLT-C, the authors also report moderate-to-high estimates of internal consistency (see source). Standard errors of measurement and confidence intervals (corresponding to the 68, 90, and 95 percent levels of confidence) are also provided for List A Trials 1–5. Score stability was examined by evaluating a sample of 106 children twice, with an average retest interval of about 1 month. Overall improvement was seen on retest, with gains of about 1–2 words per trial, depending upon the age of the child. Test–retest correlations were, however, modest and ranged from a low of .17 (cued-recall intrusions for 12 year olds) to a high of .90 (perseverations for 8 year olds). Thus, retesting, at least over the short term, may well yield a different pattern of results.

It is also worth noting that different examiners may produce somewhat different results on the CVLT (Weins et al., 1994). The exact characteristics that elicit best performance from subjects is currently not known. Examiner differences may, however, be large enough to be of concern in test-retest situations.

Validity. There is evidence (Schmidt, 1997) that the recall consistency index is substantially confounded with number of words recalled, raising concerns regarding its interpretation. The Category clustering index may be interpreted with confidence but some caution is warranted in interpreting the Serial Clustering index, because it will increase somewhat with number of words recalled.

The results of factor analyses conducted on 19 CVLT indices of normal children and adults indicate that the multiple indices assessed by the CVLT-CVLT-C cluster into six factors that reflect General Verbal Learning, Response Discrimination, Learning Strategy, Proactive Effect, Serial Position Effect, and Acquisition Rate (Delis et al., 1988; 1994). Wiens et al. (1994) reported a similar factor structure in a large sample of job applicants. In adult neurological populations, a five-factor solution tends to emerge (Delis et al., 1987). The factors represent General Verbal Learning, Response Discrimination, Serial Position Effect, Learning Strategy, and Retroactive/Short-Delay Effect. Vanderploeg et al. (1994) found a similar factor structure in a mixed group of neurological patients. Millis (1995) found a comparable six-factor solution in a sample of 75 patients with moderate to severe head injury. Differences between this study's findings and other previous investigations may be due to this study's small subject-to-variable ratio.

When the nine-word CVLT is considered, Libon et al. (1996) found that a three-factor solution emerged in normal elderly. Separate factors related to immediate free recall, delayed recall, and recognition, and the production of intrusion responses. In contrast to studies with the 16-item CVLT, measures of immediate recall tended to load on a separate factor from measures of delay recall and recognition. This difference may have been due to the restricted number of CVLT indices used in their analysis (11 vs. 15). In demented sub-

jects, a two-factor solution emerged. The first factor comprised all List A and List B test conditions as well as the recognition discriminability condition. The second factor was comprised of the intrusion error measures from the free and cued recall test trials. However, the recognition discriminability condition also loaded on this factor.

The CVLT was modeled after the Rey Auditory Verbal Learning Test (see Source). There are, however, important differences between the tests (Reeves & Wedding, 1994). In particular, the RAVLT list consists of 15 unrelated words whereas the CVLT list consists of 16 words drawn from four different semantic categories. Not surprisingly, moderate correlations are found between respective test variables (Crossen & Wiens, 1994). In normal individuals, slightly higher *raw* scores obtain on the CVLT than the RAVLT and likely reflect the slightly longer CVLT list (Crossen & Wiens, 1994) or the possibility that the CVLT list is easier. In patients with moderate-to-severe head injuries, no significant between test differences have been reported with regard to *raw* scores and correlations between raw scores ranged from .49 (Trial 1) to .83 (Trials 1–5 Total) (Stallings et al., 1995). When both tests are given in one day with an interval of about 2 to 4 hours between administrations, there are no significant effects for order of presentation (Crossen & Weins, 1994). Stallings et al. (1995) also noted no order effects in patients with moderate-to-severe head injuries. The interval between test administrations ranged from 4 hours to 3 days.

The CVLT also correlates moderately well with other standard measures of learning and memory including the Wechsler Memory Scale, the Wechsler Memory Scale—Revised, the Buschke Selective Reminding Test, and the Recognition Memory Test (see source; Delis et al., 1988a,b; Millis, 1995; Perrine 1994; Randolph et al., 1994; Shear & Kraft, 1989). The implication is that while CVLT indices share a degree of commonality with other memory tests, they may not be measuring identical cognitive processes (Shear & Kraft, 1989; Perrine et al., 1994; Stallings et al., 1995). Some researchers (Randolph et al., 1994; Stallings et al., 1993; Stallings et al.,

1995) have reported that when *standard* scores are considered, memory-impaired patients routinely perform worse on the CVLT than on other tests such as RAVLT or the WMS-R, perhaps due to differences in the composition of the standardization samples. In this context, it is important to note that the CVLT normative sample consisted of individuals of above-average intellectual functioning (see below). The CVLT, however, may also be slightly more sensitive to memory impairment than the WMS-R (Randolph et al. 1994) or the RAVLT because of its demands on semantic clustering (Stallings et al., 1995). Thus, use of the CVLT will result in a higher frequency of patients' being classed as memory-impaired and their memory impairments will appear more severe (Stallings et al., 1995).

Visual object naming (Visual Naming from the MAE) and auditory verbal comprehension (Token Test) are moderately related to various CVLT indices (Crossen et al., 1993b). Indexing delayed-recall performance to original learning (i.e., percent recall) provides a measure that is less influenced by language (Crosson et al., 1993b). Thus measures of naming and comprehension should be given when attempting to understand a patient's performance on the CVLT.

The CVLT memory scores also show modest correlations with the number of perseverative responses on the Wisconsin Card Sorting Test, Trails (part B), and Digit Span (Perrine, 1994; Vanderploeg et al., 1994; but see Paolo et al., 1995). Thus, certain aspects of executive function (e.g., attention, mental tracking) may play a role in learning and memory. Correlations between the CVLT/CVLT-C indices and Wechsler IQ scores are modest (.22–.53), suggesting that the CVLT is not simply measuring some dimension of general intellectual ability (Delis et al., 1994; Shear & Kraft, 1989; Wiens et al., 1994).

There is some evidence that the CVLT/CVLT-C multivariate scoring system is useful in characterizing the unique learning and memory profiles associated with a number of neurological and psychiatric disorders, including head injury (Crosson et al., 1988; Crossen et al., 1993a; Haut & Shutty, 1992;

Millis & Ricker, 1995; Yeates et al., 1995), epilepsy (Hermann et al., 1987; Hermann et al., 1994; Seidenberg et al., in press), Alzheimer's, Parkinson's and Huntington's diseases (Bondi et al., 1994; Kohler, 1994; Kramer et al., 1988b; Simon et al., 1994), probable ischemic vascular dementia (Libon et al., 1996), HIV infection and AIDS (Becker et al., 1995), depression, and schizophrenia (Cullum et al., 1989; Kareken et al., 1996; Massman et al., 1992; Otto et al., 1994; Paulsen et al., 1995). For example, Hermann et al. (1996) showed significantly reduced recall from the primacy and middle, but not recency, portions of the list in patients without left hippocampal sclerosis, who underwent resection of the hippocampus that was to a considerable degree structurally (and presumably functionally) intact. Crossen and colleagues (1993a) reported that a high number of intrusions on delayed-recall trials may occur not only following frontal lobe damage but also in the context of dominant temporal lobe dysfunction. Kohler (1994) has shown that patients with Alzheimer's disease (AD) benefit less than normal individuals from the repetition of information at the time of encoding. Simon et al. (1994) have found that patients with mild to moderate AD show little evidence of learning over the five trials, have poor retention even over short delays, and show deficits in clustering words by taxonomic category at recall. On the other hand, primary memory, measured by the mean recall from the recency portion of the list, was intact, whereas secondary memory (mean number of words recalled from the primacy and middle portions of the list) was impaired. Thus, primary memory appears resistant to the deleterious effects of AD at the earlier stages of the disease (see also Goldstein et al., 1996). Impairment in primary memory may occur as the disease progresses. Kramer et al. (1988b) found that AD patients are particularly prone to intrusion errors (perhaps reflecting a breakdown in semantic knowledge); patients with AD and Huntington's chorea tend to make more perseverations than patients with Parkinson's disease; patients with AD or Parkinson's disease tend to exhibit a faster rate of forgetting than patients with Huntington's disease. Massman et al. (1992)

observed that patients with Huntington's disease, in contrast to those with Alzheimer's, are aided significantly by a recognition format, suggesting that their deficit is primarily one of initiating systematic search (retrieval) of short- and long-term memory. There is some evidence (Bondi et al., 1994) that poor performance on certain CVLT measures (e.g., total of five trials, cued recall intrusions) may serve as preclinical cognitive markers for AD, especially in individuals with a positive family history. The cognitive deficits associated with HIV infection and AIDS also have a "subcortical" pattern, similar to that observed in Huntington's disease, reflected in relatively poor acquisition and retention on the words list, but with relatively spared recognition memory (Becker et al., 1995). While the literature suggests considerable heterogeneity in the learning and memory performances of individuals suffering from depression or schizophrenia, a substantial number of such patients also demonstrate CVLT profiles similar to those found in patients with subcortical dementias (Massman et al., 1992; Paulsen et al., 1995). Crossen and colleagues (1988; Novack et al., 1995) reported that individuals who have suffered traumatic brain injuries tend to display a slow rate of learning and poor delayed recall; they are less likely than normal people to use semantic clustering strategies to support recall (see also Stallings et al., 1995), and they commit more intrusion errors during learning and recall trials. There is also some evidence that adults with closed-head injury can be divided into neurologically meaningful subtypes based on their performance on the CVLT (Haut & Shutty, 1992; Millis & Ricker, 1994). For example, Millis and Ricker (1994) uncovered four distinct subtypes in 65 individuals with moderate-to-severe traumatic brain injuries. The Active subtype demonstrated impaired unassisted retrieval, but used active encoding strategies and showed relatively intact ability to store novel information. The Disorganized subtype demonstrated an inconsistent, haphazard learning style along with deficits in encoding. The Passive subtype was marked by an overreliance on a serial clustering strategy as well as impaired encoding and/or consolidation. The Deficient subtype

was the most impaired of all groups, exhibiting a slowed rate of acquisition, passive learning style, and significant impairment in encoding. The Active subtype showed the least impairment on the CVLT of all the groups and tended to occur in individuals with less severe injuries.

Discrepancies that favor recognition over free recall performance have been considered as markers of possible retrieval deficits. Delis et al. (1987) suggest that a standard score discrepancy favoring the Recognition Discriminability score over the Long Delay Free Recall score may be a marker for partial retrieval deficits. However, recent findings with a closed-head-injury (CHI) sample failed to support the use of this discrepancy as an indicator of retrieval deficits, at least in patients with CHI (Wilde et al., 1995). Discrepancy and nondiscrepancy groups who differed in their Recognition Discriminability performance but were equated on Long-Delay Free Recall were compared on CVLT indices hypothesized to reveal performance patterns consistent with retrieval deficits. Results showed that the discrepancy group produced fewer intrusions, but the groups did not differ in their consistency of recall or relative degree of benefit from semantic cuing. Thus, operationally defined retrieval problems may have little to do with the retrieval process itself. It may be, for example, that those who present with better recognition memory have mild encoding problems. While their encoding ability may be too weak to support free recall, it may be strong enough to allow for efficient recognition of the stimuli.

Measures from the test do appear to be useful in detecting poor effort or malingering (Millis et al., 1995; Trueblood, 1994). Trueblood (1994) found that CVLT total and recognition hits were of value in detecting incomplete effort. Mildly head-injured patients who appeared to be giving poor effort based on symptom validity testing differed from mild head-injured controls on these variables. Millis et al. (1995) compared patients with unequivocal evidence of significant traumatic brain injury with mildly injured patients who, on the basis of at-or-below-chance performance on a dichotomous forced-choice memory test (Recognition Memory Test), appeared to be demonstrating less than optimal effort, or at worst, were feigning or exaggerating impairment. The mild-head-injury group obtained significantly lower scores on CVLT total, recognition discriminability, recognition hits, and long-delay cued recall. The recognition format of discriminability and hits proved particularly useful in detecting incomplete effort (Millis, personal communication, January 1996).

In summary, the existing literature suggests that careful assessment of CVLT/CVLT-C indices can provide valuable information for distinguishing among different memory disorders in adults as well as in children. The CVLT/CVLT-C manuals are generally well-written and provide useful discussions of the theoretical foundation and interpretive guidelines for the various scores that are derived. However, information regarding test–retest reliability is currently available only for normal individuals, and these data suggest caution when making inferences regarding stability of scores. Furthermore, some of the indices have significant correlations with number of words recalled, and thus are not pure measures of the qualitative traits that they purportedly assess (Schmidt, 1997).

Normative Data

Delis et al. (1987) normed the adult version of the test on a group of 273 neurologically intact individuals (mean age = 58.93, SD = 15.35; mean educational level of 13.83 years, SD = 2.70). They present CVLT norms for seven age groups (ages 17–80) for each sex. Tables are provided in the CVLT manual for converting raw scores to standard scores. The computer scoring software automatically calculates and reports these scores. For all variables except List A Total Trials 1–5, the standard z-scores have a mean of 0 and a standard deviation of 1. Z-scores are rounded to whole numbers. A scale with a mean of 50 and a standard deviation of 10 (a "T scale") is used for List A Total Trials 1–5.

Some confusion may occur in the interpretation of these scores. First, the practice of rounding z-scores may result in an individual

appearing more impaired than he or she is. Second, a scaled score of +1 or more (that is, one or more standard deviations above the mean) on most of the test variables indicates intact performance, whereas a score of −1 or less suggests impairment. For example, a scaled score of −1 on the long-delay free-recall trials may suggest an encoding/storage deficit. Note, however, that an elevated perseveration, intrusion, or false positive rate is indicated by a scaled score of +1 or higher.

Delis and colleagues (1987) warn that their norms may not be representative for the U.S. population in terms of demographic variables such as education, race, and region, and therefore interpretation should be made with caution. In fact, the evidence (Randolph et al., 1994) indicates that the CVLT normative sample consisted of individuals who were above average in terms of their functioning. Accordingly, estimates of memory function based on the CVLT norms are more likely to suggest a deficit when performance is actually in the average range, particularly for individuals with below-average educational attainment or when performance is interpreted relative to global intelligence (Randolph et al., 1994). Wiens and colleagues (1994) recently provided normative data based on a sample of 700 job applicants. The sample was relatively young, with an average age of 29.1 years (SD = 6.0). The average education level was 14.5 years (SD = 1.6) and 81 percent were male. The data for select variables (total words recalled over five learning trials, Trial 1, List B, short- and long-delay free recall, perseverations, total intrusions, and recognition score) are presented in Table 10–11 separately for males and females, taking into account both age and FSIQ. Note that the cell sizes are generally small, particularly for women. Wiens et al. (1994) reported that the values are somewhat more lenient (that is, slightly lower) than those reported by Delis et al. (1987).

Because the CVLT normative sample has been criticized as being relatively small, Paolo et al. (1997) have provided additional data for elderly individuals and extended the normative data to persons older than 80 years of age. Their sample consisted of 212 normal individuals (92 males, 120 females), mostly Cau-

Table 10—11. California Verbal Learning Test Scores by Age and IQ

FSIQ	Males			Females		
	Age 20–29	Age 30–39	Age 40–49	Age 20–29	Age 30–39	Age 40–49

Total Words over Five Learning Trials

FSIQ	Age 20–29	Age 30–39	Age 40–49	Age 20–29	Age 30–39	Age 40–49
80–89	$n = 15$	$n = 6$		$n = 5$	$n = 1$	
Mean	50.6	54.8		57.2	46	
SD	6.4	8.7		7.3		
90–99	$n = 81$	$n = 49$	$n = 1$	$n = 21$	$n = 12$	$n = 3$
Mean	54.1	52.1	50	55.9	55.9	60.0
SD	6.5	7.9		6.0	8.1	6.1
100–109	$n = 132$	$n = 65$	$n = 9$	$n = 35$	$n = 16$	$n = 1$
Mean	57.6	52.8	46.8	60.0	58.2	64
SD	6.6	7.4	4.9	6.4	6.5	
110–119	$n = 68$	$n = 48$	$n = 9$	$n = 12$	$n = 9$	
Mean	57.8	53.4	52.9	61.6	61.3	
SD	7.1	7.6	6.8	5.5	5	
120–129	$n = 26$	$n = 31$	$n = 9$	$n = 4$	$n = 6$	$n = 3$
Mean	57.3	57.6	55.1	61.0	62.2	60.3
SD	8.3	8.3	12.3	7.1	7.2	4.0
130+	$n = 10$	$n = 3$	$n = 4$	$n = 1$	$n = 3$	
Mean	60	61.7	58.2	67	60	
SD	4.4	7.1	4.9		5.3	

Trial 1

FSIQ	Age 20–29	Age 30–39	Age 40–49	Age 20–29	Age 30–39	Age 40–49
80–89	$n = 15$	$n = 6$		$n = 5$	$n = 1$	
	Min = 4	Min = 6		Min = 5	Min =	
	Max = 10	Max = 10		Max = 8	Max =	
	Mean = 6.9	Mean = 7.8		Mean = 6.6	Mean = 6	
	SD = 1.8	SD = 1.5		SD = 1.3	SD =	
90–99	$n = 81$	$n = 49$	$n = 1$	$n = 21$	$n = 12$	$n = 3$
	Min = 5	Min = 4	Min =	Min = 4	Min = 4	Min = 8
	Max = 11	Max = 14	Max =	Max = 10	Max = 9	Max = 10
	Mean = 7.4	Mean = 7.4	Mean = 5	Mean = 7.6	Mean = 7.6	Mean = 9
	SD = 1.4	SD = 2	SD =	SD = 1.6	SD = 1.5	SD = 1
100–109	$n = 132$	$n = 65$	$n = 9$	$n = 35$	$n = 16$	$n = 1$
	Min = 4	Min = 4	Min = 5	Min = 5	Min = 6	Min =
	Max = 12	Max = 10	Max = 8	Max = 12	Max = 12	Max =
	Mean = 7.8	Mean = 6.8	Mean = 6.9	Mean = 8.3	Mean = 8.7	Mean = 10
	SD = 1.7	SD = 1.3	SD = 1	SD = 1.8	SD = 1.7	SD =
110–119	$n = 68$	$n = 48$	$n = 9$	$n = 12$	$n = 9$	
	Min = 5	Min = 5	Min = 5	Min = 5	Min = 6	
	Max = 12	Max = 10	Max = 8	Max = 11	Max = 9	
	Mean = 8.1	Mean = 7.5	Mean = 6.6	Mean = 8.8	Mean = 7.8	
	SD = 1.7	SD = 1.4	SD = .9	SD = 1.9	SD = 1.2	
120–129	$n = 26$	$n = 31$	$n = 9$	$n = 4$	$n = 6$	$n = 3$
	Min = 5	Min = 5	Min = 5	Min = 7	Min = 7	Min = 7
	Max = 12	Max = 13	Max = 13	Max = 10	Max = 11	Max = 12
	Mean = 8.1	Mean = 7.9	Mean = 8.2	Mean = 8.8	Mean = 8.7	Mean = 9.3
	SD = 1.8	SD = 1.8	SD = 3	SD = 1.3	SD = 1.5	SD = 2.5

(continued)

Table 10—11. California Verbal Learning Test Scores by Age and IQ *(Continued)*

FSIQ	Males			Females		
	Age 20–29	Age 30–39	Age 40–49	Age 20–29	Age 30–39	Age 40–49

Trial 1 *(Continued)*

130+	n = 10	n = 3	n = 4	n = 1	n = 3	
	Min = 6	Min = 7	Min = 7	Min =	Min = 7	
	Max = 11	Max = 9	Max = 8	Max =	Max = 8	
	Mean = 7.7	Mean = 8	Mean = 7.8	Mean = 12	Mean = 7.3	
	SD = 1.3	SD = 1	SD = .5	SD =	SD = .6	

List B

80–89	n = 15	n = 6		n= 5	n = 1	
	Min = 4	Min = 7		Min = 5	Min =	
	Max = 10	Max = 10		Max = 9	Max =	
	Mean = 6.4	Mean = 7.8		Mean = 7.2	Mean = 6	
	SD = 1.6	SD = 1.2		SD = 1.5	SD =	
90–99	n = 81	n = 49	n = 1	n = 21	n = 12	n = 3
	Min = 4	Min = 3	Min =	Min = 5	Min = 6	Min = 6
	Max = 11	Max = 11	Max =	Max = 11	Max = 12	Max = 9
	Mean = 7.4	Mean = 6.8	Mean = 5	Mean = 7.8	Mean = 7.7	Mean = 7.7
	SD = 1.5	SD = 1.7	SD =	SD = 1.9	SD = 1.7	SD = 1.5
100–109	n = 132	n = 65	n = 9	n = 35	n = 16	n = 1
	Min = 4	Min = 4	Min = 3	Min = 4	Min = 5	Min =
	Max = 12	Max = 12	Max = 9	Max = 12	Max = 10	Max =
	Mean = 7.3	Mean = 7.4	Mean = 6.6	Mean = 8.2	Mean = 7.4	Mean = 10
	SD = 1.7	SD = 1.8	SD = 1.9	SD = 1.7	SD = 1.4	SD =
110–119	n = 68	n = 48	n = 9	n = 12	n = 9	
	Min = 4	Min = 5	Min = 4	Min = 4	Min = 7	
	Max = 12	Max = 11	Max = 10	Max = 12	Max = 10	
	Mean = 7.7	Mean = 7.4	Mean = 6.6	Mean = 8.5	Mean = 8.1	
	SD = 1.8	SD = 1.4	SD = 2.2	SD = 2.8	SD = 1	
120–129	n = 26	n = 31	n = 9	n = 4	n = 6	n = 3
	Min = 4	Min = 5	Min = 5	Min = 7	Min = 6	Min = 6
	Max = 12	Max = 10	Max = 9	Max = 10	Max = 10	Max = 9
	Mean = 8	Mean = 7.7	Mean = 7.4	Mean = 8.5	Mean = 8.3	Mean = 7.7
	SD = 1.8	SD = 1.4	SD = 1.2	SD = 1.3	SD = 1.6	SD = 1.5
130 +	n = 10	n = 3	n = 4	n = 1	n = 3	
	Min = 6	Min = 5	Min = 7	Min =	Min = 8	
	Max = 11	Max = 8	Max = 9	Max =	Max = 9	
	Mean = 8.6	Mean = 6.7	Mean = 7.8	Mean = 10	Mean = 8.7	
	SD = 1.4	SD = 1.5	SD = 1	SD =	SD = .6	

Short Delay Free Recall

80–89	n = 15	n = 6		n = 5	n = 1	
	Min = 7	Min = 8		Min = 10	Min =	
	Max = 13	Max = 14		Max = 16	Max =	
	Mean = 10.7	Mean = 9.8		Mean = 12	Mean = 9	
	SD = 1.6	SD = 2.1		SD = 2.4	SD =	
90–99	n = 81	n = 49	n = 1	n = 21	n = 12	n = 3
	Min = 6	Min = 6	Min =	Min = 5	Min = 7	Min = 8
	Max = 16	Max = 16	Max =	Max = 15	Max = 16	Max = 13
	Mean = 11.3	Mean = 10.8	Mean = 11	Mean = 11.5	Mean = 11.9	Mean = 11
	SD = 2.1	SD = 2.5	SD =	SD = 2.3	SD = 2.9	SD = 2.6
100–109	n = 132	n = 65	n = 9	n = 35	n = 16	n = 1
	Min = 6	Min = 5	Min = 7	Min = 9	Min = 9	Min =
	Max = 16	Max = 16	Max = 13	Max = 16	Max = 16	Max =
	Mean = 12.2	Mean = 11.1	Mean = 9	Mean = 13.1	Mean = 12.6	Mean = 12
	SD = 2.1	SD = 2.5	SD = 2.1	SD = 2.2	SD = 2.1	SD =

(continued)

Table 10—11. *(Continued)*

FSIQ	Males			Females		
	Age 20–29	Age 30–39	Age 40–49	Age 20–29	Age 30–39	Age 40–49

Short Delay Free Recall *(Continued)*

FSIQ	Males Age 20–29	Age 30–39	Age 40–49	Females Age 20–29	Age 30–39	Age 40–49
110–119	$n = 68$ Min = 8 Max = 16 Mean = 12.6 SD = 2.3	$n = 48$ Min = 6 Max = 16 Mean = 11.1 SD = 2.5	$n = 9$ Min = 9 Max = 14 Mean = 11.7 SD = 1.6	$n = 12$ Min = 11 Max = 15 Mean = 13.1 SD = 1.2	$n = 9$ Min = 11 Max = 15 Mean = 13.8 SD = 1.2	
120–129	$n = 26$ Min = 8 Max = 16 Mean = 12.2 SD = 2	$n = 31$ Mkin = 7 Max = 16 Mean = 12.5 SD = 2.1	$n = 9$ Min = 7 Max = 14 Mean = 10.2 SD = 2.4	$n = 4$ Min = 11 Max = 15 Mean = 13.5 SD = 1.7	$n = 6$ Min = 10 Max = 15 Mean = 13.3 SD = 1.8	$n = 3$ Min = 11 Max = 12 Mean = 11.3 SD = .6
130 +	$n = 10$ Min = 13 Max = 16 Mean = 14.2 SD = 1.1	$n = 3$ Min = 12 Max = 16 Mean = 14.3 SD = 2.1	$n = 4$ Min = 13 Max = 15 Mean = 14.2 SD = 1	$n = 1$ Min = Max = Mean = 13 SD =	$n = 3$ Min = 13 Max = 16 Mean = 14.7 SD = 1.5	

Long Delay Free Recall

FSIQ	Males Age 20–29	Age 30–39	Age 40–49	Females Age 20–29	Age 30–39	Age 40–49
80–89	$n = 15$ Min = 7 Max = 15 Mean = 10.9 SD = 2.1	$n = 6$ Min = 8 Max = 15 Mean = 10.7 SD = 2.4		$n = 5$ Min = 10 Max = 16 Mean = 13 SD = 2.6	$n = 1$ Min Max Mean10 SD =	
90–99	$n = 81$ Min = 6 Max = 16 Mean = 11.7 SD = 2.2	$n = 49$ Min = 5 Max = 16 Mean = 11.2 SD = 2.5	$n = 1$ Min = Max = Mean = 7 SD =	$n = 21$ Min = 6 Max = 15 Mean = 12.3 SD = 2.5	$n = 12$ Min = 5 Max = 16 Mean = 12.1 SD = 3.1	$n = 3$ Min = 8 Max = 15 Mean = 12.3 SD = 3.8
100–109	$n = 132$ Min = 6 Max = 16 Mean = 12.7 SD = 2	$n = 65$ Min = 6 Max = 16 Mean = 11.8 SD = 2.3	$n = 9$ Min = 8 Max = 12 Mean = 9.7 SD = 1.3	$n = 35$ Min = 9 Max = 16 Mean = 13.6 SD = 2.1	$n = 16$ Min = 10 Max = 16 Mean = 13.1 SD = 2.1	$n = 1$ Min = Max = Mean = 14 SD =
110–119	$n = 68$ Min = 8 Max = 16 Mean = 13 SD = 2.2	$n = 48$ Min = 6 Max = 15 Mean = 11.4 SD = 2.6	$n = 9$ Min = 8 Max = 15 Mean = 12.8 SD = 2	$n = 12$ Min = 12 Max = 16 Mean = 13.8 SD = 1.2	$n = 9$ Min = 10 Max = 16 Mean = 13.7 SD = 2	
120–129	$n = 26$ Min = 9 Max = 16 Mean = 12.5 SD = 2	$n = 31$ Min = 9 Max = 16 Mean = 13 SD = 2.1	$n = 9$ Min = 6 Max = 14 Mean = 11 SD = 2.9	$n = 4$ Min = 11 Max = 16 Mean = 14 SD = 2.2	$n = 6$ Min = 9 Max = 16 Mean = 13.5 SD = 2.4	$n = 3$ Min = 12 Max = 13 Mean = 12.3 SD = .6
130 +	$n = 10$ Min = 13 Max = 16 Mean = 14.5 SD = 1.2	$n = 3$ Min = 13 Max = 16 Mean = 14 SD = 1.7	$n = 4$ Min = 14 Max = 15 Mean = 14.5 SD = .6	$n = 1$ Min = Max = Mean = 14 SD =	$n = 3$ Min = 11 Max = 16 Mean = 14 SD = 2.6	

Perseverative Responses

FSIQ	Males Age 20–29	Age 30–39	Age 40–49	Females Age 20–29	Age 30–39	Age 40–49
80–89	$n = 15$ Min = 0 Max = 16 Mean = 5.3 SD = 4.6	$n = 6$ Min = 2 Max = 18 Mean = 7.5 SD = 6.6		$n = 5$ Min = 1 Max = 10 Mean = 5.4 SD = 3.4	$n = 1$ Min = Max = Mean = 5 SD =	

(continued)

Table 10—11. California Verbal Learning Test Scores by Age and IQ *(Continued)*

FSIQ	Males			Females		
	Age 20–29	Age 30–39	Age 40–49	Age 20–29	Age 30–39	Age 40–49

Perseverative Responses (Continued)

FSIQ	Males Age 20–29	Age 30–39	Age 40–49	Females Age 20–29	Age 30–39	Age 40–49
90–99	n = 81	n = 49	n = 1	n = 21	n = 12	n = 3
	Min = 0	Min = 0	Min =	Min = 2	Min = 0	Min = 5
	Max = 23	Max = 25	Max =	Max = 13	Max = 17	Max = 19
	Mean = 7.6	Mean = 8.4	Mean = 11	Mean = 6.7	Mean = 6.7	Mean = 13.7
	SD = 5.5	SD = 5.4	SD =	SD = 3.4	SD = 6.3	SD = 7.6
100–109	n = 132	n = 65	n = 9	n = 35	n = 16	n = 1
	Min = 0	Min = 0	Min = 2	Min = 1	Min = 1	Min =
	Max = 21	Max = 21	Max = 22	Max = 23	Max = 16	Max =
	Mean = 7	Mean = 8.1	Mean = 8.1	Mean = 5.3	Mean = 6.4	Mean = 8
	SD = 4.4	SD = 5.2	SD = 6.5	SD = 4.7	SD = 4.4	SD =
110–119	n = 68	n = 48	n = 9	n = 12	n = 9	
	Min = 0	Min = 0	Min = 1	Min = 0	Min = 1	
	Max = 25	Max = 24	Max = 18	Max = 13	Max = 16	
	Mean = 5.6	Mean = 6.2	Mean = 7.1	Mean = 5.9	Mean = 7.1	
	SD = 4.6	SD = 4.5	SD = 5.4	SD = 3.8	SD = 5.2	
120–129	n = 26	n = 31	n = 9	n = 4	n = 6	n = 3
	Min = 0	Min = 0	Min = 3	Min = 1	Min = 0	Min = 3
	Max = 17	Max = 14	Max = 19	Max = 6	Max = 25	Max = 6
	Mean = 6.4	Mean = 4.5	Mean = 8.3	Mean = 3	Mean = 8.5	Mean = 4.7
	SD = 4.9	SD = 3.1	SD = 4.9	SD = 2.2	SD = 8.8	SD = 1.5
130 +	n = 10	n = 3	n = 4	n = 1	n = 3	
	Min = 2	Min = 1	Min = 0	Min =	Min = 3	
	Max = 25	Max = 13	Max = 10	Max =	Max = 10	
	Mean = 7.5	Mean = 6	Mean = 6	Mean = 3	Mean = 7.3	
	SD = 6.7	SD = 6.2	SD = 4.6	SD =	SD = 3.8	

Total Intrusions

FSIQ	Males Age 20–29	Age 30–39	Age 40–49	Females Age 20–29	Age 30–39	Age 40–49
80–89	n = 15	n = 6		n = 5	n = 1	
	Min = 0	Min =		Min = 0	Min =	
	Max = 14	Max = 11		Max = 3	Max =	
	Mean = 3.7	Mean = 5.2		Mean = .8	Mean = 14	
	SD = 4.3	SD = 4.4		SD = 1.3	SD =	
90–99	n = 81	n = 49	n = 1	n = 21	n = 12	n = 3
	Min = 0	Min = 0	Min =	Mkin = 0	Min = 0	Min = 3
	Max = 19	Max = 14	Max =	Max = 20	Max = 6	Max = 8
	Mean = 3.6	Mean = 3.4	Mean = 4	Mean = 4	Mean = 1.8	Mean = 5.7
	SD = 3.8	SD = 3.2	SD =	SD = 5.3	SD = 2.1	SD = 2.5
100–109	n = 132	n = 65	n = 9	n = 35	n = 16	n = 1
	Min = 0	Min = 0	Min = 0	Min = 0	Min = 0	Min =
	Max = 22	Max = 22	Max = 15	Max = 13	Max = 13	Max =
	Mean= 2.9	Mean = 3.5	Mean = 6.9	Mean = 1.9	Mean = 2.9	Mean = 0
	SD = 3.8	SD = 4.6	SD = 5.4	SD = 3	SD = 3.4	SD =
110–119	n = 68	n = 48	n = 9	n = 12	n = 9	
	Min = 0	Min = 0	Min = 0	Min = 0	Min = 0	
	Max = 10	Max = 25	Max = 7	Max = 12	Max = 8	
	Mean = 2.2	Mean = 5	Mean = 2.4	Mean = 2.8	Mean = 3.1	
	SD = 2.6	SD = 5.6	SD = 2.5	SD = 4.5	SD = 2.6	
120–129	n = 26	n = 31	n = 9	n = 4	n = 6	n = 3
	Min = 0	Min = 0	Min = 0	Min = 1	Min = 0	Min = 1
	Max = 9	Max = 14	Max = 7	Max = 5	Max = 14	Max = 12
	Mean = 1.9	Mean = 2.4	Mean = 2.6	Mean = 2.5	Mean = 2.5	Mean = 6
	SD = 2.9	SD = 3.2	SD = 2.2	SD = 1.9	SD = 5.6	SD = 5.6

(continued)

Table 10—11. *(Continued)*

	Males			Females		
FSIQ	Age 20–29	Age 30–39	Age 40–49	Age 20–29	Age 30–39	Age 40–49
Total Intrusions *(Continued)*						
130 +	n = 10 Min = 0 Max = 7 Mean = 1.6 SD = 2.4	n = 3 Min = 0 Max = 4 Mean = 2 SD = 2	n = 4 Min = 0 Max = 2 Mean = .8 SD = 1	n = 1 Min = Max = Mean = 1 SD =	n = 3 Min = 0 Max = 9 Mean = 4 SD = 4.6	
Recognition Score						
80–89	n = 15 Min = 12 Max = 16 Mean = 14.5 SD = 1.2	n = 6 Min = 14 Max = 16 Mean = 15.3 SD = .8		n = 5 Min = 14 Max = 16 Mean = 15.2 SD = .8	n = 1 Min = Max = Mean = 13 SD =	
90–99	n = 81 Min = 5 Max = 16 Mean = 14.6 SD = 1.6	n = 49 Min = 11 Max = 16 Mean = 14.5 SD = 1.5	n = Min Max Mean = 12 SD =	n = 21 Min = 12 Max = 16 Mean = 15 SD = 1.1	n = 12 Min = 10 Max = 16 Mean = 14.9 SD = 1.7	n = 3 Min = 13 Max = 16 Mean = 15 SD = 1.7
100–109	n = 132 Min = 11 Max = 16 Mean = 15.1 SD = 1.1	n = 65 Min = 11 Max = 16 Mean = 14.6 SD = 1.3	n = 9 Min = 13 Max = 16 Mean = 14.4 SD = .9	n = 35 Min = 12 Max = 16 Mean = 15.1 SD = 1.1	n = 16 Min = 13 Max = 16 Mean = 15.1 SD = 1.1	n = 1 Min = Max = Mean = 16 SD =
110–119	n = 68 Min = 11 Max = 16 Mean = 15 SD = 1.4	n = 48 Min = 12 Max = 16 Mean = 14.6 SD = 1.2	n = 9 Min = 10 Max = 16 Mean = 14.2 SD = 1.7	n = 12 Min = 13 Max = 16 Mean = 15.2 SD = .9	n = 9 Min = 13 Max = 16 Mean = 15.4 SD = 1	
120–129	n = 26 Min = 12 Max = 16 Mean = 14.9 SD = 1.2	n = 31 Min = 13 Max = 16 Mean = 15.1 SD = 1	n = 9 Min = 11 Max = 16 Mean = 14.3 SD = 1.7	n = 4 Min = 15 Max = 16 Mean = 15.8 SD = .5	n = 6 Min = 14 Max = 16 Mean = 15.2 SD = 1	n = 3 Min = 14 Max = 15 Mean = 14.7 SD = .6
130 +	n = 10 Min = 15 Max = 16 Mean = 15.9 SD = .3	n = 3 Min = 14 Max = 16 Mean = 15.3 SD = 1.2	n = 4 Min = 12 Max = 16 Mean = 14.2 SD = 1.7	n = 1 Min = Max = Mean = 16 SD =	n = 3 Min = 15 Max = 16 Mean = 15.7 SD = .6	

Source: Wiens, Tindall & Crossen. Reprinted with permission.

casian, ranging in age from 53 to 94 years (mean 70.58, SD = 6.98) and well educated (mean = 14.92 years, SD = 2.56). The study used nine overlapping cell tables to maximize sample size. Midpoint ages occur at 3-year intervals from midpoint ages 59 through 83. The age range around each midpoint is ± 6 years, except for the oldest age group, which has a larger age range. Their data are shown in Table 10–12. In addition to providing standard CVLT indices, six additional CVLT scores were computed: (1) Percent Perseverations— total number of perseverations divided by total response output (that is, total number of correct words plus total number of perseverations and intrusions across all free and cued recall trials (2) Percent Free Recall Intrusions— total number of intrusions committed during free recall divided by total number of words recalled across all free recall trials, including perseverations and free recall intrusions, (3) Percent Cued Recall Intrusions—total number of intrusions committed during cued recall divided by total number of words recalled with cuing, including perseverations and cued recall intrusions, (4) Percent Total Intrusions—total number of free and cued recall intrusions divided by the total response output, (5) Short-Delay Free Recall Percent Retained—total number of correct words recalled on short-delay free recall divided by the total number of correct words recalled on the last learning trials, and (6) Long-Delay Free Recall Percent Retained—total number of correct words recalled on long-delay free recall divided by the total number of correct words recalled on List A Trial 5. All of the above scores are multiplied by 100 to convert them to a percent score. To use their data, the clinician selects the table closest in midpoint age to the patient's actual age. Comparing their data with those in the CVLT manual,

Table 10—12a. CVLT Normative Data for Ages 53–65 (Midpoint Age = 59)

Score	Male (n = 14)		Female (n = 30)	
	M	SD	M	SD
Recall Measures				
Total word Trials 1–5	45.43	11.14	52.38	8.06
List A Trial 1	5.86	1.70	7.10	1.90
List A Trial 5	10.93	2.76	12.63	1.69
List B	5.71	1.82	6.97	1.79
Short-Delay Free Recall	8.86	4.11	11.07	2.29
Short-Delay Cued Recall	9.93	3.47	12.57	1.81
Long-Delay Free Recall	9.00	3.80	11.43	2.16
Long-Delay Cued Recall	9.71	3.31	12.30	1.86
Learning Characteristics				
Semantic clustering	1.39	0.88	2.03	0.83
Serial clustering	3.18	2.42	2.30	1.60
Percent primacy region	27.71	5.92	30.27	4.81
Percent middle region	38.07	7.08	41.57	6.47
Percent recency region	34.00	7.10	27.93	5.81
Slope	1.28	0.59	1.32	0.36
Recall Consistency	81.93	11.35	85.13	5.61
Recall Errors				
Perseverations	5.29	5.57	6.61	6.04
Free recall intrusions	2.71	4.51	1.70	2.38
Cued recall intrusions	2.57	3.37	1.10	1.71
Total intrusions	5.29	7.75	2.80	3.90
Recognition Measures				
Recognition hits	14.14	1.70	14.47	1.50
Discriminability	90.93	5.84	94.50	4.03
False positives	1.86	1.83	0.87	1.14
Response bias	−.03	0.37	−.06	0.33
Additional Measures				
Percent perseverations	4.48	3.75	5.67	5.17
Percent free intrusions	3.49	5.19	1.84	2.43
Percent cued intrusions	9.43	10.50	3.01	4.57
Percent total intrusions	5.30	6.90	2.37	3.15
SDFR percent retained[a]	78.76	24.05	87.63	14.63
LDFR percent retained[b]	80.46	20.45	90.64	12.98

[a]SDFR = Short-Delay Free Recall; [b]LDFR = Long-Delay Free Recall.

Source: Paolo et al, 1997. Reprinted with permission of Swets & Zeitlinger.

(Midpoint Age = 65)

Score	Male (n = 45)		Female (n = 59)	
	M	SD	M	SD
Recall Measures				
Total words Trials 1–5	43.33	9.63	50.03	9.18
List A Trial 1	5.76	1.54	6.63	1.89
List A Trial 5	10.67	2.54	11.98	2.32
List B	5.53	1.82	6.37	2.23
Short-Delay Free Recall	8.62	3.08	10.19	2.84
Short-Delay Cued Recall	9.91	2.73	11.85	2.24
Long-Delay Free Recall	8.80	2.93	10.85	2.64
Long-Delay Cued Recall	9.84	2.67	11.66	2.41
Learning Characteristics				
Semantic clustering	1.49	0.69	2.11	0.87
Serial clustering	2.54	1.87	1.73	1.49
Percent primary region	29.84	5.57	29.44	5.26
Percent middle region	38.93	7.72	41.05	6.98
Percent recency region	31.13	8.04	29.39	6.25
Slope	1.22	0.52	1.30	0.42
Recall consistency	78.80	12.66	82.07	9.88
Recall Errors				
Perseverations	4.20	4.83	6.32	5.39
Free recall intrusions	1.84	2.42	2.68	3.32
Cued recall intrusions	1.93	2.02	2.03	2.58
Total intrusions	3.78	3.95	4.71	5.44
Recognition Measures				
Recognition hits	13.80	1.73	14.63	1.43
Discriminability	90.64	6.21	93.54	5.45
False positives	1.89	2.28	1.47	1.98
Response bias	-.08	0.39	0.00	0.34
Additional Measures				
Percent perseverations	4.09	3.97	5.47	4.34
Percent free intrusions	2.75	3.75	3.19	3.65
Percent cued intrusions	9.27	9.43	8.01	9.32
Percent total intrusions	4.34	4.66	4.34	4.71
SDFR percent retained[a]	80.33	18.71	85.24	19.41
LDFR percent retained[b]	104.08	17.00	107.62	18.45

[a]SDFR = Short-Delay Free Recall; [b]LDFR = Long-Delay Free Recall.

(Midpoint Age = 62)

Score	Male (n = 28)		Female (n = 49)	
	M	SD	M	SD
Recall Measures				
Total words Trials 1–5	45.07	10.53	50.73	9.45
List A Trial 1	5.86	1.41	6.76	1.87
List A Trial 5	10.89	2.71	12.16	2.38
List B	5.61	1.69	6.63	1.97
Short-Delay Free Recall	9.07	3.35	10.24	2.81
Short-Delay Cued Recall	10.21	3.00	11.96	2.28
Long-Delay Free Recall	9.25	3.15	10.90	2.69
Long-Delay Cued Recall	10.25	2.94	11.73	2.46
Learning Characteristics				
Semantic clustering	1.49	0.83	2.03	0.89
Serial clustering	2.66	2.17	2.12	1.76
Percent primary region	28.54	5.18	29.78	5.65
Percent middle region	39.29	8.45	40.88	7.61
Percent recency region	32.11	8.00	29.24	6.39
Slope	1.25	0.54	1.29	0.45
Recall consistency	79.43	13.12	82.45	10.03
Recall Errors				
Perseverations	3.96	4.37	6.76	5.92
Free Recall Intrusions	2.04	3.56	2.69	3.55
Cued recall intrusions	1.93	2.51	1.92	2.67
Total intrusions	3.96	5.88	4.61	5.78
Recognition Measures				
Recognition hits	14.43	1.43	14.45	1.54
Discriminability	92.54	5.27	93.51	5.31
False positives	1.68	1.72	1.31	1.81
Response bias	0.01	0.34	-.04	0.34
Additional Measures				
Percent perseverations	3.57	3.13	5.77	4.86
Percent free intrusions	2.88	4.90	3.09	3.77
Percent cued intrusions	8.82	10.49	7.42	9.37
Percent total intrusions	4.31	6.01	4.11	4.83
SDFR percent retained[a]	82.48	19.15	84.41	18.30
LDFR percent retained[b]	104.10	15.35	106.80	16.60

[a]SDFR = Short-Delay Free Recall; [b]LDFR = Long-Delay Free Recall.

Table 10—12d. CVLT Normative Data for Ages 62–74 (Midpoint Age = 68)

Score	Male (n = 59)		Female (n = 77)	
	M	SD	M	SD
Recall Measures				
Total words Trials 1–5	42.46	9.54	48.65	9.15
List A Trial 1	5.71	1.65	6.32	1.89
List A Trial 5	10.39	2.65	11.69	2.28
List B	5.32	1.76	6.08	2.19
Short-Delay Free Recall	8.22	2.83	10.13	2.72
Short-Delay Cued Recall	9.61	2.68	11.60	2.30
Long-Delay Free Recall	8.51	2.87	10.61	2.51
Long-Delay Cued Recall	9.54	2.74	11.44	2.33
Learning Characteristics				
Semantic clustering	1.46	0.72	2.04	0.88
Serial clustering	2.55	1.96	1.95	1.91
Percent primary region	29.79	7.21	29.77	5.84
Percent middle region	38.41	8.44	40.87	7.06
Percent recency region	31.20	8.27	29.31	7.03
Slope	1.14	0.55	1.30	0.43
Recall consistency	78.44	11.28	80.47	10.96
Recall Errors				
Perseverations	3.76	4.25	5.65	5.30
Free Recall Intrusions	2.02	2.54	2.56	3.07
Cued recall intrusions	2.10	2.19	2.05	2.44
Total intrusions	4.12	4.31	4.61	5.06
Recognition Measures				
Recognition hits	13.66	1.83	14.49	1.52
Discriminability	89.86	6.32	93.65	5.17
False positives	2.10	2.35	1.29	1.81
Response bias	-.08	0.39	-.05	0.34
Additional Measures				
Percent perseverations	3.87	3.72	4.98	4.28
Percent free intrusions	3.05	3.84	3.12	3.47
Percent cued intrusions	10.31	10.29	8.07	8.91
Percent total intrusions	4.82	5.01	4.31	4.47
SDFR percent retained[a]	79.37	18.68	86.82	17.80
LDFR percent retained[b]	104.82	18.00	107.33	18.93

Table 10—12e. CVLT Normative Data for Ages 65–77 (Midpoint Age = 71)

Score	Male (n = 66)		Female (n = 76)	
	M	SD	M	SD
Recall Measures				
Total words Trials 1–5	41.15	9.27	47.47	8.68
List A Trial 1	5.33	1.82	6.00	1.73
List A Trial 5	10.15	2.59	11.45	2.23
List B	5.32	1.72	5.82	2.13
Short-Delay Free Recall	7.85	2.78	9.93	2.67
Short-Delay Cued Recall	9.44	2.55	11.32	2.25
Long-Delay Free Recall	8.18	2.82	10.47	2.52
Long-Delay Cued Recall	9.27	2.72	11.25	2.35
Learning Characteristics				
Semantic clustering	1.52	0.71	1.99	0.86
Serial clustering	2.28	1.78	2.00	1.91
Percent primary region	30.37	7.45	29.83	6.12
Percent middle region	38.86	8.82	40.89	7.38
Percent recency region	30.21	8.82	29.30	7.20
Slope	1.18	0.56	1.29	0.45
Recall consistency	77.65	11.33	79.51	10.87
Recall Errors				
Perseverations	3.68	4.00	5.89	5.56
Free Recall Intrusions	2.52	2.86	2.53	2.89
Cued recall intrusions	2.38	2.35	2.17	2.36
Total intrusions	4.89	4.73	4.70	4.79
Recognition Measures				
Recognition hits	13.61	1.87	14.39	1.58
Discriminability	89.41	6.13	93.32	5.25
False positives	2.24	2.36	1.36	1.91
Response bias	-.06	0.41	-.07	0.35
Additional Measures				
Percent perseverations	3.91	3.66	5.25	4.59
Percent free intrusions	3.85	4.43	3.15	3.33
Percent cued intrusions	11.71	11.17	8.69	8.71
Percent total intrusions	5.78	5.72	4.48	4.30
SDFR percent retained[a]	77.23	19.30	87.20	19.06
LDFR percent retained[b]	104.42	17.94	107.92	19.38

Table 10—12g. CVLT Normative Data for Ages 71–85 (Midpoint Age = 77)

Score	Male (n = 47) M	SD	Female (n = 56) M	SD
Recall Measures				
Total words Trials 1–5	39.62	9.38	45.71	8.34
List A Trial 1	5.09	1.98	5.66	1.81
List A Trial 5	9.70	2.58	11.13	2.06
List B	5.09	2.17	5.29	1.90
Short-Delay Free Recall	7.36	2.70	9.45	2.70
Short-Delay Cued Recall	8.98	2.63	10.96	2.28
Long-Delay Free Recall	7.70	2.96	9.89	2.65
Long-Delay Cued Recall	8.74	2.78	10.80	2.34
Learning Characteristics				
Semantic clustering	1.61	0.72	1.95	0.80
Serial clustering	2.14	1.77	2.13	1.90
Percent primary region	30.18	8.78	30.00	6.73
Percent middle region	40.00	9.02	41.04	7.27
Percent recency region	29.02	9.01	29.05	7.33
Slope	1.13	0.64	1.24	0.49
Recall consistency	77.13	10.33	78.96	10.68
Recall Errors				
Perseverations	3.72	4.45	5.02	4.95
Free Recall Intrusions	2.81	2.96	2.20	1.20
Cued recall intrusions	2.30	2.39	2.23	2.07
Total intrusions	5.11	4.99	4.43	3.58
Recognition Measures				
Recognition hits	13.45	2.01	14.07	1.76
Discriminability	88.47	6.43	93.00	4.58
False positives	2.51	2.61	1.16	1.35
Response bias	-.06	0.44	-.12	0.35
Additional Measures				
Percent perseverations	4.00	3.98	4.73	4.22
Percent free intrusions	4.25	4.37	3.02	2.63
Percent cued intrusions	11.62	11.62	9.38	8.70
Percent total intrusions	6.04	5.85	4.57	3.84
SDFR percent retained[a]	76.20	21.54	84.44	17.09
LDFR percent retained[b]	103.64	18.69	107.01	20.59

[a]SDFR = Short-Delay Free Recall; [b]LDFR = Long-Delay Free Recall.

Score	Male (n = 62) M	SD	Female (n = 71) M	SD
Recall Measures				
Total words Trials 1–5	40.50	8.76	46.77	8.40
List A Trial 1	5.34	1.82	5.97	1.76
List A Trial 5	9.92	2.51	11.21	2.16
List B	5.23	1.89	5.63	2.21
Short-Delay Free Recall	7.71	2.63	9.73	2.71
Short-Delay Cued Recall	9.19	2.43	11.31	2.28
Long-Delay Free Recall	8.00	2.77	10.28	2.63
Long-Delay Cued Recall	9.05	2.58	11.13	2.37
Learning Characteristics				
Semantic clustering	1.54	0.68	2.09	0.87
Serial clustering	2.22	1.66	1.86	1.81
Percent primary region	30.64	7.67	29.90	6.58
Percent middle region	39.48	8.84	40.75	7.52
Percent recency region	29.29	8.80	29.39	7.22
Slope	1.14	0.58	1.21	0.49
Recall consistency	77.37	10.45	79.20	10.47
Recall Errors				
Perseverations	3.81	4.12	5.24	5.08
Free Recall Intrusions	2.63	2.79	2.48	2.90
Cued recall intrusions	2.47	2.36	2.04	1.98
Total intrusions	5.10	4.65	4.52	4.51
Recognition Measures				
Recognition hits	13.44	1.88	14.20	1.71
Discriminability	88.76	5.79	93.03	5.01
False positives	2.37	2.39	1.28	1.65
Response bias	-.08	0.44	-.10	0.35
Additional Measures				
Percent perseverations	4.11	3.79	4.75	4.13
Percent free intrusions	3.95	4.17	3.16	3.34
Percent cued intrusions	12.15	11.28	8.41	7.83
Percent total intrusions	5.96	5.53	4.41	4.07
SDFR percent retained[a]	77.98	20.33	86.91	19.59
LDFR percent retained[b]	103.61	18.56	107.93	19.56

[a]SDFR = Short-Delay Free Recall; [b]LDFR = Long-Delay Free Recall.

Table 10–12h. CVLT Normative Data for Ages 74–86
(Midpoint Age = 80)

Score	Male (n = 29)		Female (n = 35)	
	M	SD	M	SD
Recall Measures				
Total words Trials 1–5	38.03	9.07	43.60	8.11
List A Trial 1	4.69	1.93	5.20	1.71
List A Trial 5	9.14	2.43	10.66	2.07
List B	4.86	2.18	4.83	1.89
Short-Delay Free Recall	7.03	2.78	8.89	2.63
Short-Delay Cued Recall	8.34	2.50	10.34	2.21
Long-Delay Free Recall	7.10	2.90	9.40	2.69
Long-Delay Cued Recall	8.07	2.66	10.17	2.27
Learning Characteristics				
Semantic clustering	1.65	0.62	1.82	0.78
Serial clustering	1.89	1.40	2.11	1.19
Percent primacy region	28.12	8.91	28.63	7.11
Percent middle region	41.07	9.61	40.91	8.15
Percent recency region	29.62	10.51	30.63	7.59
Slope	1.08	0.62	1.18	0.55
Recall consistency	77.62	10.69	77.57	11.92
Recall Errors				
Perseverations	3.86	4.27	6.00	5.62
Free Recall Intrusions	3.72	3.23	2.43	1.87
Cued recall intrusions	3.17	2.84	2.40	1.91
Total intrusions	6.90	5.66	4.83	3.48
Recognition Measures				
Recognition hits	13.52	2.05	13.89	1.81
Discriminability	88.00	5.90	91.89	5.17
False positives	2.79	2.32	1.49	1.76
Response bias	0.02	0.46	-.11	0.37
Additional Measures				
Percent perseverations	4.04	3.76	5.73	4.76
Percent free intrusions	5.61	4.66	3.47	2.78
Percent cued intrusions	15.62	13.03	10.73	8.68
Percent total intrusions	8.07	6.40	5.21	3.87
SDFR percent retained[a]	76.15	21.31	83.11	18.99
LDFR percent retained[b]	99.27	18.12	108.01	20.42

Table 10–12i. CVLT Normative Data for Ages 77–94
(Midpoint Age = 83)

Score	Male (n = 18)		Female (n = 21)	
	M	SD	M	SD
Recall Measures				
Total words Trials 1–5	37.39	8.41	42.52	6.75
List A Trial 1	4.67	1.78	5.05	1.77
List A Trial 5	9.00	1.97	10.62	2.06
List B	4.89	2.49	4.57	1.72
Short-Delay Free Recall	6.78	2.58	8.33	2.48
Short-Delay Cued Recall	8.11	2.27	10.14	2.22
Long-Delay Free Recall	6.78	2.67	8.71	2.65
Long-Delay Cued Recall	7.67	2.25	9.43	2.11
Learning Characteristics				
Semantic clustering	1.69	0.48	1.90	0.72
Serial clustering	1.92	1.57	2.18	1.17
Percent primacy region	29.28	7.46	30.95	7.81
Percent middle region	40.33	10.48	34.48	8.85
Percent recency region	30.11	10.21	30.57	6.95
Slope	1.03	0.56	1.17	0.59
Recall consistency	76.61	10.90	77.33	9.79
Recall Errors				
Perseverations	3.39	4.46	5.76	4.62
Free Recall Intrusions	3.61	3.18	2.43	1.72
Cued recall intrusions	3.22	3.14	2.62	2.09
Total intrusions	6.83	6.00	5.05	3.51
Recognition Measures				
Recognition hits	13.56	1.92	13.62	1.83
Discriminability	87.22	5.84	91.52	5.42
False positives	3.22	2.21	1.43	1.66
Response bias	0.09	0.45	-.15	0.35
Additional Measures				
Percent perseverations	3.49	4.11	5.86	4.25
Percent free intrusions	5.73	5.15	3.58	2.71
Percent cued intrusions	16.06	15.34	11.95	9.31
Percent total intrusions	8.30	7.28	5.54	3.92
SDFR percent retained[a]	75.11	24.91	77.68	14.70
LDFR percent retained[b]	96.18	15.94	106.50	20.89

Table 10—13. T-Score Equivalents of Raw Scores for List A Total Trials 1–5 By Age and Gender for a Depressed Sample

T-Scores	Females			Males		
	Age 18–34	Age 35–44	Age 45–54	Age 18–34	Age 35–44	Age 45–54
70	80	77	74	74	71	68
69	79	76	73	73	70	67
68	78	75	72	72	69	66
67	77	74	71	71	68	—
66	76	73	70	70	67	65
65	75	74	—	69	66	64
64	74	73	69	68	65	63
63	73	72	68	67	64	62
62	72	71	67	66	63	61
61	71	70	66	65	62	60
60	70	69	65	64	61	59
59	69	68	64	63	60	58
58	68	67	63	62	59	57
57	67	66	62	61	58	56
56	66	65	61	60	57	55
55	65	64	60	59	56	54
54	64	63	59	58	55	53
53	63	62	58	57	54	52
52	62	61	57	56	53	51
51	61	58	56	55	52	50
50	60	57	55	—	51	49
49	59	56	54	54	50	48
48	58	55	53	53	49	47
47	—	54	52	52	48	46
46	57	53	51	51	—	45
45	56	52	50	50	47	44
44	55	51	49	49	56	43
43	54	—	48	48	45	42
42	53	50	47	47	44	41
41	52	49	46	46	43	40
40	51	48	45	45	42	39
39	50	47	44	44	41	38
38	49	46	43	43	40	38
37	48	45	42	42	39	36
36	47	44	41	41	38	35
35	46	43	40	40	37	—
34	45	42	39	39	36	34
33	44	41	38	38	35	33
32	43	40	—	37	34	32
31	42	39	37	36	33	31
30	41	38	36	35	32	30

Source: Otto et al., 1994. Reprinted with permission of Elsevier Science Ltd.

Table 10—14. Means and Standard Deviations for the Nine-Word CVLT

	M	SD
List A		
Trial 1	5.8	1.3
Trial 2	7.5	1.1
Trial 3	7.8	.89
Trial 4	7.9	.97
Trial 5	8.0	1.2
Trials 1–5	37.1	4.3
List B	5.1	1.1
Semantic Cluster Ratio	.32	.15
Short-Delay Free Recall	7.0	1.60
Short-Delay Cued Recall	7.5	1.4
Long-Delay Free Recall	7.1	1.70
Long-Delay Cued Recall	7.4	1.5
Savings Score	88.9	20.0
Recognition Discrimination	95.5	4.8
Recognition Hits	8.3	.89
Recognition False Positives	.92	1.3
Percent Free Recall Intrusions	1.4	2.1
Percent Cued Recall Intrusions	5.3	9.0
Percent Perseverations	2.8	3.9

Source: Libon et al., 1996. Reprinted with permission.

Note: Savings Score—Percent of words recalled on List A Trial 5 that were recalled on the delayed free recall condition; Percent Free Recall Intrusions—percentage of total words recalled on all free recall trials of Lists A and B that were nontargets; Percent Cued Recall Intrusions—percentage of total words recalled on the two List A cued recall conditions that were nontargets; Percent Perseverations—percentage of total number of responses repeated on each trial summed across all free and cued trials of Lists A and B.

Paolo et al. (1997) reported a slightly lower total number of words recalled across trials 1 through 5.

At present, adequate normative data are not available for the alternate version of the CVLT and this form should probably be reserved for research purposes (Delis, personal communication).

Age, intelligence, education, and gender affect performance on the adult version (see Source; Hermann et al., 1988; Keenan et al., 1996; Kramer et al., 1988; Meehan, 1995; Paolo et al., 1997; Wiens et al., 1994). Recall performance tends to decline with increasing age. Further, total number of words recalled is positively related to IQ (Hermann et al., 1988; Meehan, 1995; Wiens et al., 1994; but see Paolo et al., 1997), the Vocabulary subtest of the WAIS-R (Keenan et al. 1996) and educa-

tion (Paolo et al., 1997; but see Keenan et al., 1996). The intrusion rate, however, is not related to the Vocabulary score (Keenan et al., 1996). With regard to gender, Kramer et al. (1988) reported that women displayed consistently higher levels of immediate and delayed recall (by about one word per trial) and made greater use of a semantic clustering strategy. Similar sex-related differences were noted by others (Otto et al., 1994; Paolo et al., 1997; Wiens et al., 1994).

Depression also affects performance on the CVLT (see above, Comments). Otto and colleagues (1994) reported that mean performance of patients with major depression were between one-half and one standard deviation below age- and sex-corrected norms for nondepressed populations. Otto et al. (1994) provide norms for the CVLT based on a sample of 156 patients with major depression tested during a drug-washout phase. These data are shown in Table 10–13. The T-scores reflect performance for patients with college education (16 years). Adjustments can be made by adding four points to the raw score of patients with a high school education, or deducting four points from the raw scores of patients at a doctoral level of education (20 years).

The CVLT-C normative data were derived from a sample representative of the U.S. population of children. The stratification variables were age, gender, race/ethnicity, geographic region, and parent educational level. The standardization sample consisted of 920 children in 12 age groups ranging from 5–16 years of age. Age, but not gender, was found to affect performance. Therefore, scaled score information for the CVLT-C indices is presented with males and females of the same age group combined.

Scaled score information for the CVLT-C List A Trials 1–5 Total is presented in a T-score metric with a mean of 50 and a standard deviation of 10, with the scaled scores ranging from 20 to 80. The scaled scores for the remaining CVLT-C indices are presented in a z-score metric with a mean of 0 and a standard deviation of 1, and with a scaled score range of −5 to +5 given in increments of .50.

For the nine-word short form, Libon et al. (1996) present data (means and SDs) derived from a group of 41 healthy well-educated elderly individuals (mean age = 74.8, SD = 7.1). The data are shown in Table 10–14.

References

Becker, J.T., Calarao, R., Lopez, O.L., Dew, M.A., Dorst, S.K., & Banks, G. (1995). Qualitative features of the memory deficit associated with HIV infection and AIDS: Cross-validation of a discriminant function classification scheme. *Journal of Clinical and Experimental Neuropsychology, 17*, 134–142.

Bondi, M.W., Monsch, A.U., Galasko, D., Butters, N., Salmon, D.P., & Delis, D. (1994). Preclinical cognitive markers of dementia of the Alzheimer's type. *Neuropsychology, 8*, 374–384.

Crossen, B., Novack, T.A., Trenerry, M.R., & Craig, P.L. (1988). California Verbal Learning Test (CVLT) performance in severely head-injured and neurologically normal adult males. *Journal of Clinical and Experimental Neuropsychology, 10*, 754–768.

Crossen, B., Sartor, K.J., Jenny III, A.B., Nabors, N.A., & Moberg, P.J. (1993a). Increased intrusions during verbal recall in traumatic and non-traumatic lesion of temporal lobe. *Neuropsychology, 7*, 193–208.

Crossen, B., Cooper, P.V., Lincoln, R.K., Bauer, R.M., & Velozo, C.A. (1993b). Relationship between verbal memory and language performance after blunt head injury. *The Clinical Neuropsychologist, 7*, 250–267.

Crossen, J.R., & Wiens, A.N. (1994). Comparison of the auditory-verbal learning test (AVLT) and California Verbal Learning Test (CVLT) in a sample of normal subjects. *Journal of Clinical and Experimental Neuropsychology, 16*, 190–194.

Cullum, C.M., Kuck, J., Delis, D.C. et al. (1989). Verbal learning characteristics in schizophrenia. *Journal of Clinical and Experimental Neuropsychology, 12*, 55.

Delis, D.C., Kramer, J.H., Kaplan, E., & Ober, B.A. (1987). *California Verbal Learning Test: Adult Version Manual.* San Antonio, TX: The Psychological Corporation.

Delis, D.C., Freeland, J., Kramer, J.H., & Kaplan, E. (1988a). Integrating clinical assessment with cognitive neuroscience: Construct validation of the California Verbal Learning Test. *Journal of Consulting and Clinical Psychology, 56*, 123–130.

Delis, D.C., Cullum, C.M., Butters, N., Cairns, P., & Prifitera, A. (1988b). Wechsler Memory Scale—Revised and California Verbal Learning Test: Convergence and Divergence. *The Clinical Neuropsychologist, 2*, 188–196.

Delis, D.C., Massman, P.J., Kaplan, E., McKee, R., Kramer, J.H., & Gettman, D. (1991). Alternate form of the California Verbal Learning Test: Development and reliability. *The Clinical Neuropsychologist, 5*, 154–162.

Delis, D.C., Kramer, J.H., Kaplan, E., & Ober, B.A. (1994). *CVLT-C: California Verbal Learning Test—Children's Version.* San Antonio, TX: The Psychological Corporation.

Goldstein, F.C., Levin, H.S., Roberts, V.J., Goldman, W.P., Winslow, M., & Goldstein, S.J. (1996). Neuropsychological effects of closed head injury in older adults: A comparison with Alzheimer's disease. *Neuropsychology, 10*, 147–154.

Haut, M.C., & Shutty, M.S. (1992). Patterns of verbal learning after closed head injury. *Neuropsychology, 6*, 51–58.

Hermann, B.P., Wyler, A.R., Richey, E.T., & Rea, J.M. (1987). Memory function and verbal learning ability in patients with complex partial seizures of temporal lobe origin. *Epilepsia, 28*, 547–554.

Hermann, B.P., Wyler, A.R., Steenman, H., & Richey, E.T. (1988). The interrelationship between language function and verbal learning/memory performance in patients with complex partial seizures. *Cortex, 24*, 245–253.

Hermann, B.P., Wyler, A.R., Somes, G., Dohan, F.C., Berry III, A.D., & Clement, L. (1994). Declarative memory following anterior temporal lobectomy in humans. *Behavioral Neuroscience, 108*, 3–10.

Hermann, B.P., Seidenberg, M., Wyler, A., Davies, K., Christensen, J., Moran, M., & Stroup, E. (1996). The effects of human hippocampal resection on the serial position curve. *Cortex, 32*, 323–334.

Kareken, D.A., Moberg, P.J., & Gur, R.C. (1996). Proactive inhibition and semantic organization: Relationship with verbal memory in patients with schizophrenia. *Journal of the International Neuropsychological Society, 2*, 486–493.

Keenan, P.A., Ricker, J.H., Lindamer, L.A., Jiron, C.C., & Jacobson, M.W. (1996). Relationship between WAIS-R Vocabulary and performance on the California Verbal Learning Test. *The Clinical Neuropsychologist, 10*, 455–458.

Kohler, S. (1994). Quantitative characterization of verbal learning deficits in patients with Alzheimer's Disease. *Journal of Clinical and Experimental Neuropsychology, 16*, 749–753.

Kramer, J.H., Delis, D.C., & Daniel, M. (1988a). Sex differences in verbal learning. *Journal of Clinical Psychology, 44*, 907–915.

Kramer, J.H., Levin, B.E., Brandt, J., & Delis, D. (1988b). Differentiation of Alzheimer's, Huntington's and Parkinson's Disease patients on the basis of verbal learning characteristics. *Neuropsychology, 3*, 111–120.

Libon, D.J., Mattson, R.E., Glosser, G., Kaplan, E., Malamut, B.M., Sands, L.P., Swenson, R., & Cloud, B.S. (1996). A nine-word dementia version of the California Verbal Learning Test. *The Clinical Neuropsychologist, 10*, 237–244.

Massman, P.J., Delis, D.C., Butters, N., Dupont, R.M., & Gillin, J.C. (1992). The subcortical dysfunction hypothesis of memory deficits in depression: Neuropsychological validation in a subgroup of patients. *Journal of Clinical and Experimental Neuropsychology, 14*, 687–706.

McCaffrey, R.J., Cousins, J.P., Westervelt, H.J., Martynowics, M., Remick, S.C., Szebenyi, A., Wagle, W.A., Botttomly, P.A., Hardy, C.J., & Haase, R.F. (1995). Practice effects with the NIMH AIDS abbreviated neuropsychological battery. *Archives of Clinical Neuropsychology, 10*, 241–250.

Meehan, G. (1995). Depression and verbal learning in complex partial epilepsy. Ph.D. dissertation. University of Victoria.

Millis, S.R., & Ricker, J.H. (1994). Verbal learning patterns in moderate and severe traumatic brain injury. *Journal of Clinical and Experimental Neuropsychology, 16*, 498–507.

Millis, S.R. (1995). Factor structure of the California Verbal Learning test in moderate and severe closed-head injury. *Perceptual and Motor Skills, 80*, 219–224.

Millis, S.R., Putnam, S.H., Adams, K.M., & Ricker, J.H. (1995). The California Verbal Learning Test in the detection of incomplete effort in neuropsychological evaluation. *Psychological Assessment, 7*, 463–471.

Millis, S.R., & Ricker, J.H. (1994). Verbal learning patterns in moderate and severe traumatic brain injury. *Journal of Clinical and Experimental Neuropsychology, 16*, 498–507.

Millis, S.R., & Ricker, J.H. (1995). Verbal learning and memory impairment in adult civilians following penetrating missile wounds. *Brain Injury, 9*, 509–515.

Novack, T.A., Kofoed, B.A., & Crossen, B. (1995). Sequential performance on the California Verbal Learning Test following traumatic brain injury. *The Clinical Neuropsychologist, 9*, 38–43.

Otto, M.W., Bruder, G.E., Fava, M., Delis, D.C., Quitkin, F.M., & Rosenbaum, J.F. (1994). Norms for depressed patients for the California Verbal Learning Test: Associations with depression severity and self-report of cognitive difficulties. *Archives of Clinical Neuropsychology, 9*, 81–88.

Paolo, A.M., Troster, A.I., & Ryan, J.J. (1997). California Verbal Learning Test normative data for the elderly. *Journal of Clinical and Experimental Neuropsychology, 19*, 220–234.

Paolo, A.M., Troster, A.I., Axelrod, B.N., & Koller, W.C. (1995). Construct validity of the WCST in normal elderly and persons with Parkinson's disease. *Archives of Clinical Neuropsychology, 10*, 463–473.

Paulsen, J.S., Heaton, R.K., Sadek, J.R., Perry, W., Delis, D.C., Braff, D., Kuck, J.J., Zisook, S., & Jeste, D.V. (1995). The nature of learning and memory impairments in schizophrenia. *Journal of the International Neuropsychological Society, 1*, 88–99.

Perrine, K. (1994). Relationship of the California Verbal Learning Test to other measures of memory, language, and frontal lobe functions. Paper presented to the International Neuropsychological Society, Cincinnati, Ohio.

Randolph, C., Gold, J.M., Kozora, E., Cullum, C.M., Hermann, B.P., & Wyler, A.R. (1994). Estimating memory function: Disparity of Wechsler Memory Scale—Revised and California Verbal Learning Test indices in clinical and normal samples. *The Clinical Neuropsychologist, 8*, 99–108.

Reeves, D., & Wedding, D. (1994). *The Clinical Assessment of Memory—A Practical Guide.* New York: Springer.

Schmidt, M. (1997). Some cautions on interpreting qualitative indices for word-list learning tests. *The Clinical Neuropsychologist, 11*, 81–86.

Seidenberg, M., Hermann, B.P., Schoenfeld, J., Davies, K., Wyler, A., & Dohan, F.C. (in press). Reorganization verbal memory function following early injury to the left mesial temporal lobe. *Brain and Cognition.*

Shear, J.M., & Craft, R.B. (1989). Examination of the concurrent validity of the California Verbal Learning Test. *The Clinical Neuropsychologist, 3*, 162–168.

Simon, E., Leach, L., Winocur, G., & Moscovitch, M. (1994). Intact primary memory in mild to moderate Alzheimer disease: Indices from the California Verbal Learning Test. *Journal of Clinical and Experimental Neuropsychology, 16*, 414–422.

Stallings, G.A., Boake, C., & Sherer, M. (1993). Correspondence between the California Verbal Learning Test and Rey Auditory Verbal Learning Test in closed-head-injury patients. *Journal of Clinical and Experimental Neuropsychology, 15*, 54.

Stallings, G., Boake, C., & Sherer, M. (1995). Comparison of the California Verbal Learning Test and the Rey Auditory Verbal Learning Test in head-injured patients. *Journal of Clinical and Experimental Neuropsychology, 17,* 706–712.

Trueblood, W. (1994). Qualitative and quantitative characteristics of malingered and other invalid WAIS-R and clinical memory data. *Journal of Clinical and Experimental Neuropsychology, 16,* 597–607.

Vanderploeg, R.D., Schinka, J.A., & Retzlaff, P. (1994). Relationship between measures of auditory verbal learning and executive functioning. *Journal of Clinical and Experimental Neuropsychology, 16,* 243–252.

Wiens, A.N., Tindall, A.G., & Crossen, J.R. (1994). California Verbal Learning Test: A norma-

tive data study. *The Clinical Neuropsychologist, 8,* 75–90.

Wilde, M.C., Boake, C., & Sherer, M. (1995). Do recognition-free discrepancies detect retrieval deficits in closed head injury? An exploratory analysis with the California Verbal Learning Test. *Journal of Clinical and Experimental Neuropsychology, 17,* 849–855.

Yeates, K.O., Blumenstein, E., Patterson, C.M., & Delis, D.C. (1995). Verbal learning and memory following pediatric closed head injury. *Journal of the International Neuropsychological Society, 1,* 78–87.

COLORADO NEUROPSYCHOLOGY TESTS (CNT)

Purpose

This personal computer software provides a number of measures of implicit and explicit memory.

Source

The manual and software can be obtained from Colorado Neuropsychology Tests, 102 E. Jefferson, Colorado Springs, CO 80907, at a cost of $595 US. Computer requirements include an IBM-compatible computer with at least 640K RAM, a hard drive with at least 4.0 megabytes free, and a mouse.

Description

The software (Davis, Bajszar, & Squire, 1995) includes 13 programs, all of which can be modified to create numerous test variations. The program is also flexible so that the examiner can give only a single test or several tasks.

Memory Cards provides an assessment of short-term and long-term memory and is reminiscent of the game "Concentration": Cards (from 4 to 24) are presented on the screen, face down, and the subject attempts to locate the matching pairs of cards by turning over two cards at a time. The initial trial provides an assessment of short-term memory. On subsequent trials, the cards remain in the same arrangement and can provide a measure of long-term memory. The examiner controls the number of trials, display time, response time, the intertrial interval, break between trials, and test figures (pictures, abstract fig-

ures, sounds, words, or numbers). A normed version is available in which the subject is given a total of six trials. The number of cards displayed per trial is 24.

Tower of Hanoi has been referred to as a measure of implicit memory and skill (procedural) memory, and a test of higher-order executive function. It requires that the subject move blocks one at a time in such a way that they end up in a particular goal configuration. The examiner can control the number of trials, number of rings, destination, the break between trials, maximum moves, and feedback on success. Other features include a graphical analysis of the subject's moves and a replay option for examining strategy development. The normed version of the task is set to four trials with a five-ring puzzle, and feedback is provided to the subject after each attempt. To make full use of the normative data, the subject should be tested on four occasions with an intersession interval between 1 and 7 days.

The software also includes the London and Toronto variations, which are simpler versions of the Tower of Hanoi. The Tower of London requires the subject to move colored beads from their initial position on upright sticks to achieve a new, predetermined arrangement in as few moves as possible. The software contains four tests: (1) 3 beads and 3 pegs, (2) 4 beads and 4 pegs, (3) 5 beads and 5 pegs, and (4) a test that includes a mixture of the 3-, 4-, and 5-peg puzzles. In the Tower of Toronto, subjects are required to move shaded rings from a start position on one ring to a goal position (identical arrangement) on another peg. Only one ring at a time can be moved, and a darker ring cannot be placed on a lighter colored ring. Norms are not provided for the Toronto and London adaptations.

Repeat (Pattern Sequence) is an implicit memory task in which the subject's acquisition of a repeating stimulus sequence is assessed. An "X" moves in a sequenced pattern to different quadrants of the computer screen. The subject provides reaction-time responses by hitting keys that correspond to the four quadrants. The test also contains a random sequence as a control measure, a split-attention test, and an explicit test to measure the subject's knowledge of the sequence. In the normed version of the task, adults were given 8 blocks of 100 trials with a pattern sequence of 10 moves. Thus, the pattern is repeated 10 times per block for a total repetition of 80 times.

Mirror Reading Triads is an implicit memory test in which subjects are presented words (triads) in mirror image on the computer screen. Timing of reading is accomplished by clicking the mouse button after the subject correctly reads the words aloud. A recognition test is also included. The normed test consists of five blocks of 10 triads presented in three consecutive daily sessions followed by a fourth session about 90 days later so that the subject's retention of the skill of mirror reading can be assessed. Each block contains five nonrepeated word triads and five repeated triads. The repeated triads are common to all sessions and each block of 10 triads. The average reading time for repeated and unique items within a session are presented along with normed scores.

Mirror Reading Test is similar to the triads test. Subjects are presented stories in mirror image, and latencies to read different or repeated stories are recorded.

Priming requires the subject to rate words on a Likert Scale in terms of how much they like or dislike the words. Later, the subject is presented with a three-letter word stem or word fragment and asked to respond with the first word that comes to mind. Priming is reflected by an increased probability of responding with a previously studied word. Explicit memory can also be accessed by using the recall and recognition tests that are included within the priming test software. The normed test is a stem completion task.

Recall allows the examiner to create free-recall tests. The examiner can control the order of word presentation, the number of words, the number of trials, the delay between trials, whether a trial assesses recall or recognition, and whether cues are presented. Normal individuals were tested using a variant of the Rey Auditory Verbal Learning Test.

Recognition is similar to the Recall test except the subject is simply asked if the word was previously presented by striking the "Y" key for yes and the "N" key for no. A study list of 15 high-imagery words is presented for five immediate trials with the presentation of words randomized for each trial. There is a 20-second break between the first five trials. Twenty minutes after the fifth immediate trial, the subject is given a final recognition test without presentation of the study list.

Paired Association allows the examiner to create a paired associate task. It is designed for subject or tester response entry, and it contains a multiple-choice option.

Temporal Order Test requires the subject to recall the presentation sequence of a list of words. In the normed version, subjects are shown one word at a time in the center of the computer screen and told that they should try to remember the words because their memory for the presented words will be tested. Ten words are presented for three seconds each. After the last word, a screen appears with the words arranged in a random order and the subject is requested to tell the examiner the order in which the words appeared. The tester arranges the order of the words as instructed by the subject.

Digit and Visual Span Tests allows the examiner to design a forward and/or a reverse digit/visual span test. A normed version is not provided.

Administration

See source. Test presentation is controlled by the computer software. The examiner should, however, ensure that the patient is properly oriented to the monitor and keyboard.

Approximate Time for Administration

The time required varies depending upon the particular test given.

Scoring

Test scoring is provided by the computer program. For normed tests, mean number correct and/or mean response time (and SDs) are reported.

Comment

In recent years, a distinction has been made between two functionally and supposedly anatomically separable memory systems. Declarative or explicit memory, the most intensively studied, reflects the ability to store and consciously recall or recognize information. Nondeclarative or implicit memory, by contrast, refers to a heterogeneous collection of learning abilities and can be assessed by the effects of experience on some measure of performance that does not involve conscious awareness of any part of the prior experience (Moscovitch, 1994; Squire, 1994; Winocur et al., 1996). Tests of general knowledge, skill (procedural) learning (with tasks such as pursuit rotor, mirror drawing, reading transformed script, Tower of Hanoi), and repetition priming in which exposure to a word biases subsequent identification in a word-completion test are common examples of implicit memory tests. Most of the standard neuropsychological tests evaluate recall and recognition—that is, declarative as opposed to implicit memory. The advantage of the CNT software is that it allows the examiner to assess both domains.

The literature suggests that damage to cortical or diencephalic parts of the hippocampal circuit prevents the formation of new explicit memories but spares old memories and implicit memory (Schacter & Tulving, 1994). Whereas declarative memory refers to a biologically meaningful category of memory dependent on a specific brain system, the neural substrates underlying nondeclarative memory tasks are less certain, but appear to depend on multiple brain systems (Moscovitch, 1994; Squire, 1994). For example, the neuroanatomical substrate underlying the procedural system

is thought to involve the neostriatal-prefrontal circuitry (e.g., Butters et al., 1985; Butters et al., 1990; Cohen, 1984; Glosser & Goodglass, 1990; Owen et al., 1990; Shallice, 1982; Saint-Cyr et al., 1988). There is also some evidence in the neuropsychological literature that completion of word-stems, but not of fragments, may be mediated by frontal-lobe regions in the brain (Winocur et al., 1996). In such tasks, the frontal lobes may play a supervisory role, in eliciting cue-appropriate responses and in monitoring and detection (Nyberg et al., 1997). Fragment completion, on the other hand, may be more perceptually driven and mediated by the posterior neocortex (Winocur et al., 1996). The randomly-organized letters afford little opportunity for directed search in the lexicon.

In general, the CNT tests are modifications of procedures used by others with normal and neurological populations (e.g., Cohen, 1984; Cohen & Squire, 1980; Graf et al., 1985; Nissen & Bullemer, 1987; Saint-Cyr et al., 1988; Shallice, 1982; Shimamura et al., 1990). Information regarding the reliability and validity of these specific measures are, however, not yet available. The flexibility of the CNT software, while advantageous in that it allows the examiner to detail specific aspects of functioning, may also be its weakness; that is, it tempts examiners to develop special forms or variants, perhaps impeding the development of systematic research and norms. In our experience, the subject should tell the examiner the word on the priming test. Allowing the examiner to enter the response reduces the possibility that poor spelling skills will affect results.

Normative Data

Normative data are provided for some versions of the tests (Memory Cards $n = 180$, Tower of Hanoi $n = 132$, Repeat Test $n = 136$, Mirror Triad Reading Test $n = 92$, Priming Test $n = 147$, Recall Test $n = 634$, Recognition Test $n = 456$, Temporal Order Test $n = 168$). In general, individuals tested ranged in age from 20 to 89, were typically well-educated and of above average IQ.

Krikorian et al. (1994) provide data on a

sample of 205 elementary school-age children on a 3-peg, 3-bead manual version of the Tower of London. Welsh et al. (1991) give data on a sample of 110 individuals, ranging in age from 3 to 28 years, on a 3- and 4-disk version of the Tower of Hanoi.

References

Butters, N., Wolfe, J., Martone, M., Granholm, E., & Cermak, L.S. (1985). Memory disorders associated with Huntington's disease: Verbal recall, verbal recognition and procedural learning. *Neuropsychologia, 23,* 729–743.

Butters, N., Heindel, W.C., & Salmon, D.P. (1990). Dissociation of implicit memory in dementia: Neurological implications. *Bulletin of the Psychonomic Society, 28,* 359–366.

Cohen, N. (1984). Preserved learning capacity in amnesia: Evidence for multiple memory systems. In L.R. Squire & N. Butters (Eds.), *Neuropsychology of Memory.* New York: Guilford.

Cohen, N.J., & Squire, L.R. (1980). Preserved learning and retention of pattern-analyzing skill in amnesia: Dissociation of knowing how and knowing that. *Science, 210,* 207–210.

Davis, H.P., Bajszar, G.M., & Squire, L.R. (1995). *Colorado Neuropsychology Tests. Version 2.0. Explicit Memory, Implicit Memory, and Problem Solving.* Colorado Springs, CO: Colorado Neuropsychology Tests Co.

Glosser, G., & Goodglass, H. (1990). Disorders in executive control functions among aphasic and other brain-damaged patients. *Journal of Clinical and Experimental Neuropsychology, 12,* 485–501.

Graf, P., Shimamura, A.O., & Squire, L.R. (1985). Priming across modalities and priming across category levels: Extending the domain of preserved function in amnesia. *Journal of Experimental Psychology: Learning, Memory, and Cognition, 11,* 386–396.

Krikorian, R., Bartok, J., & Gay, N. (1994). Tower of London procedure: A standard method and developmental data. *Journal of Clinical and Experimental Neuropsychology, 16,* 840–850.

Moscovitch, M. (1994). Memory and working with memory: Evaluation of a component process model and comparisons with other models. In D.L. Schacter & E. Tulving (Eds.), *Memory Systems.* Cambridge, MA: MIT Press.

Nissen, M.J., & Bullemer, P. (1987). Attentional requirements of learning: Evidence from performance measures. *Cognitive Psychology, 19,* 1–32.

Owen, A.M., Downes, J.J., Sahakian, B.J., Polkey, C.E., & Robbins, T.W. (1990). Planning and spatial working memory following frontal lobe lesions in man. *Neuropsychologia, 28,* 249–262.

Nyberg, L., Winocur, G., & Moscovitch, M. (1997). Correlation between frontal lobe functions and explicit and implicit stem completion in healthy elderly. *Neuropsychology, 11,* 70–76.

Saint-Cyr, J.A., Taylor, A.E., & Lang, A.E. (1988). Procedural learning and neostriatal dysfunction in man. *Brain, 111,* 941–959.

Schacter, D.L., & Tulving, E. (1994). *Memory Systems.* Cambridge, MA: MIT Press.

Shallice, T. (1982). Specific impairments of planning. *Philosophical Transactions of the Royal Society of London, B298,* 199–209.

Shimamura, A.P., Janowsky, J.S., & Squire, L.R. (1990). Memory for the temporal order of events in patients with frontal lobe lesions and amnesic patients. *Neuropsychologia, 28,* 803–813.

Squire, L. (1994). Declarative and nondeclarative memory: Multiple brain systems supporting learning and memory. In D.L. Schacter & E. Tulving (Eds.), *Memory Systems.* Cambridge, MA: MIT Press.

Welsh, M., Pennington, B., & Groisser, D. (1991). A normative-developmental study of executive function: A window on prefrontal function in children. *Developmental Neuropsychology, 7,* 131–149.

Winocur, G., Moscovitch, M., & Stuss, D.T. (1996). Explicit and implicit memory in the elderly: Evidence for double dissociation involving mediate temporal- and frontal-lobe functions. *Neuropsychology, 10,* 57–65.

RECOGNITION MEMORY TEST (RMT)

Purpose

The purpose of this test is to assess recognition memory for printed words and photographs of faces. It is also useful for symptom validity testing.

Source

The test (manual, test booklets and word card, 25 record forms) can be ordered from NFER/Nelson, Darville House, 2 Oxford Road East, Windsor, Berkshire SL4 1DF, U.K. for £73.05 or from Western Psychological Services, 12031 Wilshire Boulevard, Los Angeles, CA 90025-1251 at a cost of $145 US.

Description

The RMT (Warrington, 1984) is a brief, easily administered test that measures verbal and visual recognition. The test consists of a target list of 50 stimulus pictures (50 words or 50 unfamiliar male faces) that are shown to the patient one at a time. In order to ensure that the patient attends to each item, he or she must judge whether it is pleasant or not. Immediately after presentation of the 50 items, the patient is given a two-alternative forced-choice recognition task and must select the item that had previously been presented from the target list.

Administration

The instructions are provided in the RMT manual. The subject is presented with 50 stimulus pictures (words or unfamiliar male faces) at intervals of 3 seconds, and the patient is required to respond yes or no to each item according to whether it is judged as pleasant or not pleasant. This ensures that the patient attends to each item. Memory for words is tested immediately after the presentation of the 50 words; similarly, memory for faces is tested immediately after the presentation of the 50 faces. For both words and faces, retention is tested by a two-choice recognition task, each of the 50 stimuli being represented with one distractor item. The patient is required to point to the stimulus item (or read aloud, in the case of the word list). The examiner records recognition memory responses on the answer sheet.

Approximate Time for Administration

The time required is about 15 minutes.

Scoring

The raw score is the number of items correctly recognized on each task. Raw scores are converted to standard scores (mean = 10, SD = 3) and percentiles. One can also calculate a word/face discrepancy score in order to provide an estimate of material-specific memory impairment.

Comment

No information is provided regarding test reliability. With regard to validity, the RMT appears sensitive to presence of brain impairment. Diesfeldt (1990) found that the test (faces especially) is effective in identifying memory impairment in Alzheimer's disease, particularly in individuals below the age of 80. Warrington (1984) reported that even patients with mild brain atrophy show impairment on the RMT. Whether the test is sensitive to laterality of dysfunction is unclear. Warrington (1984) noted that patients with right-hemisphere lesions ($n = 134$) performed particularly poorly on the faces task whereas there was no impairment on the words task. Patients with left-hemisphere lesions ($n = 145$) were impaired on both the words and the faces tasks compared with normal controls. However, the left-hemisphere group was significantly worse than the right-hemisphere group on the words task, and conversely the right-hemisphere group was significantly worse than the left-hemisphere group on the faces task. Additional analyses suggested that face recognition is especially affected by right temporal and parietal lesions whereas word recognition is particularly sensitive to left temporal disturbance. Millis and Dijkers (1993), studying patients with traumatic brain injury, also suggested that the test was sensitive to lateralized impairment although the differences did not reach conventional levels of significance. However, in moderate–severe traumatically brain-injured patients, RMT scores were unrelated to hippocampal atrophy, evaluated by MRI (Bigler et al., 1996). In epilepsy surgery patients, the RMT is sensitive to lateralized temporal lobe lesions, but it is of extremely limited clinical utility in identifying laterality of temporal lobe seizure onset preoperatively (Hermann et al., 1995; Kneebone et al., 1997). Further, additional data are necessary in order to determine whether a particular deficit reflects a memory impairment *per se* or should be considered secondary to other cognitive deficits (e.g., aphasia, visual perceptual disturbance) (Diesfeldt, 1990; Warrington, 1984). Psychological distress may also affect performance. Boone et al. (1995) reported that in elderly individuals depression was associated with a subtle weakness on the face task.

The test appears to provide complementary information to that provided by traditional recall measures. Compton et al. (1992) evaluated clinic referrals with both the RMT and the Wechsler Memory Scale (WMS). Factor analysis of the scores suggested that the tests (RMT, WMS) measure relatively independent aspects of memory function.

Although not originally designed as a test of motivation, the RMT has promise in the detection of exaggerated memory impairment (Iverson & Franzen, 1994; Millis, 1992, 1994; Millis and Putnam, 1994). The test's forced two-choice procedure provides a known chance level of correct performance, that is, 50 percent. Scores at or below chance (less than 20 correct on either task) suggest the possibility of poor effort. Use of this criterion, however, may be too stringent and can result in a high false-negative rate. Based on studies of patients with severe head injuries, Millis (1992) suggests that a score of 29 correct or less on the words task should raise the issue of poor motivation. Iverson and Franzen (1994) reported that individuals instructed to malinger could be effectively discriminated from patients with moderate-to-severe head injuries using cutoff scores of 33 on the words task

and 30 on the faces task. There is some evidence that the words task may be a better procedure than the faces task for detecting exaggerated memory impairment (Millis, 1992). Use of both tasks is, however, recommended (Millis, 1994). Iverson and Franzen (1994) reported that individuals instructed to malinger often performed more poorly on the faces than the words task, whereas none of their patients with head injuries showed this pattern. One should note, however, that some patients with severe memory disorders (e.g., patients with Alzheimer's disease) may perform at chance level on the RMT (Diesfeldt, 1990). Therefore, poor performance may be considered suggestive, but not diagnostic, of poor motivation.

In short, the test has a number of positive characteristics. It includes both a verbal and nonverbal component. It measures a distinct and important aspect of memory function, namely recognition memory. It is somewhat sensitive to lateralized dysfunction, may be useful for patients with motor problems, and lends itself to symptom validity testing. On the other hand, there are some weaknesses (Adams, 1989; Kapur, 1987; Lezak, 1995; Tyler et al., 1989; Warrington, 1984). The words task has a relatively low ceiling. There are no data concerning an overall measure of recognition memory. There are no parallel forms, and no information is available regarding test reliability. In addition, the test may be insufficient for measuring memory deficits when these include a propensity for false-positive responding.

Normative Data

Normative data were collected from 310 inpatients with extracerebral disease, ranging in age from 18 to 70 years. The norms are presented for three age groups: 18–39 years, 40–54 years, and 55–70 years. For the faces test, Diesfeldt and Vink (1989) provide normative data for subjects aged 69–93 years. The data are shown in Table 10–15. Healthy elderly individuals require about 4.3 (SD = 1.3) minutes to complete the words recognition task and about 5.4 (SD = 1.7) minutes for recognition of the faces (Diesfeldt, 1990).

Table 10—15. Recognition Memory
for Faces by Age Group

Age group	n	M	SD	Range	Deficit score
69–79	29	41.8	2.7	36–48	37
80–84	32	39.1	5.1	30–49	30
85–93	28	36.3	4.3	30–49	29
69–93	89	39.1	4.7	30–49	31

Source: Diesfeldt & Vink, 1989. Reprinted with permission of British Psychological Society.

Age is negatively correlated with performance (Diesfeldt & Vink, 1989; Warrington, 1984; but see Diesfeldt, 1990). The effect of age appears negligible up to the age of 40 at which point a clear decrement in scores emerges. Intelligence shows a moderate correlation with performance (Diesfeldt & Vink, 1989; Warrington, 1984). Among Dutch subjects, neither gender nor education affect performance (Diesfeldt & Vink, 1989). Normative data, broken down by both age and intelligence, are needed.

References

Adams, R. (1989). Review of the recognition memory test. In J.L. Connoley & J.J. Kramer (Eds.), *The Tenth Mental Measurements Yearbook.* Lincoln: Buros Institute of Mental Measurements, pp. 693–694.

Bigler, E.D., Johnson, S.C., Anderson, C.V., Blatter, D.D., Gale, S.D., Russo, A.A., Ryser, D.K., Macnamara, S.E., & Abildskov, T.J. (1996). Traumatic brain injury and memory: The role of hippocampal atrophy. *Neuropsychology, 10,* 333–342.

Boone, K.B., Lesser, I.M., Miller, B.L., Wohl, M., Berman, N., Lee, A., Palmer, B., & Back, C. (1995). Cognitive functioning in older depressed outpatients: Relationship of presence and severity of depression to neuropsychological test scores. *Neuropsychology, 9,* 390–398.

Compton, J.M., Sherer, M., & Adams, R.L. (1992). Factor analysis of the Wechsler Memory Scale and the Warrington Recognition Memory Test. *Archives of Clinical Neuropsychology, 7,* 165–173.

Diesfeldt, H., & Vink, M. (1989). Recognition memory for words and faces in the very old. *British Journal of Clinical Psychology, 28,* 247–253.

Diesfeldt, H.F.A. (1990). Recognition memory for words and faces in primary degenerative dementia of the Alzheimer type and normal old age. *Journal of Clinical and Experimental Neuropsychology, 12,* 931–945.

Hermann, B.P., Connell, B., Barr, W.B., & Wyler, A.R. (1995). The utility of the Warrington Recognition Memory Test for temporal lobe epilepsy: Pre- and postoperative results. *Journal of Epilepsy, 8,* 139–145.

Iverson, G.L., & Franzen, M.D. (1994). The Recognition Memory Test, Digit Span, and Knox Cube Test as markers of malingered memory impairment. *Assessment, 1,* 323–334.

Kapur, N. (1987). Some comments on the technical acceptability of Warrington's Recognition Memory Test. *The British Journal of Clinical Psychology, 26,* 144–146.

Kneebone, A.C., Chelune, G.J., & Lüders, H.O. (1997). Individual patient prediction of seizure lateralization in temporal lobe epilepsy: A comparison between neuropsychological memory measures and the intracarotid amobarbital procedure. *Journal of the International Neuropsychological Society, 3,* 159—168.

Lezak, M.D. (1995). *Neuropsychological Assessment* (3rd ed.). New York: Oxford University Press.

Millis, S.R. (1992). The Recognition Memory Test in the detection of malingered and exaggerated memory deficits. *The Clinical Neuropsychologist, 6,* 404–414.

Millis, S.R. (1994). Assessment of motivation and memory with the Recognition Memory Test after financially compensable mild head injury. *Journal of Clinical Psychology, 50,* 601–605.

Millis, S.R., & Dijkers, M. (1993). Use of the Recognition Memory Test in traumatic brain injury. *Brain Injury, 7,* 53–58.

Millis, S.R., & Putnam, S.H. (1994). The Recognition Memory Test in the assessment of memory impairment after financially compensable mild head injury: A replication. *Perceptual and Motor Skills, 79,* 384–386.

Tyler, P., Eastmond, K., & Davies, J. (1989). Why forget the false positives? *British Journal of Clinical Psychology, 28,* 377–378.

Warrington, E.K. (1984). *Recognition Memory Test Manual.* Windsor, England: NFER-Nelson.

REY AUDITORY-VERBAL LEARNING TEST (RAVLT)

Other Test Name

The other test name is the Auditory Verbal Learning Test (AVLT).

Purpose

The purpose of this test is to assess verbal learning and memory.

Source

The original French version of the test can be ordered from Etablissements d'Applications Psychotechniques (EAP), 6 bis, rue Andre-Chenier, F-92130 ISSY-Les-Moulineaux, France. Users may also refer to the following text in order to design their material for use with English speaking populations. Schmidt (1996) has summarized the current literature on the RAVLT and has provided metanorms. The handbook is available through Western Psychological Services, 12031 Wilshire Boulevard, Los Angeles, CA 90025-1251 at a cost of $49.50 US. A package of 25 record sheets and summaries costs $18.50 US. The Mayo's Older Americans Normative Studies (MOANS) scoring software program provides age-extended normative scores from 56 to 97 years of age for the RAVLT (for IBM PC or compatible) and is available from the Psychological Corporation, 555 Academic Court, San Antonio, TX 78204-2498, or 55 Horner Avenue, Toronto, Ontario, M5Z 4X6, at a cost of $67 US or $105 Cdn.

Description

The RAVLT is a brief, easily administered pencil and paper measure that assesses immediate memory span, new learning, susceptibility to interference, and recognition memory. The original version was developed by Andre Rey (1958). Taylor (1959) and Lezak (1976, 1983) altered the test and adapted it for use with English-speaking subjects. There are many variations of the RAVLT. The most commonly used variant (see Figure 10–11) consists of 15 nouns (List A) read aloud (with a 1-second interval between each word) for five consecutive trials, each trial followed by a free-recall test. The order of presentation of words remains fixed across trials. Instructions are repeated before each trial to minimize forgetting. Upon completion of Trial 5, an interference list of 15 words (List B) is presented, followed by a free-recall test of that list. Immediately following this, delayed recall of the first list is tested without further presentation of those words. After a 20-minute delay period, each subject is again required to recall words from List A. Finally, a story that uses all the words from List A is presented, either orally or in written form (depending upon the patient's reading ability), and the patient must identify words recognized from List A. Alternatively, one can test recognition in a matrix array where the patient must identify List A words from a list of 50 words containing all items from Lists A and B and 20 words phonemically and/or semantically similar to those in Lists A and B. We test recognition with the list format since this is the more popular format, and there are good normative data for this version. The addition of a recognition trial permits the identification of people with suspected retrieval problems, who may score better on this trial than on free recall. A person with a generalized memory deficit will perform poorly on both free recall and recognition trials (Bleecker et al., 1988; Lezak, 1995). In addition, comparison of recognition of Lists A and B permits the evaluation of words that have been studied five times (List A) versus words that were studied once only, as well as source monitoring for which list contained the words (Schmidt, 1996).

Various studies suggest that the recollection of the temporal order of events may be more impaired than recall of the events themselves (e.g., Janowsky et al., 1989). Vakil and Blachstein (1994) recently introduced a supplementary measure, temporal order. Following the standard administration of the RAVLT, without any warning subjects are presented with the 15 words from List A in random order and asked to rewrite them in their original order. The temporal order score shows weak-to-

RAVLT Sample Scoring Sheet

Name: _____

Date: _____

Examiner: _____

(Note: Do not re-read List A for Recall Trial A6 or A7)

List A	Recall Trials A1	A2	A3	A4	A5	List B	Recall Trials B1	A6	A7	
drum						desk				drum
curtain						ranger				curtain
bell						bird				bell
coffee						shoe				coffee
school						stove				school
parent						mountain				parent
moon						glasses				moon
garden						towel				garden
hat						cloud				hat
farmer						boat				farmer
nose						lamb				nose
turkey						gun				turkey
color						pencil				color
house						church				house
river						fish				river
# correct										

Total   A1 to A5 = _____

Trial   A6 – A5 = _____

Recognition # targets correctly identified _____

distractors correctly identified _____

Word List for Testing RAVLT Recognition[1]

bell (A)	home (SA)	towel (B)	boat (B)	glasses (B)
window (SA)	fish (B)	curtain (A)	hot (PA)	stocking (SB)
hat (A)	moon (A)	flower (SA)	parent (A)	shoe (B)
barn (SA)	tree (PA)	color (A)	water (SA)	teacher (SA)
ranger (B)	balloon (PA)	desk (B)	farmer (A)	stove (B)
nose (A)	bird (B)	gun (B)	rose (SPA)	nest (SPB)
weather (SB)	mountain (B)	crayon (SA)	cloud (B)	children (SA)
school (A)	coffee (A)	church (B)	house (A)	drum (A)
hand (PA)	mouse (PA)	turkey (A)	stranger (PB)	toffee (PA)
pencil (B)	river (A)	fountain (PB)	garden (A)	lamb (B)

[1] Source: Lezak (1983). (A) words from list A; (B) words from list b; (S) word with a semantic association to a word on list A or B as indicated; (P) word phonemically similar to a word on list A or B.

Figure 10—11. Rey Auditory–Verbal Learning Test sample scoring sheet.

modest relations with other RAVLT measures, suggesting that this score may assess unique aspects of memory.

Administration

For Trial 1, give the following instructions: "*I am going to read a list of words. Listen carefully, for when I stop you are to repeat back as many words as you can remember. It doesn't matter in what order you repeat them. Just try to remember as many as you can.*"

Read List A words, with a 1-second interval between each of the 15 words. Check off the words recalled using numbers to keep track of the patient's pattern of recall. No feedback should be given regarding the number of correct responses, repetitions, or errors.

When the patient indicates that he or she can recall no more words, the examiner re-

reads the list following a second set of instructions: *"Now I am going to read the same words again, and once again when I stop I want you to tell me as many words as you can remember, including words you said the first time. It doesn't matter in what order you say them. Just say as many words as you can remember whether or not you said them before."*

The list is reread for Trials 3 through 5 using Trial 2 instructions each time. The examiner may praise the patient as he or she recalls more words; the examiner may tell the patient the number of words already recalled, particularly if the patient is able to use the information for reassurance or as a challenge.

After Trial 5, the examiner reads List B with instructions to perform as on the first (A) list trial. *"Now I'm going to read a second list of words. Listen carefully, for when I stop you are to repeat back as many words as you can remember. It doesn't matter in what order you repeat them. Just try to remember as many as you can."*

Immediately after the List B trial, the examiner asks the patient to recall as many words from the first list (List A) as he or she can (Trial 6) without further presentation of those words. *"Now tell me all the words that you can remember from the first list."*

After a 20-minute delay period, filled with other activity, ask the subject to recall the words from List A. *"A while ago, I read a list of words to you several times, and you had to repeat back the words. Tell me the words from that list."*

On completion of the delay trial, the recognition test should be given. The recognition task requires the patient to identify as many of the list words as he or she can and, if possible, the specific list of origin. If the patient can read at least at grade 7 level, ask the patient to read the list and circle the correct words. If the patient has difficulty with reading, the examiner should read the list to the patient. *"I will say some words that were on the word lists that I read to you, and some other words that were not on those lists. Tell me each time I say a word that was read to you. If you can remember that the word was from the word lists, tell me if the word was from the first or second list."*

In order to assess temporal order judgment, present the patient with a sheet of paper containing the 15 List A words arranged in random order. Ask the patient to rewrite the word list to match the order of words in the original list as she/he heard them.

Approximate Time for Administration

The time required is 10–15 minutes.

Scoring

See sample scoring sheet (includes correct answers) in Figure 10–11. Words that are repeated can be marked R; RC if repeated and self-corrected; RQ if the patient questions whether he or she has repeated the words but remains unsure. Words that are not on the list are errors and are marked E.

One can derive a number of different measures. Geffen et al. (1990) provide extensive indices of aspects of memory function, only some of which are reported here. The score for each trial is the number of words correctly recalled. In addition to scores on Trials 1 to 5, which may be used to plot a learning curve, the RAVLT yields scores for the total number of words recalled following interference (post-distractor trial or Trial 6), the number of words recalled after the 20-minute delay, and the total number of words recognized from each list. Other scores, including a total score (the sum of Trials 1 to 5), the number of repetitions and extra-list intrusions, and the amount of loss from Trial 5 to the post-distraction recall trial (6) can also be calculated. The percentage of words lost from Trial 5 to Trial 6 may be a particularly sensitive indicator of retroactive interference (i.e., the decremental effect of subsequent learning on the retention of previously learned material). Conversely, if learning List A significantly interferes with learning List B, then an unusually high degree of proactive interference may be occurring.

Several other summary measures have been proposed. For example, Ivnik and colleagues (1992) have suggested a Learning Over Trials Score (LOT = Total Learning over five trials − 5 (Trial 1 score)). In order to use norms provided by Ivnik and colleagues for adults older than 55 years, the examiner must convert RAVLT component scores, via tables provided in Ivnik et al. (1992) or computer scoring software (see Source), to age-corrected and normalized MOANS Scaled Scores (mean = 10, SD = 3). MOANS Scaled Scores are then grouped, and summed within groups, to allow derivation of three summary indices: the Mayo Auditory-Verbal Learning Efficiency Index (MAVLEI) reflects the sum of MOANS Trial 1 and LOT scores; the Mayo Auditory-Verbal Delayed Recall Index (MAVDRI) consists of the sum of MOANS Trials A6 and A7; and the Mayo Auditory-Verbal Percent Retention Index (MAVPRI) consists of the sum of Trials A6 and A7 expressed as percent retention scores and converted to MOANS Scaled Scores. Note, however, that Ivnik and colleagues use a 30-, as opposed to a 50-word list for their recognition trial.

Vakil and Blachstein (1994) provide several different measures of temporal order. These measures are highly correlated with one another. The easiest to score is the number of hits; i.e., the number of words correctly placed at their original serial position.

Comment

Over 1-year intervals, the test has moderate test–retest reliability (Snow et al., 1988; Uchiyama et al., 1995). Small, but significant, improvements (on average 1–2 words per trial) can be expected on successive administrations of the same form of the RAVLT (Crawford et al., 1989; Lezak, 1982; Uchiyama et al., 1995). Because of these practice effects, patients should not be tested with the same list twice in succession. A parallel form should be used since the literature suggests that practice effects are reduced when subjects are retested with a different RAVLT version (Crawford et al., 1989; Delaney et al., 1992; Geffen et al., 1994a). Several investigators have provided alternate forms of the test (Crawford et al., 1989; Geffen et al., 1994a; Majdan, Sziklas, & Jones-Gotman, in press; Ryan et al., 1986; Shapiro & Harrison, 1990). The versions by Geffen et al. (1994a) and Majdan et al. (in press) seem to produce comparable scores and are presented in Figure 10–12. In situa-

tions requiring retesting, however, Geffen et al. (1994a) recommend that the original form be used initially. Geffen et al. (1994a) found that the most reliable measures (with retest intervals of 6–14 days) were the total number of words learned over the five learning trials ($r = .77$), and performance on post-distractor (Trial A6) and delayed-recall (Trial A7) measures. Poor reliability was found for Trial 1 and for various derived scores (e.g., acquisition rate, information overload, proactive and retroactive interference, retrieval efficiency, misassignment and false positives in recognition, repeats, other list intrusions, and serial position recall). Geffen and colleagues suggest that these derived scores may have diagnostic significance in a single test session, but comparisons between sessions may not be meaningful.

In order to reduce cultural bias, the World Health Organization (WHO)/UCLA version of the AVLT was developed (Maj et al., 1993; Ponton et al., 1996). All test items were selected from five categories (body parts, animals, tools, household objects, and transportation vehicles) and presumably have universal familiarity. There are 15 items, three examples from each category (see Figure 10–13). The administration format is the same as that described for the standard version. When both forms were given to individuals in Germany, correlations were in the moderate range (.47–.55). In addition, comparison among normal subjects in Thailand, Zaire, Germany, and Italy suggested that the WHO/UCLA AVLT is freer of cultural influences than the traditional RAVLT.

With regard to the scores that can be derived from the test, there is evidence that some of the indices (e.g., percent recall from primacy, middle, and recency regions) have significant correlations (above .8) with the number of words recalled and therefore are not pure measures of the qualitative traits that they purportedly assess (Schmidt, 1997). An index based on recency minus primacy (Gainotti & Marra, 1994), however, appears not substantially confounded with number of words recalled, and appears promising (Schmidt, 1997).

With regard to the internal structure of the

Geffen et al. Alternate Form

List A	Interference List (List B)
pipe	bench
wall	officer
alarm	cage
sugar	sock
student	fridge
mother	cliff
star	bottle
painting	soap
bag	sky
wheat	ship
mouth	goat
chicken	bullet
sound	paper
door	chapel
stream	crab

Recognition List

alarm (A)	eye (SA)	soap (B)	ship (B)	bottle (B)
aunt (SA)	crab (B)	wall (A)	car (PA)	seat (SB)
bag (A)	star (A)	clock (SA)	mother (A)	sock (B)
creek (SA)	rag (PA)	sound (A)	duck (SA)	tone (SA)
officer (B)	bun (PA)	bench (B)	wheat (A)	fridge (B)
mouth (A)	cage (B)	bullet (B)	floor (SPA)	rock (SPB)
arrow (SB)	cliff (B)	night (SA)	sky (B)	bread (SA)
student (A)	sugar (A)	chapel (B)	door (A)	pipe (A)
hail (PA)	cream (PA)	chicken (A)	bridge (PB)	ball (PA)
paper (B)	stream (A)	coat (PB)	painting (A)	goat (B)

Figure 10—12. Alternate forms of the Rey Auditory–Verbal Learning Test (Geffen et al., 1994; Majdan et al. (in press)).

test, there appears to be a short-term memory component (a factor defined by Trials 1 and B), a storage component (defined primarily by recognition memory) and a retrieval component (defined by Trial 5, delayed recall trials, temporal order) (Talley, 1986; Vakil & Blachstein, 1993). Salthouse et al. (1996), however, gave the RAVLT to normal adults aged 18–94 years and found evidence of only a single factor of memory. Differences among studies likely reflect the particular combination of scores included in the analyses and the criteria used to determine the number of factors (Vakil & Blachstein, 1993).

The RAVLT correlates moderately well with other measures of learning and memory such as the CVLT (Crossen & Wiens, 1994; Stallings et al., 1995). Slightly lower raw scores obtain on the RAVLT than the CVLT,

likely reflecting the slightly shorter RAVLT list. Note that the tests are not interchangeable. The CVLT consists of words that can be categorized, with semantic clustering becoming the strategy of choice for normal adults. The RAVLT words do not show a clear semantic relationship and temporal tagging may become a more important strategy (Vakil & Blachstein, 1994). When standard, as opposed to raw, scores are considered, CVLT scores are considerably lower than those of the RAVLT in head-injured patients (Stallings et al., 1995). The discrepancies may reflect differences in the composition of the standardization samples and/or the greater sensitivity of the CVLT to memory impairment (perhaps related to the requirement of semantic clustering). Stallings et al. (1995) noted that use of the CVLT, as opposed to the RAVLT, results in

Majdan et al. Two Alternate Forms

Form 1

List A	List B	Recognition List Buffers:	BOTTLE	CALENDAR	
violin	orange	**scarf**	toad	donkey	train
tree	table	leaf	chin	pear	uncle
scarf	toad	**stairs**	**ham**	**cousin**	**violin**
ham	corn	frog	piano	grass	stars
suitcase	bus	table	**field**	**dog**	spider
cousin	chin	**banana**	soap	gloves	
earth	beach	hospital	**tree**	hotel	
stairs	soap	**suitcase**	city	**bucket**	
dog	hotel	peel	**hunter**	sofa	
banana	donkey	book	orange	**town**	
town	spider	blanket	money	beach	
radio	money	**padlock**	doctor	cork	
hunter	book	**earth**	soldier	corn	
bucket	soldier	television	**radio**	lunchbox	
field	padlock	rock	chest	bus	

Form 2

List A	List B	Recognition List Buffers:	TELEPHONE	ZOO	
doll	dish	**nail**	hill	foot	fly
mirror	jester	stall	forest	bread	dart
nail	hill	**bed**	**sailor**	**desert**	**doll**
sailor	coat	engine	pony	street	captain
heart	tool	jester	**road**	**machine**	shield
desert	forest	**milk**	ladder	jail	
face	perfume	soot	**mirror**	girl	
letter	ladder	heart	envelope	**horse**	
bed	girl	silk	**music**	joker	
machine	foot	insect	dish	**letter**	
milk	shield	screw	pie	perfume	
helmet	pie	car	song	plate	
music	insect	**face**	ball	coat	
horse	ball	armour	**helmet**	sand	
road	car	head	pool	tool	

Code for targets in recognition lists
bold: words from principle list
underline: words from interference list

Figure 10—12. Continued

a higher frequency of head-injury patients' being classed as memory-impaired, and their memory impairments appear greater. When both tests are given within a few days of one another, there are no significant effects for order of presentation (Crossen & Wiens, 1994; Stallings et al., 1995).

Factor analytic studies indicate that the RAVLT loads primarily with other verbal memory tests (e.g., those found on the Wechsler Memory Scale) (Mitrushina & Satz, 1991; Ryan et al., 1984; Strauss, Hunter, & Wada, 1995). The RAVLT, however, may measure a construct that is not singularly verbal in nature. Factor analyses of variable sets that in-

clude the RAVLT indicate that memory variables load together regardless of whether they are verbal or nonverbal measures (Malec et al., 1991; Moses, 1986; Smith et al., 1992).

The RAVLT is sensitive to neurological impairment (Powell et al., 1991), laterality of brain damage (Malec et al., 1991; Miceli et al., 1981), and verbal memory deficits in a variety of patient groups, including those suffering from left temporal lobe dysfunction, specific language impairment, Alzheimer's disease, Parkinson's disease, Huntington's disease, closed-head injury, AIDS, depression, or psychosis (Bigler et al., 1989; Geffen et al., 1994b; Lezak, 1983; Malec et al., 1991; Maj-

List A		List B	
arm		boot	
cat		monkey	
axe		bowl	
bed		cow	
plane		finger	
ear		dress	
dog		spider	
hammer		cup	
chair		bee	
car		foot	
eye		hat	
horse		butterfly	
knife		kettle	
clock		mouse	
bike		hand	

Recognition Items		
mirror	HORSE	truck
HAMMER	leg	EYE
KNIFE	DOG	fish
candle	table	EAR
motorcycle	CAT	BIKE
AXE	lips	snake
CLOCK	tree	stool
CHAIR	ARM	bus
PLANE	nose	BED
turtle	sun	CAR

Figure 10—13. World Health Organization/UCLA version of the Auditory Verbal Learning Test. Source: Satz, Chervinsky and D'Elia (1990). Code for target in recognition lists: lower case: distractors; capitals: words from principal list.

dan et al., in press; Mitrushina et al., 1994; Mungas, 1983; Powell et al., 1991; Records et al., 1995; Rosenberg et al., 1984; Ryan et al., 1992; Shimamura et al., 1987; Tierney et al., 1994; Tierney et al., 1996; Vakil et al., 1991). Information from the test can be used to differentiate clinically among different memory disorders (but see Crockett et al., 1992). For example, patients with dementia of the Alzheimer's type (AD) show more impairment on the RAVLT than patients with closed-head injury (CHI) or AIDS, along with a flat learning/retention curve that shows negligible improvement with repeated trials, recency effects only, and an excessive number of word intrusions (confabulation) on the recognition trial (Antonelli Incalzi et al., 1995; Bigler et al., 1989; Mitrushina et al., 1994). CHI patients, by contrast, show both a recency and a primacy effect along with improvement over repeated trials (positive-slope learning curve) (Bigler et al., 1989). While general impairment of verbal memory is a feature of CHI, ex-

aggerated retroactive interference effects are most characteristic (Geffen et al., 1994b). Moreover, retention of the learning list following the distractor trial appears to vary with severity of the closed-head injury; the more severe the injury (the longer the duration of post-traumatic amnesia), the fewer words are recalled after interference (Geffen et al., 1994b). AIDS patients showed relatively intact learning and recognition; however, their forgetting rates (comparing Trial 5 to Trial 6) were impaired (Mitrushina et al., 1991).

Various authors have noted that psychological distress, in the form of depression, post-traumatic stress, and other anxiety disorders, has some effect on RAVLT performance (Bleecker et al., 1988; Gainotti & Marra, 1994; Hinkin et al., 1992; Query & Megran, 1983; Uddo et al., 1993), although others have failed to observe a correlation (Gibbs et al., 1990; Vingerhoets et al., 1995; Wiens et al., 1988). The weight of evidence suggests, however, that caution is needed in interpreting RAVLT performance in patients with a past history or clinical suspicion of depression, post-traumatic stress disorder, or anxiety. Qualitative indices may prove useful in this regard. Uddo and colleagues (1993) found that veterans diagnosed with post-traumatic stress disorder exhibited less facile acquisition, were more sensitive to proactive interference, and showed greater perseveration on the RAVLT when compared to control subjects. Despite differences in learning, the two groups did not differ in the proportion of information recalled following a delay. Gainotti and Marra (1994) reported that a preservation of the recency effect and attenuation of the primacy effect, as well as extralist intrusions on delayed recall, point to a diagnosis of depressive pseudo-dementia. On the other hand, the presence of several false-positive errors on delayed recognition tends to be specific to AD patients and is rarely found in patients with depressive pseudo-dementia.

Scores on the RAVLT also appear to offer some predictive utility (Haddad & Nussbaum, 1989). AD patients who show a positive learning curve are more likely to benefit from rehabilitative group therapy compared to patients who show little learning.

There is also evidence that severe RAVLT

recognition memory impairment (scores less than 6) likely reflects motivation to exaggerate deficits, at least in patients with mild head injury with no neurological evidence of brain injury (Binder et al., 1993; Greiffenstein et al., 1994). Examination of serial position (the pattern of primacy and recency effects in recall) may also be useful in this regard. Bernard (1991) found that individuals attempting to fake injury tend to do so by suppressing recall of words from the first third of the list (absence of primacy but not recency effect).

Normative Data

There are a number of normative studies based on large samples of healthy people. The norms for Swiss people (Rey, 1964), reported in Lezak (1976, 1983) and Taylor (1959) cannot be used (see Wiens et al., 1988) because:

1. The English translations for some of the words differ from the original words.
2. The current administration differs from that used by Rey (1964) in that feedback regarding correct and incorrect words was provided, no distraction trial was given, and a different presentation rate was used.
3. Educational and cultural differences may invalidate comparison of current North American samples to those collected by Rey 40 years ago.

Schmidt (1996) has recently reviewed the available literature and developed metanorms by which to gauge RAVLT performance (see source). Alternatively, the examiner can refer to specific reference studies recommended for various age groups (see source and below).

Table 10–16 provides recently compiled normative data derived from schoolchildren, ages 7–15 years, for the procedure described above (Forrester & Geffen, 1991). Forrester and Geffen (1991) give normative data for additional summary measures, (for example: resistance to proactive interference (expressed as a ratio, List B/Trial 1 List A); resistance to retroactive interference (Trial A6/A5); forgetting over 20-minute delay (Trial A7/A6); retrieval efficiency (Trial 7/15)/p(A) List A, where the measure of recognition performance on List A (p[A] = 0.5[1 + HR − FP]) reflects the proportion of words correctly recognized (hit rate or HR) and the proportion of distractor words responded to as list words (false-positive rate or FP); information overload (Trial 1/Wechsler Digit Span Forward); and serial position effects.

Munsen (1987) also reported data for a sample of adolescents and the values were similar to those presented by Forrester and Geffen. Data by Bishop et al. (1990) for children, ages 5–16 years, should not be used because (1) they are based on referrals to a hospital clinic suffering from conditions known to af-

Table 10—16. RAVLT Scores for Children, Age 7 to 15

	Age 7 (n = 20)		Age 9 (n = 20)		Age 11 (n = 20)		Age 14 (n = 20)	
	M	(SD)	M	(SD)	M	(SD)	M	(SD)
Trial 1 List A	4.5	(1.3)	5.8	(1.2)	6.2	(1.0)	6.2	(1.5)
Trial 2 List A	6.7	(1.8)	8.9	(1.6)	8.3	(1.5)	9.1	(1.5)
Trial 3 List A	8.1	(2.2)	9.9	(1.8)	9.7	(1.9)	10.9	(1.8)
Trial 4 List A	9.4	(2.3)	10.9	(1.5)	11.4	(1.4)	11.3	(2.0)
Trial 5 List A	10.2	(2.6)	11.3	(1.3)	11.5	(1.5)	12.1	(1.7)
Total	38.9	(7.9)	46.7	(5.4)	46.9	(5.0)	49.5	(6.1)
Distractor List B	4.5	(1.6)	6.0	(2.0)	5.7	(1.5)	5.8	(1.7)
Trial A6 (Retention)	8.0	(2.8)	9.3	(2.5)	9.5	(1.7)	10.2	(2.1)
Trial A7 (Delayed Recall)	8.4	(2.6)	9.9	(2.3)	9.6	(1.4)	10.4	(2.3)
List A Recognition	14.5	(0.7)	14.2	(1.2)	14.5	(0.8)	14.3	(0.9)
List B Recognition	6.1	(2.2)	7.5	(1.9)	7.2	(2.2)	7.3	(1.8)
False Positives	1.1	(0.7)	2.4	(1.2)	2.1	(0.8)	3.2	(0.9)

Source: Forrester and Geffen (1991) provide data for 10 boys and 10 girls in each of four age groups, 7–8, 9–10, 11–12, and 14–15 years. Reprinted with permission of Swets & Zeitlinger.

Table 10—17. Males: Mean (SD) Number of Words *Recalled and Recognized* According to Age and Trial

| | Age | | | | | | | | | | | | |
| | 16–19 (n = 13) | | 20–29 (n = 52) | | 30–39 (n = 50) | | 40–49 (n = 41) | | 50–59 (n = 32) | | 60–69 (n = 12) | | 70+ (n = 11) | |
	M	(SD)	M	(SD)	M	(SD)	M	(SD)	M	(SD)	M	(SD)	M	(SD)
Trial 1 List A	6.9	(1.8)	7.1	(1.4)	6.3	(1.7)	6.2	(1.6)	6.3	(1.5)	5.2	(1.6)	3.6	(0.8)
Trial 2 List A	9.7	(1.7)	9.7	(1.9)	9.0	(2.5)	8.9	(2.1)	8.4	(1.8)	6.8	(1.9)	5.7	(1.7)
Trial 3 List A	11.5	(1.2)	11.4	(1.8)	10.4	(2.5)	10.0	(2.5)	9.9	(1.8)	7.9	(2.8)	6.8	(1.6)
Trial 4 List A	12.8	(1.6)	11.8	(1.9)	11.3	(2.5)	11.0	(2.6)	10.7	(2.0)	8.7	(2.6)	8.3	(2.7)
Trial 5 List A	12.5	(1.3)	12.2	(2.0)	11.6	(2.5)	11.3	(1.9)	11.1	(2.2)	9.0	(2.3)	8.2	(2.5)
Total	53.4	(5.4)	52.2	(7.3)	48.6	(10.3)	47.4	(8.8)	46.4	(7.6)	37.6	(9.8)	32.6	(8.3)
Distractor List B	6.9	(1.9)	6.6	(1.8)	5.8	(1.8)	5.9	(1.7)	5.4	(1.8)	4.7	(1.5)	3.5	(1.2)
Trial A6 (Retention)	11.2	(1.6)	11.0	(2.4)	9.8	(3.3)	9.6	(3.0)	9.0	(2.8)	7.0	(2.9)	6.4	(1.7)
Trial A7 (Delayed Recall)	11.3	(1.7)	11.1	(2.4)	10.0	(3.4)	9.4	(3.3)	8.7	(3.0)	6.8	(3.7)	5.6	(2.6)
Recognition														
List A	14.4	(0.9)	12.8	(2.2)	12.7	(2.5)	12.2	(2.6)	11.4	(2.7)	10.1	(3.3)	11.5	(2.6)
List B	8.4	(3.8)	7.6	(3.7)	5.7	(3.2)	6.5	(3.7)	5.1	(3.5)	3.9	(2.5)	3.0	(2.5)
P(A) (List A)	0.95	(0.09)	0.9	(0.1)	0.9	(0.1)	0.9	(0.1)	0.9	(0.1)	0.8	(0.1)	0.8	(0.1)
P(A) (List B)	0.8	(0.1)	0.7	(0.1)	0.7	(0.1)	0.7	(0.1)	0.7	(0.1)	0.7	(0.1)	0.6	(0.8)

Source: Geffen, personal communication, May 1995.

Note: p(A) = 0.5(1 + hit rate − false positive rate).

fect memory performance, and (2) they were given a different administration procedure.

Geffen et al. (1990) has published normative data for healthy adults, ages 16–84 years, of above-average IQ. She has recently compiled additional data (Geffen, personal communication, May 1995) for healthy Australian adults (n = 437), whose estimated IQ (from the NART) falls within the average range. The updated mean recall and recognition data are shown in Tables 10–17 and 10–18 for men and women, respectively, in each of seven age groups. It is important to note, however, that the sample was not representative of the general population, because of average but mostly above-average intelligence and had more than an average number of years of education. Note too that subjects tested before 1990 had a 20-minute delay (Trial A7); those tested and added later had a 30-minute delay. It is unlikely that there is an appreciable difference in performance after a 20- versus a 30-minute delay since the amount forgotten tends to be minimal. Normative data for additional summary indices are given in Geffen et al. (1990).

Bleecker et al. (1988), Mitrushina et al. (1991), Nielsen et al. (1989), Read (1986), Wiens

et al. (1988), Savage & Gouvier (1992), Selnes et al. (1991), and Uchiyama et al. (1995) also provide normative data for healthy adults. The values are similar, but not identical, to those reported here, although in some cases their administration differs from Geffen's (e.g., no 20-minute delayed-recall trial is given or story recognition procedure is used) or applies to only a segment of the population (e.g., males). There is evidence that norm sets are not interchangeable and that set selection determines the likelihood of a patient's being classed as memory-impaired. Thus, Stallings et al. (1995) have shown that selection of the Savage and Gouvier (1992) norms results in a significantly lower rate of classification of impairment than would other norms, such as those by Wiens et al. (1988). The Wiens and Geffen sets appear to produce relatively similar results (Stallings et al., 1995).

Ivnik et al. (1990) provide normative data based on 47 healthy subjects, aged 85 and older. (Trial 1: M = 4.0, SD = 1.5; Trial 2: M = 6.0, SD = 1.8; Trial 3: M = 7.4, SD = 2.2; Trial 4: M = 7.9, SD = 2.4; Trial 5: M = 9.1, SD = 2.3; List B: M = 3.1, SD = 1.4; Trial 6: M = 6.2, SD = 2.6; Delayed Recall: M = 5.4, SD

Table 10—18. Females: Mean (SD) Number of Words Recalled and Recognized
According to Age and Trial

	Age 16–19 (n = 14)		Age 20–29 (n = 49)		Age 30–39 (n = 58)		Age 40–49 (n = 45)		Age 50–59 (n = 31)		Age 60–69 (n = 18)		Age 70+ (n = 10)	
	M	(SD)	M	(SD)	M	(SD)	M	(SD)	M	(SD)	M	(SD)	M	(SD)
Trial 1 List A	8.0	(1.8)	7.2	(1.6)	7.3	(1.9)	6.6	(1.5)	6.3	(2.0)	6.3	(2.1)	5.6	(1.4)
Trial 2 List A	10.8	(2.1)	9.8	(2.0)	10.0	(2.2)	9.1	(1.9)	8.7	(2.1)	9.4	(2.0)	6.9	(2.1)
Trial 3 List A	12.6	(1.3)	11.3	(2.1)	11.5	(2.1)	10.9	(1.7)	10.5	(2.2)	10.6	(2.1)	8.9	(1.8)
Trial 4 List A	12.6	(1.6)	11.7	(2.0)	12.4	(2.1)	11.6	(2.2)	11.2	(2.2)	11.2	(1.7)	10.1	(1.9)
Trial 5 List A	13.3	(1.4)	12.3	(2.2)	12.4	(2.0)	12.4	(1.6)	11.8	(2.0)	11.9	(1.6)	10.1	(1.2)
Total	57.4	(5.9)	52.3	(8.0)	53.6	(8.3)	50.6	(7.1)	48.5	(8.4)	49.4	(7.5)	41.6	(6.6)
Distractor List B	7.5	(1.6)	6.5	(1.9)	6.6	(2.1)	5.9	(1.9)	5.2	(1.8)	5.6	(1.2)	4.2	(1.9)
Trial A6 (Retention)	12.1	(1.4)	11.2	(2.5)	11.4	(2.4)	10.4	(2.7)	10.0	(3.4)	9.4	(2.3)	7.8	(1.8)
Trial A7 (Delayed Recall)	11.8	(2.5)	11.1	(2.7)	11.2	(2.8)	10.6	(2.5)	10.0	(3.4)	10.2	(2.5)	8.3	(2.1)
Recognition														
List A	13.6	(2.1)	13.5	(1.6)	13.6	(1.9)	13.0	(2.2)	12.1	(2.7)	11.3	(2.8)	13.6	(2.0)
List B	7.9	(3.2)	7.8	(3.1)	8.5	(3.8)	7.4	(3.3)	6.0	(3.3)	6.2	(3.5)	7.5	(3.7)
P(A) (List A)	0.9	(0.01)	0.9	(0.1)	0.9	(0.1)	0.9	(0.1)	0.9	(0.1)	0.9	(0.1)	0.8	(0.1)
P(A) (List B)	0.7	(0.1)	0.7	(0.1)	0.8	(0.1)	0.7	(0.1)	0.7	(0.1)	0.7	(0.1)	0.7	(0.1)

Source: Geffen et al., personal communication, May 1995.

Note: p(A) = 0.5(1 + hit rate − false positive rate).

= 2.7; Recognition: M = 12.3, SD = 2.3). Since completing that report, Ivnik et al. (1992) extended their normative data base to a sample of 530 healthy persons, mostly well-educated caucasians. The authors provide tables that convert AVLT scores to age-corrected MOANS Scaled Scores and summary Mayo Auditory-Verbal Indices (mean = 100, SD = 15). The RAVLT MOANS Scaled Scores and Mayo Indices are comparable to similar indicators that can be derived for the WAIS-R and the WMS-R. It is important to bear in mind, however, that Ivnik and colleagues use a 30-, not a 50-word list for their recognition trial.

Tuokko and Woodward (1996) have recently provided data, based on 274 English-speaking, community-dwelling Canadians, aged 65 years and older, who had been screened for the absence of cognitive impairment. To use their tables, raw scores must be converted to demographically corrected (age, sex, education) T scores.

For Hispanic individuals living in the United States, Ponton et al. (1996) give normative data from a sample of 300 Spanish-speaking individuals (mostly monolingual) using the WHO-UCLA version. The data,

stratified by age, education, and gender are shown in Table 10–19.

Vakil and Blachstein (1994) provide normative data for evaluating temporal order judgement. The data, shown in Table 10–20, are based on a Hebrew version of the RAVLT.

Trial 1 may be considered an indication of immediate memory, with normal young adults recalling seven words on average. Note, however, that it is not identical to Digit Span (Talley, 1986). The first trial of the RAVLT is essentially a supraspan task, whereas digit span is a subspan task (Moses, 1986; Schmidt, 1996). In general, normal people learn about five words from Trial 1 to Trial 5; they recall about one to two fewer words on the Recall Trial (Trial 6) than on Trial 5. There is little forgetting over a 30-minute delay. Forgetting does, however, occur following lengthier delay periods. Geffen and her colleagues (in press) report that adults lose about one word following a 24-hour delay, and over a period of 7 days, one additional word is forgotten. A proactive interference effect is observed for all adult groups (but not in children) where recall for the second word list is inferior to initial recall of the first word list. Finally, a high inci-

Table 10—19. Mean and Standard Deviations (in parentheses) for Hispanic Persons on the Spanish Version of the WHO-AVLT by Age and Number of Years of Education

	Age 16–29		Age 30–39		Age 40–49		Age 50–75	
	<10 Years education	>10 Years education	<10 Years education	>10 Years education	<10 Years education	>10 Years education	<10 Years education	>10 Years education
Females								
n	12	30	22	44	16	11	25	20
Trial 5	13.3	13.5	12.8	13.8	12.6	13.3	11.5	13.2
	(1.6)	(1.9)	(2.2)	(1.4)	(1.0)	(2.1)	(1.9)	(1.3)
Trial A6 (Retention)	11.6	12.4	11.6	12.1	10.6	12.1	10.2	10.8
	(1.7)	(2.3)	(2.7)	(2.1)	(1.6)	(1.9)	(2.6)	(2.6)
Trial A7 (20-minute delay)	11.8	12.9	11.9	12.9	11.1	12.5	10.6	12.5
	(2.2)	(2.5)	(2.6)	(2.0)	(1.6)	(1.9)	(2.4)	(2.0)
Males								
n	11	25	13	18	12	17	18	6
Trial A5	12.7	13.1	12.2	13.3	12.9	13.5	12.1	12.7
	(1.6)	(1.9)	(1.6)	(1.3)	(1.8)	(1.4)	(1.7)	(1.5)
Trial A6 (Retention)	11.7	12.2	11.5	11.6	10.5	13.0	10.5	11.0
	(1.4)	(2.7)	(2.2)	(2.1)	(3.0)	(2.0)	(2.1)	(1.7)
Trial A7 (20-minute delay)	12.4	12.5	11.2	12.6	11.4	13.2	10.8	11.8
	(1.9)	(2.1)	(2.4)	(1.6)	(2.4)	(1.8)	(2.2)	(1.6)

Source: Ponton et al., 1996. Reprinted with permission of Cambridge University Press.

Table 10—20. Mean Hits and Standard Deviation for Temporal Order Measure by Age and Gender

	Age 18–25 (n = 57)		Age 26–35 (n = 42)		Age 36–45 (n = 48)		Age 46–55 (n = 42)	
	M	F	M	F	M	F	M	F
Mean	6.42	7.90	6.18	8.28	5.33	4.83	3.54	4.94
SD	2.78	3.41	3.37	4.60	3.68	3.42	3.15	3.64

Source: Vakil and Blachstein, 1994. Note that the norms are based on a sample of 190 normal participants, mean age = 35, with an average of 13 years of schooling (range 8–20 years), on a Hebrew version of the RAVLT. Reprinted with permission of American Psychological Association.

dence of false positives on the recognition task is quite unusual in normal adults.

It should be noted that age affects performance on the RAVLT; the influence of gender and intellectual/educational level is less consistent across studies (Bishop et al., 1990; Bleecker et al., 1988; Forrester & Geffen, 1991; Geffen et al., 1990; Graf & Uttl, 1995; Mitrushina et al., 1991; Mitrushina et al., 1994; Munsen, 1987; Nielsen et al., 1989; Query & Berger, 1980; Query & Megran, 1983; Petersen et al., 1992; Ponton et al., 1996; Read, 1986; Salthouse et al., 1996; Savage & Gouvier, 1992; Selnes et al., 1991; Wiens et al., 1988; Uchiyama et al., 1995; Vakil & Blachstein, 1994). The evidence indicates that certain RAVLT scores improve as a function of age in children and tend to decrease in adults with advancing age. In particular, temporal order judgment (Vakil & Blachstein, 1994) and rates of learning and recognition (Antonelli Incalzi et al., 1995; Mitrushina et al., 1991) show little change with age, whereas the number of free-recall words declines with advancing age (Antonelli Incalzi et al., 1995; Mitrushina et al., 1991). Antonelli Incalzi et al. (1995) found that forgetting increased with age. Contrary results, however, were reported by Mitrushina et al. (1991). Some have observed an age-related decline in the primacy and middle portions, but not the recency component, of free recall (Antonelli Incalzi et al., 1995, reported a decline in the primacy component only; Grat & Uttl, 1995), whereas others (Mitrushina et al., 1991) noted that age has no significant influence on primacy/recency effects.

The reason for the conflicting views is not apparent. Graf and Uttl (1995) suggest that the age change in free recall reflects age changes in processing rate and capacity, whereas Mitrushina et al. (1991) suggest that age changes in free recall are due to faulty retrieval mechanisms (see also Antonelli Incalzi et al., 1995).

Further, recall tends to be better at higher IQ/educational levels. Few researchers separate their data by gender. Those that do report inconsistent findings. Thus some fail to find that gender has any impact (e.g., Bishop et al., 1990; Forrester & Geffen, 1991; Ponton et al., 1996; Savage & Gouvier, 1992). When sex differences emerge, females outperform males on the recall, but not the recognition trials (Bleecker et al., 1988; Geffen et al., 1990; Vakil & Blachstein, 1994). Data for subjects grouped by age, sex, and intellectual level need to be gathered. Reliance on norms generated by males alone may attenuate the sensitivity to deficits in females. Similarly, estimates of memory function based on norms derived from individuals of average to above-average intellect may suggest a deficit when none is present, particularly in individuals of below-average intellectual attainment.

References

Antonelli Incalzi, R., Capparella, O., Gemma, A., Marra, C., & Carbonin, P.U. (1995). Effects of aging and Alzheimer's disease on verbal memory. *Journal of Clinical and Experimental Neuropsychology, 17,* 580–589.

Bernard, L.C. (1991). The detection of faked deficits on the Rey Auditory Verbal Learning Test. *Archives of Clinical Neuropsychology, 6,* 81–88.

Bigler, E.D., Rosa, L., Schultz, F., Hall, S., & Harris, J. (1989). Rey-Auditory Verbal Learning and Rey-Osterrieth Complex Figure Design Test Performance in Alzheimer's Disease and closed head injury. *Journal of Clinical Psychology, 45*, 277–280.

Binder, L.M., Villanueva, M.R., Howieson, D., & Moore, R.T. (1993). The Rey AVLT Recognition memory task measures motivational impairment after mild head trauma. *Archives of Clinical Neuropsychology*, 137–147.

Bishop, J., Knights, R.M., & Stoddart, C. (1990). Rey auditory-verbal learning test: Performance of English and French children aged 5 to 16. *The Clinical Neuropsychologist, 4*, 133–140.

Bleecker, M.L., Bolla-Wilson, K., Agnew, J., & Meyers, D.A. (1988). Age-related sex differences in verbal memory. *Journal of Clinical Psychology, 44*, 403–411.

Crawford, J.R., Stewart, L.E., & Moore, J.W. (1989). Demonstration of savings on the AVLT and development of a parallel form. *Journal of Clinical and Experimental Neuropsychology, 11*, 975–981.

Crockett, D.J., Hadjistavropoulos, T., & Hurwitz, T. (1992). Primacy and recency effects in the assessment of memory using the Rey Auditory Verbal Learning Test. *Archives of Clinical Neuropsychology, 7*, 97–107.

Crossen, J.R., and Wiens, A.N. (1994). Comparison of the auditory-verbal learning test (AVLT) and California Verbal Learning Test (CVLT) in a sample of normal subjects. *Journal of Clinical and Experimental Neuropsychology, 16*, 190–194.

Delaney, R.C., Prevey, M.L., Cramer, J., Mattson, R.H., et al. (1992). Test-retest comparability and control subject data for the Rey-Auditory Verbal Learning Test and Rey-Osterrieth/Taylor Complex Figures. *Archives of Clinical Neuropsychology, 7*, 523–528.

Forrester, G., & Geffen, G. (1991). Performance measure of 7- to 15-year-old children on the Auditory Verbal Learning Test. *The Clinical Neuropsychologist, 5*, 345–359.

Gainotti, G., & Marra, C. (1994). Some aspects of memory disorders clearly distinguish dementia of the Alzheimer's type from depressive pseudodementia. *Journal of Clinical and Experimental Neuropsychology, 16*, 65–74.

Geffen, G.M., Butterworth, P., Forrester, G.M., & Geffen, L.B. (1994b). Auditory verbal learning test components as measures of the severity of closed head injury. *Brain Injury, 8*, 405–411.

Geffen, G.M., Butterworth, P., & Geffen, L.B. (1994). Test–retest reliability of a new form of the Auditory Verbal Learning Test (AVLT). *Archives of Clinical Neuropsychology, 9*, 303–316.

Geffen, G.M., Geffen, L., & Bishop, K. (in press). Extended delayed recall of AVLT word lists: Effects of age and sex on adult performance. *Australian Journal of Psychology*.

Geffen, G., Moar, K.J., O'Hanlon, A.P., Clark, C.R., & Geffen, L.B. (1990). Performance measures of 16- to 86-year-old males and females on the Auditory Verbal Learning Test. *The Clinical Neuropsychologist, 4*, 45–63.

Gibbs, A., Andrewes, D.G., Szmuckler, G., et al. (1990). Early HIV-related neuropsychological impairment: Relationship to stage of viral infection. *Journal of Clinical and Experimental Neuropsychology, 12*, 766–780.

Graf, P., & Uttl, B. (1995). Component processes of memory: Changes across the adult lifespan. *Swiss Journal of Psychology, 54*, 113–130.

Greiffenstein, M., Baker, W., & Gola, T. (1994). Validation of malingered amnesia measures with a large clinical sample. *Psychological Assessment, 6*, 218–224.

Haddad, L.B., & Nussbaum, P. (1989). Predictive utility of the Rey Auditory-Verbal Learning Test with Alzheimer's patients. *The Clinical Gerontologist, 9*, 53–59.

Hinkin, C.H., Van-Gorp, W.G., Satz, P., et al. (1992). Depressed mood and its relationship to neuropsychological test performance in HIV-1 seropositive individuals. *Journal of Clinical and Experimental Neuropsychology, 14*, 289–297.

Ivnik, R.J., Malec, J.F., Tangalos, E.G., Petersen, R.C., Kokmen, S., & Kurland, L.T. (1990). The Auditory-Verbal Learning Test (AVLT): Norms for ages 55 years and older. *Psychological Assessment, 2*, 304–312.

Ivnik, R.J., Malec, J.F., Tangalos, E.G., Petersen, R.C., Kokmen, E., & Kurland, L.T. (1992). Mayo's Older Americans Normative Studies: Updated AVLT norms for ages 56 to 97. *The Clinical Neuropsychologist, 6*, 83–104.

Janowsky, J.S., Shimamura, A.P., & Squire, L.R. (1989). Source memory impairment in patients with frontal lobe lesions. *Neuropsychologia, 27*, 1043–1056.

Lezak, M.D. (1982). The test–retest stability of some tests commonly used in neuropsychological assessment. Paper presented to the 5th European Conference of the International Neuropsychological Society. Deauville, France.

Lezak, M.D. (1976). *Neuropsychological Assessment*. New York: Oxford University Press.

Lezak, M.D. (1983). *Neuropsychological Assess-*

ment (2nd ed.). New York: Oxford University Press.

Lezak, M.D. (1995). *Neuropsychological Assessment* (3rd ed.). NY: Oxford University Press.

Maj, M., D'Elia, L., Satz, P., Janssen, R., et al. (1993). Evaluation of two new neuropsychological tests designed to minimize cultural bias in the assessment of HIV-1 seropositive persons: A WHO study. *Archives of Clinical Neuropsychology, 8,* 123–135.

Majdan, A., Sziklas, V., & Jones-Gotman, M. (in press). Performance of healthy subjects and patients with resection from the anterior temporal lobe on matched tests of verbal and visuoperceptual learning. *Journal of Clinical and Experimental Neuropsychology.*

Malec, J.F., Ivnik, R.J., & Hinkeldey, N.S. (1991). Visual Spatial Learning Test. *Psychological Assessment, 3,* 82–88.

Miceli, G., Caltagirone, C., Gainotti, G., Masullo, C., & Silveri, M.C. (1981). Neuropsychological correlates of localized cerebral lesions in nonaphasic brain-damaged patients. *Journal of Clinical Neuropsychology, 3,* 53–63.

Mitrushina, M., & Satz, P. (1991). Changes in cognitive functioning associated with normal aging. *Archives of Clinical Neuropsychology, 6,* 49–60.

Mitrushina, M., Satz, P., Chervinsky, A., & D'Elia, L. (1991). Performance of four age groups of normal elderly on the Rey Auditory-Verbal Learning Test. *Journal of Clinical Psychology, 47,* 351–357.

Mitrushina, M., Satz, P., Drebing, C., & Van Gorp, W. (1994). The differential pattern of memory deficit in normal aging and dementias of different etiology. *Journal of Clinical Psychology, 50,* 246–252.

Moses, J.A. (1986). Factor structure of Benton's test of visual retention, visual construction, and visual form discrimination. *Archives of Clinical Neuropsychology, 1,* 147–156.

Mungas, D. (1983). Differential clinical sensitivity of specific parameters of the Rey Auditory-Verbal Learning Test. *Journal of Consulting and Clinical Psychology, 51,* 848–855.

Munsen, J. (1987). Unpublished data. University of Victoria.

Nielsen, H., Knudsen, L., & Daugbjerg, O. (1989). Normative data for eight neuropsychological tests based on a Danish sample. *Scandinavian Journal of Psychology, 30,* 37–45.

Petersen, R.C., Smith, G., Kokmen, E., Ivnik, R.J., & Tangalos, E.G. (1992). Memory function in normal aging. *Neurology, 42,* 396–401.

Ponton, M.O., Satz, P., Herrera, L., Ortiz, F., Ur-

rutia, C.P., Young, R., D'Elia, L.F., Furst, C.J., & Namerow, N. (1996). Normative data stratified by age and education for the Neuropsychological Screening Battery for Hispanics (NeSBHIS): Initial report. *Journal of the International Neuropsychological Society, 2,* 96–104.

Powell, J.B., Cripe, L.I., & Dodrill, C.B. (1991). Assessment of brain impairment with the Rey Auditory-Verbal Learning Test: A comparison with other neuropsychological measures. *Archives of Clinical Neuropsychology, 6,* 241–249.

Query, W.T., & Berger, R.A. (1980). AVLT memory scores as a function of age among general medical, neurological, and alcoholic patients. *Journal of Clinical Psychology, 36,* 1009–1012.

Query, W.T., & Megran, J. (1983). Age-related norms for the AVLT in a male patient population. *Journal of Clinical Psychology, 39,* 136–138.

Read, D.E. (1986). Unpublished data, University of Victoria.

Records, N.L., Tomblin, J.B., & Buckwalter, P.R. (1995). Auditory verbal learning and memory in young adults with specific language impairment. *The Clinical Neuropsychologist, 9,* 187–193.

Rey, A. (1958). *L'examen clinique en psychologie.* Paris: Presse Universitaire de France.

Rosenberg, S.J., Ryan, J.J., & Prifiteria, A. (1984). Rey Auditory-Verbal Learning Test performance of patients with and without memory impairment. *Journal of Clinical Psychology, 40,* 785–787.

Ryan, J.J., Geisser, M.E., Randall, D.M., & Georgemiller, R.J. (1986). Alternate form reliability and equivalency of the Rey Auditory Verbal Learning Test. *Journal of Clinical and Experimental Neuropsychology, 8,* 611–616.

Ryan, J.J., Paolo, A.M., & Skrade, M. (1992). Rey Auditory Verbal Learning Test performance of a federal corrections sample with acquired immunodeficiency syndrome. *International Journal of Neuroscience, 64,* 177–181.

Ryan, J.J., Rosenberg, S.J., & Mittenberg, W. (1984). Factor analysis of the Rey Auditory-Verbal Learning Test. *International Journal of Clinical Neuropsychology, 6,* 239–241.

Salthouse, T.A., Fristoe, N., & Rhee, S.H. (1996). How localized are age-related effects on neuropsychological measures? *Neuropsychology, 10,* 272–285.

Savage, R.M., & Gouvier, W.D. (1992). Rey Auditory-Verbal Learning Test: The effects of age and gender, and norms for delayed recall and story recognition trials. *Archives of Clinical Neuropsychology, 7,* 407–414.

Schmidt, M. (1996). *Rey Auditory-Verbal Learn-*

ing Test. Los Angeles: Western Psychological Services.

Schmidt, M. (1997). Some cautions on interpreting qualitative indices for word-list learning tests. *The Clinical Neuropsychologist, 11,* 81–86.

Selnes, O.A., Jacobson, I., Machado, A.M., Becker, J.T., Wesch, J., Miller, E.N., Visscher, B., & McArthur, B. (1991). Normative data for a brief neuropsychological screening battery. *Perceptual and Motor Skills, 73,* 539–550.

Shapiro, D.M., and Harrison, D. (1990). Alternate forms of the AVLT: A procedure and test of form equivalency. *Archives of Clinical Neuropsychology, 5,* 405–410.

Shimamura, A.P., Salmon, D.P., Squire, L.R., & Butters, N. (1987). Memory dysfunction and word priming in dementia and amnesia. *Behavioral Neuroscience, 101,* 347–351.

Smith, G.E., Malec, J.F., & Ivnik, R.J. (1992). Validity of the construct of nonverbal memory: A factor-analytic study in a normal elderly sample. *Journal of Clinical and Experimental Neuropsychology, 14,* 211–221.

Snow, W.G., Tierney, M.C., Zorzitto, M.L., Fisher, R.H., & Reid, D.W. (1988). One-year test–retest reliability of selected neuropsychological tests in older adults. Paper presented to the International Neuropsychological Society, New Orleans.

Stallings, G., Boake, C., & Sherer, M. (1995). Comparison of the California Verbal Learning Test and the Rey Auditory-Verbal Learning Test in head-injured patients. *Journal of Clinical and Experimental Neuropsychology, 17,* 706–712.

Strauss, E., Hunter, M., & Wada, J. (1995). Risk factors for cognitive impairment in epilepsy. *Neuropsychology, 9,* 457–464.

Talley, J.L. (1986). Memory in learning disabled children: Digit span and the Rey Auditory Verbal Learning Test. *Archives of Clinical Neuropsychology, 1,* 315–322.

Taylor, E.M. (1959). *The Appraisal of Children with Cerebral Deficits.* Cambridge, MA: Harvard University Press.

Tierney, M.C., Nores, A., Snow, W.G., et al. (1994). Use of the Rey Auditory Verbal Learning Test in differentiating normal aging from Alzhei-

mer's and Parkinson's dementia. *Psychological Assessment, 6,* 129–134.

Tierney, M.C., Snow, W.G., Szalai, J.P., Fisher, R.H., & Zorzitto, M.L. (1996). A brief neuropsychological battery for the differential diagnosis of probable Alzheimer's disease. *The Clinical Neuropsychologist, 10,* 96–103.

Tuokko, H., & Woodward, T.S. (1996). Development and validation of a demographic correction system for neuropsychological measures used in the Canadian Study of Health and Aging. *Journal of Clinical and Experimental Neuropsychology, 18,* 479–616.

Uchiyama, C.L., D'Elia, L.F., Dellinger, A.M., Becker, J.T., Selnes, O.A., Wesch, J.E., Chen, B.B., Satz, P., van Gorp, W., & Miller, E.N. (1995). Alternate forms of the Auditory-Verbal Learning Test: Issues of test comparability, longitudinal reliability, and moderating demographic variables. *Archives of Clinical Neuropsychology, 10,* 147–158.

Uddo, M., Vasterling, J.J., Brailey, K., & Sutker, P. (1993). Memory and attention in combat-related post-traumatic stress disorder. *Journal of Psychopathology and Behavioral Assessment, 15,* 43–51.

Vakil, E., & Blachstein, H. (1993). Rey Auditory Verbal Learning Test: Structure analysis. *Journal of Clinical Psychology, 49,* 883–890.

Vakil, E., & Blachstein, H. (1994). A supplementary measure in the Rey AVLT for assessing incidental learning of temporal order. *Journal of Clinical Psychology, 50,* 241–245.

Vakil, E., Blachstein, H., & Hoofien, D. (1991). Automatic temporal order judgement: The effect of intentionality of retrieval on closed-head-injured patients. *Journal of Clinical and Experimental Neuropsychology, 13,* 291–298.

Vingerhoets, G., De Soete, G., & Jannes, C. (1995). Relationship between emotional variables and cognitive test performance before and after open-heart surgery. *The Clinical Neuropsychologist, 9,* 198–202.

Wiens, A.N., McMinn, M.R., & Crossen, J.R. (1988). Rey Auditory-Verbal Learning Test: Development of norms for healthy young adults. *The Clinical Neuropsychologist, 2,* 67–87.

REY-OSTERRIETH COMPLEX FIGURE TEST (CFT)

Other Test Names

Other test names are Complex Figure (CF) and Rey Figure (RF).

Purpose

The purpose of this test is to assess visuospatial constructional ability and visual memory.

Source

The test (stimuli for the copy, recall, and recognition subtests and manual; Meyers & Meyers, 1995b) can be ordered from Psychological Assessment Resources, Inc. P.O. Box 998, Odessa, FL 33556, at a cost of $109 US. It also forms part of the Denman Neuropsychology Memory Scale, which can be ordered from Dr. Sidney B. Denman, 1040 Fort Sumter Drive, Charleston, SC 29412. The entire kit costs $298 US; the norms manual alone is $56 US. Users may also refer to the following description in order to design their own material.

Description

The CFT permits assessment of a variety of cognitive processes, including planning, organizational skills, and problem-solving strategies, as well as perceptual, motor, and memory functions (Waber & Holmes, 1986; Meyers & Meyers, 1995a). It was developed by Rey (1941) and elaborated by Osterrieth (1944). These two key French papers have been translated into English by Corwin and Bylsma (1993). The materials consist of blank pieces of paper and the Rey-Osterrieth figure (Figure 10–14) or an alternate version such as the Taylor figure (Taylor, 1969, 1979) (Figure 10–15) or one of the four Medical College of Georgia (MCG) complex figures (Meador et al., 1991, 1993) (Figures 10–16, 10–17, 10–18, 10–19). The basic procedure involves having the subject copy the figure and then, without prior warning, reproduce it from memory.

The test developed by Rey (1941) consisted of a copy trial, followed by a recall trial 3 minutes later. Current administration procedures vary considerably. Some investigators (e.g., Loring et al., 1988a; Chiulli et al., 1989; Meyers & Meyers, 1995b) give both immediate and delayed-recall trials of the CFT whereas others (e.g., Kolb & Whishaw, 1985; Bennett-Levy, 1984; Denman, 1987; King, 1981; Taylor, 1969, 1979) measure only delayed recall. Further, the amount of delay varies from 3 minutes (e.g., Bigler et al., 1989; Boone et al., 1993; Rey, 1941) to 45 minutes (Taylor, 1969, 1979). There is little difference in performance between immediate and 3-minute-delay recall scores (Meyers & Meyers, 1995a). The length of delay chosen (15, 30, 45, or 60 minutes) also does not affect overall recall performance, provided the delay is no longer than 1 hour (Berry & Carpenter, 1992). Most forgetting tends to occur very quickly, within the first few minutes after copying, perhaps as a result of an overloading of working memory (Berry & Carpenter, 1992; Chiulli et al., 1995; Delaney et al., 1992; Lezak, 1995). Delayed recall, however, may be more sensitive to the presence of various memory deficits than immediate recall (Loring et al., 1990). This is because very little difference is observed in normal subjects between immediate and delayed-recall trials (e.g., Chiulli et al., 1989, 1995, Loring et al., 1990). Accordingly, a decline between the immediate and delayed-recall trials is of clinical significance. Moreover, since memory impairment can assume many different forms, the inclusion of both an immediate or 3-minute recall trial and a delayed-recall trial allows for a more detailed examination of impaired and preserved aspects of memory. The measures of performance that are typically derived include a copy score, which reflects the accuracy of the original copy and is a measure of visual-constructional ability, the time required to copy the figure, as well as immediate or 3-minute and 30-minute delayed-recall scores, which assess amount of information retained over time.

Following the 30-minute recall, a recognition subtest (Meyers & Lange, 1994; Meyers & Meyers, 1995a) can be given (see Source). The recognition subtest was developed from elements of the Rey and Taylor figures.

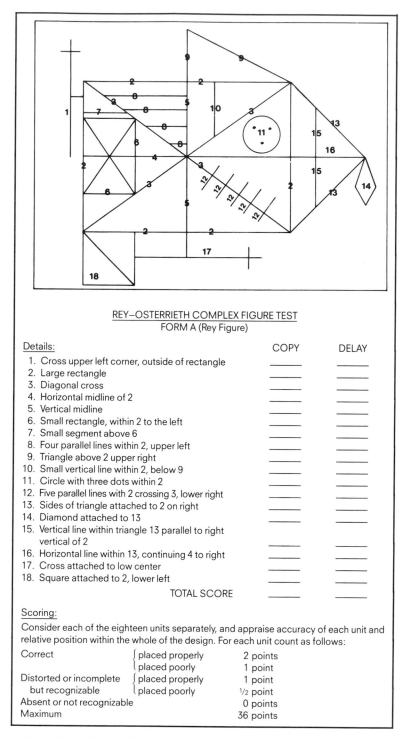

REY–OSTERRIETH COMPLEX FIGURE TEST
FORM A (Rey Figure)

Details: COPY   DELAY

1. Cross upper left corner, outside of rectangle   _____   _____
2. Large rectangle   _____   _____
3. Diagonal cross   _____   _____
4. Horizontal midline of 2   _____   _____
5. Vertical midline   _____   _____
6. Small rectangle, within 2 to the left   _____   _____
7. Small segment above 6   _____   _____
8. Four parallel lines within 2, upper left   _____   _____
9. Triangle above 2 upper right   _____   _____
10. Small vertical line within 2, below 9   _____   _____
11. Circle with three dots within 2   _____   _____
12. Five parallel lines with 2 crossing 3, lower right _____ _____
13. Sides of triangle attached to 2 on right   _____   _____
14. Diamond attached to 13   _____   _____
15. Vertical line within triangle 13 parallel to right
    vertical of 2   _____   _____
16. Horizontal line within 13, continuing 4 to right _____   _____
17. Cross attached to low center   _____   _____
18. Square attached to 2, lower left   _____   _____
                                     TOTAL SCORE   _____   _____

Scoring:

Consider each of the eighteen units separately, and appraise accuracy of each unit and
relative position within the whole of the design. For each unit count as follows:

Correct	{ placed properly	2 points
	placed poorly	1 point
Distorted or incomplete	{ placed properly	1 point
but recognizable	placed poorly	½ point
Absent or not recognizable		0 points
Maximum		36 points

Figure 10—14. Rey-Osterrieth Complex Figure Test: Form A (Rey figure) and legend.

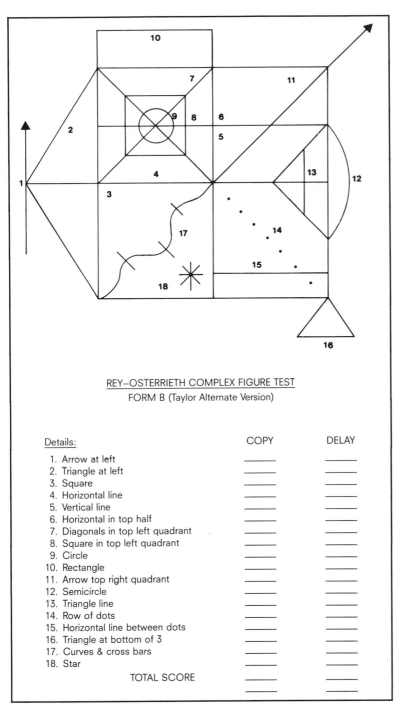

REY–OSTERRIETH COMPLEX FIGURE TEST
FORM B (Taylor Alternate Version)

Details:	COPY	DELAY
1. Arrow at left	———	———
2. Triangle at left	———	———
3. Square	———	———
4. Horizontal line	———	———
5. Vertical line	———	———
6. Horizontal in top half	———	———
7. Diagonals in top left quadrant	———	———
8. Square in top left quadrant	———	———
9. Circle	———	———
10. Rectangle	———	———
11. Arrow top right quadrant	———	———
12. Semicircle	———	———
13. Triangle line	———	———
14. Row of dots	———	———
15. Horizontal line between dots	———	———
16. Triangle at bottom of 3	———	———
17. Curves & cross bars	———	———
18. Star	———	———
TOTAL SCORE	———	———

Figure 10—15. Rey-Osterrieth Complex Figure Test: Form B (Taylor alternate version) and legend.

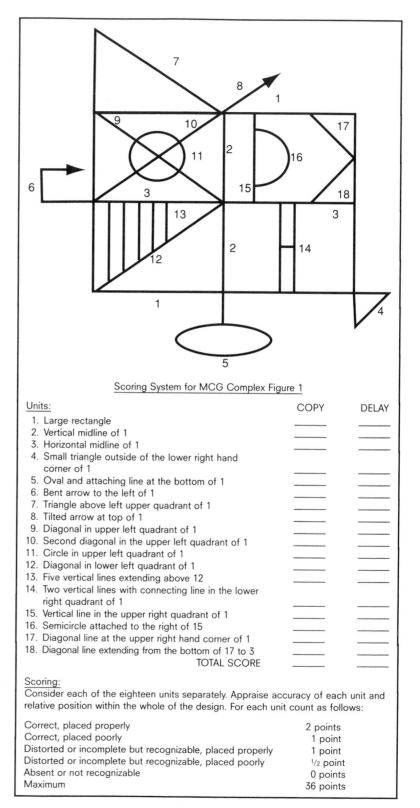

Scoring System for MCG Complex Figure 1

Units:	COPY	DELAY
1. Large rectangle	____	____
2. Vertical midline of 1	____	____
3. Horizontal midline of 1	____	____
4. Small triangle outside of the lower right hand corner of 1	____	____
5. Oval and attaching line at the bottom of 1	____	____
6. Bent arrow to the left of 1	____	____
7. Triangle above left upper quadrant of 1	____	____
8. Tilted arrow at top of 1	____	____
9. Diagonal in upper left quadrant of 1	____	____
10. Second diagonal in the upper left quadrant of 1	____	____
11. Circle in upper left quadrant of 1	____	____
12. Diagonal in lower left quadrant of 1	____	____
13. Five vertical lines extending above 12	____	____
14. Two vertical lines with connecting line in the lower right quadrant of 1	____	____
15. Vertical line in the upper right quadrant of 1	____	____
16. Semicircle attached to the right of 15	____	____
17. Diagonal line at the upper right hand corner of 1	____	____
18. Diagonal line extending from the bottom of 17 to 3	____	____
TOTAL SCORE	____	____

Scoring:
Consider each of the eighteen units separately. Appraise accuracy of each unit and relative position within the whole of the design. For each unit count as follows:

Correct, placed properly	2 points
Correct, placed poorly	1 point
Distorted or incomplete but recognizable, placed properly	1 point
Distorted or incomplete but recognizable, placed poorly	½ point
Absent or not recognizable	0 points
Maximum	36 points

Figure 10—16. Medical College of Georgia Complex Figure 1 and legend.

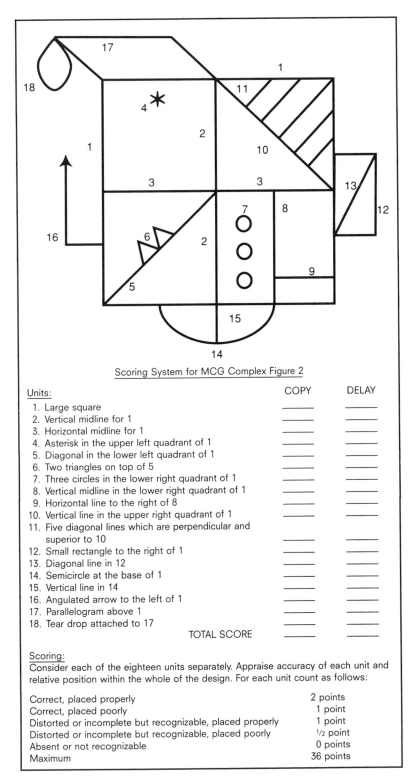

Scoring System for MCG Complex Figure 2

Units:	COPY	DELAY
1. Large square	———	———
2. Vertical midline for 1	———	———
3. Horizontal midline for 1	———	———
4. Asterisk in the upper left quadrant of 1	———	———
5. Diagonal in the lower left quadrant of 1	———	———
6. Two triangles on top of 5	———	———
7. Three circles in the lower right quadrant of 1	———	———
8. Vertical midline in the lower right quadrant of 1	———	———
9. Horizontal line to the right of 8	———	———
10. Vertical line in the upper right quadrant of 1	———	———
11. Five diagonal lines which are perpendicular and superior to 10	———	———
12. Small rectangle to the right of 1	———	———
13. Diagonal line in 12	———	———
14. Semicircle at the base of 1	———	———
15. Vertical line in 14	———	———
16. Angulated arrow to the left of 1	———	———
17. Parallelogram above 1	———	———
18. Tear drop attached to 17	———	———
TOTAL SCORE	———	———

Scoring:
Consider each of the eighteen units separately. Appraise accuracy of each unit and relative position within the whole of the design. For each unit count as follows:

Correct, placed properly	2 points
Correct, placed poorly	1 point
Distorted or incomplete but recognizable, placed properly	1 point
Distorted or incomplete but recognizable, placed poorly	½ point
Absent or not recognizable	0 points
Maximum	36 points

Figure 10—17. Medical College of Georgia Complex Figure 2 and legend.

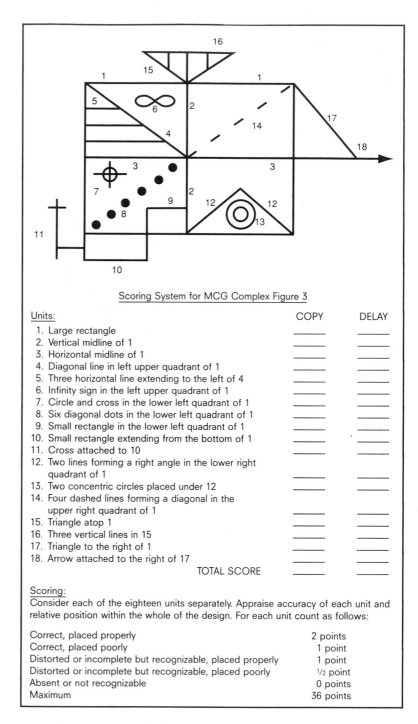

Scoring System for MCG Complex Figure 3

Units: COPY   DELAY

 1. Large rectangle
 2. Vertical midline of 1
 3. Horizontal midline of 1
 4. Diagonal line in left upper quadrant of 1
 5. Three horizontal line extending to the left of 4
 6. Infinity sign in the left upper quadrant of 1
 7. Circle and cross in the lower left quadrant of 1
 8. Six diagonal dots in the lower left quadrant of 1
 9. Small rectangle in the lower left quadrant of 1
10. Small rectangle extending from the bottom of 1
11. Cross attached to 10
12. Two lines forming a right angle in the lower right
    quadrant of 1
13. Two concentric circles placed under 12
14. Four dashed lines forming a diagonal in the
    upper right quadrant of 1
15. Triangle atop 1
16. Three vertical lines in 15
17. Triangle to the right of 1
18. Arrow attached to the right of 17
                                         TOTAL SCORE

Scoring:
Consider each of the eighteen units separately. Appraise accuracy of each unit and relative position within the whole of the design. For each unit count as follows:

Correct, placed properly	2 points
Correct, placed poorly	1 point
Distorted or incomplete but recognizable, placed properly	1 point
Distorted or incomplete but recognizable, placed poorly	½ point
Absent or not recognizable	0 points
Maximum	36 points

Figure 10—18. Medical College of Georgia Complex Figure 3 and legend.

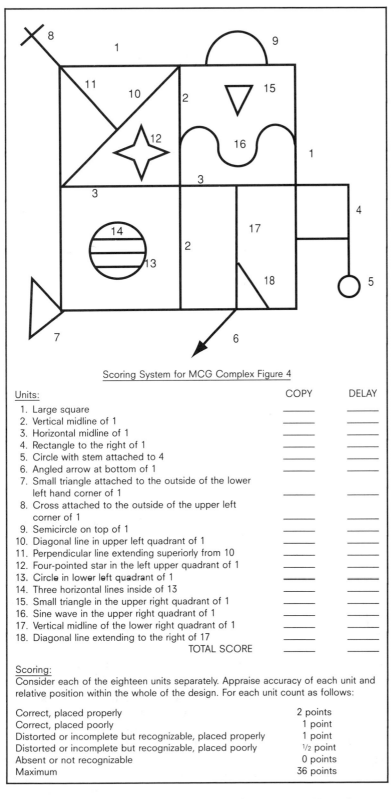

Scoring System for MCG Complex Figure 4

Units:	COPY	DELAY
1. Large square	____	____
2. Vertical midline of 1	____	____
3. Horizontal midline of 1	____	____
4. Rectangle to the right of 1	____	____
5. Circle with stem attached to 4	____	____
6. Angled arrow at bottom of 1	____	____
7. Small triangle attached to the outside of the lower left hand corner of 1	____	____
8. Cross attached to the outside of the upper left corner of 1	____	____
9. Semicircle on top of 1	____	____
10. Diagonal line in upper left quadrant of 1	____	____
11. Perpendicular line extending superiorly from 10	____	____
12. Four-pointed star in the left upper quadrant of 1	____	____
13. Circle in lower left quadrant of 1	____	____
14. Three horizontal lines inside of 13	____	____
15. Small triangle in the upper right quadrant of 1	____	____
16. Sine wave in the upper right quadrant of 1	____	____
17. Vertical midline of the lower right quadrant of 1	____	____
18. Diagonal line extending to the right of 17	____	____
TOTAL SCORE	____	____

Scoring:
Consider each of the eighteen units separately. Appraise accuracy of each unit and relative position within the whole of the design. For each unit count as follows:

Correct, placed properly	2 points
Correct, placed poorly	1 point
Distorted or incomplete but recognizable, placed properly	1 point
Distorted or incomplete but recognizable, placed poorly	½ point
Absent or not recognizable	0 points
Maximum	36 points

Figure 10—19. Medical College of Georgia Complex Figure 4 and legend.

Twenty-four figures are randomly placed on four pages in two columns per page. The subject is required to circle the figures that were part of the original design drawn. Fastenau (1996) has also developed recognition and matching trials.

In the standard procedure, the task is essentially an incidental learning test: There is no warning of the memory component until the patient is asked to recall the figure from memory. Tombaugh and his colleagues (1992) use the Taylor figure in an intentional learning paradigm. Individuals are told that they will be shown a design and will then have to draw it from memory, that they will be given four tries at this, and that they will be asked to recall it later. On each of the four trials, individuals observe the Taylor figure for 30 seconds. The figure is then removed and the subject has a maximum of 2 minutes to reproduce the figure from memory. A retention trial is given about 15 minutes after the last acquisition trial. This is followed by a copy trial where subjects are given 4 minutes to draw the figure with the model present. Specific scoring criteria (maximum score = 69 points) are provided and normative data are given for people aged 20–79 years.

Administration

See Meyers and Meyers (1995b). Alternatively, the examiner can instruct as follows:

Copy. Put a plain sheet of $8\frac{1}{2}'' \times 11''$ paper vertically on the table (Meyers & Meyers, 1995). Then say: *"I am going to show you a card on which there is a design that I would like you to copy on this sheet of paper. Please copy the figure as carefully as you can."* Begin timing as soon as you expose the drawing. Note that Meyers and Meyers (1995b) allow erasing.

One can use a system of colored pencils (pens) to record the patient's strategy. Each time the subject completes a section of the drawing, the examiner hands the patient a different colored pencil and notes the order of the colors. Use about three or four different colored pencils and switch pencils at approximately equal points in the construction of the

figure. The examiner should not switch pencils while the patient is in the middle of drawing one of the standard 18 elements. Alternatively, the examiner can reproduce the subject's drawing on a separate sheet, noting the order (by numbering) and directionality of each line as it is drawn. The latter system is preferred by some authors (Meyers & Meyers, 1995b).

It is important to supervise the drawing carefully, particularly in the early stages. If the drawing is careless, the patient should be reminded that he or she is to make the copy as accurate as possible. The card and the subject's copy are exposed for a maximum of 5 minutes and a minimum of $2\frac{1}{2}$ minutes. If by $2\frac{1}{2}$ minutes it is obvious that the patient is drawing too slowly, he or she should be told this and asked to speed up. If the patient is finished drawing before $2\frac{1}{2}$ minutes, he or she should be told to check it over carefully to make sure it is complete. After the drawing is finished, it is removed from sight along with the stimulus card.

Record the *total* time taken to complete the drawing. Subjects should normally be able to complete the drawing in no more than 5 minutes, unless they have considerable motor difficulty. It is more important, however, for a subject to complete the drawing as well as he or she can than it is to get it finished within the 5 minutes. For this reason, allow the subject as much time as needed to make the best copy that he or she is capable of.

3-Minute Recall. Following a 3-minute delay filled with talking or some other verbal task, provide a clean sheet of paper and say to the patient: *"Remember a short time ago I had you copy a figure. I would like you to draw that figure again."*

There is no time limit on this recall task. As in the copy trial, the order of approach can be recorded by using the system of colored pencils or by drawing along with the patient on a separate sheet, noting the sequence and organization of the reproduction.

Delayed Recall. The examiner waits about 30 minutes after the first administration of the CFT and then requests recall of the figure.

The interposed tests should be quite different from the CFT, in order to avoid interference. One should especially not give any tests of drawing. Then say: *"Do you remember the design I had you copy a while ago? Now I would like you to draw the figure from memory as carefully and completely as you can on this sheet of paper. If you make a mistake do not erase, just correct whatever you think is wrong."*

There is no time limit and the order of approach can be recorded by using the system of colored pencils or by drawing along on a separate sheet.

Recognition. After the 30-minute recall, the patient is provided with stimulus sheets and is instructed to circle the figures that were part of the design that was copied and drawn.

Approximate Time for Administration

The time required is about 10–15 minutes (excluding delay).

Scoring

There are several scoring systems that provide various criteria for scoring the Rey-Osterrieth Complex Figure (e.g., Bennett-Levy, 1984; Berry et al., 1991; Binder, 1982; Chervinsky et al., 1992; Chiulli et al., 1995; Duley et al., 1993; Hamby et al., 1993; Kirk & Kelly, 1986; Loring et al., 1988, 1990; Meyers & Meyers, 1995a; Osterrieth, 1994; Rapport et al., 1995; Shorr et al., 1992; Stern et al., 1994; E.M. Taylor, 1959; L.B. Taylor, 1991; Visser, 1973; Waber & Holmes, 1985, 1986; for a recent review, see Lezak, 1995). Most of the systems provide criteria for assessing accuracy of copy and recall. Some of the systems also assess quality (e.g., organization, fragmentation, symmetry, inattention) of the construction.

Accuracy. Copy and memory trials are generally scored in the same manner in terms of accuracy. The most commonly used system was proposed by Osterrieth (1944) and adapted by Taylor (1959). The figure is broken down into 18 scorable elements: 0.5–2.0 points are awarded for each element depending on accuracy, distortion, and location of its reproduction (E.M. Taylor, 1959). Two points are awarded if the unit is correct and placed properly; one point is awarded if the unit is correct but placed poorly; one point is given if the unit is distorted but placed correctly; if the unit is distorted and placed poorly, one-half point is given; and no point is awarded if the unit is absent or not recognizable. The highest possible score on each figure is 36.

These criteria are clear as to the specific elements that are to be scored; they leave considerable latitude, however, in deciding what constitutes a scorable distortion or misplacement (Duley et al., 1993). More explicit criteria have been proposed by others (e.g., Denman, 1987; Duley et al., 1993; Meyers & Meyers, 1995a; Taylor, 1991).

In order to use normative data appropriately, it is important to be attentive to both the method of administration (e.g., whether an immediate-recall trial is interposed between the copy and 30-minute delayed-recall trials) and the particular scoring criteria used to generate the norms. We generally use the normative data (ages 18–89 years) provided by Meyers and Meyers (1995b) for copy, 3-minute, 30-minute recall and recognition trials of the Rey figure. Accordingly, their explicit scoring guidelines are used for protocols within this age range (see source). Unfortunately, Meyers and Meyers have not yet provided normative data for children. Accordingly, for children aged 6–16, we use L.B. Taylor's scoring criteria for the Rey and Taylor figures shown in Figures 10–20 and 10–21. Note, however, that the normative data (see Table 10–21) were provided using only a copy and 30-minute delay trial.

One can also calculate a percent recall score [(CFT recall/CFT copy) (100)] in order to remove the effects of the level of performance on the copy administration from the memory performance (Snow, 1979). Brooks (1972) developed a percent forgetting score ((CF immediate recall − CF delayed recall)/(CF immediate recall)) (100)]. Lezak (1995) notes, however, that these scores should be interpreted cautiously since very defective copy and recall scores (immediate and delayed ones) can look good if copy (or immediate re-

Detail 1: The cross at the upper left corner, outside of the rectangle. The cross must come down to the horizontal midline of the rectangle and must extend above the rectangle. The line that joins the cross to the rectangle must be approximately in the middle of the cross and must come between Detail 7 and the top of the rectangle.

Detail 2: The large rectangle. The horizontal dimensions of the rectangle must not be greater than twice the vertical dimensions of the rectangle, nor must the rectangle resemble a square. As there are so many possibilities of distorting the rectangle and it is not possible to score for position, a score of one-half is given if the rectangle is incomplete or distorted in any way.

Detail 3: The diagonal cross must touch each of the four corners of the rectangle and intersect in the middle of the rectangle.

Detail 4: The horizontal midline of the rectangle must go clearly across from the midpoint of the left side of the rectangle to the midpoint of the right side of the rectangle in one unbroken line.

Detail 5: The vertical midline must start at the midpoint of the bottom of the rectangle and go through in one unbroken line to the midpoint at the top of the rectangle. In scoring for position of 4, 5, and 6, these details should intersect at the midpoint of the rectangle. Usually, if they do not, only one is scored as incorrect for position. Very seldom are all three scored as incorrect for not being in position.

Detail 6: The small rectangle within the large rectangle and to the left side of it. The boundaries of Detail 6 are defined by the top of the rectangle falling between lines 2 and 3 of the parallel lines that make up Detail 8, and the width of the small rectangle must be approximately one-quarter of the width of the large rectangle; that is, it should come to the midpoint between the left side of the large rectangle and the vertical midpoint of the rectangle. The cross within Detail 6 must come from the four corners of the rectangle and should intersect at the midpoint of the rectangle, i.e. words intersecting on Detail 4.

Detail 7: The straight line above Detail 6 must be shorter than the horizontal aspect of Detail 6 and must fall between the top of Detail 6 and the second line of Detail 8.

Detail 8: The four parallel lines within the rectangle in the upper left corner should be parallel, with the spaces between them approximately equal. If the lines are unduly slanted or, of course, if there are more or less than four of them, then the scoring is penalized.

Detail 9: The triangle above the rectangle on the upper right, with the height less than the base.

Detail 10: The small vertical line within the rectangle just below Detail 9. The line should be clearly shifted to the left within the upper right quadrangle in the rectangle.

Detail 11: The circle with three dots must be in the lower right half of the upper right quadrangle. It must not touch any of the three sides of the triangular area in which it is placed and the positioning of the dots should be so that there are two above and one below, so that it resembles a face.

Detail 12: The five parallel lines that are crossing the lower right aspect of Detail 3 must all be within the lower right quadrangle. They must not touch any sides of the quadrangle, and they should be approximately equidistant from one another.

Detail 13: The triangle on the right end of the large rectangle. The height of the triangle must not be greater than half of the horizontal midline of the rectangle and, as already mentioned, the slope of the sides of the triangle must not be a continuation of the slope of Detail 9.

Detail 14: The diamond attached to the end of Detail 13 should be diamond-shaped and must be attached to the end of Detail 13; it must not extend down below the bottom of the large rectangle, Detail 2.

Detail 15: The vertical line within triangle 13 must be parallel to the right vertical of Detail 2, the large rectangle, and it must be shifted to the left within Detail 13.

Detail 16: The horizontal line within 13, which is a continuation of Detail 4 to the right, must come from the midpoint of the right side of the large rectangle and extend to the top of triangle 13. If triangle 13 is slightly askew, or if Detail 4 does not meet the midpoint of the right side of the rectangle, Detail 16 should still be scored as a full two points if it went to the top of the triangle from the midpoint of the right side of the rectangle.

Detail 17: The cross attached to the lower center area of the rectangle. The right side of the cross must be clearly longer than the left side of the cross but must not extend beyond the right end of the large rectangle. It should also at its left end commence at the midpoint of the right side of the square, which is Detail 18.

Detail 18: On the lower left corner of Detail 2, must clearly be a square as opposed to the rectangular shape of Detail 6, and its sides should be the same size as the vertical aspect of Detail 6, extending half way between the left side of the rectangle and the vertical midline of the rectangle.

Figure 10—20. Taylor scoring criteria for the Rey Complex Figure (L. Taylor, personal communication, May 1989).

call) is so low that (delayed) recall cannot go much lower.

Quality. Interpretation of the CFT should consider not only the actual score but also qualitative aspects of performance. Some investigators have devised scoring systems that assess item distortion and misplacement, approach, or style and level of organization (Bennett-Levy, 1984; Binder, 1982; Chervinsky et al., 1992; Chiulli et al., 1995; Hamby et al., 1993; Kirk & Kelly, 1986; Loring et al., 1988; Rapport et al., 1995; Rapport et al., 1996; Shorr et al., 1992; Stern et al., 1994; Visser, 1973;

Detail 1: Vertical arrow at the left of the figure, extending above and below the midpoints of the upper and lower quadrants of the large square, but not extending beyond the upper and lower limits of the square, and with its midpoint meeting Detail 4.

Detail 2: Triangle whose base is the left side of the large square, with the altitude of the triangle less than half of the width of the large square.

Detail 3: Large square, which is the basic element of the figure, and which must look like a square and not a rectangle.

Detail 4: Horizontal midline of the large square, which extends outside the large square to midpoint of Detail 1.

Detail 5: Vertical midline of the large square.

Detail 6: Horizontal line bisecting the top half of large square.

Detail 7: Diagonal lines bisecting one another from the corners of the top left quadrant of the large square.

Detail 8: Small square, situated in the center of the top left quadrant, 1/4 the size of the quadrant, and with the corners of the square located on the diagonals (Detail 7).

Detail 9: Circle the centre of Detail 8, in the top left quadrant.

Detail 10: Rectangle above the top left quadrant, with its height less than 1/4 of the height of the large square.

Detail 11: Arrow extending from the center of the large square through the top right corner of the right upper quadrant, with not more than 1/3 of its length outside the large square.

Detail 12: Semicircle at the right of the figure, extending from the horizontal bisector of the top half of the base square (Detail 6) to the equivalent point in the lower half of the base square.

Detail 13: Triangle in the right half of the base square, with the same base as the semicircle (Detail 12), and with an altitude that is 1/4 the width of the large square.

Detail 14: Row of 7 dots (not circles) in the lower right quadrant, evenly spaced in a straight line from the center of the large square to the lower right corner of the quadrant.

Detail 15: Horizontal line in the lower right quadrant, between the 6th and 7th dots of Detail 14.

Detail 16: Equilateral triangle whose apex is at the lower right corner of the large square and whose altitude is not more than 1/4 of the height of the large square.

Detail 17: Curved line with a cross-bar at the centre of each of 3 sinusoids in the lower left quadrant, extending from the bottom left corner to the top right corner of the quadrant.

Detail 18: Star, composed of 8 lines radiating from a centre point, and situated in the lower left quadrant, near its lower right corner.

Figure 10—21. Scoring Guidelines of the Taylor (Alternate) Form of Rey Complex Figure (L. Taylor, personal communication, May 1989).

Waber & Holmes, 1985, 1986). Waber and Holmes (1985, 1986) devised a system that assesses organization and style, in addition to accuracy. The organizational parameter, yielding an ordinal scale, was designed to capture the "goodness" of the overall structure and focuses on such features as the integrity of the base rectangle and integration of other structures with the base rectangle. The style parameter, yielding a categorical scale, assesses the manner in which the design is executed independent of its organizational quality; it ranges from part-oriented to configurational. The system is complex but has demonstrated utility with regard to developmental issues. The most comprehensive system is by Stern et al. (1994; and its adaptation by Akshoomoff & Stiles, 1995a,b). It provides scores for various qualitative features including fragmentation, planning, organization, presence and accuracy of various features, placement, size distortions, perseveration, confabulation, rotation, neatness, symmetry,

and immediate and delayed retention. It can be used across the lifespan. Although interrater reliability is reported to be good, scoring takes from 5 to 15 minutes for a single reproduction. This decreases to about 5 minutes once the examiner is familiar with the method. The system provided by Hamby and colleagues (1993) is simpler and focuses on one aspect of production, organizational quality. It employs a 5-point Likert scale (higher ratings indicate better organization) and can be applied to both the Rey and the Taylor figures. The authors report that the system is easy to learn, quick to score (less than 1 minute per protocol), shows very good interrater reliability, and appears to have clinical utility. Organizational quality, but not copy and delay scores, on the Rey figure distinguished between symptomatic and asymptomatic HIV-positive subjects. A relatively gross approach, employed by Chiulli et al. (1995), involves categorizing the drawings as configural if the drawing begins with construction of the base

Table 10—21. Normative Data for Ages 6–85: Copy and 30-Minute Delay; L. Taylor Scoring Criteria

	Age 6	Age 7	Age 8	Age 9	Age 10	Age 11	Age 12	Age 13	Age 14	Age 15	Age 20–29	Age 30–39	Age 40–49	Age 50–59	Age 60–69	Age 70+
n	192	353	347	329	301	280	225	237	180	116	20	20	18	21	21	23
Copy	16.66	21.29	23.64	24.46	27.20	28.61	30.21	32.63	33.53	33.60	33.70	31.75	32.31	31.19	30.79	29.57
SD	7.97	7.67	8.00	6.94	7.58	7.31	6.69	4.35	3.18	2.98	1.59	3.21	2.67	3.68	4.21	3.37
30-min. recall	10.53	13.57	16.34	18.71	19.73	22.59	23.20	24.59	26.24	26.00	21.80	17.20	16.56	14.88	14.21	11.74
SD	5.80	6.28	6.77	6.61	6.71	6.65	6.38	6.29	5.40	6.35	6.56	7.08	6.69	6.95	7.50	6.11
% Recall											64.12	53.45	50.61	47.16	46.19	38.57
SD											18.39	20.13	18.77	20.59	22.91	18.22
Copy-Recall											11.95	14.58	15.75	16.31	16.57	17.83
SD											5.72	6.12	5.58	6.41	7.53	14.58

Source: Kolb and Whishaw (1990) report data that are derived from healthy schoolchildren, ages 6–15, in Lethbridge, Alberta. We provide data for healthy, well-educated (mean = 14.12 years) adults, ages 21–84.

rectangle; all other approaches are scored as nonconfigural. Reliability data, however, are not reported.

Rapport et al. (1995, 1996) have adapted the standard and Denman scoring systems to evaluate hemispatial deficits on the Rey Figure. The measures include (1) the percent of omitted items on the left or right halves of the figure, (2) attentional bias to right space as indicated when the patient begins the figure copy by drawing any portion that is rightward of the vertical midline of the large rectangle, and (3) the accuracy of the reproduction of the two sides of the figure. Rapport et al. (1996) note that when using the standard scoring system, an asymmetric error profile of two or more left-sided omissions indicates a strong likelihood of neglect.

Recognition. A correct response on the Recognition subtest (Meyers & Meyers, 1995b) is credited if the patient correctly circles a figure as having been part of the CFT; a correct score is also given if the figure was *not* part of the CFT and it was *not* circled. The maximum correct score is 24. False positive (if a figure that is not part of the CF is circled) and false negative (if a figure should have been circled but is not) are also noted.

Comment

Scoring according to Osterrieth's (1944) and E.M. Taylor's (1959) criteria (or variants of these criteria) yield adequate to high interrater and intrarater reliability for total scores (above .8; Berry et al., 1991; Boone et al., 1993; Casey et al., 1991; Delaney et al., 1992; Fastenau et al., 1996; Tupler et al., 1995). Reliabilities for the 18 individual items, however, ranged from poor (.14) to excellent (.96), suggesting that the Osterrieth system would benefit from more detailed specification of quantitative decision rules (e.g., minimal angle size required for 1 point) (Tupler et al., 1995). The strict scoring criteria described by others (e.g., Bennett-Levy, 1984; Duley et al., 1993; Fastenau et al., 1996; Loring et al., 1990; Meyers and Meyers, 1995a; Shorr et al., 1992; Stern et al., 1994; Strauss and Spreen, 1990; L.B. Taylor, 1991; Tombaugh et al.,

1992) also show high (>.90) interrater reliability for total scores. Rarely are the accuracy scoring systems compared to one another to demonstrate an advantage over similar systems. Recently, Fastenau et al. (1996) reported that their scoring system was no better than that designed by Osterrieth in terms of reliability and validity and that their system took about six times longer to apply. Troyer and Wishart (1996) compared a number of qualitative scoring systems (Bennett-Levy, 1984; Binder, 1982; Blysma et al., 1995; Hamby et al., 1993; Osterrieth, 1944; Shorr et al., 1992; Stern et al., 1994; Visser, 1973; Waber & Holmes, 1985) and found that most systems were intercorrelated ($r = .34–.84$), with the exception of the system by Waber and Holmes ($r = .25–.32$). Similarly, Rapport et al. (1997) have recently reported that interrater and internal consistency reliabilities for both the Osterrieth and Denman scoring systems were high and equivalent.

Internal consistency of the Rey figure has been evaluated by treating each detail as an item and subjecting the scores of subjects to split-half and coefficient alpha procedures (Berry et al., 1991; Fastenau et al., 1996). Both split-half and coefficient alpha reliabilities were above .60 for the copy condition and above .80 for recall conditions (immediate recall and 20/30-minute delay), suggesting that all of the details tap into a single factor.

We (unpublished data) have found that with repeated administration of the *same* figure (Rey or Taylor), practice effects occur in normal adults. In general, normal subjects show a 10 per cent improvement in percent recall scores when retested after a one-month interval. Berry and colleagues (1991) retested elderly individuals after 1 year and found that the copy condition was not reliable across this interval. Reliabilities of the immediate and 30-minute-delay recall trials were in the moderate range (.47–.59). Meyers and Meyers (1995b) noted that ranges for some of the scores (e.g., copy, recognition) are restricted due to the maximum- or near-maximum-level performance attained by most normal subjects, thus artificially reducing the magnitude of the test–retest correlation coefficients.

Moreover, the incidental learning paradigm is contaminated when a subject is retested after the original administration. Based on these considerations, Meyers and Meyers (1995b) evaluated test–retest reliability only for scores with sufficient range (Immediate Recall $r = .76$, Delayed Recall $r = .89$, Recognition Total Correct $= .87$) in a sample of 12 normal subjects following a retest interval of about 6 months. To measure the temporal stability of clinical interpretation, age-corrected T-scores for these measures were classified according to Heaton et al.'s (1991) system (e.g., average $=$ T-score 45–54, below average $=$ T-score 40–44, mildly impaired $=$ T-score 35–39). The percentage agreement in the clinical interpretation between the first and second testing sessions was high (91.7) for these same three measures (Immediate Recall, Delayed Recall, Recognition Total Correct). Meyers and Meyers (1995b) also report no significant differences for other CFT variables (Copy, Time to Copy, Recognition True Positive, False Positives, True Negatives, False Negatives) across the retest interval.

Another issue concerns the comparability of the Rey and its alternate versions. Reliability coefficients are in the moderate range when the Rey and Taylor figures are evaluated (Berry et al., 1991; Delaney et al., 1992). In children, ages 8–10 years, with and without ADHD, there is no difference between designs, both for copying and for remembering (Sadeh et al., 1996). In healthy young adults, the copy administrations of the various figures (Rey, Taylor, MCG) are of equivalent difficulty; however, recall of the Rey figure is somewhat harder (about five points in normal people) than recall of the Taylor or MCG Figures (Delaney et al., 1992; Duley et al., 1993; Hamby et al., 1993; Kuehn & Snow, 1992; Meador et al., 1993; Strauss & Spreen, 1990; Tombaugh & Hubley, 1991). There are no significant differences between the Taylor and the four MCG figures (Meador et al., 1993). The Rey figure also takes more time to both copy and reproduce from memory than does the Taylor figure (Tombaugh and Hubley, 1991). The Rey figure appears to have a more complex organizational structure (Hamby et al., 1993) and does not lend itself readily to a verbal strategy (Casey et al., 1991). As a result, individuals with visual imagery problems cannot compensate by using a verbal strategy. In contrast, with the Taylor figure deficits in visual imagery may be circumvented and therefore obscured by the use of verbal strategies. The greater recall difficulty of the Rey figure suggests that this measure may be more sensitive than the alternate versions to the presence of memory deficits, particularly nonverbal ones (Strauss & Spreen, 1990; see also Hamby et al., 1993). Even though the Taylor figure is easier to remember than the Rey figure, parallel forgetting functions occur for both figures, indicating that both reflect comparable degrees of sensitivity when they are used to measure rates of forgetting (Tombaugh & Hubley, 1991).

The precise cognitive operations required for adequate performance are thought to include visual perception, visuospatial organization, motor functioning, and, on the recall condition, memory (Chervinsky et al., 1992). Some investigators (e.g., Chiulli et al., 1995; Meyers & Meyers, 1995b; Shorr et al., 1992) argue that different information is provided by copy, immediate (or 3-minute), and 20- to 30-minute delay trials. They suggest that the copy trial reflects perceptual, visuospatial, and organizational skills; the immediate (or 3-minute) trial reflects the amount of information that is encoded; and the delay trial reflects the amount of information that is stored and retrieved from memory. Overall, the data from correlational and factor analytic studies support the validity of the CFT as a measure of visuocontructional ability (copy) and memory (recall and recognition).

Meyers and Meyers (1995b) correlated CFT scores from 601 normal individuals and found that the largest correlation was between Immediate (3-minute) and Delayed Recall ($r = .88$). The recall measures demonstrated lower, though still significant ($r = .15$), correlations with Recognition Total Correct. Time to Copy had minimal relations to the accuracy of the copy or the recall. Moderate correlations were noted between Copy raw score and Immediate (3-minute) ($r = .33$) and Delayed Recall ($r = .38$) scores, suggesting a relationship between the ability to copy the complex figure and the ability to later recall and draw the figure from memory. Similar findings emerged in a heterogeneous sample of patients with documented neurological dysfunction.

Meyers and Meyers (1995b) also conducted a principal-components factor analysis of the data for normal individuals. The analysis suggested a five-factor solution. The first factor was termed a Visuospatial Recall factor due to high loading from the 3- and 30-minute-delay trials. Factor 2 reflected a Visuospatial Recognition factor. Factor 3, labeled a Response Bias factor, demonstrated a high loading of Recognition False Positives. Factor 4 was interpreted as a Processing Speed factor because of a high loading of Time to Copy. Finally, Factor 5 reflected Visuospatial Constructional Ability with a high loading of the Copy score. Analysis of the data of brain-damaged patients ($n = 100$) revealed the same five factors.

In a heterogeneous sample of patients with neurological disorders, Meyers and Meyers (1995b) found the Copy, three- and 30-minute Recall scores, and Recognition Total Correct were significantly correlated with BVRT Total Correct, RAVLT Trial 5, Form Discrimination, Hooper, Trails B, and the Token Test. Language measures (FAS, Sentence Repetition) had no significant relationships with any CFT measures.

Other factor analytic studies of the CFT and other neuropsychological tests suggest that CFT scores load heavily on what appears to be a visuospatial perceptual/memory factor, based on common loadings with the WMS Visual Reproduction and Line Orientation tests (Berry et al., 1991). In adults and children, correlational analyses indicate that performance on the CFT is moderately related to performance on Block Design and Object Assembly subtests of the Wechsler Intelligence Test (Poulton & Moffitt, 1995; Tombaugh et al., 1992; Wood et al., 1982). Similarly, Sherman and her colleagues (1995) found that scores on the CFT (both copy and 30-minute delay) were moderately related to the Perceptual Organization factor of the WAIS-R. Scores on the CFT were not related to the Verbal Comprehension and Freedom from Dis-

tractability factors of the WAIS-R. Meyers and Meyers (1995b) also reported that in a mixed sample of patients with neurological disorders, CFT measures correlated more strongly with Performance subtests than with Verbal subtests.

Usually, older children (age 13) and literate adults copy the design from left to right (Waber & Holmes, 1985; Ardila, Rosselli, & Rosas, 1989; Poulton & Moffitt, 1995). The designs are most commonly copied in a piecemeal fashion by younger children, and they become more configurational with increasing age (but see Akshoomoff & Stiles, 1995a, who suggest that development results in change in both the nature of the parts that are identified and the way in which those parts are integrated, and that children as young as age 6 demonstrate both aspects of spatial analysis). Around age 13, a shift to the base rectangle strategy occurs, where the large central rectangle is drawn first and details are added on in relation to it. Use of a configural approach shows little decline with advancing age (Chiulli et al., 1995). In the memory production, a piecemeal strategy is very rare after age 9. In older children and adults, errors or distortions are quite common in the memory condition but are rare in the copy condition. Further, the actual act of copying and copying strategy are related to recall performance. In a study of 5th- and 8th-grade children (Waber et al., 1989), half were asked to copy the Rey figure prior to recall and half studied it visually but did not copy it. The memory productions from the 5th-graders who only studied the figure visually were more accurate and more configurational than the 5th-graders who first copied the figure. With regard to copying strategy, a disorganized piecemeal approach to copying of the figure may result in an accurate production, but recall tends to be poor. A strategy that involves clustering the elements into meaningful units is more effective than one that relies on the recall of isolated elements (Akshoomoff & Stiles, 1995b; Bennett-Levy, 1984; Chiulli et al., 1995; Hamby et al., 1993; Shorr et al., 1992).

The test does distinguish patients with probable Alzheimer's disease (AD) from normal individuals (Berry et al., 1991) and is sensitive even to mild head injury (Leininger et al., 1990). Bigler et al. (1989) reported that patients diagnosed with AD have greater difficulty both in copying and in recalling the figure than patients with moderate head trauma. Abnormally low copy and recall scores have also been reported for patients with Parkinson's disease (Cooper et al., 1991; Ogden et al., 1990) and Huntington's disease (Fedio et al., 1979). There is also evidence that the test is sensitive to individuals with a history of central nervous system health problems, such as head injury, congenital syndromes, seizure disorders (Poulton & Moffitt, 1995), cocaine and polydrug abuse (Rosselli & Ardila, 1996), and anterior communicating artery aneurysm (Diamond & DeLuca, 1996). Recently, Bigler et al. (1996) reported that degree of hippocampal atrophy in moderate-severe head-injured patients was related to percent recall on the test.

Further, information from the copy portion of the test may be useful in differentiating different disorders. For example, a piecemeal approach to the copying of the CFT is characteristic of patients with either left- or right-hemisphere lesions (Binder, 1982; Visser, 1973). However, the drawings by the right-brain-damaged patients tend to be less accurate (but see Rapport et al., 1995, Rapport et al., 1996, who find that this might apply only to patients who show neglect) and more distorted than those of their left-sided counterparts (Binder, 1982). Differences between patients with parietal-occipital lesions and patients with frontal lobe lesions have also been noted on the copy trial (Lezak, 1995; Pillon, 1981; Taylor, cited in Kolb & Whishaw, 1985). Patients with posterior lesions are more likely to have difficulty with the spatial organization of the figure. Patients with frontal lobe lesions are more likely to have difficulty planning their approach to the task. The copy task is also sensitive to hemispatial neglect. Right CVA patients identified as having neglect on a letter-cancellation task showed an increased incidence of omissions of items on the left side of the figure, a rightward attentional bias (reflected in the patient's starting point on the task), and a poorer accuracy of reproduction on the left side (Rapport et al., 1995; Rapport

et al., 1996). The measures of hemispatial deficit showed a moderate relation to the number of falls suffered by patients.

With regard to the memory trials, there is a tendency for patients with right-hemisphere lesions to perform more poorly than patients with left-hemisphere disturbances on the recall trial (Loring et al., 1988; but see Barr et al., 1997; King, 1981). The test, however, is not a perfect predictor of side of lesion (Lee et al., 1989; Loring et al., 1988). Analysis of qualitative features (e.g., distortion of overall configuration, major mislocation) may be helpful in distinguishing laterality of dysfunction (Breir et al., 1996; Loring et al., 1988). When the initial copy is performed satisfactorily, misplacement and distortion on the recall trial tend to be characteristic of patients with right-, as opposed to left-, hemisphere dysfunction.

It is important to bear in mind that poor performance on the memory trials may occur not only in the context of neurological compromise but also in individuals suffering from psychological distress. Uddo and colleagues (1993) reported that combat veterans with diagnoses of post-traumatic stress disorder performed more poorly than a healthy comparison group on the immediate recall, but not the copy, trial of the Complex Figure. Wishart and colleagues (1993) noted that in patients with epilepsy, poor recall was associated to a moderate degree with self-report of affective disturbance (depression, paranoia). Boone et al. (1995) reported that in elderly individuals, depression was associated with subtle weakness in delayed recall. Meyers and Meyers (1995b) found that patients with diffuse brain injury performed more poorly than those with chronic psychiatric disorders (schizophrenia, bipolar disorder, major depression), and the psychiatric group performed significantly poorer than the normal group on both 3- and 30-minute recall trials. For other CFT variables (e.g., Copy, Copy Time, Recognition), brain-injured patients performed significantly below psychiatric and normal groups, but the latter two groups did not differ significantly from one another. In another sample of volunteers with no history of neurological disorder, Meyers and Meyers (1995b) found moderate correlations between Beck Depression Inventory scores and Recognition Total Correct ($r = -.39$). Patients classed as depressed (Beck scores 14 or greater) scored on average 4.7 T-scores lower on 3-minute recall, 6.5 T-scores lower on 30-minute delayed recall, and 8.8 T-scores lower on Recognition Total Correct. Some (Chiulli et al., 1995; Vingerhoets et al., 1995), however, have noted that psychological distress (anxiety, depression) has no effect on CFT.

There is evidence (Berry & Carpenter, 1992; Delaney et al., 1992) that most forgetting tends to occur very quickly, within the first few minutes after copying, perhaps as a result of an overloading of working memory. This does not imply that an immediate or brief delayed recall trial will yield information comparable to longer delay periods since amnesia of different etiologies may have differing patterns of memory loss from storage (Berry & Carpenter, 1992; Loring et al., 1990; but see Lezak, 1995). Moreover, although virtually no forgetting occurs in normal subjects between immediate recall and 20- or 30-minute delay intervals, a substantial decline (of about 10 points) does occur following intervals of about 1 month (Tombaugh & Hubley, 1991).

With regard to the recognition subtest, Meyers and Lange (1994) reported that the task is effective in discriminating brain-injured individuals from normal subjects and from persons suffering from psychiatric disorders. Moreover, recognition scores correlate with overall functional ability better than recall scores. The higher the recognition subtest score, the more independently functioning were the subjects.

The CFT may also be useful in detecting malingering. Knight and Meyers (1995) found that individuals instructed to malinger could be distinguished from brain-damaged individuals by a pattern of poorer level of accuracy, slower production speed, and poorer delayed and recognition memory (see also Meyers & Meyers, 1995b).

Overall, the CFT is a useful measure providing information about a variety of cognitive processes. The addition of the recognition trial appears to be a useful addition to recall testing. Analysis of the profile or pattern of test scores on the various components (copy, recall, and recognition trials) is recommended (e.g., Meyers & Meyers, 1995b). Thus, interpretation of the recall scores must consider whether the initial copy is performed adequately. Disrupted attention may be suggested by low scores across 3-minute, 30-minute, and recognition trials. Impaired encoding may be inferred if 3- and 30-minute-delay scores are low with minimal improvement when retrieval cues are given. Disrupted storage may be suggested when 3-minute recall is higher than delayed recall and delayed recall is higher than Recognition Total Correct. One may raise the question of a retrieval problem when 3-minute recall and recognition are equivalent and higher than delayed recall or when Recognition Total Correct is higher than both 3- and 30-minute recall scores. These hypotheses, however, need to be evaluated further with additional instruments.

Normative Data

Indices that reflect the qualitative aspects of an individual's performance are still experimental, and adequate normative data are generally lacking (but see below, Chiulli et al., 1995). With respect to norms for evaluating the accuracy of the figure, wide variability exists with regard to the number and timing of recall trials (e.g., Corwin & Blysma, 1993; Lezak, 1995; Tombaugh et al., 1992). One cannot assume that normative data for immediate recall can be used to evaluate delayed recall. There is some evidence (Loring et al., 1990; Meyers & Meyers, 1995a) that inclusion of an immediate recall trial increases delayed recall performance by about two to six points in healthy young adults. Further, diverse scoring systems complicate attempts to compile norms from different sources.

We present several sets of normative data according to the copy–recall interval(s) used and the scoring criteria applied:

Administration A: A copy trial and a 30-minute-recall trial with no interposed immediate-recall trial; scoring L. B. Taylor's scoring criteria. The data for children and adults are given in Table 10–21.

Table 10—22. Normative Data for Ages 65–93: Copy, Immediate and 30-Minute Delay; E. M. Taylor's (in Lezak) Scoring Criteria

	Age 65–69	Age 70–74	Age 75–79	Age 80–84	Age 85–93
Copy	31.10	32.03	30.49	30.76	30.80
SD	3.59	3.27	4.48	4.06	2.60
N	10	50	57	35	10
Immediate	15.50	15.44	15.39	14.47	9.45
SD	5.54	6.51	6.75	6.31	3.92
N	10	49	57	35	10
30-min. Recall	15.30	15.35	15.12	13.76	9.39
SD	4.98	6.37	6.34	6.07	4.93
N	9	50	57	35	10

Source: Chiulli et al. (1989) present data for healthy adults ages 65–93, of above average IQ (Shipley estimated FSIQ = 112). Reprinted with permission.

Administration B: A copy trial followed by an immediate-recall trial and a 30-minute-delay recall trial; scoring: E.M. Taylor's (1959, in Lezak, 1995) scoring criteria. Data for healthy adults, ages 65–93, are shown in Table 10–22. These elderly subjects required on average 212 seconds (SD = 81 sec) to copy the figure (Chiulli, 1990, personal communication). Chiulli et al. (1995) also provide data on a sample of healthy, highly educated Caucasian elderly individuals using L.B. Taylor's scoring criteria. In addition, they evaluated the approach to the drawing; that is, the drawing was classed as configural or not, depending upon whether the construction began with the base rectangle. Data for accuracy and approach are shown in Table 10–23. Denman (1987) also provides data for individuals ages 10–89 years for copy, immediate- and delayed-recall trials of the Rey figure. His scoring criteria are based on a maximum score of 72 for each condition, and raw scores must be converted to scaled scores (1–19) by means of age-based normative tables. Rosselli and Ardila (1991) give normative data for copy (both accuracy and time to complete the task) and immediate memory conditions, derived from a large sample of people, ages 56 and above, from Bogota, Colombia. Scoring criteria were those of E.M. Taylor (1959, in Lezak, 1995).

Table 10—23. Mean Accuracy and Percent Adopting Configural Approach: L. B. Taylor's Scoring Criteria for Accuracy

		Age 70–74 (n = 46)	Age 75–79 (n = 58)	Age 80–91 (n = 49)
Copy	Accuracy[a]	32.6 (2.8)	31.0 (4.0)	29.8 (4.6)
Copy	Approach[b]	18 (39%)	21 (36%)	17 (35%)
Immediate	Accuracy	17.2 (6.2)	14.2 (6.6)	12.9 (6.4)
Immediate	Approach	24 (55%)	23 (41%)	19 (40%)
30-min. delay	Accuracy	16.9 (6.3)	14.2 (6.2)	12.4 (6.0)
30-min. delay	Approach	24 (55%)	29 (52%)	19 (41%)

Source: Chiulli et al. (1995) present data for 153 healthy, highly educated, noninstitutionalized elderly. The approach used to complete the drawing was classed as configural if the drawing began with construction of the large rectangle. Reprinted with permission of Swets & Zeitlinger.

[a] Mean (standard deviation).

[b] Number (%) adopting a configural approach.

Table 10—24. Normative Data for Ages 45–83: Copy and 3-Minute Delay; E. M. Taylor's (in Lezak) Scoring Criteria

	Age 45–59 (n = 38)	Age 60–69 (n = 31)	Age 70–83 (n = 22)
Copy	34.18	33.76	21.25
SD	1.8	2.8	4.7
3-min. Recall	18.88	17.33	13.77
SD	6.1	5.2	5.0
% Retention	55.03	51.16	43.77
SD	17.1	13.8	14.8

Source: Boone and colleagues (1993) give data for healthy adults of above–average education (mean = 14.5 years) and intelligence (mean WAIS-R IQ = 115.89). Reprinted with permission of Swets & Zeitlinger.

The scores for both copy and recall conditions are considerably lower than those reported by investigators working with North American populations and likely reflect cultural and educational differences.

Administration C: A copy trial followed by a 3-minute-recall trial; Scoring: E. M. Taylor's (1959) scoring criteria. Osterrieth's data (1944) should not be used because (1) the data were based on 60 adults in the 16–60 age range and no effects of age were presented, and (2) educational and cultural differences may invalidate comparison of current North American samples to those collected by Osterrieth over 50 years ago. Recently, Boone et al. (1993) obtained normative data for healthy adults, and these data are shown in Table 10–24.

Administration D: A copy trial followed by 3- and 30-minutes-recall trials as well as a recognition trial. Meyers and Meyers (1995b) provide normative data based on a sample of 601 healthy individuals, ages 18–89 years, for copy, copy time, 3- and 30-minute-recall and recognition trials of the Rey figure. Their explicit scoring guidelines must be used (see source). Normative tables are grouped into a 2-year age span for 18- and 19-year-olds, and 5-year age spans for 20–79 years of age. Caution should be used when interpreting CFT performance for patients aged 80–89 years, because of the small number of normative subjects in this age range (n = 15). Age-corrected T-scores and percentile equivalents are provided for 3-minute (called "Immedi-

ate") Recall, Delayed Recall, and Recognition Total Correct. Normative data for Copy, Time to Copy, Recognition True Positives, Recognition True and False Positives, and Recognition True and False Negatives are presented in five categories (e.g., scores greater than the 16th percentile, scores within the 16th to 11th percentile). Base rate information for CFT elements for the drawing and recognition trials is also provided.

Both age and intellectual level contribute to performance on the CFT. Inspection of the tables reveals that copy scores increase with age, with adult levels being reached at about age 13 (see also Denman, 1987). Some suggest little decrement in copy scores with advancing age (see also Chervinsky et al., 1992; Mitrushina et al., 1990). We and others, however, have found that age influences copy performance, particularly after age 70, although the changes are quite subtle (Boone et al., 1993; Chiulli et al., 1995; Denman, 1987; Meyers & Meyers, 1995b; Ponton et al., 1996; Rosselli and Ardila, 1991; Tombaugh et al., 1992). Scores on the immediate- and delayed-recall trials attain adult levels at about age 11 and show a decline with advancing age (see also Boone et al., 1993; Chervinsky et al., 1992; Chiulli et al., 1995; Denman, 1987; Meyers & Meyers, 1995b; Mitrushina, Satz, & Chervinsky, 1990; Ponton et al., 1996; Rosselli & Ardila, 1991). Rates of forgetting (copy–delay score) also show some relation with age (but see Mitrushina & Satz, 1989), suggesting that memory declines in the elderly may be attributable, at least in part, to impaired storage. Some age-related decline in organizational capacities (the way in which the person subdivides the figure into component parts) may also occur in the elderly (Chervinsky et al., 1992; Mitrushina et al., 1990). For example, Mitrushina and colleagues (1990) noted an age-related memory loss of details, particularly those that are extraneous to the main context of the figure. Recognition performance also shows a slight decline with advancing age (Meyers & Meyers, 1995b).

Scores on the CFT show a modest correlation with measures of general intellectual ability (Boone et al., 1993; Chiulli et al., 1989, 1995), particularly with nonverbal reasoning ability (Chervinsky et al., 1992; Sherman et al., 1995; Tombaugh et al., 1992). The higher the IQ, the higher the CFT scores. The fact that the correlations with IQ are only modest indicates that the CFT provides a large amount of information not given by IQ (Chervinsky et al., 1992).

The influence of education is less certain. A few (Ardila & Rosselli, 1989; Ardila et al., 1989; Berry et al., 1991; Ponton et al., 1996; Rosselli & Ardila, 1991) have reported poorer scores in individuals of lower educational levels. Some, however, have found that CFT measures are relatively unaffected by education (Chervinsky et al., 1992; Delaney et al., 1992; Meyers & Meyers, 1995b; Tombaugh et al., 1992) when the influence of IQ is partialled out (Boone et al., 1993).

The importance of gender is also controversial. Some have reported that men outperformed women (Ardila & Rosselli, 1989; Ardila et al., 1989; Bennett-Levy, 1984; King, 1981), but the differences in performance across the sexes have generally been small or nonexistent (Berry et al., 1991; Boone et al., 1993; Chiulli et al., 1995; Loring et al., 1990; Meyers & Meyers, 1995b; Ponton et al., 1996; Poulton & Moffitt, 1995; Tombaugh & Hubley, 1991; Tombaugh et al., 1992). Weinstein et al. (1990) suggest that the ambiguous and contradictory data may reflect the fact that there is considerable variability within the sexes. They argue that in addition to gender, handedness, familial handedness, and academic concentration (e.g., mathematics/science or not) need to be taken into consideration.

References

Akshoomoff, N.A., & Stiles, J. (1995a). Developmental trends in visuospatial analysis and planning: I. Copying a complex figure. *Neuropsychology, 9*, 364–377.

Akshoomoff, N.A., & Stiles, J. (1995b). Developmental trends in visuospatial analysis and planning: II. Memory for a complex figure. *Neuropsychology, 9*, 378–389.

Ardila, A., & Roselli, M. (1989). Neuropsychological characteristics of normal aging. *Developmental Neuropsychology, 5*, 307–320.

Ardila, A., & Roselli, M., & Rosas, P. (1989). Neuropsychological assessment in illiterates: Visuospatial and memory abilities. *Brain and Cognition, 11*, 147–166.

Barr, W.B., Chelune, G.J., Hermann, B.P., Loring, D., Perrine, K., Strauss, E., Trenerry, M.R., & Westerveld, M. (1997). The use of figural reproduction tests as measures of nonverbal memory in epilepsy surgery candidates. *Journal of the International Neuropsychological Society, 3*, 435–443.

Bennett-Levy, J. (1984). Determinants of performance on the Rey-Osterrieth Complex-Figure test: An analysis, and a new technique for single-case measurement. *British Journal of Psychology, 23*, 109–119.

Berry, D.T.R., Allen, R.S., & Schmitt, F.A. (1991). Rey-Osterrieth Figure: Psychometric characteristics in a geriatric sample. *The Clinical Neuropsychologist, 5*, 143–153.

Berry, D.T.R., & Carpenter, G.S. (1992). Effect of four different delay periods on recall of the Rey-Osterrieth Complex Figure by older persons. *The Clinical Neuropsychologist, 6*, 80–84.

Bigler, E.D., Rosa, L., Schultz, F., Hall, S., and Harris, J. (1989). Rey-Auditory Verbal Learning and Rey-Osterrieth Complex Figure Design test performance in Alzheimer's disease and closed head injury. *Journal of Clinical Psychology, 45*, 277–280.

Bigler, E.D., Johnson, S.C., Anderson, C.V., Blatter, D.D., Gale, S.D., Russo, A.A., Ryser, D.K., Macnamara, S.E., & Abildskov, T.J. (1996). Traumatic brain injury and memory: The role of hippocampal atrophy. *Neuropsychology, 10*, 333–342.

Binder, L.M. (1982). Constructional strategies on complex figure drawing after unilateral brain damage. *Journal of Clinical Neuropsychology, 4*, 51–58.

Boone, K.B., Lesser, I.M., Hill-Gutierrez, E., Berman, N.G., & D'Elia, L.F. (1993). Rey-Osterrieth Complex Figure performance in healthy, older adults: Relationship to age, education, sex, and IQ. *The Clinical Neuropsychologist, 7*, 22–28.

Boone, K.B., Lesser, I.M., Miller, B.L., Wohl, M., Berman, N., Lee, A., Palmer, B., & Back, C. (1995). Cognitive functioning in older depressed outpatients: Relationship of presence and severity of depression to neuropsychological test scores. *Neuropsychology, 9*, 390–398.

Breier, J.I., Plenger, P.M., Castillo, R. et al. (1996). Effects of temporal lobe epilepsy on spatial and figural aspects of memory for a complex geometric figure. *Journal of the International Neuropsychological Society, 2*, 535–540.

Brooks, D. (1972). Memory and head injury. *Journal of Nervous and Mental Disease, 155,* 350–355.

Bylsma, F.W., Bobhole, J.H., Schretlen, D., & Carreo, D. (1995). A brief reliable approach to coding how subjects copy the Rey-Osterrieth complex figure. Paper presented to International Neuropsychological Society, Seattle.

Casey, M.B., Winner, E., Hurwitz, I., & DaSilva, D. (1991). Does processing style affect recall of the Rey-Osterrieth or Taylor Complex Figures? *Journal of Clinical and Experimental Neuropsychology, 13,* 600–606.

Chervinsky, A.B., Mitrushina, M., & Satz, P. (1992). Comparison of four methods of scoring the Rey-Osterrieth Complex Figure Drawing Test on four age groups of normal elderly. *Brain Dysfunction, 5,* 267–287.

Chiulli, S.J., Yeo, R.A., Haaland, K.Y., & Garry, P.J. (1989). Complex figure copy and recall in the elderly. Paper presented to the International Neuropsychological Society, Vancouver.

Chiulli, S.J., Haaland, K.Y., LaRue, A., & Garry, P.J. (1995). Impact of age on drawing the Rey-Osterrieth figure. *The Clinical Neuropsychologist, 9,* 219–224.

Cooper, J.A., Sagar, H.J., Jordan, N., et al. (1991). Cognitive impairment in early, untreated Parkinson's Disease and its relationship to motor disability. *Brain, 114,* 2095–2122.

Corwin, J., & Bylsma, F.W. (1993). "Psychological examination of traumatic encephalopathy" by A. Rey and "The Complex Figure Copy Test" by P.A. Osterrieth. *The Clinical Neuropsychologist, 7,* 3–21.

Delaney, R.C., Prevey, M.L., Cramer, J., Mattson, R.H., et al. (1992). Test–retest comparability and control subject data for the Rey-Auditory Verbal Learning Test and Rey-Osterrieth/Taylor Complex Figures. *Archives of Clinical Neuropsychology, 7,* 523–528.

Denman, S.B. (1987). *Denman Neuropsychology Memory Scale.* Charleston: SC: S.B. Denman.

Diamond, B.J., & DeLuca, J. (1996). Rey-Osterrieth Complex Figure Test performance following anterior communicating artery aneurysm. *Archives of Clinical Neuropsychology, 11,* 21–28.

Duley, J.F., Wilkins, J.W., Hamby, S.L., Hopkins, D.G., et al. (1993). Explicit scoring criteria for the Rey-Osterrieth and Taylor Complex figures. *The Clinical Neuropsychologist, 7,* 29–38.

Fastenau, P.S. (1996). Developmental and preliminary standardization of the "Extended Complex Figure Test" (ECFT). *Journal of Clinical and Experimental Neuropsychology, 18,* 63–76.

Fastenau, P.S., Bennett, J.M., & Denburg, N.L. (1996). Application of psychometric standards to scoring system evaluation: Is "new" necessarily "improved"? *Journal of Clinical and Experimental Neuropsychology, 18,* 462–472.

Fedio, P., Cox, C.S., Neophytides, A., et al. (1979). Neuropsychological profile of Huntington's disease: Patients and those at risk. In T.N. Chase, N.S., Wexler, and A. Barbeau (Eds.). *Advances in Neurology* (Vol. 23). New York: Raven Press.

Hamby, S.L., Wilkins, J.W., & Barry, N.S. (1993). Organizational quality on the Rey-Osterrieth and Taylor Complex Figure tests: A new scoring system. *Psychological Assessment, 5,* 27–33.

Heaton, R.K., Grant, I., & Mathews, C.G. (1991). Comprehensive norms for an expanded Halsted-Reitan battery: Demographic corrections, research findings, and clinical applications. Odessa, FL: Psychological Assessment Resources.

King, M.C. (1981). Effects of non-focal brain dysfunction on visual memory. *Journal of Clinical Psychology, 37,* 638–643.

Kirk, U., & Kelly, M.S. (1986). Scoring Scale for the Rey-Osterrieth Complex Figure. Paper presented to the International Neuropsychological Society, Denver.

Knight, J.A., & Meyers, J.E. (1995). Comparison of malingered and brain-injured productions on the Rey-Osterrieth Complex Figure Test. Paper presented to the meeting of International Neuropsychological Society, Seattle.

Kolb, B., & Whishaw, I. (1990). *Fundamentals of Human Neuropsychology* (3rd ed.). New York: W.H. Freeman and Co.

Kuehn, S.M., & Snow, W.G. (1992). Are the Rey and Taylor Figures equivalent? *Archives of Clinical Neuropsychology, 7,* 445–448.

Lee, G.P., Loring, D.W., & Thompson, J.L. (1989). Construct validity of material-specific memory measures following unilateral temporal lobe ablations. *Psychological Assessment, 1,* 192–197.

Leininger, B.E., Gramling, S.E., Farrell, A.D., et al. (1990). Neuropsychological deficits in symptomatic minor head injury patients after concussion and mild concussion. *Journal of Neurology, Neurosurgery, and Psychiatry, 53,* 293–296.

Lezak, M.D. (1995). *Neuropsychological Assessment* (3rd ed.). New York: Oxford.

Loring, D.W., Lee, G.P., Martin, R.C., & Meador, K.J. (1988a). Material-specific learning in patients with partial complex seizures of temporal lobe origin: Convergent validation of memory constructs. *Journal of Epilepsy, 1,* 53–59.

Loring, D.W., Lee, G.P., & Meador, K.J. (1988b). Revising the Rey-Osterrieth: Rating right hemisphere recall. *Archives of Clinical Neuropsychology, 3*, 239–247.

Loring, D.W., Martin, R.C., Meador, K.J., & Lee, G.P. (1990). Psychometric construction of the Rey-Osterrieth Complex Figure: Methodological considerations and interrater reliability. *Archives of Clinical Neuropsychology, 5*, 1–14.

Meador, K.J., Loring, D.W., Allen, M.E., Zamrini, E.Y., Moore, E.E., Abney, O.L., & King, D.W. (1991). Comparative cognitive effects of carbamazepine and phenytoin in healthy adults. *Neurology, 41*, 1537–1540.

Meador, K.J., Moore, E.E., Nichols, M.E., Abney, O.L., Taylor, H.S., Zamrini, E.Y., & Loring, D.W. (1993). The role of cholinergic systems in visuospatial processing and memory. *Journal of Clinical and Experimental Neuropsychology, 15*, 832–842.

Meyers, J.E., & Lange, D. (1994). Recognition subtest for the Complex Figure. *The Clinical Neuropsychologist, 8*, 153–166.

Meyers, J.E., & Meyers, K.R. (1995a). Rey Complex Figure Test under four different administration procedures. *The Clinical Neuropsychologist, 9*, 63–67.

Meyers, J., & Meyers, K. (1995b). *The Meyers Scoring System for the Rey Complex Figure and the Recognition Trial: Professional Manual.* Odessa, FL: Psychological Assessment Resources.

Mitrushina, M., & Satz, P. (1989). Differential decline of specific memory components in normal aging. *Brain Dysfunction, 2*, 330–335.

Mitrushina, M., Satz, P., & Chervinsky, A.B. (1990). Efficiency of recall on the Rey-Osterrieth Complex Figure in normal aging. *Brain Dysfunction, 3*, 148–150.

Ogden, J.A., Growdon, J.H., & Corkin, S. (1990). Deficits on visuospatial tasks involving forward planning in high-functioning Parkinsonians. *Neuropsychiatry, Neuropsychology, and Behavioral Neurology, 3*, 125–139.

Osterrieth, P.A. (1944). Le test de copie d'une figure complex: Contribution a l'étude de la perception et de la mémoire. *Archives de Psychologie, 30*, 286–356.

Pillon, B. (1981). Troubles visuo-constructifs et méthodes de compensation: Résultats de 85 patients atteints de lésions cérébrales. *Neuropsychologia, 19*, 375–383.

Ponton, M.O., Satz, P., Herrera, L., Ortiz, F., Urrutia, C.P., Young, R., D'Elia, L.F., Furst, C.J., & Namerow, N. (1996). Normative data stratified by age and education for the Neuropsychological Screening Battery for Hispanics (NeSBHIS): Initial report. *Journal of the International Neuropsychological Society, 2*, 96–104.

Poulton, R.G., & Moffitt, T.E. (1995). The Rey-Osterrieth Complex Figure test: Norms for young adolescents and an examination of validity. *Archives of Clinical Neuropsychology, 10*, 47–56.

Rapport, L.J., Dutra, R.L., Webster, J.S., Charter, R., & Morrill, B. (1995). Hemispatial deficits on the Rey-Osterrieth Complex Figure drawing. *The Clinical Neuropsychologist, 9*, 169–179.

Rapport, L.J., Farchione, T.J., Dutra, R.L., Webster, J.S., & Charter, R. (1996). Measures of hemi-inattention on the Rey Figure copy by the Lezak-Osterrieth scoring method. *The Clinical Neuropsychologist, 10*, 450–454.

Rapport, L.J., Charter, R.A., Dutra, R., Farchione, T.J., & Kingsley, J.L. (1997). Psychometric properties of the Rey-Osterrieth Complex Figure: Lezak-Osterrieth versus Denman scoring systems. *The Clinical Neuropsychologist, 11*, 46–53.

Rey, A. (1941). L'examen psychologique dans les cas d'encephalopathie traumatique. *Archives de Psychologie, 28*, 286–340.

Rosselli, M., & Ardila, A. (1991). Effects of age, education, and gender on the Rey-Osterrieth Complex Figure. *The Clinical Neuropsychologist, 5*, 370–376.

Rosselli, M., & Ardila, A. (1996). Cognitive effects of cocaine and polydrug abuse. *Journal of Clinical and Experimental Neuropsychology, 18*, 122–135.

Sadeh, M., Ariel, R., & Inbar, D. (1996). Rey-Osterrieth and Taylor Complex Figures: Equivalent measures of visual organization and visual memory in ADHD and normal children. *Child Neuropsychology, 2*, 63–71.

Sherman, E.M.S., Strauss, E., Spellacy, F., & Hunter, M. (1995). Construct validity of WAIS-R factors: Neuropsychological test correlates in adults referred for possible head injury. *Psychological Assessment, 7*, 440–444.

Shorr, J.S., Delis, D.C., & Massman, P.J. (1992). Memory for the Rey-Osterrieth Figure: Perceptual clustering, encoding, and storage. *Neuropsychologia, 6*, 43–50.

Snow, W. (1979). The Rey-Osterrieth Complex Figure Test as a measure of visual recall. Paper presented at the 7th annual meeting of the International Neuropsychological Society, New York.

Stern, R.A., Singer, E.A., Duke, L.M., et al. (1994). The Boston qualitative scoring system for the Rey-Osterrieth Complex Figure: Description and interrater reliability. *The Clinical Neuropsychologist, 8,* 309–322.

Strauss, E., & Spreen, O. (1990). A comparison of the Rey and Taylor Figures. *Archives of Clinical Neuropsychology, 5,* 417–420.

Taylor, E. M. (1959). *Psychological Appraisal of Children with Cerebral Defects.* Cambridge, MA: Harvard University Press.

Taylor, L. B. (1969). Localization of cerebral lesions by psychological testing. *Clinical Neurosurgery, 16,* 269–287.

Taylor, L. B. (1979). Psychological assessment of neurosurgical patients. In T. Rasmussen & R. Marino (Eds.), *Functional Neurosurgery.* New York: Raven Press.

Taylor, L. B. (1991). Scoring criteria for the ROCF. In Spreen, O., & Strauss, E. *A Compendium of Neuropsychological Tests: Administration, Norms, and Commentary.* New York: Oxford.

Tombaugh, T. N., & Hubley, A. M. (1991). Four studies comparing the Rey-Osterrieth and Taylor Complex Figures. *Journal of Clinical and Experimental Neuropsychology, 13,* 587–599.

Tombaugh, T. N., Schmidt, J. P., & Faulkner, P. (1992). A new procedure for administering the Taylor Complex Figure: Normative data over a 60-year age span. *The Clinical Neuropsychologist, 6,* 63–79.

Troyer, A. K., & Wishart, H. (1996). A comparison of qualitative scoring systems for the Rey Osterrieth Complex Figure test. Paper presented to the International Neuropsychological Society, Chicago.

Tupler, L. A., Welsh, K. A., Asare-Aboagye, Y., & Dawson, D. V. (1995). Reliability of the Rey-Osterrieth Complex Figure in use with memory-impaired patients. *Journal of Clinical and Experimental Neuropsychology, 17,* 566–579.

Uddo, M., Vasterling, J. J., Brailey, K., & Sutker, P. B. (1993). Memory and attention in combat-related post-traumatic stress disorder (PTSD). *Journal of Psychopathology and Behavioral Assessment, 15,* 43–52.

Vingerhoets, G., De Soete, G., & Jannes, C. (1995). Relationship between emotional variables and cognitive test performance before and after open-heart surgery. *The Clinical Neuropsychologist, 9,* 198–202.

Visser, R. S. H. (1973). *Manual of the Complex Figure Test.* Lisse, Netherlands: Swets & Zeitlinger.

Waber, D. P., & Holmes, J. M. (1985). Assessing children's copy productions of the Rey-Osterrieth Complex Figure. *Journal of Clinical and Experimental Neuropsychology, 7,* 264–280.

Waber, D. P., & Holmes, J. M. (1986). Assessing children's memory productions of the Rey-Osterrieth Complex Figure. *Journal of Clinical and Experimental Neuropsychology, 8,* 565–580.

Waber, D. P., Bernstein, J. H., & Merola, J. (1989). Remembering the Rey-Osterrieth Complex Figure: A dual code, cognitive neuropsychological model. *Developmental Neuropsychology, 5,* 1–15.

Weinstein, C. S., Kaplan, E., Casey, M. B., & Hurwitz, I. (1990). Delineation of female performance on the Rey-Osterrieth Complex Figure. *Neuropsychology, 4,* 117–127.

Wishart, H., Strauss, E., Hunter, M., Pinch, D., & Wada, J. (1993). Cognitive correlates of interictal affective and behavioral disturbances in people with epilepsy. *Journal of Epilepsy, 6,* 98–104.

Wood, F. B., Ebert, V., & Kinsbourne, M. (1982). The episodic-semantic memory distinction in memory and amnesia: Clinical and experimental observations. In L. Cermak (Ed.), *Memory and Amnesia.* Hillsdale, NJ: Lawrence Erlbaum.

RIVERMEAD BEHAVIOURAL MEMORY TEST (RBMT)

Purpose

The purpose of this test is to detect impairment of everyday memory functioning and to monitor change following treatment.

Source

The kit (includes the Adult RBMT kit and supplementary children's materials) can be ordered from Western Psychological Services, 1203 Wilshire Boulevard, Los Angeles, CA 90025-1251, at a cost of $375 US.

Description

The test (Wilson, Cockburn, & Baddeley, 1985) was designed to provide analogues of everyday memory situations. The version for adults is appropriate for ages 11–95. The children's version (RBMT-C) is appropriate for use with 5- to 10-year-olds. The RBMT does not adhere to any particular theoretical model of memory; instead, it attempts to mimic the demands made on memory by normal daily life (Aldrich & Wilson, 1991). It does this through items that involve either remembering to carry out some everyday task, or retaining the type of information needed for adequate everyday functioning. For example, remembering a person's name is tested by associating a name with a photograph of a face and requiring recall of the name when the photograph is presented again later in the test session.

The RBMT consists of 12 subtests chosen following a study of memory problems typically experienced by head-injured people (Sunderland et al., 1983). The tasks include: remembering a person's first and last name, remembering a hidden belonging, remembering an appointment, picture recognition, remembering the gist of a short passage, face recognition, remembering a new route, delivering a message, answering orientation questions, and remembering the date. Two items, remembering a short passage and remembering a route around the room, have both an immediate- and delayed-recall component.

Memory for common objects and for faces is assessed using a recognition paradigm in which subjects must identify the original items among distractors. Prospective memory is assessed on three measures: (1) remembering at the end of the session to ask for a personal possession that was put away at the beginning of the session; (2) remembering when an alarm rings to ask a specific question given when the alarm was set 20 minutes earlier; and (3) remembering to take a message on the route around the room and deliver it at a specific point along the route. Orientation items assess knowledge of time, place, and person. There are four parallel versions of the RBMT so that some of the practice effects due to repeated testing with the same test can be avoided.

Administration

Instructions for administration are given in the RBMT manual. Briefly, the examiner presents stimuli, asks questions, traces a route,

and records responses. Abbreviated versions are suggested in the RBMT manual for individuals with expressive language or perceptual disorders. Where patients are unable to attempt a specific RBMT item (e.g., story recall), a filter task needs to be introduced in order to retain the time sequence of other items (Cockburn et al., 1990a). The route recall task may be difficult to administer to immobile patients. In such cases, patients may be asked to move a small figure around a line drawing of a room (Towle & Wilsher, 1989).

Approximate Time for Administration

The test can be given in about 25 minutes.

Scoring

Detailed scoring guidelines are found in the RBMT manuals. Two scoring systems are used: a Screening Score of 0 or 1 for each item and a more detailed Profile Score of 0, 1, or 2 for each item, yielding maximum scores of 12 or 24, respectively.

Comment

High interrater agreement (100%) is reported for both scoring procedures on the RBMT (Wilson, Baddeley, Cockburn, & Hiorns, 1989). Parallel-form reliability was determined by giving two versions of the test to 118 patients (all four forms were used). Correlations are moderate to high (typically above .8). Not surprisingly, the finer-grained Profile Score gave a more reliable estimate of the patient's abilities. Considering data from all 118 patients who were tested twice, the correlations between the two scores were .78 for the Screening Score and .85 for the Profile Score. Performance on the second test administration tended to be slightly better than the first, principally due to one item, remembering a belonging. Test–retest correlations are somewhat lower for the children's version and fall in the moderate range (Aldrich & Wilson, 1991).

The RBMT shows moderate correlations with various laboratory measures of memory including Warrington's Recognition Memory Test, Corsi Block Span, digit span, Wechsler

Memory Scale, recall of the Rey Figure, and the Rey Auditory Verbal Learning Test (Goldstein & Polkey, 1992; Malec et al., 1990; Wilson et al., 1989). The magnitude of the correlations is generally equal to or greater than correlations among laboratory measures (Malec et al., 1990). Malec and colleagues (1990) report that the test is not significantly correlated with the Verbal Comprehension factor of the WAIS-R, nor with measures that are thought to tap frontal lobe dysfunction (e.g., Trails B, Stroop, Mazes). It does, however, show a moderate correlation with the Perceptual Organization factor of the WAIS-R. The implication is that the RBMT does assess specific memory processes tapped by conventional laboratory memory tests (immediate learning and delayed recall of new information) but is not entirely redundant with these tasks. Further, the RBMT does not depend on remotely acquired, well-established memories, nor on measures of complex attention. Performance, however, may be confounded by visuospatial deficits (see below).

Overall, brain-damaged patients have lower scores than normal controls (Koltai et al., 1996; Lincoln & Tinson, 1989; Wilson et al., 1989a). Expressive language disorders impair performance on some of the items (memory for the name, delayed story recall, and orientation items), whereas perceptual problems impair scores on other items (the immediate and delayed route, orientation, date, and faces items) (see also Malec et al., 1990). Wilson et al. (1989) recommend that when assessing patients with language or perceptual disturbances, the examiner should omit offending items and evaluate performance on the remaining individual items. Some normative data for such modified versions are provided in the RBMT manual (see also Cockburn et al., 1990a; Cockburn et al., 1990b), allowing the clinician to detect sparing or impairment of memory despite the presence of other neuropsychological impairment (e.g., word-finding difficulties). Wilson and her colleagues (see source; Cockburn et al., 1990a) report that similar patterns of performance were shown by patients with left-hemisphere strokes without language loss as by those with right-hemisphere strokes. The implication is that side of lesion

per se may be a relatively minor factor in the measurement of preserved everyday memory ability (see also Goldstein & Polkey, 1992).

The literature suggests that the RBMT is a useful complement to more traditional memory-assessment techniques. The inclusion of prospective memory tasks (remembering to carry out actions) may make it a particularly useful measure in the elderly since such tasks may be especially susceptible to the early stages of dementia (Huppert and Beardsall, 1993). It is ecologically valid and accurately predicts everyday memory functioning. It correlates moderately well with therapist-observed rates of memory lapses and subjective ratings of memory problems by patients and relatives (Aldrich & Wilson, 1991; Goldstein & Polkey, 1992; Koltai et al., 1996; Lincoln & Tinson, 1989; Malec et al., 1990; Wilson et al., 1989). There is some evidence that prediction of everyday adaptive abilities can be improved by the use of additional tests of executive function, in particular Trails B (Malec et al., 1990). Some have suggested that it is more closely related to subjective ratings of everyday memory problems than standard psychological measures (Lincoln and Tinson, 1989; van der Feen et al., 1988). However, Koltai et al. (1996) have shown that the RBMT and other tests such as the WMS-R do not differ significantly in their relations to estimates of everyday memory functioning.

Scores on the RBMT correlate moderately with length of coma, duration of post-traumatic amnesia, employment status (Geffen et al., 1991; Schwartz & McMillan, 1989), the ability to learn a new technological skill (Wilson et al., 1989c), and the ability to live independently (Goldstein et al., 1992; Wilson, 1991b; Wilson et al., 1990). For example, Wilson and colleagues (1990; 1991b) report that people who score below 12 on the standardized profile score were unlikely to be living alone, or in paid employment, or in full-time education, whereas most of those scoring more than 12 were likely to be engaged in one or more of these. The RBMT may be better able to discriminate the independent from the dependent individuals than standard psychological measures (Wilson, 1991b), although this may hold only for certain patient populations (Goldstein et al., 1992). The test is not influenced by self-reported anxiety or depression (Wilson et al., 1989b).

One should note, however, that the RBMT has a low ceiling and may not be suitable for detecting mild forms of impairment (Wilson et al., 1989b). Further, while the test can indicate specific memory deficits, it does not appear to be particularly sensitive to such disorders (Goldstein & Polkey, 1992; Wilson et al., 1989a). More traditional laboratory methods are needed to identify the nature of the cognitive impairment.

Normative Data

The test was initially standardized on a sample of brain-damaged patients ($n = 176$, mean age = 44.4 years) and a sample of 118 healthy subjects aged 16–69 years (mean = 41.17) with a mean IQ of 106 (range = 68–136) (see source). The RBMT has since been standardized with community-dwelling elderly people ($n = 114$) aged 70 years and over (Cockburn & Smith, 1989), with healthy adolescents ($n = 85$) aged 11–14 years (Wilson et al., 1990), and with children ($n = 335$) aged 5 years to 10 years 11 months (Wilson et al., 1991).

For adults, aged 16–69, percentile tables for normal controls and brain-damaged patients can be found in the RBMT manual. These are, however, of minimal use since most of the patients scored below the 5th percentile relative to the normal control group. Accordingly, the authors suggest cutoff points for severity of memory impairment (normal, poor memory, moderately impaired, severely impaired) based on their clinical experience. Norm supplements are included in the kit to facilitate use of the RBMT with the elderly, adolescents, and children.

Scores increase with age and reach adult levels at about age 8 years. Age has little effect on performance across the age range 8–70. Subjects over the age of 70, however, are increasingly likely to show decrement on the test (see source). Modest-to-moderate correlations are reported with intelligence and general physical activity. For people over the age of 70, a table is provided in the RBMT manual so that an individual's profile score can

be compared with that expected for a person of similar age and premorbid IQ. No such table is provided for individuals below age 70. Accordingly, where IQ is low in such individuals, RBMT scores should be interpreted with caution since low scores may reflect intellectual limitation rather than impaired memory function. Gender has little influence on performance.

A modified version of the RBMT is recommended (see source, Cockburn et al., 1990a; Cockburn et al., 1990b) for patients (below age 70) who are experiencing expressive language deficits or perceptual problems. Tables are provided in the RBMT manual for evaluating such individuals. This reduces the likelihood of overestimating the severity of memory impairment. Unfortunately, tables are not provided for elderly individuals with language or perceptual difficulties. In such cases, a total score should not be calculated, but comparison of individual item scores can be made.

References

Aldrich, F.K., & Wilson, B. (1991). Rivermead Behavioural Memory Test for Children (RBMT-C): A preliminary evaluation. *British Journal of Clinical Psychology, 30,* 161–168.

Cockburn, J., & Smith, P.T. (1989). *The Rivermead Behavioural Memory Test: Supplement 3: Elderly People.* Bury St. Edmunds, England: Thames Valley Test Co.

Cockburn, J., Wilson, B., Baddeley, A., & Hiorns, R. (1990a). Assessing everyday memory in patients with dysphasia. *British Journal of Clinical Psychology, 29,* 353–360.

Cockburn, J., Wilson, B.A., Baddeley, A., & Hiorns, R. (1990b). Assessing everyday memory in patients with perceptual problems. *Clinical Rehabilitation, 4,* 129–135.

Geffen, G.M., Encel, J.S., & Forrester, G.M. (1991). Stages of recovery during post-traumatic amnesia and subsequent everyday deficits. *Cognitive Neuroscience and Neuropsychology, 2,* 105–108.

Goldstein, L.H., & Polkey, C.E. (1992). Behavioural memory after temporal lobectomy or amygdalo-hippocampectomy. *British Journal of Clinical Psychology, 31,* 75–81.

Goldstein, G., McCue, M., Rogers, J., & Nussbaum, P.D. (1992). Diagnostic differences in memory test based predictions of functional capacity in the elderly. *Neuropsychological Rehabilitation, 2,* 307–317.

Huppert, F.A., & Beardsall, L. (1993). Prospective memory impairment as an early indicator of dementia. *Journal of Clinical and Experimental Neuropsychology, 15,* 805–821.

Koltai, D.C., Bowler, R.M., & Shore, M.D. (1996). Rivermead Behavioural Memory Test and Wechsler Memory Scale-Revised: Relationship to everyday memory impairment. *Assessment, 3,* 443–448.

Lincoln, N.B., & Tinson, D. (1989). The relation between subjective and objective memory impairment after stroke. *British Journal of Clinical Psychology, 27,* 61–65.

Malec, J., Zweber, B., & DePompolo, R. (1990). The Rivermead Behavioural Memory Test, laboratory neurocognitive measures, and everyday functioning. *Journal of Head Trauma Rehabilitation, 5,* 60–68.

Schwartz, A.F., & McMillan, T.M. (1989). Assessment of everyday memory after severe head injury. *Cortex, 25,* 665–671.

Sunderland, A., Harris, B., & Baddeley, A.D. (1983). Do laboratory tests predict everyday behavior? A neuropsychological study. *Journal of Verbal Learning and Verbal Behavior, 22,* 341–357.

Towle, D., & Wilsher, C.R. (1989). The Rivermead Behavioural Memory Test: Remembering a short route. *British Journal of Clinical Psychology, 28,* 287–288.

van der Feen, van Balen, H.G.G., & Eling, P. (1988). Assessing everyday memory in rehabilitation: A validation study. *International Journal of Rehabilitation Research, 11,* 406.

Wilson, B., Cockburn, J., & Baddeley, A. (1985). *The Rivermead Behavioural Memory Test.* Bury St. Edmunds, England: Thames Valley Test Co.

Wilson, B., Baddeley, A., Cockburn, J., & Hiorns, R. (1989a). *Rivermead Behavioural Memory Test: Supplement Two.* Bury St. Edmunds, England: Thames Valley Test Co.

Wilson, B., Baddeley, A., Cockburn, J., & Hiorns, R. (1989b). The development and validation of a test battery for detecting and monitoring everyday memory problems. *Journal of Clinical and Experimental Neuropsychology, 11,* 855–870.

Wilson, B.A., Forester, S., Bryant, T., & Cockburn, J. (1990). Performance of 11–14 year olds on the Rivermead Behavioural Memory Test. *Clinical Psychology Forum,* December, 30, 8–10.

Wilson, B.A., Baddeley, A.D., & Cockburn, J.M. (1989c). How do old dogs learn new tricks: Teaching a technological skill to brain-injured people. *Cortex, 25,* 115–119.

Wilson, B.A., Ivani-Chalian, R., & Aldrich, F. (1991). *The Rivermead Behavioural Memory Test for Children Aged 5 to 10 years.* England: Thames Valley Test Co.

Wilson, B.A. (1991b). Long-term prognosis of patients with severe memory disorders. *Neuropsychological Rehabilitation, 1,* 117–134.

SENTENCE REPETITION TEST

Other Test Name

Another test name is Sentence Memory.

Purpose

The purpose of this test is to assess immediate memory for sentences of increasing length.

Source

Audiotape, manual, and scoring forms can be ordered from the Neuropsychology Laboratory, University of Victoria, Victoria, BC, V8W 2Y2, Canada at a cost of about $40 US.

Description

The test consists of two equivalent forms (A and B Figure 10–22) of 22 tape-recorded sentences, increasing in length from 1 ("Look") up to 26 syllables ("Riding his black horse, the general came to the scene of the battle and began shouting at his brave men"). To allow for sufficient material at low and high levels of performance, the length increases in one-syllable steps for the first 12 and for the last 6 sentences; sentences 13 to 16 increase in two-syllable steps. Grammatical structure and vocabulary have been held deliberately to simple, declarative sentences. The test is part (test 5) of the Neurosensory Center Comprehensive Examination for Aphasia (Spreen & Benton, 1969, 1977).

Benton, Hamsher, and Sivan (1994) use a similar test with two parallel forms of only 14 items and with varying grammatical complexity. The CELF-R contains a similar subtest

SENTENCE REPETITION—Form A—Sample Score Sheet   S# _____

1. Look	
2. Come here.	
3. Help yourself.	
4. Bring the table.	
5. Summer is coming.	
6. The iron was quite hot.	
7. The birds were singing all day.	
8. The paper was under the chair.	
9. The sun was shining throughout the day.	
10. He entered about eight o'clock that night.	
11. The pretty house on the mountain seemed empty.	
12. The lady followed the path down the hill toward home.	
13. The island in the ocean was first noticed by the young boy.	
14. The distance between these two cities is too far to travel by car.	
15. A judge here knows the law better than those people who must appear before him.	
16. There is a new method in making steel which is far better than that used before.	
17. This nation has a good government which gives us many freedoms not known in times past.	
18. The friendly man told us the directions to the modern building where we could find the club.	
19. The king knew how to rule his country so that his people would show respect for his government.	
20. Yesterday he said he would be near the village station before it was time for the train to come.	
21. His interest in the problem increased each time that he looked at the report which lay on the table.	
22. Riding his black horse, the general came to the scene of the battle and began shouting at his brave men.	

TOTAL SCORE

SENTENCE REPETITION—Form B—Sample Score Sheet   S# _____

1. See	
2. Go there.	
3. Come along.	
4. Sing the music.	
5. Winter is over.	
6. The trees began to grow.	
7. The weather can be nice here.	
8. The table was painted dark blue.	
9. The new green dress was very pretty.	
10. She washed her hair before eating supper.	
11. The boy ran quickly into that red building.	
12. He seemed happy to pay the artist for the picture.	
13. He was asked to come to their dinner party in the country.	
14. The famous doctor lived in this city for quite a number of years.	
15. The meeting of the parties took place in the famous field near the mountain pass.	
16. The valley was so dry that storms could not supply enough water to grow the wheat.	
17. The industry really needs men who are prepared to give good service for their high pay.	
18. Yesterday the clerk of the town bank opened the safe and counted the money that was there.	
19. He probably did not notice that the price of corn in the market increased much since last week.	
20. Sometimes he went down to the village to buy various supplies and hear some of the news from home.	
21. He was required to come to the late dinner even though he had some other plans for that evening.	
22. After seeing the map, we realized that we took a wrong turn when going past the college in that town.	

TOTAL SCORE

Figure 10—22. Sentence Repetition, Form A and Form B: Sample Scoring Sheets.

with 26 items, designed for children and adolescents aged 5–18 years.

Administration

The patient is seated about 2 meters from a tape recorder. Playback volume should be set at a comfortable hearing level (approximately 70 db) and may be increased for hard-of-hearing patients. Say: *"I am going to play some sentences* (point to tape recorder). *Listen carefully, and after you have heard each sentence, repeat it as well as you can. Remember? Listen carefully, and repeat the sentence right after you hear it."*

Repeat instructions if necessary and start tape recorder with Sentence Repetition Form A. Occasionally, the patient will not respond after hearing the first sentence. In this case, stop the tape and say, *"Would you repeat what you heard?"* If the patient responds, say, *"That's right. Do the same with each sentence you hear."* If the patient does not respond, say, *"Listen carefully. Then repeat what you heard."* Sentences should not be repeated during the test, although the basic instructions may be repeated. Discontinue after five consecutive failures.

Approximate Time for Administration

The test takes between 10 and 15 minutes.

Scoring

A score of 1 is given for each sentence repeated correctly. Note that since "toward" in item 12, Form A, is often repeated as "towards", "towards" is accepted as correct. On sentences 1–10, failure on a single sentence is disregarded if the following five sentences are correctly repeated. Poor articulation, if intelligible, should be noted, but not scored as an error. Record errors verbatim and note as omissions, alterations (substitution, change of tense, of location, etc.), repetitions, or additions. The maximum raw score is 22. Subtract one point from the raw score if the test was administered orally instead of by tape-playback.

The following corrections for age and educational level are applied:

Age:

<35	0
35–44	+1
45–64	+2
65+	+3

Educational level (successfully completed years of school or other formal education):

below grade 12 +2

Comment

Forms A and B appear equivalent in difficulty. Correlation between Forms A and B in an unselected group of 47 subjects in our sample was .79, and in a mentally retarded population ($n = 25$), .81 (Spreen & Benton, 1966). Brown et al. (1989) reported a test–retest correlation of .71 in 248 children (mean age = 8 years) with mixed diagnoses after an interval of 2 years, 6 months.

The test correlates .88 with the repetition of words, phrases, and sentences of the Western Aphasia Battery (Shewan & Kertesz, 1980). The correlation in adults with digit repetition forward is .75, with digit repetition reversed .66, and with Full Scale IQ (holding age constant) .62 (Lawriw, 1976).

The test is sensitive to brain damage, particularly to aphasic disturbances. In a study of 23 children and 33 adolescents with closed-head injury, 33 percent of those with severe injury and 15 percent with mild injury were found to score below the 6th percentile for their age (Ewing-Cobbs et al., 1987); the mean percentile score for mild closed-head injury patients was 48.35 and for moderate and severe injury it was 36.36.

Peck et al. (1992) reported "normative" data for 75 head-injured adults (mean age 36 years) and found a significant effect of severity of injury ($p < .05$); patients with mild injury scored at the 45th percentile, those with moderate severity at the 39th percentile; and those with severe injury at the 18th percentile. A comparison with patients 12 months post-injury did not show significantly different scores, although this may have been due to an unusually large variability (SD) of the reported means.

In brain-damaged adults between 20 and 79 years, Vargo and Black (1984) did not notice any significant decrease with age ($r = -.08$) but found significant correlations with IQ (.329) and the MQ of the Wechsler Memory Scale (.377). Their study showed the most severe impairment in patients with dementia and toxic exposure as well as with left-hemisphere lesions after CVA and closed-head injury. A comparison of aphasics, nonaphasic brain-damaged patients, and controls of low average intelligence (Lawriw, 1976), and for an aphasic population unselected as to type and severity from referral sources in New York, Iowa City, and Victoria ($n = 208$) showed means of 12.12 (SD = 3.15) for left brain-damaged patients (including aphasics) and of 15.75 (SD = 2.58) when aphasics were excluded. Fifty-six percent of the aphasics scored below the lowest score of normal controls with low average intelligence. Patients with right-hemisphere lesions had a mean of 17.64 (SD = 2.12), patients with bilateral or undetermined location of brain damage had a mean of 16.84 (SD = 5.87), and moderately mentally handicapped patients had a mean of 11.88 (SD = 3.15).

Sarno (1986) reported that among closed-head injury patients those with aphasia scored at the 35th percentile for aphasics, those with subclinical aphasia and dysarthria at the 58th percentile, and those with subclinical aphasia at the 70th percentile. Davis, Foldi, Gardner, and Zurif (1978) showed that the test is especially sensitive in cases of transcortical aphasia. The Benton and Hamsher version of the test showed significant differences between 28 young adults with specific language impairment and 28 controls (Records et al., 1995). Patients with dementia of the Alzheimer type showed moderately, but significantly, lower scores compared to normal controls matched for age, sex, and educational level (Murdoch et al., 1987).

The test score can be entered into the NCCEA profile sheet. In 353 school-age children, Sentence Repetition formed a separate factor in a factor analysis of the 20 subtests of the NCCEA, accounting for 81 percent of the total variance of this factor, and was relatively independent of digit repetition (Crockett,

1974). The test contributed to the discrimination of four empirically derived subtypes of aphasia in adults; impairment of sentence repetition was especially characteristic of individuals classed as "Type A" (good comprehension, poor attention, memory, and reproduction of speech) (Crockett, 1977).

Epstein (1982) found that dyslexics lagged behind normal reading classmates by about four syllables at age 7, three at age 8, and two at age 9. Rourke (1978), on the other hand, found that 16 dyslexic children had scores in the average range, but that syntactic comprehension was impaired. Our own data (Spreen, 1988) showed that 10-year-old learning-disabled children with neurological signs were able to repeat 10.4 syllables, while those with minimal neurological signs repeated 11.3, and those without neurological signs 15.0 syllables. At age 25, these same subjects repeated 12.8, 13.9, and 14.0 syllables, respectively, while a matched control group showed a mean of 15.5.

Children with brain damage and/or epilepsy (Hamsher, 1980, personal communication) had mean scores of 9.5 at age 6, 10 at age 7, 11 at age 8, 11.5 at age 9, 12 at age 10, 12.6 at age 10, 13.2 at age 11, 13.7 at age 12, and 14.0 at age 13.

Normative Data

Tables 10–25 and 10–26 shows normative data for students and for hospital and community volunteers, and also appropriate percentile ranks. Forms A and B produce highly similar mean scores. Williams (1965) reported that the average adult can correctly repeat sentences of 24–25 syllables in length. However, the Benton and Hamsher (1983) normative sample of 85 nonneurological patients showed an average of only 20 correctly repeated syllables.

In older, healthy, and relatively well-educated adults a small, but significant, decrease is noted after the age of 65, which justifies the correction for age (66–75 years, mean = 15.5, SD = 4.02; 76–89 years, mean = 15.0, SD = 4.49; Read & Spreen, 1986). The normative data also show a slightly better per-

Table 10—25. Normative Data for Adults

Group	n	Mean age	Form A		Form B		Est. IQ
			M	SD	M	SD	
University students	25	24.81	17.63	1.72			120
University students	24				17.83	1.96	120
Hospital and community controls	82	36.57	16.46	2.48	16.54	2.09	110

Source: Spreen & Benton, 1977.

Table 10—26. Percentile Ranks for Control Subjects

Score	Percentile rank
19–22	90+
18	80
17	70
16	58
15	36
14	14
13	2

Source: Spreen & Benton, 1977.

Table 10—27. Developmental Norms for Ages 6 to 13, Males and Females

Age	Male				Female				All normal			
	n	M	SD	Range	n	M	SD	Range	n	M	SD	Range
6	30	9.3	2.0	0–12	22	9.3	0.9	3–12	52	10.3	1.6	0–12
7	27	10.0	2.0	5–18	24	10.5	1.7	6–18	51	10.0	2.0	5–18
8	52	11.8	1.3	9–20	52	11.2	1.1	8–18	104	11.5	1.3	8–20
9	78	11.8	1.5	9–19	55	11.9	0.9	9–17	133	11.7	2.0	9–19
10	54	12.5	1.4	10–21	52	12.6	1.6	7–18	106	12.5	1.5	7–21
11	53	13.3	1.8	10–21	51	13.1	1.7	10–22	104	13.2	1.7	10–22
12	46	13.7	1.4	11–21	41	13.5	2.4	10–21	87	13.6	1.9	10–21
13	44	13.8	1.6	11–22	44	13.9	1.2	11–22	88	13.8	1.4	11–22

Source: Adapted from Carmichael & McDonald (1984), Gaddes & Crockett (1975), Spreen & Gaddes (1969).

formance in older females compared to men (approximately 1 point at each age range).

Percentile ranks for nonaphasic brain-damaged patients and for an unselected group of aphasics have been established (Lawriw, 1976).

Table 10–27 contains the norms for normal school children merged from four different sources. No education corrections are made since they would be misleading for children. If such corrections were made, adult level of performance would be reached by age 12. Table 10–28 provides percentile equivalents for each age.

The norms for children are comparable to those presented by Epstein (1982) for Swedish children (means of 13, 16, and 17 syllables for age 7, 8, and 9, respectively). The higher

Table 10—28. Sentence Repetition, Percentiles for School-Age Children

Age	Percentiles										
	0	10	20	30	40	50	60	70	80	90	100
6	1–7		8			9		10		11	12
7	1–7	8			9	10		11		12	13
8	1–9	10	11			12			13	14	15
9	1–9	10	11			12			13	14	15
10	1–9	10	11		12				13	14	15
11	1–11	12		13				14		15	16
12	1–11	12		13				14		15	16
13	1–11	12		13				14		15	16

Source: Adapted from Carmichael & MacDonald (1984), Gaddes & Crooks L (1975), Spreen & Gaddes (1969).

number of syllables repeated in that study was probably due to practice since the children repeated five sentences at each one-syllable increment in length. Epstein also found that children whose native tongue was not Swedish, but who were taught in Swedish schools, were approximately eight syllables behind native, speaking children at age 6, but that this deficit was reduced to six syllables at age 7, five at age 8, and three at age 9. This finding may have some implications for the testing of children with a mother tongue other than English.

References

Benton, A.L., Hamsher, K.deS., & Sivan, A.B. (1994). *Multilingual Aphasia Examination*. San Antonio, TX: Psychological Corporation.

Brown, S.J., Rourke, B.P., & Cicchetti, D.V. (1989). Reliability of tests and measures used in the neuropsychological assessment of children. *The Clinical Neuropsychologist, 3*, 353–368.

Carmichael, J., & McDonald, J. (1984). Developmental norms for neuropsychological tests. *Journal of Clinical and Consulting Psychology, 52*, 476–477.

Crockett, D.J. (1974). Component analysis of within correlations of language skill tests in normal children. *Journal of Special Education, 8*, 361–375.

Crockett, D.J. (1977). A comparison of empirically derived groups of aphasic patients on the Neurosensory Center Comprehensive Examination for Aphasia. *Journal of Clinical Psychology, 33*, 194–198.

Davis, L., Foldi, N.S., Gardner, H., & Zurif, E.B. (1978). Repetition in the transcortical aphasias. *Brain and Language, 6*, 226–238.

Epstein, A.G. (1982). Mastery of language measured by means of a sentence span test. Unpublished manuscript, Lyngby, Denmark.

Ewing-Cobbs, L., Levin, H.S., Eisenberg, H.M., & Fletcher, J.M. (1987). Language functions following closed-head injury in children and adolescents. *Journal of Clinical and Experimental Neuropsychology, 9*, 575–592.

Gaddes, W.H., & Crockett, D.J. (1975). The Spreen-Benton aphasia tests, normative data as a measure of normal language development. *Brain and Language, 2*, 257–280.

Lawriw, I. (1976). A test of the predictive validity and a cross-validation of the Neurosensory Center Comprehensive Examination for Aphasia. M. A. thesis. University of Victoria.

Murdoch, B.E., Chenery, H.J., Wilks, V., & Boyle, R.S. (1987). Language disorders in dementia of the Alzheimer type. *Brain and Language, 31*, 122–137.

Peck, E.A., Mitchell, S.A., Burke, E.A., & Schwartz, S.M. (1992). Post head injury normative data for selected Benton neuropsychological tests. Paper presented at the annual meeting of the American Psychological Association, Washington, D.C.

Records, N.L., Tomblin, J.B., & Buckwalter, P.R. (1995). Auditory verbal learning and memory in young adults with specific language impairment. *The Clinical Neuropsychologist, 9*, 187–193.

Rourke, B.P. (1978). Reading, spelling, arithmetic disability: A neuropsychological perspective. In H.R. Myklebust (Ed.) *Progress in Learning Disabilities*, vol. IV. New York: Wiley.

Sarno, M.T. (1986). Verbal impairment in head injury. *Archives of Physical and Medical Rehabilitation, 67*, 399–405.

Shewan, C.M., & Kertesz, A. (1980). Reliability and validity characteristics of the Western Aphasia Battery (WAB). *Journal of Speech and Hearing Disorders, 45*, 308–324.

Spreen, O. (1988). *Learning Disabled Children Growing Up*. New York: Oxford University Press.

Spreen, O., & Benton, A.L. (1966). Reliability of the Sentence Repetition Test. Iowa City, IA: Unpublished paper.

Spreen, O., & Benton, A.L. (1969, 1977). *Neurosensory Center Comprehensive Examination for Aphasia*. Victoria, BC: University of Victoria, Neuropsychology Laboratory.

Spreen, O., & Gaddes, W.H. (1969). Developmental norms for 15 neuropsychological tests age 6 to 15. *Cortex, 5*, 171–191.

Vargo, M.E. & Black, F.W. (1984). Normative data for the Spreen-Benton Sentence Repetition Test: Its relationship to age, intelligence, and memory. *Cortex, 20*, 585–590.

Williams, M. (1965). *Mental Testing in Clinical Practice*. London: Pergamon.

WECHSLER MEMORY SCALE (WMS)

Purpose

The purpose of this test is to provide measures of various aspects of memory function.

Source

The Wechsler Memory Scale can be obtained from The Psychological Corporation, P.O. Read, D.E., & Spreen, O. (1986). Normative data in older adults for selected neuropsychological tests. Unpublished manuscript, University of Victoria.

Box 9954, San Antonio, TX 78204-0954, at a cost (manual, design cards, and package of 50 response sheets) of $98 US.

Description

The Wechsler Memory Scale (WMS) (Wechsler, 1945) has undergone a major revision (WMS-R), and a new edition (WMS-III) is underway. Given the wealth of data that has accumulated with the WMS, clinicians frequently rely on the original version (Guilmette et al., 1990). We describe the original version here. The revised version is detailed in the next section.

The complete kit contains the manual, record forms, and design cards. The test consists of seven subtests. The first two subtests, Personal and Current Information (PI) and Orientation (OR), comprise simple questions that assess whether the patient is oriented to age, date of birth, government officials, time, and place. Mental Control (MC) consists of asking the patient to count backwards, recite the alphabet, and count (by 3s or 4s) under time pressure. Logical Memory (LM) examines the ability to recall the number of ideas presented in two passages read to the patient. Memory Span (MS) requires the patient to recall digits forwards and backwards. Visual Reproduction (VR) requires the subject to draw from memory simple geometric figures that were exposed briefly. Associate Learning (AL) requires the patient to listen to paired associations of words and then recall the correct response to stimulus words over three trials. The patient's raw score on each subtest is summed, and an age correction factor is added to obtain a summary score, the Memory Quotient. There are two forms of the test, Form I (Wechsler, 1945) and Form II (Stone & Wechsler, 1946), although most of the published studies deal with Form I.

The validity, standardization, and general psychometric properties of the WMS have been extensively criticized (Butters et al., 1988; Erickson & Scott, 1977; Herman, 1988; Hulicka, 1966; Larrabee et al., 1985; Lezak, 1995; Loring & Papanicolauo, 1987; Prigatano, 1977, 1978). Briefly, these criticisms refer to (1) inadequate norms; (2) the fact that scores on all subtests are combined into a summary score, the MQ, that does not differentiate among various facets of memory; (3) overreliance on immediate recall with no procedures for evaluating retention over a long time period; (4) lack of control for visuoperceptive and visuomotor abilities in measures of so-called visual memory; (5) imprecise scoring criteria; (6) the fact that the scale stresses verbal as opposed to nonverbal tasks; and (7) the fact that the test assesses constructs that, although perhaps necessary for successful memory performance (e.g., orientation, mental control), are not genuine measures of memory.

In an attempt to remedy some of the limitations of the WMS, several variations of the test have been developed. Russell's (1975) system involves the administration of only the LM and VR portions of the Scale. In addition to immediate recall, a 30-minute delayed recall is obtained for both portions. Three measures of verbal recall and three measures of nonverbal recall are obtained: immediate recall, delayed recall, and the percentage of the immediate recall produced after the 30-minute delay. Russell's revision is widely used. In addition, explicit scoring criteria have been developed (see Scoring) and good normative studies are available (see Normative Data).

The Montreal Neurological Institute's (MNI) revision (L. Taylor, personal communication) retains all the elements of the original WMS but has included a 90-minute delayed recall of LM and AL (sum of both yielding a "C" score) and VR (yielding a "D" score). According to Milner (1975), the "C" and "D" scores are useful in distinguishing laterality of brain lesion. However, no normative data are given, only rough clinical guidelines.

The Boston revision (Milberg et al., 1986) also retains all subtests from the original WMS but has added to the LM, AL, and VR subtests. LM contains an immediate recall probe asking specific questions regarding story elements (e.g., What kind of work did this person do?), in an attempt to assess retention rather than only spontaneous retrieval ability (Loring & Papanicolaou, 1987). A 20-minute delayed recall of LM is also given. Probe questions are administered for information not spontaneously recalled. However, normative data are not given. Unfortunately, one cannot simply use data for the Russell revision since the immediate probe may provide a rehearsal opportunity, which may lead to higher scores for delayed performance when compared to norms obtained without probe questioning. In the Boston revision, AL has been modified in three ways. First, immediately following the third standard trial, the order of each pair of words is reversed, and the patient is presented with the second pair member and asked to recall the first. This is done in order to measure the strength of the association. Patients who encode word pairs on a more superficial, phonetic level, rather than at a deeper semantic level, will often perform worse on this trial compared to the third trial because the phonemic sequence of the word pairs is altered (Delis, 1989). Second, 20 minutes later, free uncued recall of the pairs is assessed. Finally, the first word of each pair is provided as a cue and paired recall is measured again. The immediate VR subtest has also been altered to include recognition and copy conditions. These modifications were made in order to distinguish between retention and retrieval problems and to ensure that memory disorders are not confounded with construction difficulties. In addition to a 20-

minute delayed-recall condition, the Boston version also includes delayed multiple-choice recognition and matching tasks. Again, no normative data are given. Data available for the Russell version cannot be used because of the additional exposure with the immediate multiple-choice and copy performance (Loring & Papanicolaou, 1987).

These various innovations are useful. The Russell and MNI revisions are perhaps best used when the question is whether or not a problem exists. By contrast, the Boston version is more appropriate when one wishes to discover more about the nature of the deficit. Our procedure borrows elements from each of these approaches. All subtests in the original WMS are given. We follow Russell's procedure of interposing 30 minutes between immediate and delayed-recall conditions for LM and VR. In addition, we include a 30-minute delayed recall of AL. In general, probe questions for the LM subtest are given only after the delayed (not the immediate) recall condition. Similarly, multiple-choice recognition, matching, and copying tasks are administered only after the delayed (not the immediate) VR task. In this way, we can make use of existing normative data and, at the same time, assess different aspects of performance.

Administration

The instructions for most subtests of the WMS are the same as those in the manual (Wechsler, 1945). There are some changes in administration as follows (adapted from Russell, 1975; Milberg et al., 1986; Milner, 1975; Wechsler, 1987): The examiner waits about 30 minutes after the first administration of LM, VR, and AL subtests and then requests a second recall of the material. The interposed tests should be quite different from the memory tests in order to avoid interference. In particular, one should not give drawings or other memory tests. Subtests of the Wechsler Intelligence Scales are suitable tasks. At the end of the 30-minute period, the patient is asked to retell the stories as he or she remembers them. Say: "*Remember the stories that I read to you a few minutes ago. Tell me the stories again. Tell me*

all that you can." The stories are not read to the subject again. If either of the stories cannot be recalled at all, then say, "*Do you remember a story about a washerwoman?*" or, "*Do you remember a story about a ship?*" The examiner writes both the immediate and delayed dictated stories verbatim so that scoring can be done more accurately at a later time. If the patient does not remember all of the elements of a story accurately, then the examiner can use probe questions such as those listed in Figure 10–23 for Form II.

The patient is then asked to reproduce the designs again on a *blank* piece of paper. In order to permit evaluation of performance en route to the solution, no erasing is allowed. Say: "*A little while ago, I showed you some drawings on cards. You looked at each drawing and then drew it. Now draw them again on this sheet.*" If the subject does not remember any design, give a clue such as: "*Do you remember a design that looks like flags?*" (In Form II, substitute "*a cross*"). If the patient does not recall a design correctly, then the delayed recall task can be followed with the recognition task in which the correct design is displayed with four similar but slightly distorted distractors (see Figure 10–24). The patient should also be asked to copy the design. The matching task requires the patient to select the correct design from distractor items with the original stimulus present (see Figure 10–24). This task should be given if there is impairment on the recognition task.

For delayed recall of AL, say, "*A little while ago, I read you pairs of words. Then I read you the first word in each pair, and you were to tell me the word that went with it. Now, I want to see how well you remember the word pairs.*" Use the list for the "Second Presentation." Say, "*What word went with knife?*"

Subtest 1 of the WMS, PI, contains items that can be troublesome to Canadians. Figure 10–25 shows recommended substitutions.

The subtests of the WMS should be administered in one sitting. It is essential that the tasks of immediate and delayed recall be given in the same session. Finally, the examiner must remember to fold the answer sheet to cover up the AL subtest while the patient is performing the VR subtest.

Form II—Story 1
 1. Was it about cats, dogs, or horses? (c)
 2. Were they used in train accidents, war time, or plane crashes?
 3. Were they trained to find the enemy, the wounded, or weapons?
 4. Were dogs also trained to rescue hungry kittens, lost children, or drowning people? (c)
 5. Were they sled dogs, race dogs, or police dogs?
 6. Are they taught to run into water, making a flying leap, or ride in boats? (c)
 7. Does leaping into the water waste energy, cause problems, or save swimming strokes?
 8. Is this important for saving much money, time, or animals?
 9. Does this save 4 seconds, valuable time, or many minutes?
10. Are the best police dogs hound dogs, bull dogs or sheep dogs?
11. Are they English sheep dogs, German sheep dogs, or European sheep dogs?

Form II—Story 2
 1. Was it about adults, children, or teachers? (c)
 2. Were there a few children, many children, or 20 children?
 3. Many were uninjured, killed, or sent home?
 4. Did the accident occur in England, Spain, or France? (c)
 5. Was it Southern France, Paris, or Northern France?
 6. What was wrecked: a shopping mall, a schoolhouse, or a farmhouse? (c)
 7. What wrecked the schoolhouse: a truck, a storm, or a shell?
 8. Was the schoolhouse in a city, a village, or a Paris?
 9. Were the children thrown agains a wall, down a hill, or into a river?
10. How far were they thrown: 3 feet, a short distance, or a long distance?
11. How many children escaped uninjured? 3, none, or 2?

_____
 If the patient does not remember all of the elements of the story accurately, ask the corresponding multiple choice
questions. Correct only when indicated (c). "*If at any point you remember more of the story, please tell me.*"

Figure 10—23. Logical Memory—Delayed Cued Recall. Adapted from the Wechsler Memory Scale Logical Memory Test (Form II). Copyright 1945, renewed 1974 by The Psychological Corporation. All rights reserved. Vancouver Revision by A. Carney & K. Bate (1990).

Approximate Time for Administration

Our version of the WMS takes about 20–25 minutes, excluding the delay interval.

Scoring

The subject's raw subtest scores are summed, an age correction is added (Table 2 in WMS manual), and this corrected score may then be converted to an MQ by means of a table (Table 3 in WMS manual). For scoring of all the WMS subtests except Logical Memory, see the manual (Wechsler, 1945). A major criticism of the WMS is the imprecise scoring instructions for the LM subtest (Abikoff et al., 1987; Crosson et al., 1984; McCarty et al., 1980; Power et al., 1979; Prigatano, 1978; Schwartz & Ivnik, 1980). According to Wechsler (1945), the examiner should "record verbatim and score according to the number of ideas marked off in

selection." There have been a number of attempts to operationalize scoring of the subtest. For example, some (Power et al., 1979) suggest $1/2$-point credit for minor deviations from the fundamental idea or verbatim scoring (Abikoff et al., 1987). Others (Abikoff et al., 1987; Schwartz & Ivnik, 1980) have developed a specific set of "acceptable" responses that capture the gist or basic idea of each of the content units of the LM subtest. We use the gist-scoring criteria of Schwartz and Ivnik (1980) and Abikoff et al. (1987) because they are reliable (.99) and because norms have been developed with these systems (see Normative Data). These scoring criteria are given for Form II in Figure 10–26.

Note that on the delayed recall of the LM subtest, the prompt portion of the answer is not counted in the delay score, if the patient recalls the story but requires a prompt. Similarly, on the delayed VR task, if a prompt is

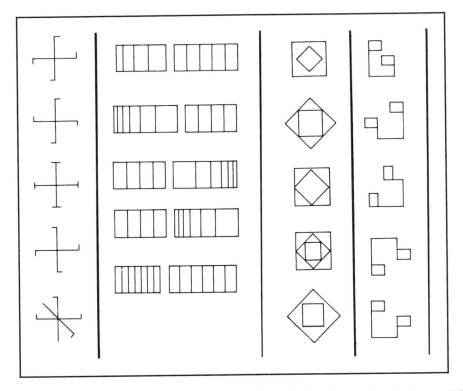

Figure 10—24. Wechsler Memory Scale: Visual Reproduction (Form II). Matching test: "POINT TO THE DESIGN THAT LOOKS LIKE THIS ONE" [point to target design]. Adapted from the Wechsler Memory Scale. Copyright 1945, renewed 1974 by The Psychological Corporation. Reproduced by permission. All rights reserved.

given, then one point is deducted from the design.

The scoring systems described above are bit-based. Webster and colleagues (1992) have developed a relationally processing-based scoring system (RPSS) for the LM subtest. In this scheme, information from the stories is classed as either essential to the plot (e.g., the protagonist was a woman) (Essential proposition) or nonessential to the plot (e.g., her name was Anna) (Detail proposition). The subject's responses are also scored for intrusion errors (Self-generated propositions). The authors found that RPSS was sensitive to prose memory deficits in left-CVA and in right-CVA patients that were not identified using a bit-based scoring system. The left-CVA subjects recalled significantly fewer essential propositions than did the right-CVA and normal control group, but also produced the fewest intrusion errors. The right-CVA group recalled significantly fewer detail propositions and produced significantly more self-generated propositions than did the normal control group. In contrast, these groups recalled approximately the same number of essential propositions. The authors report that this scoring system is highly reliable. Unfortunately, normative data are lacking for this scoring system.

When administering the immediate and delayed portions of the AL subtest, a patient may respond to "baby" with "cry" rather than "cries" and to "school" with "groceries" rather

4. Who is the prime minister of Canada?
5. Who is the premier of this province?
6. Who is the mayor of this city (or of the patient's home city)?

Figure 10—25. Recommended items for substitution on the Personal and Current Information Subtest of the WMS with Canadian Subjects (Adapted from the Wechsler Memory Scale. Copyright 1945, renewed 1974 by The Psychological Corporation. Reproduced by permission. All rights reserved.)

1. *Dogs*
Dog	1
Canine (s)	1

Are trained
are taught	1
are used	1
go around	0
learn	0
X	1

To find
to help	0
to rescue	1
to assist	0
to look for	1
to locate	1
X	1

The wounded
the injured	1
those hurt	1
casualties	1
people	0
soldiers	0
X	1

In the wartime
in war	1
during the war	1
in the war	1
in WWII	0
on the battlefield	1
X	1
(Police dog)s	1(A)
dogs	0
they	0

Are also trained
are trained	1
are taught	1
are used	1
can	0
can rescue	0
learn	0
X	1

To rescue
to save	1
to help	1
to assist	1
to find	0
X	1

Drowning people
drowning victims	1
the drowning	1
people in the water	0
swimmers	0
people from drowning	1
people from water	0
X	1

Instead of running
rather than running	1
by running	0
they don't run	1
instead of going	0
X	1

Down to the water
into the water	1
to the water	1
in the water	1
to the victim	0
down to the shore	1
X	1

And striking out
setting out	1
heading for the person	1
taking off	1
lighting out	1
jumping in	0
swimming out	1
diving in	0
starting to swim	1
X	1

They are taught
they are trained	1
learn how to	1
learned	0
X	1

To make
to take	1
to use	1
to do	1
X	1

A flying leap
a great leap	1
a big jump	1
a running dive	1
a jump	0
a leap	0
a dive	0
X	1

By which they save
in order to save	1
to save	1
which saves	1
X	1

Many swimming strokes
a lot of strokes	1
swimming strokes	0
some strokes	1
several strokes	1
a few strokes	0
X	1

And valuable
precious	1
crucial	1
much needed	1
important	1
and many	0
X	1

Seconds of time
seconds	1
time	1
minutes	0
X	1

The European sheep dog
European shepherd	1
European dog	0
sheep dog	0
German sheep dog	0
X	1

Makes the best
X	1

(Police)

(Dog)s

Figure 10—26. Detailed scoring criteria for the Wechsler Memory Scale, Logical Subtest (Abikoff et al., 1987).

2. Many			When a shell			And across		
a lot	1		when a bomb	1		across	1	
several	1		when a bombshell	1		and into	0	
some	1		after a bomb	1		over	1	
a few	0		rocket	0		down	0	
X	1		when an explosion	0		X	1	
			X	1				
(school)	1(A)					A ravine		
			Wrecked			ditch	1	
Children			destroyed	1		canyon	0	
students	1		hit	1		creek	0	
pupils	1		blew up	1		X	1	
kids	1		ruined	1				
people	0		damaged	0		A long distance		
babies	0		severely damaged	1		far	1	
youngsters	1		X	1		far away	1	
X	1					some distance	1	
			The (school)house	1(A)		a distance	1	
in (North)ern	1					and away	0	
			In their village			feet, yards, etc.	1	
France			in their town	1		X	1	
French	1		in their city	0				
Frenchmen	0		in their country	0		From the (school)house		
X	1		in their community	0		past the (school)house	1	
			X	1		X		
Were killed								
died	1		The children			Only two		
lost their lives	1		students	1		two	1	
were murdered	0		pupils	1		a couple	1	
perished	1		kids	1		several	0	
X	1		youngsters	1		X	1	
			people	0				
Or fatally hurt			babies	0		Children		
mortally hurt	1		they	1		student/pupils/kids	1	
died from their injuries	1		(if "they" clearly refers to			youngsters		
hurt	1		children or its synonym)			babies/people	0	
fatalities	1		X	1		of them	1	
maimed	0					(if "them" clearly refers to		
X	1		Were thrown			children or its synonym)		
			thrown	1		X	1	
And others			fell	0				
others	1		went down	0		Escaped uninjured		
additional	1		were flung	1		were not hurt	1	
some	1		X	1		avoided injury	1	
the rest	0					survived	0	
X	1		Down a hillside			were rescued	0	
			down a hill	1		escaped	0	
Seriously injured			to the bottom of the hill	1		X	1	
maimed	1		downhill	1				
hurt/wounded			across a hillside	0				
(qualified for severity)	1		over a hillside	0				
hurt/wounded	0		down	0				
X	1		X	1				

Figure 10—26. Continued

than "grocery." Give full credit for either of these responses.

Comment

Form I and Form II of the WMS are not interchangeable (Bloom, 1959; McCarty et al., 1980; Schultz et al., 1984; Stanton et al., 1984). Form II is a little easier than Form I, particularly with regard to the Logical Memory and Visual Reproduction subtests (Ivison, 1988, 1993). Abikoff et al. (1987) note that although both forms have 46 blocks or content units on the LM subtest, Form I blocks contain 15 percent more total words (120) than Form II blocks (104). Ivison (1990) reports a virtual absence of practice effects on Form II following a retest interval of about 5 months. The stability of the total score is .89, and the stabilities of the subtest scores range from .65 for Digit Span to .87 for Orientation. For Form I, correlations for the total score range from .75 to .89 over intervals of 14 days to 14 months (Ryan et al., 1981; Snow et al., 1988). Although there is adequate reliability in terms of stability of position in group distribution, individual subjects are likely to manifest a gain in MQ scores (4–7 points) across time on Form I (Franzen, 1989). McCaffrey et al. (1992) report that with short retest intervals (7–10 days), the Russell version of the Logical Memory and Visual Reproduction subtests as well as the Paired Associate subtest (Form I) show gains of about two points.

Information regarding internal consistency of the test as a whole as well as of the subtests is sparse (Franzen, 1989). Hall and Toal (1957) reported that Cronbach's coefficient alpha values ranged from .38 for Mental Control and Associate Learning to .65 for Digit Span. Cronbach's coefficient alpha for the whole test was .69. Ivinskis et al. (1971) reported that split-half reliability of the WMS is .75.

Story B from Form I (the "American liner" passage) is inherently more difficult to recall than any of the other logical memory passages used in the various versions of the Wechsler Memory Scale (WMS Form I, Story A, the "Anna Thompson" passage, WMS Form II. "Dogs are trained"; B. "Many schoolchildren" and WMS-R passages, "Anna Thompson,"

"Robert Miller"). Consequently, on Form I of the WMS, the recall of fewer Story B items relative to Story A is expected and not due to proactive interference (Henry et al., 1990). The first passages on WMS-I and WMS-II and both passages on WMS-R appear to be of equivalent difficulty (Ivison, 1993).

Scores on various subtests of the WMS and the Russell revision correlate moderately with those from other memory tests. For example, Compton and colleagues (1992) found that WMS total digits, Associate Learning hard pairs, Logical Memory—Immediate and Delay, and Visual Reproduction—Immediate and Delay correlated .19–.59 with the words and faces subtests of the Recognition Memory Test. Larrabee et al. (1985) noted that Immediate VR loaded on the same factor as the BVRT, Block Design, and Object Assembly subtests. Delayed VR was associated with the Continuous Visual Memory Test delayed-recognition score (Larabee et al., 1992). Mitrushina and Satz (1991) reported that both Immediate and Delayed VR comprised the same factor as the Rey Figure (Copy and Delay). There are also moderate-to-high correlations between the Wechsler IQ and WMS scores; in particular, MQ, Mental Control, Immediate Logical Memory, Digits Total (note that Digit Span appears on both the WAIS and WMS), and Immediate Visual Reproduction (Larrabee et al., 1983; Larrabee et al., 1985; Sherer et al., 1992). Delayed Logical Memory and Visual Reproduction are also affected by IQ level so that these scores should be interpreted with regard to patient IQ level (Sherer et al., 1992). Percent delayed recall on the Logical Memory and Visual Reproduction subtest appear less affected by IQ (Ivnik et al., 1991; Sherer et al., 1992).

Factor analytic studies of the original WMS have generally revealed three components: Factor I (immediate learning and recall) has loadings from LM, VR, and AL; Factor II (attention and concentration) has loadings from MC and MS; Factor III (orientation and long-term information recall) has loadings from PI and OR (for review see Wechsler, 1987). Some, however, have failed to find evidence of the third factor (Ivison, 1993b).

The factor analytic studies do not support

the unidimensional factor of memory implied in the single MQ score of the WMS. Nonetheless, because the MQ and Wechsler FSIQ are linked in normal people (e.g., Ivison, 1993b), substantial IQ–MQ discrepancies are indicative of memory impairment (Milner, 1975; Oscar-Berman et al., 1993; Prigatano, 1978). Several authors (Milner, 1975; Prigatano, 1978) have suggested that WAIS–IQ–MQ differences of 12 or more points may indicate a verbal memory deficit. However, WAIS-R IQs are about 7–8 points below their WAIS counterparts, calling into question the validity of the 12-point discrepancy as an indicator of memory impairment (Larrabee, 1987; Prifitera & Barley, 1985). A more defensible intelligence-versus-memory contrast (Oscar-Berman et al., 1993) with which to identify specific memory deficits is provided by comparison with base rates of IQ versus memory indices (see Bornstein et al., 1989, for WAIS-R versus GM, DM in section on WMS-R). Note, however, that the MQ is not sensitive to distinctive patterns of deficits, nor is it adequate in detecting mild memory problems (Butters, 1986; Squire, 1986).

Scores on the original WMS do tend to fall with increasing age, as might be predicted theoretically (Prigatano, 1978). Further, the test is sensitive to memory deficit. However, the scale is not sensitive to distinctive patterns of deficits found in specific types of amnesic and demented patients (Butters, 1986). It is affected most by left-hemisphere disturbances but does not detect memory disturbances that occur with right-hemisphere lesions (Prigatano, 1978). Addition of delayed-recall tasks (LN, VR, AL) improves validity. The Russell revision is not strongly related to psychopathology, as measured by the MMPI, and is less strongly related to intelligence than has been reported for the original WMS (O'Grady, 1988; Sherer et al., 1992). The revision is sensitive to a variety of conditions, including dementia, closed-head injury, obstructive sleep apnea syndrome, chronic cocaine and polydrug abuse, and to laterality of the disturbance (Bedard et al., 1991; Bornstein, 1982; Delaney et al., 1980; Dikmen et al., 1995; Hom, 1992; Lencz et al., 1992; Milner, 1975; Rosselli & Ardila, 1996; Russell, 1975; Solo-

mon et al., 1990). Although not all studies (e.g., Mayeux et al., 1980; Saling et al., 1993) report laterality differences in patients with epilepsy, some have found significant correlations between measures of the integrity of the left hippocampus and the Logical Memory percent retention scores (Lencz et al., 1992; Sass et al., 1992). Moreover, there may be a specificity with regard to the relationship between hippocampal integrity and measures of neuropsychological function. Left-hippocampal neuron loss in CA3 and the hilar area correlates only with the LM percent retention score, but not with language competency (assessed via the BNT) or verbal intellectual ability (VIQ) (Sass et al., 1992). Note, however, that in patients with diffuse damage the VR tests show more impairment than the verbal ones (Levin & Larrabee, 1983), a finding that must be noted in order to prevent the false attribution to right hemisphere damage in diffuse cases (Russell, 1988).

There is evidence that dementia of the Alzheimer's type (AD) can be distinguished from normality and from other neurological disorders using qualitative analysis. Jacobs and colleagues (1990), using the Visual Reproduction subtest of the WMS, found that patients with AD made significantly more prior-figure intrusion errors (i.e., the inclusion of characteristics unique to one figure in the reproduction of a subsequent figure) than did Huntington's disease (HD) patients, although both of these patient groups generated more of these errors than did intact control subjects. Patients with alcoholic Korsakoff's syndrome, but not patients with bilateral hippocampal damage, made significantly more intrusion errors than did normal controls. The WMS was more likely to elicit intrusion errors from AD and HD patients than was the WMS-R version, likely due to the lack of similarity between sequential stimuli on the latter version.

Psychological distress has a limited effect on WMS performance. Davidoff et al. (1990) demonstrated statistically significant correlations between subtests of the WMS (Delay VR, Delay PA) and Zung depression scores in acute spinal-cord injury patients, but the overall variance in WMS performance explained by depression scores was less than 10 percent.

Some have suggested that poor motivation can be detected by analyzing qualitative errors made on the WMS (Rawlings & Brooks, 1990). Unfortunately, such errors are not specific enough to motivational defects to be of clinical use (Milanovich et al., 1996).

The WMS can be considered as a fairly quick first step in the assessment of memory. Examination of the subtests may offer clues about spared and impaired functions. More detailed assessment with other tests (e.g., Buschke, CVLT, Rey Figure, RAVLT), however, is necessary in order to establish which facets of memory are impaired. One should also note that the WMS relies heavily on verbal skills. Consequently, patients with verbal expressive problems will be penalized (Erickson & Scott, 1977). Finally, it should not be used to make major decisions regarding an individual's functional capacity (Loewenstein et al., 1995).

Normative Data

Wechsler's (1945) original normative base was inadequate (D'Elia et al., 1989; Lezak, 1995; Prigatano, 1978) in that it was small, about 100 Ss, drawn from a restricted age range (25–50, although his correction scores for age extend from 20 to 64), and the information provided on that population was very sketchy. This deficiency has been remedied to some extent. Age, education, and IQ affect most WMS measures (other than percent retention scores), and several investigators have derived procedures for correcting the scores for age and education/IQ (e.g., Alekoumbides et al., 1987; Russell, 1988), while others have provided tentative norms for children and the elderly (e.g., Abikoff et al., 1987; Cauthen, 1977; Curry et al., 1986; Haaland et al., 1983; Halperin et al., 1989; Hulicka, 1966; Ivinskis et al., 1971; Ivison, 1977; Ivnik et al., 1991; Kear-Colwell & Heller, 1978; Klonoff & Kennedy, 1965, 1966; Russell, 1975, 1988; Schaie & Strother, 1968). One should note that age corrections for these younger and older subjects have typically not been made and, as a result, one cannot derive a MQ for these younger and older people.

This is not necessarily a disadvantage since the concept of MQ, as reflecting a unidimensional measure of memory function, has been severely criticized (see above).

Tables 10–29 to 10–36 allow the clinician to evaluate subtest performance with reference to age-group norms. In general, the norms are based on non-neurological populations of normal intelligence. The samples, however, may not be representative of the North American population. Table 10–29 compiles data from three different studies (Hulicka, 1966; Ivinskis, 1971; Wechsler, 1945) for the following subtests on Form I: PI, OR, MC, MS. Ivnik et al. (1991) provide normative data, stratified by IQ and education, for these subtests based on a sample of 99 healthy, Caucasian persons aged 65–97 years. The data are presented in Table 10–30. Education did not account for as much variance as IQ, and Ivnik et al. suspect that the significant correlation between education and WMS performance arises from the correlation of both with IQ. In cases where IQ scores are not available, the education–WMS association can be used to approximate the relationship between IQ and WMS performance. However, using education to estimate IQ introduces error. Therefore, when reliable IQ and education data are both available, the clinician should rely on the norms that are based on IQ.

For LM, we use the detailed gist-scoring criteria developed by Abikoff et al. (1987) and Schwartz and Ivnik (1980) (see Scoring). Normative data, broken down by age (18–80+) and education, have been generated for this scoring system (Abikoff et al., 1987) and are given in Table 10–31. The norms can be used with Form I or II. Ivison (1993) also provides normative data, but only for the immediate condition of LM and only for Form II. The values derive from a hospitalized sample and are somewhat lower than those reported here. Age and IQ/education have a significant impact on recall, and an accurate measure must correct for these variables. Prediction equations, presented in Table 10–32, can be used to compare obtained scores against expected scores. Abikoff et al. (1987) provide the following illustration: A 40-year-old with 12 years of schooling and an immediate gist-recall score

Table 10—29. Mean Scores on PI, OR, MC and MS Subtests by Age Group—Form I

Age	n	PCI	OR	MC		MS
16–18	44	5.4	4.9	7.1	fwd	6.7
SD		0.8	0.4	2.0		1.2
					bwd	5.0
						1.2
20–29	50	5.92		7.5	fwd	7.04
SD		0.02		1.9		1.2
					bwd	5.26
						1.13
30–39	53	5.56				
SD		0.72				
40–49	46	5.7		6.61	fwd	5.98
SD		0.4		1.9		1.12
					bwd	4.3
						1.11

Source: Ivinskis et al. (1971) give norms based on a population of 16–18-year-old Australian schoolchildren of average intelligence. Hulicka (1966) gives norms based on a non-neurological population of hospitalized veterans. These Ss were of average intelligence and aged 30–39. Wechsler's (1945) norms are derived from non-hospitalized subjects of average intelligence, ages 20–29, 40–49. These norms apply to Form I only. Note that for the Orientation subtest, for ages 20–29 and 40–49, Wechsler reported mean scores as 6 (SD = 0). However, the total points possible on the Orientations subtest is 5.0, making a mean of 6.0 impossible (M. Lucero, personal communication, 1997).

of 17 would have an expected recall score of 21.08. This expected score is obtained by entering the person's age and education into the prediction equation for immediate gist recall [Expected gist immediate = $6.72 + .20(40) + .93(12) - .003(40^2) = 21.08$]. Given a SD of 6.01, then the person's actual score of 17 is within 1 SD of the expected score. The equations can also be used to compare recall scores across individuals by generating standard z scores (see Abikoff et al., 1987). These equations are useful; however, for individuals aged 65–97 years, the clinician can refer to normative data provided by Ivnik et al. (1991) which are stratified according to education and WAIS-R FSIQ. These data are shown in Table 10–33. Russell (1988) also provides age and education/FSIQ corrections based on a sample of 188 normals (referred because of suspicion of neurological disorder but received a negative neurological examination) and 502 brain-damaged subjects. The norms from his study are somewhat lower than those reported by Abikoff et al. (1987). Curry et al. (1986) provide data for adolescents, aged 9.5–15.5, for the immediate and 30-minute delayed versions of the LM subtest. Age and sex differences were documented. Table 10–31 also shows these data, separately for males and fe-

Table 10—30. Means and Standard Deviations on Select WMS Subtests by Wechsler FSIQ and Years of Education in People Aged 65–97 Years

		Information		Orientation		Mental control		Digit span	
	n	M	SD	M	SD	M	SD	M	SD
IQ Group									
<90	27	4.5	1.3	4.7	.5	4.9	2.2	9.0	1.5
90–100	22	5.2	.7	4.8	.5	6.0	1.5	10.2	1.5
101–110	34	5.5	.6	4.9	.3	6.8	1.6	11.0	1.8
>110	15	5.7	.7	6.0	.0	7.9	1.4	10.9	2.0
Education									
<12	29	4.6	1.3	4.8	.5	5.6	2.3	9.6	1.9
12–15	48	5.3	.7	4.9	.4	6.3	1.8	10.6	1.7
>15	22	5.5	.7	5.0	.2	7.0	1.8	10.6	1.9

Source: Ivnik et al., 1991. Within this age-restricted sample, age was found to contribute little to the overall variance in WMS performance or to specific subtests. Reprinted with permission of the American Psychological Association.

Table 10—31. Mean Immediate and 30-Min. Delayed Recall Scores on Logical Memory Subtest by Age Group

Age	n	Immediate		Delayed	
		Score	SD	Score	SD
10–11 (male)	35	17.71	(5.02)	14.94	(4.20)
10–11 (female)	41	14.61	(4.36)	12.05	(3.96)
12—13 (male)	48	18.48	(5.09)	15.50	(4.98)
12–13 (female)	49	17.14	(4.19)	14.79	(4.01)
14–15 (male)	37	19.19	(5.08)	16.81	(4.76)
14–15 (female)	37	17.67	(4.84)	15.67	(4.95)
18–29	74	22.99	(6.66)	19.84	(6.67)
30–39	67	24.57	(6.97)	22.16	(7.57)
40–49	41	23.44	(5.01)	21.07	(5.91)
50–59	54	23.63	(6.14)	20.13	(6.48)
60–69	56	20.48	(6.42)	17.34	(6.71)
70–80+	46	19.11	(6.74)	15.33	(7.57)

Note that the scores for the two stories have not been averaged.

Source: Curry et al. (1986) provide norms for 10–15 year olds that are based on a population of U.S. schoolchildren of low to high-average verbal intelligence. Note that the scores are based on the half-point scoring system developed by Power et al. (1979) and apply only to the stories on Form I. Norms for adults (ages 20+) are taken from Abikoff et al. (1987) and are derived from a normal adult U.S. population. The participants were volunteers, 95 percent were Caucasian, and the mean education was 14.21 years. They are based on detailed gist scoring criteria (see Scoring) and can be used with Form I or II.

Table 10—32. Prediction Equations for Gist Recall Scores

Measure	Equation	SD
Immediate	$6.72 + .20(\text{age}) + .93(\text{education}) - .0026(\text{age sq.})$	6.01
Delayed	$3.40 + .26(\text{age}) + .90(\text{education}) - .0034(\text{age sq.})$	6.56

Source: Abikoff et al., 1989. Data apply to Forms I and II.

Table 10—33. Means and Standard Deviations on LM and VR by Wechsler FSIQ and Years of Education in People Aged 65–97 Years

	n	LM		LM Delay		VR		VR Delay	
		M	SD	M	SD	M	SD	M	SD
IQ Group									
<90	27	5.6	2.3	3.8	2.5	3.4	2.1	2.8	2.3
90–100	22	7.9	2.6	6.3	2.6	6.1	2.6	5.0	3.2
101–110	34	9.1	2.7	7.0	2.8	7.1	3.0	6.1	3.3
>110	15	10.5	2.9	8.1	3.1	9.3	2.6	8.1	3.5
Education									
<12	29	6.8	3.3	5.1	3.4	4.4	2.4	3.5	3.6
12–15	48	8.5	3.1	6.4	3.1	6.4	3.3	5.5	3.2
>15	22	8.6	2.3	6.8	2.5	8.0	3.2	6.9	3.8

Source: Ivnik et al., 1991. Within this age-restricted sample, age was found to contribute little to the overall variance in WMS performance or to specific subtests. Note LM is scored using the gist-scoring criteria described in Scoring. Reprinted with permission of the American Psychological Association.

Table 10—34. Mean Immediate and 30-Min. Delayed Recall Scores
on the Visual Reproduction Subtest by Age Group—Form I

Age	n	Immediate		Delayed	
		Score	SD	Score	SD
10–11 (male)	35	8.86	(2.72)	7.48	(3.09)
10–11 (female)	41	8.17	(2.87)	7.24	(3.06)
12—13 (male)	48	9.19	(2.74)	7.79	(3.03)
12–13 (female)	49	9.98	(1.94)	9.20	(1.95)
14–15 (male)	37	10.00	(2.32)	8.81	(3.03)
14–15 (female)	37	9.29	(2.42)	8.73	(2.56)
18–29	97	10.48	(1.93)	9.84	(2.21)
30–49	81	10.10	(2.55)	9.26	(2.74)
50–64	51	8.73	(2.59)	7.35	(2.46)
65–69	49	6.0	(2.1)	5.4	(2.5)
70–74	74	5.1	(2.0)	4.3	(2.3)
75–79	40	4.9	(2.0)	4.2	(1.9)
80+	13	3.3	(2.3)	2.8	(1.9)

Source: Curry et al. (1986) provide normative data for children and adolescents, based
on a population of normal U.S. schoolchildren, ages 9.5–15.5. Trahan et al. (1988) present data derived from healthy nonhospitalized adults, ages 18–69. Haaland et al.
(1983) provide norms based on a population of superior elderly individuals without
chronic medical problems, ages 65+. These normative data apply to Form I only.

males. Note, however, that the data apply
only to Form I and that Curry et al. did not use
the gist-scoring criteria developed by Abikoff
et al. (1987). Rather, LM was scored according
to the method proposed by Power et al. (1979).
This system allows ½ point credit for minor
deviations of gist (i.e., for the substitution of
one or more synonyms that do not alter the
fundamental idea; for the deletion of an adjective, adverb, or article that alters the idea to
only a slight degree).

Table 10–34 presents age-related norms for
the immediate and 30-minute delayed versions of the Form I Visual Reproduction subtest. Age and education/IQ also affect performance on this test (Ivnik et al., 1991; Russell,
1988; but see Trahan et al., 1988, who report
no correlation between VR performance and
years of education). For individuals aged 65–
97 years, the clinician can refer to normative
data provided by Ivnik et al. (1991) which are
stratified according to education and WAIS-R
FSIQ. These data are shown in Table 10–33.
Russell (1988) has developed norms for adults
(aged 20+) that also take age and educa-
tion/IQ into account. However, the data are
based on clinic referrals and are somewhat
lower than values reported here. Trahan and

Table 10—35. Mean Immediate and 30-Min.
Delayed Recall Scores on the Associate Learning
Subtest by Age Group—Form 1

Age	n	AL		Delayed AL	
		Score	SD	Score	SD
6	34	13.71	(3.21)		
7	40	15.33	(2.8)		
8	38	15.40	(3.3)		
9	44	17.15	(2.5)		
10	38	16.17	(2.8)		
11	36	16.44	(2.6)		
12–13	10	16.3	(1.9)		
16–18	44	16.9	(2.2)		
20–29	23	18.33	(1.45)	9.91	(.29)
30–39	14	18.21	(2.28)	9.92	(.28)
40–49	14	18.29	(2.82)	9.71	(.61)
50–59	10	17.30	(3.34)	8.92	(1.17)
60–69	10	14.30	(2.52)	8.64	(1.74)
70+	14	15.89	(3.10)	8.77	(1.01)

Source: Halperin et al. (1989) provide norms based on
normal lower-middle-class schoolchildren in U.S., aged
6–15. Ivinskis et al. (1971) give norms based on a population of 16- to 18-year-old Australian school children of average intelligence. We (Strauss & Spreen, unpublished
data, 1989) have compiled norms based on healthy adult
volunteers, aged 20–84. Note that AL = A/2 + B (maximum = 21). For delay, 1 point is given for each of the word
pairs (maximum = 10).

Table 10—36. Subtest Means and Standard Deviations Broken Down by Age and Sex on Form II

Subtest	Age 20–29		Age 30–39		Age 40–49		Age 50–59		Age 60–69		Age 70–79	
	M	SD	M	SD	M	SD	M	SD	M	SD	M	SD
PCI												
Male	5.06	(1.04)	5.26	(0.78)	5.56	(0.61)	5.30	(0.74)	5.44	(0.64)	5.00	(0.95)
Female	5.10	(0.86)	5.06	(0.96)	5.10	(0.68)	5.26	(0.69)	5.18	(0.72)	5.01	(0.89)
Orient												
Male	4.80	(0.49)	4.92	(0.34)	4.98	(0.14)	4.94	(0.24)	4.82	(0.39)	4.74	(0.49)
Female	4.88	(0.33)	4.96	(0.20)	4.98	(0.14)	4.94	(2.24)	4.90	(0.30)	4.74	(0.56)
MC												
Male	7.40	(1.74)	6.82	(2.02)	6.88	(1.90)	7.06	(2.03)	7.38	(1.69)	6.52	(2.16)
Female	7.42	(1.47)	6.72	(1.98)	6.78	(1.99)	6.62	(2.01)	6.50	(1.83)	5.46	(2.11)
DSp												
Male	11.04	(1.92)	10.76	(1.97)	10.56	(1.86)	10.50	(1.58)	10.02	(1.85)	9.26	(1.54)
Female	10.96	(1.70)	10.48	(1.94)	10.22	(2.16)	10.24	(1.87)	10.12	(1.71)	9.46	(1.37)
VR												
Male	12.24	(1.59)	11.82	(2.09)	11.42	(2.22)	10.98	(2.48)	9.60	(2.87)	7.24	(3.16)
Female	11.42	(2.08)	10.66	(2.12)	10.78	(2.31)	10.30	(2.31)	9.06	(2.39)	7.24	(3.39)
PAL												
Male	14.35	(3.12)	12.33	(3.52)	11.95	(2.92)	11.73	(3.67)	9.84	(4.33)	7.91	(3.74)
Female	15.10	(3.23)	13.21	(3.89)	12.29	(3.14)	12.34	(3.04)	11.21	(3.22)	9.27	(3.07)

Source: Ivison, 1993b. The data are based on 600 subjects, ages 20–79, with 100 subjects (50 males, 50 females) in each of the six age bands. The subjects are Australians, generally of lower socioeconomic status, hospitalized for non-neurological or nonpsychiatric disorders. For LM., see Table 10—31.

Quintana (1990) have analyzed data for healthy male and female adults on the visual memory test. No sex differences were noted on the delayed task, although the male–female difference on the immediate task was significant. The mean difference (in favor of the males) was less than one point, and therefore of limited significance clinically.

Solomon and colleagues (1990) provide data for a group of head-injured patients using Russell's version of the WMS. Their norms should be used with considerable caution given the vague description of their subject population.

Some normative date are available for use with children for the AL subtest on Form I (Halperin et al., 1989; Ivinskis et al., 1971). These data are shown in Table 10–35 along with norms for adults that we compiled (Strauss & Spreen, 1989) for the immediate and 30-minute-delay versions of the AL sub-

test. For the delayed version, one point is given for each of the word pairs (maximum = 10).

Normative data, shown in Table 10–36, have recently been made available for Form II (Ivison, 1993b). The norms are derived from a rather large ($n = 600$) sample of hospitalized patients, aged 20–79, with no known neurological or psychiatric impairment. The scores may be somewhat lower than those of community-dwelling people. Ivison (1993b) also provides normalized distributions for each subtest (mean = 10, SD = 3) and for the "memory quotient" total score (mean = 100, SD = 15), and the correlations among subtest scores and factorial analyses of the subtests.

Several patterns emerge from examination of the tables. In general, children score below the level of adults (Curry et al., 1986; Ivinskis et al., 1971). The exception appears to be the Associate Learning subtest where adult levels are reached by about age 7 (Halperin et al.,

1989). For adults, memory function declines with age, although not all dimensions change equally (e.g., Bak & Greene, 1981; Haaland et al., 1983; Hulicka, 1966; Ivnik et al., 1991; Margolis & Scialfa, 1984; Mitrushina & Satz, 1991; Zagar et al., 1984). In general, elderly subjects perform best on PI, OR, and MC. By contrast, VR, LM, and AL prove most difficult with advancing age. Note, however, that on the delayed recall tasks, regardless of age, normal people retain more than 80 percent of their original recollections. The implication is that age differences observed on delayed recall tasks may simply reflect differences in learning during the acquisition phase, rather than an accelerated rate of forgetting in older adults (Trahan, 1992). There is also some evidence (at least in elderly individuals) that percent retained on the LM and VR subtests is not correlated with years of education and Full Scale IQ (Ivnik et al., 1991). The implication is that savings scores may be measures of special clinical and diagnostic significance because they are relatively unaffected by benign age-related memory decline and other demographic variables (Troster et al., 1993).

References

Abikoff, H., Alvir, J., Hong, G., Sukoff, R., Orazio, J., Solomon, S., & Saravay, S. (1987). Logical Memory subtest of the Wechsler Memory Scale: Age and education norms and alternate-form reliability of two scoring systems. *Journal of Clinical and Experimental Neuropsychology, 9,* 435–448.

Abikoff, H., Alvir, J., Hong, G., Sukoff, R., Orazio, J., Solomon, S., & Saravay, S. (1989). Logical Memory subtest of the Wechsler Memory Scale: Age and education norms and alternate-form reliability of two scoring systems; A correction. *Journal of Clinical and Experimental Neuropsychology, 11,* 783.

Alekoumbides, A., Charter, R.A., Adkins, T.G., & Seacat, G.F. (1987). The diagnosis of brain damage by the WAIS, WMS, and Reitan battery utilizing standardized scores corrected for age and education. *The International Journal of Clinical Neuropsychology, 9,* 11–28.

Bak, J.S., & Greene, R.L. (1981). A review of the performance of aged adults on various Wechsler Memory Scale subtests. *Journal of Clinical Psychology, 37,* 186–188.

Bedard, M-A., Montplaisir, J., Richer, F., Rouleau, I., & Malo, J. (1991). Obstructive sleep apnea syndrome: Pathogenesis of neuropsychological deficits. *Journal of Clinical and Experimental Neuropsychology, 13,* 950–964.

Bloom, B.L. (1959). Comparison of the alternate Wechsler Memory Scale forms. *Journal of Clinical Psychology, 15,* 72–74.

Bornstein, R.A. (1982). Effects of unilateral lesions on the Wechsler Memory Scale. *Journal of Clinical Psychology, 6,* 17–36.

Bornstein, R.A., Chelune, G.J., & Prifitera, A. (1989). IQ-memory discrepancies in normal and clinical samples. *Psychological Assessment, 1,* 203–206.

Butters, N. (1986). The clinical aspects of memory disorders. In T. Incognoli, G. Goldstein & C. Golden (Eds.) *Clinical Application of Neuropsychological Test Batteries.* New York: Plenum Press. pp. 361–382.

Butters, N., Salmon, D.P., Cullum, C.M. et al. (1988). Differentiation of amnesic and demented patients with the Wechsler Memory Scale-Revised. *The Clinical Neuropsychologist, 2,* 133–148.

Cauthen, N.R. (1977). Extension of the Wechsler Memory Scale norms to older age groups. *Journal of Clinical Psychology, 33,* 208–211.

Compton, J.M., Sherer, M., & Adams, R.L. (1992). Factor analysis of the Wechsler Memory Scale and the Warrington Recognition Memory Test. *Archives of Clinical Neuropsychology, 7,* 165–173.

Crosson, B., Hughes, C.W., Roth, D.L., & Monkowski, P.G. (1984). Review of Russell's (1975) norms for the Logical Memory and Visual Reproduction subtests of the Wechsler Memory Scale. *Journal of Consulting and Clinical Psychology, 52,* 635–641.

Curry, J.F., Logue, P.E., & Butler, B. (1986). Child and adolescent norms for Russell's revision of the Wechsler Memory Scale. *Journal of Clinical Child Psychology, 15,* 214–220.

Davidoff, G., Roth, E., Thomas, P., Doljanac, R., Dijkers, M., Berent, S., Morris, J., & Yarknoy, G. (1990). Depression and neuropsychological test performance in acute spinal cord injury patients: Lack of correlation. *Archives of Clinical Neuropsychology, 5,* 77–88.

Delaney, R.C., Rosen, A.J., Mattson, R.H., & Novelly, R.A. (1980). Memory function in focal epilepsy: A comparison of nonsurgical, unilateral temporal lobe and frontal lobe samples. *Cortex, 16,* 103–117.

D'Elia, L.D., Satz, P., & Schretlen, D. (1989).

Wechsler Memory Scale: A critical appraisal of the normative studies. *Journal of Clinical and Experimental Neuropsychology, 11*, 551–568.

Delis, D.C. (1989). Neuropsychological assessment of learning and memory. In *Handbook of Neuropsychology*, Vol. 3. F. Boller & J. Grafman (Eds.) Topic Editor: L. Squire. Amsterdam: Elsevier.

Dikmen, S.S., Machamer, J.E., Winn, H.R., & Temkin, N.R. (1995). Neuropsychological outcome at 1 year post head-injury. *Neuropsychology, 9*, 80–90.

Erickson, R.A., & Scott, M.L. (1977). Clinical memory testing: A review. *Psychological Bulletin, 84*, 1130–1149.

Franzen, M.D. (1989). *Reliability and Validity in Neuropsychological Assessment*. New York: Plenum Press.

Guilmette, T.J., Faust, D., Hart, K., & Arkes, H.R. (1990). A national survey of psychologists who offer neuropsychological services. *Archives of Clinical Neuropsychology, 5*, 373–392.

Haaland, K.Y., Linn, R.T., Hunt, W.C., & Goodwin, J.S. (1983). A normative study of Russell's variant of the Wechsler Memory Scale in a healthy elderly population. *Journal of Consulting and Clinical Psychology, 51*, 878–881.

Hall, J.C., & Toal, R. (1957). Reliability (internal consistency) of the Wechsler Memory Scale and correlation with the Wechsler—Bellevue Intelligence Scale. *Journal of Consulting Psychology, 21*, 131–135.

Halperin, J.M., Healey, J.M., Zeitchik, E., Ludman, W.L., & Weinstein, L. (1989). The development of linguistic and mnestic abilities in school-age children. *Journal of Clinical and Experimental Neuropsychology, 11*, 518–528.

Henry, G.K., Adams, R.L., Buck, P., Buchanan, W.I., & Altpeter, T.A. (1990). The American Liner New York and Anna Thompson: An investigation of interference effects on the Wechsler Memory Scale. *Journal of Clinical and Experimental Neuropsychology, 12*, 502–506.

Herman, D.O. (1981). Development of the Wechsler Memory Scale—Revised. *The Clinical Neuropsychologist, 2*, 102–106.

Hom, J. (1992). General and specific cognitive dysfunctions in patients with Alzheimer's disease. *Archives of Clinical Neuropsychology, 7*, 121–133.

Hulicka, I.M. (1966). Age differences in Wechsler Memory Scale scores. *Journal of Genetic Psychology, 109*, 135–145.

Ivinskis, A., Allen, S., & Shaw, E. (1971). An extension of the Wechsler Memory Scales to lower age groups. *Journal of Clinical Psychology, 27*, 354–357.

Ivison, D.J. (1977). The Wechsler Memory Scale: Preliminary findings towards an Australian standardization. *Australian Psychologist, 12*, 303–313.

Ivison, D.J. (1988a). The Wechsler Memory Scale: Relations between Form I and II. *Australian Psychologist, 23*, 219–224.

Ivison, D.J. (1988b). Normative study of the Wechsler Memory Scale, Form 2. Paper presented the 24th International Congress of Psychology, Sydney, Australia.

Ivison, D. (1990). Reliability (stability) study of the Wechsler Memory Scale, Form 2. *The Clinical Neuropsychologist, 4*, 375–378.

Ivison, D. (1993a). Logical memory in the Wechsler Memory Scales: Does the order of passages affect difficulty in an university sample? *The Clinical Neuropsychologist, 7*, 215–218.

Ivison, D. (1993b). Towards a standardization of the Wechsler Memory Scale, Form 2. *The Clinical Neuropsychologist, 7*, 268–280.

Ivnik, R.J., Smith, G.E., Tangalos, E.G., Peterson, R.C., Kokmen, E., & Kurland, L.T. (1991). Wechsler Memory Scale: IQ dependent norms for persons ages 65 to 97 years. *Psychological Assessment: A Journal of Consulting and Clinical Psychology, 3*, 156–161.

Jacobs, D., Troster, A.I., Butters, N., Salmon, D.P., & Cermak, L.S. (1990). Intrusion errors on the visual reproduction test of the Wechsler Memory Scale and the Wechsler Memory Scale—Revised: An analysis of demented and amnesic patients. *The Clinical Neuropsychologist, 4*, 177–191.

Kear-Colwell, J.J., & Heller, M. (1978). A normative study of the Wechsler Memory Scale. *Journal of Clinical Psychology, 34*, 437–444.

Klonoff, H., & Kennedy, M. (1965). Memory and perceptual functioning in octogenarians in the community. *Journal of Gerontology, 20*, 328–333.

Klonoff, H., & Kennedy, M. (1966). A comparative study of cognitive functioning in old age. *Journal of Gerontology, 21*, 239–243.

Larrabee, G.J. (1987). Further caution in interpretation of comparisons between the WAIS-R and the Wechsler Memory Scale. *Journal of Clinical and Experimental Neuropsychology, 9*, 456–460.

Larrabee, G.J., Kane, R., & Schuck, J.R. (1983). Factor analysis of the WAIS and Wechsler Memory Scale: An analysis of the construct validity of the Wechsler Memory Scale. *Journal of Clinical Neuropsychology, 5,* 159–168.

Larrabee, G.J., Kane, R.L., Schuck, J.R., & Francis, D.J. (1985). Construct validity of various memory testing procedures. *Journal of Clinical and Experimental Neuropsychology, 7,* 497–504.

Larrabee, G.J., Trahan, D.E., & Curtiss, G. (1992). Construct validity of the Continuous Visual Memory Test. *Archives of Clinical Neuropsychology, 7,* 395–406.

Lencz, T., McCarthy, G., Bronen, R.A., Scott, T.M., Inserni, J.A., Sass, K.J., Novelly, R.A., Kim, J.H., & Spencer, D.D. (1992). Quantitative magnetic resonance imaging in temporal lobe epilepsy: Relationship to neuropathology and neuropsychological function. *Annals of Neurology, 31,* 629–637.

Levin, H.S., & Larabee, G.J. (1983). Disproportionate decline in visuospatial memory in human aging. *Society for Neuroscience Abstracts, 9,* 21.

Lezak, M.D. (1995). *Neuropsychological Assessment* (3rd Ed.). New York: Oxford University Press.

Loewenstein, D.A., Rupert, M.P., Arguelles, T., & Duara, R. (1995). Neuropsychological test performance and prediction of functional capacities among Spanish-speaking and English-speaking patients with dementia. *Archives of Clinical Neuropsychology, 10,* 75–88.

Loring, D.W., & Papanicolauo, A.C. (1987). Memory assessment in neuropsychology: Theoretical considerations and practical utility. *Journal of Clinical and Experimental Neuropsychology, 9,* 340–358.

Margolis, R.B., & Scialfa, C.T. (1984). Age differences in Wechsler Memory Scale performance. *Journal of Clinical Psychology, 40,* 1442–1449.

Mayeux, R., Brandt, J., Rosen, J., & Benson, D.F. (1980). Interictal memory and language impairment in temporal lobe epilepsy. *Neurology, 30,* 120–125.

McCaffrey, R.J., Ortega, A., Orsilla, S.M., Nelles, W.B., & Haase, R.F. (1992). Practice effects in repeated neuropsychological assessments. *The Clinical Neuropsychologist, 6,* 32–42.

McCarty, S.M., Logue, P.E., Power, D.G., Zeisat, H.A., & Rosenstiel, A.K. (1980). Alternate form reliability and age-related scores for Russell's Revised Wechsler Memory Scale. *Journal of Consulting and Clinical Psychology, 48,* 296–298.

Milanovich, J.R., Axelrod, B.N., & Millis, S.R. (1996). Validation of the Simulation Index—Revised with a mixed clinical population. *Archives of Clinical Neuropsychology, 11,* 53–59.

Milberg, W.P., Hebben, N., & Kaplan, E. (1986). The Boston process approach to neuropsychological assessment. In I. Grant & K.M. Adams (Eds.), *Neuropsychiatric Disorders.* New York: Oxford University Press.

Milner, B. (1975). Psychological aspects of focal epilepsy and its neurosurgical management. *Advances in Neurology, 8,* 299–321.

Mitrushina, M., & Satz, P. (1991). Changes in cognitive functioning associated with normal aging. *Archives of Clinical Neuropsychology, 6,* 49–60.

O'Grady, K.E. (1988). Convergent and discriminant validity of Russell's revised Wechsler Memory Scale. *Personality and Individual Differences, 9,* 321–327.

Oscar-Berman, M., Clancy, J.P., & Weber, D.A. (1993). Discrepancies between IQ and memory scores in alcoholism and aging. *The Clinical Neuropsychologist, 7,* 281–296.

Power, D.G., Logue, P.E., McCarty, S.M., Rosenstiel, A.K., & Zeisat, H.A. (1979). Interrater reliability of the Russell Revision of the Wechsler Memory Scale: An attempt to clarify some ambiguities in scoring. *Journal of Clinical Neuropsychology, 1,* 343–345.

Prigatano, G.P. (1977). Wechsler Memory Scale is a poor screening test for brain dysfunction. *Journal of Clinical Psychology, 33,* 772–777.

Prigatano, G.P. (1978). Wechsler Memory Scale: A selective review of the literature. *Journal of Clinical Psychology, 34,* 816–832.

Prifitera, A., & Barley, W.D. (1985). Cautions in interpretation of comparisons between the WAIS-R and the Wechsler Memory Scale. *Journal of Consulting and Clinical Psychology, 53,* 564–565.

Rawling, P.J., & Brooks, D.N. (1990). Simulation Index: A method for detecting factitious errors on the WAIS-R and WMS. *Neuropsychology, 4,* 223–238.

Rosselli, M., & Ardila, A. (1996). Cognitive effects of cocaine and polydrug abuse. *Journal of Clinical and Experimental Neuropsychology, 18,* 122–135.

Russell, E.W. (1975). A multiple scoring method for the assessment of complex memory functions. *Journal of Consulting and Clinical Psychology, 43,* 800–809.

Russell, E.W. (1988). Renorming Russell's version of the Wechsler Memory Scale. *Journal of Clinical and Experimental Neuropsychology, 10,* 235–249.

Ryan, J.R., Morris, J., Yaffa, S., & Peterson, L. (1981). Test–retest reliability of the Wechsler Memory Scale, Form I. *Journal of Clinical Psychology, 37,* 847–848.

Saling, M.M., Berkovic, S.F., O'Shea, M.F., Kalnins, R.M., Darby, D.G., & Bladin, P.F. (1993). Lateralization of verbal memory and unilateral hippocampal sclerosis. *Journal of Clinical and Experimental Neuropsychology, 15,* 608–616.

Sass, K.J., Sass, A., Westerveld, M., Lencz, T., Novelly, R.A., Kim, J.H., & Spencer, D.D. (1992). Specificity in the correlation of verbal memory and hippocampal neuron loss: Dissociation of memory, language, and verbal intellectual ability. *Journal of Clinical and Experimental Neuropsychology, 14,* 662–672.

Schaie, K.W., & Strother, G.R. (1968). Cognitive and personality variables in college graduates of advanced age. In G.A. Talland (Ed.), *Human Aging and Behavior.* New York: Academic Press.

Schultz, E.E., Keesler, T.Y., Friedenberg, L., & Sciara, A.D. (1984). Limitations in equivalence of alternate subtests for Russell's revision of the Wechsler Memory Scale: Causes and solutions. *Journal of Clinical Neuropsychology, 6,* 220–223.

Schwartz, M.S., & Ivnik, R.J. (1980). Wechsler Memory Scale I: Toward a more objective and systematic scoring system of Logical Memory and Visual Reproduction subtests. Paper presented to the meeting of the American Psychological Association, Montreal.

Sherer, M., Nixon, S.J., Anderson, B.L., & Adams, R.L. (1992). Differential sensitivity of the WMS to the effects of IQ and brain damage. *Archives of Clinical Neuropsychology, 7,* 505–514.

Snow, W.G., Tierney, M.C., Zorzitto, M.L., Fisher, R.H., & Reid, D.W. (1988). One-year test–retest reliability of selected neuropsychological tests in older adults. Paper presented to the International Neuropsychological Society, New Orleans.

Solomon, G.S., Thackston, L., Stetson, B.A., Greene, R.L., & Farr, S.P. (1990). Normative data for closed head injured adults on Russell's version of the Wechsler Memory Scale. *International Journal of Clinical Neuropsychology, 12,* 173–174.

Squire, L.R. (1986). The neuropsychology of memory dysfunction and its assessment. In I. Grant and K. Adams (Eds.), *Neuropsychological Assessment of Neuropsychiatric Disorders.* New York: Oxford University Press.

Stanton, B.A., Jenkins, C.D., Savageau, J.A., & Zyzanski, S.J. (1984). Age and educational differences on the Trail Making Test and Wechsler Memory Scales. *Perceptual and Motor Skills, 58,* 311–318.

Stone, C., & Wechsler, D. (1946). *Wechsler Memory Scale Form II.* San Antonio, TX: The Psychological Corporation.

Strauss, E. & Spreen, D. (1985). Unpublished data.

Trahan, D.E., & Quintana, J.W. (1990). Analysis of gender effects upon verbal and visual memory performance in adults. *Archives of Clinical Neuropsychology, 5,* 325–334.

Trahan, D.E. (1992). Analysis of learning and rate of forgetting in age-associated memory differences. *The Clinical Neuropsychologist, 6,* 241–246.

Trahan, D.E., Quintana, J., Willingham, A.C., & Goethe, K.E. (1988). The visual reproduction subtest: Standardization and clinical validation of a delayed recall procedure. *Archives of Clinical Neuropsychology, 2,* 29–39.

Troster, A.I., Butters, N., Salmon, D.P., Cullum, C.M., Jacobs, D., Brandt, J., & White, R. (1993). The diagnostic utility of saving scores: Differentiating Alzheimer's and Huntington's diseases with the Logical Memory and Visual Reproduction test. *Journal of Clinical and Experimental Neuropsychology, 15,* 773–788.

Webster, J.S., Godlewski, C., Hanley, G.L., & Sowa, M.V. (1992). A scoring method for Logical Memory that is sensitive to right-hemispheric dysfunction. *Journal of Clinical and Experimental Neuropsychology, 14,* 222–238.

Wechsler, D. (1945). A standardized memory scale for clinical use. *Journal of Psychology, 19,* 87–95.

Wechsler, D. (1987). *Wechsler Memory Scale—Revised.* San Antonio, TX: The Psychological Corporation.

Zagar, R., Arbit, J., Stuckey, M., & Wengel, W. (1984). Developmental analysis of the Wechsler Memory Scale. *Journal of Clinical Psychology, 40,* 1466–1473.

WECHSLER MEMORY SCALE—REVISED (WMS-R)

Purpose

The purpose of this test is to provide measures of various aspects of memory function.

Source

The complete WMS-R kit can be obtained from The Psychological Corporation, P.O. Box 9954, San Antonio, TX 78204-0954 at a cost of $309 US or from The Psychological Corporation, 55 Horner Avenue, Toronto, Ontario M5Z 4X6 at a cost of $465 Cdn. The Psychological Corporation provides scoring software with age-extended norms at a cost of $67 US or $105 Cdn for the disk. A new edition (WMS-III) is due in 1997.

Description

The complete kit of the WMS-R (Wechsler, 1987), includes a manual, stimulus cards, record forms, and carrying case. The revision has altered many of the test items: administration and scoring procedures; broadened its coverage of nonverbal and visual memory; and made delayed recall a standard technique. The scale is intended for individuals aged 16–74. The first subtest, Information and Orientation Questions, contains simple questions covering biographical data, orientation, and informational questions such as "Who is the President of the U.S.?" Mental Control requires the subject to recite a series of numbers or letters. On Figural Memory, the subject looks briefly at abstract designs, and then must identify them from an array. Logical Memory I examines the ability to recall ideas in two orally presented stories. On Visual Paired Associates I, the subject is shown six abstract line drawings, each paired with a different color, and is then asked to indicate the appropriate color associated with each figure. Up to six trials are provided to learn the pairs. Verbal Paired Associates I is similar: The subject is read a group of eight word pairs. Subsequently, the first word of each pair is read and the subject must say the second word. Up to six trials are provided to learn the pairs. On

Visual Reproduction I, the subject must draw geometric designs that are exposed briefly. Digit Span consists of two parts and requires the subject to repeat digits forward and in reverse order. The two parts of the Visual Memory Span subtest, Tapping Forward and Tapping Backward, are administered separately. The examiner uses a card printed with colored squares and touches the squares in sequences of increasing length. The subject must reproduce the sequences, forward and in reverse order. Following the administration of the above nine subtests, two verbal and two nonverbal subtests (Logical Memory II, Visual Paired Associates II, Verbal Paired Associates II, and Visual Reproduction II) are given a second time, thus providing 30-minute delayed-recall measures. The first subtest, Information and Orientation Questions, is included on the scale for screening purposes. The remaining 12 subtests yield five age-corrected summary indices, each with a mean of 100 and a SD of 15: One for general immediate memory, separate indexes for immediate verbal and visual memory, one for attention/concentration, and one for general delayed memory.

The Logical Memory (LM) and Visual Reproduction (VR) subtests provide scores only on free recall and lack a measure that assesses storage and retrieval. Gass (1995) has developed a 21-item five-option multiple-choice recognition test for LM (LM-REC) and a cuing technique for VR. The LM-REC questionnaire is presented following the LMII (delay) subtest. It is shown in Figure 10–27. For VR, the examiner provides a visual cue by slowly drawing a small segment of the design to prime recall of the forgotten design(s). Fastenau (1996) has also designed recognition items for LM and added recognition, matching and copy trials for VR.

Administration

The instructions for the WMS-R are given in the manual (see source). Unfortunately, there are no guidelines for speed of presentation of the LM subtest. There is some evidence that a

STORY I

1. The main character in this story was a woman.
   What was her name?
   _____   Nancy Grant
   _____   Annie Thomas
   _____   Mary Jones
   _____   Anna Thompson
   _____   Cathy Taylor

2. Where was this woman from?
   _____   South Boston
   _____   Baltimore
   _____   London
   _____   New York
   _____   West Los Angeles

3. What kind of work did she do?
   _____   house cleaner
   _____   out-of-work (unemployed)
   _____   cook in a cafeteria
   _____   secretary
   _____   waitress

4. What was the main event in this story?
   _____   she went shopping
   _____   she was hospitalized
   _____   she got married
   _____   she had an accident

5. She told the details of this event
   _____   to a friend
   _____   to a doctor
   _____   at the City Hall Station
   _____   in Nashville
   _____   to a newspaper reporter

6. When did the event take place?
   _____   Wednesday
   _____   early afternoon
   _____   the night before
   _____   on the weekend
   _____   during the holiday season

7. Her household included
   _____   her parents
   _____   two little kids
   _____   her husband
   _____   four children
   _____   several pets

8. Who else was mentioned in the story?
   _____   the police
   _____   neighbours
   _____   her parents
   _____   the fire department
   _____   people at church

9. People in the story
   _____   visited her
   _____   were touched by her story
   _____   became friends
   _____   were not able to help her
   _____   gave gifts to her

10. What happened at the end of the story?
    _____   she was given a ride
    _____   a collection was taken up for her
    _____   she got government assistance
    _____   she went on a trip
    _____   she was given flowers

Figure 10—27. Logical Memory Recognition. (Gass 1995. Reprinted with permission of Elsevier Science Ltd.)

slow rate of presentation leads to better performance (Shum et al., 1997). Fastenau (1996) adds 20 multiple-choice recognition items for LM after the delay-recall trial. VRII is also followed by recognition, matching, and copy trials, in that order. Gass' (1995) LM-REC questionnaire is also presented immediately following completion of the LMII subtest. In order to ensure that instructions are understood, the patient is asked to read and respond to the first item aloud and to mark the answer on the questionnaire form.

For VR cuing, instruct as follows: *"You have left out one (two, three, four) of the designs. Now I will try to jog your memory by starting the design for you. I will begin drawing very slowly the design(s) that you were unable to remember. Your task is to stop me as soon as you think you may recall the design. At that point, I will let you complete it. The important point is that I want to see how much you can remember."*

The examiner, using a pencil of a color different than that used by the patient, slowly draws the missing design(s), beginning with the earliest design in the sequence. Design 1 is drawn beginning with the top right-side of the diagonal and drawing downward. This is followed, if necessary, by the second diagonal, again starting at the top. Design 2 is initiated with the larger of the three circles, followed by the second largest circle. Design 3 is started with the upper segment of the large square, drawing left to right, then completing the square in a clockwise manner if necessary. This is followed by drawing its two intersecting vertical and horizontal lines if necessary. The last design starts with the largest rect-

STORY 2

11. The main character in the second story was
_____ Bob Milner
_____ Captain Jack
_____ Robert Miller
_____ Jan Thompson
_____ Rod Mills

12. This person was
_____ driving a taxi
_____ fishing
_____ driving a truck
_____ riding a bus
_____ going to school

13. The story took place in
_____ New Orleans
_____ Mississippi Delta
_____ Rocky Mountains
_____ Massachusetts
_____ a small town

14. The main thing that happened was
_____ he left to go on vacation
_____ he lost his money
_____ he won a contest
_____ he fell and hurt himself
_____ he ran off the road

15. The event occurred
_____ at sunset
_____ the day before
_____ early in the morning
_____ at night
_____ during a vacation

16. What else happened?
_____ friends joined him
_____ his axle broke
_____ he bought a used car
_____ he was given money
_____ he went to a party

17. He was also
_____ badly shaken
_____ robbed
_____ helped by the police
_____ taken to the hospital
_____ rewarded

18. The man was going
_____ to Nashville
_____ home
_____ to Grasshopper Key
_____ to Louisville
_____ to South Boston

19. One problem he had was
_____ he hadn't eaten in 2 days
_____ there was no traffic around to get help
_____ a flat tire
_____ he had no money
_____ he was out of gas

20. At the end of the story
_____ he was rescued
_____ he got his money back
_____ his two-way radio buzzed
_____ he returned home
_____ he found his money

21. What did the man say at the end?
_____ he said nothing
_____ he said, "Great trip"
_____ he said, "This is Grasshopper"
_____ he said, "I need help"
_____ he said, "Thanks a lot"

Figure 10—27. Continued

angle, followed by the upper, and finally the lower of the two smaller rectangles. If the right side of design 4 is omitted, either on free recall or after cuing the left side (rectangles), it is cued beginning with the curved portion of the half circle and followed, if necessary, by the straight vertical line. No direct cuing is performed on the small triangle attached to the semicircle.

The WMS-R is somewhat lengthy to administer. Woodard and Axelrod (1995), using a sample of 308 patients (largely with psychiatric diagnoses) developed regression equations to predict General Memory and Delayed Recall indices based on Logical Memory I, Visual Reproduction I, Verbal Paired Associates I, Logical Memory II, Visual Reproduction II, and Verbal Paired Associates II. The regression equations are provided below, in the section entitled Scoring.

Approximate Time for Administration

The time required is about 45 minutes for the entire test.

Scoring

The WMS-R manual (see source) provides detailed scoring procedures. Briefly, after obtaining the total raw scores on each WMS-R subtest, the examiner must multiply each raw score (except for scores on Information and Orientation questions) by a weight provided on the front of the Record Form. Weighted scores of subtests are summed and then transformed into their corresponding indices by means of an age-graded table in the WMS-R manual (Table C-1). Each index has a mean of 100 and an SD of 15.

The utility of the WMS-R is enhanced by the provision of percentile scores (relative to a sample of healthy control subjects) for a number of subtests including Digit Span, Visual Memory Span, Logical Memory, and Visual Reproduction (Tables C-4 and C-5 in the WMS-R manual).

Scores on the Information and Orientation questions are intended primarily to identify persons for whom the meaning of scores on the rest of the scale may be questionable. Frequency distributions for raw scores on this subtest are given in Table C-2 of the WMS-R manual.

For Gass' (1995) LM-REC, the scoring procedure involves counting the number of correct items (range 0–21). Scoring of cued VR recall is based on the same criteria that the WMS-R manual applied to scoring free recall. However, points are not allotted for any criteria that were reached or otherwise given away by the examiner in the cuing process. Education affects performance on these tasks. Gass (1995) recommends adding 1 point for persons with less than 11 years of education, and subtracting 1 point for those with more than 14 years of education.

Woodard and Axelrod (1995) provide regression equations in order to predict General Memory and Delayed Recall indices from a subset of WMS-R subtests. For each index, estimated weighted raw score sums are calculated by multiplying the unstandardized regression weights (b weights) by the raw subtest scores and adding the constant for each equation, rounding the final result. The equations are as follows: General Memory raw score sum = $2.1 \times$ LMI + $1.19 \times$ VRI + $1.45 \times$ VEPAI + 3.14. Delayed Recall raw score sum = $0.99 \times$ LMII + $1.07 \times$ VRII + $2.67 \times$ VePAII + 4.31. The index scores are obtained

by converting the estimated sum of weighted raw scores to an age-corrected index equivalent through Table C-1 in the WMS-R manual. Woodard and Axelrod (1995) reported that predicted GM and DR scores fell within 6 points of obtained scores for 92 percent and 96 percent of their sample who typically carried psychiatric diagnoses. Cross-validation with a sample of patients referred for evaluation of possible traumatic brain injury yielded similar results (Axelrod et al., 1996). It is also worth noting that Woodard and Axelrod (1995) found that there was a slight tendency for the regression equation for the General Memory index to underpredict younger patients' actual performance and overpredict performance for older patients. The regression equation for predicting the Delayed Recall index did not reflect such a pattern and tended to be slightly more accurate overall.

Comment

Wechsler (1987) presents test–retest correlation coefficients for five of the subtests and internal consistency estimates for the remaining seven subtests. The average reliability coefficients across age groups for individual subtests ranged from only .41 (Verbal Paired Associates II) to .88 (Digit Span), with a median reliability coefficient of .74. Mittenberg et al., (1992) reported that reliability coefficients for the Logical Memory (Spearman-Brown) and Visual Reproduction (coefficient alpha) subtests ranged from .71 (LMI) to .87 (VR 1 and 2). Reliability coefficients for the summary indices ranged from .70 (Visual Memory) to .90 (Attention/Concentration) (see source). Although the reliability of the summary indices is better than that of the individual subtests, the standard errors of measurement are quite large, ranging from about 5 points for the Attention/Concentration Index to about 8.5 points across age levels for the Visual Memory Index. Thus, for an individual with a true Visual Memory Index of 100, the individual's observed score would fall between 91 and 109 approximately two-thirds of the time over a large number of testing trials of that individual. The low reliabilities (and consequently larger SEMs) of individual subtests and composite scores limit interpretation of sub-tests, composites, and their differences (except for the Attention/Concentration and General Memory composites, which achieved acceptable reliability coefficients) (Chelune et al., 1989; Huebner, 1992). Similarly, correlations between WMS-R scores and other cognitive test measures should also be interpreted in light of the reliability of the measures being correlated.

A number of authors use percent retention scores by comparing the amount of information recalled after a half-hour delay (e.g., on LM and VR) with the amount recalled immediately. Although these savings scores have been found to be useful (see below), it is important to bear in mind that no formal reliability study has been conducted with these measures and that they are based on the ratio of test scores that, themselves, have less-than-perfect reliabilities (Chelune et al., 1989).

With regard to temporal stability, Wechsler (1987) used a retest interval of 4 to 6 weeks and noted that there was an increase in scores on most of the subtests and composites from the first to the second testing. There appears to be an inverse relationship between age and magnitude of practice effect (Chelune et al., 1989; Mittenberg et al., 1991). For example, individuals aged 20–24 demonstrated a net gain of about 12 raw score points on the Delayed Memory Index if retested within a 6-week interval, whereas older individuals, aged 70–74 years, showed an average gain of about 6 raw score points on retesting. Table 10–37 (Mittenberg et al., 1991) is provided in order to evaluate results obtained following short retest intervals (4–6 weeks). Table values for critical ranges indicate the differences obtained by less than 5 percent of the standardization sample for a directional hypothesis only. For example, an average 20-year-old can be expected to show a 15.04 point (SD = 10.39) retest gain on the General Memory Index. A decline of at least 2.11 points or an improvement of 32.19 points would fall outside the normal range. Two-tailed ($p < .05$) critical values can be computed by multiplying the standard deviation by 1.96 and bounding the mean improvement with this value. Mittenberg et al. point out that some decline, particularly on the Attention/Concentration, Visual Memory, and Visual Reproduction subtests, was common in the standardization sample and is therefore not likely to be of practical relevance.

Bowden et al. (1995) reassessed alcohol dependent clients (mean age = 39.3 years, SD = 10.0) following an interval of about 137 days. Test–retest correlations were high (above .8) across the five indices. Improvement in scores was noted on the second administration, but the magnitude of the differences was relatively modest (ranging from 2 to 6 points), and scores at retest typically fell within the predicted 95 percent confidence interval.

Scoring for most of the WMS-R is relatively simple and straightforward. Extensive scoring rules were developed for the Logical Memory and Visual Reproduction subtests. Wechsler (1987) reports that interscorer reliability coefficients for the Logical Memory and Visual Reproduction were .99 and .97, respectively (see also Sullivan, 1996, for independent confirmation with regard to interrater reliability for LM). Accurate administration and scoring of the Visual Memory Span subtest is problematic, however, because accuracy depends upon the experience and concentration of the examiner (Demsky & Sellers, 1995). Reliability can be increased substantially by using a cue-card method that displays a reduced facsimile of the stimulus card along with the order, in numbers, of the correct tapping sequence (Demsky & Sellers, 1995).

In terms of validity, Delis et al. (1988) report numerous strong correlations between the WMS-R and the California Verbal Learning Test. The highest correlation was between the WMS-R Delayed Memory Index and the CVLT Long Delay Free Recall score (.93). Randolph et al. (1994) recorded the correlations between the WMS-R indices and the CVLT score for the sum of trials 1–5. All correlations were significant and the highest correlation (.79) was between the CVLT Total T score and the General Memory Index. The tests, however, cannot be used interchangeably to provide estimates of degree of impairment (Randolph et al., 1994). Although both tests appear equally sensitive to memory impairment, memory-impaired patients routinely score lower on the CVLT than on the WMS-R,

Table 10—37. Standard Deviation of Differences and Critical Levels for Abnormality of Differences on Retest for Wechsler Memory Scale–Revised Subscales

Scale	Age 20–24		Age 55–64		Age 70–74		Average	
	Mean difference ± SD	95% limit lower/upper	Mean difference ± SD	95% limit lower/upper	Mean difference ± SD	95% limit lower/upper	Mean difference ± SD	95% limit lower/upper
General Memory	15.04 ± 10.39	−2.11/32.19	15.03 ± 10.17	−1.76/31.82	9.70 ± 7.94	−3.40/22.80	13.27 ± 9.49	−2.38/28.92
Attention/Concentration	5.13 ± 9.25	−10.13/20.39	1.01 ± 8.75	−13.42/15.44	2.75 ± 5.61	−6.51/12.01	2.90 ± 7.65	−9.72/12.01
Verbal Memory	14.85 ± 12.37	−5.56/35.26	13.60 ± 12.00	−6.20/33.40	7.95 ± 8.49	−6.05/21.95	12.13 ± 10.82	−5.72/29.98
Visual Memory	6.64 ± 10.61	−10.87/24.15	10.08 ± 13.91	−12.87/33.03	7.98 ± 9.49	−7.67/23.63	8.29 ± 11.23	−10.23/26.81
Delayed Recall	15.00 ± 11.42	−3.84/33.84	10.21 ± 9.25	−5.05/25.47	7.72 ± 8.49	−6.28/21.72	10.91 ± 9.49	−4.74/26.56
Logical Memory	15.21 ± 12.19	−4.90/32.30	13.81 ± 12.73	−7.19/34.81	6.58 ± 8.75	−7.58/21.01	11.86 ± 11.02	−6.33/30.05
Visual Reproduction	2.02 ± 9.49	−13.64/17.68	5.77 ± 14.07	−17.45/28.99	2.88 ± 10.17	−13.91/19.67	3.62 ± 11.02	−14.57/21.81
Logical Memory 2	18.55 ± 11.23	−0.02/37.08	17.00 ± 11.62	−2.17/36.17	7.50 ± 9.00	−7.35/22.35	14.35 ± 10.61	−3.15/31.85
Visual Reproduction 2	5.16 ± 13.75	−17.53/27.85	1.88 ± 12.08	−17.92/21.68	3.07 ± 9.49	−12.59/18.73	3.32 ± 11.81	−16.17/22.81

Source: Mittenberg et al. 1991. Reprinted with permission of the American Psychological Association.

perhaps reflecting the fact that the CVLT normative sample was higher functioning and more homogeneous than the population-based standardization sample of the WMS-R. Alternatively, the WMS-R standardization sample may suffer from less-than-stringent screening for cognitive deficits.

Crossen and Wiens (1988b) administered the WMS-R to 13 patients who had suffered moderate to severe head injuries. The scores for the five WMS-R indices were compared to performance on the RAVLT, Rey-Osterrieth Complex Figure, and the PASAT. The construct validity of the Verbal, Visual, and Delayed Memory indices was supported by impaired performance on the other tests of verbal and visual memory and delayed recall. On the other hand, more severe deficits were observed on the PASAT than on the Attention/Concentration Index. The implication is that additional measures of attention and concentration should be used to supplement the WMS-R in clinical practice.

Factor analyses of the WMS-R have found evidence of one (Elwood, 1991), two (general memory and attention/concentration) (Wechsler, 1987; Bornstein & Chelune, 1988; Roid et al., 1988; Smith et al., 1992a), or three factors (Attention/concentration, visual memory, and verbal memory: Bornstein & Chelune, 1989; Attention, general memory, and percent retention: Smith et al. 1992a; Attention, immediate, and delayed memory: Burton et al., 1993; Roth et al., 1990; Woodard, 1993), rather than the five-factor model that guided the construction of the WMS-R.

There have been a number of factor analytic studies of the WMS-R that included other measures (Bornstein & Chelune, 1988; Franzen et al., 1995; Leonberger et al., 1991, 1992; Nicks et al., 1992; Smith et al., 1992a; Smith et al., 1992b; Wechsler, 1987). The WMS-R manual (Wechsler, 1987) reports the results of principal components factor analyses of the age-corrected raw scores on the WMS-R immediate recall subtests with WAIS-R Full Scale IQ scores, computed separately for the standardization sample and a mixed clinical sample. In each analysis, two factors emerged, a general memory and an attention/concentration factor with FSIQ scores

loading on the latter factor. Similar results were obtained by Bornstein and Chelune (1988). However, when the delay scores were included, a three-factor solution emerged. Attention/Concentration tasks loaded together along with VIQ and PIQ, but the remaining subtests loaded on what were interpreted to be verbal and nonverbal memory dimensions. Franzen et al. (1995) reported that when the WMS-R Index scores were factor analyzed with the Knox Cube Test, the Trailmaking Test, and the Stroop, all index scores with the exception of the Attention/Concentration Index, loaded on the same factor. Using individual subtest scores, Franzen et al. (1995) found a distinction between verbal (Logical Memory I and II, Verbal Paired Associates I and II, and Information) and nonverbal memory (Visual Paired Associates I and II, Visual Reproduction I and II, and Figural Memory). Immediate and delayed recall, however, loaded on the same factor. By contrast, Leonberger et al. (1991, 1992) found that when the WMS-R data were factor analyzed along with the WAIS-R and Halstead-Reitan data, separate verbal and nonverbal components failed to emerge. The Attention/Concentration Index received some support in that two of three measures that make up the index (Digit Span and Mental Control) factored with other attention and concentration measures from the WAIS-R (Arithmetic) and Halstead-Reitan Battery (Speech Sounds Perception Test and Rhythm Test). However, the Visual Memory Span test loaded on a spatial reasoning factor and only loaded weakly with other measures of attention and concentration. None of the Halstead-Reitan measures loaded substantially on the memory factors defined by the WMS-R subtests. Nicks et al. (1992) reported the results of a principal components factor analysis of the WMS-R and WAIS subtest. Six factors emerged labeled as: Perceptual Organization, Verbal Comprehension, Attention/Concentration, Complex Verbal Memory, Verbal Paired-Associate Memory, and Visual Paired Associate Memory. Two of the three subtests that make up the Visual Memory Index (Figural Memory and Visual Reproduction I) loaded with the Performance subtests of the WAIS, suggesting that a good measure of nonverbal memory, apart from general measures of visuospatial abilities, remains elusive (see also Leonberger et al., 1992; Smith et al., 1992b). In a confirmatory factor analysis of combined WAIS-R, WMS-R, and RAVLT measures, Smith and colleagues (1992b) found support for a five-factor model that included Verbal Comprehension, Perceptual Organization, Attention, Learning, and Retention. The Retention factor included Logical Memory, Visual Reproduction, and RAVLT percent retention scores. They also found that Visual Reproduction I may relate more to visuoperceptual abilities than to learning or memory. In an exploratory factor analysis that included the WAIS-R, the WMS-R, the RAVLT, and Visual Spatial Learning Test, Smith et al. (1992b) found evidence only of a single general memory factor; no modality or time-specific factors were found.

In reviewing these factor-analytic studies, there is relatively consistent evidence to support interpretation of the WMS-R General Memory and Attention/Concentration Indices. Tentative support exists for the reporting of a retention or a delayed-memory factor. There is less consistent support for verbal and nonverbal dimensions. The reasons for the discrepant findings among studies likely reflect a number of sources of variation, including differences in factor-analytic procedures (e.g., the treatment of measurement error; whether delayed-recall tasks were included), differences in the composition of samples used (e.g., health status, nature, and location of lesions, age, education), the particular WMS-R measures evaluated (e.g., Logical Memory II vs. percent retention) and what other test data have been included. The clinical utility of the WMS-R, however, need not depend upon a reliable multifactorial structure (Elwood, 1991). For example, comparisons between General Memory and Delayed Recall indices (Butters et al., 1988) and Delayed Recall and IQ (Bornstein et al., 1989a) have been found to discriminate subgroups of neurologic patients even though the evidence for corresponding factors is conflicting.

There is evidence that the test is sensitive to memory disorders and may characterize the learning and memory disorders in a number of different patient groups including those with Alzheimer's disease, Huntington's disease (HD), multiple sclerosis, closed head injury, Kosakoff's, long-term alcoholism, anterior communicating artery aneurysm, exposure to neurotoxins, schizophrenia, and depression (Butters et al., 1988; Chelune & Bornstein, 1988a,b; Crossen & Wiens, 1988a; Gold et al., 1992; Fischer, 1988; Kixmiller et al., 1995; Oscar-Berman et al., 1993; O'Mahony & Doherty, 1993; Ryan & Lewis, 1988; Wechsler, 1987). For example, Crossen and Wiens (1988b) reported that the performance of moderate-to-severe head-injury patients was well below normal on all composite indices with the exception of the Attention/Concentration Index. In schizophrenia, attention and memory were equally impaired (Gold et al., 1992). Janowsky et al. (1989) found that in patients with frontal lobe lesions, the Attention/Concentration Index was lower than the memory indices. By contrast, patients with Korsakoff's disease performed within the average range on the Attention/Concentration Index but very poorly on the other indices.

Savings scores [% = (delayed recall/immediate recall) × 100] are related to the extent of hippocampal atrophy in traumatically brain-injured patients (Bigler et al., 1996). Trenerry et al. (1996) examined savings scores on the Visual Reproduction subtest and found that extirpation of a relatively large right hippocampus produces a decline in visual memory, but only in female epileptics. Savings scores also appear to be especially good detectors of AD (Dementia of Alzheimer's Type) (Butters et al., 1988; Troster et al., 1993). Troster et al. (1993) found that patients with AD showed more rapid forgetting (that is, poorer savings scores for Logical Memory and Visual Reproduction) than patients with Huntington's disease (HD). These saving scores had satisfactory-to-excellent sensitivity and specificity in differentiating AD and HD patients from healthy control subjects. The savings scores also had good sensitivity in differentiating AD from HD in the early stages of the diseases. Although these indices of forgetting continue to be sensitive in the middle stages of the disease, their increased variability, and the attendant decrease in specificity, limits their utility in distinguishing between moderately demented AD and HD patients.

Although there is some evidence that the WMS-R is somewhat sensitive to lateralized dysfunction (e.g., Barr et al., 1997; Bornstein, Pakalnis, & Drake, 1989; Chelune & Bornstein, 1988a,b; Naugle et al., 1993; Strauss et al., 1995), the Verbal and Visual Memory Indices cannot be used with any confidence to infer lateralized brain dysfunction. For example, Loring et al., (1989) found that the discrepancy between WMS-R Verbal and Visual Memory Indices was insensitive to the material-specific memory deficits associated with temporal lobectomy, and often incorrectly identified the laterality of resection (see also Kneebone et al., 1997).

Depression has been associated with attentional and memory difficulties. Some have reported that the WMS-R attention and concentration measures are affected by depression (King et al., 1995) whereas others have reported that these measures are least affected by depressed mood (Wechsler, 1987). Depression (as measured on the MMPI) may lower Logical Memory (LM I and LM II) (Blackwood, 1996; Fox, 1994; Gass, 1996; King et al., 1995) and Visual Reproduction (VR I, VR II, and percent retention) (Boone et al., 1995; Gass, 1996) scores, and thus reflect or mimic neuropsychological impairment. Claimants in litigation, especially if they report depressive complaints, may be particularly prone to misdiagnosis. Savings scores (the percent of memories retained) seems to be less affected by, but are not immune to, psychological distress.

Discrepancies between Wechsler IQ and WMS Memory Quotients of 10 to 12 points have been suggested to be indicative of specific memory disturbances (Milner, 1975). The WMS-R memory indices provide the potential for examining general as well as material-specific deficits in relation to WAIS-R IQ scores. Recall that these IQ scores appear to be relatively independent of the memory dimensions (see discussion of factor-analytic studies above). Simple IQ-Memory index discrepancies, however, cannot be used in isolation to identify memory deficits. Bornstein et

al., (1989a) reported that in a sample of patients who had diagnoses associated with memory disorders (e.g., Alzheimer's, epilepsy), discrepancy scores based on IQ and scales reflecting immediate memory (Verbal, Visual Memory) were not effective for clinical documentation of memory deficits. Discrepancies between FSIQ and Delayed Memory Index scores did differentiate patients from normal controls (see also Oscar-Berman et al. 1993). However, only one-third had FSIQ-Delayed Memory Index discrepancies that were greater than 15 points (see also Gold et al, 1992). That is, the majority of patients obtained scores that were more similar to those of normal controls (see Table 10–38 for prevalence data regarding IQ-Memory Index discrepancies).

It is important to keep in mind that the Attention/Concentration Index correlates highly with general intelligence whereas memory, as measured by the WMS-R, appears to be largely independent of IQ, as measured by the WAIS-R (Bornstein & Chelune, 1988). This difference between the Attention/Concentration and General Memory Indices may be useful in distinguishing among certain memory disorders; e.g., amnesia vs. dementia (Butters et al., 1988).

While patients' subjective experience of memory disturbance shows little correlation with actual performance on the WMS-R, there is a modest association of WMS-R scores with rating of memory disturbance by caregivers and health-care professionals (Chelune et al., 1989; Ryan & Lewis, 1988). The WMS-

Table 10—38. Percentage of Normal Subjects Exceeding IQ-Memory Index Discrepancies at Various Levels

Score	FSIQ-DMI (%)	VIQ-VbMI (%)	PIQ-VsMI (%)
12	18.2	24	25
15	10	15	18
21	7.3		
22	5.5	5	5
28	0		

Source: Bornstein et al. (1989). Copyright 1945, 1974, 1987, 1992 by The Psychological Corporation. Reprinted with permission.

R also appears to relate to work status. Crossen and Wiens (1988a) examined WMS-R performance among a sample of painters with a history of solvent exposure. Employed painters obtained higher WMS-R scores than those that were unemployed.

Information from the WMS-R may be useful in detecting incomplete effort. Bernard (1991) reported that malingerers showed inconsistent performance, while Mittenberg et al. (1993) found that individuals instructed to malinger tended to do worse on measures of attention relative to their performance on measures of memory. The average malingerer in the study earned a General Memory Index score that was one standard deviation below average and an attention/Concentration index score that was two standard deviations below normal. A difference score of 32, favoring the General Memory Index corresponded to a 95 percent chance of malingering. Recently, Iverson and Franzen (1996) have developed a two-alternative forced-choice supplement to the Logical Memory subtest. A cutting score of 18 out of 24 correctly classified all of the control and memory-impaired subjects and yielded an 85 percent correct classification rate for experimental malingerers.

The WMS-R is an improvement over the original standard version. It does, however, have limitations. The WMS-R is lengthier to administer although a shortened version is available (Woodard & Axelrod, 1995; see Administration and Scoring). There is no parallel form. Norms for certain age groups (18–19, 25–34, 45–54) were interpolated, and normative data for children and adolescents are unavailable. The WMS-R was also not standardized for subjects older than 74 years—a significant gap since memory complaints are overrepresented in this population (Franzen, 1989). It does not allow the awarding of scores below 50 and, as a result, some patients' scores may be inflated (Butters et al., 1988). It is still primarily a test of verbal learning (Chelune & Bornstein, 1988b; Loring, 1990). The new "nonverbal" subtests are not pure measures of visual learning/memory. Moreover, when calculating the indices (General, Verbal, and Visual), verbal memory performance continues to contribute more heavily. The Delayed

Memory Index represents the delayed-recall trials of both verbal and nonverbal tasks and thus confounds any potential for examination of material-specific memory deficits (Bornstein et al., 1989b; Chelune et al., 1989). Construction of the Delayed Memory Index also failed to recognize the importance of examining delayed recall as a percentage of initially learned information (Chelune et al., 1989; Cullum et al., 1990; Smith et al., 1992a). The lack of reliability of the subtests and some of the index scores, the rather large standard errors of measurement for the summary index scores, as well as the lack of support for the construct validity of some of the indices (e.g., Verbal Memory, Visual Memory) restrict interpretation (Chelune et al., 1989; Huebner, 1992). The absence of recognition tasks also limits the capacity of the scale to differentiate among patient populations (Butters et al., 1988; Chelune & Bornstein; 1988b), although this may be rectified to some extent by the inclusion of the adaptations provided recently by Gass (1995) and Fastenau (1996). Further, rate of acquisition is ignored (Chelune & Bornstein, 1988b), as are olfactory and tactile memory and memory for previously learned skills (Holden, 1988). Rigid adherence to the scoring rules for the Visual Reproduction designs may place an emphasis on drawing accuracy rather than amount of information learned. Deficits in visual perception may also confound interpretation on this task (Haut et al., 1994). Clinicians need to use measures of perception (e.g., matching) and construction (e.g., copying) on the VR test to control for deficits in these areas (Fastenau, 1996). Finally, the figural changes in the Visual Reproduction Test may limit qualitative analyses that might prove useful in differentiating patient populations. Jacobs et al. (1990) reported that the introduction of circular figures, especially the concentric circles on Card B, may reduce the tendency of demented patients to intrude characteristics of previous figures into their current reproduction of stimuli; that is, the circular figures may release patients from the effects of proactive interference between the linear figures, thereby decreasing the number of intrusion errors.

Despite these limitations, the Scale (WMS-

R) is an improvement over its predecessor, the WMS, in terms of task content, adequacy of scoring criteria, and normative data. Accordingly, it may offer a fairly quick first step in the assessment of memory. Examination of the subtests may offer clues about spared and impaired functions. More detailed assessment, however, will be needed.

In an effort to address some of the concerns, the WMS-R is being updated. The WMS-III (due out in 1997) includes individuals in each age group, an extension of the normative sample to include older adults (e.g., 74–89), and co-norming with the WAIS-III, allowing clinicians to better assess IQ/MQ discrepancy scores and multiple domains of cognitive functioning. Recognition and learning tasks have been added. Two subtests have been deleted (Figural Memory and Visual Paired Associates) and a number of new subtests have been provided (e.g., Word List Learning, Memory for Faces).

Normative Data

The test was standardized on a sample considered representative of the U.S. population. The WMS-R manual provides norms for individuals aged 16:0–74:11. Norms are based on about 50 cases in each of six age groups (ages 16–17, 20–24, 35–44, 55–65, 65–69, 70–74). Norms were estimated for ages 18–19, 25–34, and 45–54. D'Elia et al. (1989) recommend the original WMS for individuals in these latter age groups (but see Bowden & Bell, 1992, who argue that the use of interpolated normative data provided in the WMS-R manual does not violate the necessary assumptions, and that use of the WMS-R as opposed to the WMS is likely to provide more accurately scored and interpretable information regarding memory function.) Mittenberg et al. (1992) provide WMS-R norms for individuals in the 25- to 34-year-old range, based on a sample considered representative of 1980 U.S. census data. The empirically obtained values were compared to those in the manual for adjacent age groups. The group of 25–34-years old earned higher scores on the Visual Memory Span, VR II, and Information/Orientation subtests than did the group of 35-

to 44-year olds and higher Information/Orientation scores than did the group of 20- to 24-year olds. Differences between the empirically derived and published index scores appeared to be clinically significant. In certain instances the estimated and empirical index scores differed by 15–18 points. The normative data for clients aged 25–34 years presented by Mittenberg et al. (1992) for the WMS-R subtests and index equivalents of sums of weighted raw scores are shown in Tables 10–39 and 10–40. Comparison between the general and delayed indices indicated that differences of ≥12.4 points in favor of the General Memory Index were sufficiently rare in the sample to be considered significantly different from normal at the .05 level. Differences of 8.5 points in favor of the Delayed Recall index occurred in less than 5 percent of the sample. Comparisons between the Verbal and Visual Memory indices showed that Verbal greater than Visual index scores of ≥32 points and Visual greater than Verbal index scores of ≥26 points were sufficiently rare in the sample to be considered significantly different from normal at the .05 level. With regard to the General Memory and Attention/Concentration indices, differences of ≥18 points in either direction could be considered abnormal at the .05 level. Given the finding of

Table 10—39. Raw-Score Means and Standard Deviations for the Wechsler Memory Scale—Revised, Ages 25–34

Subtest	M	SD	Range
Information/Orientation	13.88	0.33	13–14
Mental Control	4.98	1.13	2–6
Figural Memory	7.20	1.49	4–10
Logical Memory 1	26.04	6.81	11–40
Visual Paired Associates 1	15.12	3.39	5–18
Verbal Paired Associates 1	20.80	3.16	12–24
Visual Reproduction 1	34.52	5.39	16–41
Digit Span	14.96	3.71	7–22
Visual Memory Span	17.66	3.62	10–25
Logical Memory 2	22.38	7.38	9–37
Visual Paired Associates 2	5.60	0.95	2–6
Verbal Paired Associates 2	7.62	0.86	4–8
Visual Reproduction 2	32.88	6.59	13–41

Source: Mittenberg et al., 1992. Reprinted with permission of American Psychological Association.

Table 10—40. Index Equivalents of Sums of Weighted Raw Scores, Ages 25–34 Years

Index score	Raw scores				
	Verbal memory	Visual memory	General memory	Attention/ concentration	Delayed recall
50	22	27	61–62	25	30
51	23	—	63	26	31
52	24	28	64	27	32
53	25	—	65–66	28	33
54	26	29	67	—	34
55	27	30	68	29	35
56	28	—	69–70	30	36
57	29	31	71	31	37
58	30	—	72–73	32	38
59	31	32	74	33	39
60	32	—	75	34	40
61	33	33	76–77	35	41
62	34	34	78	36	42
63	35	—	79	—	43
64	36	35	80–81	37	44
65	37	36	83	38	45
66	38	36	83	39	46
67	39	37	84–85	40	47
68	40	—	86	41	48
69	41	38	87	42	49
70	42	—	88–89	43	50
71	43	39	90	44	51
72	44	40	91	45	52
73	45	—	92–93	—	53
74	46	41	94	46	54
75	47	—	95	47	55
76	48	42	96–97	48	56
77	49	43	98	49	57–58
78	50	—	99–100	50	59
79	51	44	101	51	60
80	52	—	102	52	61
81	53	45	103–104	53	62
82	54	46	105	—	63
83	55	—	106	54	64
84	56	47	107–108	55	65
85	57	—	109	56	66
86	58	48	110	57	67
87	59	49	111–112	58	68
88	60	—	113	59	69
89	61	50	114	60	70
90	62	—	115–116	61	71
91	63	51	117	—	72
92	64	52	118	62	73
93	65	—	119–120	63	74
94	66	53	121	64	75
95	67	—	122	65	76
96	68–69	54	123–124	66	77
97	70	—	125	67	78
98	71	55	126–127	68	79
99	72	56	128	69	80

(*continued*)

Table 10—40. *(Continued)*

Index score	Raw scores				
	Verbal memory	Visual memory	General memory	Attention/ concentration	Delayed recall
100	73	—	129	70	81
101	74	57	130–131	—	82
102	75	—	132	71	83
103	76	58	133	72	84
104	77	59	134–135	73	85
105	78	—	136	74	86
106	79	60	137	75	87
107	80	—	138–139	76	88
108	81	61	140	77	89
109	82	62	141	78	90
110	83	—	142–143	—	91
111	84	63	144	79	92
112	85	—	145	80	93
113	86	64	146–147	81	94
114	87	65	148	82	95
115	88	—	149	83	96
116	89	66	150–151	84	97
117	90	—	152	85	98
118	91	67	153–154	86	99
119	92	68	155	—	100
120	93	—	156	87	101
121	94	69	157–158	88	102
122	95		159	89	103
123	96		160	90	104
124	97		161–162	91	105
125	98		163	92	106
126	99		164	93	107
127	100		165–166	94	108
128	101		167	95	109
129	102		168	—	110
130	103		169–170	96	111
131	104		171	97	112
132	105		172	98	113
133	106		173–174	99	114
134	107		175	100	115
135	108		176	101	116
136	109		177–178	102	117
137	110		179	103	118
138	111		180–181	—	119
139	112		182	104	
140	113+		183+	105–106	

Source: Mittenberg et al., 1992. Reprinted with permission of American Psychological Association.

differences between estimated and empirical scores in the 25- to 34-year age group, normative studies in the age ranges of 18 to 19 and 45 to 54 years would appear to be useful.

Wechsler (1987) did not give data for elderly individuals. Cullum et al. (1990) provided some preliminary normative data based on a small sample ($n = 32$) of highly educated individuals between the ages of 75–95. Lichtenberg and Christensen (1992) presented data on the Logical Memory subtest, based on a sample of 66 cognitively intact medical patients. The average educational level was lower in this study, and scores for Logical Memo-

moans

Table 10—41. MOANS Scaled Scores, Midpoint Age = 76 (Age Range = 71–81, n = 160)

	WMS-R Subtests—Immediate Recall Measures								
MOANS Scaled Scores	Mental Control	Figural Memory	Logical Memory I	Visual Paired Assoc. I	Verbal Paired Assoc. I	Visual Reprod. I	Digit Span	Visual Span	Percentile Ranges
2	0–1	0	0–3	0	0–6	0–13	0–4	0–3	<1
3	—	1–2	4–5	—	7	14–15	5–7	4–5	1
4	—	—	6–7	1	8	16	—	6–7	2
5	2	3	8–12	2	9	17–18	8	8–9	3–5
6	3	—	13–14	3	10–11	19–20	—	10	6–10
7	—	4	15–16	4–5	12	21–22	9–10	11	11–18
8	4	—	17–18	6	13	23–24	11	—	19–28
9	—	5	19	7	14	25–26	12	12	29–40
10	5	—	20–22	8–10	15–17	27–29	13	13	41–59
11	—	6	23–25	11–12	—	30–32	14	14	60–71
12	6	—	26–27	13	18–19	33	15	15	72–81
13	—	7	28–29	14–15	20	34	16	16	82–89
14	—	—	30–31	16	21	35	17	17	90–94
15	—	8	32–34	—	—	36	18–19	—	95–97
16	—	9	35–37	17	22	37	—	18	98
17	—	—	38	18	23	38	20	19	99
18	—	10	39–50	—	24	39–41	21–24	20–26	>99

	WMS-R Subtests—Delayed Recall Measures						
					Percent Retention		
MOANS Scaled Scores	Logical Memory II	Visual Paired Assoc. II	Verbal Paired Assoc. II	Visual Reprod. II	Logical Memory Percent	Visual Reprod. Percent	Percentile Ranges
2	0–1	—	0–1	0–1	0–7	0–10	<1
3	—	—	—	2–3	8–15	11–18	1
4	2	—	—	4	16–29	19–24	2
5	3–4	0	2	5–6	30–40	25–32	3–5
6	5–8	—	3	7–9	41–47	33–40	6–10
7	9–10	1	4	10–11	48–61	41–48	11–18
8	11–12	—	—	12–15	62–66	49–61	19–28
9	13–14	2	—	16–17	67–72	62–66	29–40
10	15–17	3	5–6	18–20	73–81	67–73	41–59
11	18–21	4	—	21–24	82–84	74–83	60–71
12	22–23	5	—	25–28	85–89	84–91	72–81
13	24–25	6	7	29–31	90–93	92–97	82–89
14	26–28	—	8	32–33	94–96	98–100+	90–94
15	29–30	—	—	34–35	97–99	—	95–97
16	31	—	—	36	100+	—	98
17	32–35	—	—	37–39	—	—	99
18	36–50	—	—	40–41	—	—	>99

Note: MOANS = Mayo's Older Americans Normative Studies, WMS-R = Wechsler Memory Scale—Revised. MOANS Scaled scores are corrected for age influences.

Source: Ivnik et al. (1992). Reproduced with permission of the Mayo Clinic.

ry I and II were also considerably lower than those reported by Cullum et al. (1990). Recently, Ivnik et al. (1992) published normative (Mayo Older Adult Normative Study, MOANS) data based on a sample of 441 cog-nitively normal older Americans, aged 56–97 years, on the WMS-R. Memory indices derived from these norms are called MAYO Verbal Memory (MVeMI), MAYO Visual Memory (MViMI), MAYO General Memory (MGMI),

Table 10—42. MOANS Scaled Scores, Midpoint Age = 79 (Age Range = 74–84, *n* = 151)

MOANS Scaled Scores	WMS-R Subtests—Immediate Recall Measures								
	Mental Control	Figural Memory	Logical Memory I	Visual Paired Assoc. I	Verbal Paired Assoc. I	Visual Reprod. I	Digit Span	Visual Span	Percentile Ranges
2	0–1	0	0–3	0	0–6	0–12	0–4	0–3	<1
3	—	1–2	4	—	7	13–15	5	4–5	1
4	—	—	5	1	8	—	6	6–7	2
5	2	3	8–10	2	9	16	7	8–9	3–5
6	3	—	11–12	3	10–11	17–18	8	10	6–10
7	—	4	13–14	4	12	19–20	9	11	11–18
8	—	—	15–17	5	13	21–23	10	—	19–28
9	4	5	18	6–7	14	24–25	11	12	29–40
10	5	—	19–21	8–9	15–16	26–28	12–13	13	41–59
11	—	6	22–24	10–11	17	29–30	14	14	60–71
12	6	—	25–26	12	18	31–32	15	—	72–81
13	—	7	27	13–14	19–20	33	16	15	82–89
14	—	—	28–29	15	21	34–35	17	16	90–94
15	—	—	30–31	16	—	36	18–19	17	95–97
16	—	8	32–33	17	22	—	—	18	98
17	—	9	34–36	18	23	37	20	19	99
18	—	10	37–50	—	24	38–41	21–24	20–26	>99

MOANS Scaled Scores	WMS-R Subtests—Delayed Recall Measures				Percent Retention		
	Logical Memory II	Visual Paired Assoc. II	Verbal Paired Assoc. II	Visual Reprod. II	Logical Memory Percent	Visual Reprod. Percent	Percentile Ranges
2	0	—	0–1	0–1	0–7	0–10	<1
3	1	—	—	2	8–14	11–13	1
4	—	—	—	—	15–21	14	2
5	2–4	0	2	3–4	22–39	15–20	3–5
6	5–6	—	3	5–6	40–45	21–31	6–10
7	7–9	—	—	7–10	46–55	32–41	11–18
8	10–11	1	4	11–13	56–64	42–53	19–28
9	12–13	2	—	14–16	65–70	54–64	29–40
10	14–15	3	5	17–20	71–79	65–72	41–59
11	16–19	4	6	21–22	80–84	73–81	60–71
12	20–22	5	—	23–26	85–89	82–89	72–81
13	23–25	6	7	27–29	90–93	90–95	82–89
14	26	—	8	30–31	94–96	96–97	90–94
15	27–29	—	—	32–34	97–99	98–100+	95–97
16	—	—	—	35–36	100+	—	98
17	30–32	—	—	37–38	—	—	99
18	33–50	—	—	39–41	—	—	>99

Note: MOANS = Mayo's Older Americans Normative Studies, WMS-R = Wechsler Memory Scale—Revised. MOANS Scaled scores are corrected for age influences.

MAYO Attention/Concentration (MACI), MAYO Delayed Recall (MDRI), and MAYO Percent Retention (MPRI) indices. The MPRI is a new index designed to evaluate delayed recall as a function of the amount of data originally learned. The Logical Memory and Visual Reproduction II subtests' raw scores are converted to percent retention (PR) scores (i.e., LM-PR = 100 (LMII/LMI); VR-PR = 100 (VRII/VRI]. These scores are assigned MOANS-scaled scores, and their sum is converted to a MAYO index value. Note, how

Table 10—43. MOANS Scaled Scores, Midpoint Age = 82 (Age Range = 77–87, n = 123)

MOANS Scaled Scores	WMS-R Subtests—Immediate Recall Measures								
	Mental Control	Figural Memory	Logical Memory I	Visual Paired Assoc. I	Verbal Paired Assoc. I	Visual Reprod. I	Digit Span	Visual Span	Percentile Ranges
2	0–1	0	0–3	0	0–6	0–10	0–4	0–3	<1
3	—	1–2	—	—	7	11	5	4–5	1
4	—	—	4–5	1	8	12	6	6–7	2
5	2	3	6–8	—	9	13–15	7	8–9	3–5
6	3	—	9–10	2	10	16	8	10	6–10
7	—	—	11–13	3	11–12	17–19	9	11	11–18
8	—	4	14–16	4	—	20	10	—	19–28
9	4	—	17	5–6	13–14	21–22	11	12	29–40
10	5	5	18–20	7–9	15	23–26	12–13	13	41–59
11	—	6	21–22	10	16	27–28	14	14	60–71
12	6	—	23–25	11–12	17	29–31	—	—	72–81
13	—	7	26–27	13	18–19	32–33	15–16	15	82–89
14	—	—	28	14	20	34–35	—	—	90–94
15	—	—	29–31	15	21	—	17	16	95–97
16	—	8	32–33	16	22	36	18–19	17	98
17	—	9	34–36	17	23	37	20	18	99
18	—	10	37–50	18	24	38–41	21–24	19–26	>99

MOANS Scaled Scores	WMS-R Subtests—Delayed Recall Measures						
					Percent Retention		
	Logical Memory II	Visual Paired Assoc. II	Verbal Paired Assoc. II	Visual Reprod. II	Logical Memory Percent	Visual Reprod. Percent	Percentile Ranges
2	0	—	0	0	0–7	0–10	<1
3	1	—	1	1	8–14	11–13	1
4	—	—	—	2	15–21	14	2
5	2–3	—	2	3	22–39	15–17	3–5
6	4	0	3	4–5	40–45	18–25	6–10
7	5–7	—	—	6	46–50	26–36	11–18
8	8–10	1	4	7–9	51–60	37–45	19–28
9	11–12	—	—	10–13	61–69	46–59	29–40
10	13–14	2–3	5	14–17	70–78	60–71	41–59
11	15–16	—	6	18–20	79–82	72–78	60–71
12	17–19	4	—	21–24	83–87	79–87	72–81
13	20–23	5	7	25–27	88–92	88–94	82–89
14	24–25	6	8	28–29	93–96	95–97	90–94
15	26–27	—	—	30–31	97–99	98–100+	95–97
16	28–29	—	—	32–35	100+	—	98
17	30–31	—	—	36	—	—	99
18	32–50	—	—	37–41	—	—	>99

Note: MOANS = Mayo's Older Americans Normative Studies, WMS-R = Wechsler Memory Scale—Revised. MOANS Scaled scores are corrected for age influences.

ever, that Ivnik et al.'s administration of both Paired Associates I and Visual Associates I differed from standard WMS-R administration in that they limited the number of trials on these subtests to three administrations, rather than continuing until criterion performance or the maximum of six trials. As such, MOANS data for Delayed Paired and Visual Associates (and therefore the Delayed Recall Index) are not comparable to scores from the standard administration. A different methodology was used to compute MAYO indices than is used to

Table 10—44. MOANS Scaled Scores, Midpoint Age = 85 (Age Range = 80–90, n = 84)

MOANS Scaled Scores	WMS-R Subtests—Immediate Recall Measures								
	Mental Control	Figural Memory	Logical Memory I	Visual Paired Assoc. I	Verbal Paired Assoc. I	Visual Reprod. I	Digit Span	Visual Span	Percentile Ranges
2	0–1	0	0–2	0	0–6	0–8	0–4	0–3	<1
3	—	1–2	3	—	7	9–10	5	4–5	1
4	—	—	4–5	—	8	11–12	6	6–7	2
5	2	3	6–8	1	9	13	7	8–9	3–5
6	3	—	9–10	2	10	14–15	8	10	6–10
7	—	—	11–12	3	11	16–17	—	11	11–18
8	—	4	13–15	4	12	18–19	9	—	19–28
9	4	—	16–17	5–6	13–14	20–21	10	12	29–40
10	5	5	18–19	7–9	15	22–24	11–12	13	41–59
11	—	—	20–21	10	16	25–27	13	—	60–71
12	6	6	22	11	17	28–29	14	14	72–81
13	—	—	23–25	12	18–19	30–32	15	—	82–89
14	—	7	26–27	13–14	20	—	16	15	90–94
15	—	—	28–29	—	21	33–35	17	—	95–97
16	—	8	30	15	22	36	18–19	—	98
17	—	9	31	16	23	37	20	16	99
18	—	10	32–50	17–18	24	38–41	21–24	17–26	>99

MOANS Scaled Scores	WMS-R Subtests—Delayed Recall Measures				Percent Retention		
	Logical Memory II	Visual Paired Assoc. II	Verbal Paired Assoc. II	Visual Reprod. II	Logical Memory Percent	Visual Reprod. Percent	Percentile Ranges
2	0	—	0	—	—	—	<1
3	1	—	1	0	0–13	0–9	1
4	2	—	—	1	14–21	10–13	2
5	3	—	2	2	22–37	14–15	3–5
6	4	0	3	3–5	38–41	16–19	6–10
7	5–7	—	—	6	42–50	20–35	11–18
8	8–9	1	4	7–9	51—58	36–44	19–28
9	10–11	—	—	10–12	59–64	45–50	29–40
10	12–14	2–3	5	13–15	65–77	51–68	41–59
11	15	—	6	16–19	78–81	69–77	60–71
12	16–17	4	—	20–21	82–87	78–86	72–81
13	18–19	5	7	22–25	88–92	87–92	82–89
14	20–25	6	8	26	93–96	93–97	90–94
15	26–27	—	—	27–28	97–98	98–100+	95–97
16	28–29	—	—	29	99–100+	—	98
17	30–31	—	—	30	—	—	99
18	32–50	—	—	31–41	—	—	>99

Note: MOANS = Mayo's Older Americans Normative Studies, WMS-R = Wechsler Memory Scale—Revised. MOANS Scaled scores are corrected for age influences.

compute WMS-R indices. Concordance rates suggest, however, that the performance characterstics of the comparable MAYO and WMS-R Verbal Memory, Visual Memory, General Memory, and Attention/Concentration indices are similar at ages where both can

be calculated. For clients aged 74 years and older, Tables 10–41 to 10–46 allow the examiner to convert WMS-R subtest raw scores to percentile ranges and age-corrected scaled scores (M = 10, SD = 3) and to determine the summary MAYO Indices. A worksheet is in-

Table 10—45. MOANS Scaled Scores, Midpoint Age = 88 (Age Range = 83 and above, n = 53)

MOANS Scaled Scores	WMS-R Subtests—Immediate Recall Measures								
	Mental Control	Figural Memory	Logical Memory I	Visual Paired Assoc. I	Verbal Paired Assoc. I	Visual Reprod. I	Digit Span	Visual Span	Percentile Ranges
2	0–1	0	0–2	—	0–4	0–6	—	0–3	<1
3	—	1	3	0	5–6	7–8	0–4	4–5	1
4	—	2	4–5	—	7–8	9–10	5	6–7	2
5	2	—	6–8	1	9	11	6	8–9	3–5
6	3	3	9–10	—	10	12–13	7–8	10	6–10
7	—	—	11–12	2	11	14–16	—	—	11–18
8	—	—	13–15	3–4	12	17–19	9	11	19–28
9	4	4	16	5	13–14	20	10	12	29–40
10	—	5	17–19	6–8	15	21–24	11–12	—	41–59
11	5	—	20	9	—	25–26	13	13	60–71
12	6	6	21–22	10	16–17	27	14	14	72–81
13	—	—	23–24	11–12	18–19	28–30	15	—	82–89
14	—	7	25–27	13–14	—	31–32	16	15	90–94
15	—	—	28–29	—	20–21	33–34	17	—	95–97
16	—	8	30	15	—	35	18–19	—	98
17	—	9	31	16	22–23	36	20	16	99
18	—	10	32–50	17–18	24	37–41	21–24	17–26	>99

MOANS Scaled Scores	WMS-R Subtests—Delayed-recall Measures				Percent Retention		Percentile Ranges
	Logical Memory II	Visual Paired Assoc. II	Verbal Paired Assoc. II	Visual Reprod. II	Logical Memory Percent	Visual Reprod. Percent	
2	—	—	—	—	—	—	<1
3	—	—	0	—	—	—	1
4	0	—	1	—	0–21	—	2
5	1–3	—	2	—	22–35	—	3–5
6	4	0	3	0–3	36–41	0–10	6–10
7	5–7	—	—	4–5	42–50	11–19	11–18
8	8–9	1	4	6	51—55	20–39	19–28
9	10	—	—	7–9	56–63	40–47	29–40
10	11–13	2	5	10–13	64–75	48–55	41–59
11	14–15	3	6	14–15	76–79	56–69	60–71
12	16	4	—	16–19	80–87	70–79	72–81
13	17–18	5	7	20–22	88–92	80–82	82–89
14	19–20	6	8	23–25	93–94	83–93	90–94
15	21	—	—	26	95	94–97	95–97
16	22–29	—	—	27–28	96–98	98–100+	98
17	30–31	—	—	29–30	98–100+	—	99
18	32–50	—	—	31–41	—	—	>99

Note: MOANS = Mayo's Older Americans Normative Studies, WMS-R = Wechsler Memory Scale—Revised. MOANS Scaled scores are corrected for age influences.

cluded in Figure 10–28 for calculating MOANS Scaled Scores, weighted MOANS Scale Score Sums and MAYO indices. The scoring program offered by the Psychological Corporation also computes MAYO cognitive factor scaled scores (MCFS) if the WAIS-R and RAVLT have also been given. Recently, Smith et al. (1997) have presented separate norms for persons aged 56–93 for each story from the Logical Memory subtest. Since MOANS data area based almost exclusively on Caucasians who live in an economically stable region, the

Table 10—46. Table for Converting Weighted MOANS Scaled Score Sums to MAYO Indices

MAYO Index Score	Weighted MOANS Scaled Sums						MAYO Index Score
	Verbal Sum	Visual Sum	General Sum	Atten./Concen. Sum	Delayed Recall Sum	Percent Reten. Sum	
<65	≤7	≤9	≤23	≤25	≤27	≤5	<65
65			24			6	65
66	8	10		26	28		66
67			25	27	29		67
68	9		26	28	30	7	68
69		11	27		31		69
70	10		28	29			70
71	11	12	29	30	32	8	71
72			30		33		72
73	12	13	31	31	34		73
74				32		9	74
75	13	14	32	33	35		75
76			33		36		76
77	14	15	34	34	37		77
78	15		35	35		10	78
79		16	36	36	38		79
80	16		37		39		80
81		17		37	40	11	81
82	17		38	38			82
83			39		41		83
84	18	18	40	39	42	12	84
85	19		41	40	43		85
86		19	42	41	44		86
87	20		43			13	87
88		20		42	45		88
89	21		44	43	46		89
90		21	45	44	47	14	90
91	22		46				91
92	23	22	47	45	48		92
93			48	46	49	15	93
94	24	23	49		50		94
95			50	47			95
96	25	24		48	51	16	96
97			51	49	52		97
98	26	25	52		53		98
99	27		53	50			99
100			54	51	54	17	100
101	28	26	55		55		101
102			56	52	56		102
103	29	27		53	57	18	103
104			57	54			104
105	30	28	58		58		105
106	31		59	55	59	19	106
107		29	60	56	60		107
108	32		61	57			108
109		30	62		61	20	109
110	33			58	62		110
111		31	63	59	63		111
112	34		64	60		21	112
113		32	65		64		113
114	35		66	61	65		114
115	36		67	62	66	22	115
116		33	68	63			116

(continued)

Table 10—46. Table for Converting Weighted MOANS Scaled Score Sums to MAYO Indices *(Continued)*

MAYO Index Score	Weighted MOANS Scaled Sums						MAYO Index Score
	Verbal Sum	Visual Sum	General Sum	Atten./ Concen. Sum	Delayed Recall Sum	Percent Reten. Sum	
117	37		69		67		117
118		34		64	68	23	118
119	38		70	65	69		119
120		35	71		70		120
121	39		72	66			121
122	40	36	73	67	71	24	122
123			74	68	72		123
124	41	37	75		73		124
125				69		25	125
126	42	38	76	70	74		126
127			77	71	75		127
128	43	39	78		76	26	128
129	44		79	72			129
130		40	80	73	77		130
131	45		81		78	27	131
132				74	79		132
133	46	41	82	75			133
134			83	76	80	28	134
135	47	42	84		81		135
>135	≥48	≥43	≥85	≥77	≥82	≥29	>135

Note: MOANS = Mayo's Older Americans Normative Studies; Attn./Concen. = Attention/Concentration; Percent Reten. = Percent Retention.

validity of indices computed for persons of other ethnic, cultural, and economic backgrounds may be questioned.

Norms for the WMS-R extend down to 16 years of age. Recently, Paniak et al. (in press) provided norms for Logical Memory (I and II) and Visual Reproduction (I and II) based on data from 716 students (327 males, 389 females) aged 9–15 years who attended Edmonton Public Schools. Their estimated verbal intelligence, based on the WISC-III Vocabulary subtest, was similar to that of the WISC-III normative sample. The data are shown in Table 10–47. Scores on these subtests improved with age and reached adult levels by about age 15 years. They did not differ according to gender. Percentage recall scores did not vary by gender, but the Visual Reproduction percentage recall score improved with age. The Logical Memory and Visual Reproduction percentage recall scores across ages 9–15 were similar to adult WMS-R percentage recall scores.

Examination of differences among standard WMS-R indices may provide valuable information about the patient's strengths and weaknesses. In order to determine whether the difference between two index scores is reliable (i.e., significant at $p < .05$), the examiner should refer to the table (based on the standard error of measurement − SEM) in the WMS-R manual or see Atkinson (1991), who provided a SEE (standard error of estimation) and SEP (standard errors of prediction)—based table of differences at the 10, 5, and 1 percent significance levels. It is worth bearing in mind that for all age groups, scatter between indices was large: Differences of less than 15 points were not significant for any pairing of indices. Note that the confidence intervals given (.15 and .05) refer to the reliability of the difference score as due to something other than

WMS-R Subtest	Raw Score	MOANS Score	Weight		Weighted MOANS Scale Score Sums	MAYO Indices
Immediate						
MC	_____ = _____		X 1 = _____		Verbal	MVeMI
FM	_____ = _____		X 1 = _____		+	
LM-I	_____ = _____		X 2 = _____			
ViPa-I	_____ = _____		X 4 = _____	= _____ 1/3 =	Visual	MViMI
VePA-I	_____ = _____		X 1 = _____		||	
VR-I	_____ = _____		X 4 = _____		General	MGMI
DSpan	_____ = _____		X 2 = _____		A/C	MACI
VSpan	_____ = _____		X 2 = _____	=		
Delayed						
LM-II	_____ = _____		X 1 = _____			
ViPA-II	_____ = _____		X 2 = _____			
VePA-II	_____ = _____		X 2 = _____	=	Delayed Recall	MDRI
VR-II	_____ = _____		X 1 = _____			
Percent Retention						
LM-PR	_____ = _____		X 1 = _____			
VR-PR	_____ = _____		X 1 = _____	=	Percent	MPRI

Figure 10—28. Worksheet for Calculating MOANS Scaled Scores and MAYO Indices. Note: MOANS = Mayo's Older Americans Normative Studies; WMS-R = Wechsler Memory Scale—Revised; A/C = Attention/Concentration; PR = Percent Retention; MC = Mental Control; FM = Figural Memory; LM-I = Logical Memory immediate; ViPA-I = Visual Paired Associates immediate; VePA-I = Verbal Paired Associates immediate; VR-I = Visual Reproduction immediate; DSpan = Digit Span; VSpan = Visual Span; LM-II Logical Memory delayed; ViPA-II = Visual Paired Associates delayed: VePa-II = Verbal Paired Associates delayed; VR-II = Visual Reproduction delayed; LM-PR = Logical Memory Percent Retention = $100 \times (LM\text{-}II/LM\text{-}I)$; VR-PR = Visual Reproduction Percent Retention = $100 \times (VR\text{-}II/VR\text{-}I)$; MVeMI = MAYO Verbal Memory Index; MViMI = MAYO Visual Memory Index; MGMI = MAYO General Memory Index; MACI = MAYO Attention/Concentration Index; MDRI = MAYO Delayed Recall Index; MPRI = MAYO Percent Retention Index.

Table 10—47. Performance of Children and Adolescents

Age	LM I M (SD)	LMII M (SD)	LMII/I % M (SD)	VRI M (SD)	VRII M (SD)	VRII/I % M (SD)
9	19.7	17.3	88.0	29.3	23.8	81.6
(n = 81)	(7.7)	(7.6)	(21.2)	(4.3)	(6.1)	(18.0)
10	21.2	18.6	86.6	29.8	26.3	88.8
(n = 140)	(7.3)	(7.5)	(14.5)	(4.3)	(5.5)	(16.8)
11	23.2	20.2	86.4	31.2	27.1	87.0
(n = 132)	(7.4)	(6.9)	(13.3)	(4.7)	(5.8)	(15.0)
12	24.9	22.3	89.5	33.3	30.7	92.4
(n = 123)	(6.8)	(6.8)	(11.6)	(3.6)	(4.5)	(11.1)
13	25.3	22.2	86.7	34.4	31.4	91.1
(n = 96)	(6.9)	(6.9)	(12.5)	(3.3)	(5.1)	(11.9)
14	27.8	24.7	88.3	35.5	33.7	94.5
(n = 116)	(6.4)	(6.8)	(11.3)	(2.6)	(3.8)	(9.1)
15	28.8	25.6	87.7	35.4	33.4	94.1
(n = 28)	(6.9)	(7.5)	(12.9)	(2.4)	(4.0)	(8.9)

Source: Paniak et al. (in press).

Table 10—48. Standard Deviation of Differences and Critical Levels for Abnormality of Differences Between

| | Age = 16–17 Years | | | Age = 20–24 Years | | | Age = 35–44 Years | | |
| | 95% limit | | | 95% limit | | | 95% limit | | |
Scale	One-Tailed Limit	Two-Tailed Limit	SD	One-Tailed Limit	Two-Tailed Limit	SD	One-Tailed Limit	Two-Tailed Limit	SD
General Memory Attention/Concentration	26.20	31.13	15.88	23.48	27.89	14.23	20.41	24.25	12.37
Verbal Memory Visual Memory	32.65	38.79	19.79	30.72	36.50	18.62	20.71	25.60	12.55
General Memory Delayed Recall	13.10	15.56	7.94	15.65	18.60	9.49	9.90	11.76	6.00
Logical Memory Logical Memory 2	11.07	13.15	6.71	13.56	16.11	8.22	9.90	11.76	6.00
Visual Reproduction Visual Reproduction 2	22.14	26.30	13.42	17.85	21.21	10.82	14.85	17.64	9.00
Logical Memory Visual Reproduction	34.85	41.40	21.12	34.47	40.94	20.89	25.00	29.70	15.15
Logical Memory 2 Visual Reproduction 2	32.08	38.10	19.44	28.86	34.28	17.49	24.50	29.11	14.85

Source: Mittenberg et al. (1991). Reproduced with permission of the American Psychological Association.

measurement error. They do not refer to the probability of base-rate occurrence in the normal population. That is, a discrepancy may be reliable in that it is unlikely to have occurred by chance, but it may be found with some frequency in the normal population. Table 10–48 is provided here (Mittenberg et al., 1991) in order to evaluate the clinical significance of discrepancies between scales. For example, a 16-year-old who obtains a difference between General Memory and Attention/Concentration index scores of ±15.88 points has shown a discrepancy of 1 standard deviation between the indices. If the clinican suspects abnormal memory, then a difference between General Memory and Attention/Concentration of −26.20 Index points will be needed at the .05 level (directional hypothesis). If the clinician wonders whether Attention/Concentration is different from General Memory, a difference of at least ±31.13 index score points will be necessary at the .05 level (bidirectional hypothesis). Note that there appear to be instances in which differences that would be

considered abnormal (having occurred in less than 5 percent of the standardization sample) appear unreliable. For example, a Delayed Recall index that is 12.62 points lower than the General Memory index is rare in the standardization sample. However, such a difference would not be considered reliable. The confidence interval for a reliable difference between the two indices of 19.75 points (Wechsler, 1987) would appear too conservative. Note that all table values apply to standardized scales with means of 100 and standard deviations of 15. Raw scores for the Logical Memory and Visual Reproduction subtests must be transformed first to percentile ranks (see Table C-5 in WMS-R manual) and then translated into the corresponding standardized score.

Bornstein et al. (1989a) examined the distribution of IQ–Memory Index scores in a sample of 100 normal subjects from the WMS-R standardization sample who were administered all subtests of the WAIS-R (mean age = 52.5, SD = 14.6; FSIQ = 103.5, SD = 15;

Pairs of Wechsler Memory Scale—Revised Subscales

Age = 55–64 Years			Age = 65–69 Years			Age = 70–74 Years			Average		
95% limit			95% limit			95% limit			95% limit		
One-Tailed Limit	Two-Tailed Limit	SD	One-Tailed Limit	Two-Tailed Limit	SD	One-Tailed Limit	Two-Tailed Limit	SD	One-Tailed Limit	Two-Tailed Limit	SD
26.20	31.13	15.88	24.50	29.11	14.85	25.00	29.69	15.15	24.50	29.11	14.85
25.48	30.26	15.44	24.26	28.81	14.70	26.20	31.13	15.88	24.75	29.40	15.00
14.85	17.64	9.00	12.13	14.41	7.35	12.13	14.41	7.35	12.62	14.99	7.76
12.11	14.39	7.34	11.07	13.15	6.71	13.10	15.56	7.94	11.62	13.80	7.04
20.11	23.89	12.19	16.04	19.05	9.72	16.78	19.93	10.17	17.85	21.21	10.82
26.19	31.11	15.87	26.19	31.11	15.87	30.11	35.77	18.25	29.50	35.05	17.88
28.00	33.26	16.97	23.74	28.20	14.39	30.11	35.77	18.25	27.79	33.01	16.84

General Memory Index = 100.9, SD = 17.3). Table 10–38 shows the percentages of subjects who obtained scores at various levels of IQ-Memory discrepancy. Note that the FSIQ-Memory index discrepancy does not account for overall level of performance. It is possible that at lower levels of performance, smaller discrepancies might have greater clinical significance.

Age has a significant effect on performance (e.g., Chelune et al., 1989; Cullum et al., 1990; Marcopulos et al., 1997; Mittenberg et al., 1991; Paniak et al., in press; Smith et al., 1992a; Wechsler, 1987). The Attention/Concentration Index appears the most impervious to the deleterious effects of aging. While absolute performance on the Logical Memory seems to decline at a steady pace with advancing age, performance on the Visual Reproduction trials is relatively stable from the age of 16 to 40 years and then declines in an exponential manner. WMS-R percent retention scores for LM and VR are also age-dependent, especially among individuals aged 65 years and above. Prifitera and Ledbetter (1992) exam-

ined the WMS-R standardization sample and found percent retention scores of about 65 percent for individuals aged 70–74 years, compared to about 90 percent for people aged 16–17 years. Note that although healthy elderly individuals show an increased rate of forgetting, their percent retention of material (percent retention of LM and VR) remains relatively high (Cullum et al., 1990; Smith et al., 1992). This is in marked contrast to AD patients who show extremely low savings scores (less than 20 percent) (Butters et al., 1988). Tables 10–49 and 10–50 show LM and VR percent retention scores for selected percentile points by age group (Prifitera & Ledbetter, 1992).

No relation has been found between WMS-R scores and gender (see source; Fox, 1994; Paniak et al., in press) or race (Marcopulos et al., 1997). One should note, however, that level of education is significantly correlated (.42 to .49) with all five indices (see source; Mittenberg et al., 1992; Ryan & Lewis, 1988). The average scores of subjects with less than 12 years of education and those with more

Table 10—49. Percentiles for Logical Memory Percent Retention Scores
for the Six Standardization Age Groups

	Percent Retention Score by Age Group					
Percentile	16–17	20–24	35–45	55–64	65–69	70–74
5%	54.9%	58.4%	45.5%	51.8%	26.0%	23.1%
10%	77.3%	63.3%	54.2%	59.8%	46.8%	33.3%
15%	80.0%	64.5%	59.4%	64.4%	52.8%	37.2%
20%	82.8%	68.1%	62.5%	70.8%	56.0%	41.7%
25%	84.2%	71.0%	72.3%	74.8%	59.3%	47.5%
30%	85.3%	72.1%	75.4%	75.0%	64.7%	52.9%
35%	85.7%	76.5%	77.6%	76.6%	70.8%	57.3%
40%	87.8%	82.7%	80.8%	78.9%	74.0%	65.2%
45%	89.0%	83.3%	83.2%	80.0%	75.7%	66.7%
50%	89.7%	87.7%	84.2%	81.1%	80.0%	68.8%
55%	90.3%	89.7%	85.0%	82.3%	81.0%	71.2%
60%	92.4%	91.8%	87.5%	84.0%	84.2%	73.3%
65%	93.4%	93.2%	90.6%	85.0%	86.4%	75.0%
70%	94.3%	95.8%	93.1%	87.0%	88.3%	76.2%
75%	96.4%	<100.0%	96.8%	87.6%	89.7%	81.8%
80%	97.8%		<100.0%	88.9%	90.3%	84.8%
85%	<100.0%			92.6%	92.9%	94.4%
90%				97.8%	94.2%	<100.0%
95%				<100.0%	<100.0%	

Source: Prifitera and Ledbetter (1992). Copyright 1992 © by The Psychological Corporation. All Rights Reserved. Reproduced with permission.

Note: These percent retention scores are non-normalized and are not smoothed to compensate for sampling irregularities across age groups. Estimates of percent retention equivalents for the age groups not sampled in the standardization group (i.e., 18–19, 25–34, 45–54) can be computed by utilizing a midpoint interpolation procedure.

than 12 years of education differed significantly, sometimes by nearly a full standard deviation. Consequently, years of education is an important factor to consider and may temper interpretation of any given index score (Chelune et al., 1989; Fastenau, 1996; Reinehr, 1992; also see source). Note, too, that in the standardization sample, education level and age were highly correlated ($r = -.98$), thereby introducing bias in the interpretation of WMS-R scores (Chelune et al. 1989). For example, a 23-year-old male with 12 years of education who obtains a Verbal Memory Index of 100 is probably doing somewhat better than his educationally matched peers, since the average male in his age group has a mean educational level of more than 12 years. Similarly, a 72-year-old with 12 years of education who obtains a Verbal Memory Index of 100 is likely performing below expecta-

tion, since the average individual in this age group had less than a high school education.

As might be expected, the revised version yields lower scores than the original WMS; these differences are especially prominent in older subjects (Oscar-Berman et al. 1993). Accordingly, clinicians must be cautious when interpreting differences between patient's WMS MQs and their WMS-R Index scores (Chelune et al., 1989).

With regard to Gass' (1995) adaptations, LM-REC and Visual Reproduction Cuing, normative data based on a sample of healthy individuals are lacking. He provides some data based on a sample of 99 patients with neurological diagnoses of traumatic brain injury and stroke (mean age = 52, SD = 15; education = 12 years, SD = 3.0; Full Scale IQ = 89.6, SD = 11.8) and 94 psychiatric inpatients who were diagnosed with an emotional disorder

Table 10—50. Percentiles for Visual Reproduction Percent Retention Scores
for the Six Standardization Age Groups

Percentile	Percent Retention Score by Age Group					
	16–17	20–24	35–45	55–64	65–69	70–74
5%	70.4%	67.2%	62.2%	45.0%	25.5%	10.6%
10%	76.3%	76.3%	66.7%	58.5%	51.4%	21.9%
15%	77.3%	79.3%	77.1%	66.7%	60.0%	36.9%
20%	78.8%	82.4%	80.6%	67.9%	65.2%	48.4%
25%	81.2%	86.4%	81.6%	76.7%	68.4%	51.6%
30%	83.6%	88.1%	81.9%	79.5%	70.9%	53.3%
35%	87.1%	90.5%	83.7%	83.8%	75.5%	57.1%
40%	91.3%	91.8%	85.7%	86.2%	77.5%	61.5%
45%	93.9%	92.6%	88.9%	87.0%	79.2%	66.6%
50%	97.0%	93.7%	91.2%	91.0%	80.8%	68.7%
55%	97.2%	96.5%	94.5%	92.8%	81.7%	70.7%
60%	97.5%	97.4%	97.1%	94.4%	87.4%	75.8%
65%	<100.0%	<100.0%	97.5%	96.7%	88.7%	78.2%
70%			<100.0%	98.6%	91.3%	80.8%
75%				<100.0%	96.4%	85.7%
80%					99.5%	86.1%
85%					<100.0%	93.1%
90%						99.4
95%						<100.0%

Source: Prifitera and Ledbetter (1992). Copyright 1992 © by The Psychological Corporation. All Rights Reserved. Reproduced with permission.

Note: These percent retention scores are non-normalized and are not smoothed to compensate for sampling irregularities across age groups. Estimates of percent retention equivalents for the age groups not sampled in the standardization group (i.e., 18–19, 25–34, 46–54) can be computed by utilizing a midpoint interpolation procedure.

and did not have a history of neurological disorder. The psychiatric sample had a mean age of 49 years (SD = 13), education of 12.7 years (SD = 2.4) and Full Scale IQ of 99.6 (SD = 13.8). On LM-REC, the psychiatric sample identified an average of 16.4 items (SD = 2.9) whereas the brain-damaged patients correctly identified 14.7 items (SD = 4.1). For VR Delayed with Cue, the psychiatric sample obtained an average score of 26.4 (SD = 8.3), while the brain-damaged group scored 19.1 (SD = 10.8). Gass (1995) also derived scaled scores using a global neuropsychological impairment rating as a predictive criterion. In order to use the scaled scores, raw scores must be first adjusted for education (see scoring). Fastenau (1996) collected data for his modifications from a sample of 81 community-dwelling adults (mean age = 52.9 years, SD = 13.6; mean education = 15.6 years, SD = 2.8). The sample was subdivided into three

age groups (30–45, 46–62, 63–80) and two levels of education (12–15 years, ≥16 years).

References

Atkinson, L. (1991). Three standard errors of measurement and the Wechsler Memory Scale-Revised. *Psychological Assessment, 3*, 136–138.

Axelrod, B.N., Putnam, S.H., Woodard, J.L., & Adams, K.M. (1996). Cross-validation of predicted Wechsler Memory Scale—Revised scores. *Psychological Assessment, 8*, 73–75.

Barr, W.B., Chelune, G.J., Hermann, B.P., Loring, D., Perrine, K., Strauss, E., Trenerry, M.R., & Westerveld, M. (1997). The use of figural reproduction tests as measures of nonverbal memory in epilepsy surgery candidates. *Journal of the International Neuropsychological Society, 3*, 435–443.

Bernard, L.C. (1991). Prospects for faking believable memory deficits on neuropsychology tests and the use of incentives in simulation research.

Journal of Clinical and Experimental Neuropsychology, 12, 715–728.

Bigler, E.D., Johnson, S.C., Anderson, C.V., Blatter, D.D., Gale, S.D., Russo, A.A., Ryser, D.K., Macnamara, S.E., & Abildskov, T.J. (1996). Traumatic brain injury and memory: The role of hippocampal atrophy. *Neuropsychology, 10,* 333–342.

Blackwood, H.D. (1996). Recommendation for test administration in litigation: Never administer the Category Test to a blindfolded subject. *Archives of Clinical Neuropsychology, 11,* 93–95.

Boone, K.B., Lesser, I.M., Miller, B.L., Wohl, M., Berman, N., Lee, A., Palmer, B., & Back, C. (1995). Cognitive functioning in older depressed outpatients: Relationship of presence and severity of depression to neuropsychological test scores. *Neuropsychology, 9,* 390–398.

Bornstein, R.A., & Chelune, G.J. (1988). Factor structure of the Wechsler Memory Scale—Revised. *The Clinical Neuropsychologist, 2,* 107–115.

Bornstein, R.A., & Chelune, G.J. (1989). Factor structure of the Wechsler Memory Scale—Revised in relation to age and education level. *Archives of Clinical Neuropsychology, 4,* 15–24.

Bornstein, R.A., Chelune, G.J., & Prifitera, A. (1989a). IQ-memory discrepancies in normal and clinical samples. *Psychological Assessment, 1,* 203–206.

Bornstein, R.A., Pakalnis, A., & Drake, M.E. (1989b). Verbal and nonverbal memory learning in patients with complex partial seizures of temporal lobe origin. *Journal of Epilepsy, 1,* 203–208.

Bowden, S.C., Whelan, G., Long, C.M., & Clifford, C.C. (1995). Temporal stability of the WAIS-R and WMS-R in a heterogeneous sample of alcohol dependent clients. *The Clinical Neuropsychologist, 9,* 194–197.

Bowden, S.C., & Bell, R.C. (1992). Relative usefulness of the WMS and WMS-R: A comment on D'Elia et al. (1989). *Journal of Clinical and Experimental Neuropsychology, 14,* 340–346.

Burton, D.B., Mittenberg, W., & Burton, C.A. (1993). Confirmatory factor analysis of the Wechsler Memory Scale—Revised standardization sample. *Archives of Clinical Neuropsychology, 8,* 467–475.

Butters, N., Salmon, D.P., Cullum, C.M., Cairns, P., Troster, A.I., Jacobs, D., Moss, M., & Cermak, L.S. (1988). Differentiation of amnesic and demented patients with the Wechsler Memory Scale—Revised. *The Clinical Neuropsychologist, 2,* 133–148.

Chelune, G.J., & Bornstein, R.A. (1988a). Memory characteristics of patients with unilateral temporal and nontemporal lesions. *The Clinical Neuropsychologist, 2,* 275.

Chelune, G.J., & Bornstein, R.A. (1988b). WMS-R patterns among patients with unilateral brain lesions. *The Clinical Neuropsychologist, 2,* 121–132.

Chelune, G.J., Bornstein, R.A., & Prifitera, A. (1989). The Wechsler Memory Scale—Revised: Current status and application. In J. Rosen, P. McReynolds, & G.J. Chelune (Eds.). *Advances in Psychological Assessment.* New York: Plenum Press.

Crossen, J.R., & Wiens, A.N. (1988a). Wechsler Memory Scale—Revised: Deficits in performance associated with neurotoxic solvent exposure. *The Clinical Neuropsychologist, 2,* 181–187.

Crossen, J.R., & Wiens, A.N. (1988b). Residual neuropsychological deficits following head injury on the Wechsler Memory Scale—Revised. *The Clinical Neuropsychologist, 2,* 393–399.

Cullum, C.M., Butters, N., Troster, A.I., & Salmon, D.P. (1990). Normal aging and forgetting rates on the Wechsler Memory Scale—Revised. *Archives of Clinical Neuropsychology, 5,* 23–30.

D'Elia, L., Satz, P., & Schretlen, D. (1989). Wechsler Memory Scale: A critical appraisal of the normative studies. *Journal of Clinical and Experimental Neuropsychology, 11,* 551–568.

Delis, D.C., Kramer, J.H., Kaplan, E., & Ober, B.A. (1987). *The California Verbal Learning Test.* San Antonio TX: The Psychological Corporation.

Delis, D.C., Cullum, C.M., Butters, N., Cairns, P., & Prifitera, A. (1988). Wechsler Memory Scale-Revised and California Verbal Learning Test: convergence and divergence. *The Clinical Neuropsychologist, 2,* 188–196.

Demsky, Y.I., & Sellers, A.H. (1995). Improving examiner reliability on the Visual Memory Span subtest of the Wechsler Memory Scale—Revised. *The Clinical Neuropsychologist, 9,* 79–82.

Elwood, R.W. (1991). Factor structure of the Wechsler Memory Scale—Revised (WMS-R) in a clinical sample: A methodological reappraisal. *The Clinical Neuropsychologist, 5,* 329–337.

Fastenau, P.S. (1996). An elaborated administration of the Wechsler Memory Scale—Revised. *The Clinical Neuropsychologist, 10,* 425–434.

Fischer, J.S. (1988). Using the Wechsler Memory Scale-Revised to detect and characterize memory deficits in Multiple Sclerosis. *The Clinical Neuropsychologist, 2,* 149–172.

Fox, D.D. (1994). Normative problems for the Wechsler Memory Scale—Revised Logical Memory test when used in litigation. *Archives of Clinical Neuropsychology, 9*, 211–214.

Franzen, M.D. (1989). *Reliability and Validity in Neuropsychological Assessment*. New York: Plenum Press.

Franzen, M.D., Wilhelm, K.L., & Haut, M.C. (1995). The factor structure of the Wechsler Memory Scale—Revised and several brief neuropsychological screening instruments in recently detoxified substance abusers. *Archives of Clinical Neuropsychology, 10*, 193–204.

Gass, C.S. (1995). A procedure for assessing storage and retrieval on the Wechsler Memory Scale—Revised. *Archives of Clinical Neuropsychology, 10*, 475–487.

Gass, C.S. (1996). MMPI-2 variables in attention and memory test performance. *Psychological Assessment, 8*, 135–138.

Gold, J.M., Randolph, C., Carpenter, C.J., Goldberg, T.E., & Weinberger, D.R. (1992). The performance of patients with Schizophrenia on the Wechsler Memory Scale—Revised. *The Clinical Neuropsychologist, 6*, 367–373.

Haut, M.W., Weber, A.M., Wilhelm, K.L., Keefover, R.W., & Rankin, E.D. (1994). The Visual Reproduction subtest as a measure of visual perceptual/constructional functioning in dementia of the Alzheimer's type. *The Clinical Neuropsychologist, 8*, 187–192.

Herman, D.O. (1988). Development of the Wechsler Memory Scale—Revised. *The Clinical Neuropsychologist, 2*, 102–106.

Holden, R.H. (1988). Wechsler Memory Scale—Revised. In D.J. Keyser & R.C. Sweetland (Eds.) *Test Critiques*, Vol. 7, Missouri: Test Corporation of America.

Huebner, E.S. (1992). Review of the Wechsler Memory Scale—Revised. *The 11th Mental Measurement Yearbook*, Lincoln, NB: Buros Institute, pp. 1023–1024.

Iverson, G.L., & Franzen, M.D. (1996). Using multiple-object memory procedures to detect simulated malingering. *Journal of Clinical and Experimental Neuropsychology, 18*, 38–51.

Ivnik, R.J., Malec, J.F., Smith, G.E., Tangalos, E.G., Petersen, R.C., Kokmen, E., & Kurland, L.T. (1992). Mayo's older Americans normative studies: WMS-R norms for ages 56 to 94. *The Clinical Neuropsychologist, 6*, 49–82.

Jacobs, D., Troster, A.I., Butters, N., Salmon, D.R., & Cermak, L.S. (1990). Intrusion errors on the Visual Reproduction Test of the Wechsler Memory Scale and the Wechsler Memory Scale—Revised: An analysis of demented and amnesic patients. *The Clinical Neuropsychologist, 4*, 177–191.

Janowsky, J.S., Shimamura, A.P., Kritchevsky, M., & Squire, L.R. (1989). Cognitive impairment following frontal lobe damage and its relevance to human amnesia. *Behavioral Neuroscience, 103*, 548–560.

King, D.A., Cox, C., Lyness, J.M., & Caine, E.D. (1995). Neuropsychological effects of depression and age in an elderly sample: A confirmatory study. *Neuropsychology, 9*, 399–408.

Kixmiller, J.S., Verfaellie, M., Chase, K.A., & Cermak, L.S. (1995). Comparison of figural intrusion errors in three amnesic subgroups. *Journal of the International Neuropsychological Society, 1*, 561–567.

Kneebone, A.C., Chelune, G.J., & Lüders, H.O. (1997). Individual patient prediction of seizure lateralization in temporal lobe epilepsy: A comparison between neuropsychological memory measures and the Intracarotid Amobarbital procedure. *Journal of the International Neuropsychology Society, 3*, 159–168.

Leonberger, F.T., Nicks, S.D., Goldfader, P.R., & Munz, D.C. (1991). Factor analysis of the Wechsler Memory Scale—Revised and the Halstead-Reitan Neuropsychology Battery. *The Clinical Neuropsychologist, 5*, 83–88.

Leonberger, F.T., Nicks, S.D., Larrabee, G.J., & Goldfader, P.R. (1992). Factor structure of the Wechsler Memory Scale—Revised within a comprehensive neuropsychological battery. *Neuropsychology, 6*, 239–249.

Lichtenberg, P.A., & Christensen, B. (1992). Extended normative data for the Logical Memory subtests of the Wechsler Memory Scale—Revised: Responses from a sample of cognitively intact elderly medical patients. *Psychological Reports, 71*, 745–746.

Loring, D.W., Lee, G.P., Martin, R.C., & Meador, K.J. (1989). Verbal and visual memory index discrepancies from the Wechsler Memory Scale—Revised: Cautions in interpretation. *Psychological Assessment, 1*, 198–202.

Loring, D.W. (1990). The Wechsler Memory Scale—Revised, or The Wechsler Memory Scale—Revisited? *The Clinical Neuropsychologist, 3*, 59–69.

Marcopulos, B.A., McLain, C.A., & Giuliano, A.J. (1997). Cognitive impairment or inadequate norms? A study of healthy, rural, older adults with limited education. *The Clinical Neuropsychologist, 11*, 111–131.

Milner, B. (1975). Psychological aspects of focal

epilepsy and its neurosurgical management. *Advances in Neurology, 8,* 299–321.

Mittenberg, W., Azrin, R., Millsaps, C., & Heilbronner, R. (1993). Identification of malingered head injury on the Wechsler Memory Scale—Revised. *Psychological Assessment, 5,* 34–40.

Mittenberg, W., Burton, D.B., Darrow, E., & Thompson, G.B. (1992). Normative data for the Wechsler Memory Scale—Revised: 25- to 34-year-olds. *Psychological Assessment, 4,* 363–368.

Mittenberg, W., Thompson, G.B., & Schwartz, J.A. (1991). Abnormal and reliable differences among Wechsler Memory Scale—Revised subtests. *Psychological Assessment, 3,* 492–495.

Naugle, R.F., Chelune, G.J., Cheek, R., Luders, H., & Awad, I. (1993). Detection of changes in material-specific memory following temporal lobectomy using the Wechsler Memory Scale—Revised. *Archives of Clinical Neuropsychology, 8,* 381–395.

Nicks, S.D., Leonberger, F.T., Munz, D.C., & Goldfader, P.R. (1992). Factor analysis of the WMS-R and WAIS. *Archives of Clinical Neuropsychology, 7,* 387–393.

O'Mahony, J.F., & Doherty, B. (1993). Patterns of intellectual performance among recently abstinent alcohol abusers on WAIS-R and WMS-R subtests. *Archives of Clinical Neuropsychology, 8,* 373–380.

Oscar-Berman, M., Papalopoulos Clancy, J., & Altman Weber, D. (1993). Discrepancies between IQ and memory scores in alcoholism and aging. *The Clinical Neuropsychologist, 7,* 281–296.

Paniak, C.E., Murphy, D., Miller, H.B., & Lee, M. (in press). Wechsler Memory Scale—Revised Logical Memory and Visual Reproduction subtest norms for 9 to 15 year olds. *Developmental Neuropsychology.*

Prifitera, A., & Ledbetter, M. (1992) Normative delayed recall rates based on the Wechsler Memory Scale—Revised standardization sample. Unpublished paper.

Randolph, C., Gold, J.M., Kozora, E., Cullum, C.M., Hermann, B.P., & Wyler, A.R. (1994). Estimating memory function: Disparity of Wechsler Memory Scale—Revised and California Verbal Learning Test indices in clinical and normal samples. *The Clinical Neuropsychologist, 8,* 99–108.

Reinehr, R.C. (1992). Review of the Wechsler Memory Scale—Revised. *The 11th Mental Measurement Yearbook,* Lincoln, NB: Buros Institute, pp. 1024–1025.

Roid, G.H., Prifitera, A., Ledbetter, M. (1988). Confirmatory analysis of the factor structure of the Wechsler Memory Scale—Revised. *The Clinical Neuropsychologist, 2,* 116–120.

Roth, D.L., Conboy, T.J., Reeder, K.P., & Boll, T.J. (1990). Confirmatory factor analysis of the Wechsler Memory Scale—Revised in a sample of head-injured patients. *Journal of Clinical and Experimental Neuropsychology, 12,* 834–842.

Ryan, J.J., & Lewis, C.V. (1988). Comparison of normal controls and recently detoxified alcoholics on the Wechsler Memory Scale—Revised. *The Clinical Neuropsychologist, 2,* 173–180.

Shum, D.H.K., Murray, R.A., & Eadie, K. (1997). Effect of speed of presentation on administration of the Logical Memory subtest of the Wechsler Memory Scale-Revised. *The Clinical Neuropsychologist, 11,* 188–191.

Smith, G.E., Ivnik, R.J., Malec, J.F., Kokmen, E., Tangalos, E.G., & Kurland, L.T. (1992a). Mayo's older Americans normative studies (MOANS): Factor structure of a core battery. *Psychological Assessment, 4,* 382–390.

Smith, G.E., Malec, J.F., & Ivnik, R.J. (1992b). Validity of the construct of nonverbal memory: A factor-analytic study in a normal elderly sample. *Journal of Clinical and Experimental Neuropsychology, 14,* 211–211.

Smith, G.E., Wong, J.S., Ivnik, R.J., & Malec, J.F. (1997). Mayo's Older American Normative Studies: Separate norms for WMS-R Logical Memory stories. *Assessment, 4,* 79–86.

Strauss, E., Loring, D., Chelune, G., Hunter, M., Hermann, B., Perrine, K., Westerveld, M., Trenerry, M., & Barr, W. (1995). Predicting cognitive impairment in epilepsy: Findings from the Bozeman Epilepsy Consortium. *Journal of Clinical and Experimental Neuropsychology, 17,* 909–917.

Sullivan, K. (1996). Estimates of interrater reliability for the Logical Memory subtest of the Wechsler Memory Scale—Revised. *Journal of Clinical and Experimental Neuropsychology, 18,* 707–712.

Trenerry, M.R., Jack Jr., C.R., Cascino, G.D., Sharbrough, F.W., & Ivnik, R.J. (1996). Sex differences in the relationship between visual memory and MRI hippocampal volumes. *Neuropsychology, 10,* 343–351.

Troster, A.I., Butters, N., Salmon, D.P., Cullum, C.M., Jacobs, D., Brandt, J., & White, R.F. (1993). The diagnostic utility of saving scores: Differentiating Alzheimer's and Huntington's diseases with the Logical Memory and Visual Reproduction Tests. *Journal of Clinical and Experimental Neuropsychology, 15,* 773–788.

Wechsler, D. (1987). *Wechsler Memory Scale–Revised.* San Antonio TX: The Psychological Corporation.

Woodard, J.L. (1993). Confirmatory factor analysis of the Wechsler Memory Scale—Revised in a

mixed clinical population. *Journal of Clinical and Experimental Neuropsychology, 15,* 968–973.

Woodard, J.L., & Axelrod, B.N. (1995). Parsimonious prediction of Wechsler Memory Scale—Revised memory indices. *Psychological Assessment, 7,* 445–449.

WIDE RANGE ASSESSMENT OF MEMORY AND LEARNING (WRAML)

Purpose

The test was designed to evaluate the ability of children, aged 5–17 years, to learn and memorize verbal and visual information.

Source

The complete WRAML kit (including 25 examiner and response forms) can be obtained from Jastak Associates, Inc., 1526 Gilpin Avenue, Wilmington, DE 19806, at a cost of $305 US.

Description

The complete kit of the WRAML (Adams & Sheslow, 1990) includes a manual, stimulus sets, and response and record forms. There are three verbal, three visual, and three learning subtests, yielding a Verbal Memory Index, a Visual Memory Index, and a Learning Index. Combined, these nine subtests yield a General Memory Index. For each of the nine subtests, a scaled score can be obtained. For the Verbal, Visual, and Learning Indices, as well as the General Memory Index, standard scores and percentiles can be derived. Four optional delayed recall tasks and one recognition subtest are also available with guidelines provided to determine whether the level of performance was "Bright Average, Average, Low Average, Borderline, or Atypical" compared to age-mates.

Subtests on the Verbal Memory Scale assess the patient's capabilities on auditorily presented tasks increasing in semantic complexity. The child is asked to repeat series of mixed numbers and letters (Number/Letter Memory subtest: e.g., 2–S), to repeat meaningful sentences (Sentence Memory: e.g., I like pizza), and to recall two short stories that vary

in interest and linguistic complexity (Story Memory). The three visual subtests also increase in meaningfulness. The child is asked to recall a series of spatial patterns (Finger Windows), to recall the elements and locations of designs (Design Memory), and to recall parts of pictures displaying scenes (Picture Memory).

The three learning subtests assess the ability to retain information presented over trials. Thus, one subtest (Verbal Learning) examines the ability to recall a list of unrelated words (13 words for ages 8 and younger, 16 words for ages 9 and older). Another (Visual Learning) examines the ability to recall locations of designs. A third subtest (Sound Symbol) requires the child to recall sounds associated with various abstract symbols.

Delayed-recall subtests are included for Verbal Learning, Visual Learning, Sound Symbol, and Story Memory procedures in order to assess forgetting. Also available is a recognition format for delayed retention of the Story Memory subtest so that the examiner can explore issues of storage versus retrieval.

A Screening, or short, form is available and comprises Picture Memory, Design Memory, Verbal Learning, and Story Memory. Space is provided on the Examiner Form following the administration of the first four subtests to calculate a Memory Screening Index score.

Administration

The instructions for the WRAML are given in the manual (see source). Generally, the subtests are arranged so as to alternate between visual, verbal, and learning subtests. The examiner is encouraged to administer the subtests in the order presented in the manual.

Approximate Time for Administration

The time required to administer the WRAML is about 45 minutes and may extend to 1 hour if all Delayed Recall tasks are presented. The short form takes about 10–15 minutes to administer.

Scoring

The WRAML manual (see source) provides detailed scoring procedures. Briefly, after obtaining the raw scores on each subtest, the examiner must convert each raw score into a scaled score (mean = 10, SD = 3) using age-based tables provided in the WRAML manual. The sum of the scaled scores comprising the Verbal Memory Index, Visual Memory Index, and Learning Index are also computed using age-based tables. The General Memory Index is obtained by adding the sum of all scaled scores. Each Index has a mean of 100 and a standard deviation of 15. If only eight subtests have been given, a prorated General Memory Index can be calculated using a table provided in the WRAML manual. If the short form is given, the sum of the scaled scores for the four subtests is converted to a Memory Screening Index (mean = 100, SD = 15), using age-based tables provided in the manual.

A measure of forgetting can be obtained for Verbal Learning, Story Memory, Sound Symbol, and Visual Learning subtests by calculating difference scores (subtracting the Delay trial score from the Trial IV score). The examiner is provided with a descriptive ranking (Atypical, Borderline, Low Average, Average, Bright Average) based on standard deviations from the mean. Similar rankings are provided to judge the Story Memory Recognition scores.

Comment

Adams and Sheslow (1990) reported coefficient alpha measures of WRAML subtests and indices by age. Median coefficients for the subtests ranged from .78 (Verbal Learning) to .90 (Sound Symbol), and median coefficients for the various indices ranged from .90 (Visual Memory) to .96 (General Memory). Eighty-seven individuals from the normative sample were given the WRAML a second time with intervals ranging from 61 to 267 days; this second testing yielded stability coefficients for the indices ranging from .61 (Visual Memory) to .84 (General Memory). The subtest scaled score standard error of measurements (SEMs) ranges from .9 to 1.3. The Index median standard score SEMs are 3.9, 4.7, and 4.5 for Verbal Memory, Visual Memory, and Learning, respectively. The median General Memory Index standard score SEM is 3.0. Using these SEMs, confidence bands can be determined for each test score and significant differences determined between subtests or indices. When the respective two SEM bands of two obtained scores do not overlap, there is a 95 percent chance that the two "true scores" are actually different. Interscorer reliability for the Design Memory subtest was reported as .996 (Adams & Sheslow, 1990).

Although the correlation between the General Memory Index (GMI) and Screening Memory Index (MSI) is high (above .8), the MSI tends to overestimate the GMI by nearly five points, and thus may produce a false negative bias (Kennedy & Guilmette, 1997).

The WRAML is related to other memory measures. Adams and Sheslow (1990) found that the WRAML General Memory Index correlated .72 with the memory index from the McCarthy Scales, .54 with the WMS-R General Memory Index, and .80 with the Stanford-Binet Short Term Memory Index. Both the WRAML and the WMS-R can be given to individuals in the 16- to 17-year age group. The WRAML Verbal Memory Index correlated .44 with the WMS-R Verbal Memory Index. The WRAML Visual Memory Index correlated .47 with the WMS-R Visual Memory Index. The WRAML General Memory Index correlated .54 with the WMS-R General Memory Index, but .61 with the WMS-R Attention/Concentration Index, raising the concern that the test is more a measure of attention than of memory.

As might be expected based on the developmental nature of memory, scores improve with age (Adams & Sheslow, 1990). Correlations among the subtests tend to be low to moderate, although positive, indicating that the various measures of memory incorporated in the WRAML are related to one another.

The authors reported that principal components analysis yielded three factors that corresponded generally to the verbal memory, visual memory, and learning divisions suggested by them. Visual Learning, however, loaded more strongly on the visual memory than the learning component, and the Story Memory subtest loaded more on learning than verbal memory.

Subsequent work has called into question the validity of the Learning Memory Index and has suggested an attention/concentration dimension. Burton et al. (1996) examined the construct validity of the WRAML summary indices in the standardization sample using structural equation analysis. Findings supported a 3-factor model including Verbal Memory (Story Memory, Verbal Learning, Sound Symbol subtests), Visual Memory (Finger Windows, Design Memory, Picture Memory, Visual Learning subtests) and Attention/Concentration (Number/Letter, Sentence Memory, and to a lesser extent, Finger Windows). A distinct Learning Index was not found.

Williams and Dykman (1994) explored nonverbal abilities in 104 children, aged 7:10 to 16:6 years, referred for learning, emotional, and/or behavioral difficulties. The subtests composing the Visual Memory Index were given along with the WISC-R, the Beery, Benton's Form Discrimination, Trails, Grooved Pegboard, and Finger Tapping. Both Design Memory and Finger Windows loaded on the same factor as Block Design and the Beery, suggesting that these subtests contain significant visuo-spatial components. Picture Memory loaded on the same factor as Picture Completion and Picture Arrangement, suggesting the importance of the ability to attend to visual details.

The factor-analytic studies by Burton et al. (1996) and Williams and Dykman (1994) imply that the Finger Windows subtest contains both attentional and visuoperceptual components. As such, clinical interpretations of this subtest should include a consideration of both sources of variability.

The WRAML shows a moderate relation to general intellectual status and academic achievement. The test was given to forty children along with the WISC-R (Adams & Sheslow, 1990). The Verbal Memory Index correlated more strongly (.44) with Verbal IQ than with PIQ (.22). By contrast, the Visual Memory Index correlated more strongly (.51) with PIQ than with VIQ (.26). The General Memory Index showed a moderate relation (.56) with Full Scale IQ. The General Memory Index also is moderately related (.35–.46) to WRAT-R measures of reading, spelling, and arithmetic in children aged 6 to 8 years of age; in older children (aged 16 to 17 years), however, only the correlation (.38) with arithmetic was significant (Adams & Sheslow, 1990).

The WRAML has a number of advantages. It is relatively easy to administer and score. There is no evidence that sexual or racial bias significantly affects the test (Adams & Sheslow, 1990). In addition, Medway (1992) suggests that the WRAML is superior to the WMS-R in the 16–17 year age range since the latter was standardized on a smaller number of adolescents ($n = 50$) and has a lower reliability coefficient.

The instrument is relatively new and has not been subjected to necessary research or neuropsychological studies. We still do not know if data from the WRAML provide adequate information for making differential diagnoses (Clark, 1992). Moreover, based on current factor-analytic studies, it would appear that clinicians should be cautious when using the published WRAML indices. Reorganizing the subtests in order to provide Verbal Memory, Visual Memory, and Attention/Concentration indices might increase the utility of the scale (Burton et al., 1996).

Normative Data

The test was standardized on a sample of 2,363 children, ages 5:0 through 17:11, considered representative of the U.S. population in terms of age, sex, race, regional, and metropolitan/nonmetropolitan residence. Norms are based on about 110 cases in each of 21 age groups. There were half-year intervals for each age group through the age of 13. For the 14- and 15-year olds, there was a full year interval, while there was a 2-year interval for 16- and 17-year-olds. Children were selected from regular school classrooms. To reflect a representative population, children with special needs were also included "in appropriate proportions." However, children with specific disabilities that made it impossible to respond to the items were excluded.

References

Adams, W., & Sheslow, D. (1990). *WRAML* Manual. Wilmington, DE: Jastak Associates.

Burton, D.B., Donders, J., & Mittenberg, W. (1996). A structural equation analysis of the Wide Range Assessment of Memory and Learning in the standardization sample. *Child Neuropsychology, 2*, 39–49.

Clark, R.M. (1992). Review of the Wide Range As-

sessment of Memory and Learning. In J.J. Kramer & J. Close Conoley (Eds.) *The Eleventh Mental Measurements Yearbook*. Lincoln, NB: Buros Institute.

Kennedy, M.L., & Guilmette, T.J. (1997). The relationship between the WRAML Memory Screening and General Memory indices in a clinical population. *Assessment, 4*, 69–72.

Medway, F.J. (1992). Review of the Wide Range Assessment of Memory and Learning. In J.J. Kramer & J. Close Conoley (Eds.) *The Eleventh Mental Measurements Yearbook*. Lincoln, NB: Buros Institute.

Williams, J., & Dykman, R.A. (1994). Nonverbal factors derived from children's performances on neuropsychological test instruments. *Developmental Neuropsychology, 10*, 19–26.

11

Language Tests

Because of the central importance of verbal communication deficits after brain lesions as well as delays in language development in children, numerous tests of language function have been developed, including brief as well as detailed (Benton et al., 1989; Code et al., 1990; Eisenson, 1994; Goodglass & Kaplan, 1987; Huber et al., 1984; Kertesz, 1982; Porch, 1971; Schuell, 1973; Spreen & Benton, 1977) "aphasia screening tests" and bedside examinations (Fitch-West & Sands, 1986; Reitan, 1984; Reitan and Wolfson, 1992; Williams & Shane, 1986). In addition, tests directed more at the ability of the patient to communicate in daily life have been developed (Holland, 1980; Sarno, 1969).

While readers may wish to make their own choice among these batteries (see review by Spreen & Risser, 1991), we present here three comprehensive batteries: The relatively brief Multilingual Aphasia Examination (MAE), the more detailed and lengthy Boston Diagnostic Aphasia Examination (BDAE), and the Communication Abilities in Daily Living Test (CADL); these three are suitable if more than a screening of language abilities in test performance and in daily life is desirable. In addition, we review a selection of highly sensitive, but brief individual tests: Boston Naming Test, Controlled Oral World Association, Peabody Picture Vocabulary Test, Sentence Repetition Test [described in the memory section of this book] and the Token Test. In addition, two relatively new, specialized tests aimed

at specific patient populations, should be mentioned: the Boston Assessment of Severe Aphasia (BASA; Helm-Estabrooks et al., 1989), and the Arizona Battery for Communication Disorders in Dementia (ABCD; Bayles & Tomoeda, 1990). We include the first of these, but not the second, which includes examinations of mental status, memory, and other functions for the use by speech therapists, but which neuropsychologists probably would prefer to assess with other, better validated instruments.

Several comprehensive tests are available for children, notably the Test of Language Development (TOLD, Newcomer & Hamill, 1988) for the age range from 4 years to 12 years 11 months, the Clinical Evaluation of Language Fundamentals—Revised (CELF-3; Semel, Wiig, & Secord, 1995) for the age range from 5 years to 21 years 11 months, and the now somewhat dated Illinois Test of Psycholinguistic Abilities (Kirk et al., 1995). All three are based on a linguistic rather than neuropsychological model and show extensive psychometric sophistication. We selected the CELF-3 because of its coverage of language functions tested which may also be useful in adult aphasia examinations. Among tests of individual language functions, the new Comprehensive Receptive and Expressive Vocabulary Test, covering the range between 4 years and 17 years 11 months (CRVET; Wallace & Hammill, 1994) may be of interest to the reader, but is not reviewed here because it overlaps with the vocabulary subtest of the Wechsler tests and with the Boston Naming Test.

References

Bayles, K.A., & Tomoeda, C.K. (1990). *Arizona Battery for Communication Disorders of Dementia (ABCD)*. Tucson, AZ: Canyonlands Publishing Inc.

Benton, A.L., Hamsher, K. deS., & Sivan, A.B. (1994). *Multilingual Aphasia Examination* (3rd ed.) San Antonio, TX: Psychological Corporation.

Code, C., Heer, M., & Schofield, M. (1990). *The Computerized Boston (BDAE)*. San Antonio, TX: Psychological Corporation.

Eisenson, J. (1994). *Examining for Aphasia* (3rd ed.). Austin, TX; Pro-Ed.

Fitch-West, J., & Sands, E.S. (1986). *Bedside Evaluation and Screening Test of Aphasia*. Austin, TX: Pro-Ed.

Goodglass, H., & Kaplan, E. (1987). *Boston Diagnostic Aphasia Examination (BDAE)* (2nd ed.). Philadelphia: Lea & Febiger.

Helm-Estabrooks, N., Ramsberger, G., Morgan, A.R., & Nicholas, M. (1989). *BASA: Boston Assessment of Severe Aphasia*. Chicago: Riverside Publishing Co.

Holland, A.L. (1980). *Communicative Abilities of Daily Living: Manual*. Baltimore: University Park Press.

Huber, W., Poeck, K., & Willmes, K. (1984). The Aachen Aphasia Test. In F.C. Rose (Ed.) *Progress in Aphasiology*. Advances of Neurology, Vol. 42. New York: Raven Press. pp. 291–303.

Kertesz, A. (1982). *Western Aphasia Battery*. San Antonio, TX: Psychological Corporation.

Kertesz, A. (1993). *Western Aphasia Battery Scoring Assistant*. San Antonio, TX: Psychological Corporation.

Kirk, S.A., McCarthy, J., & Kirk, W. (1968). *The Illinois Test of Psycholinguistic Abilities*. Urbana: Illinois University Press.

Newcomer, P.L., & Hammill, D.D. (1988). *Tests of Language Development* (2nd ed.). Austin, TX: Pro-Ed.

Porch, B. (1971). *The Porch Index of Communicative Ability*. Vol. 2. *Administration and Scoring*. Palo Alto, CA: Consulting Psychologists Press.

Reitan, R.M. (1984). *Aphasia and Sensory-Perceptual Deficits in Adults*. Tucson, AZ: Reitan Neuropsychology Laboratory.

Reitan, R.M., & Wolfson, D. (1992). A short screening examination for impaired brain functions in early school-age children. *Clinical Neuropsychologist, 6*, 287–294.

Sarno, M.T. (1969). *The Functional Communication Profile*. Manual of Directions. New York: New York University Medical Center, Institute of Rehabilitation Medicine.

Schuell, H. (1973). *Differential Diagnosis of Aphasia with the Minnesota Test* (2nd ed.). Minneapolis: University of Minnesota Press.

Semel, E., Wiig, E.H., & Secord, W. (1987). *Clinical Evaluation of Language Fundamentals*. San Antonio, TX: Psychological Corporation.

Spreen, O., & Benton, A.L. (1977). *Neurosensory Center Comprehensive Examination for Aphasia*. Victoria, BC: Neuropsychology Laboratory, University of Victoria.

Spreen, O., & Risser, A. (1990). Assessment of aphasia. In M.T. Sarno (Ed.), *Acquired Aphasia* (2nd ed.). New York: Academic Press.

Wallace, G., & Hammill, D.D. (1994). *Comprehensive Receptive and Expressive Vocabulary Test (CREVT)*. Austin, TX: Pro-Ed.

Williams, J.M., & Shane, B. (1986). The Reitan-Indiana Aphasia Screening Test: Scoring and factor analysis. *Journal of Clinical Psychology, 42*, 156–160.

BOSTON ASSESSMENT OF SEVERE APHASIA (BASA)

Purpose

The purpose of the BASA is to provide a full assessment of language and other communicative functions in severely aphasic patients.

Source

The test is available from Riverside Publishing Company, 8420 Bryn Mawr Ave., Chicago, IL 60631, at a price of $210 US for the complete set of material, including manual and briefcase.

Description

The BASA (Helm-Estabrooks et al., 1989) consists of 61 items in 15 subtests:

1. Social Greetings and Simple Conversation. Responding appropriately to greeting ("Good afternoon," "How are you feeling to-

day?"), name, statement of purpose of visit, etc. Four items.

2. Personally Relevant Yes/No Questions. ["Is this (wrong name) hospital?"]. The patient responds verbally or by using a yes/no knob. Five items.

3. Orientation to Time and Place. The patient responds verbally or by pointing to a calendar (for month, part of month), or map ("Where do you live"?). Three items.

4. Bucco-Facial Praxis. The patient is requested to make mouth movements on command. Four items.

5. Sustained "Ah" and Singing. Two items.

6. Repetition. Single words and short sentences ("I love you") are repeated. Six items.

7. Limb Praxis. Patient is asked to show how to salute and shake a finger at a naughty child. Two items.

8. Comprehension of Number Symbols. Point to the appropriate number on a four-choice card, or indicate the number of fingers shown by the examiner. Three items.

9. Object Naming. Patient is asked to name, describe the use, or demonstrate the use of objects (e.g., toy gun). Two items.

10. Action Picture Items. Patient is asked to choose a picture of an activity demonstrated or verbalized by the examiner (e.g., sleeping), and name the activity. Ten items.

11. Comprehension of Coin Names. Patient indicates the correct coin or coins named by the examiner. Six items.

12. Famous Faces. Name, describe, or otherwise indicate identity of Hitler, W.C. Fields, and Marilyn Monroe. Three items.

13. Emotional Words, Phrases, and Symbols. Reading or otherwise indicating comprehension of words (e.g., "pain"). Five items.

14. Visuospatial Items. Free-hand drawing of a man, visual matching, and visual memory for a drawing or stick design. Four items.

15. Signature. Patient is asked to sign, and leaves the session with appropriate greeting. Two items.

Administration

See source. Note that several items can be administered in a relatively informal manner or as part of a conversation.

Approximate Time of Administration

Approximately 30–40 minutes are required for the administration of the full test.

Scoring

See source. Items are scored at several levels of performance, dependent on the task demands: NR = no verbal or gestural response; GR = gestural refusal; G0 = noncommunicative gestural response; G1 = partially communicative gestural response; G2 = fully communicative gestural response; A = gestural response with affective quality; P = perseverative gestural response; VR = verbal refusal; V0 = noncommunicative verbal response; V1 = partially communicative verbal response; V2 = fully communicative verbal response; A = verbal response with affective quality; and P = perseverative verbal response. For each subtest, exact scoring criteria are provided. Correct responses (V2) are summed across five item clusters (auditory comprehension, praxis, oral-gestural expression, reading comprehension, gesture recognition + writing + visuospatial tasks). The grand total of correct responses forms the BASA total score. The total of other responses can also be summed across clusters and for the total test.

Comment

Internal consistency is high (between .72 and .89) for the five areas and .94 for the total score, slightly lower in global aphasics. Test–retest reliability for 39 severe aphasics after an average of 3.7 months ranged from .52 to .73 for the area scores, and was .74 for the total score. Reliability was similar for 23 global aphasics. Interrater reliability ranged from 80 to 100 percent in two patients.

Concurrent validity studies with the Boston Diagnostic Aphasia Examination (BDAE; described elsewhere in this section) show modest to adequate correlations. This is probably to be expected because of the low range of the BASA subtests and the wide range of the BDAE. The correlation for 43 patients between BASA total score and BDAE aphasia severity rating was .67.

Cluster-total score correlations ranged from .44 to .76, suggesting some independence of each area score. A factor analysis showed an expressive, a visuospatial, and a comprehensive language factor.

The BASA samples a wide range of communicative functions at a relatively low level and lends itself to bedside examination of severely language-impaired patients. The authors state that a number of items were inappropriate or ineffective when testing (presumably non-aphasic) closed-head injury patients. The test has many qualities that make it comparable to the Communication Abilities in Daily Living test (CADL), but is shorter and perhaps not suitable for the wider range of aphasia severity covered by the CADL. It has, however, demonstrated significant improvement in 31 global, 5 severe Wernicke's and 5 other severe aphasics over a 2-year period (Nicholas et al., 1993); the authors noted that initial test scores were less accurate than 6-months post-onset cluster scores for the prediction of the total BASA score after 24 months.

The scoring of affect, perseveration, and of partial verbal and gestural responses can provide useful information for the examiner and others, but so far these have not been further investigated.

Normative Data

Norms are presented as preliminary and are based on the performance of 111 patients with severe and 47 with global aphasia. To use the norms, raw scores for the five areas are converted into standard scores, which in turn can be used to assign a percentile rank within this aphasic population. Norms for normal healthy speakers are not provided, because they would presumably achieve a perfect score. Effects of age, gender, or education are not reported.

References

Helm-Estabrooks, N., Ramsberger, G., Morgan, A.R., & Nicholas, M. (1989). *BASA: Boston Assessment of Severe Aphasia*. Chicago: Riverside Publishing Co.

Nicholas, M., Helm-Estabrooks, N., Ward-Lonergan, J., & Morgan, A.R. (1993). Evolution of severe aphasia in the first two years post onset. *Archives of Physical Medicine and Rehabilitation, 74*, 830–836.

BOSTON DIAGNOSTIC APHASIA EXAMINATION (BDAE)

Purpose

The purpose of the BDAE is to provide a full assessment of an aphasic patient's language functioning with special reference to the classic, anatomically based aphasia syndromes.

Source

The test is available from the Psychological Corporation, 555 Academic Court, San Antonio, TX 78204-2498, at a price of $72 US for the complete set, including manual. A Spanish (Goodglass & Kaplan, 1986), a French (Mazaux & Orgogozo, 1985), and a Hindi version (Kacker et al., 1991) are available. Computerized scoring and interpretation software is also available (Code et al. 1990).

Description

The test is described in "The Assessment of Aphasia and Related Disorders" (Goodglass & Kaplan, 1983b) and includes 16 stimulus cards, a scoring booklet for naming, and the spiral-bound 60 picture-cards of the Boston Naming Test described separately in this section. The text includes a description of the nature of aphasic deficits, common clusters of defects, and information on reliability and validity, standardization, administration, and scoring, as well as illustrative test profiles for major aphasia syndromes.

The first part of the test covers conversational and expository speech in response to seven questions, a brief open-ended conversation, and the description of the "cookie-theft card." On the basis of these speech samples, a 5-point aphasia severity rating, ranging from "minimal discernable speech handicap" to "no usable speech or auditory comprehension" is made, followed by a 7-point rating on specific aspects of speech (melodic line, phrase length, articulatory agility, grammatical form, paraphasia, repetition, word-finding, and auditory comprehension). In addition, neologisms, literal, verbal, and extended paraphasias as well as articulation are rated on the basis of errors that occurred during Automated Sequences, Reciting, Word Repetition, and Repetition of Phrases and Sentences as described below.

The second part of the BDAE consists of formal testing of:

1. Auditory Comprehension, which tests for

   a. Word Discrimination (pointing to objects, actions, forms, numbers, letters, colors on cards as requested by the examiner; 36 items);

   b. Body-Part Identification ("Show me your . . . ," including right-left discrimination; 26 items);

   c. Commands (including 1 to 5 informational units, e.g., "make a fist"; 5 items.);

   d. Complex Ideational Material (yes or no responses to questions like "Will a stone sink in water?" and questions indicating that the patient has comprehended four different paragraphs; 24 items).

2. Oral Expression, including

   a. Oral Agility (six different mouth movements);

   b. Verbal Agility (rapid repetition of seven different words; number of repetitions and parahasias are coded);

   c. Automated Sequences (e.g., recite days of the week; 4 items);

   d. Recitation, Singing, and Rhythm (e.g., reciting nursery rhyme, pledge of allegiance, singing familiar song, repeating a rhythm tapped on the table; 10 items);

   e. Repetition of Words (of increasing length and difficulty; 10 items);

   f. Repeating Phrases and Sentences (of high and low probability; 16 items);

   g. Word Reading;

   h. Responsive Naming ("What do we tell time with?");

   i. Visual Confrontational Naming (38 items);

   j. Animal Naming (controlled oral word association for 90 seconds);

   k. Oral Sentence Reading (10 items).

3. Understanding Written Language, including

   a. Symbol and Word Discrimination (10 items);

   b. Word Recognition (point to the word spoken by the examiner; 8 items);

   c. Comprehension of Oral Spelling (by saying the word; 8 items);

   d. Word-Picture Matching (10 items);

   e. Reading Sentences and Paragraphs (using a multiple-choice sentence-completion technique; 10 items).

4. Writing, including

   a. A 4-point rating of the Mechanics of Writing;

   b. Serial Writing (alphabet and numbers);

   c. Primer-Level Dictation (letters, numbers, and words);

   d. Spelling to Dictation (10 items);

   e. Written Confrontation Naming (10 items);

   f. Narrative Writing ("Cookie-theft" picture);

   g. Sentences to Dictation.

In addition, several optional supplementary language tests explore psycholinguistic aspects of language; comprehension of prepositions of location, passive subject-object discrimination, and possessive relationships; expression of indicative, interrogative, and conditional verb and tense usage; specific repetition tasks for conduction aphasia; naming by touch; instructions for exploring minor hand agraphia; and the Boston Naming Test (described separately in this volume) as an extended vocabulary test.

Supplementary nonlanguage tests (spatial-quantitative tests, also called the "Boston Parietal Lobe Battery") are included as a separate chapter as well as on the profile summary. These include constructional apraxia (drawing to command—including clock drawing, stick construction copying, stick construction from memory, three-dimensional block design— similar to Benton's test), finger agnosia, right-left orientation, acalculia, and ideational apraxia, as well as commands to test for bucco-facial apraxia.

Administration

See source. For the novice user, the differences in order of presentation in the manual compared to the answer booklet and the profile summary can be confusing. It should be kept in mind that the manual follows a convenient order of administration in a clinical setting, whereas the booklet is provided for scoring convenience, and the summary profile reorganizes the results in a logical fashion for interpretation purposes.

Approximate Time of Administration

Approximately 90–120 minutes are required for the administration of the full test, although Kertesz (1989) suggested that the test may take up to 8 hours in some patients.

Scoring

See source. Ratings are used for the first part of the test as described above. For all other tests, scoring instructions are provided in the manual (Chapter 4 of Goodglass & Kaplan, 1983b) and are only partly repeated in the answer booklet. The profile summary automatically translates raw scores into percentile ranks, based on 242 aphasic patients.

Comment

The BDAE is one of the more popular (Beele et al., 1984) comprehensive aphasia batteries. As the title implies, it attempts to cover all areas of language function that are relevant to the diagnosis of the classic anatomically based subtypes of aphasia rather than following a specific model of language.

A unique feature of the test is the inclusion of ratings of free speech samples. Agreement between three judges rating 99 aphasic speech samples was .85 or better, except for word-finding difficulties and paraphasias (.78 and .79, respectively). Other interrater agreement studies have also shown satisfactory results (Davis, 1993).

Internal consistency ranges from .98 for visual confrontation naming to .68 for body-part identification. Test–retest reliability is not reported.

Knowledge of the "Boston school" approach to aphasia classification is necessary to interpret the BDAE. The test is lengthy and probably more useful for assessments in the context of detailed studies of aphasia and aphasia rehabilitation than as a routine language test included in a general neuropsychological assessment. The somewhat unwieldy, large number of tasks is clearly the result of trying to fit classical clinical-neurological testing into a psychometric format. In addition, the test includes useful directions for observing and recording many specific types of errors (e.g., paraphasias) found in aphasia, demonstrating the Boston process approach. However, even if the full-length test is not used, a number of subtests can be useful additions to neuropsychological assessment depending on the presenting symptoms of the patient. The inclusion of the "parietal lobe battery" and tests of apraxia, dyscalculia, and articulation is unusual in a language examination; it indicates that the authors developed the BDAE from the richness of the clinical "process" rather than from a specific model of language; most of these tests are sufficient for screening purposes, although many are also available (in somewhat different format) as separate tests described elsewhere in this manual.

Borod et al. (1984) applied the parietal lobe battery to 163 right-handed aphasics and found four factors: construction, visual schemata, verbal components of the Gerstmann syndrome, and visual finger recognition. Impairment was strongest in patients with lesions in both left parietal and frontal areas. The spatial-quantitative tests (formerly called the parietal lobe battery) together with the WAIS was applied to right- and left-handed aphasics: Left-handed aphasics were significantly poorer on both, especially on tasks involving visuo-spatial construction, suggesting that in left-handers, the left hemisphere is typically dominant for tasks usually considered as right-hemisphere specific (Borod et al., 1985).

Construct validity has been examined by reviewing the intercorrelation matrix of the 43 language and 23 nonlanguage measures of the BDAE and by factor analysis. In an earlier analysis (Goodglass & Kaplan, 1972), a strong general language factor emerged, as expected, with other factors covering spatial-quantitative-somatognostic, articulation-grammatical fluency, auditory-comprehension, and paraphasia domains. A second factor analysis (Goodglass & Kaplan, 1983b), omitting ratings and non-language tests, resulted in five factors (comprehension/reading/naming, recitation/repetition, writing, oral agility/singing/rhythm, auditory comprehension). When rating scales were included, three additional factors (fluency, reading, paraphasia) were found. The addition of the spatial-quantitative tests resulted in a 10-factor solution including a strong spatial-quantitative factor, a finger identification factor, and a factor labeled "freedom from paraphasia." Discriminant validity between cases of Broca, Wernicke, conduction, and anomic aphasia was optimal when the following tests were entered into the equation: body-part identification, repetition of high-probability sentences, paraphasia rating, word-finding rating, phrase-length rating, and verbal paraphasias.

Divenyi and Robinson (1989) reported correlations of .86 and .93 of the auditory comprehension measured in the BDAE with the Token Test and with the respective part of the Porch Index of Communication Ability. The BDAE and the oral apraxia task specifically were found to be related to other articulation tasks (Sussman et al., 1986).

However, the BDAE auditory comprehension subtest was not an adequate predictor of auditory paragraph comprehension in independent standardized material (Brookshire & Nicholas, 1984); a second study (Nicholas et al., 1986) showed that both aphasic and healthy subjects were able to answer a similar number of questions about a paragraph without having actually read the passage, suggesting a high passage dependency of this test. Dyadic interaction measures of nonverbal

communication also did not correlate well with the BDAE (Behrman & Penn, 1984).

Decision rules for the "diagnosis" of the individual subtypes are not always clearly defined, although a paper by Reinvang and Graves (1975) attempted such clarification. Crary et al. (1992) tried to isolate subtypes of aphasia empirically by means of a Q-type factor analysis for the BDAE and the closely related Western Aphasia Battery (WAB); the resulting seven patient clusters (labeled Broca, anomic, global, Wernicke, conduction, and two unclassified clusters) agreed only poorly (in 38 percent of 47 patients) with the classification obtained using the classification rules of the test itself; the results were even worse for the WAB. The study, aside from its limited subject population for factor-analytic studies and the use of a somewhat dated cluster-analysis technique, suggests that BDAE classification rules are based on clinical rather than construct validity. Similarly, Naeser and Hayward (1978) and Reinvang (1985) pointed out that scale profiles can aid in the classification, but do not firmly classify patients into subtypes of aphasia. The test authors acknowledge that 30 to 80 percent of aphasic patients are not classifiable; this is also consistent with clinical experience that a majority of aphasic patients show mixed rather than pure symptomatology.

In other studies of aphasia, Li and Williams (1990) showed that in the Repeating Phrases and Sentences subtest, conduction aphasics showed a greater number of phonemic attempts, word revisions, and word and phrase repetitions; Broca's aphasics showed more phonemic errors and omissions; and Wernicke's aphasics produced more unrelated words and jargon. The BDAE also predicted progress in therapy well (Helms-Estabrooks & Ramsberger, 1986; Davidoff & Katz, 1985). In aphasics, word reading (Selnes et al., 1984) and confrontation naming (Knopman et al., 1984) showed striking improvement after 6 months had elapsed since time of insult.

In dementia of the Alzheimer type (AD), Kirshner (1982) found language to be fluent with normal prosody, syntax, and phrase length; few paraphasias were found, but word-finding problems and poor repetition of low-probability phrases were present. Sentence comprehension, but not letter and word reading, were found to be related to severity of AD patients (Cummings et al., 1986). Whitworth and Larson (1989) compared 25 AD patients, 25 patients with other dementias, and 58 age-matched controls: They found significant differences compared to controls on all but four of 38 BDAE scores (paraphasia, articulation, primer dictation, word reading). Discriminant function analysis produced correct classification for 95 percent of the three groups. Nineteen test scores contributed to the discrimination of four levels ("stages") of severity of dementia, resulting in correct classification of 100 percent of 22 dementia patients. Gorelick et al. (1993) found also that scores on the BDAE Commands and Responsive Naming subtests were lower in 66 patients with multi-infarct dementia as compared to a group of 86 patients with infarcts without dementia. In a comparison of multi-infarct, AD, and normal control subjects, Mendez and Ashla-Mendez (1991) found that the unstructured cookie-theft description discriminated better than structured tests between groups: The multi-infarct group produced fewer words per minute and constructional assemblages.

In an acute trauma center study, Gruen et al. (1990) found that 218 patients with closed head-injury showed significantly poorer word-fluency skills than normal subjects; although their strategies were similar to those used by normal subjects, some qualitative differences in semantic associations were found that were related to severity of cognitive disruption.

Normative Data

The BDAE was standardized on 147 healthy normal adult subjects (Borod et al., 1984) to provide cutoff scores at 2 SD below the mean, and age and education corrections are included. These means, ranges, and suggested cutoff scores are included in the manual. Means, standard deviations, and ranges for the subtests, based on 147–193 patients in the 1972 sample, and on 97–232 patients in the 1983 sample, including many with cerebrovascular accidents, but also those with other neurological disorders, are presented to provide an index of severity of aphasia in the various areas tested. These norms are useful only for neuropsychologists who work with patient populations similar to those of the test authors.

Emery (1986) found only minimal, insignificant decline of scores on all subtests when comparing 20 healthy adults aged 30–42 years with a similar group aged 75–93 years. Whitworth and Larson (1989) found no significant effects for gender and education in their sample. Heaton, Grant, and Matthews (1991) present norms for the comprehension of complex material task of the BDAE in scaled scores, corrected for gender, education, and age, that are based on 553 normal subjects. However, these norms should be used with caution because the number of subjects in some of the

Table 11–1. Norms for the Parietal Lobe Battery in Older Adults

Age	40–49	50–59	60–69	70–79	80–89
n	16	16	16	12	8
Drawings	10.4	10.9	10.4	9.6	8.4
Stick Designs	11.2	10.8	10.8	10.4	8.4
Finger Gnosis	148.2	146.8	148.5	145.1	142.4
R-L Orientation	30.4	31.7	33.0	31.2	30.4
Arithmetic	30.4	29.9	30.7	30.0	30.0
Clock Setting	11.1	11.2	11.5	10.9	7.9
Map Orientation	12.3	12.7	12.6	11.9	10.0
Block Construction	9.5	9.4	9.5	8.0	4.3

Source: Farver & Farver (1982).

cells is quite small. Norms based on 180 normal Spanish speakers from Colombia, broken down by educational level and three age ranges (16–39, 31–50, 51–65 years) were presented by Rosselli et al. (1990). These data show a significant effect of educational level for most tasks, and an age effect for some of the tasks, e.g., word discrimination, confrontation and animal naming, oral sentence reading, high- and low-probability repetition, symbol discrimination, oral spelling, word-picture matching, sentence-paragraph comprehension, and serial, primer-level dictation, written confrontation, spelling to dictation writing, all showed a significant drop in the oldest age group.

Norms for the parietal lobe battery in older subjects (ages 40–89) were presented by Farver and Farver (1982) and are shown as Table 11–1.

References

Beele, K.A., Davies, E., & Muller, D.J. (1984). Therapists' views on the clinical usefulness of four aphasia tests. *British Journal of Disorders of Communication, 19,* 169–178.

Behrman, M., & Penn, C. (1984). Non-verbal communication of aphasic patients. *Journal of Disorders of Communication, 19,* 169–178.

Borod, J.C., Carper, M., Goodglass, H., & Naeser, M. (1984). Aphasic performance on a battery of constructional, visuo-spatial, and quantitative tasks: Factorial structure and CT scan localization. *Journal of Clinical Neuropsychology, 6,* 189–204.

Borod, J.C., Carper, M., Naeser, M., & Goodglass, H. (1985). Left-handed and right-handed aphasics with left hemisphere lesions compared on nonverbal performance measures. *Cortex, 21,* 81–90.

Brookshire, R.H., & Nicholas, L.E. (1984). Comprehension of directly and indirectly stated main ideas and details in discourse by brain-damaged and non-brain-damaged listeners. *Brain and Language, 21,* 21–36.

Code, C., Heer, M., & Schofield, M. (1990). *The Computerized Boston.* Malvern, PA: Lea & Febiger.

Crary, M.A., Wertz, R.T., & Deal, J.L. (1992). Classifying aphasias: Cluster analysis of Western Aphasia Battery and Boston Diagnostic Aphasia Examination. *Aphasiology, 6,* 29–36.

Cummings, J.L., Houlihan, J.P., & Hill, M.A. (1986). The pattern of reading deterioration in dementia of the Alzheimer type: Observations and implications. *Brain and Language, 29,* 315–323.

Davidoff, M., & Katz, R. (1985). Automated telephone therapy for improving comprehension in aphasic adults. *Cognitive Rehabilitation, 3,* 26–28.

Davis, A.G. (1993). *A Survey of Adult Aphasia* (2nd ed.). Englewood Cliffs, NJ: Prentice-Hall.

Divenyi, P.L., & Robinson, A.J. (1989). Non-linguistic auditory capabilities in aphasia. *Brain and Language, 37,* 290–326.

Emery, O.B. (1986). Linguistic decrement in normal aging. *Language and Communication, 6,* 47–64.

Farver, P.F., & Farver, T.B. (1982). Performance of normal older adults on tests designed to measure parietal lobe function (constructional apraxia, Gerstmann's syndrome, visuospatial organization). *American Journal of Occupational Therapy, 36,* 444–449.

Goodglass, H., & Kaplan, E. (1972). *The Assessment of Aphasia and Related Disorders.* Malvern, PA: Lea & Febiger.

Goodglass, H., & Kaplan, E. (1983a). *Boston Diagnostic Aphasia Examination.* Philadelphia: Lea & Febiger.

Goodglass, H., & Kaplan, E. (1983b). *The Assessment of Aphasia and Related Disorders* (2nd ed.). Malvern, PA: Lea & Febiger.

Goodglass, H., & Kaplan, E. (1986). *La evaluacion de la afasia y de transfornos relacionados* (2nd ed.). Madrid: Editorial Medical Panamericana.

Gorelick, P.B., Brody, J., Cohen, D., & Freels, S. (1993). Risk factors for dementia associated with multiple cerebral infarcts: A case-control analysis in predominantly African-American hospital-based patients. *Archives of Neurology, 50,* 714–720.

Gruen, A.K., Frankle, B.C., & Schwartz, R. (1990). Word fluency generation skills of head-injured patients in an acute trauma center. *Journal of Communication Disorders, 23,* 163–170.

Heaton, R.K., Grant, I., & Matthews, C.G. (1991). *Comprehensive Norms for an Expanded Halstead-Reitan Battery: Demographic Corrections, Research Findings, and Clinical Applications.* Odessa, FL: Psychological Assessment Resources.

Helms-Estabrook, N., & Ramsberger, G. (1986). Treatment of agrammatism in long-term Broca's aphasia. *British Journal of Disorders of Communication, 21,* 39–45.

Kacker, S.K., Pandit, R., & Dua, D. (1991). Reliability and validity studies of examination for aphasia test in Hindi. *Indian Journal of Disability and Rehabilitation, 5*, 13–19.

Kertesz, A. (1989). Assessing aphasic disorders. In E. Perecman (Ed.), *Integrating Theory and Practice in Clinical Neuropsychology.* Hillsdale, NJ: Laurence Erlbaum.

Kirshner, H.S. (1982). Language disorders in dementia. In F. Freeman & H.S. Kirshner (Eds.), *Neurolinguistics,* Vol. 12. *Neurology of Aphasia.* Amsterdam: Swets & Zeitlinger.

Knopman, D.S., Selnes, O.A., Niccum, N., & Rubens, A.B. (1984). Recovery of naming in aphasia: Relationship to fluency, comprehension, and CT findings. *Neurology, 34,* 1461–1470.

Li, E.C., & Williams, S.E. (1990). Repetition deficits in three aphasic syndromes. *Journal of Communication Disorders, 23,* 77–88.

Mazaux, J.M., & Orgogozo, J.M. (1985). *Echelle d'évaluation de l'aphasie.* Issy-les-Moulineaux, France: EAP.

Mendez, M.F., & Ashla-Mendez, M. (1991). Differences between multi-infarct dementia and Alzheimer's disease on unstructured neuropsychological tasks. *Journal of Clinical and Experimental Neuropsychology, 13,* 923–932.

Naeser, M.A., & Hayward, R.W. (1978). Lesion localization in aphasia with cranial computed tomography and the Boston Diagnostic Aphasia Exam. *Neurology, 28,* 545–551.

Nicholas, L.E., MacLennan, D.L., & Brookshire, R.H. (1986). Validity of multiple sentence reading of comprehension tests for aphasic adults. *Journal of Speech and Hearing Disorders, 51,* 82–87.

Reinvang, I. (1985). *Aphasia and Brain Organization.* New York: Plenum Press.

Reinvang, I., & Graves, R. (1975). A basic aphasia examination: Description with discussion of first results. *Scandinavian Journal of Rehabilitation Medicine, 7,* 129–135.

Rosselli, M., Ardila, A., Florez, A., & Castro, C. (1990). Normative data on the Boston Diagnostic Aphasia Examination in a Spanish-speaking population. *Journal of Clinical and Experimental Neuropsychology, 12* 313–322.

Selnes, O.A., Niccum, N.E., Knopman, D.S., & Rubens, A.B. (1984). Recovery of single word comprehension: CT-scan correlates. *Brain and Language, 21,* 72–84.

Sussman, H., Marquardt, T., Hutchinson, J., & MacNeilage, P. (1986). Compensatory articulation in Broca's aphasia. *Brain and Language, 27,* 56–74.

Whitworth, R.H., & Larson, C.M. (1989). Differential diagnosis and staging of Alzheimer's disease with an aphasia battery. *Neuropsychiatry, Neuropsychology, and Behavioral Neurology, 1,* 255–265.

BOSTON NAMING TEST (BNT)

Purpose

The purpose of the test is to assess the ability to name pictured objects.

Source

The test can be ordered from Lea & Febiger, 600 Washington Square, Philadelphia, PA 19106, or from Psychological Assessment Resources (PAR), Box 998, Odessa, FL, at a cost of about $40 US, including scoring booklets.

Description

Because of the high incidence of naming problems in aphasia as well as in other neuropathological conditions, virtually all aphasia examinations contain a naming task. This popular test, originally published by Kaplan et al. (1978) as an experimental version with 85 items and now revised to a 60-item test (Kaplan et al., 1983), provides a detailed examination of naming abilities, well standardized across age, which is preferred when more than a brief examination is desired. It is an addition to, rather than part of, the Boston Diagnostic Aphasia Examination (BDEA, Goodglass & Kaplan, 1987). Sixty line drawings ranging from simple, high-frequency vocabulary ("tree") to rare words ("abacus") are presented one at a time on cards, and two prompting cues (phonemic cue, stimulus cue) are given if the patient does not produce the word spontaneously. A Spanish adaptation is available (Taussig et al., 1988; Ponton et al., 1992), and Morrison et al., (1996) used the test with normal French-speaking subjects in Quebec, Canada. This test may also be suitable for children from age 5 years to 14 years 11 months.

Administration

For young children and all aphasics, begin with item 1 and discontinue after six successive failures. For all other adult subjects, begin with item 30 (harmonica). If any of the next eight items are failed, proceed backward from item 29 until a total of eight consecutive preceding items are passed; then resume in a forward direction and discontinue the test when the patient makes six consecutive errors. Credit is given if the item is correctly named in 20 seconds. Only in those instances where the patient has clearly misperceived the picture is the subject told that the picture represents something else, and the patient is supplied with the bracketed stimulus cues that appear on the record form.

For example, if the response for mushroom is "umbrella," the patient is given the first (semantic) stimulus cue, "something to eat." If the subject then correctly names the item within 20 seconds, a check is entered in the stimulus cue correct column. If the subject is unable to name the picture correctly within 20 seconds, a second (phonemic) cue (i.e., the underlined initial phoneme(s) of the name of the item, e.g., "m") is offered. The response is recorded and entered in the appropriate column (phonemic cue correct, incorrect), but no credit is given.

Time for Administration

The test requires approximately 10–20 minutes.

Scoring

Recorded are (1) the number of spontaneously given correct responses, (2) the number of stimulus cues given, (3) the number of correct responses following a stimulus cue, (4) the number of phonemic cues, and (5) the number of correct and incorrect responses following phonemic cues.

A total naming score is derived by summing the number of correct responses [(1) and (3)]

between the baseline item and the ceiling item, and adding that total to the number of test items that precede the baseline.

Azrin et al. (1996) warned that in Southern African-American subjects some regionally correct words should be scored, e.g., "snake," "worm" (pretzel), "tomwalkers," "walkers" (stilts), "falseface" (mask), and "harp," "mouth organ" (harmonica), although on average the inclusion of these responses as correct increased the total score only by .32 points. Tombaugh and Hubley (1996) noted "mouth organ" and other incorrect responses ("lock" or "bold" for latch, "dice" for dominoes, "toadstool" for mushroom) and suggested that in these and similar cases a follow-up question should be asked ("What is another name for this?"). Worall et al. (1995) found scores to be 2 to 5 points lower than U.S. norms in elderly Australian subjects, and warn that word-frequency differences between cultures should be taken into account when interpreting scores of non-American subjects.

Comment

Test–retest reliability after 8 months in 51 adult intractable epileptics is reported as .94 (Sawrie et al., 1996). Henderson et al. (1990) reported an 80 percent response consistency for both uncued and cued responses in Alzheimer disease patients after 6 months. Huff et al. (1986) divided the original version of the test into two equivalent forms and obtained between-forms correlations of .81 in healthy control subjects, and of .97 in patients with Alzheimer's disease. The coefficient alpha between the two forms was .96. Thompson and Heaton (1989) compared the old experimental version of 85 items, with the standard 60-item, and with the two non-overlapping 42-item versions (Huff et al., 1986), in 49 clinical patients. The correlations between the 85-, the 60-, and the 42-items versions ranged from .96 to .92, whereas the two non-overlapping short forms correlated .84. The authors recommend the use of the short forms, especially since they may be more suitable if repeat testing is required. Another study constructed an "odd-item" and "even-item" as well as an experimental version of the

BNT and found that all three short versions discriminated well between Alzheimer's disease, other dementing diseases, and normal older (mean age 73.7) subjects (Williams et al., 1989). Another 30-item version, developed for a Chinese population, showed a sensitivity between 56 and 80 percent and specificity between 54 and 70 percent in separating demented and nondemented subjects of low and high educational background (Salmon et al., 1995).

Mack et al. (1992) developed four 15-item forms for subjects who may be so impaired that even a 30-item version may be burdensome. Franzen et al. (1995) evaluated the various short forms with 320 subjects with various neuropsychiatric disorders, including 194 patients with dementia: They found internal consistency ranging from .96 for the full version to .58 and .34 for two of the 15-item versions. Correlations of short and full versions were between .99 and .93. However, misclassification rates were fairly high when compared to the full version and differed between the various short forms. The authors suggest caution in the use of shortened forms of the BNT. However, Wilson et al. (1996) found that an unspecified 15-item short form was the only one of seven tests that correlated significantly with volumetric MRI measures of the temporal cortex (.43), the parahippocampal gyri (.30), and the hippocampal formation (.33) in 47 AD patients. Most recently, Lansing et al. (1996) examined various short forms with a population of 717 controls and 237 AD subjects in the age range of 50–98 years. They found significant correlations with age and education as well as gender effects for all forms, including the original full-length version. Correct classification rates varied from 58 to 69 percent for AD patients, and from 77 and 87 percent for normal controls. Based on a discriminant function analysis, the authors developed a new empirical 15-item version balanced for gender equity. If a shortened version is used, we recommend the 30-item version (using odd or even items) because of its better internal consistency and high correlation with the full-length BNT.

Construct validity in children was investigated by Halperin et al. (1989). The test loaded highly on a word knowledge, or vocabulary factor together with the PPVT-R, but showed low loadings on a verbal fluency or a memory factor, suggesting that it is a relatively pure measure in children. Axelrod et al. (1994) also found loadings on the three major factors of intelligence in adults: Verbal comprehension, perceptual organization, and freedom from distractibility. Kirk (1992) found a relatively high number of aphasic-like errors (especially circumlocution and semantic errors) in school-age children. She provides details on items that apparently are not yet part of the working vocabulary of school children, and she suggests a revised children's BNT based on her error analysis. Gioia, Isquith, and Kenworth (1996) found BNT test scores in a clinical sample were below those on the Beery Picture Vocabulary Test and other measures of verbal ability in the same group; they warn that the items of the BNT may be too difficult for children; in particular, African-American children scored an average of 21 points below the scores obtained with the Beery Test. Cooper and Rosen (1997) found that the BNT identified children with language disorder, and with language and reading disorder successfully, with a sensitivity of 76 percent, using a 1 SD cutoff criterion.

Concurrent validity with the Visual Naming Test of the Multilingual Aphasia Examination (Benton, Hamsher, & Sivan, 1994) was described by Axelrod et al. (1994). Hawkins et al. (1993) also found correlations between .74 and .87 between the Gates-McGinite Reading Vocabulary Test and the BNT across normal and clinical adult populations; they demonstrated that norms for the test may lead to many false-positive rates for naming deficit, and that corrections should be applied, especially for subjects with lower-than-average reading level.

Jordan et al. (1992) found no differences on the BNT between 14 children who had sustained mild closed-head injury 10 years earlier and a matched control group; this finding obtained also for other language tests, e.g., the NCCEA and TOAL-2. Weyandt and Willis (1994) found that test results did not differ between children with and without ADHD. Children with dysphonetic dyslexia (Cohen et al., 1988) and with developmental dyscalculia (Shalev et al., 1988) showed impairment on the BNT.

The manual provides means for aphasics with a severity level from 0 to 5 as determined by the BDAE, all of which are well below the level for normal adults. However, the range for aphasics with severity levels 2 to 5 extends well into the range for normals. This is not surprising since naming is not necessarily impaired in all types of aphasia. Sandson and Albert (1987) found that aphasic patients made more perseverative errors than patients with right-hemisphere lesions; further, perseverations were more frequent in patients with posterior rather than frontal lesions.

With regards to all types of errors made, Kazniak et al. (1988) found that normal elderly subjects make one error, whereas patients with Alzheimer's dementia (AD) with a mild degree of impairment obtain a mean of 5.5 errors, and those with moderate impairment make about 7.5 errors. Eighty percent of AD patients showed anomia with 11 or more errors on the BNT (Freedman et al., 1995). Welsh et al. (1995a) found that African-American subjects with AD scored lower than white subjects even when age and education level were controlled for. Poor naming has also been singled out as a poor prognostic sign in AD with a more rapidly progressive course (Knesevich et al., 1986). LaBarge et al. (1992), Petrick et al. (1992), and Zec et al. (1992) found the test highly sensitive to very mild AD; it also discriminated well between AD and vascular dementia (Barr et al., 1992). Cahn et al. (1995) found that the test discriminated well between 238 normal elderly subjects, 77 at-risk for AD, and 45 AD patients. The test also was one of four contributors to a regression equation designed to obtain optimal group discrimination among a total of 17 test scores. In a subsequent qualitative error analysis, Cahn et al. (1997) found that both semantic and lexical naming errors discriminated between the three groups, but sensitivity was poor, indicating that these two types of errors occur also in normal elderly people.

Poor performance of patients with AD can exceed the impairment shown in patients with anomia (Margolin et al., 1990); the authors explain this on the basis of the amount of semantic processing required for the BNT, as compared to phonological processing in the COWA. Lindman (1996) came to similar conclusions in a comparison of BNT and animal fluency data of 68 AD patients and 80 control subjects, and, in addition, found that female AD patients performed significantly worse than males. Loewenstein et al. (1992) compared the performance of 33 AD patients on the BNT and seven other tests with eight functional tasks (reading a clock, telephone skills, preparing a letter for mailing, counting currency, writing a check, balancing a checkbook, shopping with a written list); the BNT only correlated (.40) with the ability to shop with a written list, but did not contribute to a stepwise regression analysis of the eight tests in predicting functional competence. All tests combined accounted for less than 50 percent of the explained variance. However, Baum et al. (1996) conducted a canonical analysis of a variety of measures of activities of daily living and a set of neuropsychological tests in AD patients. The BNT had a loading of .88 on the first canonical variate, indicating good ecological validity in this population.

The test is sensitive to subcortical disease (multiple sclerosis and Parkinson's disease) even if global mental status is only mildly affected; in addition, responses were slower than in normal controls (Beatty & Monson, 1989; Lezak et al., 1990). Knopman et al. (1984) reported good measurement of recovery of naming after strokes of small volume in the left posterior temporal/inferior parietal and the insula-putamen areas. Scores in 87 patients with temporal lobe epilepsy were impaired (mean = 42.4) compared to 719 normal controls (mean = 52.3), but better than for 325 patients with AD (mean = 34.4) (Randolph et al., 1996). Welsh et al. (1995b) found that semantic errors and circumlocutions in AD patients were associated with left mesial and lateral temporal lobe metabolism as measured by PET and FDG emission techniques. In addition, the left anterior temporal area has also been implicated (Tranel, 1992). However, Trenerry et al. (1995) reported that carefully limited anterior right or left temporal lobectomy in 31 left and 24 right lobectomy patients with left-hemisphere language lateralization did not impact positively or negatively on BNT performance. The BNT was also not sensitive to side of epileptic focus in a study of patients with idiopathic epilepsy (Haynes & Bennett, 1990) and in patients with anterior temporal lobectomy (Cherlow & Serafetinides, 1976).

The test did not discriminate between 10 fluent aphasics and 10 speech-disordered schizophrenics (Landre et al., 1992). Depressives (mean = 48.50, $n = 14$) as well as depressives with reversible cognitive dysfunction (mean = 45.64, $n = 11$) did differ significantly from AD patients (mean = 27.23, $n = 13$) (Hill et al., 1992). While mild and even moderate depression has little effect on the test performance of elderly subjects (Boone et al., 1995), poor naming performance in depression has been described as a poor prognostic sign in a 6-months treatment study (King et al., 1991).

As with other tests that rely on pictorial material (e.g., Peabody Picture Vocabulary Test, PPVT), visual-perceptual integrity should be checked if errors occur. Kaplan et al. (1983) noted that, particularly in patients with right frontal damage, "fragmentation responses" may be made (e.g., the mouthpiece on a har-

monica is interpreted as a line of windows in a bus; Lezak, 1995).

Normative Data

The norms accompanying the test are based on small groups of adults aged 18–59. No age-related changes or differences between adults with 12 years of schooling or less and those with more than 12 years of education were noted. However, other normative data (Table 11–2, Albert et al., 1988; Mitrushina & Satz, 1989; Ross et al., 1995; van Gorp et al., 1986) show a significant effect of both age and education when older subjects are included; the major age effect (a decrease of approximately 5 points) is found in the 70- to 80-year-old group. These norms are almost identical with those presented by Ivnik, Malec, and Smith (1996), who also include data for older age groups from a major normative data collection. Tombaugh and Hubley (1996), however, found a much smaller age effect (70–74: 52.5, SD 4.6, $n = 18$; 75–79: 51.7, SD 5.5, $n = 24$; 80–88: 53.1, SD 4.0, $n = 29$) in community-dwelling volunteers in Ottawa, Canada. Subjects with less than 8 years of education score approximately 10 points lower, and subjects

Table 11—2. Boston Naming Test: Norms for Adults

Age	n	M	SD	Suggested Cut-Off
25–34	22[b]	55.9	2.8	
35–44	28[b]	55.5	3.9	
45–54	33[b]	54.8	4.1	
55–59	24[b]	55.2	3.6	
57–65	28[a]	55.6	3.5	51
66–70	45[a]	55.8	3.1	47
71–75	57[a](10)	53.0 (48.9)	7.3 (6.3)	44
75–79	247[a]	52.5[d]		
76–85	26[a](7)	50.8 (42.0)	7.0 (7.6)	37
80–84	255[a]	50.5[d]		
85+	138[a]	49.0[d]		
90–97	78[c]	45.5[d]		

[a]Ross et al., 1995, 1997 with permission of the authors and Swets Publishing Service.

[b]Tombaugh & Hubley, 1996.

[c]Mitrushina & Satz, 1989 with permission of Karger AG, Basel. Based on volunteers with a mean education level of 14 years from an independent retirement community. Data in parentheses from Lichtenberg et al. (1994), based on less-educated (mean education = 11.1 years) patients without cognitive deficit admitted to a geriatric rehabilitation unit. Means for African-Americans were between 1.5 (70–74) and 6 points (80 +) lower.

[d]Extrapolated from Ivnik, Malec, & Smith, 1996

Table 11—3. Adult Norms Corrected for Reading Vocabulary Level

Reading level[a]	Percentile rank[b]	Estimated BNT Total
4.1	01	34.4
5.0	03	37.2
6.1	05	39.9
7.0	08	42.0
8.0	13	44.7
9.2	21	47.5
10.1	29	49.6
11.1	40	51.6
12.2	45	52.3
Post high school	58	53.7
	66	54.3
	82	55.7
	90	56.4

[a]Estimated on the basis of Gates-McGinite Reading Vocabulary.

[b]Based on Gates-McGinite Reading Vocabulary, Level 7–9, Form K.

Source: Hawkins et al. (1993), based on a mixed psychiatric and normal sample ($n = 88$) with permission of the authors and from Elsevier Science Ltd.

with 15 or more years of education about 3 points higher. Wilkins et al. (1996) warn that normative data should not be applied to subjects with a WAIS-R vocabulary score of 7 or less, because such subjects scored much lower than the norms provided in the manual. Our norms in Table 11–2 are very similar to those presented by Welch et al. (1996) for subjects aged 60 to 80+ years; these authors found that in this age range males scored about four points higher than females. The norms are also consistent with those published by Russell and Starkey (1993) and Taussig, Henderson and Mack (1988) for the current version; the preliminary norms based on a French-Canadian population (Morrison et al., 1996; by LaBarge et al. (1986) and Montgomery and Costa (1983) for the 85-item version; and by Villardita et al. (1985), by Rich (1993), and by Lansing et al. (1996); for 15-item versions. Lichtenberg et al. (1994) report values for a small sample of 70- to 80+-year-old subjects with lower education level (included in Table 11–2). Ross et al. (1995, 1997) warn that for elderly subjects hospitalized for non-neurological disorders in a demographically diverse medical setting (mean education 10.6 years, 56 percent African-Americans) considerably lower values and higher SDs can be expected (shown as means across education levels in Table 11–2). Some of these exceed even the cutoff points suggested by Satz and Mitrushina; subjects with education below grade 12 scored about 7 points lower than those with an education of grade 12 and better, a difference that expanded to 12 points in the highest age group. Finally, Hawkins et al. (1993) found that education corrections based on reading level are needed for the full adult range (18–68 years) and presented appropriate norms shown in Table 11–3. They did not find a correlation with age within the age range sampled. We also present percentile norms for adults, broken down by age and education level (Tombaugh & Hubley (in press) (Table 11–4).

Heaton, Grant, and Matthews (1991) present norms for the 85-item version in scaled scores, corrected for gender, education, and age, and based on 553 normal subjects; these norms should be used with caution because

Table 11—4. 60-Item BNT Norms Expressed as Percentiles for Age and Education: Total Correct

Percentiles	Age 25–69 yrs		Age 70–88 yrs		Total ($n = 219$)
	9–12 yrs. ed. ($n = 78$)	13–21 yrs. ed. ($n = 70$)	9–12 yrs. ed. ($n = 45$)	13–21 yrs. ed. ($n = 26$)	
90	59	60	59	59	60
75	58	60	58	58	58
50	56	58	55	56	57
25	54	56	52	53	54
10	51	53	47	49	51

Source: Tombaugh & Hubley (in press).

Table 11—5. Norms for Normal School Children on the Boston Naming Test

Age	Male			Female			Compiled[a]		
	n	M	SD	n	M	SD	n	M	SD
5							62	27.76	5.9
6	16	35.69	6.1	18	32.50	5.6	150	33.56	4.9
7	18	39.94	4.9	22	37.91	6.7	153	36.87	5.2
8	23	41.17	3.0	15	39.93	4.1	147	38.99	4.6
9	20	43.20	4.7	25	42.92	5.2	152	41.74	4.6
10	16	45.56	5.9	22	46.41	4.4	167	45.10	4.5
11	16	46.44	3.5	20	46.90	5.2	146	46.84	4.8
12	2	51.50	3.5	8	47.00	3.9	80	48.55	3.9
13							22	49.55	4.7

Source: From Halperin et al., 1989.

[a]Yeates, 1994 with permission from Swets Publishing Service.

the individual cell size is not provided and may be quite small.

Albert et al. (1988) and Nicholas et al. (1985) point out that errors in older subjects consist mainly of substitutions of semantically related associates and circumlocutions on object rather than action names. An error analysis by Goodglass et al. (1997) suggests that, on the other hand, success in naming for aphasics and normals is best predicted by phonetically correct initial responses.

Norms for small groups of children from kindergarten to grade 5 accompany the test. The progression with age corresponds to the data presented by Kindlon and Garrison (1984). The Kindlon and Garrison study also shows gender differences at younger ages, with females scoring about 5 points higher at ages 6 and 7, whereas Halperin et al. (1989) and other researchers failed to find gender effects. Other norms for school-age children were presented by Cohen et al. (1988) and Guilford and Nawojczyk (1988). Halperin and colleagues reported that scores increase by 2–3 points after phonemic cuing. A meta-analysis of five normative studies by Yeates (1994) provided compiled norms for ages 5 to 13, weighted for n and SD (Table 11–5). The norms published by Kirk (1992) are very similar but showed no significant gender differences. This still leaves a gap in the normative data for the BNT for adolescents between 14 and 17.

References

Albert, M.S., Heller, H.S., & Milberg, W. (1988). Changes in naming ability with age. *Psychology and Aging, 3,* 173–178.

Axelrod, B.N., Ricker, J.H., & Cherry, S.A. (1994). Concurrent validity of the MAE visual naming test. *Archives of Clinical Neuropsychology, 9,* 317–321.

Azrin, R.L., Mercury, M.G., Millsaps, C., et al. (1996). Cautionary note on the Boston Naming Test: Cultural considerations. *Archives of Clinical Neuropsychology, 11,* 365–366 (abstract).

Barr, A., Benedict, R., Tune, L., & Brandt, J. (1992). Neuropsychological differentiation of Alzheimer's disease from vascular dementia. *International Journal of Geriatric Psychiatry, 7,* 621–627.

Baum, C., Edwards, D., Yonan, C., & Storandt, M. (1996). The relation of neuropsychological test performance to performance on functional tasks in dementia of the Alzheimer type. *Archives of Clinical Neuropsychology, 11,* 69–75.

Beatty, W.W., & Monson, N. (1989). Lexical processing in Parkinson's disease and multiple sclerosis. *Journal of Geriatric Psychiatry and Neurology, 2,* 145–152.

Benton, A.L., Hamsher, K., & Sivan, A.B. (1994). *Multilingual Aphasia Examination* (3rd ed.). Iowa City, IA: AJA.

Boone, K.B., Lesser, I.M., Miller, B.L., Wohl, M., Berman, N., Lee, A., Palmer, B., & Back, C. (1995). Cognitive functioning in older depressed outpatients: Relationship of presence and severity of depression to neuropsychological test scores. *Neuropsychology, 9,* 390–398.

Borod, J.C., Goodglass, H., & Kaplan, E. (1980). Normative data on the Boston Diagnostic Aphasia Examination, Parietal Lobe Battery, and the Boston Naming Test. *Journal of Clinical Neuropsychology, 2,* 209–215.

Cahn, D.A., Salmon, D.P., Bondi, M.W. et al. (1997). A population-based analysis of quantitative features of the neuropsychological test performance of individuals with dementia of the Alzheimer type: Implications for individuals with questionable dementia. *Journal of the International Neuropsychological Society, 3,* 387–393.

Cahn, D.A., Salmon, D.P., Butters, N., Wiederholt, W.C., Corey-Bloom, J., Edelstein, S.L., & Barrett-Connor, E. (1995). Detection of dementia of the Alzheimer type in a population-based sample: Neuropsychological test performance. *Journal of the International Neuropsychological Society, 1,* 252–260.

Cherlow, D.G., & Serafetinides, E.A. (1976). Speech and memory assessment in psychomotor epileptics. *Cortex, 12,* 21–26.

Cohen, M., Town, P., & Buff, A. (1988). Neurodevelopmental differences in confrontational naming in children. *Developmental Neuropsychology, 4,* 75–81.

Cooper, M.E., & Rosen, W.G. (1977). Utility of the Boston Naming Test as a screen for language disorders in children. *Archives of Clinical Neuropsychology, 12,* 303 (abstract).

Franzen, M.D., Haut, M.W., Rankin, E., & Keefover, R. (1995). Empirical comparison of alternate forms of the Boston Naming Test. *Clinical Neuropsychologist, 9,* 225–229.

Freedman, L., Snow, W.G., & Millikin, C. (1995). Anomia in Alzheimer's disease. *Journal of the International Neuropsychological Society, 1,* 386 (abstract).

Gioia, G.A., Isquith, P.K., & Kenworthy, L. (1996). The Boston Naming Test with children: Is it time to re-engineer? *Journal of the International Neuropsychological Society, 2,* 29 (abstract)

Goodglass, H., & Kaplan, E. (1987). *The Assessment of Aphasia and Related Disorders* (2nd ed.) Philadelphia: Lea & Febiger.

Goodglass, H., Wringfield, A., Hyde, M.R., Gleason, J.B., Bowles, N.L. & Gallagher, R.F. (1997). The importance of word-initial phonology: Error patterns in prolonged naming efforts by aphasic patients. *Journal of the International Neuropsychological Society, 3,* 128–138.

Guilford, A.M., & Nawojczyk, D.C. (1988). Standardization of the Boston Naming Test at the kindergarten and elementary school levels. *Language, Speech, and Hearing Services in the Schools, 19,* 395–400.

Halperin, J.M., Healy, J.M., Zeitschick, E., Ludman, W.L., & Weinstein, L. (1989). Developmental aspects of linguistic and mnestic abilities in normal children. *Journal of Clinical and Experimental Neuropsychology, 11,* 518–528.

Hawkins, K.A., Sledge, W.H., Orleans, J.F., Quinland, D.M., Rakfeldt, J., & Hoffman, R.E. (1993). Normative implications of the relationship between reading vocabulary and Boston Naming Test performance. *Archives of Clinical Neuropsychology, 8,* 525–537.

Haynes, S.D., & Bennett, T.L. (1990). Cognitive impairment in adults with complex partial seizures. *International Journal of Clinical Neuropsychology, 12,* 74–81.

Heaton, R.K., Grant, I., & Matthews, C.G. (1991). *Comprehensive Norms for an Expanded Halstead-Reitan Battery: Demographic Corrections, Research Findings, and Clinical Applications.* Odessa, FL: Psychological Assessment Resources.

Henderson, V.W., Mack, W., Freed, D.M., Kemper, D., & Andersen, E.S. (1990). Naming consistency in Alzheimer's Disease. *Brain and Language, 39,* 530–538.

Hill, C.D., Stoudemire, A., Morris, R., Martino-Saltzman, D., Markwalter, H.R., & Lewison, B.J. (1992). Dysnomia in the differential diagnosis of major depression, depression-related cognitive dysfunction, and dementia. *Journal of Neuropsychiatry and Clinical Neuroscience, 4,* 64–69.

Huff, F.J., Collins, C., Corkin, S., & Rosen, T.J. (1986). Equivalent forms of the Boston Naming Test. *Journal of Clinical and Experimental Neuropsychology, 8,* 556–562.

Ivnik, R.J., Malec, J.F., & Smith, G.E. (1996). Neuropsychological test norms above age 55: COWAT, MAE Token, WRAT-R Reading, AMNART, Stroop, TMT, and JLO. *The Clinical Neuropsychologist, 10,* 262–278.

Jordan, F.M., Cannon, A., & Murdoch, B.E. (1992). Language abilities of mildly closed head injured (CHI) children 10 years post-injury. *Brain Injury, 6,* 39–44.

Kaplan, E.F., Goodglass, H., & Weintraub, S. (1978, 1983). *The Boston Naming Test.* Experimental edition (1978), Boston: Kaplan & Goodglass. 2nd ed., Philadelphia: Lea & Febiger.

Kazniak, A.W., Bayles, K.A., Tomoeda, C.K., & Slauson, T. (1988). Assessing linguistic communicative functioning in Alzheimer's dementia: A theoretically motivated approach. *Journal of*

Clinical and Experimental Neuropsychology, 10, 53 (abstract).

Kindlon, D., & Garrison, W. (1984). The Boston Naming Test: Norm data and cue utilization in a sample of normal 6- and 7-year-old children. *Brain and Language, 21,* 255–259.

King, D.A., Caine, E.D., Conwell, Y., & Cox, C. (1991). Predicting severity of depression in the elderly at six-months follow-up: A neuropsychological study. *Journal of Neuropsychiatry and Clinical Neuroscience, 3* 64–66.

Kirk, U. (1992). Confrontation naming in normally developing children: Word-retrieval or word knowledge? *The Clinical Neuropsychologist, 6,* 156–170.

Knesevich, J.W., LaBarge, E., & Edwards, D. (1986). Predictive value of the Boston Naming Test in mild senile dementia of the Alzheimer type. *Psychiatry Research, 19,* 155–161.

Knopman, D.S., Selnes, O.A., Niccum, N., & Rubens, A. (1984). Recovery of naming in aphasia: Relationship to fluency, comprehension, and CT findings. *Neurology, 34,* 1461–1470.

LaBarge, E., Balota, D.A., Storandt, M., & Smith, D. (1992). An analysis of confrontation naming errors in senile dementia of the Alzheimer type. *Neuropsychology, 6,* 77–95.

LaBarge, E., Edwards, D., & Knesevich, J.W. (1986). Performance of normal elderly on the Boston Naming Test. *Brain and Language, 27,* 380–384.

Landre, N.A., Taylor, M.A., & Kearns, K.P. (1992). Language functioning in schizophrenic and aphasic patients. *Neuropsychiatry, Neuropsychology, and Behavioral Neurology, 5,* 7–14.

Lansing, A.E., Randolph, C., Ivnik, R.J., & Cullum, C.M. (1996). Short forms of the Boston Naming Test. *Journal of the International Neuropsychological Society, 2,* 2 (abstract).

Lezak, M.D. (1995). *Neuropsychological Assessment* (3rd ed.). New York: Oxford University Press.

Lezak, M.D., Whitham, R., & Bourdette, D. (1990). Emotional impact of cognitive insufficiencies in multiple sclerosis (MS). *Journal of Clinical and Experimental Neuropsychology, 12,* 50 (abstract).

Lichtenberg, P.A., Ross, T., & Christensen, B. (1994). Preliminary normative data on the Boston Naming Test for an older urban population. *The Clinical Neuropsychologist, 8,* 109–111.

Lindman, K.K. (1996). Gender differences in dementia of the Alzheimer's type: Evidence for differential semantic memory degradation. Paper presented at the meeting of the International Neuropsychological Society, Chicago.

Loewenstein, D.A., Rubert, M.P., Berkowitz-Zimmer, N., Guterman, A., Morgan, R., & Hayden, S. (1992). Neuropsychological test performance and prediction of functional capacities in dementia. *Behavior, Health, and Aging, 2,* 149–158.

Mack, W.J., Freed, D.M., Williams, B.W., & Henderson, V.W. (1992). Boston Naming Test: Shortened version for use in Alzheimer's disease. *Journal of Gerontology, 47,* 164–168.

Margolin, D.I., Pate, D.S., Friedrich, F.J., & Elia, E. (1990). Dysnomia in dementia and in stroke patients: Different underlying cognitive deficits. *Journal of Clinical and Experimental Neuropsychology, 12,* 597–612.

Mitrushina, M., & Satz, P. (1989). Differential decline of specific memory components in normal aging. *Brain Dysfunction, 2,* 330–335.

Montgomery, K., & Costa, L. (1983). Neuropsychological test performance of a normal elderly sample. Paper presented at the meeting of the International Neuropsychological Society, Mexico City.

Morrison, L.E., Smith, L.A., & Sarazin, F.F.A. (1996). Boston Naming Test: A French-Canadian normative study (preliminary analyses). *Journal of the International Neuropsychological Society, 2,* 4 (abstract).

Nicholas, M., Obler, L., Albert, M., & Goodglass, H. (1985). Lexical retrieval in healthy aging. *Cortex, 21,* 595–606.

Petrick, J.D., Kunkle, J., & Franzen, M.D. (1992). Confontational and productive naming in depression and dementia. *The Clinical Neuropsychologist, 6,* 323 (abstract).

Ponton, M.O., Satz, P., Herrera, L., Young, R., Ortiz, F., d'Elia, L., Furst, C., & Namerow, N. (1992). A modified Spanish version of the Boston Naming Test. *The Clinical Neuropsychologist, 6,* 334 (abstract).

Randolph, C., Lansing, A., Ivnick, R.J., Cullum, C.M., & Hermann, B.P. (1996). Determinants of confrontation naming performance. *Journal of the International Neuropsychological Society, 2,* 6 (abstract).

Rich, J.B. (1993). Pictorial and verbal implicit and recognition memory in aging and Alzheimer's disease: A transfer-appropriate processing account. Ph.D. dissertation, University of Victoria.

Ross, R.P., Lichtenberg, P.A., & Christensen, K. (1995). Normative data on the Boston Naming Test for elderly adults in a demographically diverse medical sample. *The Clinical Neuropsychologist, 9*, 321–325.

Ross, T.P., & Lichtenberg, P.A. (1997). Expanded normative data for the Boston Naming Test in an urban medical sample of elderly adults. Paper presented at the meeting of the International Neuropsychological Society, Orlando, FL.

Russell, E.W., & Starkey, R.I. (1993). *Halstead Russell Neuropsychological Evaluation System.* Los Angeles: Western Psychological Services.

Salmon, D.P., Jin, H., Zhang, M., Grant, I., & Yu, E. (1995). Neuropsychological assessment of Chinese elderly in the Shanghai Dementia Survey. *The Clinical Neuropsychologist, 9*, 159–168.

Sandson, J., & Albert, M.L. (1987). Varieties of perseveration. *Neuropsychologia, 22*, 715–732.

Sawrie, S.M., Chelune, G.J., Naugle, R.I., & Luders, H.O. (1996). Empirical methods for assessing meaningful change following epilepsy surgery. *Journal of the International Neuropsychological Association, 2*, 556–564.

Shalev, R.S., Weirtman, R., & Amir, N. (1988). Developmental dyscalculia. *Cortex, 24*, 555–561.

Taussig, I.M., Henderson, V.W., & Mack, W. (1988). Spanish translation and validation of a neuropsychological battery: Performance of Spanish- and English-speaking Alzheimer's Disease patients and normal comparison subjects. Paper presented at the meeting of the Gerontological Society of America, San Francisco.

Thompson, L.L., & Heaton, R.K. (1989). Comparison of different versions of the Boston Naming Test. *The Clinical Neuropsychologist, 3*, 184–192.

Tombaugh, T.N., & Hubley, A. (in press). Normative data for the Boston Naming Test. *Journal of Clinical and Experimental Neuropsychology.*

Tranel, D. (1992). Functional neuroanatomy: Neuropsychological correlates of cortical and subcortical changes. In S.C. Yudofski & R.E. Hales (Eds.), *Textbook of Neuropsychiatry.* Washington, DC: American Psychiatric Press. pp. 57–88.

Trenerry, M.R., Cascino, G.D., Jack, C.R., Sharbrough, F.W., So, F.L., & Lagerlund, T.D. (1995). Boston Naming Test performance after temporal lobectomy is not associated with laterality of cortical resection. *Archives of Clinical Neuropsychology, 10*, 399 (abstract).

Van Gorp, W.G., Satz, P., Kiersch, M.E., & Henry, R. (1986). Normative data on the Boston Naming Test for a group of normal older adults. *Journal of Clinical and Experimental Neuropsychology, 8*, 702–705.

Villardita, C., Cultrera, S., Cupone, V., & Meija, R. (1985). Neuropsychological test performances and normal aging. *Archives of Gerontology and Geriatrics, 4*, 311–319.

Wallace, G., & Hammill, D.D. (1994). *Comprehensive Receptive and Expressive Vocabulary Test.* Austin, TX: Pro-Ed.

Welch, L.W., Doineau, D., Johnson, S., & King, D. (1996). Education and gender normative data for the Boston Naming Test in a group of older adults. *Brain and Language, 53*, 260–266.

Welsh, K.A., Fillenbaum, G., Wilkinson, W., et al. (1995a). Neuropsychological test performance in African-American and white patients with Alzheimer's disease. *Neurology, 45*, 2207–2211.

Welsh, K.A., Watson, M., Hoffman, J.M., Lowe, V., Earl, N., & Rubin, D.C. (1995b). The neural basis of visual naming errors in Alzheimer's disease: A positron emission tomography study. *Archives of Clinical Neuropsychology, 10*, 403 (abstract).

Weyandt, L.L., & Willis, W.G. (1994). Executive functions in school children: Potential efficacy of tasks in discriminating clinical groups. *Developmental Neuropsychology, 10*, 27–38.

Wilkins, J.W., Hamby, S.L., & Thompson, K.L. (1996). Difficulties with Boston Naming norms in individuals with below average WAIS-R vocabulary. *Archives of Clinical Neuropsychology, 11*, 464 (abstract).

Williams, B.W., Mack, W., & Henderson, V.W. (1989). Boston naming test in Alzheimer's disease. *Neuropsychologia, 27*, 1073–1079.

Wilson, R.S., Sullivan, M., Toledo-Morrell, L.d., et al. (1996). Association of memory and cognition in Alzheimer's disease with volumetric estimates of temporal lobe structures. *Neuropsychology, 10*, 459–463.

Worrall, L.E., Yiu, E.M.L., Hickson, L.M.H., & Barnett, H.M. (1995). Normative data for the Boston Naming Test for Australian elderly. *Aphasiology, 9*, 541–551.

Yeates, K.O. (1994). Comparison of developmental norms for the Boston Naming Test. *The Clinical Neuropsychologist, 8*, 91–98.

Zec, R.F., Vicari, S., Kocis, M., & Reynolds, T. (1992). Sensitivity of different neuropsychological tests to very mild DAT. *The Clinical Neuropsychologist, 6*, 327 (abstract).

CLINICAL EVALUATION OF LANGUAGE FUNDAMENTALS—THIRD EDITION
(CELF-3)

Purpose

The aim is to provide a comprehensive assessment of language development in school-age children.

Source

The test kit includes an examiner's manual, a technical manual, two stimulus manuals, and record forms in a briefcase, and can be purchased from the Psychological Corporation, 555 Academic Court, San Antonio, TX 78204-2498 for $325 US, or the Psychological Corporation, 55 Horner Ave., Toronto, ON M82 4X6 for $515 Cdn. A "clinical assistant," a "communication checklist" and a screening version are in preparation. A preschool version (CELF-Preschool) for ages 3 years to 6 years, 11 months is available (Wiig et al., 1992).

Description

The test battery (Semel et al., 1995) consists of three receptive and three expressive language tests which differ by age group (6 to 8 years; 9 years to 21 years 11 months). In addition, the test includes two supplementary tests. The tests are as follows:

Ages 6 to 8—Receptive:

Sentence Structure: The child must point to one of four line drawings that corresponds to the statement read by the examiner (e.g., "The man comes home from work"). This subtest measures comprehension of negative, passive, infinitive, and other phrase structures. 20 items.

Concepts and Directions: The child must follow instructions by pointing to white or black circles, triangles, or squares, increasing in length and complexity of modifiers, similar to the Token Test; e.g., "Point to the last large black triangle to the left of the small black circle." 30 items.

Word Classes: The child must identify two words that "go together best" out of three or four read by the examiner; e.g., chair, table, plant, dog. Relationships include semantic, opposite, spatial, and temporal. 34 items.

Ages 6 to 8—Expressive:

Word Structure: The child must complete sentences requiring regular and irregular plurals, pronominalization, and other derivational forms; e.g., "John said, 'I want this candy, and I want. . . .' 32 items.

Recalling Sentences: The child must repeat phrases similar to the Sentence Repetition Test, but increasing not only in length but also in syntactical complexity. 26 items.

Formulated Sentences: The child must make up a sentence containing a given word, either describing the stimulus card or making up a sentence of his or her own. Words range from "car" to "unless." 22 items.

Ages 6 to 8—Supplementary:

Listening to Paragraphs: The child listens to two stories read by the examiner and then answers four questions about the content of each story.

Word Associations: The task requires generating as many words from a given category (animals, ways to get from one place to another, work people do) as possible in 60 seconds. The task is identical with category Controlled Word Association. 3 trials.

For ages 9 years to 21 years 11 months the following tests are given:

Receptive: Concepts and Directions, Word Classes, Semantic Relationships.

Expressive: Formulated Sentences, Recalling Sentences, Sentence Assembly.

Supplementary: Listening to paragraphs, Word Associations.

Optional: Rapid Automatic Naming: The child must name as rapidly as possible colors, then shapes, then colors and shapes ("green triangle"). 36 items each.

The stimulus material is presented in two stimulus manuals that fold up into easel form.

The screening version uses a shortened selection of items from each of the subtests.

Administration

Administration for all tests is described in detail in the manual, but essential instructions are also provided on the Record Form. Age-appropriate entry points and discontinuation rules allow considerable time-saving.

Time for Administration

Approximately 30–45 minutes are required for the complete test.

Scoring

See source. The Record Form provides scoring not only for each answer and each subtest's raw score, but also for major types of errors, depending on the stimulus material (e.g., Concepts and Directions for time, location, sequence, condition, inclusion/exclusion). Raw scores are entered on the front page and are translated into standard scores by referring to tables in one-year age intervals up to 16 years, 11 months in the examiner's manual. The final age interval (17 to 21 years, 11 months) shows no further gain for most subtests. The standard scores are summed to provide a receptive, expressive, and total standard language score with a mean of 100 and a SD of 15, as well as an age equivalent. For each subtest, points above or below the mean, a confidence interval, percentile range (with its own confidence interval) are also entered on the Record Form; the form also provides for calculation of receptive/expressive differences with a notation of the prevalence of such differences. The manual recommends that scores from the supplementary expressive or receptive language tests be used to replace scores that may be questionable or missing in the main test.

Comment

This is the third, revised edition of the *Clinical Evaluation of Language Functions* (1980). The Technical Manual provides full details of the revision of the test, and information regarding reliability and validity. The test is designed primarily for use by the school psychologist and child speech therapist.

Internal consistency ranged from .55 to .91 for subtests, and from .83 to .95 for expressive/receptive/total language scores, depending on age. Retest reliability after 4–8 weeks for a subsample of 152 children ranged from .50 (for word associations at age 7) to .90 (for recalling sentences at age 7), and from .77 (for receptive language score in 13-year-olds) to .93 (for total language score in 7-year-olds).

Criterion-related validity was based on the comparison of 136 students with language learning disability and 136 matched normal learning age peers at 6, 7, 9, 11, 15, and 16 years. Correct classification was 71.3%, using a cutoff of 85 or less (1 SD) for the total language score. Concurrent validity, as measured against the CELF-R ranged from .42 to .75 for subtests, and from .72 to .79 for language scores. CELF-3 scores were approximately 5 points higher than CELF-R scores. Concurrent validity of the CELF-R had previously been reported as .68 against the PPVT-R ($n = 53$), .52 (receptive .44, expressive .46); against an intelligence test (WISC-R, $n = 48$), .42 (receptive .32, expressive .37). Intercorrelations between CELF-R subtests ranged from .23 to .61 for a sample of 918 students. The CELF-3 correlated .75 with the Full Scale IQ of the WISC-III ($n = 203$, receptive language score .71, expressive language score .71). A factor analysis done with the CELF-3 extracted four factors, although a general language ability factor accounted for most of the variance.

Semel et al. (1987) changed the name of the test from "Functions" to "Fundamentals" to avoid the implication that it covers all aspects of language development. They emphasize that it does not necessarily measure language use in communicative contexts.

No studies of specific neuropsychological

interest have been presented so far. However, the test provides downward extensions or modifications of at least three tests that have been extensively used with neurological populations: Word Associations (Category Word Fluency, Controlled Oral Word Association), Recalling Sentences (Sentence Repetition), and Concepts and Directions (Token Test). When testing children, neuropsychologists may wish to use these as welcome substitutes with a good normative data base. The full-length CELF-3 is suitable for the exploration of both developmental and acquired language deficits in children. While it may not satisfy everybody's model of language functions, it covers the major areas of syntax and semantics in both the receptive and expressive mode. It does not cover phonological (articulatory) problems.

One particular strength of the manual is the provision of sources for additional testing and instructional resources throughout the Examiner's Manual for each subtest. The constant reminders of confidence intervals for each test and for differences between tests on the summary page are also a welcome addition to this test.

Normative Data

The test has been well standardized on 2,450 children representative of the United States in terms of region, age, sex, and ethnicity. White–black and male–female differences are reported and discussed in the technical manual but are not used in the standard-score transformations. However, rules on the interpretation of dialectical variants (including "black English") for Word Formation (morphology) and Sentence Structure (syntax) are provided in the manual. The authors stress the need for local norms to be developed by the test user since they can differ considerably from the norms presented in the manual.

References

Semel, E., Wiig, E. H., & Secord, W. (1987, 1995). *Clinical Evaluation of Language Fundamentals—Third Edition.* San Antonio, TX: Psychological Corporation.

Wiig, E. H., Secord, W. A., Semel, E. (1992). *Clinical Evaluation of Language Fundamentals—Preschool.* San Antonio, TX: Psychological Corporation.

COMMUNICATIVE ABILITIES IN DAILY LIVING (CADL)

Purpose

The purpose is to examine communicative abilities (including nonverbal communication) in normal living situations for aphasic adults and similar language-handicapped populations.

Source

The complete kit, including manual, scoring forms, and cassette training tape can be obtained from University Park Press, 300 North Charles Street, Baltimore, MD 21201, for approximately $170 US.

Description

This test, developed by Holland (1980), differs from other tests designed for the evaluation of language impairment in that it measures the ability of the patient to comprehend and communicate in daily living situations by what

ever means remain available to him or her, including gestures, pointing, writing, drawing, etc. However, it does not include rating scales, another means of measuring "functional communication" (Sarno, 1969). The 68 items of this test, which are shown in pictures, take the patient through a variety of situations, including actual questions, "staged" situations in a doctor's office, making telephone calls, and situations in a store and while driving. An Italian version (Pizzamiglio et al., 1984), a Spanish version developed in Spain (Martin et al., 1990), and a Japanese version (Watamori et al., 1987) are available. While the test items follow a "natural" sequence, they can be grouped into 10 categories:

1. Reading, writing, and using numbers to estimate, calculate, and judge time. There are 21 items which include reading signs, directions, making change, setting dates; e.g., stating from a clock drawing how long the pa-

tient has to wait for an appointment with "Dr. Clark" at 3 pm.

2. Speech acts, comprising 21 items, including pragmatic interchanges in which speech, gesture, or writing are used to convey information or intent; e.g., stating one's age within a 5-year margin.

3. Utilizing verbal and nonverbal context, consisting of 17 items involving responding to an item in the context supplied by the examiner; e.g., viewing a picture of a waiting room with a nonsmoking sign and a person smoking—"What's happening in this picture?"

4. Role playing consists of 10 items that require a cognitive shift to an "as if" state; e.g., visiting a doctor's office.

5. Sequenced and relationship-dependent communicative behavior comprises 9 items that require the ability to perform a sequence of behaviors; e.g., dialing a phone number.

6. Social conventions consists of 8 items; e.g., greeting, accepting apologies, leave taking.

7. Divergencies comprises 7 items that require responding to misleading information or proverbs; i.e., the generation of logical possibilities with a ready flow of ideas.

8. Nonverbal symbolic communication consists of 7 items; e.g., recognizing playing cards and facial expressions of emotion.

9. Deixis consists of 6 items with movement-related or movement-dependent communicative behavior; e.g., "Show me the mens/womens room."

10. Humor, absurdity, metaphor consists of 4 items, similar to divergencies and requiring the recognition of a humorous, absurd, or metaphoric situation in pictures.

Administration

The test situation is deliberately informal, and the examiner is instructed to act in various roles as much as possible, e.g., by changing his or her voice, by introducing humor, etc., to increase the "contextual richness" of the situations created during the test.

Approximate Time of Administration

The test requires approximately 30–90 minutes.

Scoring

Each item is scored as 0, 1, or 2 following detailed instructions in the manual, which also contains scoring booklets for two sample cases. Zero indicates an incorrect response or no response, 2 a correct response, while 1 is scored if repeating the question or rephrasing the question elicits a response. Since the ability to communicate, not the quality of the verbal or written response, is the subject of investigation, spontaneous requests for repeating a question or grammatically incorrect but comprehensible responses are scored as correct.

The total score is the sum of all points scored on the 68 items (maximum score = 136). No subscores are used, although the breakdown into areas of communication as listed above can be used as a qualitative guide to interpretation.

Comment

Reliability for 20 subjects retested after 1–3 weeks by a different examiner is reported by the author as .99, internal consistency as .97.

Concurrent validity (see source) with the Boston Diagnostic Aphasia Examination was .84, with the Porch Index of Communication Ability .93, and with the Functional Communication Profile .87. Correlation with 23 ratings by staff and family was .67. The CADL has also been shown to correlate with the number of communicative exchanges initiated by aphasics (Linebaugh et al., 1982), but not with measures of dyadic nonverbal communication (Behrmann & Penn, 1984).

Criterion validity was established by testing aphasic patients. The mean scores for different types of aphasia in a population matched for age and whether or not they were in an institution are reported in Table 11–6 together with the appropriate scores from an Italian study (Pizzamiglio et al., 1984).

This distribution of scores for different types of aphasia follows the clinical impression of their severity. However, it should be noted that the anomic group had near-normal scores (see normative data). Aphasics living in a home situation consistently had higher scores than those living in an institution. The Italian

Table 11—6. Criterion Validity of the CADL in Two Studies

Type of aphasia	Holland (1980)			Pizzamiglio et al. (1984)		
	n	M	SD	*n*	M	SD
Anomic	14	127.21	5.57	8	104.12	28.91
Conduction	4	112.00	16.06	4	87.75	7.13
Broca's	47	106.29	22.48	42	82.55	30.27
Wernicke's	17	94.88	21.92	12	77.00	34.45
Mixed	26	79.67	28.59	—	—	—
Transcortical sensory	2	55.50	33.23	1	91.00	—
Global	20	44.25	21.38	23	41.00	18.22

study also showed somewhat different scores for the various types of aphasia as well as generally lower scores. This may be the result of sample selection and classification criteria, but it also suggests that scores, especially a suggested cutoff score of 120, should be interpreted with caution. Correlation between the severity of aphasia and the CADL score in Holland's sample was .73. It should also be noted that Sarno, Buonaguro, and Levita (1987) found that scores for fluent (Wernicke's) and nonfluent (Broca's) aphasics on the Functional Communication Profile were highly similar after age, education, and time of onset had been controlled.

A comparison of 26 Wernicke's aphasia patients with 26 normal controls, 48 patients with Alzheimer's disease (AD), and 15 depressive patients (Fromm & Holland, 1989) showed impairment on the CADL corresponding to the severity of AD; patients with depression also showed lower scores than controls but tended to show incomplete responses rather than irrelevant, vague, or rambling responses seen in AD; aphasics had markedly different profiles compared to AD. A group of adult mentally retarded subjects with IQs between 50 and 80 obtained scores in the aphasic range; IQ and CADL score correlated .72 (Holland, 1980). In contrast, a group of hearing-impaired subjects (with hearing aids) showed near-normal scores (Holland, 1980).

The CADL is an excellent supplement to other aphasia examinations since it allows an estimate of the patient's communication ability rather than his or her accuracy of language. In a review, Skenes and McCauley (1985) consider the CADL as one of the few tests that meet fairly stringent requirements for test construction. The "staged" quality of some sets of items requires a certain acting ability on the part of the examiner and may not always be successful with patients who refuse or cannot enter into such interactions; it is not clear from the manual how this affects scores, but it is probably wise to take note of a patient's inability to follow the play-acting and to make allowance for this in the interpretation of the total score. Davis (1993) warns that the CADL is "still a test and does not provide for observing natural interactions." The test should also be used with caution in apraxic patients, although it may serve as a supplementary instrument in such a population (Wertz et al., 1984).

Users may wish to consider the communication portion of some of the adaptive behavior tests, like the Vineland (see section on Adaptive Behavior and Personality Tests), for a relatively brief evaluation of day-to-day communication problems.

Normative Data

Based on a total population of 130 normal adults (fluent English speakers without history of mental disorder or brain damage, and with adequate vision and hearing), the manual presents means for professionals (130.34); for self-employed, clerical, and sales- and craftspersons (128.76); for operatives, homemakers, and service personnel (128.40); and for farmers and laborers (128.76). The differences between the four groups, between institutionalized and noninstitutionalized, and between males and females were not significant.

However, a slight decline with age over 65 years was significant.

References

Behrmann, M., & Penn, C. (1984). Non-verbal communication of aphasic patients. *British Journal of Disorders of Communication, 19,* 155–168.

Davis, A.G. (1993). *A Survey of Adult Aphasia* (2nd ed.). Englewood-Cliffs, NJ: Prentice-Hall.

Fromm, D., & Holland, A.L. (1989). Functional communication in Alzheimer's disease. *Journal of Speech and Hearing Disorders, 54,* 535–540.

Holland, A. (1980). *The Communicative Abilities in Daily Living.* Manual. Austin, TX: Pro-Ed.

Holland, A. (1984). *Language Disorders in Adults: Recent Advances.* San Diego: College-Hill Press.

Linebaugh, C.W., Kryzer, K.M., Oden, S.E., & Myers, P.S. (1982). Reapportionment of communicative burden in aphasia. In R.H. Brookshire (Ed.), *Clinical Aphasiology: Conference Proceedings.* Minneapolis: BRK Publishers.

Martin, P., Manning, L., Munoz, P., & Montero, I. (1990). Communicative Abilities in Daily Living: Spanish standardization. *Evaluacion Psicologica, 6,* 369–384.

Pizzamiglio, L., Laicardi, C., Appicciafuoco, A., Gentili, P., Judica, A., Luglio, L., Margheriti, M., & Razzano, C. (1984). Capacita communicative di pazienti afasici in situationi di vita quotidiana: addatamento italiano. *Archivio di Psicologia Neurologia e Psichiatria, 45,* 187–210.

Sarno, M.T. (1969). *Functional Communication Profile.* New York: Institute of Rehabilitation Medicine.

Sarno, M.T., Buonaguro, A., & Levita, E. (1987). Aphasia in closed head injury and stroke. *Aphasiology, 1,* 331–338.

Skenes, L.L., & McCauley, R.J. (1985). Psychometric review of nine aphasia tests. *Journal of Communication Disorders, 18,* 461–474.

Watamori, T., Takauechi, M.I., Fukasako, Y., Suzuki, K., Takahashi, M., & Sasanuma, S. (1987). Development and standardization of Communication Abilities in Daily Living (CADL) test for Japanese aphasic patients. *Japanese Journal of Rehabilitation Medicine, 24,* 103–112.

Wertz, R., LaPointe, L., & Rosenbek, J. (1984). *Apraxia of Speech in Adults.* Orlando, FL: Grune & Stratton.

CONTROLLED ORAL WORD ASSOCIATION (COWA)

Other Test Names

Word Fluency, FAS-Test, Letter Fluency, Category Fluency.

Purpose

The purpose of the test is to evaluate the spontaneous production of words beginning with a given letter or of a given class within a limited amount of time (verbal association fluency).

Source

No specific material is required. The FAS-test is also included in the Neurosensory Center Comprehensive Examination for Aphasia (NCCEA, Spreen & Benton, 1969, 1977) distributed by the Psychology Clinic of the University of Victoria ($120 US for the complete test). A similar version is offered as part of the Multilingual Aphasia Examination (Benton, Hamsher & Sivan, 1994) described elsewhere in this volume. Category (animal) naming is also part of the Boston Diagnostic Aphasia Examination and the Stanford-Binet test described elsewhere in this volume. Another version of category fluency is included in the CELF-3, described elsewhere in this section.

Description

For letter (phonetic association) fluency, the subject is asked to produce orally as many words as possible beginning with a given letter in a limited period of time. As Marshall (1986) has pointed out, the label "Word Fluency" for this test is misleading, since verbal productivity in conversation or in continuous sentences is not measured. Instead, the test measures production of individual words under restricted search conditions (i.e., a given letter of the alphabet).

F, A, and S are the most commonly used letters for this popular test, although Benton, Hamsher & Sivan (1994) use C, F, L, and P, R, W. This affects the results to some extent because of differences in vocabulary size for each letter (Borkowski et al., 1967). In the

FAS set, F has the lowest, and S has the highest dictionary frequency; in the Benton and Hamsher sets, the first letter has the highest, and the last letter the lowest dictionary frequency. Overall, FAS allows more vocabulary choices than CFL and PRW, but the last two sets are approximately equivalent in the amount of choices offered. For younger children, words beginning with "sh" have been used to avoid the reliance on spelling skills.

Written word fluency was first used by Guilford (1967; J.P. Guilford & J.S. Guilford, 1980), allowing 3 minutes for each letter. Since the test is somewhat lengthy and dependent on basic spelling skills and intact motor abilities, the test is not suitable for younger children or patients with motor impairment.

For category (semantic association) fluency, the subject is asked to produce as many animal names as possible within a limited period of time. Food names and "things in the kitchen," "things in a supermarket," "things to wear," "things that get you from one place to another," etc. have also been used. Other versions of this test require alternating naming of colors and birds (Newcomb, 1969), alternating between phonetic and semantic association, or a combination of semantic and phonetic association fluency ("animal names that begin with a 'c'", Heller & Dobbs, 1993).

Administration

Use a stopwatch and have the patient comfortably seated before giving the following instructions: "*I will say a letter of the alphabet. Then I want you to give me as many words that begin with that letter as quickly as you can. For instance, if I say "B," you might give me "bad, battle, bed. . . . " I do not want you to use words which are proper names such as 'Boston, Bob, or Buick (Brylcreem).' Also, do not use the same word again with a different ending such as 'eat' and 'eating.' Any questions?*" (Pause) "*Begin when I say the letter. The first letter is F. Go ahead.*" Begin timing immediately.

Allow 1 minute for each letter (F, A, and S). Say "*Fine*" or "*Good*" after each 1-minute performance. If patients discontinue before the end of the minute, encourage them to try to think of more words. If there is a silence of 15 seconds, repeat the basic instructions, and the letter. For scoring purposes, write down the actual words in the order in which they are produced, or make plus-signs if production is too rapid for verbatim recording. If repetitions occur that may be accepted if an alternate meaning was intended by the patient ("four" and "for", "son" and "sun"), then ask what was meant by this word at the end of the 1-minute period.

Administer all three letters: F, A, and S.

Immediately following, say: "*I am going to tell you the names of some things you can find in the kitchen: spoons, knives, forks, plates, faucet. Can you think of other things in the kitchen?*" Allow the patient to name other things, and correct if he or she produces incorrect responses, explaining the task once again. Then say: "*Now tell me the names of as many animals as you can. Name them as quickly as possible.*" Allow 1 minute. If the patient discontinues before the end of the period, encourage him or her to produce more names. Repeat the basic instruction and give the starting word "dog" if there is a pause of 15 seconds or more. Start timing immediately after the instructions have been given, but allow extra time for the period when instructions are repeated. Write down the actual words in the order in which they were produced.

Approximate Time for Administration

The administration takes about 5–10 minutes.

Scoring

The scores are (1) the sum of all admissible words for the three letters. Slang terms and foreign words that are part of standard English ("faux pas, lasagna") are acceptable; (2) the sum of all admissible words for the animal category. For animal category fluency, names of extinct, imaginary, or magic animals are admissable, but given names for animals like "Fido," and "Morris" are not. Inadmissible words produced under these instructions (i.e., proper nouns, wrong words, variations, repetitions) are not counted as correct.

Errors should be reviewed carefully because they may provide clues to certain types of disorders; e.g., repetitions (perseverations), intrusions (of other letters or from another category), paraphasias, spelling errors. Often the order of words produced also suggests clues to the search strategy of the patient, e.g., words starting with the same two-letter combination ("factor, facilitate, factory, fabric") or the same semantic cluster (pets, animals in a zoo).

Comment

Reliability. Interscorer reliability is near perfect; 1-year retest reliability in older adults has been reported as .70 (.7 for F, .6 for A, and .71 for S; Snow et al., 1988), retest reliability after 19–42 days in adults as .88 (des Rosiers and Kavanagh, 1987), and in 51 adult intractable epileptic patients after 8 months as .65 (Sawrie et al., 1996) with an average gain of 1 point. Practice effects for short-term retests remain to be explored. Brown et al. (1989) report a retest reliability of .54 in 248 8-year-old children after 2½ years (using only the letters P and C); three retests over an 18-month period in HIV+ adults showed a reliability ranging from .76 to .87 (Bardi et al., 1995).

Validity. Concurrent validity has been established in several studies, generally indicating better validity for letters than for concrete category names such as "food" (Coelho, 1984). Correlation of letter association fluency with age was −.19 and with education .32; correlation with Wechsler Adult Intelligence Scale (WAIS) Verbal IQ (VIQ) was .14 and with Performance IQ (PIQ) .29 (Yeudall et al., 1986). Tombaugh and Rees (1996) report a correlation of .15 with WAIS-R Vocabulary.

In studies of construct validity, the test contributed mainly to Factor 1 (reading-writing) and Factor 6 (reading-writing-sentence construction) in a factor-analytic study with children's data (Crockett, 1974). This finding is probably due to the still-developing spelling skills at that age. In adults, desRosiers and Kavanagh (1987) found that the test loaded mainly on a "verbal knowledge" factor (together with Verbal IQ and Vocabulary); Roudier et al.

(1991, quoted in Lezak, 1995) found that it loaded on an "abstract mental operations" factor, which was characterized by other tests such as oral spelling, digit span, and mental calculations; and Crockett (1996) found the test related to naming, problem solving, sequencing, resisting distraction, perseveration, and several measures of memory. The difference in factor-analytic constructs is probably due to the fact that such studies are highly dependent on the number and type of measures included in the data. In adults, written letter fluency did not correlate with reaction time in various tasks of verbal information processing (Schweizer, 1993). One study (Schutz & Schutz, 1996) also reported validity of the COWA in predicting of several measures of driving a motor vehicle after postacute rehabilitation.

Troyer, Moscovitch and Winocur (1997) attempted to isolate the components involved in COWA tasks. They found that 'clustering,' the ability to produce words within phonetic and semantic subcategories, and 'switching,' the ability to shift between clusters, were both correlated with the number of words generated in semantic fluency tasks, and that switching was more correlated than clustering with the number of words generated on phonemic fluency. Younger healthy adults generated more words and switched more frequently on semantic fluency than older adults, whereas older adults produced larger clusters on phonemic fluency. Divided attention (for example, producing words while finger tapping at the same time) decreased the number of words produced and the number of switches for phonemic fluency only.

Neuropsychological Studies. Welsh et al. (1988) claim that functions assessed by COWA are one of the latest of prefrontal measures to mature (i.e., it develops beyond age 12 while other measures attain adult level as early as age 6). Sandler et al. (1993) found poor COWA in hyperactive children with peer problems; Barkley and Grodzinsky (1994) reported that the FAS-COWA did discriminate between ADD, ADD-H, and learning disabled children at the 90 percent level, but the number of misclassifications (60 percent) was high.

Spellacy and Brown (1984) found poor COWA (together with poor achievement test scores) to be a significant predictor of recidivism in adolescent offenders. COWA and animal fluency, however, did not show significant impairment in 62 high-functioning autistic adolescents (Minshew et al., 1995).

Ewing-Cobbs and colleagues (1987) studied discriminant validity in children with closed-head injury; 15 percent of those with mild, and 35 percent of those with moderate or severe injury scored below the 6th percentile for age and sex. Taylor and Schatschneider (1992) note that in 113 mildly impaired post-meningitis children with normal hearing the COWA was more related to social rather than medical factors; the test did, however, contribute to the prediction of outcome. Category fluency was significantly impaired in children with early hydrocephalus and spina bifida regardless of side of shunt (Holler et al., 1995).

Scores on letter fluency for a mixed group of 200 aphasic adults ranged from 3 to 46 with a mean of 11.5; unselected brain-damaged non-aphasic patients showed scores ranging from 5 to 46+ with a mean of 28.2 (Spreen & Benton, 1977). Adults with closed-head injury had mean scores of 23.8 (desRosiers & Kavanagh, 1987), and scored at the 51st percentile of the normative data for aphasics of the NCCEA (Sarno, 1986). Sarno et al. (1985) found no significant difference between male and female aphasic stroke victims nor in their rate of recovery over a 2-year period. A study of stroke victims with anomia (Margolin et al., 1990) showed more impairment on the PRW COWA (mean = 16.38) than patients with Alzheimer's dementia (AD) (mean = 29.64), while scores on the Boston Naming Test showed the reverse pattern.

Mutchnick et al. (1991) found letter fluency to be among the five best significant discriminators (out of 18 Halstead-Reitan tests) between 298 brain damaged (unspecified) and 193 pseudoneurological (referred for neuropsychological evaluation but without neurological impairment) controls. Crockett et al. (1990) also found significantly better performance in a mixed psychiatric group than in groups with verified brain dysfunction. A study of 218 patients (age 17–50) with acute

brain trauma and a minimum cognitive level (confused-inappropriate-agitated) found significant decrease in COWA, using four rather than three letters (S, T, P, C, mean 28.9; Gruen et al., 1990). Peck et al. (1992) reported "normative" data for 366 head-injured patients and found significant effects of severity of injury ($p < .003$). Mild head-injury patients scored at the 46th percentile, patients with moderate injury at the 39th percentile, and patients with severe injury at the 27th percentile; in comparison, patients tested 12 months post-injury showed relatively little, statistically nonsignificant recovery. Patients with right-hemisphere lesions did not show serious impairment on this test (Cavalli et al., 1981), although Joanette and Goulet (1986) showed a reduction in category, but not in letter fluency. Varley (1995) did not find impairment of category fluency in patients with right-hemisphere lesions, except those with "broader cognitive failures."

Miceli et al., (1981) and Bruyer and Tuyumbu (1980) report high sensitivity of COWA to frontal lobe damage regardless of side of lesion, while Parks et al. (1988), Perret (1974), Ramier and Hecaen (1970), Regard (1981), and Ruff et al. (1994) found more impairment in patients with left- and bi-frontal lesions. Benton (1986) reported the most severe impairment for bilateral frontal lesions, and Crowe's (1992) study implicated primarily the medial and orbital frontal lobe areas. Shoqueirat et al. (1990) found similar results in patients with ruptured aneurysms of the anterior communicating artery, particularly if extensive frontal damage was present (D'Esposito et al., 1996). A study by Pozzilli et al., (1991) also implicated the anterior portion of the corpus callosum in patients with multiple sclerosis and radiologically demonstrated corpus callosum atrophy. Patients with left pulvinotomy showed a 45 percent loss in COWA (Vilkki & Laittinen, 1976). Left temporal lobectomy postoperatively reduced letter as well as category (animals) fluency dramatically compared to preoperative levels, although right lobectomy showed only minimal effects; after 1 year, performance was back to the preoperative level or better (Loring et al., 1994). A recent study (Pachana et al., 1996) also found more severely impaired FAS-COWA (mean = 17.3, SD = 15.1) in patients with fronto-temporal dementia as compared to Alzheimer's dementia (mean = 26.5, SD = 11.6), presumably because of the demands of this test on "executive abilities."

In 22 healthy volunteers, Cantor-Graae et al. (1993) found that regional cerebral blood flow was primarily augmented in the dorsolateral prefrontal Cortex during the FAS-COWA task, but not during the performance of the WCST; a similar augmentation was demonstrated by Warkentin et al. (1991). A positron-emission tomography (PET) study (Parks et al., 1988) with normal volunteers indicated, however, that COWA activates bilateral temporal and frontal lobes. A recent study (Cardebat et al., 1996) used both category (animals, fruit) and letter (P, R) fluency tasks in 19 volunteers, and found increased cerebral blood flow in the right dorsolateral and medial frontal region only for the semantic (category) fluency task, but no increase compared to baseline measures for formal (letter) fluency. Finally, Coben et al. (1995) found a strong relationship between FAS-COWA and unawareness of deficit in brain-damaged patients, which they attribute to impaired frontal-mediated executive functions.

Patients with organic amnesia (Korsakoff's disease, encephalitis) showed impairment on the FAS-COWA (Shoqueirat et al., 1990), and Hewitt et al. (1991) found similar findings in female alcoholics. On the other hand, in 11 subjects, seen 1 year after hypoxia that affected primarily the hippocampal areas, COWA was not impaired (mean = 43.09, matched controls mean = 45.09) (Hopkins et al., 1995).

HIV-positive men with neuropsychological impairment showed deficits on the phonemic association task (Di Sclafini et al., 1997), and Monsch et al. (1994b) showed impairment on both tasks in HIV positive men, similar to the impairment of Huntington disease (HD) patients. Monsch et al. concluded that this may represent a pattern typical for subcortical disease. This conclusion is supported by Auriacombe et al. (1993) and Bayles et al. (1993) who found similar results in Parkinson's disease (PD) patients, and by Hanes et al. (1996)

who found significant differences between controls and patients with HD, PD, or schizophrenia (but not between patient groups) on semantic fluency and other executive control tasks (Tower of London, Stroop Test). However, Hanley et al. (1990) argued that the poor performance of PD patients was mainly due to impaired verbal ability and age. Beatty and Monson (1989) compared PD and multiple sclerosis (MS) patients with normal and impaired naming ability with an age- and education-matched control group: in both patient groups both letter (FAS) and category (animals, fruits, parts of the body) fluency was only minimally impaired in the normal-naming group, but severely impaired in the impaired-naming group; a similar impairment was found in definition vocabulary (WAIS-R). Hence it would appear that PD and MS patients show impairment not as a function of age, but consistent with name-finding ability.

Although an earlier study (Ober et al., 1986) did not find differences between letter (FAS) and category (fruits) tasks in mild and moderately severe AD patients, a number of recent studies of AD patients showed significant differences. Adams (personal communication) did not find reduced FAS-COWA in either AD or Huntington's disease patients; however, AD patients showed more intrusion (wrong letter), perseveration (repeats), and variation (fish, fishy, fishing) errors. However, Miller and Hague (1975) and Murdoch et al. (1987) did find reduced COWA in AD patients. Lafleche and Albert (1995) found significant differences between patients with mild AD and controls on FAS and three other "executive function tests" (Self-Ordering Test, Trails, and Hukok, a test somewhat similar to the Raven Progressive Matrices). Lacy (1994) reported that there were significant differences for both letter and category fluency between medical controls and psychiatric patients, but that the worst performance was found in patients with AD, and with left-hemisphere damage whereas patients with right-hemisphere damage and subcortical lesions were not significantly different from controls. Patients with AD were also found to show better performance on the Trail Making Test, Part B, if semantic (category) naming was good, while others showed good performance on writing to dictation in association with good letter fluency (Bayles et al., 1989); the authors ascribed this difference between the two tasks to the existence of two subsystems of memory on which each relies. A series of studies by Butters and colleagues (Butters et al., 1987; Monsch et al., 1992, 1994a) compared COWA (FAS) with category fluency (animals, fruits, vegetables), and found that both tasks discriminated significantly between Huntington disease patients and demographically matched normal middle-aged controls, while AD patients did poorly on the category rather than the letter fluency task. This was confirmed in a study by Cahn et al. (1995) that attempted to separate normal elderly, at-risk for AD, and AD patients; category fluency contributed better than letter fluency to group separation. However, both category and letter fluency did not add to group separation in a regression formula after the contribution of Trails B, Word List delayed recall, Boston Naming, and Wechsler Memory visual retention had been entered. Other contributors to group separation in this study were the occurrence of intrusion and perseverative errors (Cahn et al., 1997). Mickanin et al. (1994), Rich (1993), and Taussig (personal communication) reported similar results. In the Bronx Aging Study (Aronson et al., 1990; Masur et al., 1994) 442 healthy elderly subjects (mean age 79.2 years) were followed annually over 4 years. Low values for category fluency at the time of entry into the study was found to be a significant predictor ($p < .00001$) of dementia during the course of the follow-up; in combination with other measures, the prediction of occurrence of dementia was correct in 68 percent, and the prediction of absence of dementia was correct in 88 percent. Small et al. (1997) found significant differences for both letter (N,S) and category (foods) fluency between patients with incident dementia and without dementia. Letter fluency contributed significantly to the prospective prediction of AD. Goldstein et al. (1996) found that semantic, but not letter fluency contributed to the discrimination between patients with AD and elderly patients with closed-head injury; the two groups were matched for demographic features and Mini-

Mental State Examination scores. Category fluency (animals, fruits, vegetables) showed a sensitivity of 67 and 86 percent and a specificity of 70 and 78 percent in distinguishing uneducated and educated Chinese subjects with and without dementia (Salmon et al., 1995). Rich (1993) found a letter fluency mean of 16.15 in AD patients (mean age 75 years) as compared to a mean of 34.05 for healthy controls of the same age; animal fluency means were 6.90 and 15.45, respectively. Statistically, category fluency discriminated better than letter fluency between the two groups as well as between young–old and old–old age groups. It is likely that category fluency makes more demands on semantic cognitive abilities than letter fluency, which relies on well-established spelling knowledge; this may explain the relatively intact letter fluency in AD. As a study by Binetti et al. (1995) showed, AD patients not only produced fewer animal names, but were limited in producing clusters (e.g., farm animals) and used words with higher lexical frequencies. A recent study by Barr and Brandt (1996) found semantic fluency more impaired than phonetic fluency; however, this finding held for several forms of dementia, i.e. AD, HD, and vascular dementia.

Loewenstein et al., (1992) compared the performance of 33 AD patients on the FAS-COWA and seven other tests with functional tasks (reading a clock, telephone skills, preparing a letter for mailing, counting currency, writing a check, balancing a checkbook, shopping with a written list); the COWA correlated (.40) with the ability to use a telephone, and to balance a checkbook (.45), and contributed (.21) to a stepwise regression analysis of the tasks in predicting functional competence. However, all tasks combined accounted for less than 50 percent of the explained variance.

Stebbins et al. (1995) found no impairment in adults with Tourette's syndrome for both COWA and category (supermarket) fluency, which they considered as measures of semantic memory; in contrast, these patients showed impairment on measures of working and procedural memory presumably related to frontal-striatal functioning.

Mild or moderate depression appears to have no or only a minor effect on COWA:

Boone et al. (1995) found significant differences between elderly controls, patients with mild or moderate depression, and controls (means 40.45, 37.41, and 32.42, respectively), but they stress that these differences were not clinically significant. Kronfol et al. (1978) also reported that in patients with symptoms of depression mimicking dementia, word fluency showed little change, and Petrick et al. (1992) reported that COWA did not discriminate between patients with AD and patients with depression. However, elderly depressed patients (ages 62–81) with psychosis had significantly lower FAS scores than those without (Kunik et al., 1994). Gourovitch et al., (1996) reported that schizophrenics produced more phonemic (letter) associations than category words, whereas a group of normal subjects matched for premorbid intelligence showed the reverse pattern.

Both letter and category fluency can be affected by post-traumatic stress disorder (PTSD): Uddo et al. (1993) found means of 33.31 (SD = 9.08) for the letters C, F, and L, and of 9.08 (SD = 4.25) for the animal category in Vietnam combat veterans with PTSD (mean age = 41.6 years) compared to healthy National Guardsmen (mean age = 32.9 years; means = 39.73 and 13.77, SDs = 18.53 and 4.50, respectively).

Normative Data

Comparison of Different Forms of COWA. Few results are available to compare the different forms of letter and category fluency tasks. As mentioned in the description section, FAS has somewhat higher (a ratio of 1.3:1.0) dictionary frequency than CFL and PRW (which are equivalent). For this reason, Ruff et al. (1996) conclude that "the raw scores on the two versions are not comparable." However, as some studies have shown, the number of words produced with a given letter is not directly related to dictionary volume: For example, the letter F has lower dictionary frequencies than A, yet normative studies that report raw scores for individual letters (Tombaugh, Kozak & Rees, 1996; Table 11–7), consistently find the letter A more difficult than F. In addition, the ceiling imposed by the time limit of this task seems to prevent the individual from making full use of dictionary-driven opportunities for generating words.

A first study of the equivalence of the letters FAS and CFL (Lacy et al., 1996) showed that the two paradigms were comparable across two different settings and two different diagnostic groups (psychiatric vs. suspected CNS dysfunction) with correlations between .87 to .94. However, normative studies with different letter sets are not directly comparable because samples with different education and intelligence levels were used In general, however, the differences between the three letter sets appear to be small, as suggested by a comparison of Tables 11–7 and 11–8. We present available norms for both FAS and CFL separately. Written letter fluency norms are available from a few studies and appear to produce somewhat lower scores than the oral production task.

No studies of the equivalence of different categories for semantic COWA are available. However, small differences between such categories as animal names, means of transporta-

Table 11–7. COWA (FAS) by Education Level in Adults

Education	n	F		A		S		Total	
		M	SD	M	SD	M	SD	M	SD
0–8 years	32	13.1	4.5	9.8	4.0	13.9	4.5	36.5	10.7
9–12 years	479	13.7	4.5	11.2	4.3	14.4	4.6	39.3	11.6
13–16 years	332	15.1	4.4	12.9	4.3	15.7	4.6	43.7	11.6
17–21 years	51	16.2	4.1	13.5	4.4	17.1	5.1	46.9	11.6
All Education Levels	894	14.4	4.5	11.9	4.4	15.0	4.7	46.9	11.8

From Tombaugh, Kozak, and Rees (1996), based on adult volunteers in the Ottawa, Ontario area.

Table 11–8. Controlled Word Association (CFL) in Adults, Age 16–70 Years by Education Level

Education	Men (n = 180)		Women (n = 180)		Both genders (n = 360)	
	M	SD	M	SD	M	SD
12 years or less	36.9	9.8	35.9	9.6	36.5	9.9
13 to 15 years	40.5	9.4	39.4	10.1	40.0	9.7
16 years and more	41.0	9.3	46.5	11.2	43.8	10.6
All education levels	39.5	9.8	40.6	11.2	40.1	10.5

Source: Ruff et al., 1996 with permission of the authors and the National Academy of Neuropsychology.

tion, and things in the supermarket are likely to be found. We only present available norms for animals names, supermarket items, and foods.

Effects of Age, Gender, Education, and IQ. Age effects have been shown only for subjects in the higher age range (Read, 1987; Tombaugh, Kozak, & Rees, 1996, Table 11–9), whereas Ruff et al. (1994) found no age effect in the 16–70 age range. Other authors have found both smaller and larger decreases of productivity with age: Schaie and Parham (1977) showed an age-related drop in speeded productivity on this test beginning at age 53, and they found that normal adults at age 67 showed only 74 and 60 percent productivity compared to age 25 in the repeated measurement and in the independent random samples, respectively. Benton et al. (1981) stated that letter fluency shows little decline with age up to the age of 80 but applies a correction of three points to subjects over 55 years of age, a finding supported by Bolla et al. (1990) in a study of 199 healthy subjects between 39 and 89 years of age. Parkin et al. (1995) found no decline in community-dwelling adults between the age of 21 and 81 (means 43.7 and 43.9, respectively). Axelrod and Henry (1992) found on the FAS-COWA an average decline from younger adult levels of four words for healthy, independently living adults in their 70s and 80s. Only Albert et al. (1988) reported a gradual decline of letter fluency from 49.19 in 30- to 39-year-olds to 39.65 for 70- to 80-year-old healthy adults, although the sharpest drop (from 45 to 39 words) occurred between

the 60–69 and 70–79 age groups. Mittenberg et al. (1989) confirm a weak correlation with age (−.14) in normal control subjects between 20 and 75 years; Heller and Dobbs (1993) found only an insignificant decrease of letter association up to age 76 in well-educated adults, whereas that association was significant for category association (mean = 9.29 for age 28–39, 7.07 for age 60–76, using only a 30-second test period). Kozora and Cullum (1995) confirm that for normal elderly subjects with good education (mean = 14.3 years) FAS-COWA does not show age effects (means for the 6th, 7th, 8th, and 9th decade of life: 41.23, 45.76, 46.49, 40.74), whereas category fluency does (means for animal category = 20.95, 21.07, 18.96, 15.81, respectively). Tomer and Levin (1993) also found a decline of category, but not letter fluency with age (75–91 years). Tombaugh, Kozak, & Rees (personal communication, 1996) found that education was a better predictor of FAS-COWA than age; for category COWA (animals) only age and gender contributed significantly in an analysis of variance.

Crawford et al. (1992) found a correlation of .67 between controlled oral word association (FAS) and the National Adult Reading Test (NART), but not with age, in a normal sample representative for Britain. They suggested that expected scores in letter fluency could be predicted on the basis of NART scores [predicted VF = 57.5 − (0.76 × NART errors), SE (est). = 9.09)]. The comparison of their normal group with a neurological sample showed a significantly better discrimination when expected verbal fluency scores were used. A ta-

Table 11—9. Norms for FAS COWA Stratified for Age and Years of Education

	Age 16–59			Age 60–79			Age 80–95		
Percentile score	0–8 yrs. ed. (n = 12)	9–12 yrs. ed. (n = 268)	13–21 yrs. ed. (n = 242)	0–8 yrs. ed. (n = 12)	9–12 yrs. ed. (n = 268)	13–21 yrs. ed. (n = 242)	0–8 yrs. ed. (n = 12)	9–12 yrs. ed. (n = 268)	13–21 yrs. ed. (n = 242)
90	48	56	61	39	54	59	33	42	56
80	45	50	55	36	47	53	29	38	47
70	42	47	51	31	43	49	26	34	43
60	39	43	49	27	39	45	24	31	39
50	36	40	45	25	35	41	22	29	36
40	35	38	42	22	32	38	21	27	33
30	34	35	38	20	28	36	19	24	30
20	30	32	35	17	24	34	17	22	28
10	27	28	30	13	21	27	13	18	23
Mean	38.5	40.5	44.7	25.3	35.6	42.0	22.4	29.8	37.0
(SD)	(12.0)	(10.7)	(11.2)	(11.1)	(12.5)	(12.1)	(8.2)	(11.4)	(11.2)

Source: Tombaugh, Kozak & Rees (1996).

ble to convert NART errors to predicted COWA (FAS) scores is presented in Figure 11–1. The user should keep in mind that this table is based on a study with the British NART and healthy British subjects; however, a similar relationship is likely to apply for North-American subjects and the NAART.

Normative Data for Adults. Table 11–9 presents norms for the age range 16–95 years (Tombaugh, Kozak, & Rees, 1996). Spreen and Benton's (1977) normative data showed considerably lower scores (mean = 33); however, these norms were based on a poorly educated/low intelligence rural sample. Monsch et al.'s (1994) means for a normal middle-aged sample for COWA were very close to those shown in Table 11–9. Data published by Yeudall et al. (1986) were also very similar. Gender differences were insignificant in the two major normative studies (male/female Yeudall: 42.8/41.5, Tombaugh, Kozak & Rees: 40.1/41.6). Johnson et al. (1995) found that mean scores for FAS were slightly higher (about two points) for white as compared to black subjects, who, in turn, scored about two points better compared to Hispanic subjects after covarying all groups for income and education. For animal naming, white subjects scored about two points higher than black or Hispanic subjects. Caution should be used

when testing clients with a first language other than English: Taussig et al. (1988) reported a mean of 24.5 for FAS for healthy Hispanics, even when tested in Spanish; English speakers obtained a mean of 41.5, similar to the norms presented here. Norms for Hispanics presented by Ponton et al. (1996) were similar (ranging from 26.4 in 16- to 29-year-olds to 33.0 in 50- to 75-year-olds with education better than grade 10). This task may be more difficult for Spanish speakers because the *s*-sound can be produced by the letters Z, S, and C in Spanish—hence asking for words starting with S only may be a more demanding task.

Recently published norms by Ruff et al. (1996) for CFL-COWA were based on 360 subjects with equal cell size for sex and education groups (Table 11–8). These norms are an average of five points lower than Yeudall et al.'s (1986) norms for FAS. This difference may be due to the relatively high education level of Yeudall et al.'s subjects and to the use of the somewhat easier FAS letters. Rosen's (1980) norms, based on 30 healthy nursing home residents with an average age of 84 years, are much lower (Mean for CFL = 27.9, for animal naming = 11.3), although even at that age mild and moderate-to-severe AD patients showed a considerable loss in the ability to perform both COWA tasks (Mean for CFL = 13.2 and 4.2, for animal naming = 8.4 and 1.7 respectively).

N–WF	N–WF	N–WF	N–WF	N–WF	N–WF
0–57	9–51	18–44	27–37	36–30	45–23
1–57	10–50	19–43	28–36	37–29	46–23
2–56	11–49	20–42	29–35	38–29	47–22
3–55	12–48	21–42	30–35	39–28	48–21
4–54	13–48	22–41	31–34	40–27	49–20
5–54	14–47	23–40	32–33	41–26	50–19
6–53	15–46	24–39	33–32	42–26	
7–52	16–45	25–38	34–32	43–25	
8–51	17–45	26–38	35–31	44–24	

Note: Error scores refer to the NART, not the NAART. The NAART has 61 rather than 50 items; hence, if the NAART is used, appropriate adjustments should be made.

Figure 11—1. Conversion of NART(N) errors to predicted FAS-COWA(WF) scores (Crawford et al., 1992).

Table 11–8 includes norms for oral production on the FAS test for relatively well-educated, healthy elderly persons. These norms agree closely with those produced by Ivnik, Malec, and Smith (1996) and by Montgomery and Costa (1983); Rich's data (1993, using the letters C, F, and L, are only slightly higher. Steenhuis and Ostbye (1995) report somewhat lower values (mean = 25.80) for a sample of 591 normal subjects in the Canadian Study of Health and Aging with a mean age of 78.5. Table 11–10 contains similar values broken down by education level from the Cana-dian study for 265 subjects between the ages of 65 and 90 years for both written FAS COWA and category (animal) fluency (Tuokko & Woodward, 1996). Table 11–11 contains norms for animal naming based on community volunteers in Ottawa, Ontario (Tombaugh, Kozak & Rees, 1996), and Table 11–12 contains norms for animal naming stratified by age and education. In the high age range most studies report no gender differences.

Gruen et al. (1990) studied typical response strategies on letter fluency in head-injured adults: Most frequent were responses with

Table 11–10. Norms for Written FAS-COWA and Animal Naming for Subjects Aged 65 to 90 years

Age, in Years, and Gender	Education					
	8 years		12 years		16 years	
	COWA	Animal	COWA	Animal	COWA	Animal
65 male	28.8	17.3	33.8	18.9	38.9	20.3
65 female	28.7	17.3	33.6	18.9	39.0	20.4
70 male	27.8	16.5	32.8	18.2	38.0	19.8
70 female	27.7	16.5	32.9	18.2	38.0	19.8
75 male	26.8	15.4	31.9	17.4	37.0	18.9
75 female	26.8	15.5	31.6	17.4	37.0	18.9
80 male	25.3	14.9	30.8	16.7	35.9	18.2
80 female	25.8	14.9	30.9	16.8	35.9	18.2
85 male	24.3	14.3	29.8	15.7	34.8	17.4
85 female	22.0	13.4	29.7	15.6	34.9	17.4
90 male	23.8	13.3	28.7	14.9	33.8	16.7
90 female	23.8	13.4	28.8	14.9	33.8	16.7

Source: Tuokko & Woodward, 1996 with permission of the authors and Swets Publishing Service.

Note: Overall mean: Age = 78.4 (SD = 6.2), COWA = 31.4 (SD = 10.7), Category Fluency (animals) = 15.4 (SD = 3.9).

Table 11—11. Mean (SD) Numbers of Animals Named in One Minute by Education, Age, and Gender

Category	n	Animal Naming M	(SD)
Education, years			
0–8	140	13.9	(3.9)
9–12	377	16.7	(4.6)
13–16	173	19.0	(5.2)
17–21	44	19.5	(5.2)
Age, years			
16–19	19	21.5	(4.4)
20–29	41	19.9	(5.0)
30–39	43	21.5	(5.5)
40–49	45	20.7	(4.2)
50–59	43	20.1	(4.9)
60–69	92	17.6	(4.7)
70–79	228	16.1	(4.0)
80–89	200	14.3	(3.9)
90–95	24	13.0	(3.8)
Gender			
male	310	17.4	(5.1)
female	425	16.5	(5.0)
Total	735	16.9	(5.0)

Source: Tombaugh, Kozak & Rees (1996).

the same initial consonant-vowel syllable, followed by responses with the same initial consonant-consonant cluster, the same initial and final consonant with different vowel, homonyms, semantic associations, responses within the same semantic category, and with the semantically related same initial consonant-vowel syllable. These strategies did not change appreciably across subjects with various degrees of cognitive impairment. Raskin and Rearick (1996) found that adults with mild traumatic brain injury, though showing lower production rates and more errors, showed an equal proportion of semantic and phonemic clusters, similar to that found in matched normal controls. Montgomery and Costa (1983) also reported that 82 percent of their healthy elderly sample repeated one or more words, and that 40 percent used "wrong words" (e.g., "phone" for F, "Susan for S).

Heaton, Grant, & Matthews (1991) present scaled score norms for written word fluency. These norms are corrected for gender, education, and age, and are based on 553 normal subjects. However, caution in the use of these norms is recommended because the size of individual cells is not provided and may be quite small.

Normative Data in Children. Normative data for an unselected group of normal learning school children on FAS-COWA are presented in Table 11–13 (Gaddes & Crockett, 1975). These data agree closely with those published by Crockett (1974). They also agree both in terms of means as well as percentile distribution with those for children with epilepsy, brain damage, and learning disability in a multidisciplinary outpatient center in Milwaukee (Hamsher, 1980), and for children with insulin-dependent diabetes (Northam et

Table 11—12. Norms for Animal Naming Stratified for Age and Years of Education

Percentile score	Age 16–59		Age 60–79			Age 80–95		
	9–12 yrs. ed. (n = 109)	13–21 yrs. ed. (n = 78)	0–8 yrs. ed. (n = 61)	9–12 yrs. ed. (n = 165)	13–21 yrs. ed. (n = 94)	0–8 yrs. ed. (n = 75)	9–12 yrs. ed. (n = 103)	13–21 yrs. ed. (n = 46)
90	26	30	20	22	25	18	19	24
75	23	25	17	19	22	16	17	20
50	20	23	14	17	19	13	14	16
25	17	18	12	14	16	11	12	14
10	15	16	11	12	13	9	11	12
Mean	19.8	21.9	14.4	16.4	18.2	13.1	13.9	16.3
(SD)	(4.2)	(5.4)	(3.4)	(4.3)	(4.2)	(3.8)	(3.4)	(4.3)

Source: Tombaugh, Kozak & Rees (1996).

Table 11–13. Norms for School-Age Children (FAS)

	Female			Male			Total		
Age	n	M	SD	n	M	SD	n	M	SD
6	30	4.6	5.0	22	4.1	4.1	52	4.4	4.6
7	24	16.0	7.3	27	14.1	6.5	51	15.0	6.9
8	23	23.1	5.7	25	22.5	7.7	48	22.8	6.8
9	30	25.0	7.3	23	22.6	6.4	53	24.0	6.9
10	25	27.4	7.1	25	23.8	8.2	50	25.6	7.8
11	22	31.1	6.8	22	28.2	8.1	44	29.7	7.6
12	13	32.0	6.8	13	29.4	8.1	26	30.7	7.4
13	12	37.3	5.8	17	28.8	8.3	29	32.3	8.4

Source: Gaddes & Crockett, 1975.

Table 11—14. Performance of Normal School Children on Naming of Animals, Foods, and Words Beginning with "sh"

Age (years)	n	Animals		Foods		"Sh words"	
		M	SD	M	SD	M	SD
6	34	10.74	2.4	9.74	3.3	4.24	1.6
7	40	12.43	2.9	11.88	2.7	5.53	1.6
8	32	12.31	2.7	11.11	3.4	5.21	2.1
9	38	13.76	3.7	14.05	3.9	5.95	2.4
10	22	14.27	3.7	13.97	2.2	6.00	2.0
11	28	15.50	3.8	14.80	4.6	6.28	2.4
12	10	18.90	6.2	17.70	4.0	6.10	1.8

Source: Halperin et al. (1989).

Table 11—15. Children's Written Word Fluency

	Total			Female			Male		
Age	n	M	SD	n	M	SD	n	M	SD
6	80	9.28	4.47	40	9.85	4.58	40	8.70	4.33
7	133	15.87	8.22	72	17.22	8.20	61	14.26	8.00
8	197	21.52	9.29	85	23.72	10.34	112	19.85	8.05
9	208	25.93	10.18	90	28.41	9.93	118	24.03	10.01
10	189	29.98	11.92	86	33.16	11.83	103	27.32	11.39
11	146	37.08	11.98	75	39.03	10.57	71	35.01	13.07
12	140	40.58	13.00	84	44.52	12.98	56	34.61	10.61
13	167	45.07	14.10	76	51.37	13.65	91	39.81	12.26
14	175	48.46	14.72	85	52.64	14.30	90	44.52	14.08
15	120	47.35	15.22	51	51.57	13.28	69	44.23	15.88
16	69	48.28	13.69	28	53.43	10.54	41	44.76	14.56
17	79	49.65	17.51	37	53.65	17.63	42	46.12	16.83
18	30	61.47	15.29	18	64.22	14.98	12	57.33	15.42

Note: This test requires the subject to write as many words as possible beginning with the letter "s" in five minutes, and as many four-letter words as possible beginning with the letter "c" in four minutes. Means are totals for both sets of responses.

Source: Kolb & Whishaw (1985).

al., 1995), suggesting that such impairments have relatively little influence on controlled word association performance in children. In most studies a slightly lower score was found for females compared to males. A study by Mann et al. (1990) confirmed this finding in high school students (written FAS-COWA; mean for females 39.14, for males 40.08) and in a cross-cultural comparison with Japanese students. The reported means are very close to those for young adults in Table 11–10.

Norms for the production of animal names, food names, and words beginning with "sh" in children are shown in Table 11–14. Vargha-Khadem (unpublished) obtained animal naming norms for 20 children each at the age of 6 to 12, which are very similar to those shown in Table 11-14 (approximately 1 point higher). In contrast to these data, Goodglass and Kaplan (1983) suggested a norm of 12 animal names in 12-year-olds, and of 18 in the average adult. Additional norms for children age 5 years to 16 years 11 months for naming fluency in three categories (animals, transportation, types of work) can be found in the CELF-3. Table 11-15 presents norms for *written* word fluency in children, age 6 to 18 years (Kolb and Whishaw, 1985).

References

Albert, M.S., Heller, H.S., & Milberg, W. (1988). Changes in naming ability with age. *Psychology and Aging, 3*, 173–178.

Aronson, M.K., Ooi, W.L., Morgenstern, H., Hafner, A., Masur, D., Crystal, H., Frishman, W.H., Fisher, D., & Katzman, R. (1990). Women, myocardial infarction, and dementia in the very old. *Neurology, 40*, 1102–1106.

Auriacombe, S., Grossman, M., Carvell, S., & Gollomp, S. (1993). Verbal fluency deficits in Parkinson's disease. *Neuropsychology, 7*, 182–192.

Axelrod, B.N., & Henry, R.R. (1992). Age-related performance on the Wisconsin Card Sorting, Similarities, and Controlled Oral Word Association Tests. *Clinical Neuropsychologist, 6*, 16–26.

Bardi, C.A., Hamby, S.L., & Wilkins, J.W. (1995). Stability of several brief neuropsychological tests in an HIV+ longitudinal sample. *Archives of Clinical Neuropsychology, 10*, 195 (abstract).

Barkley, R.A., & Grodzinsky, G.M. (1994). Are tests of frontal lobe function useful in the diagnosis of attention deficit disorders? *The Clinical Neuropsychologist, 8*, 121–139.

Barr, A. & Brandt, J. (1996). Word-list generation deficits in dementia. *Journal of clinical and Experimental Neuropsychology, 18*, 810–822.

Bayles, K.A., Salmon, D.P., Tomoeda, C.K. & Jacobs, D. (1989). Semantic and letter category naming in Alzheimer's patients: A predictable difference. *Developmental Neuropsychology, 5*, 335–347.

Bayles, K.A., Trosset, M.W., Tomoeda, C.K., & Montgomery, E.B. (1993). Generative naming in Parkinson's disease. *Journal of Clinical and Experimental Neuropsychology, 15*, 547–562.

Beatty, W.W., & Monson, N. (1989). Lexical processing in Parkinson's disease and multiple sclerosis. *Journal of Geriatric Psychiatry and Neurology, 2*, 145–152.

Benton, A.L. (1968). Differential behavioral effects in frontal lobe disease. *Neuropsychologia, 6*, 53–60.

Benton, A.L., Eslinger, P.J., & Damasio, A.R. (1981). Normative observations on neuropsychological test performances in old age. *Journal of Clinical Neuropsychology, 3*, 33–42.

Benton, A.L., Hamsher, K., and Sivan, A.B. (1983). *Multilingual Aphasia Examination.* (3rd ed.) Iowa City, IA: AJA Associates.

Binetti, G., Magni, E., Cappa, S.F., Padovani, A., Bianchetti, A., & Trabucchi, M. (1995). Semantic memory in Alzheimer's disease: An analysis of category fluency. *Journal of Clinical and Experimental Neuropsychology, 17*, 82–89.

Bolla, K.I., Lindgren, K.N., Bonaccorsy, C., & Bleeker, M.L. (1990). Predictors of verbal fluency in the healthy elderly. *Journal of Clinical Psychology, 46*, 623–628.

Boone, K.B., Lesser, I.M., Miller, B.L., Wohl, M., Berman, N., Lee, A., Palmer, B., & Back, C. (1995). Cognitive functioning in older depressed outpatients: Relationships of presence and severity of depression to neuropsychological test scores. *Neuropsychology, 9*, 390–398.

Borkowski, J.G., Benton, A.L., & Spreen, O. (1967). Word fluency and brain damage. *Neuropsychologia 5*, 135–140.

Brown, S.J., Rourke, B.P., & Cicchetti, D.V. (1989). Reliability of tests and measures used in the neuropsychological assessment of children. *The Clinical Neuropsychologist, 3*, 353–368.

Bruyer, R., & Tuyumbu, B. (1980). Fluence verbale et lesions du cortex cerebrale: performances et types d'erreurs. *Encephale, 6*, 287–297.

Butters, N., Granholm, E., Salmon, D.P., Grant, I., & Wolfe, J. (1987). Episodic and semantic memory: A comparison of amnesic and demented patients. *Journal of Clinical and Experimental Neuropsychology, 9*, 479–497.

Cahn, D.A., Salmon, D.P., Bondi, M.W., Butters, N., Johnson, S.A., Wiederholt, W.C. & Barrett-Connor, E. (1997). A population-based analysis of qualitative features of the neuropsychological test performance of individuals with dementia of the Alzheimers type: Implications for individuals with questionable dementia. *Journal of the International Neuropsychological Society, 3*, 387–393.

Cahn, D.A., Salmon, D.P., Butters, N., Wiederholt, W.C., Corey-Bloom, J., Edelstein, S.L., & Barrett-Connor, E. (1995). Detection of dementia of the Alzheimer type in a population-based sample: Neuropsychological test performance. *Journal of the International Neuropsychological Society, 1*, 252–260.

Cantor-Graae, E., Warkentin, S., Franzen, G., & Risberg, J. (1993). Frontal lobe challenge: A comparison of activation procedures during rCBF measurement in normal subjects. *Neuropsychiatry, Neuropsychology, and Behavioral Neurology, 6*, 83–92.

Cavalli, M., De Renzi, E., Faglioni, P., & Vitale, A. (1981). Impairment of right brain-damaged patients on a linguistic cognitive task. *Cortex, 17*, 545–556.

Coben, R.A., Boksenbaum, S.I., & Kulberg, A.M. (1995). Cognitive determinants of unawareness of deficits: The importance of specific frontal-mediated executive functions. *Archives of Clinical Neuropsychology, 10*, 309 (abstract).

Coelho, C.A. (984). Word fluency measures in three groups of brain-injured subjects. Paper presented at the meeting of the American Speech-Language-Hearing Association, San Francisco.

Crawford, J.R., Moore, J.W., & Cameron, I.M. (1992). Verbal fluency: A NART-based equation for estimation of premorbid performance. *British Journal of Clinical Psychology, 31*, 327–329.

Crockett, D.J. (1974). Component analysis of within correlations of language-skill tests in normal children. *Journal of Special Education, 8*, 361–375.

Crockett, D.J. (1977). A comparison of empirically derived groups of aphasic patients on the Neurosensory Center Comprehensive Examination for Aphasia. *Journal of Clinical Psychology, 33*, 194–198.

Crockett, D.J., Hurwitz, T., & Vernon-Wilkinson, R. (1990). Differences in neuropsychological performance in psychiatric, anterior- and posterior-cerebral dysfunctioning groups. *International Journal of Neuroscience, 52*, 45–57.

Crowe, S.F. (1992). Dissociation of two frontal lobe syndromes by a test of verbal fluency. *Journal of Clinical and Experimental Neuropsychology, 14*, 327–339.

D'Esposito, M., Alexander, M.P., Fischer, R., et al. (1996). Recovery of memory and executive function following anterior communicating artery aneurysm rupture. *Journal of the International Neuropsychological Society, 2*, 565–570.

desRosiers, G., & Kavanagh, D. (1987). Cognitive assessment in closed head injury: Stability, validity and parallel forms for two neuropsychological measures of recovery. *International Journal of Clinical Neuropsychology, 9*, 162–173.

Di Sclafini, V., MacKay, R.D.S., Meyerhoff, D.J., Norman, D., Weiner, M.W., & Fein, G. (1997). Brain atrophy in HIV infection is more strongly associated with CDC clinical stage than with cognitive impairment. *Journal of the International Neuropsychological Society, 3*, 276–287.

Ewing-Cobbs, L., Levin, H.S., Eisenberg, H.M., & Fletcher, J.M. (1987). Language functions following closed-head injury in children and adolescents. *Journal of Clinical and Experimental Neuropsychology, 9*, 575–592.

Gaddes, W.H., & Crockett D.J. (1975). The Spreen-Benton aphasia tests, normative data as a measure of normal language development. *Brain and Language, 2*, 257–280.

Goldstein, F.C., Levin, H.S., Roberts, V.J., et al. (1996). Neuropsychological effect of closed head injury in older adults: A comparison with Alzheimer's disease. *Neuropsychology, 10*, 147–154.

Goodglass, H., & Kaplan, E. (1983). *The Assessment of Aphasia and Related Disorders* (2nd ed.). Philadelphia: Lea & Febiger.

Gourovitch, M.L., Goldberg, T.E., & Weinberger, D.R. (1995). Differential verbal fluency deficits in schizophrenic patients as compared to normal controls. *Journal of the International Neuropsychological Society, 1*, 357.

Gourovitch, M.L., Goldberg, T.E., & Weinberger, D.R. (1996). Verbal fluency deficits with schizophrenia: Fluency is differentially impaired as compared with phonological fluency. *Neuropsychology, 10*, 573–577.

Gruen, A.K., Frankle, B.C., & Schwartz, R. (1990). Word fluency generation skills of head-injured patients in an acute trauma center. *Journal of Communication Disorders, 23*, 163–170.

Guilford, J.P. (1967). *The Nature of Human Intelligence.* New York: McGraw-Hill.

Guilford, J.P., & Guilford, J.S. (1980). *Christensen-Guilford Fluency Tests. Manual of Instructions and Interpretations.* Palo Alto, CA: Mind Garden.

Halperin, J.M., Healy, J.M., Zeitchik, E., Ludman, W.L., & Weinstein, L. (1989). Developmental aspects of linguistic and mnestic abilities in normal children. *Journal of Clinical and Experimental Neuropsychology, 11,* 518–528.

Hanley, J.R., Dewick, H.C., Davies, A.D., & Playfer, J. (1990). Verbal fluency in Parkinson's disease. *Neuropsychologia, 28,* 737–741.

Heaton, R.K., Grant, I., & Matthews, C.G. (1991). *Comprehensive Norms for an Expanded Halstead-Reitan Battery: Demographic Corrections, Research Findings, and Clinical Applications.* Odessa, FL: Psychological Assessment Resources.

Heller, R.B., & Dobbs, A.R. (1993). Age differences in word finding in discourse and non-discourse situations. *Psychology and Aging, 8,* 443–450.

Hewett, L.J., Nixon, S.J., Glenn, S.W., & Parsons, O.A. (1991). Verbal fluency deficits in female alcoholics. *Journal of Clinical Psychology, 47,* 716–720.

Holler, K.A., Fennell, E.B., Crosson, B., Boggs, S.R., & Mickle, J.P. (1995). Neuropsychological and adaptive functioning in younger versus older children shunted for early hydrocephalus. *Child Neuropsychology, 1,* 63–73.

Hopkins, R.O., Kesner, R.P., & Goldstein, M. (1995). Memory for novel and familiar spatial and linguistic temporal distance information in hypoxic subjects. *Journal of the International Neuropsychological Society, 1,* 454–468.

Ivnik, R.J., Malec, J.F., & Smith, G.E. (1996). Neuropsychological test norm above age 55: COWAT, MAE Token, WRAT-R Reading, AMNART, Stroop, TMT and JLO. *The Clinical Neuropsychologist, 10,* 262–278.

Joanette, I., & Goulet, P. (1986). Criterion-specific reduction of verbal fluency in right brain-damaged right-handers. *Neuropsychologia, 24,* 875–879.

Johnson, M.T., Zalewski, C., & Abourdarham, J.F. (1995). The relationship between race and ethnicity and word fluency. Paper presented at the meeting of the American Psychological Association, New York.

Kolb, B., & Whishaw, I.Q. (1985). *Fundamentals of Human Neuropsychology* (2nd ed.). New York: W.H. Freeman.

Kozora, E., & Cullum, C.M. (1995). Generative naming in normal aging: Total output and qualitative change using phonemic and semantic constraints. *The Clinical Neuropsychologist, 9,* 313–320.

Kronfol, Z., Hamsher, K., Digre, K., & Waziri, R. (1978). Depression and hemispheric function change associated with unilateral ECT. *British Journal of Psychiatry, 132,* 560–567.

Kunik, M.E., Champagne, L., Harper, R.G., & Chacko, R.C. (1994). Cognitive functioning in elderly depressed patients with and without psychosis. *International Journal of Geriatric Psychiatry, 9,* 871–874.

Lacy, M.A., Gore, P.A., Pliskin, N.H., & Henry, G.K. (1996). Verbal fluency task equivalence. *The Clinical Neuropsychologist, 10,* 305–308.

Lacy, M.A., Ferman, T.J., Hamer, D.P., & Pliskin, N.H. (1994). Letter and category fluency across various clinical populations. Paper presented at the meeting of the International Neuropsychological Society, Cincinnati, OH.

Lafleche, G., & Albert, M.S. (1995). Executive function deficits in mild Alzheimer's disease. *Neuropsychology, 9,* 313–320.

Lezak, M.D. (1995). *Neuropsychological Assessment* (3rd ed.), New York: Oxford University Press.

Loewenstein, D.A., Rubert, M.P., Berkowitz-Zimmer, N., Guterman, A., Morgan, R., & Hayden, S. (1992). Neuropsychological test performance and prediction of functional capacities in dementia. *Behavior, Health, and Aging, 2,* 149–158.

Loring, D.W., Meador, K.J., & Lee, G.P. (1994). Effects of temporal lobectomy on generative fluency and other language functions. *Archives of Clinical Neuropsychology, 9,* 229–238.

Mann, V.A., Sasanuma, S., Sakuma, N., & Masaki, S. (1990). Sex differences in cognitive abilities: A cross-cultural perspective. *Neuropsychologia, 28,* 1063–1077.

Margolin, D.I., Pate, D.S., Friedrich, F.J. & Elia, E. (1990). Dysnomia in dementia and in stroke patients: Different underlying cognitive deficits. *Journal of Clinical and Experimental Neuropsychology, 12,* 597–612.

Marshall, J.C. (1986). The description and interpretation of aphasic language disorder. *Neuropsychologia, 24,* 5–24.

Masur, D.M., Sliwinski, M. Lipton, R.B., & Blau, A.D. (1994). Neuropsychological prediction of dementia and the absence of dementia in healthy elderly persons. *Neurology, 44,* 1427–1432.

Miceli, G., Caltagirone, C., Gainotti, G., Masullo, C., & Silveri, M.C. (1981). Neuropsychological correlates of localized cerebral lesions in non-aphasic brain-damaged patients. *Journal of Clinical Neuropsychology, 3,* 53–63.

Mickanin, J., Grossman, M., Onishi, K., Auriacombe, S., & Clark, C. (1994). Verbal and nonverbal fluency in patients with probable

Alzheimer's disease. *Neuropsychology, 8,* 385–394.

Miller, E., & Hague, F., (1975). Some characteristics of verbal behaviour in presenile dementia. *Psychological Medicine, 5,* 255–259.

Minshew, N.J., Goldstein, G., & Siegel, D.J. (1995). Speech and language in high-functioning autistic individuals. *Neuropsychology, 9,* 255–261.

Mittenberg, W., Seidenberg, M., O'Leary, D.S., & DiGiulio, D.V. (1989). Changes in cerebral functioning associated with normal aging. *Journal of Clinical and Experimental Neuropsychology, 11,* 918–932.

Monsch, A.U., Bondi, M.W., Butters, N., & Salmon, D.P. (1992). Comparison of verbal fluency tasks in the detection of dementia of the Alzheimer type. *Archives of Neurology, 49,* 1253–1258.

Monsch, A.U., Bondi, M.W., Butters, N., Paulsen, J.S., Salmon, D.P., Brugger, P., & Swenson, M.R. (1994a). A comparison of category and letter fluency in Alzheimer's disease and Huntington's disease. *Neuropsychologia, 8,* 25–30.

Monsch, A.U., Bondi, M.W., Paulsen, J.S., Butters, N., Brugger, P., Salmon, D.P., Heaton, R.K., Grant, I., Wallace, M.R., & Swenson, M.R. (1994b). Verbal fluency performance of HIV+ men: A comparison to patients with Alzheimer's and Huntington's diseases. Paper presented at the meeting of the International Neuropsychological Society, Cincinnati, OH.

Montgomery, K., & Costa, L. (1983). Neuropsychological test performance of a normal elderly sample. Paper presented at the Meeting of the International Neuropsychological Society, Mexico City.

Murdoch, B.E., Chenery, H.J., Wilks, V., & Boyle, R.S. (1987). Language disorders in dementia of the Alzheimer type. *Brain and Language, 31,* 122–137.

Mutchnick, M.G., Ross, L.K., & Long, C.J. (1991). Decision strategies for cerebral dysfunction IV: Determination of cerebral dysfunction. *Archives of Clinical Neuropsychology, 6,* 259–270.

Newcombe, F. (1969). *Missile wounds of the brain.* London: Oxford University Press.

Northam, E., Anderson, P., Werther, G., Adler, R., & Andrewes, D. (1995). Neuropsychological complications of insulin dependent diabetes in children. *Child Neuropsychology, 1,* 74–87.

Ober, B.A., Dronkers, N.F., Koss, E., Delis, D.C., & Friedland, R.P. (1986). Retrieval from semantic memory in Alzheimer-type dementia. *Journal of Clinical and Experimental Neuropsychology, 8,* 75–92.

Pachana, N.A., Boone, K.B., Miller, B.L., et al. (1996). Comparison of neuropsychological functioning in Alzheimer's disease and frontotemporal dementia. *Journal of the International Neuropsychological Society, 2,* 505–510.

Parkin, A.J., & Walter, B.M. (1991). Aging, short-term memory, and frontal dysfunction. *Psychobiology, 19,* 175–179.

Parkin, A., Walter, B., & Hunkin, N. (1995). Relationship between normal aging, frontal lobe function, and memory for temporal and spatial information. *Neuropsychology, 9,* 304–312.

Parks, R.W., Loewenstein, D.A., Dodrill, K.L., Barker, W.W., Yoshii, F., Chang, J.Y., Emran, A., Apicella, A., Sheramata, W.A., & Duara, R. (1988). Cerebral metabolic effects of a verbal fluency test: A PET scan study. *Journal of Clinical and Experimental Neuropsychology, 10,* 565–575.

Peck, E.A., Mitchell, S.A., Burke, E.A., & Schwartz, S.M. (1992). Post head injury normative data for selected Benton neuropsychological tests. Paper presented at the meeting of the American Psychological Association, Washington, DC.

Perret, E. (1974). The left frontal lobe of man and the suppression of habitual responses in verbal categorical behavior. *Neuropsychologia, 12,* 323–330.

Petrick, J.D., Kunkle, J., & Franzen, M.D. (1992). Confrontation and productive naming in depression and dementia. *Clinical Neuropsychologist, 6,* 323.

Ponton, M.O., Satz, P., Herrera, L. et al. (1996). Normative data stratified by age and education for the Neuropsychological Screening Battery for Hispanics (NeSBHIS). *Journal of the International Neuropsychological Society, 3,* 53–63.

Pozzilli, C., Batianello, S., Padovani, A., & Passifiume, D. (1991). Anterior corpus callosum atrophy and verbal fluency in multiple sclerosis. *Cortex, 27,* 441–445.

Ramier, A.-M., & Hecaen, H. (1970). Role respectif des attaintes frontales et la lateralisation lésionelle dans les deficits de la "fluence verbale." *Revue Neurologique,* Paris, *123,* 17–22.

Raskin, S.A., & Rearick, E. (1996). Verbal fluency in individuals with mild traumatic head injury. *Neuropsychology, 10,* 416–422.

Read, D.E. (1987). Neuropsychological assessment of memory in early dementia: Normative data for a new battery of memory tests. Unpublished manuscript. University of Victoria.

Regard, M. (1981). Cognitive rigidity and flexibility, a neuropsychological study. Ph.D. dissertation. University of Victoria.

Rich, J.B. (1993). Pictorial and verbal implicit and recognition memory in aging and Alzheimer's disease: A transfer-appropriate processing account. Ph.D. dissertation. University of Victoria.

Rosen, W.G. (1980). Verbal fluency in aging and dementia. *Journal of Clinical Neuropsychology, 2,* 135–146.

Ruff, R.M., Allen, C.C., Farrow, C.E., Niemann, H., & Wylie, T. (1994). Figural fluency: Differential impairment in patients with left versus right frontal lobe lesions. *Archives of Clinical Neuropsychology, 9,* 41–55.

Ruff, R.M., Light, R.H., & Parker, S.B. (1996). Benton controlled word association test: Reliability and updated norms. *Archives of Clinical Neuropsychology, 11,* 329–338.

Salmon, D.P., Jin, H., Zhang, M., Grant, I., & Yu, E. (1995). Neuropsychological assessment of Chinese elderly in the Shanghai Dementia Survey. *Clinical Neuropsychologist, 9,* 159–168.

Sandler, A.D., Hooper, S.R., Watson, T.E., & Coleman, W.L. (1993). Talkative children: Verbal fluency as a marker for problematic peer relationships in clinical-referred children with attention deficit. *Perceptual and Motor Skills, 76,* 943–951.

Sarno, M.T. (1986). Verbal impairment in head injury. *Archives of Physical and Medical Rehabilitation, 67,* 400–405.

Sarno, M.T., Buonaguro, A., & Levita, E. (1985). Gender and recovery from aphasia after stroke. *Journal of Nervous and Mental Disease, 173,* 605–609.

Sawrie, S.M., Chelune, G.J., Naugle, R.I., & Luders, H.O. (1996). Empirical methods for assessing meaningful change following epilepsy surgery. *Journal of the International Neuropsychological Society, 2,* 556–564.

Schaie, K.W., & Parham, I.A. (1977). Cohort-sequential analyses of adult intellectual development. *Developmental Psychology, 13,* 649–653.

Schutz, L.E., & Schutz, J.A. (1996). Neuropsychological correlates of driving recovery after postacute rehabilitation. *Archives of Clinical Neuropsychology, 11,* 446 (abstract).

Schweizer, K. (1993). Verbal ability and speed of information-processing. *Personality and Individual Differences, 15,* 645–652.

Shoqueirat, M.A., Mayes, A., MacDonald, C., &

Meudell, P. (1990). Performance on tests sensitive to frontal lobe lesions by patients with organic amnesia: Leng & Parkin revisited. *British Journal of Clinical Psychology, 29,* 401–408.

Small, B.J., Herlitz, A., Fratiglioni, L., Almkvist, O., & Bäckman, L. (1997). Cognitive predictors of incident Alzheimer's disease: A prospective longitudinal study. *Neuropsychology, 11,* 413–420.

Snow, W.G., Tierney, M.C., Zorzitto, M.L., Fisher, R.H., & Reid, D.W. (1988). One-year test–retest reliability of selected tests in older adults. Paper presented at the meeting of the International Neuropsychological Society, New Orleans.

Spellacy, F.J., & Brown, W.G. (1984). Prediction of recidivism in young offenders after brief institutionalization. *Journal of Clinical Psychology, 40,* 1070–1074.

Spreen, O., & Benton, A.L. (1969, 1977), *Neurosensory Center Comprehensive Examination for Aphasia* (NCCEA). Victoria: University of Victoria Neuropsychology Laboratory.

Steenhuis, R.E., & Ostbye, T. (1995). Neuropsychological test performance of specific groups in the Canadian Study of Health and Aging (CSHA). *Journal of Clinical and Experimental Neuropsychology, 17,* 773–785.

Stebbins, G.T., Singh, J., Weiner, J., Wilson, R.S., Goetz, C.G., & Gabrieli, J.D.E. (1995). Selective impairment of memory functioning in unmediated adults with Gilles de la Tourette's syndrome. *Neuropsychology, 9,* 329–337.

Taussig, I.M., Henderson, V.W., & Mack, W. (1988). Spanish translation of a neuropsychological battery: Performance of Spanish- and English-speaking Alzheimer's disease patients and normal comparison subjects. *Clinical Gerontologist, 2,* 95–108.

Taylor, G.H.G., & Schatschneider, C. (1992). Child neuropsychological assessment: A test of basic assumptions. *The Clinical Neuropsychologist, 6,* 259–275.

Tombaugh, T.N., Kozak, J., & Rees, L. (1996). Normative data for the controlled oral word association test. Personal communication.

Tomer, R., & Levin, B.E. (1993). Differential effects of aging on two verbal fluency tasks. *Perceptual and Motor Skills, 76,* 465–466.

Troyer, A.K., Moscovitch, M., & Wincour, G. (1997). Clustering and switching as two components of verbal fluency: Evidence from younger and older healthy adults. *Neuropsychology, 11,* 138–146.

Tuokko, H., & Woodward, T.S. (1996). Development and validation of the demographic correction system for neuropsychological measures used in the Canadian Study of Health and Aging. *Journal of Clinical and Experimental Neuropsychology, 18,* 479–616.

Uddo, M., Vasterling, J.J., Brailey, K., & Sutker, P. (1993). Memory and attention in combat-related post-traumatic stress disorder (PTSD). *Journal of Psychopathology and Behavioral Assessment, 15,* 43–52.

Varley, R. (1995). Lexic-semantic deficits following right hemisphere damage. *European Journal of Communication Disorders, 30,* 362–371.

Vilkki, J., & Laittinen, L.V. (1976). Effects of pulvinotomy and ventrolateral thalamotomy on some cognitive functions. *Neuropsychologia, 14,* 67–78.

Warkentin, S., Risberg, J., Nilsson, A., Karlson, S., & Graae, E. (1991). Cortical activity during speech production: A study of regional cerebral blood flow in normal subjects performing a word fluency task. *Neuropsychiatry, Neuropsychology, and Behavioral Neurology, 4,* 305–316.

Welsh, M.C., Groisser, D., & Pennington, B.F. (1988). A normative-developmental study of measures hypothesized to tap prefrontal functioning. *Journal of Clinical and Experimental Neuropsychology, 10,* 79.

Yeudall, L.T., Fromm, D., Reddon, J.R., & Stefanyk, W.O. (1986). Normative data stratified by age and sex for 12 neuropsychological tests. *Journal of Clinical Psychology, 42,* 918–946.

MULTILINGUAL APHASIA EXAMINATION (MAE)

Purpose

The MAE provides a relatively brief but detailed examination of the presence, severity, and qualitative aspects of aphasic language disorders for patients between 6 and 69 years of age.

Source

The MAE is available from the Psychological Corporation, 555 Academic Court, San Antonio, TX, 78204-2498, and from Psychological Assessment Resources, P.O. Box 998, Odessa, FL 33556, at a price of $188 US for the complete set, including manual, Visual Naming stimulus booklet, Reading Comprehension stimulus booklet, Block Spelling test letters, Token Test tokens, and 100 record forms, as well as 100 each of record forms A, B, C, D, and E. A Spanish version (Examen de afasia multilingue-S) is available from the same sources for $188. US.

Description

The MAE has been revised (Benton, Hamsher, Rey, & Sivan, 1994) and includes nine subtests and two rating scales in five domains:

1. *Oral Expression:* visual naming, sentence repetition in two equivalent forms, controlled word association;

2. *Spelling:* oral spelling, written spelling, block spelling;

3. *Oral Verbal Understanding:* token test, aural comprehension of words and phrases;

4. *Reading:* reading comprehension of words and phrases;

5. *Rating Scales:* rating of articulation, and rating of praxic features of writing. The Spanish form (Rey & Benton, 1991) contains the same subtests, but items and wordings were rephrased appropriately for subjects of Cuban, Mexican, and Puerto Rican origin. For example, Controlled Oral Word Association uses the letters P, T, and M, reflecting similar levels of difficulty in Spanish.

Administration

See source. Visual Naming requires the naming of line drawings or parts thereof (e.g., telephone, telephone dial; 30 items). Sentence Repetition asks for the repetition of 14 sentences of increasing length up to 22 syllables; vocabulary and syntax are deliberately simple, but interrogative, negative, and other forms are included. Controlled Word Association is identical to the one presented in this volume, but uses the letters C, F, and L (P, R, and W for Form 2). Oral, written, and Block Spelling uses three interchangeable lists of 11 words; for Oral Spelling the word is presented, then presented again in a sentence, and the patient must spell it orally; for Written Spelling, the word must be written; for Block Spelling, plastic letters are spread in front of the patient who then must use these letters to spell the word. The MAE token test is similar to the one presented in this volume, but uses only 22 commands in each of two forms, and a two-point scoring (2 for correct on first trial, 1 for correct on second trial). Aural Comprehension of Words and Phrases asks the patient to point to one of four choices of line drawings on six plates corresponding to the word or phrase (e.g., "dog under the table"). For written comprehension, another set of words or phrases is presented in written (capital block letters) form; the patient must point to the appropriate choice on the same six plates used in the previous test. No discontinuation rules are provided.

Articulation is rated immediately on completion of the other tests on a nine-point scale. Praxic features of writing are rated after completion of the written spelling test for imprecision, distortions, and legibility on a nine-point scale.

Approximate Time for Administration

Approximately 40 minutes or less are required. The Spanish manual suggests an administration time of 20 minutes in nonaphasic subjects.

Scoring

Scoring is fully described in the source and is relatively simple and straightforward. Of the nine tests, two (Sentence Repetition, Controlled Oral Word Association) require corrections for age and education level, six for education only; the MAE Token Test does not require corrections, according to the authors. The test comes with scoring sheets for each subtest and a summary sheet that provides space for percentiles compared to controls as well as to aphasics.

Comment

The test does not claim to follow a specific model of language function, although it covers the most common aspects of language function affected in aphasia. The inclusion of reading, writing, praxis of writing, and articulation in a language test covers important territory in the clinical examination of aphasic patients. A practical and distinctive feature is that alternate versions of Sentence Repetition, Controlled Oral Word Association, and the Token Test are available when repeat testing is required; Hermann and Wyler (1988) provided a research example of the utility of the MAE alternate forms in an examination of epileptic patients prior to and after temporal lobectomy.

No reliability data are presented. Comments on the clinical interpretation of each subtest can be found at the end of each section, but only some are discussed at the end of the manual. Thus we learn that Controlled Word Association is most impaired in patients with left frontal lobe lesions (no documentation given); that Visual Naming and Sentence Repetition showed a correlation of .39 in a patient group otherwise undefined; that Visual Naming and Controlled Word Association showed a correlation of .56 in 42 patients. The question whether Aural Comprehension adds significantly to the information provided by the Token Test is raised and argued, but not answered with documentation.

Validity rests primarily on the discrimination between 115 normal and 48 aphasic subjects with six of the MAE tests. Using the suggested cutoff scores, between 2.6 and 7.0 percent of normal subjects, and between 14.4 and 64.6 percent of aphasics were misclassified by individual subtests. Using failure on one subtest as a cutoff, 15 percent of controls and no aphasics were misclassified; with failure on two or more subtests, the misclassification rates were 3 and 4 percent, respectively (Jones & Benton, 1995). Patients with left temporal lobe epilepsy also showed significant impairment on the MAE (and on tests of verbal learning) compared to epileptics with right hemisphere impairment (Hermann & Wyler, 1988; Hermann et al., 1992). The MAE Token Test has been shown to be a sensitive indicator of acute confusional states (delirium) in nonaphasic medical patients (Lee & Hamsher, 1988). Levin et al. (1976, 1981) examined the linguistic performance of patients with closed-head injuries, reporting a high frequency of naming errors, defective associative word-finding, and impaired comprehension on the Token Test; these findings were correlated with severity of head injury. Goldstein et al. (1996) found a near-significant trend for Visual Naming to discriminate between normal controls, AD patients and patients with closed head injury (means = 26.1, 23.2, and 21.7, SDs = 2.7, 4.5, and 6.7 respectively), but naming of low-frequency and high frequency words was similar in all three groups.

Concurrent validity of the Visual Naming test with the Boston Naming Test in 100 consecutive neuropsychological referrals was .86; a regression analysis indicated that both naming tests showed significant relations (R2 = .53) to the WAIS-R verbal-comprehension factor, but only minimal relations to the perceptual-organization and distractibility factors (Axelrod et al., 1994).

The norms presented for MAE Controlled Word Association also correspond closely to those presented for the COWA (using different letters) in this volume. A factor analysis of 16 aphasia battery subtests (including subtests of the MAE, NCCEA and the Western Aphasia Battery) given to healthy Taiwanese volunteers (Hua et al., 1997) suggested a major factor of comprehension (including Token Test, Sentence Repetition, Digit Repetition, Visual Naming, Reading, and Aural Comprehension). A second factor was labelled effortful writing; a third factor involved mainly verbal expression and word production.

In a study of 26 children (Schum et al., 1989), 13 of 15 dyslexics performed defectively on the reading and spelling tests, six on Controlled Oral Word Association; one of four stutterers was defective on Visual Naming, and two on Controlled Word Association and MAE Token; six of seven children with expressive language disorder performed defectively on the MAE.

Normative Data

The MAE is a relatively short but comprehensive aphasia battery. It was standardized on a sample of 360 healthy Iowa adults, aged 16–69 years, stratified for age, education, and gender. As in other tests by Benton, MAE norms are presented by percentile rank with cutpoints for high average, average, borderline, defective, and very defective performance; means and standard deviations are presented for children only. Roberts and Hamsher (1984) found lower norm values of Visual Naming in an urban inner-city black population, and they found that separate educational adjustments should be made with minority subjects. Schum et al. (1989) published norms on all MAE subtests except articulation and writing-praxis ratings for 229 normal learning children, aged 6.3–12.3 years, drawn from three Iowa elementary schools. Borderline adult norms were reached at age 12.3, although values for the Token Test and Controlled Oral Word Association approached plateau values starting at age 10. These norms are included in the manual.

The manual discusses studies of norms for elderly subjects and concludes that up to age 79, no noteworthy decline in performance has been found (Benton, Eslinger, & Damasio, 1981), but that for subjects between 80 and 89 years of age subnormal performance, especially on the Sentence Repetition and Token tests, are "not rare." These studies were conducted with well-educated adults; the authors speculate that subjects with less education may show a steeper decline with age.

The Spanish version was constructed for North American (not Spanish) speakers of Spanish or Central American origin and was standardized on 234 subjects between 18 and 70 years of age, with education levels ranging from below grade 4 to 16+.

References

Axelrod, B.N., Ricker, J.H., & Cherry, S.A. (1994). Concurrent validity of the MAE Visual Naming Test. *Archives of Clinical Neuropsychology, 9,* 317–321.

Benton, A.L., Eslinger, P.J., & Damasio, A.R. (1981). Normative observations in neuropsychological test performances in old age. *Journal of Clinical Neuropsychology, 3,* 33–42.

Benton, A.L., Hamsher, K. de S., Rey, G.J., & Sivan, A.B. (1994). *Multilingual Aphasia Examination* (3rd ed.). Iowa City, IA: AJA Associates.

Goldstein, F.C., Levin, H.S., Roberts, V.J. et al. (1996). Neuropsychological effects of closed head injury in older adults: A comparison with Alzheimer's disease. *Neuropsychology, 10,* 147–154.

Hermann, B.P., Seidenberg, M., Haltiner, A., & Wyler, A.R. (1992). Adequacy of language function and verbal memory performance in unilateral temporal lobe epilepsy. *Cortex, 28,* 423–433.

Hermann, B.P., & Wyler, A.R. (1988). Effects of anterior temporal lobectomy on language function. *Annals of Neurology, 23,* 585–588.

Hua, M.S., Chang, S.H., & Chen, S.T. (1997). Factor structure and age effects with an aphasia test battery in normal Taiwanese adults. *Neuropsychology, 11,* 156–162.

Jones, R.D., & Benton, A.L. (1995). Use of the Multilingual Aphasia Examination in the detection of language disorders. *Journal of the International Neuropsychological Society, 1,* 364 (abstract).

Lee, G.P., & Hamsher, K. (1988). Neuropsycho-

logical findings in toxicometabolic confusional states. *Journal of Clinical and Experimental Neuropsychology, 10,* 769–778.

Levin, H., Grossman, R.G., & Kelly, P.J. (1976). Aphasic disorders in patients with closed-head injury. *Journal of Neurology, Neurosurgery, and Psychiatry, 39,* 1062–1070.

Levin, H., Grossman, R.G., Sarwar, M., & Meyers, C.A. (1981). Linguistic recovery after closed head injury. *Brain and Language, 12,* 360–374.

Rey, G.J., & Benton, A.L. (1991). *Examen de Afasia Multilingue.* Iowa City, IA: AJA Associates.

Roberts, R.J., & Hamsher, K. (1984). Effects of minority status on facial recognition and naming performance. *Journal of Clinical Psychology, 40,* 539–545.

Schum, R.L., Sivan, A.B., & Benton, A.L. (1989). Multilingual Aphasia Examination: Norms for children. *The Clinical Neuropsychologist, 3,* 375–383.

PEABODY PICTURE VOCABULARY TEST—REVISED (PPVT-R)

Purpose

The purpose of this test is to assess auditory comprehension of picture names.

Source

The complete test (including both forms) can be ordered from American Guidance Service, Publisher's Blvd., Circle Pines, MN 55014, at a cost of $98 US, or from Psycan, P.O. Box 290, Station U, Toronto, Ontario H6R 3A5, at a cost of $160 Cdn. The new edition ("PPVT-III", Dunn and Dunn, 1997) has two forms and cost $219.95 US, or $400 Cdn. for the complete set.

Description

This popular test (Dunn & Dunn, 1981), also part of the Florida Kindergarten Screening Battery (Satz & Fletcher, 1982), is a revision of the original 1965 edition. It was initially constructed as a test of hearing vocabulary in children but has since been standardized for adults and has been used with a variety of clinical populations. The test requires the subject to choose one of four items displayed on a card as depicting the word spoken by the exam-

iner. After five training items, 175 items of increasing difficulty can be given, but usually only 35–45 items need to be administered if a suitable entry point (six consecutive correct) is chosen; the test is discontinued after consecutive failures on six out of eight items. Two equivalent alternate forms (L and M) are available. Also, a Spanish version is available.

The new PPVT-III was not yet available for review, but includes 204 items and improved illustrations to provide gender and ethnic balance. It has been re-standardized for the age range from 2 years, 6 months to 90+ years of age.

Administration

See source. The test booklets fold out into an easel. The examiner explains to the subject that one of the four picture corresponds to a word which the examiner will say and that the subject should point to the appropriate picture. The examiner should be able to pronounce all words correctly according to the dictionary. If hearing is a problem, the word can be shown on a printed card. Responses can be gestural, making the test appropriate for severely impaired patients. Entry points can be chosen by a preliminary estimate of the subject's age-equivalent level and by consulting the appropriate table in the manual.

Approximate Time for Administration

The time required is 10–20 minutes.

Scoring

The score on this test is simply the number of items passed, including the items prior to the entry point. The manual allows translation of these scores into "age equivalent" (previously called "mental age"), "standard score equivalent" (previously called "IQ"), stanines, and percentiles. The new terms are intended to discourage the use of the test as a measure of "verbal intelligence" (as claimed in the 1965 edition). The authors have added a "true confidence band," indicating the range of scores in which the subject's true score can fall 68 times out of 100.

Comment

Split-half reliability has been reported (see source) as ranging from .61 to .88 in children and adolescents, and as .82 for Form L in adults. The reliability of alternate forms ranged from .73 to .91 (source, Stoner, 1981; Tillinghast et al., 1983). Retest reliability with the alternate form after a minimum of 9 days showed a median coefficient of .78. In children, retest stability over 11 months has been reported as .84 for the revised PPVT (Bracken & Murray, 1984), as .81 in retarded children over a period of 7 months (Naglieri & Pfeiffer, 1983), and as .71 in a mixed clinical neuropsychiatric population after 2 years 6 months (Brown et al., 1989). Internal consistency (coefficient alpha) ranged from .96 to .98 in children 6–11 years old (Kamphaus & Lozano, 1984).

A number of items have been revised or added to correspond well to the negatively accelerating growth curve of vocabulary with age. Construct validity of the test as a measure of scholastic aptitude is good (Hinton & Knights, 1971). Bracken and Murray (1984) report a predictive validity of .30 with spell-

ing, .54 with reading recognition, .58 with reading comprehension, and .59 with the total Peabody Individual Achievement Test (PIAT) for the revised PPVT; similar values were reported for the first edition (Naglieri, 1981) and for mentally handicapped children with the revised edition (Naglieri & Pfeiffer, 1983). Concurrent validity with similar tests—the Bracken Basic Concept Scale, the preschool version of the Boehm Test of Basic Concepts, and its revised version—were .68, .65, and .62, respectively (Zucker & Riordan, 1988); predictive validities of the PPVT with the K-ABC and the Metropolitan Readiness Test after one year were .55 and .51, respectively (Zucker & Riordan, 1990). Since vocabulary is the single most important subtest of most intelligence tests, the test also correlates with the WISC-R, although the results of several studies are somewhat contradictory. Correlations with measures of verbal (.87), performance (.80), and full scale IQ (.88) have been reported (Crofoot & Bennett, 1980). Similar results were obtained by Altepeter (1989), who stresses that this indicates that the test is a good screening instrument for general intellectual function, but not an index of psycholinguistic functioning. Altepeter and Johnson (1989) found only modest correlations in healthy adults with the WAIS-R (.47 with Full-Scale IQ) and warn that in this age range the test tends to overestimate IQ in the lower ability ranges and to underestimate IQ in the higher ability ranges; in a cross-tabulation of IQs in 10-point steps, less than half of the clients were classified correctly; Price et al. (1990) reported similar discrepancies in adult psychiatric inpatients. The PPVT also correlates highly with the McCarthy Scales in children (Naglieri, 1981), with the 1986 Stanford-Binet Intelligence Scale (Carvajal et al., 1987), and with the achievement scale of the Kaufman Assessment Battery for Children in a learning-disabled population (.78, D'Amato et al., 1987). However, Faust and Hollingsworth (1991) found only a correlation of .34 with the WPPSI-R Full-Scale IQ, and of .30 and .31 with the PIQ and VIQ, respectively, in normal preschoolers; and Williams, Marks, and Bialer (1977) warn that the PPVT is not an adequate measure of hearing vocabulary in mentally handicapped subjects because it is also closely related to visual decoding ability as measured with the Illinois Test of Psycholinguistic Ability (ITPA), and that the use of the PPVT as a measure of intelligence in mentally handicapped persons may be misleading.

Hollinger and Sarvis (1984) also stress the role of perceptual-organizational ability in PPVT performance of school-age children, and Taylor (1975) reached the same conclusion for preschool children based on a factor analysis of the WPPSI and the ITPA as well as the PPVT. In a factor analysis of PIAT, WISC-R, and PPVT results with a sample of child psychiatry patients, however, the PPVT loaded mainly on the first factor (verbal comprehension), and only minimally on factors of verbal achievement, perceptual organization, and arithmetic (Culbert et al., 1989; also Zagar, 1983). Children with impaired oral language production (Rizzo & Stephens, 1981) and nonpsychotic, emotionally disturbed adolescents (Dean, 1980) tend to produce variable results. Elliott et al. (1990) found also that the PPVT results in children between 6 and 11 years of age with normal pure-tone hearing were strongly influenced by the ability to make fine-grained auditory discriminations with consonant-vowel stimuli varying in timing and place of articulation.

Connolly, Byrne, and Dywan (in press) used an experimental version of the PPVT in which the pictures were presented on a computer screen, and either a correct or an incorrect word was produced electronically. The subject had to press one of two keys, indicating whether the word was correct or incorrect. The study showed that response latency (time until the appropriate key was pressed) was longer for correct than incorrect words, and that the P-400 evoked response potential (ERP) was higher for correct than incorrect words. These differences were also found in children, age 9–11 years (Byrne, Dywan, & Connolly, 1995), but in both adults and children these differences did not occur for words that were not part of the subject's regular vocabulary. The authors conclude that both response latency and ERP are related to the amount of cognitive processing required, and

they suggest the technique as a measure suitable for subjects with motor/articulatory problems such as cerebral palsy.

The test showed significant differences between 28 young adults with specific language impairment and 28 controls (means 82.36 and 92.79, respectively) (Records et al., 1995). Das et al. (1995) demonstrated that the PPVT is sensitive to the mental decline (dementia) in older (age >50 years) Down syndrome patients, with results parallel to those in a dementia rating scale.

Quattrochi and Golden (1983) found only small correlations with the children's version of the Luria-Nebraska Battery (Receptive Speech Scale, Visual, Arithmetic, Memory, and Intellectual Processes scales). Thirty-six children with ADHD did not differ from 45 controls on the PPVT-R (Weyandt & Willis, 1994). Stone et al. (1989) reported beta weights and multiple correlation coefficients of both the oral and the written (printed on cards) format of the PPVT with the WISC-R and tests selected from the Halstead-Reitan Neuropsychological Battery (HRNB) for 934 learning-disabled children, ranging from .001 for location on the Tactual Performance Test to .377 for the Speech Sound Perception Test; 43 percent of the PPVT variance could be explained by the HRNB–WISC-R combination. Whether this demonstrates that "much of the information offered by the PPVT may be attributed to neuropsychological constructs" (p. 65) remains questionable.

The test is relatively nonthreatening and requires little verbal interaction; since it allows also for gestural or pointing responses, the test is suitable for language-impaired as well as autistic or withdrawn individuals. Considering the warnings mentioned above, the auditory and visual-perceptual integrity of the patient should be carefully considered in interpreting the results of this test.

Normative Data

The revised edition has been standardized on a sample of people considered representative of the 1970 U.S. census ranging in age from 2 years 6 months to 40 years. Normative data based on 4,200 subjects, including 828 adults, are available. Canadian norms are available from the distributor (Psycan). Kamphaus and Lozano (1984) note that in 6- to 11-year-old children with Spanish surnames (about half of whom spoke Spanish at home), standard scores were about 12–13 points below the national norms, although they showed regular, expected increases with age. Sattler (1988) recommends special care in the interpretation of scores of ethnic minority children because their scores tend to be lower, reflecting their verbal and experiential differences rather than their ability. No norms for elderly subjects are available (Lezak, 1987), but the PPVT-III contains norms for ages 2 years 6 months to 90 years, based on a sample of 2,725 subjects representative of the 1994 U.S. census.

References

Altepeter, T.S. (1989). The PPVT-R as a measure of psycholinguistic functioning: A caution. *Journal of Clinical Psychology, 45*, 935–941.

Altepeter, T.S., & Johnson, K.A. (1989). Use of the PPVT-R for intellectual screening with adults: A caution. *Journal of Psychoeducational Assessment, 7*, 39–45.

Bracken, B.A., & Murray, A.M. (1984). Stability and predictive validity of the PPVT-R over an eleven-month interval. *Educational and Psychological Research, 4*, 41–44.

Brown, S.J., Rourke, B.P., & Cicchetti, D.V. (1989). Reliability of tests and measures used in the neuropsychological assessment of children. *The Clinical Neuropsychologist, 3*, 353–368.

Byrne, J.M., Dywan, C.A., & Connolly, J.F. (1995). Assessment of children's receptive vocabulary using event-related potentials: Development of a clinically valid test. *Child Neuropsychology, 1*, 211–223.

Connolly, J.F., Byrne, J.M., & Dywan, C.A. (in press). Assessment of receptive vocabulary with event-related brain potentials: An investigation of cross-modal and cross-form priming. *Journal of Clinical and Experimental Neuropsychology.*

Carvajal, H., Gerber, J., & Smith, P.D. (1987). Relationship between scores of young adults on Stanford-Binet IV and Peabody Picture Vocabulary Test–Revised. *Perceptual and Motor Skills, 65*, 721–722.

Crofoot, M.J., & Bennett, T.S. (1980). A comparison of three screening tests and the WISC-R in special education evaluations. *Psychology in the Schools, 17*, 474–478.

Culbert, J.P., Hamer, R., & Klinge, V. (1989). Factor structure of the Wechsler Intelligence Scale for Children—Revised, Peabody Picture Vocabulary Test, and the Peabody Individual Achievement Test in a psychiatric sample. *Psychology in the Schools, 26*, 331–336.

D'Amato, R.C., Gray, J.W., & Dean, R.S. (1987) Concurrent validity of the PPVT-R with the K-ABC for learning problem children. *Psychology in the Schools, 24*, 35–39.

Das, J.P., Mishra, R.K., Davison, M., & Naglieri, J.A. (1995). Measurement of dementia in individuals with mental retardation: Comparison based on PPVT and Dementia Rating Scale. *Clinical Neuropsychologist, 9*, 32–37.

Dean, R.S. (1980). The use of the Peabody Picture Vocabulary Test with emotionally disturbed adolescents. *Journal of School Psychology, 18*, 172–175.

Dunn, L.M., & Dunn, E.S. (1981). *Peabody Picture Vocabulary Test—Revised.* Circle Pines, MN: American Guidance Service.

Dunn, L.M., & Dunn, E.S. (1997). *Peabody Picture Vocabulary Test—III.* Circle Pines, MN: American Guidance Service.

Elliott, L., Hammer, M.A., & Scholl, M.E. (1990). Fine-grained auditory discrimination and performance on tests of receptive vocabulary and receptive language. *Annals of Dyslexia, 40*, 170–179.

Faust, D.S., & Hollingsworth, J.O. (1991). Concurrent validation of the Wechsler Preschool and Primary Scale of Intelligence—Revised (WPPSI-R) with two criteria of cognitive abilities. *Journal of Psychoeducational Assessment, 9*, 224–229.

Hinton, G.G., & Knights, R.M. (1971). Children with learning problems. Academic history, academic prediction, and adjustment three years after assessment. *Exceptional Children, 37*, 513–519.

Hollinger, C.L., & Sarvis, P.A. (1984). Interpretation of the PPVT-R: A pure measure of verbal comprehension? *Psychology in the Schools, 21*, 34–41.

Kamphaus, R.W., & Lozano, R. (1984). Developing local norms for individually administered tests. *School Psychology Review, 13*, 491–498.

Lezak, M.D. (1987). Norms for growing older. *Developmental Neuropsychology, 3*, 1–12.

Naglieri, J.A. (1981). Concurrent validity of the revised Peabody Picture Vocabulary Test. *Psychology in the Schools, 18*, 286–289.

Naglieri, J.A., & Pfeiffer, S.I. (1983). Stability, concurrent and predictive validity of the PPVT-R. *Journal of Clinical Psychology, 39*, 965–967.

Price, D.R., Herbert, D.A., Walsh, M.L., & Law, J.G. (1990). Study of the WAIS-R, Quick Test and PPVT IQs for neuropsychiatric patients. *Perceptual and Motor Skills, 70*, 1320–1322.

Quattrochi, M.M., & Golden, C.J. (1983). Peabody Picture Vocabulary Test–Revised and Luria-Nebraska Neuropsychological Battery for Children: Intercorrelations for normal youngsters. *Perceptual and Motor Skills, 56*, 632–634.

Records, N.L., Tomblin, J.B., & Buckwalter, P.R. (1995). Auditory verbal learning in young adults with specific language impairment. *Clinical Neuropsychologist, 9*, 187–193.

Rizzo, J.M., & Stephens, M.I. (1981). Performance of children with normal and impaired oral language production on a set of auditory comprehension tests. *Journal of Speech and Hearing Disorders, 46*, 150–159.

Sattler, J.M. (1988). *Assessment of Children* (3rd ed.). San Diego: Jerome M. Sattler.

Satz, P., & Fletcher, J. (1982). *Manual for the Florida Kindergarten Screening Battery*. Odessa, FL: Psychological Assessment Resources.

Stone, B.J., Gray, J.W., Dean, R.S., & Strom, D.A. (1989). Neuropsychological constructs of the PPVT with learning-disabled children: Printed stimulus cards versus oral administration. *Developmental Neuropsychology, 5*, 61–67.

Stoner, S.B. (1981). Alternate form reliability of the revised Peabody Picture Vocabulary Test for Head Start children. *Psychological Reports, 49*, 628.

Taylor, L.J. (1975). The Peabody Picture Vocabulary Test: What does it measure? *Perceptual and Motor Skills, 41*, 777–778.

Tillinghast, B.S., Morrow, J.E., & Uhlig, G.E. (1983). Retest and alternate form reliability of the PPVT-R with fourth, fifth, and sixth grade pupils. *Journal of Educational Research, 76*, 243–244.

Weyandt, L.L., & Willis, W.G. (1994). Executive functions in school-aged children: Potential efficacy of tasks in discriminating clinical groups. *Developmental Neuropsychology, 10*, 27–38.

Williams, A.M., Marks, C.J., & Bialer, I. (1977). Validity of the Peabody Picture Vocabulary Test as a measure of hearing vocabulary in mentally retarded and normal children. *Journal of Speech and Hearing Research, 20*, 205–211.

Zagar, R. (1983). Analysis of short test batteries for children. *Journal of Clinical Psychology, 39*, 590–597.

Zucker, S., & Riordan, J. (1988). Concurrent validity of new and revised conceptual language measures. *Psychology in the Schools, 25*, 252–256.

Zucker, S., & Riordan, J. (1990). One-year predictive validity of new and revised conceptual language measurements. *Journal of Psychoeducational Assessment, 8*, 4–8.

TOKEN TEST

Purpose

The purpose of this test is assessment of verbal comprehension of commands of increasing complexity.

Source

The manual for the 39-item form, answer sheets, and plastic tokens can be ordered from the Psychology Clinic, University of Victoria, Victoria, BC V8W 3P5, at a cost of $70 US.

Description

The test as originally developed by De Renzi and Vignolo (1962) and by Boller and Vignolo (1966) had 62 commands. Our version uses 20 plastic tokens in five colors (red, white, yellow, blue, green), two sizes (small: approx. 2 cm in diameter; large: approx. 3 cm in diameter), and two shapes (circles and squares—squares replacing the rectangles in the original version) arranged in a fixed order in front of the patient. Thirty-nine commands of increasing length are listed on the answer sheet. An expanded linguistic version was presented by McNeil and Prescott (1978). Short versions have also been presented (De Renzi & Faglioni, 1978; Orgass, 1976; Spellacy & Spreen, 1969; van Harskamp & van Dongen, 1977). A 22-item version is described as part of the Multilingual Aphasia Examination (Benton et al., 1994). Wood et al. (1997) presented odd-item selections of the MAE Token Test as a screening test. A form of the Token test is also part of the CELF-3. The Spellacy and Spreen 16-item version and the De Renzi and Faglioni short form have been specifically rec-

---

Row 1
Large circles in order: red, blue, yellow, white, green

Row 2
Large squares in order: blue, red, white, green, yellow

Row 3
Small circles in order: white, blue, yellow, red, green

Row 4
Small squares in order: yellow, green, red, blue, white

Figure 11—2. Token Test arrangement of tokens in front of subject.

ommended for the screening of receptive language in children (Cole & Fewell, 1983; Lass et al., 1975). A 21-item children's version (age range 5 years to 11 years 11 months; DiSimoni, 1978), a visual presentation mode (Kiernan, 1986; Poeck & Hartje, 1979), and a concrete object form (Martino et al., 1976) have also been described. Our version of the Token Test is also part of the Neurosensory Center Comprehensive Examination for Aphasia (Test 11) (Spreen & Benton, 1969, 1977) and can be used with children as well as adults.

Administration

Present tokens in the order shown in Figure 11–2, and ask the first question *"Show me a circle."* Pronounce clearly and slowly, but avoid deliberate stretching of speech. Instructions for parts A and B may be repeated once. No other instructions may be repeated. If the patient makes no response, he or she should be encouraged to give at least a partial response. For example, if the patient says that he or she does not remember or asks for repetition of instructions, say: *"Do it as I said. Do as much as you remember."* Discontinue after three consecutive failures (i.e., on sections A, B, and C, if no part of the questions received credit; on section D, if only one part; and on sections E and F if only two parts received credit).

The first section (questions 1 through 7) also provides a gross check on color blindness, which might affect performance on this test. If difficulties in color recognition are noticed, further examination with the Ishihara plates

or a similar test of color blindness is necessary. If gross color blindness is established both on this test and by a color-vision test, the test should be omitted.

Scoring

The questions are listed on the Score Sheet (Figure 11–3). Give one point for each part of a question correctly performed. For example, the correct performance of questions 1 to 7 receives 1 point each, the correct performance of questions 12 through 15 (*"small, white circle"*) receives three points each. For questions 24 to 39, the verb and the preposition as well as the correct token receive credit (e.g., *"Put the red circle on the green square"* = 6 points). Occasionally a preposition may be interpreted in several ways; for example, item 25 (i.e., "behind" may be viewed as away from the patient or as to the right of the yellow circle). In these instances, any reasonable interpretation of the preposition is accepted and scored as correct. Similarly, if the subject puts the green circle behind the red square, she or he receives 5 points, since the performance shows that the five parts of the command (i.e., put, red, green, circle, square) were comprehended, but the relationship (on) was not. If the test is discontinued, prorate the remaining items of that section on the basis of the subject's performance on the administered items. For example, if the test is discontinued after item 26 (three items of part F), and items 24 to 26 received 2 points, the remaining 13 items would also receive 2 points, for a total of 32 points for part F. If all or most items of sections B, C, D, E, and/or F have not been given because of previous failures, add a score of 3 for part B, 5 points for part C, 6 points for Part D, 9 points for Part E, and 18 Points for part F. No correction for age and educational level is necessary (but see notes on age effects below). Maximum score = 163.

Comment

This popular test was listed by 31 percent of speech therapists as one of their "frequently used tests" (Beele et al., 1984). Boller and Dennis (1979) reviewed the extensive literature of

Name _____ Date _____ Age _____ Examiner _____

Score Sheet 7–20
IDENTIFICATION BY SENTENCE (TOKEN TEST)

A. Present tokens as in Table 7–12. Instructions may be repeated once	
1. Show me a circle	
2. Show me a square	
3. Show me a yellow one	
4. Show me a red one	
5. Show me a blue one	
6. Show me a green one	
7. Show me a white one	
TOTAL A(7)	

B. Present only large tokens. Instructions may be repeated once	
8. Show me the **yellow square**	
9. Show me the **blue circle**	
10. Show me the **green circle**	
11. Show me the **white square**	
TOTAL B(8)	

C. Present all tokens as in Table 7–12. Do not repeat instructions	
12. Show me the **small white circle**	
13. Show me the **large yellow square**	
14. Show me the **large green sqaure**	
15. Show me the **small blue square**	
TOTAL C(12)	

D. Present large tokens only. Do not repeat instructions	
16. Take the **red circle** and the **green square**	
17. Take the **yellow square** and the **blue square**	
18. Take the **white square** and the **green circle**	
19. Take the **white circle** and the **red circle**	
TOTAL D(16)	

E. Present all tokens as in Table 7–12. Do not repeat instructions	
20. Take the **large white circle** and the **small green square**	
21. Take the **small blue circle** and the **large yellow square**	
22. Take the **large green sqaure** and the **large red square**	
23. Take the **large white square** and the **small green circle**	
TOTAL E(24)	

F. Present large tokens only. Do not repeat instructions	
24. **Put** the **red circle on** the **green square**.	
25. **Put** the **white square behind** the **yellow circle**.	
26. **Touch** the **blue circle with** the **red square**.	
27. **Touch** the **blue circle and** the **red square**.	
28. **Pick up** the **blue circle OR** the **red square**.	
29. **Move** the **green square away from** the **yellow square**.	
30. **Put** the **white circle in front of** the **blue square**.	
31. **If** there is a **black circle, pick up** the **red square**.	
32. **Pick up all squares except** the **yellow one**.	
33. **Put** the **green square beside** the **red circle**.	
34. **Touch** the **squares slowly and** the **circles quickly**.	
35. **Put** the **red circle between** the **yellow square** and the **green square**.	
36. **Touch all circles, except** the **green one**.	
37. **Pick up** the **red circle—no—** the **white square**.	
38. **Instead of** the **white square, pick up** the **yellow circle**.	
39. **Together with** the **yellow circle, pick up** the **blue circle**.	
TOTAL F(96)	
TOTAL A-F (163)	

Figure 11—3. NCCEA Subtest 11 (Token Test) sample scoring sheet.

clinical and experimental studies. The current version of the Token Test uses a scoring system that credits almost *every word* of each item rather than assigning a score of 1 point for the *entire item*. The first four parts of the test were found to be homogenous in a test of a probabilistic test model, whereas the last part was different because of the greater syntactic/semantic variability that was introduced (Willmes, 1981).

For normal children above age 11 and for adults with average intelligence, ceiling scores can be expected. For this reason, one-year retest reliability in older adults has been reported as only .50 (Snow et al., 1988). Three-day retest reliability in 30 aphasics was between .92 and .94 (Gallagher, 1979). Orgass (1976) reported a retest reliability of .96.

The scoring is sensitive to even minor impairments of receptive language: Spellacy and Spreen (1969) reported a correct classification rate of 89 percent for unselected aphasics and of 72 percent for nonaphasic brain-damaged patients, using a cutoff score of 156. De Renzi and Faglioni (1978) and Cavalli et al. (1981) found virtually no difference between patients with right-hemisphere lesions and normal controls. Our own data do show a mild impairment of right-hemisphere nonaphasic patients. The difference between these two findings is probably due to our more sensitive scoring system. This contention is borne out by the findings of Swisher and Sarno (1969) that patients with right-hemisphere lesions without aphasia had significantly poorer scores than controls in parts E and F of the test, although left brain-damaged aphasics showed the highest number of errors. However, care should be taken to not deliberately stretch speech during the presentation of the test since this may lead to improvement of test performance in aphasics (Poeck & Pietron, 1981).

De Renzi and Faglioni (1978) reported correct classification rates of 93 percent for aphasics as compared to 95 percent for patients without damage to the central nervous system. Good discrimination between aphasic and nonaphasic adults was also reported by Cohen et al. (1976), Orgass (1976), Sarno (1986), and Woll et al. (1976). Sarno, Buonaguro, and

Levita (1985) found no sex differences on the Token Test for moderately and severely aphasic patients, either 4–6 months after stroke or in their course of recovery over a period of 2 years. Lang (1981) reported that the test was most sensitive to global and sensory aphasia, whereas the error percentage was lower in motor aphasia and relatively minor in amnestic aphasia. The test was also sensitive to changes in patients after ventrolateral thalamotomy, but not after pulvinotomy (Vilkki & Laitinen, 1976). An extended version of the test also discriminated well between 28 young adults with specific language impairment and 28 controls (Records et al., 1995).

Validation studies have pointed out that the Token Test measures other factors of cognitive performance in addition to the obvious one of oral language comprehension. McNeil (1983), for example, claimed that the variability of performance as well as nonverbal deficits shown by aphasics reflect general brain damage and "oscillating biological systems" and attention deficits rather than specific linguistic or focal neurological damage. Similarly, Riedel and Studdert-Kennedy (1985) maintained that impairment on the Token Test and similar perceptual tasks in aphasics reflects a general cognitive rather than a language-specific deficit. This was confirmed in a study of 100 patients with dementia of the Alzheimer type (AD) (Swihart et al., 1989), which found a high correlation between the Token Test and the MMSE ($r = .74$) and a correct classification rate of 83 percent between AD and control patients, which was as good as the discrimination achieved by the MMSE (82 percent). Rich (1993) also reported severe impairment in AD patients compared to elderly controls. Swihart et al. (1989) concluded that for this patient group, the Token Test measures not only auditory comprehension but also severity of cognitive impairment. The effect of short-term memory on the Token Test has been investigated in several studies, but the reported correlations with various short-term memory tests are small to moderate ($r = .14$ to $.60$; Wold & Reinvang, 1990).

The test is not only sensitive to language impairment in adults; Ewing-Cobbs et al. (1987) reported that about 25 percent of children and adolescents with closed head injury showed impaired scores on the Token Test. Mean centile scores (using age-appropriate norms) for 5- to 10-year-olds with mild injury were 47.5 and for moderate-to-severe injury 46.8; for 11- to 15-year-olds the respective scores were 58.9 and 51.9. Gutbrod and Michel (1986) found good discriminative validity for aphasic children and adolescents. Lenhard (1983) found that 100 6-year-old children who had hyperbilirubinemia as infants performed significantly more poorly than normal subjects on the Token Test, and that children who had received phototherapy in infancy did more poorly than those who had not. Harris et al. (1983) found that in 104 6- to 8-year-old children who were followed up for the effects of different ranges of birthweight and bilirubin, poor scores on birth variables were related to low scores on the Token Test as well as a smaller right-ear advantage on a dichotic consonant-vowel and a dichotic staggered spondaic word test. They interpreted these results as indicating a "lack of pronounced hemispheric dominance for language." Tallal, Stark, and Mellits (1985) found the Token Test as well as other auditory comprehension tests to be sensitive to developmental aphasia. The test also showed significant differences between 62 high-functioning autistic adolescents and matched controls (Minshew et al., 1995). Naeser et al. (1987) claimed that the Token Test performance of 3-year-old children

resembled that of severe Wernicke's aphasia, and that the performance of 6-year-olds was similar to that of aphasics with mild comprehension deficits and frontal-parietal perisylvian lesions (i.e., the notion of comprehension deficit in aphasia as a regression to earlier developmental stages). A similar regression hypothesis was proposed in a comparison of pre-middle-aged, young-old, and old-old adults (Emery, 1986).

A correlation of .63 between the Token Test and the Northwestern Syntax Screening Test in 5- to 8-year-old children has been interpreted as an indicator for the validity of the Token Test for receptive language (Cartwright & Lass, 1974). Similarly, Lass and Golden (1975) reported a correlation of .71 between the Token Test and the PPVT in normal children 5–12 years old.

Table 11—16. Percentile Ranks for the Token Test for Normal Adults ($n = 82$)

Score	Percentile ranks
162	70
161	50
158	30
157	18
156	14
154	10
153	6
151	—

Table 11—17. Token Test: Norms for School-Age Children

Age	Female			Male			Total		
	n	M	SD	n	M	SD	n	M	SD
6	30	147.0	15.9	22	142.7	10.9	52	145.2	14.1
7	24	153.5	8.9	27	152.9	7.9	51	153.1	8.3
8	23	158.2	4.6	25	158.8	4.1	48	158.5	4.3
9	30	157.1	5.3	23	157.7	3.7	53	157.4	4.6
10	25	160.6	1.8	25	158.3	4.5	50	159.4	3.6
11	22	160.4	2.5	22	159.9	3.5	44	160.1	3.0
12	13	160.2	2.2	13	160.4	3.0	26	160.3	2.6
13	12	161.0	1.0	17	160.3	2.2	29	160.6	1.8

Source: Gaddes & Crockett, 1975.

Table 11—18. Token Test Norms in Percentiles for Children Ages 6–13

Score	Centiles in children of age: 6	7	8	9	10	11	12	13	Centiles in adults
163	90	90	90	90	84	84	84	84	75+
162	88	86	86	86	75	75	75	75	70
161	86	84	81	78	65	61	61	57	50
160	84	78	78	72	57	50	47	39	40
159	84	75	68	65	47	35	32	19	35
158	81	72	65	53	35	25	19	8	30
157	78	68	61	47	25	16	10	2	18
156	78	61	57	39	19	8	4	0.9	14
155	75	57	53	28	12	4	2		12
154	72	53	43	22	7	2	1		10
153	72	50	35	16	4	1	0.7		6
152	68	47	28	10	2	0.8			
151	65	39	22	8	1	0.3			
150	61	35	16	4	0.9				
149	61	32	12	2	0.5				
148	57	28	7	1					
147	53	25	4	1					
146	53	19	3	0.8					
145	50	16	2	0.5					
144	47	14	1						
143	43	12	1						
142	43	10	0.7						
141	39	7							
140	35	5							
139	35	4							
138	32	4							
137	28	3							
136	25	2							
135	25	1							
134	22								
133	19								
132	19								
131	16								
130	14								
129	14								
128	12								
127	10								
126	8								
125	8								
124	7								
123	5								
122	5								
121	4								
120	4								
119	3								
118	3								
117	2								
116	2								
115	2								
114	1								

Source: Hamsher (personal communication, 1981) and Gaddes and Crockett (1975).

Elliott et al. (1990) found a relationship between Token Test performance and fine-grained auditory discrimination of rapidly presented consonant-vowel stimuli (e.g., pa–da–ba) in younger children (age 6–7 years, r = .64), but not in older children (age 9–11, r = .37); this may be related to the developmental stage of the child, or, as the authors point out, to the increasing influence of the written mode of language learning. A study by Whitehouse (1983) reported significant differences between dyslexic and normal reading adolescents (grades 7–12), but emphasized that 55 percent of the dyslexics did not make more errors than normal readers. She concluded that errors on Part E of the Token Test reflected impaired ability to process cognitive information. The Token Test also did not predict paragraph comprehension scores in adult aphasics (Brookshire & Nicholas, 1984), although comprehension of written commands of the Token Test is very similar to the oral version of the test in aphasic patients (Kiernan, 1986). The test has shown modest relationship to intelligence, especially with severe intellectual impairment: Coupar (1976) reported a correlation of .35 with the Raven Progressive Matrices. Correlation with the WISC-R Verbal and Performance IQs were reported as .42 and .47, respectively (Kitson, 1985). Fusilier and Lass (1984) reported that the Token Test showed significant correlations only with the grammatical closure and sound blending tasks of the 12 tasks of the ITPA, suggesting that the two tests measure relatively different aspects of language. Examining 113 postmeningitis children, Taylor and Schatschneider (1992) found that the test related significantly to sociobehavioral outcome measures, e.g., the Vineland Scales, as well as to other neuropsychological tests.

Factor–analytic validity in children was established by Niebergall et al. (1978) and Remschmidt et al. (1977), who found strong loadings on a verbal communication and language development factor as well as high correlations with age in children 6–14 years old. The authors interpreted the factor-analytic findings as indicating that the Token Test measures more complex language abilities in addition to comprehension.

Normative Data

Table 11–16 provides our normative data for 82 adult community volunteers. The mean score for adults (and adolescents 14 years and over) is 161. Scores below 157 are virtually absent in a normal adult population. Tuokko and Woodward (1996) reported that this cutoff also holds for elderly subjects between 60 and 85 years of age, and De Renzi and Faglioni (1978) reported a correlation with age of only −.03. Swisher and Sarno (1969), Rich (1993), and Ivnik, Malec, and Smith (1996) also found only minimal nonsignificant age effects; in the latter study scores dropped by about 2 points for old-old (78–97 years) subjects in a large sample of 399 subjects. However, Emery (1986) found a mean of 159.90 (SD = 6.7) for 20 healthy adults aged 30–42 years, and of 142.40 for 10 healthy adults aged 72–83 years; this mean dropped to 117.30 (SD = 21.2) for 10 old-old adults (age 84–93). De Renzi and Faglioni did recommend a correction for education [+ 2.36 − (.30) (years of schooling)] for an item-by-item scoring, but our experience has been that such a correction is not needed for subjects with a grade 8+ education.

Normative data for children, presented in Tables 11–17 and 11–18, are based on studies by Gaddes and Crockett (1975) and Hamsher (personal communication, 1981). The progression of scores is quite similar to that reported by DiSimoni (1978), Noll (1970), and Whitaker and Noll (1972). Remschmidt et al. (1977), using a pass-fail score system for each item, also found a leveling off of the error score after age 8.

Zaidel (1977) reported mean scores of 143.7 for children 5 years 5 months old, and of 125.4 for children 4 years 6 months old, suggesting a consistent downward extension of these norms in young children.

References

Beele, K.A., Davies, E., & Muller, D.J. (1984). Therapists' views on the clinical usefulness of four aphasia tests. *British Journal of Disorders of Communication*, 19, 169–178.

Benton, A.L., Hamsher, K. de S., & Sivan A.B. (1994). *Multilingual Aphasia Examination* (3rd ed.). Iowa City, IA: AJA Associates.

Boller, F., & Dennis, M. (1979). *Auditory Comprehension. Clinical and Experimental Studies with the Token Test.* New York: Academic Press.

Boller, F., & Vignolo, L. (1966). Latent sensory aphasia in hemisphere-damaged patients: An experimental study with the Token-Test. *Brain, 89,* 815–831.

Brookshire, R.H., & Nicholas, L.E. (1984). Comprehension of directly and indirectly stated main ideas and details in discourse by brain-damaged and non-brain-damaged patients. *Brain and Language, 21,* 21–36.

Cartwright, L.R., & Lass, N.J. (1974). A comparative study of children's performance on the Token Test, Northwestern Syntax Screening Test, and Peabody Picture Vocabulary Test. *Acta Symbolica, 5,* 19–29.

Cavalli, M., De Renzi, E., Faglioni, P., and Vitale, A. (1981). Impairment of right brain-damaged patients on a linguistic cognitive task. *Cortex, 17,* 545–556.

Cohen, R., Kelter, S., Engel, D., List, G., & Strohner, H. (1976). Zur Validität des Token-Tests. *Nervenarzt, 47,* 357–361.

Cole, K.N., & Fewell, R.R. (1983). A quick language screening test for young children. *Journal of Speech and Hearing Disorders, 48,* 149–153.

Coupar, M. (1976). Detection of mild aphasia: A study using the Token Test. *British Journal of Medical Psychology, 49,* 141–144.

De Renzi, E., & Faglioni, P. (1978). Development of a shortened version of the Token Test. *Cortex, 14,* 41–49.

De Renzi, E., & Vignolo, L. (1962). The Token Test: A sensitive test to detect receptive disturbances in aphasics. *Brain, 85,* 665–678.

DiSimoni, F. (1978). *The Token Test for Children.* Hingham, MA: Teaching Resources Corporation.

Elliott, L.L., Hammer, M.A., & Scholl, M.E. (1990). Fine-grained auditory discrimination and performance on tests of receptive vocabulary and receptive language. *Annals of Dyslexia, 40,* 170–179.

Emery, O.B. (1986). Linguistic decrement in normal aging. *Language and Communication, 6,* 47–64.

Ewing-Cobbs, L., Levin, H.S., Eisenberg, H.M., & Fletcher, J.M. (1987). Language functions following closed-head injury in children and adolescents. *Journal of Clinical and Experimental Neuropsychology, 9,* 575–592.

Fusilier, F.M., & Lass, N.J. (1984). A comparative study of children's performance on the Illinois Test of Psycholinguistic Abilities and the Token Test. *Journal of Auditory Research, 24,* 9–16.

Gaddes, W.H., & Crockett, D.J. (1975). The Spreen-Benton aphasia test; normative data as a measure of normal language development. *Brain and Language, 4,* 257–280.

Gallagher, A.J. (1979). Temporal reliability of aphasic performance on the Token Test. *Brain and Language, 7,* 34–41.

Gutbrod, K., & Michel, M. (1986). Zur klinischen Validität des Token Tests bei hirngeschädigten Kindern mit und ohne Aphasie. *Diagnostica, 32,* 118–128.

Harris, V.L., Keith, R.W., & Novak, K.K. (1983). Relationship between two dichotic listening tests and the Token test for children. *Ear and Hearing, 6,* 278–282.

Ivnik, R.J., Malec, J.F., & Smith, G.E. (1996). Neuropsychological test norms above age 55: COWAT, MAE Token, WRAT-R Reading, AMNART, Stroop, TMT and JLO. *The Clinical Neuropsychologist, 10,* 262–278.

Kiernan, J. (1986). Visual presentation of the Revised Token Test: Some normative data and use in modality independence testing. *Folia Phoniatrica, 37,* 216–222.

Kitson, D.L. (1985). Comparison of the Token Test of language development and the WISC-R. *Perceptual and Motor Skills, 61,* 532–534.

Lang, C. (1981). Token-Test und Drei-Figuren-Test; ein Vergleich zwischen zwei psychometrischen Kurztesten zur Sprachverständnisprüfung. *Diagnostica, 27,* 39–50.

Lass, N.J., DePaolo, A.M., Simcoe, J.C., & Samuel, S.M. (1975). A normative study of children's performance on the short form of the Token Test. *Journal of Communication Disorders, 8,* 193–198.

Lass, N.J., & Golden, S.S. (1975). A comparative study of children's performance on three tests for receptive language abilities. *Journal of Auditory Research, 15,* 177–182.

Lenhard, M.L. (1983). Effects of neonatal hyperbilirubinemia on Token Test performance of six-year-old children. *Journal of Auditory Research, 23,* 195–204.

Martino, A.A., Pizzamiglio, L., & Razzano, C. (1976). A new version of the Token Test for aphasics: A concrete objects form. *Journal of Communication Disorders, 9,* 1–5.

McNeil, M.M., & Prescott, T.E. (1978). *Revised Token Test.* Austin, TX: Pro-Ed.

McNeil, M.R. (1983). Aphasia: Neurological considerations. *Topics in Language Disorders, 3,* 1–19.

Minshew, N.J., Goldstein, G., & Siegel, D.J. (1995). Speech and language in high-functioning autistic individuals. *Neuropsychology, 9*, 255–261.

Naeser, M.A., Mazurski, P., Goodglass, H., & Peraino, M. (1987). Auditory syntactic comprehension in nine aphasic groups (with CT scan) and children: Differences in degree, but not order of difficulty observed. *Cortex, 23*, 359–380.

Niebergall, G., Remschmidt, H., Geyer, M., & Merschmann, W. (1978). Zur faktoriellen Validität des Token-Tests in einer unausgelesenen Stichprobe von Schulkindern. *Praxis der Kinderpsychologie und Kinderpsychiatrie, 27*, 5–10.

Noll, J.D. (1970). The use of the Token Test with children. *Program of the American Speech and Hearing Association*. New York.

Orgass, B. (1976). Eine Revision des Token Tests II. Validitätsnachweis, Normierung und Standardisierung. *Diagnostica, 22*, 141–156.

Poeck, K., & Hartje, W. (1979). Performance of aphasic patients in visual versus auditory presentation of the Token Test: Demonstration of a supramodal deficit. In F. Boller, & M. Dennis (Eds.), *Auditory Comprehension: Clinical and Experimental Studies with the Token Test*. New York: Academic Press.

Poeck, K., & Pietron, H.P. (1981). The influence of stretched speech presentation on Token Test performance in aphasic and right brain damaged patients. *Neuropsychologia, 19*, 133–136.

Records, N.L., Tomblin, J.B., & Buckwalter, P.R. (1995). Auditory verbal learning and memory in young adults with specific language impairment. *Clinical Neuropsychologist, 9*, 187–193.

Remschmidt, H., Niebergall, G., Geyer, M., & Merschmann, W. (1977). Die Bestimmung testmetrischer Kennwerte des Token-Testes bei Schulkindern unter Berücksichtigung der Intelligenz, des "Wortschatzes" und der Händigkeit. *Zeitschrift für Kinder- und Jugendpsychiatrie, 5*, 222–237.

Rich, J.B. (1993). Pictorial and verbal implicit and recognition memory in aging and Alzheimer's disease: A transfer-appropriate processing account. Ph.D. dissertation. University of Victoria.

Riedel, K., & Studdert-Kennedy, M. (1985). Extending formant transitions may not improve aphasic's perception of stop consonant place of articulation. *Brain and Language, 24*, 223–232.

Sarno, M.T. (1986). Verbal impairment in head injury. *Archives of Physical and Medical Rehabilitation, 67*, 399–404.

Sarno, M.T., Buonaguro, A., & Levita, E. (1985). Gender and recovery from aphasia after stroke. *Journal of Nervous and Mental Disease, 173*, 605–609.

Snow, W.G., Tierney, M.C., Zorzitto, M.L., Fisher, R.H., & Reid, D.W. (1988). One-year test–retest reliability of selected neuropsychological tests in older adults. *Journal of Clinical and Experimental Neuropsychology, 10*, 60 (abstract).

Spellacy, F., & Spreen, O. (1969). A short form of the Token Test. *Cortex, 5*, 390–397.

Spreen, O., & Benton, A.L. (1969, 1977). *The Neurosensory Center Comprehensive Examination for Aphasia*. Neuropsychology Laboratory, University of Victoria.

Swihart, A.A., Panisset, M., Becker, J.T., Beyer, J.T., Beyer, J.R., & Boller, F. (1989). The Token Test: Validity and diagnostic power in Alzheimer's disease. *Developmental Neuropsychology, 5*, 71–80.

Swisher, L.P., & Sarno, M.T. (1969). Token Test scores of three matched patient groups: Left brain-damaged with aphasia; right brain-damaged without aphasia; non-brain-damaged. *Cortex, 5*, 264–273.

Tallal, P., Stark, R.E., & Mellits, D. (1985). The relationship between auditory temporal analysis and receptive language development: Evidence from studies of developmental language disorder. *Neuropsychologia, 23*, 527–534.

Taylor, H.G., & Schatschneider, C. (1992). Child neuropsychological assessment: A test of basic assumptions. *The Clinical Neuropsychologist, 6*, 259–275.

Tuokko, H., & Woodward, T.S. (1996). Development and validation of a demographic system for neuropsychological measures used in the Canadian Study of Health and Aging. *Journal of Clinical and Experimental Neuropsychology, 18*, 479–616.

Van Harskamp, F., & Van Dongen, H.R. (1977). Construction and validation of different short forms of the Token Test. *Neuropsychologia, 15*, 467–470.

Vilkki, J., & Lattinen, L.V. (1976). Effects of pulvinotomy and ventrolateral thalamotomy on some cognitive functions. *Neuropsychologia, 14*, 67–78.

Whitaker, H.A., & Noll, J.D. (1972). Some linguistic parameters of the Token Test. *Neuropsychologia, 10*, 395–404.

Whitehouse, C.C., (1983). Token Test performance by dyslexic adolescents. *Brain and Language, 18*, 224–235.

Willmes, K. (1981). A new look at the Token Test using probabilistic test models. *Neuropsychologia, 19*, 631–645.

Wold, A.H., & Reinvang, I. (1990). The relation between integration, sequence of information, short-term memory, and Token Test performance in aphasic subjects. *Journal of Communication Disorders, 23,* 31–59.

Woll, G., Naumann, E., Cohen, R., & Kelter, S. (1976). Kreuzvalidierung der Revision des Token Tests durch Orgass. *Diagnostica, 22,* 157–162.

Wood, K.R., Duis, C. & Schefft, B.K. (1997). The use of short forms of the MAE Token Test in neuropsychological screening. *Archives of Clinical Neuropsychology, 12,* 429 (abstract).

Zaidel, E. (1977). Unilateral auditory language comprehension on the Token Test following cerebral commissurotomy and hemispherectomy. *Neuropsychologia, 15,* 1–18.

12

Visual, Visuomotor, and Auditory Tests

Numerous tests of visual-perceptual and visuo-motor performance have been developed, especially stimulated by the notion that such tests may contribute to the riddle of dyslexia, but also aimed at subtle disorders of spatial recognition, orientation, visual neglect, and forms of agnosia; in addition to visual perception, many require a considerable amount of cognitive processing. We include only a small selection of such tests in an attempt to avoid duplication. Our selection was also guided by clinical experience as well as correlational studies indicating that each of these tests makes a unique contribution to the examination of the patient.

From among the visual-perceptual tests without a motor component we selected the Hooper Visual Organization Test, the more detailed Test of Visual-Perceptual Skills, standardized mainly for children and adolescents, and the Facial Recognition Test. Motor responses are required in the Embedded Figures Test, the Developmental Test of Visuo-Motor Integration, and the more specialized Bells Visual Neglect, Right-Left Orientation, and Trail Making tests. Researchers and clinicians may also wish to consider the Visual Object and Space Perception Battery (Warrington & James, 1991) which, however, needs further psychometric development and a clearer definition of the specific strengths of each of its eight subtests. A newcomer, the WRAVMA (Adams & Sheslow, 1997), designed and nationally standardized for chil-

dren between 3 and 17 years, covers visuo-spatial, visuo-motor, and fine motor skills in one battery, but was not yet available for review.

We also included only two visuoconstructional tests (Clock Drawing, Three-Dimensional Constructional Praxis) although constructional praxis is also included in other tests, such as the WAIS-R Block Design Test, the Rey-Osterrieth Figure, and many other drawing tasks are available [e.g., bicycle (Greenberg et al., 1994), house, tree]. As Benton (1994) points out, the concept of constructional apraxia still needs more operational definitions to be optimally useful. Other tests of apraxia (e.g., symbolic and nonsymbolic finger, hand, and body movements) have been available for some time (e.g., DeRenzi et al., 1980) but have not found adequate psychometric development to be included in this volume. The reader may wish to refer to the apraxia test contained in the Boston Diagnostic Examination for Aphasia, described elsewhere in this volume.

Some tests require basic abilities of color recognition. Color blindness *per se* is sometimes of interest in neuropsychology (see Kolb & Whishaw, 1995), and screening for color blindness may be necessary if any doubt arises about the patient's ability to distinguish colors. The most frequently used tests for color blindness consist of pseudo-isochromatic plates (i.e., letters, numbers, or shapes printed in color on a grey background of matching darkness; these cannot be traced by color-blind persons). The tests by Ishahara (1982) and Dvorine (1953) appear to be optimal under different viewing conditions (Long et al., 1985). As pointed out in the section on face recognition, poor vision (20/50 or poorer) can also impair the results of tests using visual processing or visual stimuli in general (Kempen et al., 1994).

Only a few specific auditory tests have been developed; however, in a wider sense many of the auditory comprehension tests described in the language section could have been included in this section, but they are more appropriately placed in the context of the language section of the book.

We did not include a number of other tests derived from the Seashore Tests of Musical Ability—for example, the Seashore Rhythm Test (Reitan & Wolfson, 1989), the Wepman Speech Sound Perception Test, the phoneme discrimination test (Benton et al., 1983) or the Meikle Consonant Perception Test developed in our laboratory—because in our experience these tests fail to add important specific information to the patient's disability profile, because of their limited usefulness and/or inadequate standardization.

Prior to the administration of any of the auditory tests, a screening for auditory acuity of the patient is necessary. There is no need for a full audiologic evaluation, unless the screening indicates hearing loss. We use a standard Maico audiometer, that generates a pure-tone signal calibrated in decibels (dB); for each ear, frequencies (pitch) of 500, 1000, 2000, 4000, and 6000 Hz are tested with one ascending and one descending trial. Hearing levels between 0 and 15 dB are considered normal; hearing levels of 35 dB and higher indicate impairment and tend to invalidate auditory tests unless the impairment is bilateral and uni-

formly affects all frequencies (in this case a stronger amplification of the test signals is indicated).

References

Adams, W., & Sheslow, D. (1997). *Wide Range Assessment of Visual Motor Abilities* (WRAVMA). Wilmington, DE: Wide Range Inc.

Benton, A.L. (1994). Neuropsychological assessment. *Annual Review of Psychology, 45*, 1–23.

Benton, A.L., Hamsher, K. de S., Varney, N.R., & Spreen, O. (1983). *Contributions to Neuropsychological Assessment*. New York: Oxford University Press.

DeRenzi, E., Motti, F., & Nichelli, P. (1980). Imitating gestures: A quantitative approach to ideomotor apraxia. *Archives of Neurology, 37*, 6–10.

Dvorine, I. (1953). *Dvorine Pseudo-Isochromatic Plates*. New York: Psychological Corporation.

Greenberg, G.D., Rodriguez, N.M., & Sesta, J.J. (1994). Revised scoring, reliability, and validity investigations of Piaget's bicycle drawing test. *Assessment, 1*, 89–101.

Ishahara, S. (1982). *The Series of Plates Designed as a Test for Color-Blindness*. Tokyo: Kanehara.

Long, G.M., Lyman, B.J., & Tuck, J.P. (1985). Distance, duration, and blur effects on the perception of pseudoisochromatic stimuli. *Ophthalmic and Physiological Optics, 5*, 185–194.

Kempen, J.H., Kritchevsky, M., & Feldman, S.T. (1994). *Journal of Clinical and Experimental Neuropsychology, 16*, 223–231.

Kolb, B., & Whishaw, I.Q. (1990). *Fundamentals of Human Neuropsychology* (3rd ed.). New York: Freeman.

Reitan, R.M., & Wolfson, D. (1989). The Seashore Rhythm Test and brain functions. *The Clinical Neuropsychologist, 3*, 70–78.

Warrington, E.K., & James, M. (1991). *Visual Object and Space Perception Battery*. Bury St. Edmunds, Suffolk, England: Thames Valley Test Co.

CLOCK DRAWING

Purpose

This test is a clinical screening task for visuo-spatial and constructional disabilities.

Source

No specific test material is required. Tuokko et al. (1995) offer a commercial version, The Clock Test, published by Multi-Health Systems (65 Overlea Blvd., Suite 210, Toronto, ON M4H 1P1; in the United States, 908 Niagara Falls Blvd., Tonawanda, NY 14120-2060) for $225 Cdn.

Description

The simple free-hand drawing of a clock face, together with the drawing of a daisy, a house—also of a person, a bicycle—has been part of the brief mental status examination in neurology for a long time (Battersby et al., 1956; Critchley, 1953; Goodglass & Kaplan, 1972; Strub & Black, 1977) and is frequently recommended as a screening test for dementia. In contrast to the primarily verbal content of most dementia scales, clock drawing relies on visuospatial, constructional, as well as higher-order cognitive abilities. The test requires merely a sheet of paper and a pencil and can be given as part of a bedside examination, or in other instances when lengthy neuropsychological testing is not possible. Free-hand drawing is preferred to Wolf-Klein et al.'s (1989) procedure, which uses a sheet with a printed circle, representing the shape of the clock face. Freedman et al. (1994) recommend the use of free-hand drawing, followed by a predrawn circle, and of three predrawn clocks with numbers into which the correct time settings (hands) have to be inserted. Clock-setting is also part of the parietal lobe battery in the Boston Diagnostic Aphasia Examination described elsewhere in this book. The Clock Test (Tuokko et al., 1995) uses three tasks: clock drawing (with predrawn circles), clock reading, and clock setting. Microcog (Powell et al., 1993) includes clock reading as one of its computerized sub-tests and provides measures of both accuracy and response time.

Administration

Place upright a standard unlined letter-size sheet of paper and a pencil in front of the patient and say: "*I want you to draw the face of a clock with all the numbers on it. Make it large.*" After completion of the clock face, instruct as follows: "*Now, draw the hands pointing at 20 to 4.*" Instructions may be repeated or rephrased if the patient does not understand, but no other help should be given. The time taken to complete the task may be noted.

Pre-drawn circles are not part of our standard administration, but may be used if the patient fails to make a connected drawing (score of three or less according to the scoring criteria below) in order to explore specific aspects of number placements and hand settings.

Approximate Time for Administration

Approximately 5 minutes are required.

Scoring

A 10-point scoring system, adapted from Sunderland et al. (1989) and Wolf-Klein et al. (1989), is used as follows:

10 Normal drawing, numbers and hands in approximately correct positions, hour hand distinctly different from minute hand and approaching 4 o'clock.

9 Slight errors in placement of hands (not exactly on 8 and 4, but not on one of the adjoining numbers) or one missing number on clock face.

8 More noticeable errors in placement of hour and minute hand (off by one number); number spacing shows a gap.

7 Placement of hands significantly off course (more than one number); very inappropriate spacing of numbers (e.g., all on one side).

6 Inappropriate use of clock hands (use of digital display or circling of numbers de-

spite repeated instructions); crowding of numbers at one end of the clock or reversal of numbers.

5   Perseverative or otherwise inappropriate arrangement of numbers (e.g., numbers indicated by dots). Hands may be represented, but do not clearly point at a number.

4   Numbers absent, written outside of clock or in distorted sequence. Integrity of the clock face missing. Hands not clearly represented or drawn outside of clock face.

3   Numbers and clock face no longer connected in the drawing. Hands not recognizably present.

2   Drawing reveals some evidence of instructions received, but representation of clock is only vague; inappropriate spatial arrangement of numbers.

1   Irrelevant, uninterpretable figure or no attempt.

Roman numerals and embellishments of the clock (clock feet, bells) are acceptable.

Tuokko et al. (1992, 1995) score systematically for several types of errors (e.g., omission, perseveration, rotation) in the drawing part, and they use a 15-point system for clock reading and clock setting, but each subtest provides only a single score for interpretative purposes; others award one point for each individual part of the drawing up to a maximum of 30 points (Mendez et al., 1992) or 15 points (Freedman et al., 1994).

For the clinical interpretation of the clock face drawing, special features should be noted, such as crowding of the drawing into one corner of the page, "closing-in" (i.e., placing lines too close to each other), oblique shape, tremulousness, inaccurate meeting of the circle line. The most common errors are omissions and misplacements of the numbers on the clock face (Tuokko et al., 1992). Rouleau et al. (1992) developed a qualitative scoring system that includes stimulus-bound, conceptual, perseverative, planning, and neglect types of errors in addition to the quantitative score.

Comment

Retest reliability for clock drawing after 12 weeks was .78 for Alzheimer's disease patients

(Mendez et al., 1992). Tuokko et al. (1995) found similar values when Alzheimer's disease (AD) patients were retested after 4 days. A practice effect has not been reported. Interrater reliability for drawings by elderly normal subjects and Alzheimer's disease patients was .97 and did not differ between clinicians and nonclinicians (Kozora & McCullum, 1994; Mendez et al., 1992; Rouleau et al., 1992; Sunderland et al., 1989; Tuokko et al., 1995). Nussbaum et al. (1992) reported interrater agreement of .79 to .93 for three different scoring methods in a neuropsychiatric sample. Kozora and McCullum (1994) found a moderately high correlation between 3-point, 10-point, and 16-point scoring systems (.67 to .70).

Construct validity was examined by Freedman et al. (1994), who found that clock drawing loaded on a nonverbal visuoconstructional factor together with the copy form of the Rey-Osterrieth test, WAIS-R Block Design, and perseverative responses on the Wisconsin Card Sorting Test, but only marginally on a verbal factor.

Construct validity has also been demonstrated by correlations with the Mini-Mental Scale, ranging from .41 to .58, with the Mattis Dementia Rating Scale from .38 to .45, with the Global Impression of Neuropsychological Impairment scale from .49 to .60, and with the Block Design test under extended time conditions .41 (Kozora & McCullum, 1994; Mendez et al., 1992; Nussbaum et al., 1992; Shulman et al., 1993). Tuokko et al. (1995) found moderate correlations (.41 to .57) of clock drawing with the information, similarities, digit span, and block design subtests of the WAIS-R in AD patients; correlations with clock reading were slightly higher (.54 to .64), and correlations with clock setting were highest (.58 to .77) for these subtests. Mendez et al. also report a moderately strong correlation with the Rey Complex Figure (.66) and the Symbol Digits Modalities Test (.65). The test did not correlate with the Beery Test in children (Kirk et al., 1996). Libon et al. (1993) found the test correlated with tests presumed to measure executive functions (e.g., Block Design, Go-No-Go Test, Trail Making Test) in dementia. Huntzinger et al. (1992) found only a modest correlation (.30) with a six-item orientation/memory/concentration test; it also does not correlate significantly with the Raven Progressive Matrices (Kozora & McCullum, 1994), suggesting that this test measures different aspects of cognitive performance. In a 6-, 12-, and 18-month follow-up, Shulman et al. (1993) noted deterioration of clock-drawing performance to correlate with deterioration on other tests; patients who showed deterioration were also more likely to be institutionalized than those who did not.

Discriminant validity has been investigated in differentiating groups of normal elderly subjects and patient groups with AD, multi-infarct dementia, and depression (Wolf-Klein et al., 1989), with a mean age of 76 years. Correct classification in normal subjects was 97 percent, for AD patients 87 percent, for multi-infarct dementia 62 percent, and for depression 97 percent. Tuokko et al. (1992) report a correct classification rate of 86 percent for Alzheimer's disease and of 92 percent for normal elderly controls. A new study (O'Rourke et al., 1997) also found good predictive validity; sensitivity was 91 percent at time of first testing for clients later diagnosed with AD, and specificity was 95 percent. Kozora and McCullum (1994) reported a mean score of 6.61 (range 2–10) in AD patients as compared to 9.59 for normal age-matched control subjects. Barr et al. (1992) found, however, that the test does not discriminate between AD and vascular dementia patients; this finding was also replicated by Libon et al. (1993), but the authors found that in the copy condition, patients with cerebrovascular dementia performed worse than patients with AD. A second study (Libon et al., 1996) with a different population of 31 AD and 27 cerebrovascular dementia patients confirmed this result. In addition, rescoring of the clock drawings by summing all errors, by graphomotor, hand/number placement, and "executive control" errors (e.g., turning the page while writing numbers, writing numbers counterclockwise, perseverations) suggested that patients with cerebrovascular dementia made more graphomotor errors in the drawing-on-command condition, and more executive control and more total errors in the copy condition than AD patients. Executive control errors also correlated with other tests presumed to measure executive functions (e.g., WMS-

Mental Control, COWA-FAS, WAIS-R Block Design) and loaded on the same factor in a factor analysis. Dastoor et al. (1991) and Watson et al. (1993) also report significant differences between patients with Alzheimer's disease and those with depression and other disorders that do not meet the criteria for probable dementia. Lee and Lawler (1995) found that clock drawing may be abnormal in geriatric populations because of depression, and that scores improved when the depression resolved, i.e., that poor scores may be state dependent. Freedman et al. (1994) found impaired scores in demented patients with Parkinson's disease, but near-normal scores in nondemented Parkinson's patients. Cahn et al. (1996) found a sensitivity of 81 percent and a specificity of 72 percent using both quantitative and qualitative measures, although the test did not contribute significantly to a regression formula to separate normal elderly, at-risk for AD, and AD patients when the test was administered together with Trail Making, Boston Naming, and Wechsler Visual Retention tasks (Cahn et al., 1995); the authors warn that the test is not suitable as a single screening measure, and that other measures such as verbal fluency and memory must be considered in the screening process. Cahn et al. (1994) also reported that the test discriminated with a sensitivity of 66 percent and a specificity of 90 percent between cognitivity impaired and normal elderly Spanish-speaking individuals.

While the test may be useful in the diagnosis of AD and other forms of dementia, it should be noted that this test serves many purposes. Basically, it provides an estimate of visuospatial as well as cognitive skills. The test results are affected by hemianopsia and right visual neglect (Ogden, 1985), which is apparent in corresponding unilateral errors. However, Ishiai et al. (1993) did not find a strong relation between clock-drawing errors and unilateral errors on line bisection, drawing of a daisy, and letter cancellation in patients with specific *left* unilateral neglect syndrome; rather, clock drawings were related to Wechsler IQ. The test is reported to be sensitive to visuospatial disorders or constructional apraxia, such as those found in right or bilateral temporo-parietal lesions (Critchley, 1953).

Kozora and McCullum (1994) consider the poor clock-drawing performance of AD patients and of older normal subjects as support for a "frontal dysfunction" hypothesis of aging (Albert & Kaplan, 1980; Hecaen & Albert, 1978). Based on case studies, Freedman et al. (1994) point out that in focal right parietal lesions, major spatial disorganization (sometimes with retention of the essential elements of the clock) can be expected; patients with frontal lesions often show difficulty in integrating the multiple task demands of clock drawing (number sequence and spatial layout); patients with left posterior lesions may show difficulty with numbers and time settings because of receptive aphasia; similar problems may occur with left anterior lesions (e.g., setting the clock *after* instead of *before*). Unless such lesion-specific effects can be firmly established, the interpretation of the test should be made in the context of other test results; Freedman et al. also warn that such "signs" can only be used for generating hypotheses for interpretation. Tuokko et al. (1992) stress that clock drawing is also dependent on the individual's ability to use time concepts as shown in similar deficits in clock setting and clock reading tasks that do not require visuospatial and constructive skills. Verbally mediated planning difficulties were invoked to explain the poor clock-drawing performance of some schizophrenics who showed poor results on verbal tests regardless of severity of psychopathology (Tawfik-Reedy et al., 1995).

Other time settings ("20 after 8", "10 after 11") have been used; the identification of hemilateral neglect or hemianopia is facilitated if the two hands of the clock are in different halves of the clock face. Use of time settings like "10 after 11" may help in identifying the "pull" of frontal pathology since the 10 is right beside the 10, pulling the minute hand toward the 11, and because it requires recoding of 10 minutes into 2 hourly segments; i.e., setting the minute hand at 2 o'clock (Freedman et al., 1994).

For clinicians who wish to use clock drawing (with predrawn circles), reading, and setting in geriatric practice, the Clock Test (Tuokko et al., 1995) may be preferable because it pro-vides templates for accurate measurement of deviations, and a prepared set of test material is supplied. However, interrater and retest reliability, sensitivity, and specificity in AD (93 and 94 percent, respectively) are similar to those reported for other versions, and the "profile" is merely a printed conversion of the three test scores into T-scores for five age groups over 65 years. According to the manual, two of the test scores should be above the age-appropriate cutoff when dementia is considered.

Normative Data

Currently available normative data (Sunderland et al., 1989; Wolf-Klein, 1989) suggest that scores between 7 and 10 should be considered normal; a score of 6 is borderline (achieved by 13 percent of normal subjects and 88 percent of Alzheimer's disease patients); scores of 5 or less are rare in normal subjects (.8 percent), but frequent in Alzheimer's disease (83 percent). Kozora and Mc-Cullum (1994) examined 100 older adults and found a normal range from 7 to 10 points up to the age of 69 with a 10-point scoring system, but in normal subjects between 70 and 95 years of age the range dropped to 4 to 10 points; a similar drop for the highest age group (80–89 years), but not earlier (age 70–79), has been reported for clock drawing by Marcopulos, McLain, and Giuliano (1997), and for clock setting by Farver and Farver (1982). Marcopulos et al. (1997) found a moderate education effect (less than 2 points between 0–4 and 6–10 years of education), and no effect of race in an elderly rural U.S. sample. Cahn and Kaplan (1995) found no further decrease in either the quantitative or qualitative score between three "old-old" age groups (67–74, 75–84, 85+ years) in a healthy community-living sample.

Freedman et al. (1994) used a 15-point ordinal cumulative scoring system in which each feature was awarded 1 point. These features ("critical items") were selected only if healthy subjects had a near-perfect success rate, and they include such features as acceptable contour, correct numbers, numbers in correct order, minute hand longer than hour hand, correctly drawn or extrapolated center, etc. With this system, normal subjects between 20 and 69 years of age ($n = 348$) had near-perfect scores (mean = 14.7, SD = .60); the mean score for age 70–79 was 13.68 (SD = 1.84), and for age 80–90, it was 13.34 (SD = 2.09). Thus, this study reflects similar age-related decline in old age.

The Clock Test (Tuokko et al., 1995) presents an excellent standardization for five age groups from 65 to 85+ years, based on a Canadian cross-section of 1,753 healthy elderly subjects and 269 clinical cases. Age effects are noticeable particularly in the older age groups. Norms for younger age groups or for geographic or ethnic differences are not available.

Kirk, McCarthy, and Kaplan (1996) reported data on the development of clock-drawing skills in 220 children between the age of 6 and 15 years and found that total accuracy increased significantly at age 7 and again at age 10. No gender differences were noted. Similarly, Edmonds et al. (1994) examined 434 normal public school children, aged 6 to 12 years. They also reported that the ability to draw a clock correctly was established by age 8 in a significant majority of children, that number reversals disappeared by age 7, and that 9-year olds could correctly indicate time to the minute. This study suggests that the test can be used with school-age children if adequate norms become available.

References

Albert, M.S., & Kaplan, E. (1980). Organic implication of neuropsychological deficits in the elderly. In W. Poon, J.L. Fozard, L.S. Cermak, D. Arenberg, & L.W. Thompson (Eds.), *New Directions in Memory and Aging*. Hillsdale, NJ: Erlbaum.

Barr, A., Benedict, R., Tune, L., & Brandt, J. (1992). Neuropsychological differentiation of Alzheimer's disease from vascular dementia. *International Journal of Geriatric Psychiatry, 7*, 621–627.

Battersby, W.S., Bender, M.B., Pollack, M., & Kahn, R.L. (1956). Unilateral "spatial agnosia" ("inattention") in patients with cortical lesions. *Brain, 79*, 68–93.

Cahn, D.A., & Kaplan, E. (1995). Clock drawing in the oldest old. *The Clinical Neuropsychologist, 9*, 274–275 (abstract).

Cahn, D.A., Salmon, D.P., Butters, N., Wiederholt, W.C., Corey-Bloom, J., Edelstein, S.L., & Barrett-Connor, E. (1995). Detection of dementia of the Alzheimer type in a population-based sample: Neuropsychological test performance. *Journal of the International Neuropsychological Society, 1*, 252–260.

Cahn, D.A., Salmon, D.P., Monsch, A.U., et al. (1996). Screening for dementia of the Alzheimer type in the community: The utility of the Clock Drawing Test. *Archives of Clinical Neuropsychology, 11*, 529–539.

Cahn, D.A., Wiederholt, W.C., Salmon, D.P., et al. (1994). Detection of cognitive impairment in Spanish-speaking elderly with the clock drawing test. *Archives of Clinical Neuropsychology, 9*, 112 (abstract).

Critchley, M. (1953). *The Parietal Lobes* (reprinted 1966). New York: Hafner.

Dastoor, D.P., Schwartz, G., & Kurzman, D. (1991). Clock-Drawing—An assessment technique in dementia. *Journal of Clinical and Experimental Gerontology, 13*, 69–85.

Edmonds, J.E., Cohen, M.J., Riccio, C.A., et al. (1994). The development of clock face drawing in normal children. *Archives of Clinical Neuropsychology, 9*, 125 (abstract).

Farver, P.F., & Farver, T.B. (1982). Performance of normal older adults on tests designed to measure parietal lobe functions. *American Journal of Occupational Therapy, 36*, 444–449.

Freedman, M., Kaplan, E., Delis, D., & Morris, R. (1994). *Clock Drawing: A Neuropsychological Analysis*. New York: Oxford University Press.

Goodglass, H., & Kaplan, E. (1972). *The Assessment of Aphasia and Related Disorders*. Philadelphia: Lea & Fibiger.

Hecaen, H., & Albert, M.L. (1978). *Human Neuropsychology*. New York: Wiley.

Huntzinger, J.A., Rosse, R.B., Schwartz, B.L., Ross, L.A., & Deutsch, S.I. (1992). Clock drawing in the screening assessment of cognitive impairment in an ambulatory care setting: A preliminary report. *General Hospital Psychiatry, 14*, 142–144.

Ishiai, S., Suishita, M., Ichikawa, T., Gono, S., & Watabiki, S. (1993). Clock-drawing test and unilateral spatial neglect. *Neurology, 43*, 106–110.

Kirk, U., McCarthy, C., & Kaplan, E. (1996). The development of clock-drawing skills: Implications for neuropsychological assessment of children. Paper presented at the meeting of the International Neuropsychological Society, Chicago.

Kozora, E., & McCullum, M. (1994). Qualitative features of clock drawing in normal aging and Alzheimer's disease. *Assessment, 1,* 179–187.

Lee, H., & Lawler, B.A. (1995). State-dependent nature of the Clock Drawing Test in geriatric depression. *Journal of the American Geriatric Society, 43,* 796–798.

Libon, D.J., Malamut, B.L., Swenson, R., Sands, L.P., & Cloud, B.S. (1996). Further analyses of clock drawings among demented and non-demented older subjects. *Archives of Clinical Neuropsychology, 11,* 193–205.

Libon, D.J., Swenson, R.A., Barnoski, E.J., & Sands, L.P. (1993). Clock drawing as an assessment tool for dementia. *Archives of Clinical Neuropsychology, 8,* 405–415.

Marcopulos, B.A., McLain, C.A., & Giuliano, A.J. (1997). Cognitive impairment or inadequate norms? *The Clinical Neuropsychologist, 11,* 111–131.

Mendez, M.F., Ala, T., & Underwood, K.L. (1992). Development of scoring criteria for the clock drawing task in Alzheimer's disease. *Journal of the American Geriatrics Society, 40,* 1095–1099.

Nussbaum, P.D., Fields, R.B., & Starrat, C. (1992). Comparison of three scoring procedures for the clock drawing. *Journal of Clinical and Experimental Neuropsychology, 14,* 44 (Abstract).

Ogden, J.A. (1985). Anterior–posterior interhemispheric differences in the loci of lesions producing visual hemineglect. *Brain and Cognition, 4,* 59–75.

O'Rourke, N., Tuokko, H., Hayden, S., & Beattie, B.L. (1997). Early identification of dementia: Predictive validity of the clock test. *Archives of Clinical Neuropsychology, 12,* 257–267.

Powell, D., Kaplan, E., Whitla, D., Weintraub, S., & Catlin, R. (1993). *Microcog: Assessment of Cognitive Functioning.* San Antonio, TX: Psychological Corporation.

Rouleau, I., Salmon, D.P., Butters, N., Kennedy, C., & McGuire, K. (1992). Quantitative and qualitative analyses of clock face drawings in Alzheimer's and Huntington's diseases. *Brain and Cognition, 18,* 70–87.

Shulman, K.I., Gold, D.P., Cohen, C.A., & Zucchero, C.A. (1993). Clock drawing and dementia in the community: A longitudinal study. *International Journal of Geriatric Psychiatry, 8,* 487–496.

Strub, R.L., & Black, F.W. (1977). *The Mental Status Examination in Neurology.* Philadelphia: F.A. Davis.

Sunderland, T., Hill, J.L., Mellow, A.M., Lawlor, B.A., Gundersheimer, J., Newhouse, P.A., & Grafman, J.H. (1989). Clock drawing in Alzheimer's disease; a novel measure of dementia severity. *Journal of the American Geriatric Association, 37,* 725–729.

Tawfik-Reedy, Z., Zuker, T., Paulsen, J.S., Sadek, J.R., Heaton, R.K., Butters, N., & Jeste, D.V. (1995). Clock drawing in schizophrenia: A qualitative analysis of impairment. *Archives of Clinical Neuropsychology, 10,* 396.

Tuokko, H., Hadjistavropoulos, T., Miller, J.A., & Beattie, B.L. (1992). The clock test: A sensitive measure to differentiate normal elderly from those with Alzheimer's disease. *Journal of the American Geriatrics Society, 40,* 579–584.

Tuokko, H., Hadjistavropoulos, T., Miller, J.A., Horton, A., & Beattie, B.L. (1995). *The Clock Test. Administration and Scoring Manual.* Toronto, ON: Multi-Health Systems.

Watson, Y.I., Arfken, C.L., & Birge, S.J. (1993). Clock completion: An objective screening test for dementia. *Journal of the American Geriatrics Society, 41,* 1235–1240.

Wolf-Klein, G.P., Silverstone, F.A., Levy, A.P., & Brod, M.S. (1989). Screening for Alzheimer's disease by clock drawing. *Journal of the American Geriatric Association, 37,* 730–734.

DICHOTIC LISTENING: WORDS

Purpose

This test can provide an indicator of language lateralization. It is also a measure of divided attention.

Source

Cassette tape with dichotic words, instructions, and recording sheets can be obtained from the Neuropsychology Laboratory, University of Victoria, Victoria, BC V8W 3P5 for $50 US (Music $50 US). The original Kimura stimuli (including digits, melodies, and words) are available from DK Consultants, 412 Duffrin Ave., London, ON N6B 1Z6, for $160 Cdn. (with additional children's digits $200 Cdn.). Graves and Allan (1995) describe hardware requirements and offer software for the generation of new dichotic listening tasks (e-mail:rgraves@.uvic.ca).

Description

This test was originally developed by Broadbent (1958) to investigate the ability to attend to two signals simultaneously, one to each ear. Kimura (1961) modified the task by using spoken one-syllable numbers in sets of three pairs, after which the subject was requested to repeat as many of the numbers as possible. Kimura noted that in epileptic patients with documented left-hemisphere speech dominance, right-ear recall was better than recall from the left ear. Patients with right-hemisphere speech showed the reverse. These findings are consistent with the notion that the crossed auditory connections are stronger than ipsilateral pathways. Her subsequent studies also suggested a left-ear preference for the recognition of nonverbal information such as music. Numerous experimental investigations with a wide variety of stimulus material and subject populations followed these initial studies. There are a number of different methods available, including the free-recall technique (e.g., Kimura, 1961), the dichotic monitoring test (Geffen et al., 1978), and the fused-rhyme procedure (Wexler & Halwes, 1983). There is no clear evidence that one procedure is better than another in predicting speech lateralization (Strauss, 1988). More recently, the test has also been used as a measure of stimulus processing speed, assuming that the results are influenced by limitations of the immediate processing channel (Spellacy & Ehle, 1990).

We use a free-recall technique similar to the one developed by Kimura (1961) in which six one-syllable words are presented, three to each ear. The tape prepared in our laboratory is synchronized for stimulus onset and calibrated for equal loudness in both ears. Both right- and left-ear stimuli begin with the same consonant to control voice onset time.

The apparatus consists of a high-quality stereo tape-player and amplifier, a pair of earphones plugged into the appropriate outlets, and the dichotic words tape. The right and left channel on the tape may be connected to the right or left earphone of the subject. They can be used alternately, or reversed after half of the test (to avoid bias created by poor earphone calibration), but care should be taken to note on the answer sheet which channel goes to which ear.

A sound-level meter (Scott or similar product) should be used in order to calibrate and balance the earphones before starting the test. The earphones should be calibrated to produce exactly equal loudness of 65–70 dB for both ears, the "most comfortable loudness level" reported by Riegler (1980).

Before administering the test the examiner should check the subject with an audiometer to determine whether there is satisfactory hearing in both ears. Dichotic listening effects are fairly robust in the presence of minor hearing impairment (discrepancy of 5–10 decibels between right and left ears), but with higher discrepancies, the results should be interpreted with caution. If the discrepancy between ears is beyond 20 dB, the test should not be given.

Administration

The subject is seated with earphones on, with the earphone marked "*Right*" on the right ear and that marked "*Left*" on the left ear. Say: "*You are going to hear some words, and I want you to repeat as many of these words as possible*". On the tape are two three-word sets of single words. The first set is heard on the right ear. After the subject repeats these words correctly, play the second set, which is heard by the left ear. These practice sets can be repeated if the subject fails to understand the instructions. If the subject completes the practice trials correctly, say: "*You will now hear words which will come into both ears at the same time. I want you to repeat all the words you hear. Each time you will hear three sets of words, and when I stop the tape, you must start repeating the words immediately, as many as you can remember.*"

After each set of three word pairs, stop the tape and wait for the subject to respond. Reverse earphones half-way through the test. Circle the words the subject remembers on the answer sheet (Figure 12–1). Dubious responses should be written above the word they resemble, but *only the words on the answer sheet are accepted as correct.*

Dichotic Listening–Words

Name _____
DOB _____
Date Tested _____
Examiner _____

	Right Ear			**Left Ear**			**Other**
Trial 1	pack	test	hat	port	tea	cow	_____
Trial 2	fame	sum	bond	fur	sale	bee	_____
Trial 3	duck	ship	gas	deck	shoe	gun	_____
Trial 4	vine	zone	mob	vane	zoo	meal	_____
Trial 5	nose	pride	track	name	plate	trail	_____
Trial 6	coast	flight	sake	corn	fleet	sunk	_____
Trial 7	bowl	damp	good	bell	deed	game	_____
Trial 8	shine	vent	zest	sheep	vast	zeal	_____
Trial 9	mass	nine	pin	mill	nail	pace	_____
Trial 10	tin	cloth	faith	torn	clock	fresh	_____
Trial 11	speak	bark	need	spit	belt	night	_____

REVERSE HEADPHONES

Trial 12	shore	guest	vault	shell	guard	vote	_____
Trial 13	though	map	note	there	mad	nick	_____
Trial 14	pal	tongue	cream	pig	teeth	crust	_____
Trial 15	flag	send	blown	fault	sand	brain	_____
Trial 16	dawn	give	shift	ditch	glow	shirt	_____
Trial 17	vim	then	mink	view	this	month	_____
Trial 18	noun	pan	top	noon	pork	tan	_____
Trial 19	coop	fog	style	cord	fit	stamp	_____
Trial 20	birth	neck	grain	band	noise	glove	_____
Trial 21	shame	verb	that	shoot	voice	than	_____
Trial 22	male	nudge	coop	mine	nice	cord	_____

Right Total _____   Left Total _____   Other Total _____

GRAND TOTAL _____
Z SCORE _____
% ILE _____

Figure 12—1. Dichotic listening (Words) sample answer sheet.

If the subject responds with only one or two words, you may say once: *"Is that all?"* or *"Are those all the words that you can remember?"* before proceeding with the next set.

Approximate Time for Administration

About 10–20 minutes are required.

Scoring

Count one point for each word that is listed on the record sheet. Total each side.

Comment

Test–retest reliability is good (.75 to .92; Strauss et al., 1987). Bruder (1988) reports reliability coefficients ranging from .60 to .80. However, other results have not been as favorable. For example, Hatta (1988) found that in 37 Japanese right-handed university students, ear advantage changed for 35 percent for a vowel-consonant test, and in 17.7 percent for a CVC test, with changes most frequent for subjects with deviant scores on the first test. No significant practice effects need be expected.

Intertest correlations between free recall of digits, free recall of consonant–vowel syllables, consonant–vowel syllable monitoring, and Morse code recall were low (.01 to .51) for both right- and left-handers, and direction of ear preference changed in 23–62 percent of the sample (Jancke et al., 1992). On the other hand, using a fused-word technique with 5-, 8-, and 11-year-old children, Christianson et al. (1992) found good agreement between ear advantage and visual-half-field advantage for letter and picture naming.

The test agrees reasonably well with speech localization as determined by the sodium amytal test (Strauss et al., 1987). In that study, patients with left-hemisphere speech lateralization obtained scores of 29.03 for the right ear, 12.95 for the left ear; the corresponding scores for patients with right-hemisphere speech were 15.20 and 21.48, and for patients with bilateral speech the scores were 19.88 and 13.24. However, the percentage of patients with right-ear advantage in each of the three groups was 86, 50, and 71 percent. Failure to obtain a right–left ear difference suggests that language lateralization may not follow the normal pattern, but it should not be used as definite evidence regarding hemispheric dominance. Based on a study of 106 patients for whom language lateralization was determined by the intracarotid amobarbital test, Lee et al. (1994) warn that DL is not a valid indicator of language dominance in the individual case, and that even group differences between left, right, and bilateral language-dominant patients may not be statistically significant. Hence firm statements about language lateralization cannot be made; the test provides clues only. In normal right-handers the test seems to underestimate the incidence of left-hemisphere speech lateralization (74 percent right-ear advantage, REA) (Lee et al., 1994), which is consistent with Lake and Bryden's (1976) finding of 75 percent REA in right-handed males. Right-handed females apparently show even lower incidence rates for REA (62 percent, Lake & Bryden, 1976). In a sample of 126 6- to 9-year-old left-handed children, Hugdahl and Andersson (1989) found REA in 65 percent, left-ear advantage in 25.4 percent, and no ear advantage in 9.6 percent.

Richardson et al. (1990) investigated DL in 275 control, 50 head-injured, 35 malaria-encephalitis, and 16 Parkinson patients. They found significantly lower DL scores in a substantial number of patients in all three clinical groups, and they recommend DL as a "useful diagnostic tool with populations who are at risk for disruption of subcortical white matter pathways either by transient electrical discharges (i.e., seizure disorders) or structural changes at the subcortical level" (p. 426). Springer et al. (1991) also found that DL distinguishes between dysphoric patients with complaints of seizure-like phenomena and other depressives, and that DL scores improved after carbamazepine treatment. Studies of patients with documented white matter disease have shown similar impairment (Jerger & Jerger, 1975; Levin et al., 1989; Pujol et al., 1991; Rao et al., 1989). Deficits in DL have also been found in Alzheimer's disease patients (Mohr et al., 1990) and in patients who had suffered from high fever (hyperpyrexia) without direct brain involvement (e.g., encephalitis) (Varney et al., 1994).

A shift to left-ear advantage in aphasics (Papanicolaou et al., 1987) has been interpreted as evidence of increased right-hemisphere involvement during recovery from aphasia, of attentional factors, or a lesion effect in the left hemisphere (Moore & Papanicolaou, 1991; Niccum & Speaks, 1991). In a study of 49 seizure patients, Grote et al. (1995) reported that in patients with left-hemisphere speech dominance a reduced right-ear score was always predictive of a left-hemisphere seizure focus, but that left-ear extinction can be associated with unilateral lesions in either hemisphere. A study by Niccum et al. (1983) indicated that integrity of the left posterior superior area is essential for the perception of right-ear stimuli. Strauss et al. (1985) reported that epileptic patients who showed a right-ear advantage on a verbal dichotic listening test were likely to have a wider left posterior sylvian region (as measured on carotid arteriograms). Patients who showed a left-ear advantage were more likely to have a wider right poste-

Table 12—1. Verbal Dichotic Listening: Norms for Children and Adults

Grade/Age	Sex	*n*	Right ear	Left ear	Total
Preschool					
Age 2	f	2	13.0	5.0	18.0
	m	3	12.0	2.0	14.0
Age 3	f	9	19.1	5.6	24.7
	m	5	15.3	4.8	20.0
Age 4	f	7	24.1	8.0	31.9
	m	7	25.3	9.8	35.2
Kindergarten					
Age 5	f	10	19.6	13.1	32.7
	m	9	20.2	16.9	37.1
Elementary school					
Grade 1	f	15	24.7	12.7	37.4
	m	12	26.8	16.0	42.8
Grade 2	f	29	29.0	12.4	41.3
	m	16	30.4	13.2	43.6
Grade 3	f	19	29.6	16.9	46.5
	m	11	29.1	19.2	48.3
Grade 4	f	15	32.5	16.9	48.7
	m	16	30.0	22.6	52.6
Grade 5	f	23	33.3	20.0	53.3
	m	15	31.0	20.6	51.5
Grade 6	f	12	30.5	19.6	50.1
	m	18	32.5	20.2	52.9
Adult					
Right-handers		175	M 24.95	16.23	41.18
			SD 9.60	8.30	10.12

Note: Kosaka and Kolb used the Victoria tape for adults, reversing the headphones after half of the trials.

Source: [Children's norms] Kosaka & Kolb (unpublished data, 1977); [adult right-hander norms] Strauss et al. (1987).

rior sylvian region. Roberts et al. (1990) demonstrated generally reduced DL scores in a series of 24 patients with complex partial seizures due to electrophysiological dysfunction that interfered with normal signal transmission from the left or right ear to the perisylvian language zone. The scores improved significantly after anticonvulsant medication had been instituted.

The role of the corpus callosum in dichotic listening is not clear: Reinvang et al. (1994) found reduced left-ear scores in multiple sclerosis patients with left hemisphere dominance and narrowing of the corpus callosum, pre-

sumably because of a lessening of interhemispheric transfer. Wishart et al. (1995) found in MS patients a pattern of left-sided suppression and/or right-sided enhancement, consistent with impairment of interhemispheric transfer. Lassonde and collaborators (1981, 1990) found enhanced rather than reduced lateral differences in acallosal children, and they suggested that the corpus callosum inhibits rather than promotes interhemispheric transfer. Sugishita et al. (1995) studied five patients with partial section of the corpus callosum and compared them to 50 normal controls: Patients with section of the posterior part of the corpus callosum showed no left-ear suppression, whereas those with lesions of the splenium did, suggesting that the splenium is the crucial part of the corpus callosum for transfer of auditory information. Daniel et al. (1995) compared ear preference with handedness, footedness, and eyedness in 42 dyslexic and 30 normal control Danish subjects; they found left-ear preference (but not preference for hand, foot, or eye) more often in the dyslexic group, and they considered discordance of laterality, a "noisy mismatch" between hemispheres, as an underlying cause of dyslexia.

Both total score and difference score have been investigated as a measure of stimulus processing speed (Levine et al., 1987, Saccuso et al., 1986, Strayer et al., 1987). However, there is only a moderate correlation with tests that measure similar abilities; e.g., Test D2, Trail Making, PASAT, and the right–left difference score loads on a factor separate from an information processing factor (Spellacy & Ehle, 1990).

Normative Data

Normative data are shown in Table 12–1. In general, the total score for recall on the full tape is approximately 40 words. Sex differences, suggesting a stronger left-hemisphere lateralization for males, have been reported in some experimental studies. However, a meta-analysis of 49 experiments by Hiscock et al. (1994) confirmed Bryden's (1988) conclusion that "there are sex differences in dichotic listening performance, although they are small and of marginal significance" (pp. 31–32).

The proportion of words recalled from the right ear versus the left ear is of primary interest. Failure to obtain a right-ear advantage suggests that language lateralization may not follow the normal pattern.

Normative data for children from preschool to regular kindergarten up to grade 6 (Table 12–1) suggest that children of kindergarten age already show right-ear superiority, and that right–left ear differences reach adult levels by grade 3. Overall recall scores in fact exceeded those of normal adults, possibly owing to lack of clarity of the tape used in the Strauss et al. study as well as to differences in attention. Rodriguez et al. (1990) found that the total recall score declines in normal-hearing, cognitively intact elderly adults (aged 60–85 years) for this and for a synthetic-sentence-identification/ipsilateral-competing-message test; they interpret this finding as evidence of declining central auditory processing ability without concomitant decline in peripheral hearing sensitivity and linguistic competence. Further normative studies in elderly subjects would be desirable.

DICHOTIC LISTENING: MUSIC

Purpose

The purpose of this test is to determine ear advantage for musical stimuli.

Source

The dichotic listening tape for music was developed by Spellacy (1970) in our laboratory and is available, together with instructions and recording sheets, through the Neuropsychology Laboratory, University of Victoria, Victoria, BC V8W 3P5. The price is $50 US. The original Kimura (1964) version is available from DK Consultants, 412 Duffrin Avenue, London, ON N6B 1Z6, at a cost of $160 Cdn. including digits, words, and melodies.

Description

Dichotic listening with musical stimuli was first introduced by Kimura (1964), who used commonly known melodies. Other nonverbal dichotic procedures use chords (Gordon, 1980), complex tones (Sidtis, 1981), and click stimuli (Ruff et al., 1981). We use taped (short 2-second excerpts) musical stimuli (original compositions for the violin, excerpted from the musical aptitude test by Gordon, 1965) that are synchronized for onset and offset and simultaneously presented to the two ears. Since subjects cannot be expected to repeat the stimuli by singing, each pair of musical stimuli is followed by a recognition foil; the subject merely indicates whether the foil is the same melody as one of the two just heard. This technique unfortunately requires a large number of trials (46) and hence makes the test somewhat lengthy.

Administration

The apparatus is similar to the dichotic listening words test. Care must be taken to see that the *Right* channel is coming to the *Right* ear, and the *Left* to the *Left* ear. As in the verbal test, the subject's hearing should be tested first and the earphones calibrated. Instruct the subject as follows: *"You are going to hear two pieces of music, one in each ear. After a short pause, you will hear one piece of music. I want you to tell me whether the second piece that you heard was the same as either one of the previous two, or whether it was completely different from either of the first two pieces."*

Scoring

The answer sheet consists of a sheet of paper numbered from 1 to 46; the examiner records Same or Different as the response to each trial.

Comment

Information regarding reliability and validity is not available.

We use this test only occasionally when speech and music laterlization are of importance in the assessment. DL has been used extensively in the study of patients with commissurotomy. However, the test may also be useful in patients with white matter lesions as described under DL-Words. Failure to recognize melodies correctly may also be indicative of right temporal lobe lesions (Lezak, 1995) and of amusia, but such suspicions should be checked out further using common tunes or similar material.

Normative Data

Spellacy (1970) reports means of 19.5 correct for the left ear and of 17.0 for the right ear in 32 young adults, for a total of 36.5 correct out of 48. Richardson et al. (1990) found that women show better scores than men, and that subjects older than 40 years of age perform more poorly and show a greater degree of asymmetry than younger adults.

References

Broadbent, D.E. (1958). *Perception and Communication*. Oxford: Pergamon Press.

Bruder, G.E. (1988). Dichotic listening in psychiatric patients. In K. Hugdahl (Ed.), *Handbook of Dichotic Listening: Theory, Methods, and Research*. New York: Wiley.

Bryden, M.P. (1988). An overview of the dichotic listening procedure and its relation to cerebral organization. In K. Hugdahl (Ed.), *Handbook of Dichotic Llistening: Theory, Methods and Research*. New York: Wiley.

Christianson, S.A., Saisa, J., Hugdahl, K., & Asbjornsen, A. (1992). Hemispheric asymmetry effects in children studied by dichotic listening and visual half-field testing. *Scandinavian Journal of Psychology, 33*, 238–246.

Daniel, W.F., Naeslund, J.C., & Johansen, K.V. (1995). Dyslexia and human laterality: Evidence for a dissociation between handedness and earedness. *Journal of the International Neuropsychological Society, 1*, 369 (abstract).

Geffen, G., Traub, E., & Stierman, I. (1978). Language laterality assessed by unilateral ECT and dichotic monitoring. *Journal of Neurology, Neurosurgery and Psychiatry, 41*, 354–360.

Gordon, E. (1965). *Musical Aptitude Profile*. Boston: Houghton Mifflin.

Gordon, H.W. (1980). Degree of asymmetry for perception of dichotic chords and for illusary chord localization in musicians of different levels of competence. *Journal of Experimental Psychology (Human Perception), 6*, 516–527.

Graves, R.E., & Allen, T. (1995). Utilizing the Sound Blaster 16 board for dichotic listening studies. Unpublished Manuscript, Department of Psychology, University of Victoria.

Grote, C.L., Pierre-Louis, S.J.C., Smith, M.C., Roberts, R.J., & Varney, N.R. (1995). Significance of unilateral ear extinction on the dichotic listening test. *Journal of Clinical and Experimental Neuropsychology, 17*, 1–8.

Hatta, T. (1988). Reliability of laterality effects in dichotic listening. *Psychologia—An International Journal of Psychology in the Orient, 31*, 84–90.

Hiscock, M., Inch, R., Jacek, C., Hiscock-Kalil, C., & Kalil, K. M. (1994). Is there a sex difference in human laterality? I. An exhaustive survey of laterality studies from six neuropsychology journals. *Journal of Clinical and Experimental Neuropsychology, 16,* 423–435.

Hugdahl, K., & Andersson, B. (1989). Dichotic listening in 126 left-handed children: Ear advantage, familial sinistrality and sex differences. *Neuropsychologia, 27,* 999–1006.

Jancke, L., Steinmetz, H., & Volkmann, J. (1992). Dichotic listening: What does it measure? *Neuropsychologia, 30,* 941–950.

Jerger, J., & Jerger, S. (1975). Clinical validity of central auditory tests. *Scandinavian Audiology, 4,* 147–163.

Kimura, D. (1961). Cerebral dominance and the perception of verbal stimuli. *Canadian Journal of Psychology, 15,* 166–171.

Kimura, D. (1964). Left–right differences in the perception of melodies. *Quarterly Journal of Psychology, 15,* 166–171.

Kosaka, B., & Kolb, B. (1977). Unpublished normative data.

Lake, D.A., & Bryden, M.P. (1976). Handedness and sex differences in hemispheric asymmetry. *Brain and Language, 3,* 266–282.

Lassonde, M., & Bryden, M.P. (1990). Dichotic listening, callosal agenesis and cerebral laterality. *Brain and Language, 39,* 475–481.

Lassonde, M., Lortie, J., Ptito, M., & Geoffroy, G. (1981). Hemispheric asymmetry in callosal agenesis as revealed by dichotic listening performance. *Neuropsychologia, 19,* 455–458.

Lee, G.P., Loring, D.W., Newell, J.R., & Meador, K.J. (1994). Is dichotic word listening a valid predictor of cerebral language dominance? *The Clinical Neuropsychologist, 8,* 429–438.

Levin, H.S., High, W.M., Williams, D.H., Eisenberg, H.M., Amparo, E.G., Guinto, F.C., & Ewert, J. (1989). Dichotic listening and manual performance in relation to magnetic resonance imaging after closed head injury. *Journal of Neurology, Neurosurgery, and Psychiatry, 52,* 1162–1169.

Levine, G., Preddy, D., & Thorndike, R. (1987). Speed of information processing and level of cognitive ability. *Personality and Individual Differences, 8,* 599–607.

Lezak, M. (1995). *Neuropsychological Assessment* (3rd ed.). New York: Oxford University Press.

Mohr, E., Cox, C., Williams, J., Chase, T.N., & Fedio, P. (1990). Impairment of central auditory function in Alzheimer's disease. *Journal of Clinical and Experimental Neuropsychology, 12,* 235–246.

Moore, B.D., & Papanicolaou, A.C. (1991). Dichotic listening in aphasics: Response to Niccum and Speaks. *Journal of Clinical and Experimental Neuropsychology, 14,* 641–645.

Niccum, N., Rubens, A.D., & Selnes, O.A. (1983). Dichtoic listening performance, language impairment, and lesion localization in aphasic listeners. *Journal of Speech and Hearing Research, 26,* 42–49.

Niccum, N., & Speaks, C. (1991). Interpretation of outcome on dichotic listening tests following stroke. *Journal of Clinical and Experimental Neuropsychology, 13,* 614–628.

Papanicolaou, A.C., Moore, B.D., Levin, H.S., & Eisenberg, H.M. (1987). Evoked potential correlates of right hemisphere involvement in language recovery following stroke. *Archives of Neurology, 44,* 521–524.

Pujol, J., Junque, C., Vendrell, P., Garcia, P., Capdevila, A., & Marti-Vilalta, J.L. (1991). Left-ear extinction in patients with MRI periventricular lesions. *Neuropsychologia, 29,* 177–184.

Rao, S.M., Bernadin, L., Leo, G.J., Ellington, L., Ryan, S.B., & Bung, L.S. (1989). Cerebral disconnection in multiple sclerosis: Relationship to atrophy of the corpus callosum. *Archives of Neurology, 46,* 918–920.

Reinvang, I., Bakke, S.J., Hugdahl, K., Karlsen, N.R., & Sundet, K. (1994). Dichotic listening performance in relation to callosal area on the MRI scan. *Neuropsychology, 8,* 445–450.

Richardson, E.D., Springer, J.A., Varney, N.R., Struchen, M.A., & Roberts, R.J. (1990). Dichotic listening in the clinic: New neuropsychological applications. *The Clinical Neuropsychologist, 8,* 416–428.

Riegler, J. (1980). Most comfortable loudness level of geriatric patients as a function of Seashore Loudness Discrimination scores, detection threshold, age, sex, setting, and musical background. *Journal of Music Therapy, 17,* 214–222.

Roberts, R.J., Varney, N.R., Paulsen, J.S., & Dickinson, E.D. (1990). Dichotic listening and complex partial seizures. *Journal of Clinical and Experimental Neuropsychology, 12,* 448–458.

Rodriguez, G.F., DiSarno, N.J., & Hardiman, C.J. (1990). Central auditory processing in normal-hearing elderly adults. *Audiology, 29,* 85–92.

Ruff, R.M., Hersh, N.A., & Pribram, H. (1981). Auditory spatial deficits in the personal and intrapersonal frames of reference due to cortical lesions. *Nueropsychologia, 19,* 435–443.

Saccuzzo, D., Larson, G., & Rimland, B. (1986). Visual, auditory and reaction time approaches to the measurement of speed of information processing and individual differences in intelligence. *Personality and Individual Differences, 7,* 659–667.

Sidtis, J.J. (1981). The complex tone test: Implications for the assessment of auditory laterality effects. *Neuropsychologia, 19,* 103–112.

Spellacy, F. (1970). Lateral preferences in the identification of patterned stimuli. *Journal of the Acoustical Society of America, 47,* 574–578.

Spellacy, F., & Ehle, D.L. (1990). The dichotic listening test as a measure of stimulus processing speed following mild to moderate concussion. Unpublished manuscript, University of Victoria.

Springer, J.A., Garvey, M.J., Varney, N.R., & Roberts, R.J. (1991). Dichotic listening failure in dysphoric neuropsychiatric patients who endorse multiple seizure symptoms. *Journal of Nervous and Mental Disease, 179,* 459–467.

Strauss, E. (1988). Dichotic listening and sodium amytal: Functional and morphological aspects of hemispheric asymmetry. In K. Hugdahl (Ed.), *Handbook of Dichotic Listening.* New York: Wiley.

Strauss, E., Gaddes, W.H., & Wada, J. (1987). Performance on a free-recall verbal dichotic listening task and cerebral dominance determined by the carotid amytal test. *Neuropsychologia, 25,* 747–753.

Strauss, E., Lapointe, J.S., Wada, J.A., Gaddes, W., & Kosaka, B. (1985). Language dominance: Correlation of radiological and functional data. *Neuropsychologia, 23,* 415–420.

Strayer, D., Wickens, C., & Braune, R. (1987). Adult age differences in the speed and capacity of information processing: 2. An electrophysiological approach. *Psychology and Aging, 2,* 99–110.

Sugishita, M., Otomo, K., Yamasaki, K., & Yoshioka, M. (1995). Dichotic listening in patients with partial section of the corpus callosum. *Brain, 118,* 417–427.

Varney, N.R., Campbell, D., & Roberts, R.J. (1994). Long-term neuropsychological sequelae of fever associated with amnesia. *Archives of Clinical Neuropsychology, 9,* 347–352.

Wexler, B.E., & Halwes, R.K. (1983). Increasing power of dichotic methods: The fused rhymed words test. *Neuropsychologia, 21,* 59–66.

Wishart, H.A., Strauss, E., Hunter, M., & Moll, A. (1995). Interhemispheric transfer in multiple sclerosis. *Journal of Clinical and Experimental Neuropsychology, 17,* 937–940.

DEVELOPMENTAL TEST OF VISUAL-MOTOR INTEGRATION (VMI)

Other Test Name

This test is also called the Beery Test.

Source

The manual and 25 booklets each of the long and short forms of the 1989 version of this test can be ordered from Pro-Ed, 8700 Shoal Creek Blvd., Austin, TX 78757-6897, for $169 US; or from M.D. Angus Assoc., 2639 Kingsway Ave., Port Coquitlam, B.C., Canada, V3C 1T5, for $190 Cdn.

Description

This copying test (Beery, 1967; Beery & Buktenica, 1967) was restandardized in 1982; the 1989 edition introduced a new scoring system; the 1997 edition provides new norms representative of the U.S. census. The VMI was adopted as part of the Florida Kindergarten Screening Battery (Fletcher & Satz, 1982). It was originally modeled after the visual perception test of Frostig et al. (1966) and was designed primarily for the child of preschool and elementary school age. It is similar to the Bender-Gestalt Test or the copying form of the Benton Visual Retention Test, but it presents the geometric designs to be copied in clearly delineated squares of space equal to the original; moreover, the 24 designs are intended to follow a developmental gradient of difficulty starting with a vertical line for 2-year-olds and progressing to three-dimensional cube and star designs for 14- and 15-year-olds. The long form allows testing up to age 14 years 11 months and, according to the author, retains validity for older age groups and adults (Beery, 1982). The short form includes the first 15 designs for children ages 2–8 years.

Administration

See source. Briefly, the subject is asked: *"Make one like that,"* and *"Make yours right here"* (i.e., in the square below the stimulus figure). The test is discontinued after three consecutive failures. There are no time limits or time scores. Group administration is possible, although in that case discontinuation rules cannot be applied.

Approximate Time for Administration

About 15–20 minutes are required for this test.

Scoring

The 1989 manual provides explicit scoring criteria and examples of acceptable and unacceptable responses together with a number of "developmental comments" on typical drawings in children of different age levels. "Lenient" scoring is recommended; that is, when in doubt about the correctness of an individual drawing, credit should be given. The raw score for the original test was obtained by counting the number of acceptable drawings up to the discontinuation of the test (Maximum: 24 points). The 1989 manual expands the scoring to 1 to 4 points for the items for older children with a maximum of 50 points. However, virtually all published research still uses the old 24-point scoring system.

The raw score can be converted into an age-equivalent score, a percentile, and a standard score by use of the tables in the manual. Consultation of tables in the source based on a restandardization (Beery, 1989) is recommended. Scoring requires some training. The test author's comment that scoring can be done by classroom teachers with minimal training has been criticized (Pryzwansky, 1977), but other studies confirm good interrater reliability ($>.90$) both in experienced raters and teachers with no experience with the test (Lepkin & Pryzwansky, 1983).

Comment

Interrater reliability for the original form has been reported to range from .58 to .99, with a median of .93 across a number of studies (Cosden, 1985). Retest reliability ranges from .63 after 7 months to .92 after 2 weeks, and split-half reliability was .74 (Ryckman & Rentfrow, 1971) for various populations, whereas the test manual reports a median split-half reliability of .78.

An item analysis by Abbatiello and Kpo (1988), based on data from 1,940 normal school children between the ages of 6 and 17 years, found that items did not show the expected gradual increase of difficulty: rather, two clusters of items with similar levels of difficulty were found, with a large gap between clusters, mainly due to the change from two-dimensional to three-dimensional drawings. The authors also noted a ceiling effect at age 12 and questioned the test's utility in older children. The 50-point scoring system introduced in 1989 remedies some of these problems. Shapiro and Simpson (1994) report that the three-dimensional scores showed good sensitivity to visuomotor development in emotionally and behaviorally disturbed adolescents between age 12 years and 17 years 11 months; these scores also correlated with cognitive ability subtests, accounting for 57 percent of the variance.

The validity studies with the VMI focus on correlations with the Bender Gestalt test and the predictive validity for academic success. Correlations with the Bender Gestalt test range from .79 in mentally handicapped males (Liemohn & Wagner, 1975), to .74 for learning-disabled students, to .36 for normal students (Armstrong & Knopf, 1982; Breen, 1982). The VMI tends to produce somewhat lower age-equivalent scores (7 months) than the Bender, although this may be a function of the relatively low ceiling (11 years) of the Bender compared to the Beery, which is presumed to provide challenging items up to age 15. However, Breen (1982) reported no differences in mean scores between the two tests in emotionally disturbed boys between ages 5 years 9 months and 12 years 1 month, and with learning-disabled children (Spirito, 1980). Spirito also found significant correlations between the two tests only up to age 9, but not for 9- to 11-year-olds. Porter and Binder (1981) found a correlation of .62 between the two tests in a 9- to 12-year-old clinic sample, and they suggest that, though sharing some common variance, the two tests measure different constructs of visual-motor development. A similar conclusion is reached by DeMers and Wright (1981), who compared results with the two tests in mentally retarded children. The test also correlated (.60) with the WPPSI-R geometric design subtest (Aylward & Schmidt, 1986).

As part of the Florida Kindergarten Screening Battery, the VMI, given at kindergarten age, predicted school achievement in grade 5 (Gates, 1984). Whereas one study did not find good prediction in grade 2 (Flynn & Flynn, 1978), another study confirmed good predictive validity for a cohort of 299 school children (LaTorre, 1985). Prediction of school achievement on the basis of the VMI alone has been poor (Duffy et al., 1976) or moderate (Klein, 1978; Reynolds et al., 1980); correlation with school achievement has been reported as .65 (Curtis et al., 1979). Richardson et al. (1980) suggested that the VMI is more closely correlated with the Wechsler Intelligence Scale for Children (WISC) IQ than with achievement tests such as the Wide Range Achievement Test (WRAT). In this study, the VMI did not contribute significantly to the prediction of achievement when the WISC-IQ had been partialed out. It also still remains to be clarified whether the VMI is more related to achievement in arithmetic, language skills, or spelling. Studies by Ysseldyke et al. (1981) suggest that the test loads most strongly on an arithmetic and a reasoning factor and predicts composite achievement scores (Colarusso et al., 1980).

The test discriminated between normal children and children with visual-perceptual dysfunction referred to an optometric clinic (Wesson & Kispart, 1986). A significant impairment was also found in hydrocephalic children with spina bifida whose intelligence was not in the retarded range (Holler et al., 1995). The performance of physically handicapped children on the Beery is likely to be impaired (Zeitschel et al., 1979). A useful chapter on remediation is included in the test manual.

In the context of a neuropsychological evaluation, the VMI would seem to be particularly useful for the exploration of visual-perceptual and motor skills in children, especially those with learning disabilities, but also those with other neuropsychological deficits, although studies of such populations are not available. Use with very young children (ages 2–3 years)

may be questionable since only three items cover the development during this age span. Use with adult patients may be appropriate, but in the absence of norms, especially for elderly subjects, any deviation from near-perfect scores (raw scores of 23 or 24 are expected for children 14 years 11 months old) may have to be considered as an indication of deficit. Hall et al. (1996) found the test sensitive to aging effects, and one study applied the VMI to elderly patients (mean age 74 years) with vascular dementia and dementia of the Alzheimer type (Barr et al., 1992). Mean scores for vascular dementia ($n = 31$) were 13.2 (SD = 4.9) and for Alzheimers disease 11.9 (SD = 5.4). The test did not significantly contribute to the discrimination between the two patient groups, but the results suggest that the VMI may be sensitive to dementia generally.

Normative Data

The restandardization (Beery, 1982) is based on 3,090 children, stratified according to the 1980 U.S. census with respect to ethnic origin, income, residence, and sex, and seems to eliminate problems of ethnic and socioeconomic distribution of normative data raised for the original (1969) edition. It provides norms for ages 2 years 11 months through 14 years 6 months. No sex differences were found. The new edition (Beery, 1997) provides further updated norms.

Norms for older adolescents and adults are not available. The author (Beery, 1982) suggests, however, that for practical purposes the norms for 13- and 14-year-olds can be used for older age groups.

References

Abbatiello, A., & Kpo, W. (1988). Test of visuomotor integration: Evaluation of test effectiveness for practitioners. *Special Services in the Schools, 5,* 77–88.

Armstrong, B.B., & Knopf, K.F. (1982). Comparison of the Bender-Gestalt and Revised Developmental Test of Visual-Motor Integration. *Perceptual and Motor Skills, 56,* 164–166.

Aylward, E.H., & Schmidt, S. (1986). An examination of three tests of visuomotor integration. *Journal of Learning Disabilities, 19,* 328–330.

Barr, A., Benedict, R., Tune, L., & Brandt, J. (1992). Neuropsychological differentiation of Alzheimer's disease from vascular dementia. *International Journal of Geriatric Psychiatry, 7,* 621–627.

Beery, K.E. (1967). *Developmental Test of Visual-Motor Integration.* Administration and Scoring Manual. Chicago: Follett Publishing Company.

Beery, K.E. (1982). *Revised Administration, Scoring, and Teaching Manual for the Developmental Test of Visual-Motor Integration.* Cleveland: Modern Curriculum Press.

Beery, K.E. (1989). *The Visual-Motor Integration Test. Administration, Scoring, and Teaching Manual.* Cleveland: Modern Curriculum Press.

Beery, K.E. (1997). *The Visual-Motor Integration Test* (4th ed.). *Administration, Scoring, and Teaching Manual.* Austin, TX: Pro-Ed.

Beery, K.E., & Buktenica, N.A. (1967). *Developmental Test of Visual-Motor Integration.* Student Test Booklet. Chicago: Follett Publishing Co.

Breen, M.J. (1982). Comparison of educationally handicapped students' scores on the Revised Developmental Test of Visual-Motor Integration and Bender Gestalt. *Perceptual and Motor Skills, 54,* 1227–1230.

Colarusso, R., Gill, S., Plankenhorn, A., & Brooks, R. (1980). Predicting first-grade achievement through formal testing of 5-year-old high-risk children. *Journal of Special Education, 14,* 355–363.

Cosden, M. (1985). Developmental Test of Visual-Motor Integration. In D.J. Keyser & R.C. Sweetland (Eds.), *Test Critiques.* Vol. IV, pp. 229–237. Kansas City: Test Corporation of America.

Curtis, C.J., Michael, J.J., & Michael, W.B. (1979). The predictive validity of the Developmental Test of Visual-Motor Integration under group and individual modes of administration relative to academic performance measures of second-grade pupils without identifiable major learning disabilities. *Educational and Psychological Measurement, 39,* 401–410.

DeMers, S.T., & Wright, D. (1981). Comparison of scores on two visual-motor tests for children referred for learning or adjustment difficulties. *Perceptual and Motor Skills, 53,* 863–867.

Duffy, J.B., Ritter, D.R., & Fedner, M. (1976). Developmental Test of Visual-Motor Integration and the Goodenough Draw-A-Man Test as predictors of academic success. *Perceptual and Motor Skills, 43,* 543–546.

Fletcher, J.M., & Satz, P. (1982). Kindergarten prediction of reading achievement: A seven-year longitudinal follow-up. *Educational and Psychological Measurement, 39,* 681–685.

Flynn, T.M., & Flynn, L.A. (1978). Evaluation of the predictive ability of five screening measures administered during kindergarten. *Journal of Experimental Education, 46,* 65–70.

Frostig, M., Lefever, D.W., & Whittlesey, J.R.B. (1966). *Administration and Scoring Manual for the Frostig Developmental Test of Visual Perception.* Palo Alto, CA: Consulting Psychologists Press.

Gates, R.D. (1984). Florida Kindergarten Screening Battery. *Journal of Clinical Neuropsychology, 6,* 459–465.

Hall, S., Pinkston, S.L., Szalda-Petree, A.C., & Coronis, A.R. (1996). The performance of healthy older adults on the Continuous Visual Memory Test and the Visual-Motor Integration Test: Preliminary findings. *Journal of Clinical Psychology, 52,* 449–454.

Holler, K.A., Fennell, E.B., Crosson, B., Boggs, S.R., & Mickle, J.P. (1995). Neuropsychological and adaptive functioning in younger versus older children shunted for early hydrocephalus. *Child Neuropsychology, 1,* 63–73.

Klein, A.E. (1978). The validity of the Beery Test of Visual-Motor Integration in predicting achievement in kindergarten, first, and second grade. *Educational and Psychological Measurement, 38,* 457–461.

LaTorre, R.A. (1985). Kindergarten screening: A cross-validation of the Florida Kindergarten Screening Battery. *Alberta Journal of Educational Research, 31,* 174–190.

Lepkin, S.R., & Pryzwansky, W. (1983). Interrater reliability of the original and the revised scoring system for the Developmental Test of Visual-Motor Integration. *Psychology in the Schools, 20,* 284–288.

Liemohn, W., & Wagner, P. (1975). Motor and perceptual determinants of performance on the Bender-Gestalt and the Beery Developmental Scale by retarded males. *Perceptual and Motor Skills, 40,* 524–526.

Porter, G.L., & Binder, D.M. (1981). A pilot study of visual-motor developmental inter-test reliability: The Beery Developmental Test of Visual-Motor Integration and the Bender Visual Motor Gestalt Test. *Journal of Learning Disabilities, 14,* 124–127.

Pryzwansky, W.B. (1977). The use of the Developmental Test of Visual-Motor Integration as a group screening instrument. *Psychology in the Schools, 14,* 419–422.

Reynolds, C.R., Wright, D., & Wilkinson, W.A. (1980). Incremental validity of the test for Auditory Comprehension of Language and the Developmental Test of Visual-Motor Integration. *Educational and Psychological Measurement, 40*, 503–507.

Richardson, E., DiBenedetto, B., Christ, A., & Press, M. (1980). Relationship of auditory and visual skills to reading retardation. *Journal of Learning Disabilities, 13*, 77–82.

Ryckman, D.B., & Rentfrow, R.K. (1971). The Beery Developmental Test of Visual-Motor Integration: An investigation of reliability. *Journal of Learning Disabilities, 4*, 333–334.

Shapiro, S.K., & Simpson, R.G. (1994). Patterns and predictors of performance on the Bender-Gestalt and the Developmental test of Visual-Motor Integration in a sample of behaviorally and emotionally disturbed adolescents. *Journal of Psychoeducational Assessment, 12*, 254–263.

Spirito, A. (1980). Scores on Bender-Gestalt and Developmental Test of Visuo-Motor Integration of learning-disabled children. *Perceptual and Motor Skills, 50*, 1214.

Wesson, M.D., & Kispert, C. (1986). The relationship between the test for Visual Analysis Skills (TVAS) and standardized visual-motor tests in children with visual perception difficulties. *Journal of the American Optometric Association, 57*, 844–849.

Ysseldyke, J.E., Algozzine, B., & Shinn, M. (1981). Validity of the Woodcock-Johnson Psychoeducational Battery for learning disabled youngsters. *Learning Disability Quarterly, 4*, 244–249.

Zeitschel, K.A., Kalish, R.A., & Colarusso, R. (1979). Visual perception tests used with physically handicapped children. *Academic Therapy, 14*, 565–576.

EMBEDDED FIGURES TEST

Other Test Names

This test is also called the Hidden Figures Test and the Figure-Ground Test.

Purpose

The purpose of the test is to examine visual search and tracing of figures embedded in the background.

Source

The test (manual, 20 forms, 20 answer sheets) can be obtained from the Neuropsychology Laboratory, University of Victoria, Victoria, BC V8W 3P5, at a cost of approximately $75 Cdn. Twenty forms for left-handers cost $35 Cdn. A different version by Witkin is available from Consulting Psychologists Press, Palo Alto, CA and the Ontario Institute for Studies in Education, 712 Gordon Baker Road, Toronto, ON M2H 3R7, for $93 Cdn. (which also distributes children and group administration forms). A similar test is also included as a subtest of the Test of Visual-Perceptual Skills, described elsewhere in this volume.

Description

Experimental versions of this test have been in use since 1960. The test (Spreen & Benton, 1969) consists of 16 straight-line drawings used as stimulus figures and presented in the left half of 5½ × 8½ inch sheets of paper assembled in a test booklet. The right half of each sheet contains a complex figure drawing in which the stimulus figure is embedded. Subjects are required to search for and trace the stimulus figure in the embedded design. An ordinary soft pencil is used for the tracings. The test is preceded by two demonstration items.

For left-handed subjects, placement of stimulus figure and embedded design is reversed; that is, the stimulus figure is shown in the right half and the embedded design in the left half of the test booklet. An equivalent parallel form of this test, Form B, is also available.

Administration

Show the subject the first demonstration item and say: *"Do you see this figure, this shape?"* (pointing to stimulus figure). *You can find it in this larger figure"* (point to embedded design). Trace the stimulus figure in the embedded design with firm strokes so that the outline is clearly visible. *"Now let us look at another one* (expose second demonstration item). *You draw this figure in the larger figure."* If the subject draws correctly, tell the subject: *"That's right."* If the subject draws the figure too lightly, have him or her go over it and say: *"Draw it darker. Press down with your pencil."* If the subject fails to trace the figure correctly, say: *"No, that is not quite right. Let me show you* (draw the embedded figure). *See, this figure is just like the one over here."*

Other, more detailed instructions or demonstrations are permissible if the subject fails to understand the task.

The test items are then presented individually with the instruction *"Now do this one."* Begin timing after presentation of each stimulus figure and record the time needed to complete the item in seconds. If the subject has not started to draw within 20 seconds after the presentation of an item, turn the page in the booklet to expose the next item. If the subject has begun drawing, allow him or her to finish and record the time.

After the subject finishes an item, present the next design with the appropriate instructions. Avoid commenting on the subject's performance, except for noncommittal remarks (*"All right, let's try the next one"*).

Discontinue after five consecutive failures to draw the designs correctly.

Approximate Time for Administration

The test requires approximately 5–15 minutes.

Scoring

One point is given for every design correctly completed within 30 seconds (Point score). One additional point is given if the design is completed within 20 seconds (Credit points). Maximum score for all 16 items is 16 points; maximum credit score is 32 points.

No credit is given for incorrect reproductions or for correct tracings not completed within 30 seconds. All parts of the stimulus figure have to be traced correctly in the embedded design. Poor drawing (rounded corners, sloppiness in tracing, incomplete con-nections between lines) are disregarded if the stimulus figure is clearly recognizable.

Special scoring rules are as follows: Design 11 is scored as correct if the K-figure is repeated. Design 15 is scored as correct if the squares are drawn with interrupted lines (as in the stimulus figure).

Comment

Embedded (or "hidden") figures have been used in many experimental studies since the time of Gottschaldt (1928). Their clinical use goes back to Poppelreuter's (1917) overlapping figures test. Some tests use shading, grids, or strong distractor figures as overlay or masking. Similar abilities are required by incomplete figures (visual closure), described by Thurstone (1944). The figures by Witkin et al. (1971) have been used in studies of "cognitive style": i.e., field dependence and independence. Witkin's test does not involve drawing, but tracing with the finger, and timed performance. The simple form is exposed for 15 seconds and then taken away, but may be shown again. Two forms with 12 items each and a simplified version for children 10 and younger are available. Reliability coefficients were between .9 and .61. No studies with neurological patients have been conducted with the Witkin test, but schizophrenics, asthmatic children, diabetics, alcoholics, enuretics, patients with borderline personality disorder (O'Leary et al., 1991), and obsessive-compulsives have been shown to have stronger field dependence. However, in recent studies, the relationship with ability level has been shown to be stronger than with cognitive style (Widiger et al., 1980). Other tests have been published by Ayres (1966), Coates (1972), Mahlios and D'Angelo (1983), Thompson and Melancon (1987), and Talland (1965), all designed primarily for children of preschool and school age.

Odd–even reliability and retest reliability for most tests, including the EFT described here, are usually reported as high (r = .90). Validity studies suggest that patients with right-hemisphere lesions do more poorly than patients with left-hemisphere lesions on tests

Table 12—2. Embedded Figures Test: Normative Data for Adults

Age groups	n	Total correct		Total credit	
		M	SD	M	SD
16–20	10	15.3	1.0	30.4	2.1
20–29	23	14.5	1.0	31.78	0.85
30–39	14	15.7	1.0	31.64	0.74
40–49	14	14.1	1.0	31.14	1.46
50–59	10	15.4	0.9	31.60	0.80
60–69	10	14.5	0.8	30.30	2.50
70–79	14	15.5	0.5	30.36	2.41

Source: Spreen & Benton, 1969.

of this type (De Renzi & Spinnler, 1966). Patients with anterior lesions do better than those with posterior lesions if no time limit is imposed (Egelko et al., 1988; Masure & Tzavaras, 1976), although most patients with brain damage have some difficulty with the test, depending on the size of lesion (Corkin, 1979). This is confirmed in our own data where a mixed group of brain-damaged patients at all age levels was significantly inferior to normal subjects (average score 3 points, 6 credit points below normals); this was even more pro-

Table 12—3. Embedded Figures Test: Normative Data for Children (in Percentiles)

	Percentiles										
	0	10	20	30	40	50	60	70	80	90	100
Age 6 (Max. score = 16)	1–4	5–6	7	8	9	10	11	12	13–14	15–16	
Age 7 (Max. score = 16)	1–4	5–6	7	8	9	10	11	12	13–14	15–16	
Age 8 (Max. score = 16)	1–9	10	11	12		13		14	15	16	
(Max. credit = 32)	0–16	17–18	19–20	21	22–23	24	25	26	27–28	29–30	
Age 9 (Max. score = 16)	1–9	10	11	12		13		14	15	16	
(Max. credit = 32)	0–16	17–18	19–20	21	22–23	24	25	26	27–28	29–32	
Age 10 (Max. score = 16)	1–10	11	12		13	14		15	16		
(Max. credit = 32)	1–19	20–21	22–23	24	25	26–27	28–29	30–31	32		
Age 11 (Max. score = 16)	1–10	11	12		13	14		15	16		
(Max. credit = 32)	1–19	20–21	22–23	24	25	26–27	28–29	30–31	32		
Age 12 (Max. score = 16)				questionable < 15 > normal							
(Max. credit = 32)				questionable < 30 > normal							
Age 13 (Max. score = 16)				questionable < 15 > normal							
(Max. credit = 32)				questionable < 30 > normal							

Source: Spreen & Gaddes (1969).

Note: Credit scores are not calculated below age 9.

nounced in the older (60+) age group where the differences between brain-damaged and normal performance reached 6–9 points. Sala et al. (1995) also found significant impairment in patients with AD and with right-hemisphere lesions.

The test does not discriminate between mentally retarded children with and without demonstrated brain damage (Horne & Justiss, 1967).

Normative Data

Healthy adults make very few errors on this test, as indicated in Table 12–2. The idea that older adults tend to make more errors ("return to field dependence," Witkin et al., 1971) is not supported by our preliminary normative data for this test. Differences between males and females are negligible. Fogliani and Messina (1983) also found no significant sex difference for the Witkin test in older subjects (60–74 years). Sala et al. (1995) found a significant influence of age and education, but not sex, in an investigation of 237 healthy Italian adults with a Poppelreuter-Ghent version of the test. Mahlios and D'Angelo (1983) also found no sex differences in 10- to 12-year-old children.

The rapid progression both in correct solutions and in time credits in children (Spreen & Gaddes, 1969) is discernible from Table 12–3. Differences between males and females are negligible. Deegener (1981) reports a strong relationship to IQ and a minor effect of visual acuity on a similar test in a population of 5-year-olds.

References

Ayres, A.J. (1966). *Southern California Figure-Ground Visual Perception Test*. Manual. Los Angeles: Western Psychological Services.

Coates, S.W. (1972). *Preschool Embedded Figures Test*. Manual. Palo Alto, CA: Consulting Psychologists Press.

Corkin, S. (1979). Hidden-Figures-Test performance: Lasting effects of unilateral penetrating head injury and transient effects of bilateral cingulotomy. *Neuropsychologia, 17*, 585–605.

Deegener, G. (1981). Ergebnisse mit dem Preschool Embedded Figures Test bei fünfjährigen deutschen Kindergartenkindern. *Praxis der Kin-*

derpsychologie und Kinderpsychiatrie, 30, 144–150.

De Renzi, E., & Spinnler, H. (1966). Visual recognition in patients with unilateral cerebral disease. *Journal of Nervous and Mental Disease, 142*, 515–525.

Egelko, S., Gordon, W.A., Hibbard, M.R., Diller, L., Lieberman, A., Holliday, R., Ragnarson, K., Shaver, M.S., & Orazem, J. (1988). Relationship among CT scans, neurological exam, and neuropsychological test performance in right-brain-damaged stroke patients. *Journal of Clinical and Experimental Neuropsychology, 10*, 539–564.

Fogliani, F., & Messina, D. (1983). Embedded figures test in old age, a psychometric note. *Perceptual and Motor Skills, 56*, 284–286.

Gottschaldt, K. (1928). Über den Einfluss der Erfahrung auf die Wahrnehmung von Figuren. *Psychologische Forschung, 8*, 18–317.

Horne, B.M., & Justiss, W.A. (1967). Clinical indicators of brain damage in mentally retarded children. *Journal of Clinical Psychology, 23*, 464–465.

Mahlios, M.C., & D'Angelo, K. (1983). Group embedded figures test: Psychometric data on children. *Perceptual and Motor Skills, 56*, 423–426.

Masure, M.C., & Tzavaras, A. (1976). Perception de figures entrecroisées par des sujets atteints de lésions corticales unilaterales. *Neuropsychologia, 14*, 371–374.

O'Leary, K.M., Browers, P., Gardner, D.L., & Cowdry, R.W. (1991). Neuropsychological testing of patients with borderline personality disorder. *American Journal of Psychiatry, 148*, 106–111.

Poppelreuter, W. (1917). *Die psychischen Schädigungen durch Kopfschuss im Kriege 1914/18*. Leipzig: Leopold Voss.

Sala, S.D., Laiacona, M., Trivelli, C., & Spinnler, H. (1995). Poppelreuter-Ghent Overlapping Figures Test: Its sensitivity to age, and its clinical use. *Archives of Clinical Neuropsychology, 10*, 511–534.

Spreen, O., & Benton, A.L. (1969). Embedded Figures Test. Neuropsychological Laboratory, University of Victoria, Victoria, BC.

Spreen, O., & Gaddes, W.H. (1969). Developmental norms for 15 neuropsychological tests age 6 to 15. *Cortex, 5*, 171–191.

Talland, G.A. (1965). *Deranged Memory*. New York: Academic Press.

Thompson, B., & Melancon, J.G. (1987). *Finding Embedded Figures Test*. New Orleans, LA: Psychometrics Group.

Thurstone, L.L. (1944). *A Factorial Study of Per-*

ception. Chicago, IL: University of Chicago Press.

Widiger, T.A., Knudson, R.M., & Rorer, L.G. (1980). Convergent and discriminant validity of measures of cognitive style and abilities. *Journal of Personality and Social Psychology, 39,* 116–129.

Witkin, H.A., Oltman, P.K., Raskin, E., & Karp, S.A. (1971). *A Manual for the Embedded Figures Test.* Palo Alto, CA: Consulting Psychologists Press.

FACIAL RECOGNITION TEST

Purpose

The purpose of this test is to assess the ability to recognize unfamiliar human faces.

Source

The test can be ordered from Oxford University Press, 2001 Evans Rd., Cary, NC, at a cost of $45 US. The manual (which includes 11 other tests) costs $23.95 US.

Description

The test (Benton et al., 1994), developed by Benton and Van Allen (1968), requires the subject to discriminate photographs of unfamiliar human faces. Clothing and hair are shaded out so that only facial features can be used. The full test ("Long Form") consists of 54 items, the Short Form (for use as a brief screening of face recognition; Levin et al., 1975) of 27 items. The test consists of three parts:

1. *Matching of identical front-view photographs.* The subject is presented with a single front-view photograph of a face and is instructed to identify it (by pointing to it or calling its number) in a display of six front-view photographs appearing below the single photograph. In both the short and the long version of the test, three male and three female faces are presented for matching, calling for a total of six responses.

2. *Matching of front-view with three-quarter-view photographs.* The subject is presented with a single front-view photograph of a face and is instructed to locate it three times in a display of six three-quarter views, three being of the presented face and three being of other faces. In the Long Form of the test, four male and four female faces are presented for matching, calling for a total of 24 responses. In the Short Form, one male face and three female faces are presented, calling for a total of 12 responses.

3. *Matching of front-view photographs under different lighting conditions.* The subject is presented with a single front-view photograph of a face taken under full lighting conditions and is instructed to locate it three times in a display of six front views taken under different lighting conditions; three photographs in the display are of the presented face and three are of other faces. In the Long Form, four male and four female faces are presented for matching, calling for a total of 24 responses. In the Short Form, two male faces and one female face are presented, calling for a total of nine responses.

Administration

See source. Intact vision is important for this test. Kempen et al. (1994) reported significantly poorer scores on this test with patients whose Jaeger near-vision was J5 (equivalent to 20/50) or worse due to refractory error, as compared to subjects with normal vision. For this reason, a standard vision test should be administered before an interpretation of the results is attempted.

The test is assembled in a spiral-bound booklet. Each stimulus picture and its corresponding response choices are presented in two facing pages with the single stimulus picture above the six response-choice pictures ("*You see this woman? Show me where she is on this picture*"). If they are able to do so, subjects are encouraged to hold and manipulate the test material to their best visual advantage.

The test is arranged so that the first 13 stimulus and response display pictures, which comprise the Short Form, are presented first.

Following this is a page that identifies the remaining items of the 54 items of the Long Form.

Scoring

Record correct responses by checking the appropriate item; record errors by circling the appropriate numbers on the right side of the record form. Each correct response is assigned a score of one. A minimum score of 25 may be expected on the basis of chance alone. Hence the effective range of Long Form scores may be considered to be 25–54. For the Short Form, the effective range may be considered to be 11–27 points.

Utilization of the record sheet will facilitate recording and scoring. If the Short Form is used, the number of correct responses on the record sheet needs to be converted to Long Form scores following a conversion table in the manual. The test manual also provides age and education corrections for the Long Form and the converted Short Form scores.

Comment

Test–retest reliability after one year in elderly controls has been reported as .60 (Levin et al., 1991); correlations between Long and Short Form range from .88 in normals to .92 in brain-damaged subjects (Benton et al., 1994). Internal consistency (coefficient alpha) in 206 undergraduates was only .57 (Hoptman & Davidson, 1993); however, the authors recalculated the coefficient omitting the first six pages of the test (identity matches) as .66.

Although the inability to recognize familiar faces (prosopagnosia) has been recognized for some time as a special form of agnosia, standardized tests have not been available so far. The use of unfamiliar faces (as opposed to faces of actors or public figures, Warrington & James, 1967) eliminates the long-term memory component and the need for name finding, but it changes the nature of the task to a primarily perceptual one. Benton et al. (1994) also warn that patients with serious difficulties in the recognition of unfamiliar faces may well be able to recognize familiar faces since cases of true prosopagnosia are rare. The dissocia-

tion of these two abilities may suggest separate loci of brain damage (Benton & Van Allen, 1972; Benton, 1980, 1994). The test is sensitive to right parietal lobe damage, and, to a lesser extent, right temporal lobe damage (Dricker et al., 1978; Hamsher et al., 1979). Recent studies with cerebral blood flow and positron emission tomography in normal subjects have indicated the importance of the right inferior occipito-temporal region for face recognition (Haxby et al., 1991). Egelko et al. (1988) also report scores in the lowest percentile range for right-hemisphere stroke patients. The correlation between hemianopic field cut and face recognition was .49. The computed tomography (CT) scan damage correlated highest with face-recognition performance if the damage was in the right parietal area. Trahan (1997) found that 53 percent of 85 patients with right-hemisphere CVA were impaired on the Face Recognition Test (FRT), as opposed to only 27 percent of 45 patients with left-hemisphere CVA. In particular, patients with left visual neglect showed impaired FRT scores. Vilkki and Laitinen (1976) reported serious deficits in face recognition after right thalamotomy. Some patients with left anterior and posterior lesions and with aphasia and comprehension deficits also do poorly on this test, suggesting that the test relies on linguistic functions to some extent (Hamsher et al., 1979). Tzavaras et al. (1970) found face recognition deficits also in patients with spatial agnosia, dyslexia, and dysgraphia. Impaired performance on this test has also been reported for children with hemispherectomy regardless of the side of removal (Strauss & Verity, 1983), in patients with Parkinson's disease (Bentin et al., 1981; Hovestadt et al., 1987), and in patients with severe closed-head injury (Levin et al., 1977). This was confirmed in a study of 128 head-injured patients by Risser and Andrikopoulos (1997) for severe head injury with post-traumatic dementia, although patients without dementia performed within the lower range of normal limits. Patients with mild head injury and psychiatric patients scored within the normal range. Similarly, Peck et al. (1992) found mean scores in the "low average" range for 107 patients with mild, moderate, and severe head injury, both

Table 12—4. Benton Test of Face Recognition: Normative Standards after Correction for Age and Education

Corrected score	Percentile rank	Classification
53–54	98+	very superior
50–52	88–97	superior
47–49	72–85	high average
43–46	33–59	average
41–42	16–21	low average
39–40	8–11	borderline
37–38	3–6	defective
<37	1	severely defective

Source: Benton et al. (1983).

Table 12—5. Normative Data for Children with Normal Intelligence (IQ 85 to 116)

Age	n	Long Form mean
6	22	33.0
7	59	37.2
8	33	37.6
9	27	38.1
10	50	40.6
11	33	41.3
12	—	—
13	23	43.0
14	19	45.1

Source: Benton et al., 1994.

during and after the first year post-injury. A study of 42 AD patients, matched with 37 controls for overall level of performance found that matching of front-view with three-quarter view photographs provided the best discrimination between groups. This task appears to require the ideal level of performance for this group (Andrikopoulos, 1997).

Whereas Levin and Benton (1977) reported that face recognition scores in psychiatric patients were indistinguishable from those of normal subjects, Echternacht (1986) found more defective scores in such patients and in a matched chronic psychiatric inpatient group than would be expected in normal subjects, but less than would be expected from specific brain-damaged populations. Hence, impaired performance on this test should not be interpreted, in and of itself, as evidence of neurological disturbance.

Normative Data

Benton et al. (1994) provide score distributions for 286 normal adults with age and education correction. Test performance in old age showed some decline (Benton et al., 1981). Mittenberg et al. (1989) report a correlation of −.25 with age in normal control subjects 20–75 years of age. Table 12–4 provides a guide for test score interpretation in adults. The mean of 45.6 for 206 undergraduates reported by Hoptman and Davidson (1993) fits well into this distribution. The mean for 115 normal Italian adults was 46.2 (Ferracuti & Ferracuti, 1992), and the mean for 94 inner-city African-

Americans was 44.7 (Roberts & Hamsher, 1984), suggesting that the test is relatively independent from ethnic-cultural factors. Gilbert (1973) reported somewhat lower scores for weakly left-handed compared to strongly right- or left-handed persons. Norms for children with average intelligence indicate a gradual improvement of face recognition ability from age 6 (mean = 33 correct) to age 14 (mean = 45 correct) when adult performance level is reached (Table 12–5).

References

Andrikopoulos, J. (1997). Qualitative facial recognition test performance in Alzheimer's disease. *Archives of Clinical Neuropsychology, 12,* 282 (abstract).

Bentin, S., Silverberg, R., & Gordon, H.W. (1980). Asymmetrical cognitive deterioration in demented and Parkinsonian patients. *Cortex, 17,* 533–544.

Benton, A.L. (1980). The neuropsychology of facial recognition. *American Psychologist, 35,* 176–186.

Benton, A.L. (1994). Neuropsychological assessment. *Annual Review of Psychology, 45,* 1–23.

Benton, A.L., Eslinger, P.J., & Damasio, A.R. (1981). Normative observations on neuropsychological test performances in old age. *Journal of Clinical Neuropsychology, 3,* 33–42.

Benton, A.L., Sivan, A.B., Hamsher, K. de S., Varney, N.R., & Spreen, O. (1994). *Contributions to Neuropsychological Assessment. A Clinical Manual* (2nd ed.). New York: Oxford University Press.

Benton, A.L., & Van Allen, M.W. (1968). Impairment in facial recognition in patients with cerebral disease. *Cortex, 4,* 344–358.

Benton, A.L., & Van Allen, M.W. (1972). Prosopagnosia and facial discrimination. *Journal of the Neurological Sciences, 15,* 167–172.

Dricker, J., Butters, N., Berman, G., Samuels, I., & Carey, S. (1978). The recognition and encoding of faces by alcoholic Korsakoff and right hemisphere patients. *Neuropsychologia, 16,* 683–695.

Echternacht, R. (1986). The performance of pseudoneurological chronic psychiatric inpatients on the test of Facial Recognition. Judgment of Line Orientation, and Aphasia Screening Test. Paper presented at the 7th Annual Meeting of the Midwest Neuropsychology Group, Rochester, MN.

Egelko, S., Gordon, W.A., Hibbard, M.R., Diller, L., Lieberman, A., Holliday, R., Ragnarsson, K., Shaver, M.S., & Orazem, J. (1988). Relationship among CT scans, neurologic exam, and neuropsychological test performance in right-brain-damaged stroke patients. *Journal of Clinical and Experimental Neuropsychology, 10,* 539–564.

Ferracuti, F., & Ferracuti, S. (1992). Taratura del campione Italiano. In *Test de Riconoscento di Volti Ignoti.* Florence: Organizzazione Speciali, pp. 26–29.

Gilbert, J.G. (1973). Thirty-five year follow-up study of intellectual functioning. *Journal of Gerontology, 28,* 68–72.

Hamsher, K. de S., Levin, H.S., & Benton, A.L. (1979). Facial recognition in patients with focal brain lesions. *Archives of Neurology, 36,* 837–839.

Haxby, J.V., Grady, C.L., Ungerleider, L.G., & Horwitz, B. (1991). Mapping the functional anatomy of the intact human brain with brain work imaging. *Neuropsychologia, 29,* 539–555.

Hoptman, M.J., & Davidson, R.J. (1993). Benton's Facial Recognition Task: A psychometric evaluation. Paper presented at the meeting of the International Neuropsychological Society, Galveston, TX.

Hovestadt, A., de Jong, G.J., & Meerwaldt, J.D. (1987). Spatial disorientation as an early symptom of Parkinson's disease. *Neurology, 37,* 485–487.

Kempen, J.H., Kritchevsky, M., & Feldman, S.T. (1994). Effect of visual impairment on neuropsychological test performance. *Journal of Clinical and Experimental Neuropsychology, 16,* 223–231.

Levin, B.E., Llabre, M.M., & Reisman, S. (1991). Visuospatial impairment in Parkinson's disease. *Neurology, 41,* 365–369.

Levin, H.S., & Benton, A.L. (1977). Facial recognition in "pseudoneurological" patients. *Journal of Nervous and Mental Disease, 164,* 135–138.

Levin, H.S., Grossman, R.G., & Kelly, J. (1977). Impairment in facial recognition after closed head injuries of varying severity. *Cortex, 13,* 119–130.

Levin, H.S., Hamsher, K. de S., & Benton, A.L. (1975). A short form of the test of facial recognition for clinical use. *Journal of Psychology, 91,* 223–228.

Mittenberg, W., Seidenberg, M., O'Leary, D.S., & DiGiulio, D.V. (1989). Changes in cerebral functioning associated with normal aging. *Journal of Clinical and Experimental Neuropsychology, 11,* 918–932.

Peck, E.A., Mitchell, S.A., Burke, E.A., & Schwartz, S.M. (1992). Post head injury normative data for selected Benton neuropsychological tests. Paper presented at the meeting of the American Psychological Association, Washington, DC.

Risser, A.H. & Andrikopoulos, J. (1997). Facial Recognition Test performance in traumatic brain injury. Paper presented at the meeting of the International Neuropsychological Society, Orlando, FL.

Roberts, R.J., & Hamsher, K. (1984). Effects of minority status on facial recognition and naming performance. *Journal of Clinical Psychology, 40,* 539–545.

Strauss, E., & Verity, L. (1983). Effects of hemispherectomy in infantile hemiplegics. *Brain and Language, 20,* 1–11.

Trahan, D.E. (1997). Relationship between facial discrimination and visual neglect in patients with unilateral vascular lesions. *Archives of Clinical Neuropsychology, 12,* 57–62.

Tzavaras, A., Hecaen, H., & Le Bras, H. (1970). La problème de la specifité du déficit de la reconnaisance du visage humain lors des lésions hémispherique unilaterales. *Neuropsychologia, 8,* 403–416.

Vilkki, J., & Laitinen, L.V. (1976). Effects of pulvinotomy and vetrolateral thalamotomy on some cognitive functions. *Neuropsychologia, 14,* 67–78.

Warrington, E.K., & James, M. (1967). An experimental investigation of facial recognition in patients with unilateral cerebral lesions. *Cortex, 3,* 317–326.

HOOPER VISUAL ORGANIZATION TEST (VOT)

Purpose

This is a test of the ability to conceptually rearrange pictures that have been disarranged.

Source

The Hooper Visual Organization Test can be ordered from Western Psychological Services, 12031 Wilshire Blvd., Los Angeles, CA 90025, at a cost of $87.50 US.

Description

This test consists of 30 drawings of common objects on 4″ × 4″ cards in a ringbinder (test booklet). Each object is cut into two or more parts and illogically arranged in the drawing. The task is to name the object. The test is similar to other fragmented figures tests. Although originally designed to differentiate adult subjects with and without brain damage (Hooper, 1958), several studies have attempted to delimit its use more closely. The 1983 edition ("developed by the staff of Western Psychological Services," no author) is based on Hooper's original studies but adds references to more recent studies, age- and education-corrected raw score tables, and a T-score conversion table.

Approximate Time for Administration

The time required is about 10–15 minutes.

Administration

See source. With individual administration, the correct naming of each object is required. Group administration relies on written responses. The test manual stresses that in addition to the simple correct/incorrect scoring, the quality of the responses may be important. Wetzel and Murphy (1991) found that discontinuing the test after five consecutive failures does not significantly change the scoring of this test.

Scoring

The score is simply the total number of correct responses, although half credit is given for some of the items for partially correct responses (e.g., "tower" or "castle" instead of lighthouse). Qualitative scoring includes the distinction between isolate, perseverative, bizarre, and neologistic responses.

Comment

Lezak (1982) reported a coefficient of concordance of .86, indicating good test–retest reliability after 6 and again after 12 months; however, 8-months reliability in 51 adult intractable epileptics was .75 (Sawrie et al., 1996) and one-year retest reliability in elderly subjects was only .68 (B. E. Levin et al., 1991). Split-half reliability was reported as .82 (Hooper, 1948) in college students, and .80 in hospitalized adults (Gerson, 1974). Seidel (1994) also found that internal consistency (.72) in children was similar to that obtained for adults. Kirk (1992) suggested a reordering of items based on item difficulty in 5- and 13-year-old boys.

Seidel (1994) found significant correlations with four WISC-R performance subtests (Block Design, Picture Arrangement, Object Assembly, Picture Completion); the test loaded primarily on a visuospatial/visuomotor factor in a factor analysis of 13 tests. This was confirmed in a recent study by Paolo et al. (1996) who stressed that the test is more dependent on perceptual-organizational abilities than on confrontation naming as measured with the Boston Naming Test.

Ricker and Axelrod (1995), found that in 100 consecutive neuropsychological referrals without dysnomia, the test was relatively independent of confrontation naming ability measured with the Multilingual Aphasia Examination, and of the ability to name the VOT objects themselves; a perceptual organization factor accounted for 48 percent of the VOT variance.

The validity of this test for "general screening for brain damage" has been hotly debated (Boyd, 1982a, 1982b; Rathbun & Smith, 1982;

Woodward, 1982). Although correct classification rates of 74 percent between unselected brain-damaged subjects and healthy controls with a cutoff score of 25 have been reported (Boyd, 1981), and Lezak (1995) states that "more than 11 failures usually indicate organic brain pathology," Wetzel and Murphy (1991) found that many brain-injured persons perform well on the VOT. The validity of the test in detecting specific deficits as well as the localization of brain lesions would seem to be of greater importance. The face validity of the test lies in its demand on perceptual differentiation and conceptual reorganization (including mental rotation) of the fragmented objects. Rathbun and Smith (1982) point out that such functions are frequently spared in patients with right-frontal or left-hemisphere lesions, whereas impairment is most pronounced in right-posterior lesions. Wang (1977) found only a trend toward lower scores in right-hemisphere-lesion patients; Fitz et al. (1992) found differences between 11 patients with right-parietal-lobe lesions and 13 right non-parietal lesions; however, this difference was significant only after adjustment for age and education. In a comparison of 44 right-hemisphere with 23 left-hemisphere geriatric VA patients, Nadler et al. (1996) found significantly poorer VOT performance in patients with right-hemisphere CVA; also, in scoring this test for qualitative error types, right CVA patients made more part and unformed/unassociated errors, whereas left-hemisphere CVA patients made more language-based errors. Boyd (1981), however, found no difference that was due to lateralization of lesion. Zec et al. (1992) found the test sensitive to patients with very mild dementia of the Alzheimer type compared to age-matched controls. McCaffrey et al. (1988) reported significantly lower scores in a substance-abuse population.

Farver and Farver (1982) and Tamkin and Hyer (1984) interpreted age-related decline on this test in normal subjects, aged 40–88 years, together with six other parietal lobe tests of the BDAE, as evidence of cognitive dysfunction related to right-parietal-lobe/right-hemisphere functional decline with age. However, Libon et al. (1994) compared the performance of young-old (64–74) and old-old (75–94) normal healthy subjects and found a decline of 3.2 points on the test, which was strongly related to decline of other executive function tests (e.g., semantic and phonemic controlled word association, Wisconsin Card Sorting Test), but not to tests that did not have an integrative component (e.g., judgment of line orientation, copy of the Rey Complex Figure). The authors concluded that decline on this test is more likely associated with decline of frontal lobe rather than right-hemisphere functions. Sohlberg and Mateer (1989) found the test useful for the examination of temporal lobe dysfunction. Richardson et al. (1995) found that the test was the best of five neuropsychological tests in the prediction of performance-based activity of daily living ratings in a geriatric population.

Comparing the VOT to other tests, Tamkin et al. (1984) and Tamkin and Kunce (1985) found that the Weigl Color-Form Sorting Test was most sensitive to brain dysfunction, but that the addition of the Benton Visual Retention Test and the VOT increased predictive validity. Sterne (1973), on the other hand, found that the addition of the VOT did not add to the discrimination between Veterans Administration patients classified as normal, organic, and indeterminate based on the Wechsler Adult Intelligence Scale, the Benton Visual Retention Test, and the Porteus Maze Test, whereas the addition of the Trail Making Test did.

Tamkin and Jacobsen (1984) reported that scores for 211 male psychiatric inpatients were approximately 2.5 points below average, and Gerson (1974) concluded that the test is "not sensitive to . . . thought disorders" (p. 98) and that neologisms and bizarre responses did not occur in this population at all.

We use this test only with individual patients to explore further any difficulties in perceptual organization, but not as a test confirming the presence of brain damage. Lezak (1995) notes that the test elicits perceptual-fragmentation-type responses in some patients who view the world in that manner; for example, when only the center piece of item 21 is focused on, it may be interpreted as "desert island," and the tail of the mouse in item 22 may be viewed as "a pipe." Since the test

Table 12—6. Performance of Normal School Children on the Hooper VOT

| | Kirk | | | | | | Seidel | | |
| | Boys | | | Girls | | | Boys & girls | | |
age	*n*	M	SD	*n*	M	SD	*n*	M	SD
5	17	17.59	3.13	7	17.57	4.45	21	18.4	3.1
6	24	21.60	2.52	32	21.13	2.54	34	19.4	3.8
7	22	21.75	3.32	32	21.31	2.36	32	21.1	3.1
8	23	22.19	3.59	19	21.95	3.10	28	23.4	2.0
9	20	23.23	3.16	32	22.61	2.56	28	23.7	2.9
10	36	24.07	2.55	25	23.76	2.61	34	24.0	2.5
11	37	24.22	2.77	38	24.00	2.07	30	24.1	2.9
12	21	25.74	2.56	22	23.80	2.54			
13	18	25.94	3.51	9	23.11	3.30			

Source: Kirk, 1992: Seidel, 1994. With permission of the authors and Swets Publishing Company.

requires naming, results in even mildly aphasic patients may be questionable.

Normative Data

See source. The published norms still seem to rely mainly on the original studies reported by Hooper (1958), although age corrections (up to age 69) and education corrections have been added. A score of 26 corresponds to a T-score of 50 (average); a score of 21 to a T-score of 60 (1 SD below average); and a score of 16 to a T-score of 70 (2 SD below average). Hooper maintained that the test is invalid for subjects with below-average intelligence. The Victoria norms (*n* = 40; 22 females, 18 males; 34 right-handed, 6 left-handed; mean age 24.7, SD = 4.55) agree closely (mean = 26.75, SD = 1.97).

Lezak (1982) found no significant correlation with sex, education, age (except in old age), or intelligence (except at borderline defective and lower levels). However, Wentworth-Rohr et al. (1974) report correlations with intelligence of .31 and .50, and with age of .04 to .28 for younger subjects, and of .37 to .69 for populations including subjects up to 85 years of age. Tamkin and Jacobsen (1984) found similar results. Farver and Farver (1982) report a drop of one point for subjects 60–69 years of age, of two points for the 70–79 years age group, and of four points for the 80–89 year age group compared to younger

adults. This is consistent with the results of Montgomery and Costa (1983) who reported a mean of 22.5 (SD = 4.1) for 82 healthy adults 65–89 years of age, and with Farver and Farver (1982) in Boston. However, Lichtenberg et al. (1995) reported a mean of only 18.6 (SD = 11.7) for 32 non-neurologic low-education inpatients (mean age 73.2) in an inner-city hospital. A significant drop in scores of "old-old" (age 76–92) healthy subjects was reported by Whelihan and Lesher (1985). Richardson and Marottoli (1996) found means of 17.9 (SD = 4.0) and 21.7 (SD = 4.0) for subjects in the 76–80 year age group with less than 12 and 12 or more years of education respectively. For ages 81–91 the corresponding means were 17.6 (SD = 6.2) and 19.7 (SD = 3.0).

Norms for children were presented by Kirk (1992) and are listed in Table 12–6. Norms collected in Eastern Canada by Seidel (1994) are very similar; they are included in the table because of their better fit with a developmental gradient. In Kirk's study, 13-year-old boys approached adult levels of performance, while scores for girls were significantly lower and did not approach adult levels. Seidel did not find a differences between genders up to age 11.

References

Boyd, J.L. (1981). A validity study of the Hooper Visual Organization Test. *Journal of Consulting and Clinical Psychology, 49*, 15–19.

Boyd, J.L. (1982a). Reply to Rathbun and Smith: Who made the Hooper blooper? *Journal of Consulting and Clinical Psychology, 50,* 284–285.

Boyd, J.L. (1982b). Reply to Woodward. *Journal of Consulting and Clinical Psychology, 50,* 289–290.

Farver, P.F., & Farver, T.B. (1982). Performance of normal older adults on tests designed to measure parietal lobe functions. *American Journal of Occupational Therapy, 36,* 444–449.

Fitz, A.G., Conrad, P.M., Hom, D.L., & Sarff, P.L. (1992). Hooper Visual Organization Test performance in lateralized brain injury. *Archives of Clinical Neuropsychology, 7,* 243–250.

Gerson, A. (1974). Validity and reliability of the Hooper Visual Organization Test. *Perceptual and Motor Skills, 39,* 95–100.

Hooper, H.E. (1948). A study in the construction and preliminary standardization of a visual organization test for use in the measurement of organic deterioration. Unpublished M.A. thesis, University of Southern California.

Hooper, H.E. (1958). *The Hooper Visual Organization Test.* Manual. Beverly Hills, CA: Western Psychological Services.

Kirk, U. (1992). Evidence for early acquisition of visual organization ability: A developmental study. *The Clinical Neuropsychologist, 6,* 171–177.

Levin, B.E., Llabre, M.M., & Reisman, S. (1991). Visuospatial impairment in Parkinson's disease. *Neurology, 41,* 365–369.

Lezak, M.D. (1982). The test–retest stability and reliability of some tests commonly used in neuropsychological assessment. Paper presented at the meeting of the International Neuropsychological Society, Deauville, France.

Lezak, M.D. (1995). *Neuropsychological Assessment* (3rd ed.). New York: Oxford University Press.

Libon, D.J., Glosser, G., Malamut, B.L., Kaplan, E., Goldberg, E., Swenson, R., & Sands, L.P. (1994). Age, executive functions, and visuospatial functioning in healthy older adults. *Neuropsychology, 8,* 38–43.

Lichtenberg, P.A., Manning, C.A., Vangel, S.J., & Ross, T.P. (1995). Normative and ecological validity data in older urban medical patients: A program of neuropsychological research. *Advances in Medical Psychotherapy, 8,* 121–136.

McCaffrey, R.J., Krahula, M.M., Heimberg, R.G., Keller, K.E., & Purcell, M.J. (1988). A comparison of the Trail Making Test, Symbol Digits Modalities Test, and the Hooper Visual Organization Test in an inpatient substance abuse population. *Archives of Clinical Neuropsychology, 3,* 181–187.

Montgomery, K., & Costa, L. (1983). Neuropsychological test performance of a normal elderly sample. Paper presented at the meeting of the International Neuropsychological Society, Mexico City.

Nadler, J.D., Grace, J., White, D.A., Butters, M.A., & Malloy, P.F. (1996). Laterality differences in quantitative and qualitative Hooper performance. *Archives of Clinical Neuropsychology, 11,* 223–229.

Paolo, A.M., Cluff, R.B., & Ryan, J.J. (1996). Influence of perceptual organization and naming abilities on the Hooper Visual Organization Test. *Neuropsychiatry, Neuropsychology, and Behavioral Neurology, 9,* 254–257.

Rathbun, J., & Smith, A. (1982). Comment on the validity of Boyd's validation study of the Hooper Visual Organization Test. *Journal of Consulting and Clinical Psychology, 50,* 281–283.

Richardson, E.D., & Marottoli, R.A. (1996). Education-specific normative data on common neuropsychological indices for individuals older than 75 years. *The Clinical Neuropsychologist, 10,* 375–381.

Richardson, E.D., Nadler, J.D., & Malloy, P.F. (1995). Neuropsychologic prediction of performance measures of daily living skills in geriatric patients. *Neuropsychology, 9,* 565–572.

Ricker, J.H., & Axelrod, B.N. (1995). Hooper Visual Organization Test: Effects of object naming ability. *Clinical Neuropsychologist, 9,* 57–62.

Sawrie, S.M., Chelune, G.J., Naugle, R.I., & Luders, H.O. (1996). Empirical methods for assessing meaningful neuropsychological changes following epilepsy surgery. *Journal of the International Neuropsychological Society, 2,* 556–564.

Seidel, W.T. (1994). Applicability of the Hooper Visual Organization Test to pediatric populations: Preliminary findings. *Clinical Neuropsychologist, 8,* 59–68.

Sohlberg, M.M., & Mateer, C.A. (1989). *Introduction to Cognitive Rehabilitation.* New York: Guilford Press.

Sterne, D.M. (1973). The Hooper Visual Organization Test and the Trail Making Test as discriminants of brain injury. *Journal of Clinical Psychology, 29,* 212–213.

Tamkin, A.S., & Hyer, L.A. (1984). Testing for cognitive dysfunction in the aging population. *Military Medicine, 149,* 397–399.

Tamkin, A.S., & Jacobsen, R. (1984). Age-related norms for the Hooper Visual Organization Test. *Journal of Clinical Psychology, 40,* 1459–1463.

Tamkin, A.S., & Kunce, J.T. (1985). A comparison

of three neuropsychological tests: The Weigl, Hooper, and Benton. *Journal of Clinical Psychology, 41*, 660–664.

Tamkin, A.S., Kunce, J.T., Blount, J.B., & Magharious, W. (1984). The effectiveness of the Weigl Color-Form Sorting Test in screening for brain dysfunction. *Journal of Clinical Psychology, 40*, 1454–1459.

Wang, P.L. (1977). Visual organization ability in brain-damaged adults. *Perceptual and Motor Skills, 45*, 723–728.

Wentworth-Rohr, I., Mackintosh, R.M., & Fialkoff, B.S. (1974). The relationship of Hooper VOT score to sex, education, intelligence and age. *Journal of Clinical Psychology, 30*, 73–75.

Wetzel, L., & Murphy, S.G. (1991). Validity of the use of a discontinue rule and evaluation of discriminability of the Hooper Visual Organization Test. *Neuropsychology, 5*, 119–122.

Whelihan, W.M., & Lesher, E.L. (1985). Neuropsychological changes in frontal functions with aging. *Developmental Neuropsychology, 1*, 371–380.

Woodward, C.A. (1982). The Hooper Visual Organization Test: A case against its use in neuropsychological assessment. *Journal of Consulting and Clinical Psychology, 50*, 286–288.

Zec, R.F., Vicari, S., Kocis, M., & Reynolds, T. (1992). Sensitivity of different neuropsychological tests to very mild DAT. *Clinical Neuropsychologist, 6*, 327 (abstract).

REACTION TIME

Purpose

The purpose of this test is to measure the speed of reaction time (RT) by finger pressing after an auditory or visual signal.

Source

The equipment can be easily constructed (see description) or purchased from Lafayette Instruments, Health Science Department, P.O. Box 5729, Lafayette, IN 47903 (in Canada from Technolab, 8531 Delmeade, Montreal, PQ H4T 1M1). Norland Software (P.O. Box 84499, Los Angeles, CA 90073-0499) offers CALCAP, a computerized simple and choice reaction time program developed by Miller et al. (1991) in English or Spanish for $495 US and provides T-scores based on normative data derived from 600 subjects. Simple auditory and visual RT is also computer-administered in Microcog, described elsewhere in this volume. Life Science Associates (1 Fenimore Rd., Bayport, NY 11705) offers a program with numbers appearing in different parts of the screen, thus allowing measurement of RT in the right and left half of the visual field. RT are also measured in the Continuous Performance Test.

Description

RT is a classical psychophysics experiment with a long history (Woodworth & Schlossberg, 1954), first adapted for neuropsychological use by Blackburn and Benton (1955). Our equipment consists of a solid-state electronic timer that is activated at the same time as a light (5-mm red light-emitting diode) or sound (60 dB 1000 Hz sound generator transmitted via earphones) signal that is started by the examiner. The subject's task is to press a touchplate as soon as the light or sound appears. Touching the plate closes an electrical circuit and stops the timer as well as the signal. There is no key depression involved to avoid variability associated with spring tension.

Because of the variable rise time, incandescent lights or mechanically driven timers should not be used. Note also that size and brightness of the visual stimulus and the intensity of the auditory signal affect RT.

Administration

The subject is seated comfortably on a chair with a back rest and is asked to rest his or her hand on the touch board with the index finger raised above the plate and to watch for the light. For some subjects it may be necessary to apply a light coating of electronic jelly to the palm of the hand and to the index finger to improve conductance. Instruct the subject as follows:

"You see a small light bulb here. As soon as the light comes on, you can turn it off by touching the plate with your finger. Do it as fast as you can. Get ready."

Two practice trials are given for each hand, beginning with the dominant hand. More practice trials can be added to ensure that the subject's attention is completely on the task and that he or she is reacting as fast as possible. Discontinue this task if the subject fails to attend after repeated practice.

The examiner should be seated so that his or her hand activating the sound/light and timer are fully concealed, and so that she or he can watch the subject's eyes. The stimulus should not be activated until the subject appears to be focusing on the light.

A warning signal ("*Ready?*") is used. With children it is better to say "*Ready? Watch the light*" because on the word "*Ready*" alone some children tend to shift their attention and nod or answer rather than adopt a response set.

The interval between saying "*Ready*" and activating the light/sound and timer should be varied between 2 and 4 seconds to avoid anticipation, which may lead to spuriously short RTs. If for any one trial the subject's attention wanders from the task during the interval, the trial should be discarded and a new trial substituted.

Three trials each are given for the dominant and the nondominant hand, followed by two trials for the dominant and the nondominant hand.

For auditory RT, the same instructions are used, except that the subject is told that she or he will hear a tone in both ears. Three plus two trials each are given for responses made with the dominant and the nondominant hand.

Approximate Time for Administration

Visual RT takes bout 5–10 minutes. Approximately 15 minutes are required if both visual and auditory reaction times are administered.

Scoring

RT for each trial is recorded in milliseconds. A total for each set of five trials and a mean RT for each set are calculated.

Comment

Benton (1977) found a split-half reliability of .90 for an 18-trial task. Benton and Blackburn (1957) found no practice effects for simple or choice RTs across a set of 30 trials in brain-damaged and control subjects. Ranfft (1980) also reported no significant improvement of scores when comparing first and second sets of trials, suggesting that five-trial sets may be satisfactory.

In a study by Ranfft (1980) auditory signals were given to the left, right, and both ears. The results showed minimally shorter RTs for both ears (mean = 182.8 msec) compared to either the right or the left ear (mean = 185.9 msec).

Bagshaw (1990) factor-analyzed RTs for visual and auditory (right, left, and both ears) stimuli performed with the right and left hand by 728 subjects with brain damage, for emotional disorders, and without neuropsychiatric findings; he found that all conditions could be accounted for by a single factor, labeled psychomotor speed. This result is similar to that obtained by Seashore et al. (1940). While this argues for the use of a single measure of RT, a breakdown by modality and hand use remains of interest in clinical neuropsychological investigations.

Brain-damaged subjects frequently show slower reaction time; in addition, intragroup and intrasubject variability is high (Stuss et al., 1989b). Slow reaction times can be found after head injuries of all grades of severity and show maximal recovery after one year (van Zomeren, 1981). Bolla and Rignani (1997) found no further change of simple visual RT between 12 and 28 months after chronic lead exposure; subjectively, subjects reported that their symptoms became more severe. A study by Lavach et al. (1996) showed that improvement after training of closed-head injury patients in auditory and visual reaction time was associated with improved scores on the Halstead-Reitan Neuropsychological Deficit Scale and with improved functional outcome. A heterogenous group of 388 brain-damaged individuals showed a mean visual RT of 328 msec (compared to 252 msec in clinic-referred controls) and an auditory RT of 265 msec (compared to 196 msec in controls) (Bagshaw, 1990). Western and Long (1996; Collins & Long, 1996) reported that in 426 subjects with traumatic brain injury both simple and choice RT showed "hit rates" (approximately 85 percent) comparable to that of other neuropsychological tests. Strauss et al. (1994) compared 28 patients (age 16–35) 2 years after mild-to-moderate closed-head injury (CHI) with eight age-matched controls and found a mean auditory reaction time of 224.1 msec for patients with CHI compared to a mean of 175.9 in controls. Nine undergraduate students instructed to pretend they were head-injured in a car accident achieved a mean of 515.5 msec. The authors found that the test correctly predicted group membership for 71 percent of the CHI patients, for 75 percent of the controls, and for 89 percent of the "malingerers." Patients with lesions in the right hemisphere have been shown to have slower RT than patients with left-hemisphere damage (Howes & Boller, 1975), but a study by Bub et al. (1990) did not confirm this; instead, these authors reported marked deterioration of performance over time in patients with right-hemisphere strokes, whereas patients with left-hemisphere stroke showed a small amount of improvement.

Benton (1977) compared younger (mean age 35 years) and older (mean age 55 years) controls and brain-damaged patients; he found an interaction of brain-damage and age; i.e., the difference between controls and brain-damaged subjects increased (from 44 to 68 msec for auditory, from 39 to 95 msec for visual RT) with age. He ascribed this difference to the differential impact of a lesion on the brain of the older person with already existing "diffuse cerebral changes characterized by neuronal degeneration and loss" (p. 369). Korteling (1990) found similar results: He used choice RT with 10 patients 2 or more years after traumatic head injury (mean age 30 years) compared to 10 control subjects matched for age and driving mileage during the past 3 years. In a study of ten 61- to 73-year-old subjects, he found even longer RTs on this task. In an attempt to validate the results against car-driving skills as tested with more complex RTs in simulated and actual driving, however, he found that brain-damaged subjects made more errors than both the young and old control subjects. Teng et al. (1990) reported that simple RT may be among the most sensitive tests in a test battery when testing dementing patients. Similar results were obtained by Sano et al. (1995), who also found that AD patients benefited less from the administration of the warning signal at consistent intervals. Arena et al. (1979) reported slower simple and complex reaction times in patients with epilepsy compared to matched controls.

Choice RT (e.g., instructions to respond with the right hand to a red, and with the left hand to a white light, or to respond only to one stimulus ("airplane") out of five recurring stimuli) or to a target at a cued or uncued location with variable cue-to-target delays (Townsend et al., 1996) invariably leads to longer RTs because it introduces an element of decision making. While retesting on five consecutive days showed no practice effect for simple RT, choice RT did improve with practice; degree of slowing was related to severity of closed-head injury (Gronwall, 1987; Stuss et al., 1989; van Zomeren, 1981). The slowing is particularly pronounced in patients with superior temporal lobe lesions when processing and discrimination of patterns is required (Lamb et al., 1990).

The increase of RT in patients with traumatic head injury (TBI) was confirmed by Segalowitz et al. (1997). The authors attempted to relate RT to evoked potential (p300) latencies, which reflect stimulus evaluation time (attention). This relationship was found in normal controls whereas in TBI patients p300 latency was related to variability rather than speed of RT.

Schweinberger et al. (1993) found practice effects (shorter RT and less variability) in 30 stroke patients on a choice RT task, but not in control subjects. Choice RT also allows further separation of right- vs. left-hand response, but Benton and Joynt (1959), using the two-lights/right-left hand paradigm, found only faster RT with the right hand in patients with right-hemisphere lesions; patients with lesions of the left hemisphere showed no difference between right- and left-hand RT. Another variation was used by Benton et al. (1962):

No warning signal was given, but the stimuli were systematically varied [light preceded by sound (crossmodal), red light preceded by green light, high tone preceded by low tone (ipsimodal)]. Under these conditions, crossmodal RTs were slower for both controls and brain-damaged subjects, but a significant difference was found only in a comparison of controls with diffuse brain-damaged subjects; subjects with focal lesions did not display a significant difference compared to controls. Cross-hemispheric RTs (right hand–left field, left hand–right field) were three times longer in acallosal patients and a patient with callosotomy than in IQ-matched controls, although even controls showed somewhat longer RTs in the cross-hemispheric as compared to the within-hemisphere conditions (Di Stefano et al., 1992). Patients with right-hemisphere lesions and left hemispatial neglect were faster when stimuli were presented in the right visual field, as expected, but patients with right-hemisphere lesions without neglect were faster in the left visual field (Ladavas et al., 1990). A recent study (Schmitter-Edgecombe, 1996) also used a dual-task paradigm (choice RT to two- or four-tone sequences while, at the same time, rating a list of names on the computer screen for likability). Under these conditions, RT showed considerable increase in patients with closed-head injury as well as a higher error percentage compared to controls.

In a study similar to Benton et al. (1962), Sutton et al. (1961) obtained significant crossmodal retardation also for schizophrenic subjects. Both simple and choice reaction times are also slowed in depressed patients (Cornell et al., 1984) and hence may not contribute to the differential diagnosis between dementia and pseudodementia (Lezak, 1995). Liotti and Tucker (1992) found that women (but not men) showed slower RT to left visual field stimuli after depression mood suggestions; they ascribe this result to the notion that depression interferes with right-hemisphere arousal mechanisms. A group of 289 patients with heterogenous mild emotional disorders also showed significantly slower RT (auditory 220 msec compared to 196 msec in controls; visual 274 msec compared to 252 msec in controls), but

these values were lower than those found for brain-damaged patients (Bagshaw, 1990). Van Hegewald et al. (1996) point out that in their reaction time study means did not differ significantly between pseudoneurologic and traumatic breain-injured subjects, but that intraindividual variability was significantly higher in the head-injured group.

Normative Data

Table 12–7 presents data for normal healthy subjects between the age of 20 and 79 years on simple reaction time tasks. Sex differences were not significant. A second study from our laboratory with 83 normal controls (age 16–49), conducted at the Psychology Clinic and in the Gorge Road Rehabilitation Hospital, found very similar results. This study also found only minimal and nonsignificant differences between male and female subjects, between age groups (16–29 years vs. 30–49 years), and between test location (hospital vs. university clinic). A third study (Bagshaw, 1990) with 57 clinic-referred controls (no neuropsychological or emotional disorder) confirmed our norms but showed a significant sex effect persistent across age groups: Females were approximately 10 msec slower than males.

Changes in experimental equipment and conditions may lead to slightly different norms. For example, in a study of 163 healthy community-dwelling adults age 16–84 years, Graf and Uttl (1995) found means that were highly similar to the age distribution shown in Table 12–7, but approximately 50 msec longer at all age levels; however, this study used RT measured by depressing a computer key in response to the appearance of an X in the center of the monitor suggesting that the differences were due to differences in equipment.

Another study of simple auditory RT using a computer setup (Bub et al., 1990) reported means of 475 msec for 66- to 74-year-old control subjects (compared to means between 217 and 236 msec in Table 12–7). In a study of 20 controls (mean age 36.7, mean education 10.1 years), Benton and Joynt (1959) found a mean of 208 msec (SD = 37 msec) for visual RT. As pointed out above, larger light sources and

Table 12—7. Visual and Auditory Reaction Time: Norms for Right and Left Hand by Age

		Auditory				Visual			
		Left hand		Right hand		Left hand		Right hand	
Age	n	M	(SD)	M	(SD)	M	(SD)	M	(SD)
20–29	20	184.67	(35.64)	189.99	(42.15)	229.04	(36.70)	233.05	(35.77)
30–39	20	194.79	(58.53)	184.68	(38.31)	237.15	(51.36)	227.52	(39.03)
40–49	18	225.95	(58.23)	209.27	(41.76)	247.94	(47.44)	232.44	(39.09)
50–59	20	189.91	(44.20)	184.41	(39.26	240.00	(45.40)	230.82	(47.04)
60–69	21	221.74	(86.54)	217.94	(83.25)	258.88	(46.20)	241.83	(42.24)
70–79	23	239.71	(79.92)	236.07	(60.83)	276.39	(45.85)	272.57	(47.87)
All subjects	122	209.63	(65.72)	203.99	(56.38)	249.02	(47.57)	240.65	(44.41)

higher intensity have been related to faster RTs, although such differences are not large (<50 msec) when compared to differences between clinical and normal groups. Cordo and Nashner (1982) pointed out that in EMG studies, RT was reduced by as much as 50 msec when the subject was allowed to lean against a chest support, i.e., that standing or sitting unsupported during a reaction time task may lead to longer reaction times.

RT is also longer in older subjects: Benton (1977) compared twelve 16- to 43-year-old subjects with twelve 47- to 63-year-old controls and found a difference of 14 msec for visual and of 20 msec for auditory RT. Our norms (Table 12–7) show a slight but significant age effect, although the increase is only minimal until the 7th decade of life. Similar though minimal age-related slowing ($r = .36$) was reported by Graf and Uttl (1995).

References

Arena, R., Menchetti, G., Tassinari, G., & Tognetti, M. (1979). Simple and complex reaction time to lateralized visual stimuli in groups of epileptic patients. XIth Epilepsy Symposium. Florence, Italy.

Bagshaw, J. (1990). Redundancy in reaction time measures. Unpublished paper; University of Victoria.

Benton, A.L. (1977). Interactive effects of age and brain disease on reaction time. *Archives of Neurology, 34,* 369–370.

Benton, A.L., & Blackburn, H.L. (1957). Practice effects in reaction-time tasks in brain-injured patients. *Journal of Abnormal and Social Psychology, 54,* 109–113.

Benton, A.L., & Joynt, R.J. (1959). Reaction time in unilateral brain disease. *Confinia Neurologica, 19,* 247–256.

Benton, A.L., Sutton, S., Kennedy, J.A., & Brokaw, J.R. (1962). The crossmodal retardation in reaction time of patients with cerebral disease. *Journal of Nervous and Mental Disease, 135,* 413–418.

Blackburn, H.L., & Benton, A.L. (1955). Simple and choice reaction time in cerebral disease. *Confinia Neurologica, 15,* 327–338.

Bolla, K., & Rignani, J.E. (1997). Clinical course of neuropsychological functioning after chronic exposure to organic and inorganic lead. *Archives of Clinical Neuropsychology, 12,* 123–131.

Bub, D., Audet, T., & Lecours, A.R. (1990). Reevaluating the effect of unilateral brain damage on simple reaction time to auditory stimulation. *Cortex, 26,* 227–237.

Collins, L.F., & Long, C.J. (1996). Visual reaction time and its relationship to neuropsychological test performance. *Archives of Clinical Neuropsychology, 11,* 613–623.

Cordo, P.J., & Nashner, L.M. (1982). Properties of postural adjustments associated with rapid arm movements. *Journal of Neurophysiology, 47,* 287–302.

Cornell, D.G., Suarez, R., & Berent, S. (1984). Psychomotor retardation in melancholic and non-melancholic depression: Cognitive and motor components. *Journal of Abnormal Psychology, 93,* 150–157.

Di Stefano, M., Sauerwein, H., & Lassonde, M. (1992). Influence of anatomical factors and spatial compatibility on the stimulus-response relationship in the absence of the corpus callosum. *Neuropsychologia, 30,* 177–185.

Graf, P., & Uttle, B. (1995). Component processes of memory: Changes across the adult lifespan. *Swiss Journal of Psychology, 54,* 113–130.

Gronwall, D. (1987). Advances in the assessment of attention and information processing after head injury. In H.S. Levin, J. Grafman, & H.M. Eisenberg (Eds.), *Neurobehavioral Recovery from Head Injury.* New York: Oxford University Press.

Howes, D., & Boller, F. (1975). Simple reaction time: Evidence for focal impairment from lesions of the right hemisphere. *Brain, 98,* 317–332.

Korteling, J.E. (1990). Perception-response speed and driving capabilities of brain-damaged and older drivers. *Human Factors, 52,* 95–108.

Ladavas, E., Petronio, A., & Umilta, C. (1990). The development of visual attention in the intact field of hemineglect patients. *Cortex, 26,* 307–317.

Lamb, M.R., Robertson, L.C., & Knight, R.T. (1990). Component mechanisms underlying the processing of hierarchically organized patterns: Inferences from patients with unilateral cortical lesions. *Journal of Experimental Psychology: Learning, Memory, and Cognition, 16,* 471–483.

Lavach, J.F., Black, N., Gailey, P., & Solomon, R. (1996). Simple and conditional reaction time training and the prognosis for functional outcome in head injured adults. *Archives of Clinical Neuropsychology, 10,* 418 (abstract).

Lezak, M.D. (1995). *Neuropsychological Assessment* (3rd ed.). New York: Oxford University Press.

Liotti, M., & Tucker, D.M. (1992). Right hemisphere sensitivity to arousal and depression. *Brain and Cognition, 18,* 138–151.

Miller, E.N., Staz, P., & Visscher, B.V. (1991). Computerized and conventional neuropsychological assessment of HIV-1 infected homosexual men. *Neurology, 41,* 1608–1616.

Ranfft, M. (1980). Equipment modification: Simple visual and auditory reaction time and finger tapping measures in the right and left hand. B.A. thesis, University of Victoria.

Sano, M., Rosen, W., Stern, Y., & Rosen, J. (1995). Simple reaction time as a measure of global attention in Alzheimer's disease. *Journal of the International Neuropsychological Society, 1,* 56–61.

Seashore, R.H., Buxton, C.E., & McCollom, I.N. (1940). Multiple factorial analysis of fine motor skills. *American Journal of Psychology, 53,* 251–259.

Schmitter-Edgecombe, M. (1996). Effects of divided attention on implicit and explicit memory performance following severe closed head injury. *Neuropsychology, 10,* 155–167.

Schweinberger, S.R., Buse, C., & Sommer, W. (1993). Reaction time improvements with practice in brain-damaged patients. *Cortex, 29,* 333–340.

Segalowitz, S.J., Dywan, J., & Unsal, A. (1997). Attentional factors in response time variability: An ERP study. *Journal of the International Neuropsychological Society, 3,* 95–107.

Strauss, E., Spellacy, F., Hunter, M., & Berry, T. (1994). Assessing believable deficits of attention and information processing capacity. *Archives of Clinical Neuropsychology, 9,* 483–490.

Stuss, D.T., Stethem, L.L., & Picton, T.W. (1989a). Traumatic brain injury, aging, and reaction time. *Canadian Journal of Neurological Sciences, 16,* 161–167.

Stuss, D.T., Stethem, L.L., & Hugenholtz, H. (1989b). Reaction time after head injury: Fatigue, divided and focused attention, and consistency of performance. *Journal of Neurology, Neurosurgery, and Psychiatry, 52,* 742–748.

Sutton, S., Hakerem, G., & Zubin, J. (1961). The effect of shift in sensory modality on serial reaction time: A comparison of schizophrenics and normals. *American Journal of Psychology, 74,* 224–232.

Teng, E.L., Chui, H.C., & Saperia, D. (1990). Senile dementia: Performance on a neuropsychological test battery. *Recent Advances in Cardiovascular Disease, 11,* 27–34.

Townsend, J., Harris, N.S., & Courchesne, E. (1996). Visual attention abnormalities in autism: Delayed orienting to location. *Journal of the International Neuropsychological Society, 2,* 541–550.

van Hegewald, W.M., Ginsberg, J., Long, C.J., & Collins, L. (1996). Within-subject variability of reaction time an indication of impairment. *Archives of Clinical Neuropsychology, 10,* 460 (abstract).

Van Zomeren, A.H., & Deelman, B.G. (1978). Long-term recovery of visual reaction time after closed head injury. *Journal of Neurology, Neurosurgery, and Psychiatry, 41,* 452–457.

Van Zomeren, A.H. (1981). *Reaction Time and Attention after Closed Head Injury.* Lisse, Netherlands: Swets & Zeitlinger.

Western, S.L., & Long, C.J. (1996). Relationship between reaction time and neuropsychological test performance. *Archives of Clinical Neuropsychology, 11,* 557–571.

Woodworth, R.S., & Schlossberg, H. (1954). *Experimental Psychology* (2nd ed.). New York: Methuen.

RIGHT-LEFT ORIENTATION

Purpose

The purpose of this test is to assess the discrimination of left from right.

Source

Test material and scoring forms for the Benton and Culver forms are available from the Psychology Clinic, University of Victoria, BC V8W 3P5, at a cost of $70 US. A shortened (20-item) version of Benton's test is available from Oxford University Press (record forms $21.95 US); the manual (including 12 other tests) is published under the title *Contributions to Neuropsychological Assessment: A Clinical Manual* (Benton et al., 1994, Oxford University Press, $23.95 US). Another version is included in the parietal lobe battery of the Boston Diagnostic Aphasia Examination, described elsewhere in this volume.

Description

We use two forms: The Benton form was developed from items in Forms A and V in Benton (1959, pp. 14–15) and consists of 32 commands progressing from *"Show me your left hand"* to the indication of *"Which hand is on which ear."* on pictures (untimed). Since the test is fairly easy, it can be used with children and produces deficits only in seriously injured adults. A different form, derived from Culver (1969), requires the indication of right or left for each of 20 pictures of hands and feet in various positions; this test is timed.

Administration-Benton Form

The subject is seated across a table from the examiner and given the instructions as laid out in the answer sheet (Figure 12–2). Emphasis should be given to the words *right* and *left*.

For the first 12 commands, subjects are asked to show that they know left from right on their own bodies; for example: *"Touch your right eye with your left hand."*

The following twelve items utilize a 5" wide × 7½" high black-ink, full-length drawing of a boy. This picture is laid flat in front of the subject, who is not allowed to manipulate it in any way. The subject is asked: *"Put your left hand on the boy's right ear,"* etc.

The last eight items on the test use eight (5" wide × 7½" high) black-ink drawings of the head and torso of a man. These are laid flat in front of the subject in the same manner as the drawing of the boy.

Any item may be repeated once if the subject appears hesitant or requests the examiner to do so. No time limit is imposed.

Administration-Culver Form

Present the patient with the form showing 20 pictures of hands or feet in different positions (Figure 12–3) and say: *"The hands and feet on this page are either rights or lefts. On the top are two examples, A and B, which are marked correctly. Starting with the number one, as I point to each of these figures, tell me whether it is the right or the left hand or foot."*

Stress accuracy rather than time on this test, but record time until completion of the last item.

Approximate Time for Administration

The Benton form requires 5–10 minutes; the Culver form about 2 minutes.

Scoring-Benton Form

Number Correct. A score of one is assigned to each item performed exactly as it appears on the answer sheet (Fig. 12–3). Partially correct responses (e.g., item 17: right hand on right ear) receive no credit. If the subject changes his or her answer before the next item is given, the changed answer is recorded. For erroneous responses, the subject's error is noted in the margin, next to the item. For example, if the picture shows the left hand to be on the right eye, and the subject says that the left hand is on the left eye, LL would be placed in the margin.

Answer Sheet (Benton Form)

Name: _____ Age _____ Date _____ Examiner _____

Examiner to subject	Response
1. Show me your LEFT hand	1.
2. Show me your RIGHT eye	2.
3. Show me your LEFT ear	3.
4. Show me your RIGHT hand	4.
5. Touch your LEFT ear with your RIGHT hand	5.
6. Touch your RIGHT eye with your LEFT hand	6.
7. Touch your RIGHT knee with your RIGHT hand	7.
8. Touch your LEFT eye with your LEFT hand	8.
9. Touch your RIGHT ear with your LEFT hand	9.
10. Touch your LEFT knee with your RIGHT hand	10.
11. Touch your RIGHT ear with your RIGHT hand	11.
12. Touch your LEFT eye with your RIGHT hand	12.

THIS BOY (Picture 1) IS FACING YOU JUST AS I AM.
REMEMBER, HE IS FACING YOU.

	Response	Reversal Score
13. Point to the boy's RIGHT eye	13.	
14. Point to the boy's LEFT leg	14.	
15. Point to the boy's LEFT ear	15.	
16. Point to the boy's RIGHT hand	16.	
17. Put your RIGHT hand on the boy's LEFT ear	17.	
18. Put your LEFT hand on the boy's LEFT eye	18.	
19. Put your LEFT hand on the boy's RIGHT shoulder	19.	
20. Put your RIGHT hand on the boy's RIGHT eye	20.	

Naming:

21. E points to the boy's right hand. Which hand is this?	21.
22. E points to the boy's left ear. Which ear is this?	22.
23. E points to the boy's left hand. Which hand is this?	23.
24. E points to the boy's right eye. Which eye is this?	24.

NOW LOOK AT THESE PICTURES. I WANT YOU TO TELL ME:

25. Picture 2 (left hand–left ear). Which hand is on which ear?	25.
26. Picture 3 (right hand–left eye). Which hand is on which eye?	26.
27. Picture 4 (right hand–right ear). Which hand is on which ear?	27.
28. Picture 5 (left hand–right eye). Which hand is on which eye?	28.
29. Picture 6 (right hand–left ear). Which hand is on which ear?	29.
30. Picture 7 (right hand–right eye). Which hand is on which eye?	30.
31. Picture 8 (left hand–left eye). Which hand is on which eye?	31.
32. Picture 9 (left hand–right ear). Which hand is on which ear?	32.

Total Correct _____

Total Reversal Score _____

Figure 12—2. Right–Left Orientation (Benton Form) sample answer and scoring sheet.

Reversal Score. A reversal score of one is assigned to each item completely reversed in orientation on confrontation testing (e.g., item 17: left hand on right ear). Reversal scores can be given to items 17–20 and items 25–32. For items 13–16 and 21–24, a reversal score is given only if right and left are consistently reversed; that is, if all four items in either of these sections are reversed in orientation. No reversal scores are assigned for orientation on the subject's own person (items 1–12). The rationale for scoring reversals is that the subject (especially a child) shows some consistent side discrimination, although the names ("right" and "left") are reversed.

Total Score. The total score is either the number of items performed correctly or the reversal score, whichever is higher.

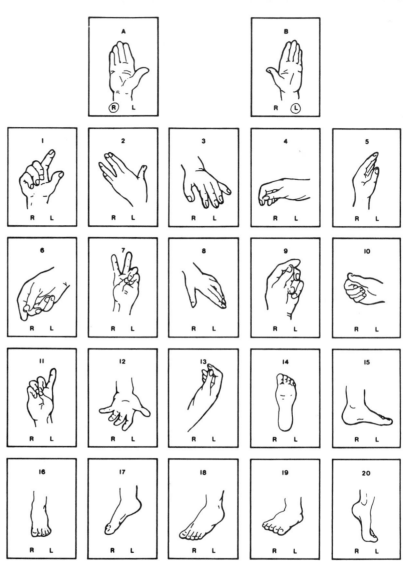

Figure 12—3. Right–Left Orientation: Culver Form, Test 1, showing hands and feet.

Scoring-Culver Form

Total number correct and total time in seconds are recorded. Correct answers are (in order from item 1 to 20): R, L, L, R, L; R, L, L, L, R; R, L, R, L, L; L, R, L, R, L.

Comment

Few studies have investigated reliability; Sarazin and Spreen (1986) report a 15-year (age 10–25) stability of .27 in learning-disabled subjects for the Benton Form. This low value, however, should be considered minimal since it covers a large time span during development in an exceptional group.

Only a few studies have investigated the validity of right–left discrimination. Correlation with intelligence is only minimal in children (Clark & Klonoff, 1990). Using a number of different tests, McFie and Zangwill (1960) found right–left confusion in five out of eight patients with left parietal damage and none in 21 patients with right parietal damage. Kolb and Whishaw (1995) also report more impairment in patients with left parietal lobe lesions. Semmes, Weinstein, Ghent, and Teuber (1960) and Sauguet, Benton, and Hecaen (1971) showed similar findings. Most authors point out that right–left discrimination is not a unitary function, but involves spatial orientation, mental rotation, conceptual abilities, and hand preference. Benton et al. (1994) stress that if one considers only the confronting-person parts of the test, 43 percent of aphasic and only 4 percent of nonaphasic left-hemisphere patients, but also 16 percent of nonaphasic right-hemisphere patients fail this part. Hence, the left parietal lobe hypothesis does not seem to apply to opposing-body parts of the test, which require more mental rotation and spatial thinking. The relationship to the Gerstmann syndrome and to visual neglect has been pointed out (Benton, 1979). In comparison with the 20- to 30-year-old control group of normal learners (17.8 correct in 60.3 sec), formerly learning-disabled subjects of

the same age and normal intelligence obtained 15 correct in an average of 74.8 seconds on the Culver form, and formerly learning-disabled subjects with minimal or definite brain damage showed a mean of 16.2 in 89.5 seconds (Spreen, 1988).

In short, the Benton form is sensitive to developmental delay but may be useful in adults only if moderate-to-severe impairment is present. Performance may be affected by parietal lobe lesions in both forms, but time scores in the Culver form tend to be delayed in the presence of any CNS impairment.

Normative Data-Benton Form

Table 12–8 shows normative data on the Benton form. Benton (1959) reports that for 7-year-olds the average performance is approximately one point (SD = 2.81) and for 6-year-olds another three points (SD = 3.09) lower, although Klonoff and Low (1974) found even lower values. It is obvious that basic right–left orientation develops rapidly during early school age and that generalization of right and left to the external environment is

Table 12—8. Right–Left Orientation in Children and Adults (Benton Form)

Age	Male			Female			All normals		
	n	M[a]	SD	n	M[a]	SD	n	M[a]	SD
6	(est.)							16.7	
7	(est.)							19.7	
8	7	24.1	6.7	8	17.6	5.5	15	20.7	6.9
9	19	24.4	7.4	24	22.2	7.2	43	23.2	7.4
10	21	26.4	5.4	21	26.9	6.2	42	26.7	5.8
11	26	27.9	5.2	19	25.1	6.2	45	26.7	5.8
12	24	27.9	3.9	23	25.5	6.0	47	26.7	5.2
13	16	28.1	4.8	22	27.4	5.6	38	27.7	5.3
14	21	27.7	5.3	23	24.8	6.8	44	26.2	6.3
15	7	27.9	4.9				7	27.9	4.9
16–20	6	28.5	8.1	8	29.9	5.2	14	29.1	7.0
21–25	8	31.7	0.7	4	32.0	0.0	12	31.8	0.3
26–30				4	31.7	0.55	4	31.7	0.0
31–50	4	32.0	0.0	6	32.0	0.0	10	32.0	0.0
51–60	6	31.2	1.6	1	32.0	0.0	7	31.4	1.2
61–70	5	31.6	0.5	3	31.7	0.6	8	31.6	0.5
71–80	5	31.0	1.0	3	25.7	6.0	8	28.1	3.1

Note: Sample consists of unselected group of school children in the Greater Victoria area.

[a]Mean of the total number correct out of 32 items or the total number of reversals—whichever is higher.

Source: Spreen & Gaddes (1969).

Table 12—9. Normative Data for Right–Left Orientation (Culver Form)

Age	n	No. correct		Time	
		M	SD	M	SD
20–30	20	17.82	2.40	60.31	15.2
50–59	19	17.16	2.89	40.79	16.2
60–69	27	16.78	2.98	52.74	23.9
70–79	23	15.17	2.66	67.17	31.9
80+	15	15.00	2.70	69.07	26.4

Note: Sample consists of healthy adult volunteers in Greater Victoria.

not reached before the age of 8 years and older (Clark & Klonoff, 1990). Reversal scores occur in 5- to 10-year-olds at an average of 14.0 (females) and 8.8 (males) points; scores drop off to 12.5 (females) and 7.5 (males) points in children 11–15 years old, and they reach an adult level of almost 0 in 16- to 20-year-old females, while males reach this level at 21–25 years of age (Spreen & Gaddes, 1969). Scores for women and for persons with less than grade 12 education are minimally lower [although Snyder (1991) found no significant gender differences]. Data on small samples of adults show that performance on this test remains stable and at ceiling level until old age.

Normative Data-Culver Form

As Table 12–9 shows, errors are relatively rare in normal, healthy volunteers. Children show a rapid increase in performance between the age of 5 and 15 years; the 15-year age group reaches almost adult levels on a similar test (Kolb & Whishaw, 1990; Snyder & Jarrat, 1989). Sex differences in children are clearly in favor of males, although this difference becomes minimal in adults (Kolb & Whishaw, 1990; Snyder & Jarratt, 1989). Differences between handedness groups are also minimal but seem to favor right-handers. In an elderly population the number of correct answers drops only slightly while the time score rises. Mittenberg et al. (1989) reported a correlation of .37 with age for this form in a sample of normal control subjects between 20 and 75 years of age. On the other hand, Farver and Farver (1982) found no change in total score with age

in populations ranging from 40 to 89 years for a right–left orientation test that included elements of the Benton and the Culver forms.

References

Benton, A.L. (1959). *Right–Left Discrimination and Finger Localization.* New York: Hoeber.

Benton, A.L. (1979). Body-schema disturbances: Right–left orientation and finger localization. In K.M. Heilman & E. Valenstein (Eds.), *Clinical Neuropsychology.* New York: Oxford University Press.

Benton, A.L., Sivan, A.B., Hamsher, K. de S., Varney, N.R., & Spreen, O. (1994). *Contributions to Neuropsychological Assessment: A Clinical Manual* (2nd ed.). New York: Oxford University Press.

Clark, C., & Klonoff, H. (1990). Right and left orientation in children aged five to thirteen years. *Journal of Clinical and Experimental Neuropsychology, 12,* 459–466.

Culver, C.M. (1969). Test of right–left discrimination. *Perceptual and Motor Skills, 29,* 863–867.

Farver, P.F., & Farver, T.B. (1982). Performance of normal older adults on tests designed to measure parietal lobe functions. *American Journal of Occupational Therapy, 36,* 444–449.

Klonoff, H., & Low, M. (1974). Disordered brain function in young children and early adolescents: Neuropsychological and electroencephalographic correlates. In R.M. Reitan & L.A. Davison (Eds.), *Clinical Neuropsychology: Current Status and Applications.* New York: Wiley.

Kolb, B., & Whishaw, I.Q. (1995). *Fundamentals of Human Neuropsychology* (3rd ed.). New York: W.H. Freeman.

McFie, J., & Zangwill, O.L. (1960). Visual-constructive disabilities associated with lesions of the left hemisphere. *Brain, 83,* 243–260.

Mittenberg, W., Seidenberg, M., O'Leary, D.S., & DiGiulio, D.V. (1989). Changes in cerebral functioning associated with normal aging. *Journal of Clinical and Experimental Neuropsychology, 11,* 918–932.

Sarazin, F., & Spreen, O. (1986). Fifteen year reliability of some neuropsychological tests in learning disabled subjects with and without neurological impairment. *Journal of Clinical and Experimental Neuropsychology, 8,* 190–200.

Sauguet, J., Benton, A.L., & Hecaen, H. (1971). Disturbances of the body schema in relation to language impairment and hemispheric locus of lesion. *Journal of Neurology, Neurosurgery and Psychiatry, 34,* 496–501.

Semmes, J., Weinstein, S., Ghent, L., & Teuber, H.L. (1960). *Somatosensory Changes after Penetrating Brain Wounds in Man.* Cambridge, MA: Harvard University Press.

Snyder, T.J. (1991). Self-rated right–left confusability and objectively measured right–left discrimination. *Developmental Neuropsychology*, 7, 219–230.

Snyder, T.J., & Jarratt, L. (1989). Adult differences in right–left discrimination according to gender and handedness. *Journal of Clinical and Experimental Neuropsychology, 11*, 70 (abstract).

Spreen, O. (1988). *Learning Disabled Children Growing Up.* New York: Oxford University Press.

Spreen, O., & Gaddes, W.H. (1969). Developmental norms for 15 neuropsychological tests age 6 to 15. *Cortex, 5,* 171–191.

SOUND RECOGNITION

Other Test Names

Other test names include the Acoustic Recognition Test and the Nonverbal Auditory Perception Test.

Purpose

The purpose of this test is to assess the ability to recognize familiar environmental sounds (auditory object recognition).

Source

The test can be ordered from the Psychology Clinic, University of Victoria, Victoria, BC V8W 3P5. The tape, instructions, norms, pictures, and words for the multiple-choice version and 20 answer sheets cost $50 US.

Description

The test was developed by Spreen and Benton (1963) as a procedure for assessing auditory object recognition analogous to tests for visual and tactile object recognition. The term *auditory agnosia* is often misapplied to denote the inability of a patient to understand spoken language. But the latter is a verbal disability, analogous to dyslexia in the visual realm and agraphesthesia or "tactile dyslexia" in the tactile realm; terms such as *word deafness* or *receptive aphasia* are more appropriate designations for this. If auditory agnosia is conceived of as being the auditory counterpart of visual object agnosia and astereognosis, it is the loss of the ability to recognize familiar nonverbal auditory stimuli. Because of the special problems posed by "amusia," such nonverbal auditory stimuli probably should not include the recognition of melodies, songs, etc.

There are two approximately equivalent forms (A and B) of the test, each consisting of 13 items. The items are listed in Figures 12–4 and 12–5 in the order in which they are presented on the sound tape. Some researchers prefer to administer both forms (26 items) to reduce the risk of false negatives (Varney & Damasio, 1986).

Administration

The subject is seated at a table. The playback loudspeaker is placed at a distance of about 7 feet in front of the subject. The sound tape is inserted into a tape deck/amplifier. For patients with normal hearing, the volume is set at a level of approximately 70 dB. For hard-of-hearing subjects, the volume may be increased or the sounds may be presented through earphones of adequate sensitivity. Instruct the subject as follows:

"We have a number of sounds recorded on this tape. I am going to play these sounds to you and I want you to guess what made these sounds, where they come from. The sounds will be loud enough for you to hear. Every time you hear a sound, listen carefully and then tell me what you think made the sound, where the sound came from. After each sound, there will be a pause so that you can think about it and tell me the answer. If you need more time after the sound, tell me so that I can stop the tape. If you do not know what made the sound, make a guess, give me your best guess."

Start the tape at the beginning of series A or B. If the subject requests it, or if it is obvious that the subject will not complete the answer within the 15-second pause between sounds, stop the tape. If the subject gives a partially

| Item | Score credits | | |
No.	3	2	0
1	cat, kitty meowing imitating a cat		
2	coughing, throat clearing, someone has cold	man*	someone's sick
3	bell, chime, church clock, outdoor clock	school bell, church*	doorbell, dinner bell
4	applause, clapping	people*, crowd*	horse walking, shoes, tap dancing
5	machine gun, automatic rifle	gun*, shooting*, bullet	
6	fog horn, boat, train whistle, ship coming in	factory whistle, whistle*	car honking
7	airplane, jet, airship	train, truck, car	factory, storm, thunder, volcano erupting
8	telephone ringing, telephone bell, calling on phone	bell*, doorbell	
9	piano, clavichord, harpsichord, organ, xylophone	chimes*, record player*, music box*, instrument*	band*, orchestra*, nursery music*, lullaby*, radio*, bells, organ grinder
10	woman, girl or boy speaking English	someone speaking English*, TV show*, church*	man or woman speaking foreign language, man speaking, people talking
11	birds (any type of bird except fowl)	animals*	ducks
12	door slamming, door closing, door closing and opening	planks falling, unloading wooden boards, car door slamming, banging*	something falling, chopping wood, hitting something, hammering
13	trumpet, fanfare, any brass instrument	band*, orchestra*, record player*, movie*, show starting*, music*, end of show*, march*, instruments*, organ, any wind instrument	piano, violin, or other string instrument

Figure 12—4. Sound Recognition Test: Scoring standards for Form A. *Note:* The underscored responses in the "3" column identify the actual source of the sound. For those items indicated by an asterisk (*), score 2 or 0 only if the answer cannot be improved upon by questioning (see Administration).

correct response or a response that is not specific enough to meet the criteria outlined in Figures 12–5 and 12–6 (responses marked with an asterisk), ask "*What was it exactly that made the sound?*", or "*Was that all you heard?*" In formulating the question, the examiner may use the information given in the subject's response; e.g., "*What kind of bell?*" or "*How did the people make the sound?*" However, the examiner should be careful not to give cues as to the correct response when posing the question. Some exceptions to this general rule are as follows: For items A 9, A 13, B 7, and B 13, if the patient indicates that it was a musical instrument, it is permissible to ask, "*What kind of an instrument was it.*" For items A10 and B11, if the patient indicates that it is "a voice" or "a person talking", it is

permissible to ask "*Was the person speaking English?*" After the subject has completed an answer, continue by pushing the release button. If more than one error occurs in the series presented first, the alternate form should also be given.

Multiple Choice Administration, Verbal

This administration should be used only with patients who have difficulty responding orally but are able to read. A multiple-choice card for each sound is used. Instructions and procedure are essentially the same as for standard administration except that the subject is required to point to the response that he or she selects from the four choices on the card.

Item No.	Score credits		
	3	2	0
1	whistling		
2	dog barking		
3	baby or child crying		
4	auto, car, truck, bus, motor starting	cars, cars won't start	lion, jet
5	knocking or tapping on door, tapping on wood	tapping cane on floor, somebody at door, pounding desk with knuckles	hammering*, walking, tap dancing
6	dialing on telephone	banging receiver*, calling wrong number*, calling somebody on phone*	phone ringing
7	drums, drum corps	band*, Indians, soldiers, men marching	music*, train
8	typewriter		
9	thunder, thunderstorm	explosion, cannons, blast, bomb, storm, rainstorm	lightning, earthquake, gun, rain, rocket, shooting, bowling
10	faucet running, faucet water, pouring bucket of water, taking bath or shower	washing, washing machine, hose spraying, rain	steam
11	man speaking foreign language	man speaking English, they are talking*	boy speaking
12	frogs and crickets, frogs, crickets, toad	insect*, swamp noises	pigs, ducks, mud turtle, grasshopper
13	organ, church music	music*, instrument*	church*, TV*, piano, band*, orchestra*, horn, record player*

Figure 12—5. Sound Recognition Test: Scoring standards for Form B. *Note:* Underscored responses in "3" column identify the actual source of the sound. For items indicated by an asterisk (*), score 2 or 0 only if the answer cannot be improved upon by questioning (see Administration).

Multiple Choice Administration, Pictures

This administration should be used only with patients who have difficulty in responding orally and who are not able to read. A multiple-choice card with four pictures for each sound is used. Instructions and procedure are essentially the same as for the standard administration except that the subject is required to point to the response he or she has selected from the four choices on the card. Correct responses are the same as for the oral multiple choice administration.

Administration Time

The time required is 10 minutes for each form.

Scoring

The responses are scored for correct identification according to the criteria presented in Figures 12–5 and 12–6. A score of 3 points is given if the sound is identified correctly or if a response is given that was found to be equivalent in normative samples (the original source of the sounds is underlined in the left column on the tables). A score of 2 points is given for responses that are correct but too general and that cannot be improved upon questioning (center columns on Figures 12–5 and 12–6). The right-hand column in the figures lists some incorrect responses for which a 0 score is given; a few very general responses are also included in this column.

Occasionally, a subject will give two responses without indicating a preference (the "or" response). In this case, the following scoring rules apply:

1. If both a 3-point and a 2-point response are given, a score of 2 is given.

2. If both a 3-point and a wrong (score 0) response are made, a score of 1 is given.

The correct responses for the multiple-choice administration Forms A and B (with A for upper left, B for upper right, C for lower left, and D for lower right) are:

1B
2D
3C
4A
5C
6D
7B
8A
9C
10B
11B
12D
13A

Comment

The product-moment correlation between the two forms in a group of 79 adult control patients was found by the authors to be .73; the correlation for all adult subjects ($n = 101$) tested (including brain-damaged patients) was .68. The correlation between the two forms for a group of 97 normal children (ages 5–10 years) was .97.

The error rate for most brain-damaged patients tends to be low. However, Merrick et al. (1989) reported that with a longer (30 stimuli) and somewhat more difficult tape, normal controls gave only 28 correct answers (SD = 1.8); 19 neurologically impaired (not specified) subjects obtained only 16 (SD = 6.1); and 6 Alzheimer's disease patients gave only 15 correct answers (SD = 5.7). The large standard deviations indicate large variability from patient to patient. Varney (1982) found a fairly close relationship between defective sound recognition and pantomime recognition in aphasics, but suggested that sound recognition is more closely related to aural comprehension (Varney, 1980, 1984b). Lezak (1995) lists defects in sound recognition as indicative of right temporal lobe lesions (Gordon, 1974; Milner, 1971). Benton (1994) also points out the association of defects in the recognition of meaningless sounds with right-hemisphere disease. Based on autopsy results, a right temporal lesion was also most likely in a case of auditory agnosia without aphasia (Spreen et al., 1965). In contrast, Varney and Damasio (1986) found sound recognition defects in aphasics with left-hemisphere lesions in the basal ganglia, the auditory cortex, the supramarginal gyrus, the angular gyrus, and area 37, although not all patients with lesions in these areas had sound recognition defects. Normal sound recognition in aphasics predicted rapid and almost complete recovery of even severe forms of aural comprehension deficits (Varney, 1984a).

Normative Data

Normal adults almost invariably obtain near-perfect scores (38 out of a maximum of 39) on

Table 12—10. Mean Sound Recognition Test Scores for Normal School Children Ages 5–10 (IQs 80–120 Inclusive)

Age	n	Form A	Form B	Mean age	Mean IQ
5	9	30.67	30.22	5.6	105.3
6	20	32.80	30.60	6.4	103.9
7	11	35.82	36.45	7.6	100.4
8	13	35.85	36.54	8.6	103.8
9	15	36.80	36.93	9.5	105.6
10	5	36.00	34.40	10.3	106.6
Total	73	34.58	34.26	—	104.1

Note: The standard administration was used.

this test. In brain-damaged patients, true sound agnosia is rare, so that even aphasic patients may obtain perfect scores if the multiple-choice (nonverbal) form is used.

Children seem to acquire the ability to recognize sounds only gradually. Table 12–10 shows the progression of scores with age in normal children. Klonoff and Low (1974) reported virtually no differences between children with higher and lower IQ and a similar progression with age. Although they used the same test, a different scoring method makes it impossible to compare age mean scores. Both their acute and chronic brain damage groups scored significantly lower than did matched controls. However, the difference between matched controls and two minimal cerebral damage groups was not significant. It should be noted that Klonoff and Low used the test with children 2–5-years old, obtaining scores only 3 points below the 6-year-old group.

References

Benton, A.L. (1994). Neuropsychological assessment. *Annual Review of Psychology, 45*, 1–23.

Gordon, H.W. (1974). Auditory specialization of the right and left hemispheres. In M. Kinsbourne & W.L. Smith (Eds.), *Hemispheric Disconnection and Cerebral Function*. Springfield, IL: C.C. Thomas.

Klonoff, H., & Low, M. (1974). Disordered brain function in young children and early adolescents: Neuropsychological and electroencephalographic correlates. In R.M. Reitan & L.A. Davison (Eds.), *Clinical Neuropsychology: Current Status and Applications*. New York: John Wiley.

Lezak, M.D. (1995). *Neuropsychological Assessment* (3rd ed.). New York: Oxford University Press.

Merrick, W.A., Moulthrop, M.A., & Luchins, D.J. (1989). Recall and recognition of acoustic semantic memories: Development of the acoustic recognition test (ART). *Journal of Clinical and Experimental Neuropsychology, 11*, 87.

Milner, B. (1971). Interhemispheric differences in the localization of psychological processes in man. *British Medical Bulletin, 27*, 272–277.

Spreen, O., & Benton, A.L. (1963). A sound recognition test for clinical use. Mimeo. University of Iowa.

Spreen, O., Benton, A.L., & Fincham, R.W. (1965). Auditory agnosia without aphasia. *Archives of Neurology, 13*, 84–92.

Varney, N.R. (1980). Sound recognition in relation to aural language comprehension in aphasic patients. *Journal of Neurology, Neurosurgery, and Psychiatry, 43*, 71–75.

Varney, N.R. (1982). Pantomime recognition defect in aphasia: Implications for the concept of asymbolia. *Brain and Language, 15*, 32–39.

Varney, N.R. (1984a). The prognostic significance of sound recognition in receptive aphasia. *Archives of Neurology, 41*, 181–182.

Varney, N.R. (1984b). Phonemic imperception in aphasia. *Brain and Language, 21*, 85–94.

Varney, N.R., & Damasio, H. (1986). CT scan correlates of sound recognition defect in aphasia. *Cortex, 22*, 483–486.

TEST OF VISUAL-PERCEPTUAL SKILLS (TVPS)

Purpose

This test measures visual recognition of various types of figures without requiring motor responses and is designed for children and adolescents.

Source

The test is available in two forms, for children (TVPS, age 4 to 12 years 11 months) and for adolescents (Upper Level, TVPS-UL, age 12–18), from Western Psychological Services, 12031 Wilshire Blvd., Los Angeles, CA 90025-1251, and costs $105 US (TVPS) and $87.50 US (TVPS-UL).

Description

The test (Gardner, 1982) consists of the seven subtests described below. They are presented in two ringbinders. Each test has one practice item and 16 test items in increasing order of difficulty. The accompanying manual describes briefly the test development, scoring, and interpretation.

The subtests are as follows:

1. Visual discrimination. The subject must point out which one of five geometric figures is identical to the one printed above the multiple-choice set of items.

2. Visual memory. The stimulus item is presented for "4 or 5 seconds" (up to 8 seconds for young children). The page is then turned to expose five geometric figures from which the subject must choose the correct one.

3. Visual-spatial relationships. The subject must choose which one of five geometric figures "is going a different way"; i.e., is different from the others.

4. Visual form constancy. The subject must point to one of five geometric figures that is identical to the one printed above. While similar to the visual discrimination subtest, the multiple-choice items here are printed in different spatial orientation and/or embedded in geometric designs of increasing complexity.

5. Visual sequential memory. Sequences of between two and nine simple geometric figures (plus or minus signs, circles, squares, triangles) are presented on the stimulus card for 5–14 seconds, depending on the number of stimulus figures. The subject must then choose the correct stimulus sequence from among four alternatives printed on the response card.

6. Visual figure-ground. The subject must find a geometric figure shown on the top of the card in one of four embedded figures printed below.

7. Visual closure. The subject must choose one of four incomplete (dashed line) figures that corresponds to the completed figure shown above.

Administration

The author suggests that all subtests be administered, although separate norms are available.

Discontinuation rules vary from 3 out of 4 to 4 out of 5 items failed.

Approximate Time for Administration

The test takes approximately 45–60 minutes, although it is shorter with young children when discontinuation rules apply earlier.

Scoring

The manual allows conversion from raw scores to scaled scores by age at quarterly intervals for ages 4–6 years, and at half-year intervals for ages 7–10, and yearly for ages 11 and 12. The Record Form also provides percentile ranks and allows the calculation of a "perceptual quotient," a "median perceptual age," and a perceptual age for each subtest.

Comment

Subtest reliability (internal consistency) is reported as ranging from .24 to .85 dependent on subtest and age, and between .83 and .91 for the perceptual quotient. Retest reliability in first- and second-grade children with learning disability after 1–2 weeks was .81 for the test as a whole, but the subtest reliability ranged from .33 to .70 (McFall, Deitz, & Crowe, 1993).

Concurrent validity coefficients ranged from .26 to .52 for the WISC-R picture completion test, from .09 to .48 with the Bender Gestalt Test, from .11 to .59 with the Beery Visual Motor Integration Test, and from .26 to .41 with the WRAT Reading and Spelling subtests. Correlations with WISC-R IQ range from .27 for Visual Form Constancy to .61 with Performance IQ. The author concludes from these data that the TVPS measures abilities that are distinctly different from those measured with the other tests. However, a factor analysis of the subtests of the TVPS with inclusion of other tests is not reported.

A group of 45 learning-handicapped students scored significantly lower than normal controls (source).

A study by Menken (1987) of 24 children with cerebral palsy (CP) with an IQ of 80 or better showed significant differences compared to a control group. The total test standard score for the CP group was 39.8, and for the control group 99.9. Similar differences were found for all subtests. Su et al. (1995) also found significant differences between an adult (45–84 year old) group of 22 patients with cerebrovascular accident and a control group of 155 controls matched for age and education. The correct classification rate was 74.4 percent. A study by the author (Gardner, 1982) appended to the manual in 1988, suggests that 104 children evaluated because of learning problems do not have a lower perceptual quo-

Table 12—11. Test of Visual-Perceptual Skills, Total Time and Accuracy Scores for Adults

	Age										
	45–54 (n = 36)		55–64 (n = 46)		65–74 (n = 40)		75–84 (n = 33)		Total (n = 155)	
TVPS	M	(SD)	M	(SD)	M	(SD)	M	(SD)	M	(SD)
Total-T	1196.44	(289.82)	1331.74	(355.72)	1746.68	(571.32)	2095.52	(546.68)	1570.01	(563.64)
Total-A	85.64	(13.89)	79.00	(13.32)	73.07	(14.31)	65.33	(16.54)	76.10	(15.98)
Vis-Discr.	13.11	(1.92)	12.87	(2.17)	11.15	(3.12)	10.33	(3.15)	11.94	(2.81)
Vis.Memory	10.97	(2.40)	10.33	(2.74)	9.40	(2.65)	8.21	(2.87)	9.79	(2.82)
V-Sp-Rel.	13.53	(2.31)	12.00	(2.58)	12.03	(2.58)	10.64	(3.18)	12.07	(2.81)
V-F-Const.	11.39	(3.27)	10.48	(2.68)	10.33	(2.44)	9.15	(2.49)	10.37	(2.81)
V-Sequ.Mem	12.33	(2.37)	10.76	(2.02)	9.85	(2.33)	8.21	(2.67)	10.35	(2.71)
V-Fig.Gr.	12.36	(2.45)	10.93	(2.52)	10.00	(2.25)	8.85	(2.72)	10.58	(2.75)
V-Closure	11.94	(2.44)	11.63	(2.70)	10.33	(2.89)	9.94	(2.87)	11.01	(2.83)

Source: Su et al., 1995. With permission of the authors.

tient (97.01 vs. 100 according to the standardization sample); for this group, the WISC-R PIQ was 99.73. Poor handwriting is related more to perceptual-motor tests, but good handwriting is significantly related to visual-perceptual skills as measured with the TVPS (Tseng & Murray, 1994).

The test is frequently used by occupational therapists (Rodger, 1994) and has been used successfully to measure progress during occupational and physical therapy for children with learning disabilities (Palisano, 1989). However, Zaide (personal communication, 1996) reported consistent overestimation of skills and poor correlation with everyday life and academic abilities.

This test presents an interesting mix of memory and discrimination tasks that are reminiscent of those available in the Bender Gestalt Test, the Poppelreuther hidden figures, the Gottschaldt embedded figures, and the BVRT-multiple choice test. It is designed for children and adolescents in an educational setting, but at least one study showed that it can be used with adults in a neuropsychological setting—this is not surprising since abilities such as those measured with the TVPS tend to peak at an early age. What is not clear from existing studies is whether all seven subtests are necessary. Subtest scores show intercorrelations ranging from .18 (Visual Sequential Memory with Visual Closure) to .40 (Visual-Spatial Relations with Visual Discrimination), suggesting that they may load on different factors.

We use this test on an experimental basis with children and adults with caution, pending further studies or norms, especially for adults, and of construct validity, which may establish whether all or only some subtests contribute to neuropsychological assessment.

Normative Data

The standardization sample consisted of 962 predominantly white children in the San Francisco Bay area enrolled in 12 private and parochial schools. Since socioeconomic demographics are not reported, the appropriate-

ness of this sample as a general North-American standard may be questionable. A study of 24 normal children in Boston (Menken, 1987) reports a mean standard score of 99.87, thus supporting the standardization. No significant sex differences were found in the standardization sample.

In healthy adults, women performed more accurately only on two subtests, visual-sequential memory and visual figure-ground (Su et al., 1995). The same study found significant effects of education, and TVPS performance decreased with age between the age of 45 and 84 years. Norms from this population are reported in Table 12–11 but should be treated as preliminary because it consisted of a relatively small sample of Taiwanese subjects with relatively low (mean 6.31 years) education level.

References

Gardner, M.F. (1982). *TVPT—Test of Visual-Perceptual Skills (non-motor)*. Los Angeles, CA: Western Psychological Services.

McFall, S.A., Deitz, J.C., & Crowe, T.K. (1993). Test–retest reliability of the Test of Visual Perceptual Skills with children with learning disabilities. *American Journal of Occupational Therapy, 47*, 819–824.

Menken, C. (1987). Evaluating the visual-perceptual skills of children with cerebral palsy. *American Journal of Occupational Therapy, 41*, 340–345.

Palisano, R.J. (1989). Comparison of two methods of service delivery for students with learning disabilities. *Physical and Occupational Therapy in Pediatrics, 9*, 79–100.

Rodger, S. (1994). A survey of assessments used by pediatric occupational therapists. *Australian Occupational Therapy Journal, 41*, 137–142.

Su, C.Y., Chien, T.H., Cheng, K.F., & Lin, Y.T. (1995). The performance of older adults with and without cerebrovascular accident on the Test of Visual-Perceptual Skills. *American Journal of Occupational Therapy, 49*, 491–499.

Tseng, M.H., & Murray, E.A. (1994). Differences in perceptual-motor measures in children with good and poor handwriting. *Occupational Therapy Journal of Research, 14*, 19–36.

THREE-DIMENSIONAL BLOCK CONSTRUCTION (3-D)

Other Test Name

The test is also known as the three-dimensional constructional praxis test.

Purpose

The purpose of this test is to assess visuoconstructional ability by how well constructions in three-dimensional space are copied.

Source

The complete test with 100 record forms can be ordered from Oxford University Press, 2001 Evans Road, Cary, NC 27513, for $185 US; the manual (together with 11 other tests) can be ordered from the same source for $23.95 US.

Description

This is a standardized and objectively scored test of visuoconstructional ability (Benton et al., 1994) requiring the subject to reproduce three block models of increasing complexity using 6, 8, and 15 blocks from an assortment of blocks on a tray. Two alternate forms (Forms A and B), equivalent in difficulty, as well as an experimental form using photographic stimuli are provided. Other versions of block construction and stick construction are included as part of the parietal lobe battery in the Boston Diagnostic Aphasia Examination, described elsewhere in this book.

Administration

See source. Briefly, 29 individual blocks of different sizes and shapes are presented in a standard arrangement on a tray placed to the right or left of the subject. Only the model to be copied is set before the subject who is instructed to *"use the blocks and put some of them together so that they look like the model as you face it."* Accuracy rather than speed is emphasized. The time taken for the construction of each model is recorded in seconds. A maximum of 5 minutes is allowed for each model.

Approximate Time for Administration

The time required is 10–15 minutes.

Scoring

One point is credited for each block placed correctly. Thus, perfect scores on the test models are 6, 8, and 15 points, respectively. A notation of the types of errors made in the construction of each model is made in addition to the overall "number correct" score.

Three types of errors are found: (1) omissions and additions; (2) substitutions; and (3) major displacements (angular deviations of 45 degrees or more, separations or lack of separation between blocks, misplacements).

An alternate scoring system counts only omissions and additions, substitutions, gross rotations, and gross misplacements. The total score is the number of blocks placed correctly on designs I, II, and III.

If the total time taken for constructing the three designs exceeds 380 seconds, 2 points are subtracted from the total score.

Comment

Reliability data for this test are not available. Constructional praxis as required in drawing, putting together a jigsaw puzzle, or assembling a model, a bicycle, or household items, is a skill required in daily life and in many occupations. It is frequently disrupted or diminished after brain lesions. Common two-dimensional tests (e.g., Kohs Block Design, stick construction, Rey Complex Figure, Draw-A-Man, etc.) have long been known to be sensitive to such lesions. The 3-D Block Construction test is the first standardized test that uses three-dimensional constructions of wooden blocks with various shapes and sizes.

Defective performance is frequently found in brain-damaged patients. Levin and Benton (1984) report that 37 out of 100 patients scored lower than 95 percent, and 26 scored lower than 98 percent of control patients; in comparison, the WAIS Block Design subtest placed 32 and 21 of these patients into the impaired ranges. Benton (1979, 1994) discussed the possible contribution of defects of both the right and left posterior areas to constructional defects: The visuoperceptive impairment may be more frequent for both frontal and parietal right-hemisphere lesions, whereas "true," "executive" constructional impairment may be attributed only to left parietal lesions. However, the findings of clinical studies have not been consistent. In either case, the defective performance is not based on primary visual or motor disorders. In Benton's study, 54 percent of right-hemisphere lesion patients had scores lower than 95 percent of normal controls, while only 23 percent of left-hemisphere lesion patients scored at that level. However, 50 percent of left-hemisphere lesion patients with receptive aphasia also performed poorly on this test. Sixty percent of patients with general mental impairment showed defective performance (Arrigoni & De Renzi, 1964, Benton & Fogel, 1962).

In addition to constructional praxis, the test often reveals visual disorders such as unilateral neglect or field defects by unusual constructions in which one side of the model is omitted or very poorly constructed whereas the other side is a perfect copy of the model. Using photographic presentations increases the difficulty of the task for brain-damaged patients, but does not appear to improve hit rates.

Welsh et al. (1995) report that African-American subjects with AD show lower scores than white subjects with AD even after correction for education level and age.

Normative Data

See source. Normal controls (nonneurologic hospital patients with a mean age of 42 years) had scores between 26 and 29 (with only one subject scoring 25). Scores for subjects over the age of 50 years are one point lower on average; specific norms for elderly subjects are not available.

In children, a steady progression of scores from age 6 (median 21) to age 12 (median 27) has been observed (Spreen & Gaddes, 1969), suggesting that adult-level scores may be reached by about age 14. Time to construct each model also decreases from 180 seconds

Table 12—12. 3D Block Construction: Time to Construct the Three Models for Children Ages 6–12 Years

Age	n	Mean	SD	Median	Range
Model I					
6	12	36.5	13.3	29.5	12–60
7	50	36.7	37.6	29.8	15–262
8	41	29.4	15.3	26.0	13–113
9	38	25.3	10.9	22.5	15–71
10	36	20.5	7.0	18.5	10–39
11	39	18.5	6.7	17.0	10–38
12	36	18.6	11.1	15.3	9–63
Model II					
6	12	77.8	32.4	70.5	36–165
7	50	75.3	47.6	67.0	21–300
8	41	62.1	25.8	56.3	35–179
9	38	57.8	21.7	52.5	25–143
10	36	47.0	21.9	40.5	25–150
11	39	48.1	21.6	40.3	19–121
12	36	43.0	18.1	40.5	25–117
Model III					
6	12	149	37	159	85–210
7	50	160	53	142	85–295
8	41	139	46	125	72–300
9	38	120	47	110	68–290
10	36	110	76	92	52–480
11	39	89	23	87	58–153
12	36	81	29	71	51–207

Source: Spreen & Gaddes, 1969.

for Model III at age 6, to 71 seconds at age 12. Because time scores (measured covertly and without stressing speed of construction) may be of interest in the evaluation of developmental delay in children, Table 12–12 presents this information in detail.

References

Arrigoni, G., & De Renzi, E. (1964). Constructional apraxia and hemispheric locus of lesion. *Cortex, 1*, 170–197.

Benton, A.L. (1979). Visuoperceptive, visuospatial, and visuoconstructive disorders. In K.M. Heilman & E. Valenstein (Eds.), *Clinical Neuropsychology.* New York: Oxford University Press, pp. 186–232.

Benton, A.L. (1994). Neuropsychological assessment. *Annual Review of Psychology, 45*, 1–23.

Benton, A.L., & Fogel, M.L. (1962). Three-dimensional constructional praxis: A clinical test. *Archives of Neurology, 7*, 347–354.

Benton, A.L., Hamsher, K. de S., Varney, N.R., & Spreen, O. (1994). *Contributions to Neuropsychological Assessment. A Clinical Manual* (2nd ed.). New York: Oxford University Press.

Levin, H.S., & Benton, A.L. (1984). Neuropsychologic Assessment. In A.B. Baker (Ed.), *Clinical Neurology.* Philadelphia: Harper & Row.

Spreen, O., & Gaddes, W.H. (1969). Developmental norms for 15 neuropsychological tests age 6 to 15. *Cortex, 5,* 170–191.

Welsh, K.A., Fillenbaum, G., Wilkinson, W., et al. (1995). Neuropsychological test performance in Afro-American and white patients with Alzheimer's disease. *Neurology, 45,* 2207–2211.

TRAIL MAKING TESTS

Other Test Names

Trail Making Test (TMT), Partington Pathways, Oral Trail Making Test, Color Trails Test (CTT).

Purpose

These are tests of speed for attention, sequencing, mental flexibility, and (except for the Oral Trailmaking Test) of visual search and motor function.

Source

The test can be purchased from Reitan Neuropsychology Laboratory, 2920 South 4th Ave., South Tucson, AZ 85713-4819. The administration manual and 100 copies of parts A and B for adults cost $40 US; for children $40 US. The Color Trails Test (CTT) is available from Psychological Assessment Resources, Box 998, Odessa, FL, for $89 US. The manual includes a Spanish administration section, and alternate forms for both Parts 1 and 2. The Oral TMT, described below, does not require specific material.

Description

The TMT, originally constructed in 1938 as "Partington's Pathways" or "Divided Attention Test" (Partington & Leiter, 1949),* was part of the Army Individual Test Battery (1944); it was added by Reitan to the Halstead Battery. It requires the connection, by making pencil lines, between 25 encircled numbers randomly arranged on a page, in proper order (Part A) and of 25 encircled numbers and letters in alternating order (Part B). The

*We are grateful to Dr. S. Lippold, Houston, TX, for providing us with information about the origin of this test.

test has two forms: the Children ("Intermediate") Form and the Adult Form. The intermediate form is used for children 9–14 years of age. This version uses 15 stimuli rather than 25 in each form. The adult form is used from age 15 years. Franzen (1992) constructed alternate forms for Trails A and B by simply reversing the order of the sequences to be used if repeat testing is necessary. Lewis and Rennick (1979) presented four equivalent alternate forms.

Ricker and Axelrod (1994, Abraham et al., 1996; Ricker et al., 1996) recommend the addition of an oral version of the TMT in which the subject is merely asked to count from 1 to 25 (Part A), and to alternate between numbers and letters progressively up to 13 (Part B); they found comparable oral-to-written ratios for three age groups, and they recommend this form as an alternative for special populations for whom the drawing form may be inappropriate.

The Color Trails Test (D'Elia et al., 1996) is designed to minimize the influence of language and covers the full children-to-adult age range. Part 1 is similar to the TMT Part A, except that all odd-numbered circles have a pink background, and all even-numbered circles have a yellow background. Part 2 shows all numbers from 1 to 25 twice, one with a pink and one with a yellow background. The subject is required to connect the numbers from 1 to 25 alternating between pink and yellow circles and disregarding the numbers in circles of the alternate color (D'Elia & Satz, 1989). An alternate form for both parts is provided.

Administration-Part A

Sample A. When ready to begin the test, place the Part A test sheet in front of the subject, give the subject a pencil, and say: "*On this page* (point) *are some numbers. Begin at number 1* (point to "1") *and draw a line from one to two,* (point to "2"), *two to three* (point to "3"), *three to four* (point to "4"), *and so on, in order, until you reach the end* (pointing to the circle marked 'END'). *Draw the lines as fast as you can. Do not lift the pencil from the paper. Ready! Begin!"*

If the subject makes a mistake on Sample A, point it out and explain it. The following explanations of mistakes are acceptable:

1. *"You started with the wrong circle. This is where you start* (point to "1")."
2. *"You skipped this circle* (point to the one omitted). *You should go from number one* (point) *to two* (point), *two to three* (point) *and so on, until you reach the circle marked 'END'* (point)."
3. *"Please keep the pencil on the paper, and continue right on to the next circle."*

After the mistake has been explained, the examiner marks out the wrong part and says: *"Go on from here"* (point to the last circle completed correctly in the sequence).

If the subject still cannot complete Sample A, take the subject's hand and guide the pencil (eraser end down) through the trail. Then say: *"Now you try it. Put your pencil, point down. Remember, begin at number one* (point) *and draw a line from one to two* (point to "2"), *two to three* (point to "3"), *three to four* (point to "4"), *and so on, in order until you reach the circle marked 'END'* (point). *Do not skip around but go from one number to the next in the proper order. If you make a mistake, mark it out. Remember, work as fast as you can. Ready! Begin!"*

If the subject succeeds this time, go on to Part A of the test. If not, repeat the procedure until the subject does succeed, or it becomes evident that he or she cannot do it.

If the subject completes the sample item correctly, and in a manner which shows that he or she knows what to do, say: *"Good! Let's try the next one."* Turn the page and give Part A of the test.

Test. Say, *"On this page are numbers from 1 to 25. Do this the same way. Begin at number*

one (point) *and draw a line from one to two* (point to "2"), *two to three* (point to "3"), *three to four* (point to "4"), *and so on, in order until you reach the end* (point). *Remember, work as fast as you can. Ready! Begin!"*

Start timing. If the subject makes an error, call it to his or her attention immediately, and have the subject proceed from the point where the mistake occurred. Do not stop timing.

If the examinee completes Part A without error, remove the test sheet. Record the time in seconds. Errors count only in the increased time of performance. Then say: *"That's fine. Now we'll try another one."* Proceed immediately to Part B, sample.

Administration-Part B

Sample. Place the test sheet for Part B, sample side up, flat on the table in front of the examinee, in the same position as the sheet for Part A was placed. Point with the right hand to the sample and say: *"On this page are some numbers and letters. Begin at number one* (point) *and draw a line from one to A* (point to 'A'), *A to two* (point to '2'), *two to B* (point to 'B'), *B to three* (point to '3'), *three to C* (point to 'C'), *and so on, in order until you reach the end* (point to circle marked 'END'). *Remember, first you have a number* (point to '1'), *then a letter* (point to 'A'), *then a number* (point to '2'), *then a letter* (point to 'B'), *and so on. Draw the lines as fast as you can. Ready! Begin!"*

If the subject makes a mistake on Sample B, point it out and explain it. The following explanations of mistakes are acceptable:

1. *"You started with the wrong circle. This is where you start"* (point to '1').
2. *"You skipped this circle* (point to the one omitted). *You should go from one* (point) *to A* (point), *A to two* (point), *two to B* (point), *B to three* (point), *and so on until you reach the circle marked 'END'"* (point). If it is clear that the subject intended to touch the circle but missed it, do not count it as an omission, but caution him or her to touch the circle.
3. *"You only went as far as this circle* (point). *You should have gone to the circle marked 'END'"* (point).

4. *"Please keep the pencil on the paper and go right on to the next circle."*

After the mistake has been explained, the examiner marks out the wrong part and says: *"Go on from here"* (point to the last circle completed correctly in the sequence).

If the subject still cannot complete Sample B, take the subject's hand and guide the pencil (eraser end down) through the circles. Then say: *"Now you try it. Remember you begin at number one* (point) *and draw a line from one to A* (point to 'A'), *A to two* (point to '2'), *two to B* (point to 'B'), *B to three* (point to '3'), *and so on until you reach the circle marked 'END'* (point). *Ready! Begin!"*

If the subject succeeds this time go on to Part B of the test. If not, repeat the procedure until the subject does succeed, or it becomes evident that he or she cannot do it.

Test. If the subject completes the sample item correctly, say: *"Good. Let's try the next one."* Turn the page over and proceed immediately to Part B, and say: *"On this page are both numbers and letters. Do this the same way. Begin at number one* (point) *and draw a line from one to A* (point to 'A'), *A to two* (point to '2'), *two to B* (point to 'B'), *B to three* (point to '3'), *three to C* (point to 'C'), *and so on, in order, until you reach the end* (point to circle marked 'END'). *Remember, first you have a number* (point to '1'), *then a letter* (point to 'B'), *and so on. Do not skip around, but go from one circle to the next in the proper order. Draw the lines as fast as you can. Ready! Begin!"*

Start timing. If the subject makes an error, immediately call it to his or her attention and have the subject proceed from the point at which the mistake occurred. Do not stop timing.

If the subject completes Part B without error, remove the test sheet. Record the time in seconds. Errors count only in the increased time of performance.

The administration of the CTT, as described briefly in the description section, is further detailed in the Source. Prompts and corrections are given as in the TMT.

Approximate Time for Administration

The time required is 5–10 minutes.

Scoring

For both forms, scoring is expressed in terms of the time in seconds required for Part A and Part B of the test. Some examiners also calculate a Trails B/Trails A ratio.

For the Color Trails Test, the time for the completion of Parts 1 and 2 is recorded in seconds. In addition, this test attempts a qualitative scoring of number errors, near-misses, corrections, and prompts; further, an "interference index" (ratio of Part 2 minus 1 over Part 1 time scores) is calculated.

Comment

For the TMT, interrater reliability has been reported as .94 for Part A and .90 for Part B (Fals-Stewart, 1991). Dye (1979) and Stuss et al. (1987) reported significant practice effects after a short interval and after one week, and Durvasula et al. (1996) found continuing improvement for both parts during repeat testing at 6-months intervals which flattened off after five administrations. In contrast, Lezak (1982) claimed that significant practice effects in the course of three administrations in 6-month intervals occur only for Part A, but not Part B. In the same study, reliability was reported as .98 for Part A and .67 on Part B (coefficient of concordance). Lezak also noted that the simplification of scoring achieved by using time scores instead of both error and time scores reduces reliability, since error correction may take a variable amount of time depending on both the examiner and the examinee's ability to comprehend. She (Lezak, 1995) recommends using the Part B–Part A difference score, which would at least partly eliminate the variability introduced by the examiner's interruptions. Snow et al. (1988) found a one-year retest reliability of .64 for Part A and of .72 for Part B in 100 older subjects (mean age 67). Goldstein and Watson (1989) found similar reliability coefficients (.69 to .94 for Part A, .66 to .86 for Part B) for various neurological groups, but not for schizophrenics (.36 for Part A, .63 for Part B).

Matarazzo et al. (1974) gave the test twice, 12 weeks apart, and reported reliability coefficients of .46 and .44 (Parts A and B) for young healthy normal males, and of .78 and .67 for 60-year-old patients with diffuse cerebrovascular disease. Bardi et al. (1995) gave the test four times over an 18-month period to cognitively stable HIV+ adults, and found retest reliability to range from .49 to .50 for Trails A, and from .54 to .62 for Trails B. Dodrill and Troupin (1975) reported 6- to 12-month reliabilities for epileptics ranging between .67 and .89 for Part A, and between .30 and .87 for Part B (the highest values were obtained at the fourth repeat administration). Stuss et al. (1989) report that the times required for Trails A and B showed steady and significant improvement in the course of five office visits within a 3-year period for patients with traumatic head injury; this improvement was beyond the practice-effect gain in controls. Charter et al. (1987) found alternate form reliability (by changing numbers and letters, but leaving the circles in place) of .89 and .92 (Parts A and B); similar studies by des Rosiers and Kavanagh (1987), Franzen (1996), Franzen et al., 1996; and Kelland and Lewis (1994) reported reliabilities of .80, .78, and .81 respectively; McCracken and Franzen (1992) showed that the original and the alternate forms contributed similar variance in factor analyses with other tests. A meta-analysis by Leckliter et al. (1992) reviewed Guilford's range/SD criterion ratios for four children studies and concluded that the TMT Part A is reliable, but that Part B may be less reliable across the 9- to 14-year age range.

Parts A and B correlate only .49 with each other, suggesting that they measure somewhat different functions (Heilbronner et al., 1991). In addition to switching between numbers and letters in Part B, the actual distances between circles are longer (Part B requires 56.9 cm more line length). Part B also includes more visual interference; there are 11 items within a 3-cm distance from the lines to be drawn in Part A, and 28 such items in Part B. Hence, Part B requires more visual-perceptual processing ability than part A (Woodruff et al., 1995). Gaudino et al. (1995) investigated these factors, and found that

using alternating numbers and letters took 11 sec. longer for Part A and 13.5 sec longer for Part B compared to using just numbers. The authors conclude that a low score on Trails B relative to A does not necessarily imply reduced cognitive efficiency, but may reflect its increased demands in motor speed and visual search.

The test loaded on both a "rapid visual search" and a "visuospatial sequencing" factor (des Rosiers & Kavanagh, 1987; Fossum et al., 1992), as well as "cognitive set-shifting" (Pontius & Yudowitz, 1980). O'Donnell et al. (1994) found in a factor analysis of Trails B, Category Test, Wisconsin Card Sorting Test, Visual Search and Attention Test (VSAT), and Paced Serial Addition Test (PASAT) in a group of neuropsychiatric patients that TMT B loaded only on a first "focused mental processing speed" factor together with VSAT and PASAT. Shum et al. (1990) also reported high loadings on a visuomotor scanning factor, the first of three factors of tests of attention; other tests loading on this factor were the digit symbol test, letter cancellation, and the Symbol-Digit Modality Test. Schmidt et al. (1994) provided a partial replication of Shum's factors, using scores from 7 other test measuring attention, together with the TMT. However, when Digit Span and Visual Memory were added, a clear one-factor solution emerged. The authors concluded that factor analysis so far has not provided adequate insight into the measurement of different aspects of attentional processes.

Construct validity for visual search was also established by correlations (.36 to .93) with an object-finding test and a hidden pattern test obtained in 92 aphasic and nonaphasic patients (Ehrenstein et al., 1982). In this study, the test did not correlate with verbal tests, for example, the Token Test, Peabody Picture Vocabulary Test (PPVT), and picture naming.

A study of 69 patients with mixed neuropsychiatric diagnoses (Schear & Sato, 1989) investigated the question of how TMT B performance was affected by near visual acuity, motor speed, and dexterity. Visual acuity was measured with a vision tester, motor speed with the finger-tapping test, and dexterity with the Grooved Pegboard Test. While visual acuity showed modest correlations (−.27) with TMT-B, and Tapping and Pegboard (−.42 and .46) showed significant correlations, only the latter two contributed to a regression analysis of the TMT as well as all performance subtests of the WAIS-R, while visual acuity did not.

The test was found to be highly sensitive to brain damage (Dodrill, 1978; Leininger et al., 1990; O'Donnell, 1983), although a study by Heilbronner et al. (1991) did not find significant differences between right- or left-hemisphere lesion patients and controls; only patients with diffuse lesions were significantly worse than controls. The test has been reported to be sensitive to closed-head injury (desRosiers & Kavanagh, 1987) and alcoholism (Grant et al., 1984, 1987) and polysubstance abuse (McCaffrey et al., 1988), but not to formaldehyde-exposure victims (Cripe & Dodrill, 1988). Performance on the TMT reflected closely the different stages of neuropsychological impairment and degree of brain atrophy in HIV-positive patients (Di Sclafani et al., 1997). A major one-year follow-up study of 436 adults with head injury compared to 132 control patients with injury to other parts of the body (Dikmen et al., 1995) found highly significant differences on both parts of the TMT, although the range of scores overlapped for the two groups, especially for TMT A. Outcome of head injury in terms of independent living was significantly predicted by a series of tests including Trails A and B (Acker & Davis, 1989). Times for a group of 586 patients with mixed psychiatric complaints exceeded even the lowest percentile norms (Warner et al., 1987), but Schmidt et al. (1994) found that, as single tests, TMT A correctly classified only 17 percent, and TMT B only 26 percent of patients with neuropsychological deficit. Prigitano et al. (1983) found significant differences between a matched control group, mildly hypoxemic patients, and patients with chronic obstructive pulmonary disease, on part B, but not on Part A. Kelland and Lewis (1994) reported significantly longer times for TMT B in normal subjects participating in a diazepam drug trial as compared to those taking a placebo. Part B contributed also to a discriminant function analysis between 298 brain-damaged patients (nature of brain damage unspecified) and 193 pseudoneurological controls (referred for testing, but no neurological findings); however, the test's contribution to the final discriminant formula based on 18 Halstead-Reitan tests was negligible. Alekoumbides et al. (1987) reported significant differences between normal subjects and three clinical groups with respect to correct classification rates: The percentages were (for Parts A and B) 80 and 74 percent for normal subjects; 26 and 20 percent for patients with diffuse lesions; 95 and 94 percent with focal lesions; and 43 and 43 percent with Korsakoff's disease. Young adult learning-disabled subjects differed from controls only on Part B, but not Part A (O'Donnell, 1983).

Lafleche and Albert (1995) found significant differences between mild AD and control patients on Trails B (means 194.4 and 131.5, respectively) in the context of several other "executive function" tests. Time scores were also very high in 37 patients with Alzheimer's disease and 31 patients with cerebrovascular dementia (Part A: 218 and 186 sec., respectively; Part B: 571 and 528 sec.), but the difference between the two groups was not significant (Barr et al., 1992). However, Cahn et al. (1995) successfully separated groups of 238 normal elderly subjects, 77 at-risk for Alzheimer's disease patients, and 45 Alzheimer's patients with TMT A (means: 47.9, 55.6, and 84.2, respectively) and TMT B (means: 123.5, 172.7, and 228.4, respectively) with a sensitivity of 69 percent, and a specificity of 90 percent for TMT A, and of 87 and 88 percent for TMT B. Trails B was also the major contributor to a regression equation for correct classification of the three groups. Further evidence for this sensitivity comes from studies by Greenlief et al. (1985), Storandt et al. (1984), and Botwinick, et al. (1988). Baum et al. (1996) conducted a canonical analysis of a variety of measures of activities of daily living and a set of neuropsychological tests. Trails A had a loading of .87 on the first canonical variate, indicating good ecological validity in this population.

Larger than normal differences between Parts A and B have been interpreted as indicative of left lateralized lesions (Lewinsohn,

1973; Wheeler & Reitan, 1963), but more recent studies have not confirmed this (Heilbronner et al., 1991; Hom & Reitan, 1990; Schreiber et al., 1976; Wedding, 1979). Another interpretation has been that such differences indicate difficulties in the ability to execute and modify a plan of action (Annlies et al., 1980, Eson et al., 1978) or to maintain two trains of thought at the same time, which may possibly be related to frontal lobe damage (Lezak, 1983; Reitan 1971). Libon et al. (1994) found that Part B was closely related to other tests of timed executive function; for this reason they also suggested that the test measures frontal lobe dysfunction. D'Esposito et al. (1996) found severe slowing on Trails B (mean = 324.5 sec, SD = 105.7) in patients with aneurysm of the anterior communicating artery and bilateral frontal, corpus callosum, and caudate damage demonstrated by postoperative CT scan as opposed to those whose lesions were limited to the basal forebrain (mean = 153.6, SD = 55.1); however, recovery within the first month after surgery eliminated this difference. In contrast, Reitan and Wolfson (1995) tested the frontal lobe hypothesis by comparing 32 patients with frontal and 32 patients with comparable nonfrontal lesions; although scores for all groups were in the impaired range, they found no significant difference between groups for the Part A–Part B normalized difference scores, nor were differences between left and right frontal lesions significant. The authors caution against unwarranted interpretations of a "frontal lobe deficit." Similarly, Anderson, Bigler, and Blatter (1995) found no significant differences on the Trail Making Test between patients with frontal and nonfrontal lesions, nor was the volume of frontal lesions related to test scores.

Significant differences between patients with cerebral dysfunction and nonpsychotic personality dysfunction (Barnes & Lucas, 1974) and psychiatric patients (Heaton, 1978) have not been established for this test, although Crockett et al. (1990) did find significant differences between groups with anterior and posterior brain dysfunction and a mixed psychiatric group for Part A, but not

Part B of the test. Harker et al. (1995) reported a minor correlation (Part A .257; Part B .333) with the somatic question portion of the Beck Depression Inventory in HIV-positive patients. Elderly patients with depression did poorly on Trails B even after the depression had lifted after 6 months of treatment (means 201.6 and 171.5, respectively, compared to 85.0 in controls) (King et al., 1991, 1995). TMT performance as part of an attention/mental tracking factor was also found to be related to depression measured with the BDI in survivors of severe deprivation in prisoners-of-war camps, but not to weight loss sustained during imprisonment (Sutker et al., 1995). Performance on this test does not seem to be affected by the presence or absence of aphasia (Ehrenstein et al., 1982).

The test is fairly robust against simulation of brain damage. When 102 adults in their early 30s were instructed to "fake brain damage," the results for Part A showed considerably faster times than those of 43 brain-damaged subjects, similar to normal controls, but this discrepancy was even more pronounced for Part B (Goebel, 1983). It seems obvious that in the fake attempt, subjects underestimated the difficulty of Part B more than that of Part A. However, Youngjohn et al. (1995) found scores in the impaired range on both parts for patients with "functional" impairment who were in litigation after concussion.

Part B is clearly the more sensitive part of the TMT. Beyond the sensitivity to brain damage, the observation of a patient's behavior on this test may be of considerable value—for example, the ability to shift course during an ongoing activity (Pontius & Yudowitz, 1980), and the ability to deal with more than one stimulus at a time (Eson et al., 1978)—but performance on Part B should not be overinterpreted given the increased complexity and length of the test (Gaudino et al., 1995; Woodruff et al., 1995).

Ricker and Axelrod (1994) and Abraham et al. (1996) recommend that the oral version of the TMT be given if the times exceed normal limits. They argue that, if oral TMT is also slow, it is likely that changing the set in a cognitive sequence is impaired. If the oral

TMT is within normal limits, the deficit is more likely to be found in the spatial-perceptual and motor components of the test. In normal subjects, oral and written TMT are strongly correlated (.68 for Part A; .72 for Part B). They also found this version particularly sensitive to anterior lesions in stroke patients, but found no difference for right and left lateralized lesions.

For the CTT, 2-week reliability is reported as .64 for Trails 1, and .79 for Trails 2. Correlations with the TMT were .41 and .5 respectively (Maj et al., 1993). Williams et al. (1995) describe a study with children between 5:11 to 16 years. They found good agreement (correlations of .74 and .69 between the respective parts) with the TMT, good discriminant validity between normal controls and children with altered neuropsychological functions, and appropriate age-progression of scores.

In a study of factorial validity using the CTT together with the TMT, the Color Figure Mazes, and the Stroop Test (Uchiyama et al., 1994) the CTT loaded primarily on a first factor, labeled "perceptual tracking and divided attention." Criterion validity was demonstrated with a sample of 63 patients with traumatic brain injury which differed significantly (.000 for CTT 1, .002 for CTT 2) from normal subjects. Significant impairment was also found in 383 HIV patients compared to 298 seronegative and 314 asymptomatic seropositive patients (Maj et al., 1993, 1994).

In summary, the TMT is a well-established, sensitive test of visual search and sequencing, backed by a solid body of research and normative data. The oral TMT is a variation of this test which omits the visual-motor component of the TMT, and is suitable for patients with visual and severe motor handicaps. The CTT is an interesting attempt to create a "culture-fair" version of the TMT by alternating between colors instead of between numbers and letters. It is backed by good standardization data and some initial clinical studies. The somewhat longer times required for the CTT may be due to the addition of a Stroop effect to the test. Curiously, the manual does not show clear evidence of culture-fairness by comparing African, Hispanic, and Caucasian-American groups nor is this point specifically discussed, although data from the WHO study in other countries appear to be available.

Normative Data

The use of cutoff scores designating "organic impairment," suggested by Reitan and Wolfson (1985, 1988) (e.g., >85/86 seconds for Part B) and Matarazzo et al. (1974) (>40 sec for Part A, >91 sec for Part B) has been abandoned by most authors (see Bornstein, 1986); instead, actual normative data are used. Drebing et al. (1994) included the TMT in a screening battery for the early detection of cognitive decline. Comparing 60 healthy volunteers and 45 subjects with neurodegenerative or cerebrovascular disease, mild closed-head injury, major depression, and alcohol or substance abuse, and the meta-analysis of another existing study (Bornstein, 1985) of the same age distribution (mean age: 43 years), they determined optimal cutoff scores of 1, 2, and 3 SD. The scores were: Part A: 45.5, 55.7, 65.9 respectively, for men; 43.4, 52.3, 61.2 for women; Part B: 104.4, 130.5, 156.6 for men; 114.5, 141.6, 168.7 for women. Russell (1980) observed that, in 158 patients with neurological disorders, more than one-third exceeded the time limit of 300 seconds, although the remainder of the group showed a fairly continuous score distribution similar to other cognitive tests.

Table 12–13 presents normative data for adults, aged 20–85 in percentiles. Table 12–14 presents the means and the SDs for this population, and Table 12–15 shows detailed data that can be used for older age groups. Sex differences in these age groups were minimal (Ivnik, Malec, & Smith, 1996; Yeudall et al., 1987). The age differences shown in Tables 12–13 to 12–15 are only minimal for the younger age groups; the increase of time, especially for the difference between Part A and Part B, becomes more pronounced with age. This has been confirmed in studies by Davies (1986), Hays (1995), and Price et al. (1980). Ivnik, Malec, and Smith (1996) found a correlation of .30 for Part A and .53 for Part B with age in a sample of 746 subjects between the age of

Table 12—13. Norms for the Trail Making Test at Different Age Levels

	Percent							
	20–29 (n = 35)	30–39 (n = 30)	40–49 (n = 45)	50–59 (n = 48)	60–69 (n = 61)	70–74 (n = 30)	75–79 (n = 31)	80–85 (n = 28)
Part A								
90	17	20	20	24	23	27	26	33
80	20	22	24	27	27	31	31	40
70	22	23	26	30	30	34	38	43
60	23	25	28	31	32	36	41	47
50	25	27	30	33	34	37	46	52
40	28	39	32	34	38	39	50	59
30	30	36	34	37	40	43	53	65
20	35	43	37	46	45	50	58	88
10	42	47	40	54	47	57	73	106
Part B								
90	40	40	40	56	55	63	58	85
80	47	46	51	60	60	72	67	94
70	50	49	55	65	65	81	88	102
60	53	53	59	67	72	84	97	111
50	57	62	62	72	75	94	116	114
40	61	64	66	74	77	102	124	138
30	65	69	73	84	84	110	142	154
20	67	83	82	93	94	125	158	217

Source: Tombaugh, Rees & McIntyre (1996), based on 308 community-dwelling adults with an average education of 12.7 years.

55 and 95+, but no effects of gender or education. Libon et al. (1994) investigated age-related decline for Part B by testing healthy young-old (64–74) and old-old (75–94 year old) controls, and they found an average increase from 87.6 to 134.4 sec (similar to the increase shown in Table 12–15), slightly higher in females. The norms agree reasonably well with those published by Cripe and Dodrill (1988), des Rosiers and Kavanagh (1987), Dodrill (1978), Ernst (1987), Harley et al. (1980), Grant et al. (1984), Russell and Starkey (1993), Stanton et al. (1984), and Stuss et al. (1988), but not with those of Alekoumbides et al. (1987) and Davies (1968), who reported much longer times in the older age range. A steady, accelerating increase in time (from 100 sec. for 20-year-olds to 400 sec. in 80-year-olds for Part B) was also reported by Salthouse and Fristoe (1995); the strikingly longer time scores were probably due to the fact that the authors used a computerized version of the test.

Scores are strongly affected by the education level and intelligence of the subject.

Heaton et al. (1986) reported that to complete Part B, normal 40- to 60-year-old adults with less than 12 years of education needed 102.2 sec., those with 12–15 years of education, 69.7 sec., and those with 16 and more years of education, 57.9 sec. Correlation coefficients

Table 12—14. Means and SDs for Adults on the Trail Making Test

Age	n	Trails A		Trails B	
		M	(SD)	M	(SD)
15–19	83[a]	25.7	(8.8)	49.8	(15.2)
20–29	35	27.4	(9.6)	58.7	(15.9)
30–39	30	30.2	(10.4)	64.0	(23.4)
40–49	45	30.7	(8.8)	64.4	(18.3)
50–59	48	35.1	(10.6)	77.7	(23.8)
60–69	61	35.8	(11.9)	81.2	(38.5)
70–74	30	41.3	(15.0)	111.4	(72.2)
75–79	31	47.2	(17.9)	119.4	(50.2)
80–85	28	60.7	(26.0)	152.2	(83.1)

[a]Extrapolated from Yeudall et al. (1987) and Tombaugh et al. (1996).

Source: Tombaugh, Rees, & McIntyre, 1996.

Table 12—15. Trail Making Test: Normative Data for Older Subjects

Percentile	56–62 ($n = 160$)		66–71 ($n = 286$)		72–77 ($n = 236$)		81–86 ($n = 162$)		87–97 ($n = 162$)	
	Part A	Part B	Part A	Part B	Part A	Part B	Part A	Part B	Part A	Part B
90	20	45	25	52	25	56	29	75	29	76
75	25	57	29	68	30	75	38	101	38	101
50	31	70	35	85	38	102	50	125[a]	47	125
25	38	90	44	120	48	156	60	172	60	165
10	50	130	60	180	75	210	79	235	80	235

[a]Richardson and Marottoli (1996) provide a further breakdown by education level based on a total of 101 subjects. For Trails B, they found means of 197.2 (SD = 71.0) and 119.2 (SD = 33.5) for age 76 to 80 with education levels of less than 12 and, 12 and better respectively. The corresponding values for age 81–91 were 195.5 (SD = 69.7) and 137.3 (SD = 55.9) respectively.

Source: Adapted from Ivnik, Malec and Smith (1996). With permission of the authors and Swets Publishing Company.

between education and TMT A and B have been reported as .19 and .33 (partialing out the effect of age; Bornstein, 1985; Ernst, 1986; see also Stanton et al., 1984; and Stuss et al., 1987; but see Ivnik et al., 1996). The effect of IQ is somewhat more pronounced but most noticeable on Part B (Dodrill, 1987). Warner et al. (1987) reported correlations with IQ between .42 and .30 for Part A and between .48 and .42 for Part B. Waldman et al. (1992) found significant IQ effects especially in the low average (mean 25.7 and 51.5, respectively, for Parts A and B) and borderline (means 47.7 and 111.6) ranges in 69 18- to 30-year-olds.

Heaton, Grant, and Matthews (1991) present norms in scaled scores, corrected for gender, education, and age, and based on 553 normal subjects. These norms should be used with caution since the cell sizes are not provided and may be quite small.

A study by Arnold et al. (1994) found no acculturation differences between Anglo-American, Mexican-American, and Mexican subjects.

Table 12–16 presents norms for normal school children, aged 6–15, using the intermediate form of the test. Values for 6-, 7-, and 14- to 15-year-old children were extrapolated from other sources as indicated. Since the test is dependent on knowledge of number and letter sequences, norms for the youngest age groups must be interpeted with caution. The norms presented here are slightly lower than those reported by Klonoff and Low (1974), but

similar to Knights (1970), Knights and Norwood (1980), and Reitan (1971). Trites (1977) reports values that are somewhat higher for all age groups, but show a similar age progression. Sex-related differences appear to be minimal in children for this test.

First normative data for the oral TMT suggest that both parts require only half the time needed for the drawing form of the TMT. Part A (counting) in particular is performed very quickly. Scores increase with age similar to the drawing form.

Normative data for the Color Trails Test (D'Elia et al., 1996) are based on the performance of 1,528 healthy volunteers, including subsamples of 182 African-Americans and 292 Hispanic-Americans between the age of 18 and 89 years 12 months. These norms are presented separately for education levels of 8 years and below, 12 years, 13–15 years, 16 years, and higher than 16 years. In general, time in seconds for the CTT is somewhat longer than for the TMT (e.g., in 20- to 30-year-olds 37 and 82 sec. for the CTT 1 and CTT 2, respectively, compared to 26 and 56 sec. for the TMT A and TMT B). The means presented for African- and Spanish-Americans suggest that these populations perform the CTT somewhat slower than Caucasian-Americans, although the tables presented in the manual are confounded by the effects of age and education level. Errors, near-misses, prompts, and an interference index of >2.0 occur only in the below 16th percentile range, i.e., they

Table 12—16. Trails Test: Normative Data for Children (Intermediate Version): Time Score in Seconds

Age	Part A					Part B				
	n	Mean	SD	Median	Range	n	Mean	SD	Median	Range
Male										
8	11	32.4	11.7	30.5	16–55	11	77.8	34.5	76.5	32–159
9	22	26.8	8.9	25.5	13–45	22	58.0	21.6	57.5	22–120
10	26	21.3	6.1	20.5	13–42	26	51.6	14.7	52.5	18–82
11	21	16.4	5.6	14.8	9–30	21	43.3	20.0	38.8	25–122
12	48	16.6	5.9	15.1	10–43	48	39.6	13.3	37.8	14–90
13	7	16.0	10.1	13.3	9–39	7	34.0	12.4	34.0	17–99
(14–15)[a]	5	16.0	12.0	16.0	8–30	5	28.6	12.0	29.0	13–45
Female										
8	12	36.4	18.7	33.5	16–86	12	71.8	39.0	77.5	26–176
9	19	23.1	8.1	21.0	13–48	19	50.7	14.5	50.8	24–76
10	25	18.2	4.6	17.8	10–28	25	43.2	15.0	42.0	25–84
11	30	18.0	6.6	17.2	9–37	30	40.6	11.8	38.5	15–62
12	44	16.0	5.4	14.7	7–32	44	33.5	11.1	31.3	20–74
13	7	13.7	1.9	13.3	12–18	7	30.7	6.9	29.3	22–43
(14–15)[a]	5	13.0	2.3	13.0	12–17	5	25.0	14.6	25.0	13–50
All Normals										
(6)[b]	99	70	40			45	133	51		
(7)	101	36	11			96	91	41		
8	88	31	12	30.5	16–86	88	72	30	76.5	26–176
9	41	25.1	8.8	23.0	13–48	41	54.6	19.0	51.3	22–120
10	51	19.8	5.7	19.4	10–42	51	47.5	15.4	45.8	18–84
11	51	17.4	6.3	16.3	9–37	51	41.7	15.8	38.8	15–122
12	92	16.3	5.7	14.9	7–43	92	35.7	12.5	34.0	14–90
13	14	14.9	7.6	13.3	9–39	14	30.0	19.5	29.5	17–99
(14–15)[a]	10	14.6	6.2	14.6	8–30	10	27.0	12.8	27.0	13–50

[a]Estimate, based on Knights & Norwood (1980).

[b]Estimate, based on Rhode Island norms and Klonoff & Low (1974).

[c]Estimate, based on Reitan (1971) and Klonoff & Low (1974).

[d]Estimate, based on Knights & Norwood (1980) and Klonoff & Low (1974).

Source: Spreen & Gaddes (1969).

are relatively rare and require special exploration if they occur. In children, age 5 years 11 months to 16, a steady age-progression was noted. Female children completed Color Trails 2 and Trail Making Part B more quickly than males (Williams et al., 1995).

References

Abraham, E., Axelrod, B.N., & Ricker, J.H. (1996). Application of the oral Trail Making Test to a mixed clinical sample. *Archives of Clinical Neuropsychology, 11,* 697–701.

Acker, M.B., & Davis, J.R. (1989). Psychology test scores associated with late outcome in head injury. *Neuropsychology, 3,* 1–10.

Alekoumbides, A., Charter, R.A., Adkins, T.G., & Seacat, G.F. (1987). The diagnosis of brain damage by the WAIS, WMS, and Reitan Battery utilizing standardized scores corrected for age and education. *International Journal of Clinical Neuropsychology, 9,* 11–28.

Anderson, C.V., Bigler, E.D., & Blatter, D.D. (1995). Frontal lobe lesions, diffuse damage, and neuropsychological functioning in traumatic brain-injured patients. *Journal of Clinical and Experimental Neuropsychology, 17,* 900–908.

Annelies, A., Pontius, A.A., & Yudowitz, L.B. (1980). Frontal lobe system dysfunction in some criminal actions as shown with the Narratives Test. *Journal of Nervous and Mental Disease, 168,* 111–117.

Army Individual Test Battery. (1944). Manual of

Directions and Scoring. Washington, DC: War Department, Adjutant General's Office.

Arnold, B.R., Montgomery, G.T., Castaneda, I., & Longoria, R. (1994). Acculturation and performance of Hispanics on selected Halstead-Reitan neuropsychological tests. *Assessment, 1,* 239–248.

Bardi, C.A., Hamby, S.L., & Wilkins, J.W. (1995). Stability of several brief neuropsychological tests in an HIV+ longitudinal sample. *Archives of Clinical Neuropsychology, 10,* 295 (abstract).

Barnes, G.W., & Lucas, G.J. (1974). Cerebral dysfunction vs. psychogenesis in Halstead-Reitan tests. *Journal of Nervous and Mental Disease, 158,* 50–60.

Barr, A., Benedict, R., Tune, L., & Brandt, J. (1992). Neuropsychological differentiation of Alzheimer's disease from vascular dementia. *International Journal of Geriatric Medicine, 7,* 621–627.

Baum, C., Edwards, D., Yonan, C., & Storandt, M. (1996). The relation of neuropsychological test performance to performance on functional tasks in dementia of the Alzheimer type. *Archives of Clinical Neuropsychology, 11,* 69–75.

Bornstein, R.A. (1985). Normative data on selected neuropsychological measures from a nonclinical sample. *Journal of Clinical Psychology, 41,* 651–659.

Bornstein, R.A. (1986). Classification rates obtained with "standard" cutoff scores on selected neuropsychological measures. *Journal of Clinical and Experimental Neuropsychology, 8,* 413–420.

Botwinick, J., Storandt, M., Berg, L., & Boland, S. (1988). Senile dementia of the Alzheimer type: Subject attrition and testability in research. *Archives of Neurology, 45,* 493–496.

Cahn, D.A., Salmon, D.P., Butters, N., Wiederholt, W.C., Corey-Bloom, J., Edelstein, S.L., & Barrett-Connor, E. (1995). Detection of dementia of the Alzheimer type in a population-based sample: Neuropsychological test performance. *Journal of the International Neuropsychological Society, 1,* 252–260.

Charter, R.A., Adkins, T.G., Alekoumbides, A., & Seacat, G.F. (1987). Reliability of the WAIS, WMS, and Reitan Battery: Raw scores and standardized scores corrected for age and education. *International Journal of Clinical Neuropsychology, 9,* 28–32.

Cripe, L.I., & Dodrill, C.B. (1988). Neuropsychological test performances with chronic low level formaldehyde exposure. *The Clinical Neuropsychologist, 2,* 41–48.

Crockett, D.J., Hurwitz, T., & Vernon-Wilkinson, R. (1990). Differences in neuropsychological performance in psychiatric, anterior- and posterior-cerebral dysfunctioning groups. *International Journal of Neuroscience, 52,* 45–57.

Davies, A. (1986). The influence of age on Trail Making Test performance. *Journal of Clinical Psychology, 24,* 96–98.

D'Elia, L., & Satz, P. (1989). *Color Trails 1 and 2.* Odessa, FL: Psychological Assessment Resources.

D'Esposito, M., Alexander, M.P., Fischer, R., et al. (1996). Recovery of memory and executive function following anterior communicating artery aneurysm rupture. *Journal of the International Neuropsychological Society, 2,* 565–570.

des Rosiers, G., & Kavanagh, D. (1987). Cognitive assessment in closed head injury: Stability, validity and parallel forms for two neuropsychological measures of recovery. *International Journal of Clinical Neuropsychology, 9,* 162–173.

Dikmen, S.S., Machamer, J.E., Winn, H.R., & Temkin, N.R. (1995). Neuropsychological outcome at 1-year post head injury. *Neuropsychology, 9,* 80–90.

Di Sclafani, V., Mackay, R.D.S., Meyerhoff, D.J., Norman, D., Weiner, M.W., & Fein, G. (1997). Brain atrophy in HIV infection is more strongly associated with CDC clinical stages than with cognitive impairment. *Journal of the International Neuropsychological Society, 3,* 276–287.

Dodrill, C.B. (1978). A neuropsychological battery for epilepsy. *Epilepsia, 19,* 611–623.

Dodrill, C.B. (1987). What's Normal? Presidential address, Pacific Northwest Neuropsychological Association. Mimeo.

Dodrill, C.B., & Troupin, A.S. (1975). Effects of repeated administration of a comprehensive neuropsychological battery among chronic epileptics. *Journal of Nervous and Mental Disease, 161,* 185–190.

Drebing, C.E., Van Gorp, W.G., Stuck, A.E., Mitrushima, M., & Beck, J. (1994). Early detection of cognitive decline in higher cognitively functioning older adults: Sensitivity and specificity of a neuropsychological screening battery. *Neuropsychology, 8,* 31–37.

Durvasula, R.S., Satz, P., Hinkin, C.H., et al. (1996). Does practice make perfect?: Results of a six-year longitudinal study with semi-annual testing. *Archives of Clinical Neuropsychology, 11,* 386 (abstract).

Dye, O.A. (1979). Effects of practice on Trail Making Test performance. *Perceptual and Motor Skills, 48,* 296.

Ehrenstein, W.H., Heister, G., & Cohen, R.

(1982). Trail Making Test and visual search. *Archiv für Psychiatrie und Nervenkrankheiten*, *231*, 333–338.

Ernst, J. (1987). Neuropsychological problem-solving skills in the elderly. *Psychology and Aging*, *2*, 363–365.

Eson, M.E., Yen, J.K., & Bourke, R.S. (1978). Assessment of recovery from serious head injury. *Journal of Neurology, Neurosurgery and Psychiatry*, *41*, 1036–1042.

Fals-Stewart, W. (1991). An interrater reliability study of the Trail Making Test (Part A and B). Unpublished manuscript.

Fossum, B., Holmberg, H., & Reinvang, I. (1992). Spatial and symbolic factors in performance on the Trail Making Test. *Neuropsychology*, *6*, 71–75.

Franzen, M.D. (1996). Cross-validation of the alternate forms reliability of the Trail Making Test. *Archives of Clinical Neuropsychology*, *11*, 390 (abstract).

Franzen, M.D., Paul, D., & Iverson, G.L. (1996). Reliability of alternate forms of the Trail Making Test. *The Clinical Neuropsychologist*, *10*, 125–129.

Fromm-Auch, D., & Yeudall, L.T. (1983). Normative data for the Halstead-Reitan tests. *Journal of Clinical Neuropsychology*, *5*, 221–238.

Gaudino, E.A., Geisler, M.W., & Squires, N.K. (1995). Construct validity in the Trail Making Test: What makes Trail B harder? *Journal of Clinical and Experimental Neuropsychology*, *17*, 529–535.

Goebel, R.A. (1983). Detection of faking on the Halstead-Reitan neuropsychological test battery. *Journal of Clinical Psychology*, *39*, 731–742.

Goldstein, G., & Watson, J.R. (1989). Test–retest reliability of the Halstead-Reitan battery and the WAIS in a neuropsychiatric population. *The Clinical Neuropsychologist*, *3*, 265–273.

Grant, I., Adams, K.M., & Reed, R. (1984). Aging, abstinence, and medical risk in the prediction of neuropsychological deficit among long-term alcoholics. *Archives of General Psychiatry*, *41*, 710–716.

Grant, I., Reed, R., & Adams, K.M. (1987). Diagnosis of intermediate-duration and subacute organic mental disorders in abstinent alcoholics. *Journal of Clinical Psychiatry*, *48*, 319–323.

Greenlief, C.L., Margolis, R.B., & Erker, G.J. (1985). Application of the Trail Making Test in differentiating neuropsychological impairment of elderly persons. *Perceptual and Motor Skills*, *61*, 1283–1289.

Harker, J.O., Satz, P., Jones, F.D., Verma, R., Gan, M.P., Poer, H.L., Gould, B.D., & Chervinsky, A.B. (1995). Measurement of depression and neuropsychological impairment in HIV-1 infection. *Neuropsychology*, *9*, 110–117.

Harley, J.P., Leuthold, C.A., Matthews, C.G., & Bergs, L.E. (1980). Wisconsin neuropsychological test battery T score norms for older Veterans Administration Medical Center Patients. Mimeo. Madison, WI: Department of Neurology. University of Wisconsin.

Hays, J.R. (1995). Trail Making Test norms for psychiatric patients. *Perceptual and Motor Skills*, *80*, 187–194.

Heaton, R.K., Baade, L.E., & Johnson, K.L. (1978). Neuropsychological test results associated with psychiatric disorders in adults. *Psychological Bulletin*, *85*, 141–162.

Heaton, R.K., Grant, I., & Matthews, C.G. (1986). Differences in neuropsychological test performance associated with age, education, and sex. In I. Grant & K.M. Adams (Eds.), *Neuropsychological Assessment of Neuropsychiatric Disorders*. New York: Oxford University Press.

Heaton, R.K., Grant, I., & Matthews, C.G. (1991). *Comprehensive Norms for an Expanded Halstead-Reitan Battery: Demographic Corrections, Research Findings, and Clinical Applications*. Odessa, FL: Psychological Assessment Resources.

Heilbronner, R.L., Henry, G.K., Buck, P., Adams, R.L., & Fogle, T. (1991). Lateralized brain damage and performance on Trail Making A and B, Digit Span Forward and Backward, and TPT memory and location. *Archives of Clinical Neuropsychology*, *6*, 251–258.

Hom, J., & Reitan, R.M. (1990). Generalized cognitive function after stroke. *Journal of Clinical and Experimental Neuropsychology*, *12*, 644–654.

Ivnik, R.J., Malec, J.F., & Smith, G.E. (1996). Neuropsychological tests norms above age 55: COWAT, MAE Token, WRAT-R Reading, AMNART, Stroop, TMT and JLO. *The Clinical Neuropsychologist*, *10*, 262–378.

Kelland, D.Z., & Lewis, R.F. (1994). Evaluation of the reliability and validity of the repeatable cognitive-perceptual-motor battery. *The Clinical Neuropsychologist*, *8*, 295–308.

Kennedy, K.J. (1981). Age effects on Trail Making Test performance. *Perceptual and Motor Skills*, *52*, 671–675.

King, D.A., Caine, E.D., Conwell, Y., & Cox, C. (1991). Predicting severity of depression in the elderly at six-months follow-up: A neuropsychological study. *Journal of Neuropsychiatry and Clinical Neurosciences*, 3, 64–66.

King, D.A., Cox, C., Lyness, J.M., & Caine, E.D. (1995). Neuropsychological effects of depression and age in an elderly sample: A confirmatory study. *Neuropsychology*, 9, 300–408.

Klonoff, H., & Low, M. (1974). Disordered brain function in young children and early adolescents: neuropsychological and electroencephalographic correlates. In R.M. Reitan & L.A. Davison (Eds.), *Clinical Neuropsychology: Current Status and Applications*. New York: Wiley.

Knights, R.M. (1970). Smoothed normative data on tests for evaluating brain damage in children. Unpublished manuscript, Department of Psychology, Carleton University, Ottawa, ON.

Knights, R.M., & Norwood, J.A. (1980). Revised smoothed normative data on the neuropsychological test battery for children. Mimeo. Department of Psychology, Carleton University, Ottawa, ON.

Lafleche, G., & Albert, M.S. (1995). Executive function deficits in mild Alzheimer's disease. *Neuropsychology*, 9, 313–320.

Leckliter, I.N., Forster, A.A., Klonoff, H., & Knights, R.M. (1992). A review of reference group data from normal children for the Halstead-Reitan Battery for older children. *The Clinical Neuropsychologist*, 6, 201–229.

Leininger, B.E., Gramling, S.E., & Farrell, A.D. (1990). Neuropsychological deficits in symptomatic minor head injury patients after concussion and mild concussion. *Journal of Neurology, Neurosurgery, and Psychiatry*, 53, 293–296.

Lewinsohn, P.M. (1973). Psychological assessment of patients with brain injury. Unpublished manuscript, University of Oregon, Eugene, OR.

Lewis, R.F., & Rennick, P.M. (1979). *Manual for the Repeatable Cognitive-Perceptual-Motor Battery*. Grosse Pointe Park, MI: Axon Publishing Company.

Lezak, M.D. (1982). The test–retest stability and reliability of some tests commonly used in neuropsychological assessment. Paper presented at the 5th European Conference of the International Neuropsychological Society, Deauville, France.

Lezak, M.D. (1983). *Neuropsychological Assessment* (2nd ed.). New York: Oxford University Press.

Lezak, M.D. (1995). *Neuropsychological Assessment* (3rd ed.). New York: Oxford University Press.

Libon, D.J., Glosser, G., Malamut, B.L., Kaplan, E., Goldberg, E., Swenson, R., & Sands, L.P.

(1994). Age, executive functions, and visuospatial functioning in healthy older adults. *Neuropsychology*, 8, 38–43.

Maj, M., D'Elia, L.F., Satz, P., et al. (1993). Evaluation of two new neuropsychological tests designed to minimize cultural bias in the assessment of HIV-1 seropositive persons: A WHO study. *Archives of Clinical Neuropsychology*, 8, 123–135.

Maj, M., Satz, P., Janssen, R., et al. (1994). WHO neuropsychiatric AIDS study, cross-sectional phase II: Neuropsychological and neurological findings. *Archives of General Psychiatry*, 51, 51–61.

Matarazzo, J.D., Wiens, A.N., Matarazzo, R.G., & Goldstein, S.G. (1974). Psychometric and clinical test–retest reliability of the Halstead Impairment Index in a sample of healthy, young, normal men. *Journal of Nervous and Mental Disease*, 158, 37–49.

McCaffrey, R.J., Krahula, M.M., Heimberg, R.G., Keller, K.E., & Purcell, M.J. (1988). A comparison of the Trail Making Test, Symbol Digit Modalities Test, and the Hooper Visual Organization Test in an inpatient substance abuse population. *Archives of Clinical Neuropsychology*, 3, 181–187.

McCracken, L.M., & Franzen, M.D. (1992). Principal-components analysis of the equivalence of alternate forms of the Trail Making Test. *Psychological Assessment*, 4, 235–238.

Mutchnick, M.G., Ross, L.K., & Long, C.J. (1991). Decision strategies for cerebral dysfunction IV: Determination of cerebral dysfunction. *Archives of Clinical Neuropsychology*, 6, 259–270.

O'Donnell, J.P. (1983). Neuropsychological test findings for normal, learning disabled, and brain damaged young adults. *Journal of Consulting and Clinical Psychology*, 51, 726–729.

O'Donnell, J.P., McGregor, L.A., Dabrowski, J.J., Oestreicher, J.M., & Romero, J.J. (1994). Construct validity of neuropsychological tests of conceptual and attentional abilities. *Journal of Clinical Psychology*, 50, 596–600.

Partington, J.E., & Leiter, R.G. (1949). Partington's Pathway Test. *The Psychological Service Center Bulletin*, 1, 9–20.

Pontius, A.A., & Yudowitz, B.S. (1980). Frontal lobe system dysfunction in some criminal actions in a Narratives Test. *Journal of Nervous and Mental Disease*, 168, 111–117.

Price, L.S., Fein, G., & Feinberg, I. (1980). Neuropsychological assessment of cognitive function in the elderly. In L.W. Poon (Ed.), *Aging in the 1980s*. Washington, DC: American Psychological Association.

Prigitano, G.P. (1983). Neuropsychological test performance in mildly hypoxemic patients with chronic obstructive pulmonary disease. *Journal of Consulting and Clinical Psychology, 51,* 108–116.

Reitan, R.M. (1971). Trail Making Test results for normal and brain-damaged children. *Perceptual and Motor Skills, 33,* 575–581.

Reitan, R.M., & Wolfson, D. (1985). *The Halstead-Reitan Neuropsychological Test Battery.* Tucson, AZ: Neuropsychology Press.

Reitan, R.M., & Wolfson, D. (1988). *Traumatic Brain Injury. Vol. II: Recovery and Rehabilitation.* Tucson, AZ: Neuropsychology Press.

Reitan, R.M., & Wolfson, D. (1995). Category Test and Trail Making Test as measures of frontal lobe functions. *Clinical Neuropsychologist, 9,* 50–56.

Richardson, E.D., & Marottoli, R.A. (1996). Education-specific normative data on common neuropsychological indices for individuals older than 75 years. *The Clinical Neuropsychologist, 10,* 375–381.

Ricker, J.H., & Axelrod, B.N. (1994). Analysis of an oral paradigm for the Trail Making Test. *Assessment, 1,* 47–51.

Ricker, J.H., Axelrod, B.N., & Houtler, B.D. (1996). Clinical validation of the oral Trail Making Test. *Neuropsychiatry, Neuropsychology, and Behavioral Neurology, 9,* 50–53.

Russell, E.W. (1980). Tactile sensation—An all-or-none effect of cerebral damage. *Journal of Clinical Psychology, 36,* 858–864.

Russell, E.W., & Starkey, R.I. (1993). *Halstead Russell Neuropsychological Evaluation System.* Los Angeles: Western Psychological Services.

Salthouse, T.A., & Fristoe, N.M. (1995). Process analysis of adult age effects on a computer-adinistered Trail Making Test. *Neuropsychology, 9,* 518–528.

Schear, J.M., & Sato, S.D. (1989). Effects of visual acuity and visual motor speed and dexterity on cognitive test performance. *Archives of Clinical Neuropsychology, 4,* 25–33.

Schmidt, M., Trueblood, W., Merwin, M., & Durham, R.L. (1994). How much do "attention" tests tell us? *Archives of Clinical Neuropsychology, 9,* 383–394.

Shum, D.H.K., McFarland, K.A., & Bain, J.D. (1990). Construct validity of eight tests of attention: Comparison of normal and closed head injury samples. *Clinical Neuropsychologist, 4,* 151–162.

Snow, W.G., Tierney, M.C., Zorzitto, M.L., Fisher, R.H., & Reid, D.W. (1988). One-year test–retest reliability of selected neuropsychological tests in older adults. *Journal of Clinical and Experimental Neuropsychology, 10,* 60 (abstract).

Schreiber, D.J., Goldman, H., Kleinman, K.M., Goldfader, P.R., & Snow, M.Y. (1976). The relationship between independent neuropsychological and neurological detection of cerebral impairment. *Journal of Nervous and Mental Disease, 162,* 360–365.

Stanton, B.A., Jenkins, C.D., Savageau, J.A., Zyzanski, S.J., & Aucoin, R. (1984). Age and education differences on the Trail Making Test and Wechsler Memory Scales. *Perceptual and Motor Skills, 58,* 311–318.

Storandt, M., Botwinick, J., & Danziger, W.L. (1984). Psychometric differentiation of mild dementia of the Alzheimer type. *Archives of Neurology, 41,* 497–499.

Stuss, D.T., Stethem, L.L., Hugenholtz, H., & Richard, M.T. (1989). Traumatic brain injury: A comparison of three clinical tests, and analysis of recovery. *The Clinical Neuropsychologist, 3,* 145–156.

Stuss, D.T., Stethem, L.L., & Poirier, C.A. (1987). Comparison of three tests of attention and rapid information processing across six age groups. *The Clinical Neuropsychologist, 1,* 139–152.

Stuss, D.T., Stethem, L.L., & Pelchat, G. (1988). Three tests of attention and rapid information processing: An extension. *The Clinical Neuropsychologist, 2,* 246–250.

Sutker, P.B., Vasterling, J.J., Brailey, K., & Allain, A.N. (1995). Memory, attention, and executive deficits in POW survivors: Contributing biological and psychological factors. *Neuropsychology, 9,* 118–125.

Tombaugh, T.N., Rees, L., & McIntyre, N. (1996). Normative data for the Trail Making Test. Personal communication.

Trites, R.L. (1977). *Neuropsychological Test Manual.* Ottawa, ON: Royal Ottawa Hospital.

Uchiyama, C.L., Mitrushina, M.N., D'Elia, L.F., et al. (1994). Frontal lobe functioning in geriatric and nongeriatric samples: An argument for multimodal analyses. *Archives of Clinical Neuropsychology, 9,* 215–227.

Waldman, B.W., Dickson, A.L., Monahan, M.C., & Kazelskis, R. (1992). The relationship between intellectual abilities and adult performance on the Trail Making Test and the Symbol Digit Modalities Test. *Journal of Clinical Psychology, 48,* 360–363.

Warner, M.H., Ernst, J., Townes, B.D., Peel, J., & Preston, M. (1987). Relationship between IQ and neuropsychological measures in neuropsychiatric populations: Within-laboratory and cross-cultural replications using WAIS and WAIS-R. *Journal of Clinical and Experimental Neuropsychology, 9,* 545–562.

Wedding, D. (1979). A comparison of statistical, actuarial, and clinical models used in predicting presence, lateralization, and type of brain damage in humans. Unpublished Ph.D. dissertation, University of Hawaii.

Wheeler, L., & Reitan, R.M. (1963). Discriminant functions applied to the problem of predicting cerebral damage from behavioral tests: A cross-validation study. *Perceptual and Motor Skills, 16,* 681–701.

Williams, J., Rickert, V., Hogan, J., Zolten, A.J., Satz, P., D'Elia, L.F., Asarnow, R.F., Zaucha, K., & Light, R. (1995). Children's Color Trails.

Archives of Clinical Neuropsychology, 10, 211–223.

Woodruff, G.R., Mendoza, J.E., Dickson, A.L., Blanchard, E., & Christenberry, L.B. (1995). The effects of configural differences on the Trail Making Test. *Archives of Clinical Neuropsychology, 10,* 408 (abstract).

Yeudall, L.T., Reddon, J.R., Gill, D.M., & Stefanyk, W.O. (1987). Normative data for the Halstead-Reitan neuropsychological tests stratified by age and sex. *Journal of Clinical Psychology, 43,* 346–367.

Youngjohn, J.R., Burrows, L., & Erdal, K. (1995). Brain damage or compensation neurosis? The controversial post-concussion syndrome. *Clinical Neuropsychologist, 9,* 112–123.

VISUAL NEGLECT

Other Test Name

This test is also known as the Bells Test.

Purpose

The purpose of this test is to detect visual hemi-inattention or "hemineglect," usually to the side contralateral to the lesion.

Source

A number of different measures have been developed by several authors. Line bisection (marking the midpoint of a horizontal line) is one of the simplest ones, requiring no specific test material. The test is also available in a computer version from Life Science Associates, 1 Fenimore Road, Bayport, NY 11705 for $40 US. Another computer program available from the same source requires the subject to "Search for the Odd Shape," the position of which is constantly varied. Cohen et al. (1995) use a colored circle presented at the center and peripheral right or left on a computer screen. Observations during clock and other drawings, block construction, writing, and right–left orientation often provide useful clues. The Visual Search and Attention Test (VSAT) and Raven's Progressive Matrices also provide some indications of visual neglect. Albert (1973) presented an array of 40 short lines randomly placed on a page which must be crossed by the patient, and Villardita et al.

(1983) increased the number of lines to be crossed to 90. Letter cancellation (including the D2-test) can be used (Diller & Weinberg, 1977); Caplan (1987) offered an indented paragraph reading test. A formally published test, offered by Wilson et al. (1987), combines subtests of line bisection, letter cancellation, star cancellation, figure copying, representational drawing, article reading, and letter copying. We use the Bells Test (Gauthier et al., 1989).

Description

The Bells Test (Gauthier et al., 1989) consists of a 21.5 × 28 cm sheet of paper on which seven lines of 35 distractor figures (bird, key, apple, mushroom, car etc.) and five target figures (bells) each are presented. The target figures are arranged so that five each appear in seven equal columns on the page. The number of distractor figures in each column also remains constant. The test is similar to that used in the Arizona Battery for Communication Disorders of Dementia (ABCD) which uses letters instead of bells.

Administration

The subject is seated at a table across from the examiner with both forearms placed comfortably on the table. He or she is presented with a demonstration sheet including the target figure at the center and all distractors (Figure 12–6) and asked to name the items as the ex-

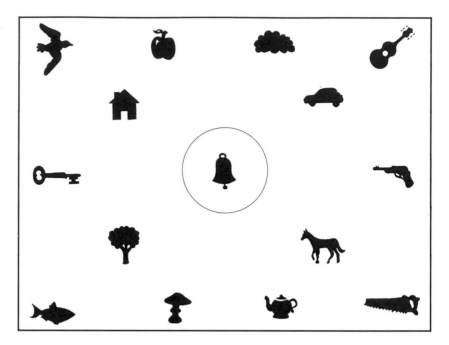

Figure 12—6. Demonstration Sheet for the Bells Test. Used to familiarize the subject with the bell figure and distractor figures. Gauthier et al. (1989).

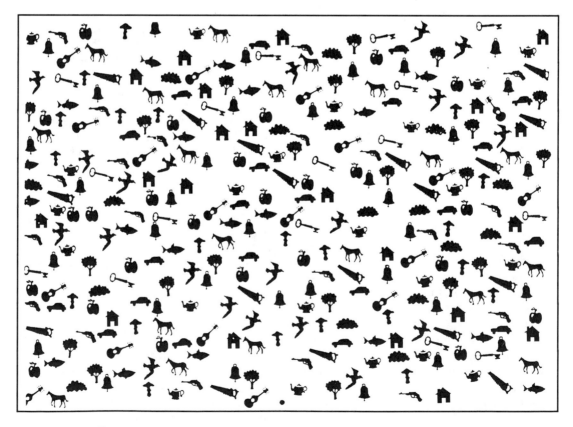

Figure 12—7. Bells Test for Visual Neglect. Gauthier et al. (1989).

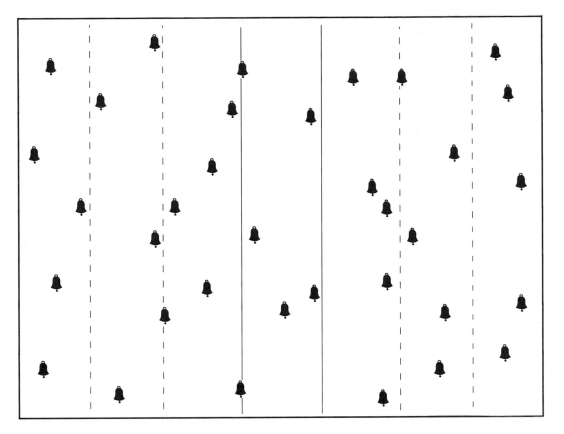

Figure 12—8. Scoring Sheet for the Bells Test, indicating bells in central location and in three left and three right sectors of the visual field. Source: Gauthier et al. (1989).

aminer points to them. If the subject is unable to name the items because of language problems, he or she is asked to place cards representing each object on top of the object to ensure proper object recognition. The examiner then presents the test copy (Figure 12–7) and provides the following instructions: *"Your task consists of circling with the pencil all the bells that you can find on this sheet. Start when I say 'GO' and stop when you have circled all the bells"* (adapted from Gauthier et al., 1989, pp. 49–50).

If the patient stops before all bells are circled, the examiner gives the following reminder only once: *"Are you sure that all bells are now circled? Please check again."* The examiner continues to check bells circled after this admonition, but marks them by underlining or circling the numbers for later identification.

Care should be taken that the sheet is placed in the center of the subject's view and that he or she does not lean to the right or left of the sheet.

Approximate Time for Administration

The test requires 1–5 minutes after instructions.

Scoring

The examiner keeps the score sheet (Figure 12–8) away from view of the subject and records by successive numbering the circling of bells by the subject as well as the circling of other elements in the approximate location. This allows analysis of the scanning pattern of the patient after the test is completed.

The score consists of the number of bells correctly circled, and the time for completion of the test.

Gauthier et al. (1989) recommend scoring only the errors in the right and left side of the visual field, and scoring omissions in the center separately. For this type of scoring, the test sheet is divided lengthwise into seven sections (three left, three right, one center, see Fig. 12–8).

Comment

Visual neglect or hemi-inattention has been viewed as a more severe form of visual extinction (by competing stimuli in the opposite field), but others (Halligan & Robertson, 1992) have pointed out that it can be viewed as a separate, and even dissociated phenomenon. A detailed symposium discussion of recent research on neglect is introduced by Cermak (1996).

The reliability of the Bells Test is not reported. To establish concurrent validity, Vanier et al. (1990) compared the test with Albert's line crossing task and found that it identifies a higher percentage of stroke patients with neglect in comparison to Albert's test. Other studies (Wilson et al., 1987) indicate that results vary when different measures of neglect are used. The use of distractor items ("background noise") instead of line crossing also tends to detect mild and moderate neglect more readily (Marsh & Kersel, 1993; Weintraub & Mesulam, 1985) because the subject has to develop a consistent search strategy: Moving across the page in either horizontal or vertical fashion. Improvement on measures of neglect during the first 90 days after stroke correlates positively with functional outcome as measured on an activities-of-daily-living scale (Marsh & Kersel, 1993).

The results by Gauthier et al. (1985) suggest that patients with right-hemisphere lesions (Parkinson's disease) are more likely to show neglect. This has been demonstrated in previous studies with other tests (Battersby et al., 1956; Costa et al., 1969; Friedland & Weinstein, 1977; Gainotti et al., 1972). Heilman and Valenstein (1972) viewed unilateral neglect as a result of a defect in the attention-arousal response relating to damage to the "corticolimbic-reticular loop." A possible effect of language problems in left-hemisphere-damaged subjects because of the use of verbalizations during the search for figures (bells)

has been ruled out in a study by Caplan (1985), who found comparable results by subjects with neglect on nonverbal and verbal cancellation tasks. Visual field defects and hemianopia appear to affect visual neglect tasks only minimally; patients with field defects appear to be able to compensate with adequate search strategies (Rosenberger, 1974). Patients with AD tend to make more errors in the center of the page due to poor search strategies (Geldmacher et al., 1995).

It has been noted that patients with right-hemisphere lesions tend to start the search process on the side ipsilateral to the lesion (i.e., the right side) (Friedman, 1992; Gainotti et al., 1990). This simple observation is fairly predictive of neglect in 83 percent of the cases during the early stages of the disorder but tends to be less frequent and less predictive after several months when adequate search strategies have been redeveloped. Patients with right-hemisphere lesions also showed crossovers and bisected lines to the left of the midline (Chatterjee, 1995) and responded more slowly to left-sided stimuli (Ladavas et al., 1994). Samuelson et al. (1996) found that neglect after right-hemisphere stroke was correctly identified in 83 percent of their cases, and in 98 percent of cases without neglect with the Behavioral Inattention Test; however, identification was less reliable when only one of the measures was used. At a 6- to 7 months follow-up they also found that only 50 percent of their patients still showed neglect, while patients without neglect were identified at the same rate (98 percent).

Kixmiller et al. (1995) note that neglect may not be unitary in nature, and that visual and tactile neglect may be dissociated, dependent on the site of the lesion; as a tactual exploration task, they asked blindfolded subjects to find a pin on a corkboard. Beschin et al. (1996) described four patients with right cerebral lesions, two of whom showed left and two who showed right tactile neglect.

Normative Data

The authors consider total time for completion of the test as irrelevant to the measurement of neglect although it may be of importance

Table 12—17. Distribution of Subjects According to the Number of Omitted Bells in Each Visual Field

	Controls (n = 20)	Brain Damaged	
		Right (n = 19)	Left (n = 20)
Left Omissions			
0	11	1	10
1–3	9	8	8
4–35	0	10	2
Right Omissions			
0	11	5	10
1–3	9	13	7
4–35	0	1	3

Source: Gauthier et al., 1989.

when test performances at different times during the recovery stage are compared.

The number of errors in the three left and the three right segments of the Bells Test for older (mean age = 71 years) hospital controls without neurological deficit and for older right- and left-CVA patients (mean age = 68 years) are shown in Table 12–17. Young control subjects (age 18–28 years) showed an organized scanning pattern either vertical or horizontal and made no more than two errors on either half of the test; normal subjects between age 50 and 81 years omitted no more than three bells; in contrast, CVA patients tended to show a more disorganized scanning pattern and higher error scores.

It should be noted that line bisection and similar tasks tend to show a tendency to bisect too far to the left in both normal right-handed and left-handed subjects (Luh et al., 1995). Fujii et al. (1995) confirmed this finding but noted that in older (61–82 years) subjects this changes to a deviation to the right side. The possibility of a similar "pseudoneglect" has not yet been investigated for the Bells Test.

Gauthier et al. (1989) report no significant effects for sex of subjects.

References

Albert, M.C. (1973). A simple test of visual neglect. *Neurology, 23,* 558–664.

Battersby, W.S., Bender, M.B., & Pollack, M. (1956). Unilateral spatial agnosia (inattention) in patients with cerebral lesions. *Brain, 79,* 68–93.

Beschin, N., Cazzani, M., Cubelli, R., et al. (1996). Ignoring left and far: An investigation of tactile neglect. *Neuropsychologia, 34,* 41–49.

Caplan, B. (1985). Stimulus effects in unilateral neglect? *Cortex, 21,* 69–80.

Caplan, B. (1987). Assessment of unilateral neglect: A new reading test. *Journal of Clinical and Experimental Neuropsychology, 9,* 359–364.

Cermak, L.S. (1996). Varieties of neglect. *Journal of the International Neuropsychological Society, 2,* 403.

Chatterjee, A. (1995). Cross-over, completion, and confabulation in unilateral spatial neglect. *Brain, 118,* 455–465.

Cohen, A., Ivry, R.B., Rafal, R.D., & Kohn, C. (1995). Activating response codes by stimuli in the neglected visual field. *Neuropsychology, 9,* 165–173.

Costa, L.D., Vaughan, H.G., Horwitz, M., & Ritter, W. (1969). Patterns of behavior deficit associated with visual spatial neglect. *Cortex, 5,* 242–263.

Diller, L., & Weinberg, J. (1977). Hemi-inattention in rehabilitation: The evolution of a rational remediation program. In E.A. Weinstein & P. Friedland (Eds.), *Hemi-Inattention and Hemisphere Specialization. Advances in Neurology,* Vol. 18. New York: Raven Press, pp. 63–68.

Friedland, R.P., & Weinstein, E.A. (1977). Hemi-inattention and hemisphere specialization: Introduction and historical review. In E.A. Weinstein & R.P. Friedland (Eds.), *Hemi-Inattention and Hemisphere Specialization. Advances in Neurology,* Vol. 18. New York: Raven Press. pp. 1–31.

Friedman, P.J. (1992). The star cancellation test in acute stroke. *Clinical Rehabilitation, 6,* 23–30.

Fujii, T., Fukatsu, R., Yamadori, A., & Kimura, I. (1995). Effect of age on the line bisection test. *Journal of Clinical and Experimental Neuropsychology, 17,* 941–944.

Gainotti, G., Giustolisi, L., & Nocentini, U. (1990). Contralateral and ipsilateral disorders of visual attention in patients with unilateral brain damage. *Journal of Neurology, Neurosurgery, and Psychiatry, 53,* 422–426.

Gainotti, G., Messerli, P., & Tissot, R. (1972). Qualitative analysis of unilateral spatial neglect in relation to laterality of cerebral lesions. *Journal of Neurology, Neurosurgery, and Psychiatry, 35,* 545–550.

Gauthier, L., DeHaut, F., & Joanette, Y. (1989).

The Bells Test: A quantitative and qualitative test for visual neglect. *International Journal of Clinical Neuropsychology, 11,* 49–54.

Gauthier, L., Gauthier, F., & Joanette, Y. (1985). Visual neglect in left, right and bilateral Parkinsonism. *Journal of Clinical and Experimental Neuropsychology, 7,* 145 (abstract).

Geldmacher, D.S., Doti, L., & Heilman, K.M. (1995). Letter cancellation performance in Alzheimer's disease. *Neuropsychiatry, Neuropsychology, and Behavioral Neurology, 8,* 259–263.

Halligan, P.W., & Robertson, I.H. (1992). The assessment of unilateral neglect. In J.R. Crawford, D.M. Partker, & W.W. McKinlay (Eds.), *A Handbook of Neuropsychological Assessment.* Hillsdale, NJ: Lawrence Erlbaum. pp. 151–175.

Heilman, K.M., & Valenstein, E. (1972). Frontal lobe neglect in man. *Neurology, 22,* 600–664.

Kixmiller, J.S., Rogers, M., & Fischer, R.S. (1995). Lesion site and different manifestations of hemispatial neglect. *Archives of Clinical Neuropsychology, 10,* 351 (abstract).

Ladavas, E., Farne, M., Carbetti, M., & Zeloni, G. (1994). Neglect determined by the relative location of responses. *Brain, 117,* 705–714.

Luh, K.E. (1995). Line bisection and perception of asymmetries in normal subjects: What you see is not what you get. *Neuropsychology, 9,* 435–448.

Marsh, N.V., & Kersel, D.A. (1993). Screening tests for visual neglect following stroke. *Neuropsychological Rehabilitation, 3,* 245–257.

Rosenberger, P. (1974). Discriminative aspects of visual hemi-inattention. *Neurology, 24,* 17–23.

Samelson, H., Hjelmquist, E., Naver, H., & Blomstrand, C. (1996). Visuospatial neglect and an ipsilateral bias during the start of performance in conventional tests of neglect. *The Clinical Neuropsychologist, 10,* 15–24.

Vanier, M., Gauthier, L., & Lambert, J. (1990). Evaluation of left visuospatial neglect: Norms and discrimination power of two tests. *Neuropsychology, 4,* 87–96.

Villardita, C., Smirni, P., & Zappala, G. (1983). Visual neglect in Parkinson's disease. *Archives of Neurology, 40,* 737–739.

Weintraub, S., & Mesulam, M.M. (1985). Mental state assessment of young and elderly adults in behavioral neurology. In M.M. Mesulam (Ed.), *Principles of Behavioral Neurology.* Contemporary Neurology Series, Vol. 26. Philadelphia: F.A. Davis Co. pp. 71–123.

Wilson, B., Cockburn, J., & Halligan, P. (1987). *Behavioural Inattention Test.* Fareham, England: Thames Valley Test Company.

13

Tactile, Tactile-Visual, and Tactile-Motor Tests

Tactile sensitivity is part of the routine examination in neurology, typically conducted with touch by gauze pad, pin prick, or von Frey hair stimulation. A small number of standardized techniques including calibrated stimulators have been developed since Bender's (1948) studies of extinction on double stimulation, Benton's (1959) work on right–left discrimination and finger localization, and Teuber's (Semmes et al., 1960) investigations of somatosensory changes after penetrating head injury, including the automated and highly technically refined stimulation technique of Carmon and Dyson (1967).

Neuropsychological examinations with standardized tests can and do surpass the accuracy of the clinical neurological examination. The main interest is usually on differences between the two sides (usually hands) of the body, although bilaterally raised thresholds may also be of significance. Our selection includes pure touch threshold measurements (aesthesiometer), the tactile extinction on double stimulation technique, two-point dis-

crimination, and the psychologically more complex functions of finger localization, stereognostic recognition (Tactile Form Perception), and the Tactual Performance Test, which includes both a localization and a memory component in addition to stereognosis. We have omitted graphaesthesia (skin writing) and similar tests that tend to overlap with the tests described here.

References

Bender, M.B., Wortis, S.B., & Cramer, J. (1948). Organic mental syndromes with phenomena of extinction and allesthesia. *Archives of Neurology and Psychiatry*, 59, 273–291.

Benton, A.L. (1959). *Right-Left Discrimination and Finger Localization.* New York: Hoeber.

Carmon, A., & Dyson, J.A. (1967). New instrumentation for research on tactile sensitivity and discrimination. *Cortex*, 3, 406–418.

Semmes, J., Weinstein, S., Ghent, L., & Teuber, H.L. (1960). *Somatosensory Changes after Penetrating Brain Wounds in Man.* Cambridge, MA: Harvard University Press.

AESTHESIOMETER

Other Test Name

Another test name is Pressure Aesthesiometer.

Purpose

The purpose of the test is to measure tactile thresholds.

Source

The Semmes-Weinstein Monofilaments can be ordered from Lafayette Instrument Company, P.O. Box 5729, Lafayette, IN 47903-5729, at a cost of $295 US.

Description

The test consists of 20 nylon filaments of uniform 3.8 cm length and of increasing thickness, each mounted at the end of a 13 cm plastic stick holder. The material comes with pressure weight labels as described in Semmes, Weinstein, Ghent, and Teuber (1960), attached to the holders but with only a minimum of instructions. Since the weight labels are on a relatively meaningless logarithmic scale, we have translated them into gram pressure in the scoring sheet (Figure 13–1).

Administration

Although tactile thresholds can be tested on any part of the body, our routine administration is to test the third finger nailbed of each hand to avoid areas of hair growth and callus. Stimuli are applied slowly with enough pressure to create a 45-degree bend in the filament out of sight of the subject (preferably under a covering box) and held in that position for about one second. The subject is asked to say "touch" or otherwise indicate when he or she feels the stimulus. Reports made when

	Aesthesiometer Sample Scoring Sheet	
Name:	Date:	Age: Examiner:
Right Hand		Left Hand
Third Finger Nailbed		Third Finger Nailbed
Ascending Descending	grams/pressure	Ascending Descending
	447.0	
	281.5	
	127.0	
	75.0	
	29.0	
	15.0	
	11.7	
	8.65	
	5.50	
	3.63	
	2.06	
	1.49	
	1.19	
	.70	
	.41	
	.17	
	.07	
	.03	
	.02	
	.004	
_____	Threshold Measure Hand Threshold	_____
_____	Mean	_____
_____	Median	_____
_____	SD	_____

Figure 13—1. Aesthesiometer sample scoring sheet.

there is no stimulus are scored as zero. If the examiner feels that the subject is merely slow in responding, the examiner repeats the admonition to report as soon as the stimulus is felt, and also repeats the stimulation if necessary.

Begin stimulation with the dominant hand using filament .004 and ascend in single steps until three successive touches have been reported. Begin descending order with the next lowest filament (i.e., the second above the ascending threshold) and decrease in single steps until two successive zero scores have been obtained.

Young children often show fear of the filament, believing that they are going to be pricked or that the stimulus is painful. It is good practice to assure all subjects that the procedure is not painful, and to accompany such assurance with a demonstration on the subject's and/or the examiner's forearm before screening the hand. Apply stimuli slowly since otherwise a velocity component is added to filament resistance and can lead to spuriously low thresholds.

With small children, accuracy of site of stimulation is restricted to the general area between the distal joint and the fingernail.

Care should be taken to avoid experimenter cues when the stimulus is applied. The subject may be asked to look away or close the eyes.

Since the objective is to obtain a relatively stable measure, there is no objection to repeating the stimulation if necessary.

Approximate Time for Administration

The time required is 5–10 minutes for both hands.

Scoring

The threshold measure for each hand is the mean of the first ascending and the last descending touch response.

If the subject reports a touch at a low level followed by zero responses at greater pressure, the trial series should be repeated. The lowest score is taken to mean the lowest of two successive positives.

Comment

Reliability data are not available. This rather expensive equipment tends to deteriorate with frequent use. Handle with care. Although similar results may be obtained with various commercial versions of "von Frey hair" stimulators on the market, we found this instrument more accurate and reliable. The main value of the test is usually in discovering unilateral elevations in threshold. Differences of three or more steps between hands raise the possibility of a pathologically increased threshold. Larger differences are fairly reli-

Table 13—1. Smoothed Normative Data for Adults by Age

Age	n	Right hand	(SD)	Left hand	(SD)
Males					
20–29	24	0.34	(0.25)	0.30	(0.21)
30–49	18	0.42	(0.25)	0.43	(0.22)
50–59	24	0.57	(0.34)	0.42	(0.30)
60–69	25	0.66	(0.39)	0.50	(0.43)
70–84	18	0.86	(0.46)	0.80	(0.53)
Females					
20–29	26	0.25	(0.20)	0.24	(0.17)
30–49	20	0.44	(0.33)	0.45	(0.50)
50–59	24	0.52	(0.37)	0.45	(0.30)
60–69	23	0.59	(0.39)	0.46	(0.38)
70–84	25	0.66	(0.45)	0.65	(0.40)

Source: Spreen & Strauss, 1990

able indicators of pathology. The possibility of peripheral lesions should be explored before central lesions are inferred. The test is surprisingly sensitive even if the standard tactile threshold examination in neurological practice yields negative results.

However, minor differences may be due to unilateral neglect rather than elevated thresholds. Specific testing for neglect may be indicated (see section on tactile extinction). In some subjects other attentional problems may interfere.

Normative Data

Semmes et al. (1960) reported data on head-injured patients. Weinstein's studies on tactile sensitivity for different parts of the body (1962, 1968), following up on Weber's classical study (1835), found minor differences showing better sensitivity for the left hand and for females for the three phalanges of each finger. A study in our laboratory (Table 13–1) with healthy adults confirmed these slight differences between hands and showed increasing thresholds with age. In addition, females had significantly lower thresholds than males.

Using a von Frey hair instrument with nine stimulators of increasing pressure, Russell (1980) found that most of 40 normal and 158 brain-damaged subjects scored on the first three stimuli; a few more of the brain-damaged subjects scored on the fourth stimulus, and only a small proportion of brain-damaged subjects on the last five stimuli. He proposed that tactile sensitivity may be an "all-or-none" function. However, threshold pressures or actual pressures for each of the nine stimuli were not reported. Although the "all-or-none" effect in patients with cerebral damage may be true, smaller pressure differences between stimuli may have detected minor differences that went unnoticed with the instrument used in this study.

Table 13—2. Aesthesiometer: Normative Data for Children Ages 6–12 Years

Age	n	Mean	SD	Median	Range
6	12	.5	0.6	0.4	0.03–2.1
7	50	.3	0.3	0.2	0.03–1.2
8	41	.2	0.2	0.2	0.02–0.7
9	38	.2	0.1	0.2	0.004–0.7
10	36	.2	0.2	0.2	0.004–0.7
11	38	.2	0.2	0.2	0.02–0.7
12	36	.2	0.2	0.2	0.02–0.7

Note: No meaningful differences between right and left hand or between boys and girls were found.

Source: Spreen & Gaddes (1969).

Children's norms developed in our laboratory (Spreen & Gaddes, 1969) are listed in Table 13–2. As can be seen from the table, fairly stable levels are reached by age 8, and they remain within the same range up to age 30.

References

Russell, E.W. (1980). Tactile sensation—An all-or-none effect of cerebral damage. *Journal of Clinical Psychology, 36,* 858–864.

Semmes, J., Weinstein, S., Ghent, L., & Teuber, H.L. (1960). *Somatosensory Changes after Penetrating Head Wounds in Man.* Cambridge, MA: Harvard University Press.

Spreen, O., & Gaddes, W.H. (1969). Developmental norms for 15 neuropsychological tests age 6 to 15. *Cortex, 5,* 171–191.

Weber, E.H. (1835). Über den Tastsinn. *Archiv für die gesamte Anatomie, Physiologie und Wissenschaftliche Medizin, 152.*

Weinstein, S. (1962). Tactile sensitivity of the phalanges. *Perceptual and Motor Skills, 14,* 351–354.

Weinstein, S. (1968). Intensive and extensive aspects of tactile sensitivity as a function of body part, sex, and laterality. In D.R. Kenchalo (Ed.), *The Skin Senses. Proceedings of the First International Symposium on the Skin Senses.* Springfield, IL: C.C. Thomas.

FINGER LOCALIZATION

Purpose

The purpose of the test is the identification, naming, and localization of fingers.

Source

The test is contained in Benton, Hamsher, Varney, and Spreen (1994): *Contributions to Neuropsychological Assessment*. Oxford University Press, 200 Madison Ave. New York, NY 10016. The manual (including 11 other tests) costs $23.95 US. The test material for finger localization is $19.95 US.

Description

This test is based on Benton's (1959) book and originally consisted of 80 items in five parts:

1. Identification by name on the subject's own hand.
2. Identification by name on the examiner's hand.
3. Naming fingers touched by the examiner by either naming or pointing to a hand chart or to the number of the stimulated finger on the chart.
4. Identification of fingers touched by the examiner while the hand is hidden under a curtained table screen.
5. Identification of two simultaneously touched fingers while the hand is hidden.

Only the last three parts are used in the Benton et al. (1994) sourcebook; the first two sets involve naming and are used in our laboratory as introductory material, especially with children. The last three parts can be performed without involving language.

Another version of finger gnosis is included as part of the parietal lobe battery in the Boston Diagnostic Aphasia Examination, described elsewhere in this volume. A somewhat similar, shorter examination is offered by Reitan and Davison (1974) as part of the Halstead-Reitan battery and by Goodglan and Kaplan as part of the Parietal Lobe Battery (see BDEA). Although other versions of tests for finger localization are available, we prefer this one because it is not likely to be affected by even mild aphasia, and it has a sufficient number of trials and extensive norms.

Administration

Five trials for each hand in Parts 1 and 2 are given as introductory material. The test itself consists of 10 trials for each hand for Parts 3, 4, and 5.

Approximate Time for Administration

Approximately 10 minutes are required for this test.

Scoring

Each of the 30 items for the left hand and the 30 items for the right hand is scored as either correct or incorrect (see source). The maximum score is 30 for each hand, with a maximum total of 60.

Comment

Attention to finger agnosia was given following Gerstmann's (1924) and Head's (1920) descriptions. It can occur with lesions on either side of the brain (Benton & Sivan, 1993). While unilateral finger agnosia clearly refers to a unilateral brain lesion, usually with sensory or motor deficit, bilateral finger agnosia is frequent in patients with general mental impairment and aphasia, although this is by no means a regular occurrence.

Reliability data are not available. Concurrent validity with finger dexterity (tapping, putting paper clips into a box) was weak (.26 and .21, Benton, 1959).

Finger localization develops steadily and rapidly with age before age 6 and continues to develop up to age 12. Failure to reach age-appropriate levels has been related to developmental delay and subsequent failure in reading achievement (Badian et al., 1990), but not with differences between right- and left-hand performance (Zung, 1986). Hutchinson (1983) found significant correlations between finger localization and matching spoken to

Table 13—3. Finger Localization: Normative Data for Children Aged 6–13 Years

Age	Normal children				Superior-IQ children			
	n	Right	Left	Total	n	Right	Left	Total
6	12	21	21	42	21	25	25	50
7	50	24	24	48	24	25	25	50
8	41	25	25	50	20	28	28	56
9	38	26	26	52	21	28	28	56
10	36	27	27	54	24	28	28	56
11	38	27	27	54	20	28	28	56
12	36	28	28	56	22	28	28	56
13	52	28	28	56				

Note: Standard deviations range from 3.0 at age 6, to 1.7 at age 13.

printed words and for silent reading and re-telling of a paragraph. Dysphasic children had significantly more difficulty on this task than normal-language children.

Normative Data

Benton et al. (1994) provide detailed norms for 104 normal adults (where errors are quite rare) in relation to educational background up to the age of 65, and for children from ages 3–12 (when adult level is reached), for both right- and left-hand performance. Differences between hands usually do not exceed one or two points (see source). Our own norms for children (Table 13–3) agree closely with those presented by Wake (unpublished, see source) but are higher than those reported by Benton et al., both for normal- and superior-IQ children.

References

Badian, N.A., McAnulty, G.B., Duffy, F.H., & Als, H. (1990). Prediction of dyslexia in kindergarten boys. *Annals of Dyslexia, 40,* 152–169.

Benton, A.L. (1959). *Right-Left Discrimination and Finger Localization. Development and Pathology.* New York: Hoeber/Harper.

Benton, A.L., Hamsher, K.deS., Varney, N.R., & Spreen, O. (1994). *Contributions to Neuropsychological Assessment* (2nd ed). New York: Oxford University Press.

Benton, A.L., & Sivan, A.B. (1993). Body schema disturbances: Finger agnosia and right-left disorientation. In K.M. Heilman & E. Valenstein (Eds.), *Clinical Neuropsychology* (3rd ed.). New York: Oxford University Press.

Gerstmann, J. (1924). Fingeragnosie: eine umschriebene Störung der Orientierung am eigenen Körper. *Wiener klinische Wochenschrift, 37,* 1010–1012.

Head, H. (1920). *Studies in Neurology.* London: Oxford University Press.

Hutchinson, B.P. (1983). Finger localization and reading ability in three groups of children ages three through twelve. *Brain and Language, 20,* 143–154.

Reitan, R.M., & Davison, L.A. (1974). *Clinical Neuropsychology: Current Status and Applications.* New York: Winston/Wiley.

Zung, B.J. (1986). Cognitive-academic correlates of finger localization in right-handed kindergarten girls. *Perceptual and Motor Skills, 62,* 227–234.

TACTILE EXTINCTION

Other Test Names

This test is also known as Double Simultaneous Stimulation.

Purpose

The purpose of this test is to examine for subtle somatosensory deficits.

Source

The test may be administered according to the administration described below or purchased in a standardized version (Centofani & Smith, 1979) from Western Psychological Services, 12031 Wilshire Blvd., Los Angeles, CA 90025, for $55 US.

Description

Extinction on double tactile stimulation (TE) refers to the inability to recognize one or both of two tactile stimuli applied to two parts of the body at the same time—the second stimulus is "extinguished" or not attended to (hemiinattention). TE was first described by Loeb in 1884 (Benton, 1956); Oppenheim (1885) described the examination procedure. Bender (1945, 1952, 1977) developed the "Face-Hand Test"; i.e., two parts of the body (e.g., hand and cheek or right and left hand) are simultaneously touched with the examiner's fingers, a cotton applicator, a gauze pad, or a similar soft or blunt instrument, and the patient is asked to report what stimulation(s) he or she has noticed. Centofani and Smith (1979) present a series of 20 trials alternating between right and left hand and/or cheek and intermixed with single stimulations of one of these parts of the body. The trials can be repeated if errors occur. Schwartz et al. (1979) developed a "Quality Extinction Test," in which they applied materials of different texture such as carpet, wire mesh, paper, or tin foil, and ask the patient whether the stimuli are the same or different.

Administration

The patient is seated with hands in palm-down position, placed on the knees, and not touching each other. He or she is asked to close the eyes and report verbally or by pointing where the patient has been touched by the examiner. We found the aesthesiometer stimuli (see description) useful for TE because they provide the opportunity to apply pressure levels just above the threshold for the body part tested. It should be noted that the thresholds for different body parts are quite different. For example, the cheeks are much more sensitive than the hands or feet (Hannay, 1986). For this reason, the TE can be refined by using suprathreshold stimuli after thresholds have been established with the aesthesiometer. However, extinction occurs even in normal subjects if one or both stimuli are barely above threshold. Hence, in clinical situations, suprathreshold should be defined as at least three steps above threshold.

We recommend three double-stimulation trials each for hand-hand (right and left), cheek-cheek, and for each hand-cheek combination with interspersed single stimulations. Centofani and Smith suggest "two simultaneous light and brisk strokes with the index fingers" as specified in their manual, to either hand and/or cheek.

Approximate Time for Administration

Depending on the number of trials, the test takes about 5–10 minutes.

Scoring

Centofani and Smith count number of extinction errors to the right and left cheek and hand, displacement errors (indicating stimulation on a body part not stimulated), and adjunction errors (indicating two stimulations when only one was applied) in 20 trials. Similar counts are used by other authors.

Comment

TE is a relatively robust measure of subtle sensory deficits. It has been described as "neglect," "allesthesia" (displacement of perceived stimulation to other body parts), and as part of an inattention syndrome (Friedland &

Weinstein, 1977). Heilman (1979) views these terms as continuous; i.e., neglect, allesthesia, and extinction occur at different stages of the patient's recovery, with extinction persisting after other manifestations of neglect can no longer be found. Others see it as different or even dissociated from "neglect" (Halligan & Robertson, 1992).

Information on reliability is not available. Since normal subjects rarely make more than one or two errors on Centofani and Smith's version of the test, any score of three or more errors is indicative of elevated thresholds, reflecting possible lesions in one or both parietal areas. Centofani and Smith (1979) note that bilateral errors are frequent in the acute stage of even a unilateral lesion, and that such bilateral errors tend to diminish in the course of recovery. They also report that TE misclassified only 2.5 percent of normal subjects, but correctly classified 56 percent of 172 patients with cerebral lesions. TE showed impairment in 56 percent of patients with acute lesions. Only 13 percent of the errors were displacements, and only 4 percent were adjunction errors. Schwartz et al. (1979) report 94 percent correct classification in patients with parietal lesions, using the Quality Extinction Test. Kolb and Whishaw (1995) argue that extinction is most common with damage to the somatic secondary cortex (areas PE and PF), especially in the right parietal lobe. Heilman (1979) specifies the inferior parietal lobule ("a multimodal secondary association area") as the primary area affected when a neglect syndrome occurs; however, dorsolateral frontal and cingulate gyrus lesions may also be involved, as well as the neostriate area and the thalamus. The syndrome occurs more often to the left side of the body with right-sided lesions (Hecaen & Albert, 1978). Hence, the test has the potential of contributing to the localization of brain lesions, and it is also sensitive to progressive dementia (Eastwood et al., 1983).

The technique can be applied in the visual or auditory, and even the olfactory and gustatory modality; e.g., by presenting two stimuli simultaneously in the visual fields. In fact, the dichotic listening and the dichhaptic (Witelson, 1974) techniques rely on the extinction phenomenon. Cross-modality studies have also been described (Bender, 1977).

Normative Data

Centofani and Smith present norms based on 431 subjects in six age groups. More than one error was found only in the age groups over 54 years. A mild increase with advancing age was also found by Kahn and Miller (1978).

References

Bender, M.B. (1945). Extinction and precipitation of cutaneous sensations. *Archives of Neurology and Psychiatry, 54,* 1–9.

Bender, M. (1952). *Disorders of Perception.* Springfield, IL: C.C. Thomas.

Bender, M.B. (1977). Extinction and other patterns of sensory interaction. In E.A. Weinstein & R.P. Friedland (Eds.), *Advances in Neurology,* Vol. 18, 197–110.

Benton, A.L. (1956). Jaques Loeb and the method of double stimulation. *Journal of the History of Medicine, 11,* 47–53.

Centofani, C.C., & Smith, A. (1979). *The Single and Double Simultaneous (Face-Hand) Stimulation Test (SDSS).* Los Angeles: Western Psychological Services.

Eastwood, M.R., Lautenschlaeger, E., & Corbin, S. (1983). A comparison of clinical methods for assessing dementia. *Journal of the American Geriatric Society, 31,* 342–347.

Friedland, R.P., & Weinstein, E.A. (1977). Hemiinattention and hemispheric specialization: Introduction and historical review. In E.A. Weinstein & R.P. Friedland (Eds.), *Advances in Neurology,* Vol. 18, pp. 1–31.

Halligan, P.W., & Robertson, I.H. (1992). The assessment of unilateral neglect. In J.R. Crawford, D.M. Parker, & W.W. McKinlay (Eds.), *A Handbook of Neuropsychological Assessment.* Hillsdale, NJ: Lawrence Erlbaum, pp. 151–175.

Hannay, H.J. (1986). *Experimental Techniques in Human Neuropsychology.* New York: Oxford University Press.

Hecaen, H., & Albert, M.L. (1978). *Human Neuropsychology.* New York: Wiley.

Heilman, K.M. (1979). Neglect and related disorders. In K.M. Heilman & E. Valenstein (Eds.), *Clinical Neuropsychology.* New York: Oxford University Press, pp. 268–307.

Kahn, R.L., & Miller, N.E. (1978). Assessment of altered brain function in the aged. In I. Storandt,

I. Siegler, & M. Ellis (Eds.), *The Clinical Psychology of Aging*. New York: Plenum Press.

Kolb, B., & Whishaw, I. (1995). *Fundamentals of Human Neuropsychology* (3rd ed.). New York: W.H. Freeman.

Oppenheim, H. (1885). Über eine durch eine klinisch bisher nicht verwertete Untersuchungsmethode ermittelte Form der Sensibilitätsstörung bei einseitigen Erkrankungen des Grosshirns. *Neurologisches Zentralblatt*, *23*, 529–533.

Schwartz, A.S., Marchok, P.L., Kreinich, C.J., & Flynn, R.E. (1979). The asymmetric lateralization of tactile extinction in patients with unilateral cerebral dysfunction. *Brain*, *102*, 669–684.

Witelson, S.F. (1974). Hemispheric specialization for linguistic and nonlinguistic tactual perception using a dichotomous stimulation technique. *Cortex*, *11*, 3–17.

TACTILE FORM PERCEPTION

Other Test Name

The test is also known as the Stereognosis Test.

Purpose

The test is used as a measure of tactile form recognition and spatial thinking.

Source

The test is contained in Benton et al. (1994). The manual for 12 tests can be obtained from Oxford University Press for $23.95 US. The Tactile Form Perception Test material and forms cost $135 US.

Description

The test consists of two equivalent sets of 10 cards on which geometric figures of fine-grade sandpaper have been pasted. The subject feels one card at a time with one hand under a box-screen with curtain and must point to the corresponding figure on a multiple-choice card with 12 ink-drawn figures which is placed on top of the box.

Administration

Ten trials are given for each hand (see source).

Approximate Time for Administration

The time required is 10–15 minutes.

Scoring

Each item is scored as either correct or incorrect (see source). One set of 10 cards is used for each hand, allowing for a maximum score of 10 correct choices for each hand. One additional card is used for practice.

Comment

Alternate form reliability is reported as showing only minimal differences when both forms were given (Benton et al., 1994), but other reliability data are not available. This test is more demanding than the usual object-naming or object-matching tasks routinely used during neurological and neuropsychological examinations because (1) the stimuli are of an abstract nature; (2) no naming is required; and (3) it adds to the task a dimension of spatial exploration by touch. It is a more rigorous examination of stereognosis than Halstead's three-dimensional tactile form recognition test in which only four objects (cross, circle, triangle, and square) are used for both hands.

Careful observation of the exploratory movements by the subject is necessary, since failure to explore may give misleading results. The test usually cannot be used in subjects with moderate sensory loss or with motor impairment.

Patients with unilateral lesions tend to show impairment on the contralateral side. The test authors also report high sensitivity of this test for right-hemisphere lesions (with bilateral impairment), although patients with left-hemisphere lesions may also show impaired

Table 13—4. Tactile Form Perception: Norms for Children

Age	Number correct			Time for 10 cards (in seconds)		
	n	M	SD	n	M	SD
8	37	8.1	1.3	16	124.1	34.8
9	86	8.1	1.3	40	119.7	41.4
10	90	8.3	1.3	44	108.8	40.6
11	61	8.6	1.2	18	83.5	32.5
12	48	9.3	0.9			
13	38	9.3	1.0			
14	44	9.5	0.9			
15	7	9.8	0.6			

Source: Spreen & Gaddes (1969).

performance (Benton, 1994), and the performance of patients with bilateral lesions is quite low.

Normative Data

The source provides detailed norms for adults, elderly adults, and children, and for a variety of performance patterns in patients with brain damage. Performance levels in children under the age of 12 years tend to vary, especially for the nonpreferred hand. The adult level of near-perfect performance (no more than one error) is usually reached by age 14, as shown by Spreen and Gaddes (1969) (Table 13–4). Differences between preferred and nonpreferred hands and between boys and girls were minimal in this study. Although under standard administration conditions no time score is taken (the trial is discontinued if the subject does not respond after 45 seconds, with prompting after 30 seconds), our table shows a rapid increase of speed of performance between the ages of 8 and 11 years.

References

Benton, A.L. (1994). Neuropsychological assessment. *Annual Review of Psychology, 45,* 1–23.

Benton, A.L., Sivan, A.B., Hamsher, K. de S., Varney, N.R., & Spreen, O. (1994). *Contributions to Neuropsychological Assessment.* New York: Oxford University Press.

Spreen, O., & Gaddes, W.H. (1969). Developmental norms for 15 neuropsychological tests age 6 to 15. *Cortex, 5,* 171–191.

TACTUAL PERFORMANCE TEST (TPT)

Other Test Names

Other test names are Form Board Test and the Seguin-Goddard Formboard.

Purpose

The purpose of this test is to assess tactile form recognition, memory for shapes and spatial location, as well as psychomotor problem solving.

Source

The test can be ordered from the Reitan Neuropsychology Laboratory, 2920 S. Fourth Ave., Tucson, AZ 85713-4819 (10- and 6-hole boards, stand, and 10 blocks) at a cost of $310 US, (without 6-hole board) $255. It is also available from Lafayette Instrument Company, P.O. Box 5729, Lafayette, IN 47903-5729 (10- and 6-hold board and blocks) for $75 US, and from Psych Tec, Inc., 6211 9th N.E., Seattle, WA 98115 (set of 2 boards, blocks, and stand in lightweight plastic) $295 US; or from Technolab Industries, Ltd., 5757 Decelles Ave., Montreal, PQ H3S 2C3 (set of 2 boards, blocks, and stand) for $432 Cdn. Psychological Assessment Resources (P.O. Box 998, Odessa, FL) offers a portable version of both boards and a brief manual for $315 US.

Description

This version of the Seguin formboard is administered according to Halstead's (1947) procedure. As a test of tactile memory, it includes two trials, one for the preferred and one for the nonpreferred hand, a third using both hands. After completion of these trials, the board is concealed, the blindfold is removed, and the subject is asked to draw from memory, indicating both the shape of the blocks and their placement relative to each other. Three scores are obtained: (1) total time on the tactile trials, (2) a memory score for the number of blocks correctly reproduced, and (3) a location score for the number of correctly located blocks in the drawing. There are two different formboards: The 10-hole formboard is used for subjects aged 15 and over, and the 6-hole formboard is used for children below the age of 15. In addition to the formboard material, a clean, comfortably fitting blindfold (eye mask) and a stopwatch are required. Scoring forms can be easily produced. The material is sturdy and hardly ever needs replacement.

Administration

For subjects 8 years old and younger, the 6-block formboard is mounted horizontally in the stand with the cross in the upper left-hand corner. With subjects aged 9 years to 14 years, 11 months, the 6-block formboard is mounted vertically in the stand with the cross in the upper right-hand corner. With subjects 15 years of age and older, the 10-block board is mounted vertically in the stand with the cross in the upper right-hand corner.

For repeat administration, the board is set upright at the same angle as above, but the long axis of the board is vertical instead of horizontal. Instructions and procedure are exactly the same, but in scoring the subject's drawing, one must remember that the face of the board has been turned 90 degrees.

The subject is seated squarely facing and close to the table. Two gauze pads are placed over the eyes and a blindfold is tied over them. The examiner questions the subject about his or her ability to see, especially downward. When the examiner is certain the subject cannot see, the board is brought out. The blocks are placed in random sequence between the board and the subject. Blocks adjacent to each other on the board should not be placed next to each other on the table. Some examiners prefer to guide the subject to each block presented in standardized order, whereas our administration allows the subject to pick blocks in random order. Chavez, Schwartz, and Brandon (1982) indicated that the two modes of presentation show no differences in the results of the test.

Ask the subject to give you the preferred (dominant) hand. Take the subject's wrist and move the hand over the board and the pieces on the table while giving the following instructions: "*In front of you on the table is a board. This is the size and shape of it.* (Move the subject's hand around the edge of the board). *On the face of the board are holes of various shapes and sizes* (move subject's hand across the face of the board), *and here in front of you are blocks of various shapes and sizes* (pass the subject's hand over the blocks, then place the subject's hand in his or her lap). *You are to fit the blocks into the spaces on the board. There is a place for each block and a block for each opening. Now I want you to do your best using only your right hand* (or left if that is the dominant hand). *You may begin whenever you are ready.*"

Start the stopwatch when the subject first touches the board or blocks and stop it when the last piece has been placed. Record the time for each hand in minutes and seconds. It is helpful to praise the subject for correctly placed blocks, and to encourage the subject if he or she is not doing well. As the blocks in front of the subject are used up, push over the others to keep a supply ready at hand. When the subject has finished, ask him or her not to remove the blindfold and suggest that the subject relax for a minute or two.

If after 10 minutes less than seven blocks are placed correctly, the trial is discontinued. If seven or more blocks have been placed, the trial should continue up to 15 minutes and then be stopped unless the patient is about to complete the task.

After laying out the blocks again in random order, say: "*Now I want you to do the test again, and this time you are to use only your left hand* (or 'right', if that is the nondominant hand). *Begin whenever you are ready."* Record the time needed for this hand.

Lay out the blocks for the third time and say: *"This time you may use both hands for the test."* When the subject is finished, ask him or her to leave the blindfold on for a few minutes. Record the time required for both hands; then put the board out of sight. Tell the subject to remove the blindfold.

Place a sheet of white paper and pencil in front of subject and say: *"Now on this sheet of paper I want you to draw an outline of the shape of the board. On your drawing, put in the shapes of the blocks in the same place as you remember them to be on the board. Note that there are three parts to your task; the shape of the board, the shapes of the blocks, and their location on the board. Be sure to label the top of your drawing. There is no time limit on this."*

Approximate Time for Administration

The time required ranges from 15 minutes to 50 minutes.

Scoring

This test is scored by calculating the total time for the three tactile placement trials (Time right, left, both hands), by counting the number of blocks correctly drawn (Memory), and by counting the number of blocks properly located in the drawings (Location). Differences between right- and left-hand performance should be noted as shown in the sample score

Seconds	Score
1–3	0.0
4–8	0.1
9–15	0.2
16–20	0.3
21–27	0.4
28–32	0.5
33–39	0.6
40–44	0.7
45–51	0.8
52–56	0.9
57–60	1.0

Figure 13—3. TPT: Converting Seconds to Decimal Parts of a Minute.

sheet (Fig. 13–2). For the total time, the seconds should be converted to decimal parts of a minute (Figure 13–3). Some authors have adopted the use of a minutes-per-block score rather than a total-time score (Heaton et al., 1986, 1991). In counting the blocks correctly reproduced, count only those that are fairly accurately drawn and indicate that the subject had a true mental picture of the block. A star of four or five points is accepted as correct. The location score is obtained by counting the right place on the drawing in relation to the other blocks and the formboard.

Before using the normative data tables for the appropriate age of the subject, the education corrections (Figure 13–4) should be applied to the raw score.

Subjects who have difficulty reproducing a shape on the drawing part of the test are given credit if they can correctly name the shape. However, they should be urged to do their best at drawing the figures. When two figures on the drawing look very similar, the examiner should ask the patient if they are the same figure. For example, the square and rectangle are often drawn very much alike. If the subject calls one a square and the other a rectangle (or a "long square"), the subject is given credit for both. If two identical figures are drawn, the examiner should give credit to the one most correctly localized even if it is not the most accurate drawing. In scoring location, the relationship of the figure to the board as well as to other shapes drawn should be considered. For example, if the triangle is drawn near the top

```
Sample Score Sheet

        Tactual Performance Test
Trial   Hand           Circle     Time
1       dominant       R  L       _____
2       nondominant    R  L       _____
3       both                      _____

        Total Time     _____
        Memory         _____
        Location       _____
```

Figure 13—2. Tactual Performance Test sample scoring sheet.

Education	Preferred hand	Nonpreferred hand	Both hands	Total time	Memory
1 year	.30	.12	.55	−1.58	1
5 years	.17	.05	.29	−.64	1
10 years	.00	−.03	.03	−.08	0
12 years	−.07	−.07	−.15	+.35	0
15 years	−.17	−.12	−.35	+.80	−1
20 years	−.34	−.20	−.67	+1.53	−1

Figure 13—4. Tactual Performance Test, Corrections for number of years of education. *Source:* Adapted from Alekoumbides et al. (1987).

of the board and the cross and half-circle are placed on each side of it, but another shape is drawn in above the triangle, then the triangle does not count as correctly localized.

Comment

Odd–even reliability for age- and education-corrected scores in 123 young adults was reported as .60 to .78 for blocks per minute, .77 to .93 for time, .64 for memory, and .69 for location (Cauthen, 1978); similar values were found for a "mixed sample" of normal and brain-damaged subjects (Charter et al., 1987). Interjudge agreement has been reported as poor for both memory and location scores (Lezak, 1995). Schludermann and Schludermann (1983) report retest coefficients of .76 for time, .55 for location, and .60 for memory scores in a sample of 174 executives after 2 years, and coefficients of .91, .53, and .72, respectively for 86 subjects in the same sample taking the test again after 3 years. Goldstein and Watson (1989) reported retest reliabilities after 4–469 weeks for 150 neuropsychiatric patients, ranging from .66 to .74 for time, .46 to .73 for memory, and from .32 to .69 for location, with similar values for alcoholics and trauma and vascular disorder patients, and somewhat lower coefficients for schizophrenics. In a review, Thompson and Parsons (1985) noted that retesting after 3 weeks led to improvement on all three scores, including a gain of more than 3 minutes on the time score. Dodrill (1987) reported that total time scores improved by about 3 minutes on retest even after 5 years. Retest reliability in a sample of 248 8-year-old children referred because of

learning disability, mental retardation, brain injury, emotional disorder, or environmental deprivation after 2.6 years was between .29 and .40 for time, .48 for location, and .43 for memory (Brown et al., 1989).

Klonoff and Low (1974), Clark and Klonoff (1988), and Russell (1985) have recommended the use of the 6-block formboard with adults, arguing that this cuts down the administration time by two-thirds (total time 4–5 minutes). Clark and Klonoff's study with 79 right-handed males (age 55.5) who had coronary bypass surgery but were without any neurological disorder found high reliability (internal consistency coefficients from .80 to .63) from presurgery to 24 months postsurgery. Memory and location scores correlated .62 with each other in brain-damaged patients (Heilbronner et al., 1991). Thompson and Parsons (1985) also reported intercorrelations between memory and location of .56 to .71, and between time and memory or location of .26 to .72.

Bornstein (1990) found that all three TPT scores loaded on the same factor with only minor loadings from a large number of other tests. Campbell et al. (1989), however, found that, in young adults, the time score loaded on a factor with other time-dependent scores, e.g., Picture Completion and Block Design; the memory score loaded on an attention factor together with digit span, digit symbol, Seashore rhythm, and Trail Making A; location scores loaded on all three of the extracted factors. The authors concluded that the test is multifactorial in nature.

Concurrent validity with the Benton Visual Retention Test and the Block Design Test was high (Clark & Klonoff, 1988). Discriminant va-

Table 13—5. Normative Data for the Tactual Performance Test by Age

		Time									
		Preferred hand			Nonpreferred hand			Both hands			
Age	n	M	SD	Range	M	SD	Range	M	SD	Range
15–17	32	4.6	1.2	2.6–6.8	3.3	1.2	1.1–6.4	17	0.5	.8–3.3
18–23	74	5.1	2.2	1.9–13.5	3.5	1.6	1.1–10.8	2.1	1.3	.4–9.3
24–32	56	4.5	1.8	1.7–9.5	3.1	1.1	1.5–7.1	1.8	0.8	.5–4.6
33–40	18	4.9	1.7	1.9–9.0	3.7	1.0	2.2–5.9	2.3	0.8	1.4–4.4
41–50	10	5.6	1.5	4.0–9.0	4.2	1.6	2.4–8.1	3.0	2.1	1.4–5.5
51–60	19	7.1	3.1	4.0–9.0	5.3	2.8	2.0–8.0	3.4	2.0	1.4–6.0
61–76	125	9.1	4.1	4.0–12.1	7.4	1.4	3.0–8.5	6.0	3.6	1.6–8.0

Note: For Location and Memory portions, all subjects placed 10 blocks in less than 15 minutes with the preferred, non-preferred, and both hands.

[a]SDs are extrapolated from Bak & Green (1980) and Fromm-Auch & Yeudall (1983). Means are extrapolated from all five sources.

Sources: Extrapolated from Bak & Greene (1980); Cauthen (1978); Ernst (1987); Fromm-Auch & Yeudall (1983); Heaton, Grant & Matthews (1986); Moore, Richards, & Hood (1984).

lidity for most Halstead-Reitan tests has traditionally been established by comparing scores for normal, "pseudoneurological" (referred for evaluation but found not neurologically impaired), and "brain-damaged" samples, using optimal cutoff scores. Significant differences between such groups have been reported for all parts of the test by many authors (e.g., O'Donnell, 1983; Reitan & Davison, 1974; Rojas & Bennett, 1995) and by Bigler and Tucker (1981) between brain-damaged and control blind subjects. Heaton, Grant, and Matthews (1991) and Mutchnick et al. (1991), however, found good discrimination only for the time and memory, but not the location score of this test. In a major study that compared 436 adults one year after head injury with 132 controls with trauma to other parts of the body, Dikmen et al. (1995) found a highly significant difference between groups for time, but the range of scores overlapped widely, depending on the severity of the head injury. Barnes and Lucas (1974) found that the TPT discriminated successfully between a group of 77 "organic" patients with varying etiologies and 39 "psychogenic" patients after age and IQ effects had been statistically controlled, whereas other tests of the Reitan battery (with the exception of the aphasia test) did not; the psychogenic group did better on these tasks. A

study by Heilbronner et al. (1991) found that both memory and location as well as the memory minus location scores of the TPT discriminated between patients with right- or left-hemisphere lesions and those with diffuse lesions, as well as healthy controls. Hom and Reitan (1982) report better scores for 50 patients with trauma compared to cerebrovascular and neoplastic lesions, and for left-hemisphere lesions, especially for ipsilateral performance. Alekoumbides et al. (1987) described a correct classification rate for normal subjects between 73 and 79 percent for blocks per minute, and 81 percent for memory scores, corrected for age and education, as compared to patients with diffuse lesions (20–24 percent for blocks per minute, and 27 percent for memory), with Korsakoff's disease (34–40 and 18 percent), and with focal lesions (31–38 and 47 percent). Such "correct classification rates," although significant, are not especially convincing, and they suggest that the test must be used with caution and in the context of other tests when diagnostic interpretations are sought. Heilbronner and Parsons (1989) present a detailed analysis of the performance of four patients and conclude that the strategies employed by the patient deserve specific consideration, and that it is incumbent upon the psychologist to investigate the qualitative aspects of the

Time			Location			Memory		
Total								
M	SD	Range	M	SD[a]	Range	M	SD[a]	Range
9.5	2.1	4.7–14.1	6.8	2.5	1–10	8.9	1.0	6–10
11.4	4.5	4.2–29.1	5.7	2.1	1–10	8.2	1.3	4–10
11.4	3.0	3.8–18.8	5.1	1.8	2–9	8.0	1.1	6–10
11.7	2.9	5.9–19.4	5.3	2.2	1–9	8.1	1.1	6–10
16.0	3.6	8.3–20.6	4.1	1.8	2–7	7.6	1.5	4–9
16.5	5.0	8.0–21.0	3.8	3.1	2–7	6.2	1.6	4–9
23.0	9.0	8.5–23.0	1.6	1.6	1–7	5.0	2.0	4–9

many different skills required for TPT performance; such a qualitative analysis may lead to specific retraining approaches.

The test appears to be sensitive also to epileptic patients with and without demonstrated neurological impairment (Klove & Matthews, 1974). Dodrill (1987) found time scores for epileptics to be twice as long as for an age-matched group of normal controls, whereas memory and location scores were only 1.5 points lower in epileptics.

Dodrill and Clemmons (1984) found the TPT predictive for overall adjustment and independent living, but not for vocational adjustment in epileptic high school students, and the differences on all scores between fully functioning and deficient functioning subjects in that population were not significant. Halstead (1947) and Reitan (1964) consider the test especially sensitive to frontal lobe lesions because of the amount of mental organization required, but patients with parietal lesions may show poor performance as well because of reduced stereognostic and tactile-kinesthetic ability, especially on the hand contralateral to the side of lesion (Teuber & Weinstein, 1954). The test results, especially time scores, are sensitive to alcoholism (Fabian et al., 1981) but appear to show little change under conditions of state and induced depression (Harris et al., 1981) or in learning-disabled young adults (O'Donnell, 1983). However, Davis et al. (1989) found that the TPT was among the most sensitive discriminators between learning-disabled and normal children between 10 and 14 years of age. Prigitano (1983)

also reported significant differences for all parts of the test between controls and patients with mild hypoxemia and chronic obstructive pulmonary disease. Boivin et al. (1995) reported that 195 5- to 12-year-old children from rural parts of Zaire scored significantly below American and Canadian control groups; this is ascribed to poorer anthropomorphic indicators of nutritional well-being rather than intercultural differences; i.e., the test may be sensitive to the effects of malnutrition.

In an examination of deliberate "faking brain damage," Goebel (1983) found that 102 subjects in their early 30s instructed to fake tended to obtain scores much more similar to normal controls than to actual brain-damaged patients on all parts of the test; they clearly underestimated the difficulty of the task for brain-damaged subjects.

Finally, Lezak (1995) points to the considerable discomfort experienced by some patients while being blindfolded for as long as 10 minutes or more; in her opinion, the test is "not worth the time and trouble" because the information obtained is "equivocal and often redundant." Our experience with the test has been more positive, especially when given to children who often enjoy the blindfolding "game," and considering the large amount of research with this test.

Normative Data

A number of authors have published or distributed normative data for the TPT for adults, for healthy elderly subjects, and for various

Table 13—6. TPT Normative Data for Children

	Range	Male M	(SD)	Female M	(SD)	All M	(SD)
Age 5 (N = 10)							
Time							
Dominant hand	12–26	7.0[a]	(7.5)	7.0	(7.5)	7.0	(7.5)
Nondominant hand	3–12	6.0	(6.5)	6.0	(6.5)	6.0	(6.5)
Both hands	2.5–19	5.8	(6.5)	5.8	(6.0)	5.8	(6.3)
Total time, all 3 trials	19–52	19.0	(12.5)	18.0	(18.4)	18.0	(15.8)
Memory	0–5	2.1	(1.9)	2.2	(1.3)	2.2	(1.8)
Location	0–3	0.7	(1.2)	1.3	(1.3)	0.9	(1.2)
Age 6 (N = 12)							
Time							
Dominant hand	2–15	7.6	(3.7)	6.3	(2.6)	7.0	(3.5)
Nondominant hand	1.5–15	5.0	(3.1)	6.6	(4.2)	5.8	(3.8)
Both hands	0.7–7.0	3.3	(2.0)	4.2	(2.4)	3.7	(2.2)
Total time, all 3 trials	5–45	15.9	(10.0)	17.1	(14.0)	16.6	(12.0)
Memory	3–6	4.0	(1.0)	3.0	(1.1)	3.5	(1.1)
Location	0–5	2.0	(1.3)	1.4	(1.0)	1.7	(1.1)
Age 7 (N = 25)							
Time							
Dominant hand	0.6–15.0	6.1	(6.0)	6.1	(4.9)	6.1	(5.5)
Nondominant hand	0.7–15.0	4.0	(3.0)	4.8	(4.9)	4.4	(4.0)
Both hands	0.5–15.0	2.0	(1.0)	1.8	(1.0)	1.9	(1.0)
Total time, all 3 trials	2–45	11.8	(9.9)	13.9	(8.9)	12.8	(9.3)
Memory	0–6	4.2	(1.3)	3.3	(1.1)	3.7	(1.2)
Location	0–6	2.5	(1.9)	2.6	(1.3)	2.6	(1.6)
Age 8 (N = 32)							
Time							
Dominant hand	0.7–15.0	4.4	(1.5)	6.5	(2.4)	5.3	(2.2)
Nondominant hand	0.7–15.0	3.1	(1.5)	4.0	(1.1)	3.8	(1.4)
Both hands	0.4–15.0	1.4	(2.0)	1.8	(2.0)	1.5	(2.0)
Total time, all 3 trials	1.7–45.0	9.7	(3.9)	12.0	(4.9)	10.8	(4.5)
Memory	2–6	4.3	(1.3)	4.3	(1.0)	4.3	(1.1)
Location	1–6	2.8	(1.3)	3.4	(2.4)	3.2	(2.1)
Age 9 (N = 71)							
Time							
Dominant hand	2–10	3.2	(3.0)	4.0	(2.0)	3.8	(2.2)
Nondominant hand	.9–10.0	3.4	(2.1)	4.1	(2.2)	3.8	(2.1)
Both hands	0.5–5.0	1.5	(0.8)	1.5	(0.8)	1.5	(0.8)
Total time, all 3 trials	3.1–20.0	9.8	(5.6)	9.9	(5.2)	9.9	(5.4)
Memory score	3–6	4.3	(1.3)	4.4	(1.0)	4.3	(1.1)
Location	1–5	2.7	(1.4)	3.3	(1.7)	8.0	(1.6)

(continued)

Table 13—6. (*Continued*)

	Range	Male		Female		All	
		M	(SD)	M	(SD)	M	(SD)
Age 10 (N = 57)							
Time							
Dominant hand	2–12	3.9	(1.6)	3.9	(2.7)	3.9	(2.2)
Nondominant hand	0.5–7.0	2.7	(1.3)	3.0	(1.6)	2.9	(1.4)
Both hands	0.5–3.5	1.3	(0.7)	1.4	(0.9)	1.4	(0.8)
Total time, all 3 trials	3.3–23.0	8.3	(2.8)	9.5	(4.8)	9.1	(3.9)
Memory	2–6	4.5	(1.1)	4.0	(1.3)	4.3	(1.2)
Location	0–6	3.1	(1.4)	3.0	(1.7)	3.0	(1.5)
Age 11 (N = 42)							
Time							
Dominant hand	1–6	3.1	(1.7)	3.0	(1.3)	3.0	(1.4)
Nondominant hand	1–6	2.2	(0.9)	2.4	(0.9)	2.3	(0.9)
Both hands	.5–3.0	1.2	(0.5)	1.2	(0.5)	1.2	(0.5)
Total time, all 3 trials	3–14	6.5	(2.5)	6.6	(2.3)	6.5	(2.4)
Memory	2–6	4.5	(1.0)	4.4	(1.1)	4.4	(1.1)
Location	0–6	3.2	(1.4)	3.1	(1.4)	3.1	(1.4)
Age 12 (N = 43)							
Time							
Dominant hand	1–8	2.9	(1.4)	3.6	(1.4)	3.3	(1.4)
Nondominant hand	0.5–6.5	2.1	(1.2)	2.3	(1.5)	2.2	(1.3)
Both hands	0.7–2.5	1.0	(0.5)	1.2	(0.5)	1.1	(0.5)
Total time, all 3 trials	3–15	6.0	(2.2)	7.1	(3.0)	6.6	(2.6)
Memory	3–6	5.2	(0.7)	4.8	(0.9)	5.0	(0.8)
Location	1–6	4.0	(1.2)	4.0	(1.3)	4.0	(1.2)
Age 13 (N = 11)							
Time							
Dominant hand	1.5–4.0	2.7	(1.0)	2.4	(1.0)	2.6	(1.0)
Nondominant hand	0.8–2.7	1.8	(0.7)	1.8	(0.5)	1.8	(0.6)
Both hands	0.5–1.5	0.9	(0.3)	1.1	(0.3)	1.0	(0.3)
Total time, all 3 trials	3.0–7.5	5.5	(1.5)	5.1	(1.0)	5.3	(1.2)
Memory	3–6	4.8	(1.1)	4.5	(1.2)	4.7	(1.1)
Location	1–5	3.5	(1.2)	3.4	(1.2)	3.5	(1.2)

Note: Children were from Victoria, B.C. and Ottawa, Ontario.

[a]Extrapolated values are in parentheses.

Sources: Knights & Norwood (1980); Spreen & Gaddes (1969); Trites (1977).

brain-damaged groups. The Wayne State norms presented by Reitan and Wolfson (1985) are very similar to those by Klove (1974) for American and Norwegian control subjects, and by Dodrill (1978, 1987) for a carefully selected representative normal sample. Age effects are quite noticeable when comparing the norms for an older sample (47 years, total time = 18.29 minutes, location = 2.62, memory = 6.28; Alekoumbides et al., 1987) with those of a younger one (28 years of age, total time = 13.65 minutes, location = 4.97, memory =

7.86; Dodrill, 1987). Norms for the higher age group are also confirmed by Cripe and Dodrill (1988), Ernst (1987), and Prigitano and Parsons (1976).

A meta-analysis of 69 studies presenting normative data over the last 20 years by Bengtson et al. (1996) suggests that scores on the TPT have improved—in parallel to the improvement found for intelligence tests—by as much as 1.0 SD for location, .72 SD for time, and .71 for memory during that period, a warning that older norms may be outdated.

Dodrill (1987) investigated effects of intelligence on TPT scores. For subjects in the 115–130 IQ range, total time was 10.8 minutes; for subjects with average IQ 13.5; and for subjects with IQs in the 70–85 range it was approximately 22 minutes. The respective means for location were 6, 5, and 3.5, for memory 8, 8, and 6.5. Similarly, Warner et al. (1987) report correlations between .28 and .49 for various TPT scores with IQ, and between .04 and .20 with number of years of education in both a U.S. (Seattle) and a British (Bristol) sample. Heilbronner et al. (1991) reported correlations between TPT Location and IQ of .36, and between Memory and IQ of .41 (Heilbronner et al., 1991). Subjects with at least a grade 9 education did better in comparison to those with less than grade 9 education (Harley et al., 1980; Schluderman & Schluderman, 1983; Thompson et al., 1987). For subjects with less than 12 years of education, location and memory scores were approximately .5 point less, and for subjects with 16 years of education or better they are approximately .5 point higher; total time for these two education groups was about 4 minutes longer and 1.5 minutes shorter, respectively (Heaton et al., 1986). Alekoumbides et al. (1987) presented correction equations for both age and education.

Dodrill (1987) has pointed out that TPT scores (like times scores for many psychological tests) are severely skewed to the left, with approximately 95 percent of normal subjects completing the test within 4–19 minutes, but with outliers taking as long as 47 minutes. The partial dependence of these scores on intelligence should be taken into account when results for an individual subject are interpreted.

Because of the effects of age and intelligence, we recommend the use of normative data stratified by age compiled from several sources (Table 13–5) after application of the education level correction extrapolated from Alekoumbides (Figure 13–4). Table 13–5 suggests a sharp drop in TPT performance in subjects 65–76 years old. Additional norms for elderly subjects are not available. Similar norms were obtained from 200 patients with a "negative neurological examination" by Russell and Starkey (1993) and from 225 normal adults by Yeudall et al. (1987). Heaton, Grant, and Matthews (1991) also presented similar norms in scaled scores, corrected for gender, education, and age, based on 553 normal subjects; caution in the use of these norms is recommended because cell sizes are not reported and may be quite small. [Norms published by Anthony et al. (1980), Klove (1974), Levine & Feinstein (1972), and Vega and Parsons (1967) show slightly better scores than those presented in Table 13–5.]

Kupke (1983) reported an interaction effect of sex with location and memory scores; subjects in that study tended to show significantly better scores with examiners of the opposite sex (approximately 1 point on memory, 1.5 points on location). Heaton, Grant, and Matthews (1986) also found that females tend to be about 2 minutes slower on the total time score compared to males, but that location and memory scores need no sex correction; Yeudall et al. (1987) found only minimal sex differences on all scores. In contrast, Chavez, Schwartz, and Brandon (1982) found that females had higher scores only on location, but did not differ on other scores. Finally, Fabian, Jenkins, and Parsons (1981) found that women were superior on recall, but poorer on location. Clearly, the issue of sex differences on this test is not settled as yet.

Differences between dominant and nondominant hand performance tend to be more pronounced in younger adults (20 percent better) than in adults over the age of 50, and higher in left-handers (30 percent) than right-handers (11.7 percent) and in "mixed right-handers" (6.3 percent) (Heaton et al., 1986). Although normally the second trial shows an improvement of about 30 percent in normal subjects (Boll, 1981), a reversal of this pattern (second trial with the nondominant hand and third trial with both hands slower than first trial) is found not infrequently, especially in older normal subjects (Thompson et al., 1987). Thompson and Heaton (1991) explored this pattern of performance in two groups of 96 matched normal subjects representing the two patterns; they found slightly poorer performance on left-hand fine motor coordination and spatial analysis (frequently attributed to right-hemisphere function) in the reversal group, and they warn that in clinical practice such reversals should not be interpreted as evidence of acquired right-hemisphere lesions, unless the differences are large and other evidence supports such an interpretation.

A study comparing Anglo-American, Mexican-American, and Mexican subjects (Arnold et al., 1994) indicated an acculturation effect (faster performance in Anglo-Americans) only for time (dominant, nondominant, total), but not for location and memory scores.

Norms for children (Table 13–6) have been compiled from our own data (including Spreen & Gaddes, 1969) and from data presented by Knights and Norwood (1980) and Trites (1977). They agree fairly well with normative data by Klonoff and Low (1974). The norms for younger children not only are based on small samples, but also indicate that performance at these ages is quite variable and does not stabilize adequately until age 10. For these reasons, norms can only provide guidelines. Leckliter et al. (1992) recommend caution also for the interpretation of scores for 9- to 14-year-olds because of large SDs, high average intelligence in the samples, and the possibility of outdated samples. The performance of the individual young child should also be evaluated qualitatively, based on the child's task organization, task orientation, attention, and apparent stereognostic deficits. Finlayson (1978) showed that the nonpreferred hand score relative to the preferred hand time score decreased significantly between the ages of 5 and 12, suggesting an increasing interhemispheric transfer effect of practice with age.

References

Alekoumbides, A., Charter, R.A., Adkins, T.G., & Seacat, G.F. (1987). The diagnosis of brain damage by the WAIS, WMS, and Reitan Battery utilizing standardized scores corrected for age and education. *International Journal of Clinical Neuropsychology, 9,* 11–28.

Anthony, W., Heaton, R., & Lehman, R. (1980). An attempt to cross-validate two actuarial systems for neuropsychological test interpretation. *Journal of Consulting and Clinical Psychology, 48,* 317–326.

Arnold, B.R., Montgomery, G.T. Castaneda, I., & Longoria, R. (1994). Acculturation and performance of Hispanics on selected Halstead-Reitan neuropsychological tests. *Assessment, 1,* 239–248.

Bak, J.S., & Greene, R.L. (1980). The effects of aging on a modified procedure for scoring localization and memory components of the Tactual Performance Test. *Clinical Neuropsychology, 2,* 114–117.

Barnes, G.W., & Lucas, G.J. (1974). Cerebral dysfunction vs. psychogenesis in Halstead-Reitan tests. *Journal of Nervous and Mental Disease, 158,* 50–60.

Bengtson, M.L., Mittenberg, W., Schneider, W., & Sellers, A. (1996). An assessment of Halstead-Reitan score changes over 20 years. *Archives of Clinical Neuropsychology, 11,* 368 (abstract).

Bigler, E.D., & Tucker, D.M. (1981). Comparison of verbal IQ, tactual performance, Seashore rhythm and finger oscillation tests in the blind and brain-damaged. *Journal of Clinical Psychology, 37,* 849–851.

Boivon, M.J., Giordani, B., & Bornefeld, B. (1995). Use of the Tactual Performance Test for cognitive ability testing with African children. *Neuropsychology, 9,* 409–417.

Boll, T.J. (1980). The Halstead-Reitan Neuropsychology battery. In S.B. Filskov & T.J. Boll (Eds.), *Handbook of Clinical Neuropsychology,* pp. 577–607. New York: Wiley.

Bornstein, R.A. (1990). Neuropsychological test batteries in neuropsychological assessment. In G.B. Baker & M. Hiscock (Eds.), *Neuromethods, Vol. 17: Neuropsychology.* Clifton, NJ: Humana Press.

Brown, S.J., Rourke, B.P., & Cicchetti, D.V. (1989). Reliability of tests and measures used in the neuropsychological assessment of children. *The Clinical Neuropsychologist, 3,* 353–368.

Campbell, M.L., Drobes, D.J., & Horn, R. (1989). Young adult norms, predictive validity, and relationship between Halstead-Reitan tests and WAIS-R scores. Paper presented at the 9th meeting of the National Academy of Neuropsychologists, Washington, DC.

Cauthen, N. (1978). Normative data for the tactual performance test. *Journal of Clinical Psychology, 34*, 456–460.

Charter, R.A., Adkins, T.G., Alekoumbides, A., & Seacat, G.F. (1987). Reliability of the WAIS, WMS, and Reitan Battery: Raw scores and standardized scores corrected for age and education. *International Journal of Clinical Neuropsychology, 9*, 28–32.

Chavez, E.L., Schwartz, M.M., & Brandon, A. (1982). Effects of sex of subject and method of block presentation on the Tactual Performance Test. *Journal of Consulting and Clinical Psychology, 50*, 600–601.

Clark, C., & Klonoff, H. (1988). Reliability and construct validity of the six-block Tactual Performance Test in an adult sample. *Journal of Clinical and Experimental Neuropsychology, 10*, 175–184.

Cripe, L.I., & Dodrill, C.B. (1988). Neuropsychological test performance with chronic low-level formaldehyde exposure. *The Clinical Neuropsychologist, 2*, 41–48.

Davis, R.D., Adams, R.E., Gates, D.O., & Cheramie, G.M. (1989). Screening for learning disabilities: A neuropsychological approach. *Journal of Clinical Psychology, 45*, 423–429.

Dikmen, S.S., Machamer, J.E., Winn, H.R., & Temkin, N.R. (1995). Neuropsychological outcome at 1-year post head injury. *Neuropsychology, 9*, 80–90.

Dodrill, C.B. (1978). A neuropsychological battery for epilepsy. *Epilepsia, 19*, 611–623.

Dodrill, C.B. (1987). *What's normal? Presidential Address.* Pacific Northwest Neuropsychological Association. Seattle.

Dodrill, C.B., & Clemmons, D. (1984). Use of neuropsychological tests to identify high school students with epilepsy who later demonstrate inadequate performances in life. *Journal of Consulting and Clinical Psychology, 52*, 520–527.

Ernst, J. (1987). Neuropsychological problem-solving skills in the elderly. *Psychology and Aging, 2*, 363–365.

Fabian, M.S., Jenkins, R.L., & Parsons, O.A. (1981). Gender, alcoholism, and neuropsychological functioning. *Journal of Consulting and Clinical Psychology, 49*, 138–140.

Finlayson, M.A.J. (1978). A behavioral manifestation of the development of interhemispheric transfer of learning in children. *Cortex, 14*, 290–295.

Fromm-Auch, D., & Yeudall, L.T. (1983). Normative data for the Halstead-Reitan neuropsychological tests. *Journal of Clinical Neuropsychology, 5*, 221–238.

Goebel, R.A. (1983). Detection of faking on the Halstead-Reitan neuropsychological test battery. *Journal of Clinical Psychology, 39*, 731–742.

Goldstein, G., & Watson, J.R. (1989). Test–retest reliability of the Halstead-Reitan battery and the WAIS in a neuropsychiatric population. *The Clinical Neuropsychologist, 3*, 265–273.

Halstead, W.C. (1947). *Brain and Intelligence. A Quantitative Study of the Frontal Lobes.* Chicago: University of Chicago Press.

Harley, J.P., Leuthold, C.A., Matthews, C.G., & Bergs, L.E. (1980). *T-Score Norms; Wisconsin Neuropsychological Test Battery (CA 55-79).* Mimeo.

Harris, M., Corss, H., & VanNieuwkerk, R. (1981). The effects of state depression, induced depression and sex on the finger tapping and tactual performance tests. *Clinical Neuropsychology, 3(4)*, 28–34.

Heaton, R.K., Grant, I., & Matthews, C.G. (1986). Differences in neuropsychological test performance associated with age, education, and sex. In I. Grant & K.M. Adams (Eds.). *Neuropsychological Assessment of Neuropsychiatric Disorders.* New York: Oxford University Press.

Heaton, R.K., Grant, I., & Matthews, C.G. (1991). *Comprehensive Norms for an Expanded Halstead-Reitan Battery. Demographic Corrections, Research Findings, and Clinical Applications.* Odessa, FL: Psychological Assessment Resources.

Heilbronner, R.L., Henry, G.K., Buck, P., Adams, R.L., & Fogle, T. (1991). Lateralized brain damage and performance on Trail Making A and B, Digit Span Forward and Backward, and TPT Memory and Location. *Archives of Clinical Neuropsychology, 6*, 252–258.

Heilbronner, R.L., & Parsons, O.A. (1989). The clinical utility of the Tactual Performance Test (TPT): Issues of lateralization and cognitive style. *The Clinical Neuropsychologist, 3*, 250–264.

Hom, J., & Reitan, R.M. (1982). Effect of lateralized cerebral damage upon contralateral and ipsilateral sensorimotor performance. *Journal of Clinical Neuropsychology, 4*, 249–268.

Klonoff, H., & Low, M. (1974). Disordered brain function in young children and early adolescents:

Neuropsychological and electrophysiological correlates. In R.M. Reitan & L.A. Davison (Eds.), *Clinical Neuropsychology: Current Status and Applications*, pp. 121–178. New York: Wiley.

Klove, H. (1974). Validation studies in adult clinical neuropsychology. In R.M. Reitan & L.A. Davison (Eds.), *Clinical Neuropsychology: Current Status and Applications*, pp. 211–236. New York: Wiley.

Klove, H., & Matthews, C.G. (1974). Neuropsychological studies of patients with epilepsy. In R.M. Reitan & L.A. Davison (Eds.), *Clinical Neuropsychology: Current Status and Applications*, pp. 237–266. New York: Wiley.

Knights, R.M., & Norwood, J.A. (1980). *Revised Smoothed Normative Data on the Neuropsychological Test Battery for Children*. Mimeo. Department of Psychology, Carleton University, Ottawa, ON.

Kupke, T. (1983). Effects of subject sex, examiner sex, and test apparatus on Halstead Category and Tactual Performance Tests. *Journal of Consulting and Clinical Psychology, 51*, 624–626.

Leckliter, I.N., Forster, A.A., Klonoff, H., & Knights, R.M. (1992). A review of reference group data from normal children for the Halstead-Reitan neuropsychological test battery for older children. *The Clinical Neuropsychologist, 6*, 201–229.

Levine, J., & Feinstein, D. (1972). Differences in test performance between brain-damaged, schizophrenic and medical patients. *Journal of Consulting and Clinical Psychology, 39*, 508–511.

Lezak, M.D. (1995). *Neuropsychological Assessment* (3rd ed.) New York: Oxford University Press.

Moore, T.E., Richards, B., & Hood, J. (1984). Aging and the coding of spatial information. *Journal of Gerontology, 39*, 210–212.

Mutchnick, M.G., Ross, L.K., & Long, C.J. (1991). Decision strategies for cerebral dysfunction. IV: Determination of cerebral dysfunction. *Archives of Clinical Neuropsychology, 6*, 259–270.

O'Donnell, J.P. (1983). Neuropsychological test findings for normal, learning disabled and brain damaged young adults. *Journal of Consulting and Clinical Psychology, 51*, 726–729.

Prigitano, G.P. (1983). Neuropsychological test performance in mildly hypoxic patients with chronic obstructive pulmonary disease. *Journal of Consulting and Clinical Psychology, 51*, 108–116.

Prigitano, G.P., & Parsons, O.A. (1976). Relationship of age and education to Halstead Test performance in different populations. *Journal of Consulting and Clinical Psychology, 44*, 527–533.

Reitan, R.M. (1964). Psychological deficit resulting from cerebral lesions in man. In J.M. Warren & K. Akert (Eds.), *The Frontal Granular Cortex and Behavior*. New York: McGraw-Hill.

Reitan, R.M., & Davison, L.A. (Eds.) (1974). *Clinical Neuropsychology: Current Status and Applications*. New York: Wiley.

Reitan, R.M., & Wolfson, D. (1985). *The Halstead-Reitan Neuropsychological Test Battery*. Tucson, AZ: Neuropsychology Press.

Rojas, D.C., & Bennett, T.L. (1995). Single versus composite score discriminative validity with the Halstead-Reitan battery and the Stroop Test in mild brain injury. *Archives of Clinical Neuropsychology, 10*, 101–110.

Russell, E.W. (1985). Comparison of the TPT-10- and 6-hole form board. *Journal of Clinical Psychology, 41*, 68–81.

Russell, E.W., & Starkey, R.I. (1993). *Halstead Russell Neuropsychological Evaluation System (HRNES)*. Los Angeles: Western Psychological Services.

Schludermann, E.H., & Schludermann, S.M. (1983). Halstead's studies in the neuropsychology of aging. *Archives of Gerontology and Geriatrics, 2*, 49–172.

Spreen, O., & Gaddes, W.H. (1969). Developmental norms for 15 neuropsychological tests age 6 to 15. *Cortex, 5*, 171–191.

Teuber, H.L., & Weinstein, S. (1954). Performance on a formboard task after penetrating brain injury. *Journal of Psychology, 38*, 177–190.

Thompson, L.L., & Heaton, R.K. (1991). Patterns of performance on the Tactual Performance Test. *The Clinical Neuropsychologist, 5*, 322–328.

Thompson, L.L., Heaton, R.K., Matthews, C.G., & Grant, I. (1987). Comparison of preferred and nonpreferred hand performance on four neuropsychological motor tasks. *The Clinical Neuropsychologist, 1*, 324–334.

Thompson, L.L., & Parsons, O.A. (1985). Contribution of the TPT to adult neuropsychological assessment. *Journal of Clinical and Experimental Neuropsychology, 7*, 430–444.

Trites, R.L. (1977). *Neuropsychological Test Manual*. Mimeo. Ottawa, ON: Royal Ottawa Hospital.

Vega, A., & Parsons, O. (1967). Cross-validation of the Halstead-Reitan tests for brain damage. *Journal of Consulting Psychology, 38*, 177–190.

Warner, M.H., Ernst, J., Townes, B.D., & Peel, J.

(1987). Relationship between IQ and neuropsychological measures in neuropsychiatric populations: Within-laboratory and cross-cultural replications using WAIS and WAIS-R. *Journal of Clinical and Experimental Neuropsychology, 9,* 545–562.

Yeudall, L.T., Reddon, J.R., Gill, D.M., & Stefanyk, W.O. (1987). Normative data for the Halstead-Reitan neuropsychological tests stratified by age and sex. *Journal of Clinical Psychology, 43,* 346–367.

TWO-POINT DISCRIMINATION

Other Test Name

Another name for this test is Two-Point Aesthesiometer.

Purpose

The purpose of this test is to measure two-point discrimination thresholds.

Source

The instrument can be ordered from Lafayette Instrument Co., P.O. Box 5729, Lafayette, IN 47903, as a 2-point or 3-point aesthesiometer, at a cost of approximately $65 US, or from Technolab, Succursale St. Laurent, C.P. 5195, Montreal, PQ H4L 4Z8, for $78.40 Cdn.

Description

The test consists of simple sharp-point calipers that can be varied in distance from each other. The instrument is calibrated in centimeters. Older versions are calibrated in $^1/_{16}$ of an inch (1 inch = 2.52 cm).

Administration

Although two-point discrimination can be tested on any part of the body, the standard administration introduced by Weinstein (1961) and by Corkin et al. (1970) uses the center of the palm of each hand. If there is a known unilateral impairment, begin with the unimpaired side; otherwise start with the preferred hand.

First, demonstrate the calipers to the subject and explain what you will be doing, that you will be touching the hand gently. Ask the subject to place the hand under a cover screen, palm up and hand open. Touch the center of the palm with the points of the instrument, taking care that for two-point stimulation both points touch simultaneously.

Start with the widest setting. Touch the hand with one or two points in the sequence given on the sample scoring sheet (Figure 13–5) for each trial. For example, for the trial of 2.85 cm between points, touch the preferred hand with two points of the calipers, then with one point, again one, then two, etc. The next trial is conducted at the same width with the nonpreferred hand. Ask the subject to indicate verbally or with his or her fingers whether one or two points have been touched. If the subject is accurate for all touches of the 2.9 cm width ($^{18}/_{16}$ inch), skip the next trial, and proceed to 2.5 cm width ($^{16}/_{16}$ inch). Continue with every alternate setting down to 1.75 cm width or until errors occur. Then give all trials in sequence until three errors have been made on two consecutive trials for each hand. Discontinuation criteria are used separately for each hand: If the subject makes three errors on two consecutive trials for the "bad" hand, continue with the other hand until you reach the discontinuation criterion.

Approximate Time for Administration

Approximately 10 minutes are required.

Scoring

Figure 13–5 shows a sample scoring sheet, indicating the width of the calipers and whether one or two points should be stimulated at each trial. The first trial refers to the preferred, and the second to the nonpreferred hand. Correct answers should be circled. The threshold is the last trial before a trial with three errors.

Scoring Sheet: Two-Point Discrimination in centimeters (fractions of inches in parentheses)

												Errors
2.85 (18/16″)	Preferred Hand	2	1	1	2	1	1	1	2	2	2	
	Non-Preferred	1	2	1	1	1	1	2	2	2	2	
2.70 (17/16″)		1	2	2	1	2	2	2	1	1	1	
		1	2	2	2	1	1	1	2	2	1	
2.54 (16/16″)		1	2	1	2	1	2	1	1	2	2	
		1	1	2	1	2	1	1	2	2	2	
2.38 (15/16″)		2	1	2	1	2	2	2	1	1	1	
		2	1	1	1	2	1	2	1	2	2	
2.22 (14/16″)		1	2	1	2	1	1	2	2	2	1	
		2	2	1	2	1	1	2	2	1	1	
2.06 (13/16″)		1	1	1	2	1	1	2	2	2	2	
		2	1	2	2	2	1	2	1	1	1	
1.90 (12/16″)		1	2	1	1	2	1	2	2	1	2	
		2	2	1	2	2	2	1	1	1	1	
1.75 (11/16″)		1	2	1	2	2	2	1	1	2	1	
		1	1	1	2	2	2	2	1	2	1	
1.59 (10/16″)		2	2	1	1	1	2	2	2	1	1	
		1	2	2	2	1	1	1	1	2	2	
1.42 (9/16″)		1	2	2	1	1	2	1	1	2	2	
		1	2	2	2	2	1	1	2	1	1	
1.27 (8/16″)		2	1	1	2	1	2	1	1	2	2	
		2	2	2	2	1	1	2	1	1	1	
1.11 (7/16″)		1	2	1	1	2	1	2	2	1	2	
		1	2	2	1	2	2	2	1	1	1	
0.95 (6/16″)		2	2	1	1	1	1	1	2	2	2	
		2	2	2	1	2	1	1	1	2	1	
0.79 (5/16″)		2	2	1	1	2	2	1	1	1	2	
		1	1	2	1	2	1	1	2	2	2	
0.64 (4/16″)		1	2	2	1	2	2	2	1	1	1	
		2	2	2	1	2	1	1	1	1	2	
0.48 (3/16″)		2	1	1	2	1	2	1	2	1	2	
		2	1	1	1	2	1	2	2	2	1	
0.32 (2/16″)		1	2	2	1	1	1	2	1	2	1	
		1	1	2	2	2	1	1	2	1	2	

Figure 13—5. Two-Point Discrimination sample scoring sheet.

Comment

Information on reliability is not available. Some examiners erroneously substitute this procedure for the Weinstein Aesthesiometer. It should be noted that it measures a different function: discrimination of two points at relatively strong pressure compared to the tactile threshold measurement. The results of the two procedures are likely to correlate highly

Table 13—7. Two-Point Discrimination Test, Normative Data for Adults, in Centimeters (and inches)

Age	n	Preferred hand	SD	Nonpreferred hand	SD
20–30	24	0.59 (3.69)	0.20 (1.24)	0.61 (3.83)	0.36 (0.91)
30–49	18	0.60 (3.70)	0.24 (1.58)	0.61 (3.82)	0.04 (0.26)
50–59	24	0.69 (4.34)	0.37 (2.34)	0.68 (4.25)	0.23 (1.49)
60–69	25	0.78 (4.87)	0.21 (1.28)	0.78 (4.87)	0.26 (1.65)
70+	23	0.80 (5.01)	0.19 (1.16)	0.89 (5.60)	0.26 (1.65)

Note: Mean Distance between two points and SDs in centimeters (¹/₁₆ = 0.16 cm).

in healthy persons, but may differ greatly if sensory functions are defective since the two functions rely on somewhat different pathways. The original procedure described by Semmes et al. (1960) included directional judgments with simultaneous or successive stimulation in two (and three) different points of an eight-spoked pattern of dots printed on the subject's palm. Defective scores were found mainly in subjects with parietal lesions invading the postcentral gyrus of the contralateral hemisphere, but were extremely rare if the postcentral gyrus was spared or if the lesion was in another area of the brain.

Normative Data

Table 13–7 shows norms (thresholds) for adults recently compiled in our laboratory. The right hand tends to have slightly lower thresholds. Thresholds tend to rise slightly in an older population. There are no significant sex-related differences in adults. The means obtained for younger adults agree closely with those reported by Corkin et al. (1970). Corkin et al. (1970) consider values of 1.0 cm as indicative of a slight defect, and of 1.6 cm as suggesting a moderate defect. Normative data for children are not available.

References

Corkin, S., Milner, B., & Rasmussen, T. (1970). Somatosensory thresholds. *Archives of Neurology*, *23*, 41–58.

Semmes, J., Weinstein, S., Ghent, L., & Teuber, H.L. (1960). *Somatosensory Changes after Penetrating Head Wounds in Man*. Cambridge, MA: Harvard University Press.

Weinstein, S. (1962). Tactile sensitivity of the phalanges. *Perceptual and Motor Skills*, *14*, 351–354.

14

Motor Tests

Tests of motor performance, usually of the hands, are an essential part of most neuropsychological examinations. A number of measures are especially useful for identifying subtle motor impairment and making inferences about the functional integrity of the two cerebral hemispheres. These include measures of somewhat separate aspects of handedness: preference (e.g., Annett, 1970), strength (e.g., Hand Dynamometer), speed (e.g., Finger Tapping), and dexterity (e.g., Purdue Pegboard). Reaction-time tasks are discussed in a separate chapter. In general, performance with the preferred hand is slightly superior to that with the nonpreferred hand; however, there is considerable variability in the normal population, and the preferred hand is not necessarily the more proficient one (e.g., Benton et al., 1962; Satz et al., 1967). Patterns of performance indicating equal or better performance with the nonpreferred hand occur with considerable regularity in the normal population, and neurological disturbance should not be inferred from an isolated lack of concordance. Further, even fairly large intermanual discrepancies on one motor task are quite common in the normal population. On the other hand, discrepant performances that are consistent across several tests are quite rare in the normal population and thus are more likely to suggest a lesion in the contralateral hemisphere (Bornstein, 1986; Thompson et al., 1987). There is some evidence (Haaland et al., 1994) that grip strength recovers more rapidly than finger tapping after neurological insult. Accordingly, finger tapping may be more sensitive to deficits in the post-acute phase.

It is also worth bearing in mind that there can be reasons other than lateralized motor defect for a neurologically impaired individual to perform poorly on skilled motor tasks. These include peripheral injury, general cognitive slowing, deterioration of attentional processes, and lack of effort. The literature suggests that the pattern of motor skill deficiency may also be useful in the diagnosis of functional disturbance. Greiffenstein et al. (1996) found that grip strength was useful in discriminating TBI patients with clinically evident motor abnormalities and compensation-seeking post-concussion patients (PCS). TBI patients showed relatively good performance on grip strength, with poorer performance on measures of finger tapping and dexterity. The PCS group showed worst performance on grip strength and relatively better performance on finger tapping and dexterity.

Because a variety of studies have shown a relationship between motor disability (e.g., hemiplegia, mobility, independence in self-care) and functional outcome, including employment, in a variety of neurological conditions (e.g., head injury, dementia), motor skills should be assessed routinely (Haaland et al., 1994).

References

Annett, M. (1970). A classification of hand preference by association analysis. *British Journal of Psychology, 61*, 303–321.

Benton, A.L., Meyers, R., & Polder, G.J. (1962). Some aspects of handedness. *Psychiatrica et Neurologica Basel, 144*, 231–337.

Bornstein, R.A. (1986). Consistency of intermanual discrepancies in normal and unilateral brain lesion patients. *Journal of Consulting and Clinical Psychology, 54*, 719–723.

Greiffenstein, M.F., Baker, W.J., & Gola, T.

(1996). Motor dysfunction profiles in traumatic brain injury and postconcussion syndrome. *Journal of International Neuropsychological Society, 2*, 477–485.

Haaland, K.Y., Temkin, N., Randahl, G., & Dikmen, S. (1994). Recovery of simple motor skills after head injury. *Journal of Clinical and Experimental Neuropsychology, 16*, 448–456.

Satz, P., Achenbach, K., & Fennell, E. (1967). Correlations between assessed manual laterality and predicted speech laterality in a normal population. *Neuropsychologia, 5*, 295–310.

Thompson, L.L., Heaton, R.K., Mathews, C.G., & Grant, I. (1987). Comparison of preferred and nonpreferred hand performance on four neuropsychological motor tasks. *The Clinical Neuropsychologist, 1*, 324–334.

FINGER TAPPING TEST

Other Test Name

This test is also called the Finger Oscillation Test.

Purpose

The purpose of this test is to measure motor speed of the index finger of each hand.

Source

The finger tapper (manual tapper) can be ordered from the Reitan Neuropsychology Laboratory, 1338 East Edison Street, Tucson, AZ 85719, at a cost of $95 US. Because children below the age of 9 years have difficulty manipulating the arm of the manual tapper, an electric finger tapper was devised that can also be ordered from the Reitan Neuropsychology Laboratory at a cost of $165 (US). There are a number of other tapping devices on the market. However, different levels of performance may be obtained when subjects are tested with devices other than the Reitan apparatus (Snow, 1987; Whitfield & Newcomb, 1992). If another device is used (e.g., computer), the examiner should ensure that comparable results are obtained with the new finger tapping unit.

Description

The Finger Tapping Test (FTT) (Reitan, 1969) was originally called the Finger Oscillation Test (FOT) and was part of Halstead's (1947) test battery. Using a specially adapted tapper, the subject is instructed to tap as rapidly as possible using the index finger of the preferred hand. A comparable set of measurements is then obtained with the nonpreferred hand.

Administration

Have the subject place the preferred hand palm down with fingers extended and the index finger placed on the key. Direct the subject to tap as quickly as he or she can, moving only the index finger, not the whole hand or arm. The subject is given five consecutive 10-second trials with the preferred hand. The procedure is then repeated with the nonpreferred hand. Five 10-second trials are given for each hand except when the results are too variable from one trial to another. Specifically, the test procedure requires that the five consecutive trials for each hand be within a five-point range from fastest to slowest. If one or more of the trials exceed this range, additional trials are given and the scores of the deviant trial(s) are discarded. This procedure is used in order to avoid instances in which a single deviant score unduly influences the score. A maximum of 10 trials with each hand is allowed (Bornstein, 1985, 1986a).

Fatigue may affect performance, and a brief rest period should be given after each trial. Even when no sign of fatigue is apparent, a rest period of 1–2 minutes is required after the third trial. A practice trial is given before the test begins so that the subject may get a "feel" for the apparatus.

Do not allow the subject to move the whole hand from the wrist. With young children and poorly coordinated adults this requirement is difficult and may be relaxed as long as it is clear that the score is obtained by index finger oscillation and not by movement of the whole hand.

Record the number on the counter when the examiner says stop, not when the subject in fact stops.

Approximate Time for Administration

The time required is 10 minutes.

Scoring

The finger tapping score is computed for each hand separately and is the mean of five consecutive 10-second trials within a range of five taps. A maximum of 10 trials with each hand is allowed, and if the above criterion is not met, the score is the mean of the best five trials.

Comment

Performance with each hand is quite stable over time, even with lengthy intervals between retest sessions (e.g., 2 years). Reliability coefficients ranging from .58 to .93 have been reported with both normal and neurologically impaired subjects (Dodrill & Troupin, 1975; Gill et al., 1986; Goldstein & Watson, 1989; Morrison et al., 1979; Provins & Cunliffe, 1972; Ruff & Parker, 1993; but see Matarazzo et al., 1974, for somewhat lower values). Haaland et al. (1994) noted a slight improvement, two taps per 10 seconds, for both normal subjects and individuals with mild head injuries who were tested at one

month and again at one year after injury. The similar, though subtle, improvement in finger tapping should alert clinicians to overinterpreting tapping improvement as evidence of recovery. Some investigators have reported that the differences between hands are consistent ($r = > .70$) (Massman & Doody, 1996; Provins & Cunliffe, 1972). Others, however, have indicated that the differences between hands are not highly reliable (.50) (Morrison et al., 1979).

Finger tapping measures are included in neuropsychological examinations to assess subtle motor and other cognitive impairment. The measure is sensitive to the presence and laterality of brain lesion (Barnes & Lucas, 1974; Bigler & Tucker, 1981; Dodrill, 1978; Haaland & Delaney, 1981; Finlayson & Reitan, 1980; Hom & Reitan, 1982, 1990; Reitan & Wolfson, 1994, 1996). Given the crossed nature of the motor system, performance tends to be worse in the hand contralateral to the lesion. Typically, the performances of the preferred and nonpreferred hands are compared to determine if there is consistent evidence of poor performance with one hand relative to the other. In general, performance with the preferred hand is superior to that with the nonpreferred hand (Bornstein, 1985, 1986a; Peters, 1990; Thompson, et al., 1987). The most frequently reported guideline is that the preferred hand should perform about 10 percent better than the nonpreferred hand (Reitan & Wolfson, 1985). However, there is considerable variability in the normal population, and the preferred hand is not necessarily the faster one, especially when left-handed people are considered (Bornstein, 1986a; Thompson et al., 1987). Patterns of performance indicating equal or better performance with the nonpreferred hand occur with considerable regularity in the normal population (about 30 percent), and neurological involvement should not be inferred from an isolated lack of concordance. Fairly large discrepancies between the hands on the Finger Tapping Test alone also cannot be used to suggest unilateral impairment since discrepancies of large magnitude are not uncommon (about 25 percent) in the normal population (Bornstein, 1986a; Thompson et al., 1987). Greater confidence in the clinical judgment of impaired motor function with one or the other hand can be gained from consideration of the consistency of intermanual discrepancies across several motor tasks since truly consistent, deviant performances are quite rare in the normal population (Bornstein, 1986a, 1986b; Thompson et al., 1987).

It is also important to note that there could be reasons other than a lateralized motor defect for an individual with brain dysfunction to perform poorly with the nonpreferred hand on skilled motor tasks. For example, if intellectual efficiency is reduced, perhaps as a result of cortical and/or subcortical involvement in both hemispheres, then performance with the nonpreferred (less practiced) hand may be affected on tasks that require adaptation and skilled movement, such as finger tapping (Lewis & Kupke, 1992).

Finally, there is evidence that tapping frequency is reduced in a number of conditions including chronic alcoholism (Leckliter & Matarazzo, 1989), closed-head injury (Haaland et al., 1994), and the mild stages of degenerative dementias (Massman & Doody, 1996; Muller et al., 1991; Ott et al., 1995), perhaps reflecting involvement of left and/or right premotor/motor regions, general cognitive slowing, or deterioration of attentional processes. That is, in addition to direct motoric effects, the speed, coordination, and pacing requirements of finger tapping could be affected by variable levels of alertness, impaired ability to focus attention, or slowing of responses. Further, the test can distinguish patients with motor dysfunctions of cerebellar, basal ganglia, and cerebral origins from normal subjects (Shimoyama et al., 1990). However, tapping frequency cannot distinguish one abnormal group from another (Shimoyama et al., 1990). Other measures (e.g., intertap variability, time in flexion and extension in the tap cycle, time-sequential histograms of tapping intervals) may, however, be able to distinguish among groups and to identify motor impairments that are not apparent in tapping rate (Roy et al., 1992; Shimoyama et al., 1990).

There is also evidence that performance on the test is moderately predictive of daily living skills in geriatric patients referred for possible dementia (Searight et al., 1989) and in trau-matic brain-injury patients (Prigatano et al., 1990).

Normative Data

Conventional cutoff scores (Reitan & Wolfson, 1985) should not be used since high false-positive rates are likely to occur (Bernard, 1989; Bornstein, 1986c). These cutoffs were based on the performance of individuals who were largely middle-aged and above average intellectually. For example, among Bornstein's sample of 365 healthy volunteers with a mean age of 43 years, use of conventional cutoff scores resulted in 80 percent being misclassified as impaired on preferred hand tapping scores.

Table 14–1 provides cross-sectional normative data for 365 adult volunteers, aged 20–69 years, stratified on the basis of age (20–39, 40–59, 60–69 years), sex, and education (<HS, ≥HS) (Bornstein, 1985). Right-handers comprised 91.5 percent of the sample. No information is provided, however, regarding the representativeness of the sample. Normative data are also available from Heaton, Grant & Mathews (1991) for use with adults between 20 and 80 years of age. The data, broken down into 10 age groups, education (6–8, 9–11, 12, 13–15, 16–17, 18+ years), and sex, were derived from healthy individuals recruited in the United States and Canada. The representativeness of their sample is also not certain. Moreover, size of their overall sample ($n =$ 486), and as a result the number of subjects within each category, is very small, in many cases less than 10 subjects per cell. Accordingly, we prefer the data provided by Bornstein (1985). Fromm-Auch and Yeudall (1983), Goldstein and Braun (1974), Trahan et al. (1987), and Ruff and Parker (1993) also give normative data for healthy men and women. Their values are somewhat higher than those reported here; however, their data were not stratified according to education.

Finlayson and Reitan (1976) give normative data for right-handed boys and girls at each of six age levels (Table 14–2). The representativeness of the sample is not discussed. A comparison with Klonoff and Low's (1974) norms shows fairly good agreement; however,

Table 14—1. Mean Performance of Adults for Finger Tapping

Age group	Education <grade 12			Education ≥grade 12		
	n	M	SD	*n*	M	SD
Males						
Preferred hand						
20–39	21	49.7	6.0	86	48.5	6.5
40–59	13	42.3	5.2	17	43.4	7.9
60–69	16	39.1	5.7	23	43.0	4.7
Nonpreferred hand						
20–39	21	47.0	5.5	86	44.8	6.4
40–59	13	39.8	3.6	17	39.5	5.8
60–69	16	35.2	5.2	23	39.3	6.2
Females						
Preferred hand						
20–39	13	45.2	6.0	49	44.3	5.8
40–59	22	36.3	7.8	43	40.5	7.1
60–69	22	29.7	6.2	34	32.2	6.0
Nonpreferred hand						
20–39	13	40.7	5.0	49	40.6	5.6
40–59	22	35.2	5.8	43	37.8	6.0
60–69	22	29.8	5.6	34	32.0	4.9

Note: The sample consisted of 365 healthy individuals from the general population of a large Canadian city.

Source: Bornstein (1985).

their data are not specified for each sex separately. Spreen and Gaddes (1969) also provide data for a small group of normal children. Their version of the test is slightly different from the one presented here in that a 50-tap warm-up period and six 10-second trials were given. Their data, however, are fairly consistent with those reported by Finlayson and Reitan (1976).

When each hand is considered separately, several trends emerge from the normative data. In general, better performance is associ-

Table 14—2. Mean Performance of Children for Finger Tapping

Age	*n*	Male				Female			
		Right hand		Left hand		Right hand		Left hand	
		M	SD	M	SD	M	SD	M	SD
6	20	35.60	(4.06)	32.00	(4.32)	33.10	(4.07)	30.10	(3.45)
7	20	37.00	(3.83)	33.40	(3.34)	36.90	(5.57)	32.50	(5.06)
8	20	39.90	(5.15)	35.20	(5.09)	38.80	(4.95)	33.30	(4.55)
12	20	41.00	(6.34)	36.40	(4.95)	41.40	(5.83)	35.50	(3.92)
13	20	45.80	(3.99)	38.90	(5.36)	40.70	(5.17)	35.40	(4.33)
14	20	47.30	(7.13)	40.70	(6.72)	44.70	(4.83)	39.30	(4.95)

Note: The data were derived from 120 normal right-handed children, 20 at each of six age levels, with boys and girls being equally represented.

Source: Finlayson & Reitan (1976).

ated with male sex (Bornstein, 1985; Carlier et al., 1993; Fromm-Auch & Yeudall, 1983; Harris et al., 1981; Heaton et al., 1991; Leckliter & Matarazzo, 1989; Nagasaki et al., 1988; Shimoyama et al., 1990; Trahan et al., 1987), younger age (Bornstein, 1985; Goldstein & Braun, 1974; Heaton et al., 1991; Leckliter & Matarazzo, 1989; Ott et al., 1995; Shimoyama et al., 1990; Trahan et al., 1987; but see Moehle & Long, 1989, who reported no age-related effect for 86 subjects aged 15 years and older), the preferred hand (Finlayson & Reitan, 1976; Shimoyama et al., 1990), increasing IQ (Leckliter & Matarazzo, 1989), and more years of education (Bornstein, 1985; Heaton et al., 1991). Bornstein (1985) reported that age and gender had a stronger effect on performance than education and that the main effects of age, gender, and education were more pronounced than their interaction effects. Ruff and Parker (1993), however, found that handedness, by itself, and education had no effect on tapping performance. Further, gender interacted with age. On the average, men (aged 16–70) experienced no significant decrements in finger tapping speeds with increasing age, whereas women's (aged 16–70) performances decreased with advancing age. In general, men outperformed women. Dodrill (1979) suggests that the observed sex difference for finger tapping may be attributed to sexual dimorphism in body and hand size rather than to a neuropsychological mechanism.

The findings regarding sex differences in intermanual difference scores are inconsistent; some studies report greater between-hand differences for males than for females (Bornstein, 1986b; From-Auch & Yeudall, 1983), and others do not (Ruff & Parker, 1993; Thompson et al., 1987). There is some evidence that right-handers show larger intermanual differences than left-handers (Thompson et al., 1987). Age and years of education do not seem to have a strong relationship with measures of intermanual difference (Bornstein, 1986b; Heaton et al., 1991; Ruff & Parker, 1993; Thompson et al., 1987).

Ethnicity appears not to affect tapping performance using the Heaton et al. (1991) norms, at least among Hispanics (Arnold et al., 1994). Thus, their norms appear appropriate for use with this population.

References

Arnold, B.R., Montgomery, G.T., Castaneda, I., & Longoria, R. (1994). Acculturation and performance of hispanics on selected Halstead-Reitan neuropsychological tests. *Assessment, 1*, 239–248.

Barnes, G.W., & Lucas, G.J. (1974). Cerebral dysfunction vs. psychogenesis in Halstead-Reitan tests. *The Journal of Nervous and Mental Disease, 158*, 50–60.

Bernard, L.C. (1989). Halstead-Reitan neuropsychological test performance of black, hispanic, and white young adult males from poor academic backgrounds. *Archives of Clinical Neuropsychology, 4*, 267–274.

Bigler, E.D., & Tucker, D.M. (1981). Comparison of verbal IQ, tactual performance, Seashore rhythm and finger oscillation tests in the blind and brain damaged. *Journal of Clinical Psychology, 37*, 849–851.

Bornstein, R.A. (1985). Normative data on selected neuropsychological measures from a nonclinical sample. *Journal of Clinical Psychology, 41*, 651–659.

Bornstein, R.A. (1986a). Normative data on intermanual differences on three tests of motor performance. *Journal of Clinical and Experimental Neuropsychology, 8*, 12–20.

Bornstein, R.A. (1986b). Consistency of intermanual discrepancies in normal and unilateral brain lesion patients. *Journal of Consulting and Clinical Psychology, 54*, 719–723.

Bornstein, R.A. (1986c). Classification rates obtained with "standard" cut-off scores on selected neuropsychological measures. *Journal of Clinical and Experimental Neuropsychology, 8*, 413–420.

Brown, S.J., Rourke, B.P., & Cicchetti, D.V. (1989). Reliability of tests and measures used in the neuropsychological assessment of children. *The Clinical Neuropsychologist, 3*, 353–368.

Carlier, M., Dumont, A.M., Beau, J., & Michel, F. (1993). Hand performance of French children on a finger tapping test in relation to handedness, sex and age. *Perceptual and Motor Skills, 76*, 931–940.

Dodrill, C.B. (1978). A neuropsychological battery for epilepsy. *Epilepsia, 19*, 611–623.

Dodrill, C.B. (1979). Sex differences on the Halstead-Reitan Neuropsychological battery and on other neuropsychological measures. *Journal of Clinical Psychology, 35,* 236–241.

Dodrill, C.B., & Troupin, A.S. (1975). Effects of repeated administrations of a comprehensive neuropsychological battery among chronic epileptics. *Journal of Nervous and Mental Disease, 161,* 185–190.

Finlayson, M.A., & Reitan, R.M. (1976). Handedness in relation to measures of motor and tactile-perceptual function in normal children. *Perceptual and Motor Skills, 43,* 475–481.

Finlayson, M.A.J., & Reitan, R.M. (1980). Effect of lateralized lesions on ipsilateral and contralateral motor functioning. *Journal of Clinical Neuropsychology, 2,* 237–243.

Fromm-Auch, D., & Yeudall, L.T. (1983). Normative data for the Halstead-Reitan neuropsychological tests. *Journal of Clinical Neuropsychology, 5,* 221–238.

Gill, D.M., Reddon, J.R., Stefanyk, W.O., & Hans, H.S. (1986). Finger tapping: effects of trials and sessions. *Perceptual and Motor Skills, 62,* 674–678.

Goldstein, S.G., & Braun, L.S. (1974). Reversal of expected transfer as a function of increased age. *Perceptual and Motor Skills, 38,* 1139–1145.

Goldstein, G., & Watson, J.R. (1989). Test–retest reliability of the Halstead-Reitan battery and the WAIS in a neuropsychiatric population. *The Clinical Neuropsychologist, 3,* 265–273.

Haaland, K.Y., & Delaney, H.D. (1981). Motor deficits after left or right hemisphere damage due to stroke or tumor. *Neuropsychologia, 19,* 17–27.

Haaland, K.Y., Temkin, N., Randahl, G., & Dikmen, S. (1994). Recovery of simple motor skills after head injury. *Journal of Clinical and Experimental Neuropsychology, 16,* 448–456.

Halstead, W.C. (1947). *Brain and Intelligence.* Chicago: University of Chicago Press.

Harris, M., Cross, H., Van Nieuwkerk, R. (1981). The effects of state depression, induced depression and sex on the finger tapping and tactual performance tests. *Clinical Neuropsychology, 3,* 28–34.

Heaton, R.K., Grant, I., & Mathews, C.G. (1991). *Comprehensive Norms for an Expanded Halstead-Reitan Battery.* Odessa: FL: Psychological Assessment Resources.

Heaton, R.K., Grant, I., & Mathews, C.G. (1996). Differences in neuropsychological test performance associated with age, education, and sex. In I. Grant & K.M. Adams (Eds.), *Neuropsychological Assessment of Neuropsychiatric Disorders.* New York: Oxford University Press.

Hom, J., & Reitan, R.M. (1982). Effect of lateralized cerebral damage upon contralateral and ipsilateral sensorimotor performances. *Journal of Clinical Neuropsychology, 4,* 249–268.

Hom, J., & Reitan, R.M. (1990). Generalized cognitive function after stroke. *Journal of Clinical and Experimental Neuropsychology, 12,* 644–655.

Klonoff, H., & Low, M. (1974). Disordered brain function in young children and early adolescents: Neuropsychological and electroencephalographic correlates. In R. Reitan and L.A. Davidson (Eds.), *Clinical Neuropsychology: Current Status and Applications.* Washington: V.H. Winston & Sons.

Leckliter, I.N., & Matarazzo, J.D. (1989). The influence of age, education, IQ, gender, and alcohol abuse on Halstead-Reitan neuropsychological test battery performance. *Journal of Clinical Psychology, 45,* 484–512.

Lewis, R., & Kupke, T. (1992). Intermanual differences on skilled and unskilled motor tasks in nonlateralized brain dysfunction. *The Clinical Neuropsychologist, 6,* 374–382.

Massman, P.J., & Doody, R.S. (1996). Hemispheric asymmetry in Alzheimer's disease is apparent in motor functioning. *Journal of Clinical and Experimental Neuropsychology, 18,* 110–121.

Matarazzo, J.D., Wiens, A.N., Matarazzo, R.G., & Goldstein, S.G. (1974). Psychometric and clinical test–retest reliability of the Halstead Impairment Index in a sample of healthy, young, normal men. *Journal of Nervous and Mental Disease, 158,* 37–49.

Moehle, K.A., & Long, C.J. (1989). Models of aging and neuropsychological test performance decline with aging. *Journal of Gerontology, 44,* 176–177.

Morrison, M.W., Gregory, R.J., & Paul, J.J. (1979). Reliability of the finger tapping test and a note on sex differences. *Perceptual and Motor Skills, 48,* 139–142.

Muller, G., Weisbrod, S., & Klingberg, F. (1991). Finger tapping frequency and accuracy are decreased in early stage primary degenerative dementia. *Dementia, 2,* 169–172.

Nagasaki, H., Itoh, H., Maruyama, H., & Hashizume, K. (1988). Characteristic difficulty in rhythmic movement with aging and its relation to Parkinson's disease. *Experimental Aging Research, 14,* 171–176.

Ott, B.R., Ellias, S.A., & Lannon, M.C. (1995). Quantitative assessment of movement in Alzheimer's disease. *Journal of Geriatric Psychiatry and Neurology, 8,* 71–75.

Peters, M. (1990). Subclassification of non-pathological left-handers poses problems for theories of handedness. *Neuropsychologia, 28,* 279–289.

Prigatano, G.P., Altman, I.M., & O'Brien, K.P. (1990). Behavioral limitations that traumatic brain-injured patients tend to underestimate. *The Clinical Neuropsychologist, 4,* 163–176.

Provins, K.A., & Cunliffe, P. (1972). The reliability of some motor performance tests of handedness. *Neuropsychologia, 10,* 199–206.

Reitan, R.M. (1969). *Manual for Administration of Neuropsychological Test Batteries for Adults and Children.* Indianapolis.

Reitan, R.M., & Wolfson, D. (1985). *The Halstead-Reitan Neuropsychological Test Battery: Theory and Interpretation.* Tucson, AZ: Neuropsychology Press.

Reitan, R.M., & Wolfson, D. (1994). Dissociation of motor impairment and higher-level brain deficits in strokes and cerebral neoplasms. *The Clinical Neuropsychologist, 8,* 193–208.

Reitan, R.M., & Wolfson, D. (1996). Relationships between specific and general tests of cerebral functioning. *The Clinical Neuropsychologist, 10,* 37–42.

Roy, E.A., Clark, P., Aigbogun, S., & Quare-Storer, P.A. (1992). Ipsilesional disruptions to reciprocal finger tapping. *Archives of Clinical Neuropsychology, 7,* 213–219.

Ruff, R.M., & Parker, S.B. (19930. Gender- and age-specific changes in motor speed and eye-hand coordination in adults: Normative values for the finger tapping and grooved pegboard tests. *Perceptual and Motor Skills, 76,* 1219–1230.

Searight, H.R., Dunn, E.J., Grisso, T., Margolis, R.B., et al. (1989). The relation of the Halstead-Reitan neuropsychological battery to ratings of everyday functioning in a geriatric sample. *Neuropsychology, 3,* 135–145.

Shimoyama, I., Ninchoji, T., & Uemura, K. (1990). The Finger Tapping Test: A quantitative analysis. *Archives of Neurology, 47,* 681–684.

Snow, W.G. (1987). Standardization of test administration and scoring criteria: Some shortcomings of current practice with the Halstead-Reitan Test Battery. *The Clinical Neuropsychologist, 1,* 250–262.

Spreen, O., & Gaddes, W.H. (1969). Developmental norms for 15 neuropsychological tests age 6 to 15. *Cortex, 5,* 170–191.

Thompson, L.L., Heaton, R.K., Mathews, C.G., & Grant, I. (1987). Comparison of preferred and nonpreferred hand performance on four neuropsychological motor tasks. *The Clinical Neuropsychologist, 1,* 324–334.

Trahan, D.E., Patterson, J., Quintana, J., & Biron, R. (1987). The finger tapping test: A re-examination of traditional hypotheses regarding normal adult performance. Paper presented at the International Neuropsychological Society, Washington, D.C.

Whitfield, K., & Newcomb, R. (1992). A normative sample using the Loong computerized tapping program. *Perceptual and Motor Skills, 74,* 861–862.

HAND DYNAMOMETER

Other Test Name

Another test name is Grip Strength.

Purpose

The purpose of this test is to measure strength or intensity of voluntary grip movements of each hand.

Source

The Smedley dynamometer can be ordered from the Stoelting Co., 1350 S. Kostner Avenue, Chicago, Illinois 60623, at a cost of $165 US.

Description

This frequently used measure of hand strength (Reitan & Davison, 1974) requires the subject to hold the upper part of the dynamometer in the palm of the hand and to squeeze the stirrup with the fingers as hard as he or she possibly can.

Administration

Briefly, the length of the dynamometer stirrup must be adjusted to the size of the subject's hand (see Instrument Manual). Demonstrate the use of the instrument to the subject. Indicate that the lower pointer will register the grip, so that the subject does not have to continue gripping while the scale is read. Then place the dynamometer in the subject's preferred hand (palm down) and instruct the subject to hold his or her arm down at the side and away from the body. The subject is then told to squeeze the dynamometer as hard as he or she can, taking as much time as needed to squeeze to the maximum. Allow one practice trial and two recorded trials with each hand, preferred and nonpreferred alternately with 10-second pauses between each trial to avoid excessive fatigue. If either an increase or a decrease of more than 5 kg occurs on the second trial for either hand, provide a third trial.

Approximate Time for Administration

The time required is approximately 5 minutes.

Scoring

The amount (in kg) registered at each trial is recorded, and the mean is calculated for each hand separately.

Comment

The performance of each hand is quite stable over test sessions, even with lengthy intervals between retest sessions (e.g., 30 months). Reliability coefficients ranging from .52 to .96 have been reported with both normal and neurologically impaired subjects (Brown et al., 1989; Dodrill & Troupin, 1975; Dunn, 1978; Matarazzo et al., 1974; Provins & Cunliffe, 1972; Reddon et al., 1985). The differences between hands, however, are not highly reliable, and variations in performance from time to time may be influenced by variations in motivation (Provins & Cunliffe, 1972; Sappington, 1980).

Within a session, grip strength does deteriorate after an extended number of grip trials (Reddon et al., 1985; Montazer & Thomas, 1992). Performance drops significantly after two trials, with grip strength decreasing to about 80 percent with 10 trials and about 40 percent in 100 trials. From trial 100 to 200, only an additional 10 percent drop occurs (Montazer & Thomas, 1992).

Grip strength measures are included in neuropsychological examinations to assess gross and subtle motor impairment. There is evidence that in stroke patients grip strength can be used as a gross index of recovery of arm function (Sunderland et al., 1989). Further, the measurement of grip strength has some prognostic value. Sunderland et al. (1989) noted that the absence of measureable grip strength one month after stroke indicated that there would be poor outcome with regard to motor function. If there was detectable grip at one month, then the clinician could be reasonably certain that there would be at least rudimentary function 5 months later. Haaland et al. (1994) found that grip strength was sensitive to recovery in the first year after head injury. Normal individuals showed no change, whereas head-injured patients showed improved performance from the one-month to the one-year evaluation.

Grip strength has also proven useful in discriminating epileptic patients with left-hemisphere speech from those with right-hemisphere speech (Strauss & Wada, 1988), in differentiating brain-damaged from normal people, and in detecting the laterality of brain lesion (Bornstein, 1986b; Dodrill, 1978; Finlayson & Reitan, 1980; Haaland & Delany, 1981; Hom & Reitan, 1982; Lewis & Kupke, 1990). Given the crossed nature of the motor system, right-hemisphere lesions tend to depress performance on the left hand, and left-hemisphere lesions tend to lower performance on the right hand. Dodrill (1978) reports that the dynamometer correctly identified the lateralization of brain lesions with higher accuracy than either the Finger Tapping Test or the Tactual Performance Test. The relative advantage of the dynamometer in making inferences regarding laterality of damage may lie, at least in part, in its relative simplicity and low demands on skill and adaptation, a function that may be compromised in brain-damaged individuals, particularly those with subcortical and/or bilateral disturbance (Haaland et al., 1994; Lewis & Kupke, 1990). Tests that require more skilled movement (e.g., tapping, Purdue) may place greater cognitive demands (e.g., in terms of speed, coordination, and pacing requirements), and patients may have more difficulty adapting to such a task, particularly with the non-preferred (less practiced) hand. In such cases, intermanual differences may reflect less a lateralized disturbance than a generalized reduction in cognitive efficiency (Lewis & Kupke, 1990).

The assumption is often made that a right-handed person should perform better on the dynamometer with the right hand and that a left-handed person should perform better with the left hand (e.g., Reitan & Wolfson, 1985). In general, performance with the preferred hand is superior to that with the nonpreferred hand (Bornstein, 1985, 1986a). However, there is considerable variability in the normal population, and the preferred hand is not necessarily the stronger one, especially when left-handed people are considered (Benton et al., 1962; Koffler & Zehler, 1985; Lewandowski et al., 1982; Satz et al., 1967; Smiljanic-Colanovic, 1974). Patterns of performance indicating equal or better performance with the nonpreferred hand occur with considerable regularity in the normal population, and neurological involvement should not be inferred from an isolated lack of concordance. Even fairly large discrepancies between the hands on the grip strength measure alone cannot be used to suggest unilateral impairment (Bornstein, 1986a; Koffler & Zehler, 1985; Thompson et al., 1987). Large-magnitude discrepancies (more than 1 SD from the mean) are not uncommon (about 25 percent) in the normal population. Greater confidence in the clinical judgment of impaired motor function with one or the other hand can be derived from consideration of the consistency of intermanual discrepancies across several motor tasks (Bornstein, 1986; Thompson et al., 1987). Consistent, deviant performances are quite rare in the normal population and thus, in the absence of peripheral injury, are likely to indicate lateralized brain dysfunction (Bornstein, 1986b; Thompson et al., 1987).

Crews and Harrison (1994) reported that depressed women (as determined by scores on the Beck Depression Inventory) displayed similar grip strength as their nondepressed counterparts. Depressed women, however, showed more accurate half-grip strength responses (subjects instructed to squeeze the dynamometer half as hard as the first time) than nondepressed women, particularly with the left hand. The authors suggest that the finding of more accurate left half-grip strength reflects right hemisphere arousal in depressed woman.

Normative Data

There are several normative studies based on relatively large samples of healthy people. Table 14–3 provides cross-sectional normative data for adults, stratified on the basis of age, sex, and education (Bornstein, 1985). Right-handers comprised 91.5 percent of the sample. Ernst (1988), Fromm-Auch and Yeudall (1983) and Koffler and Zehler (1985) also provide normative data for healthy men and women. Their values are similar to those reported here; however, their data were not stratified according to education. Table 14–4 gives normative data for right-handed boys and girls at six age levels (Finlayson & Reitan, 1976). A comparison with Spreen and Gaddes's (1969) norms and those given with the instrument (from Stoelting) show relatively good agreement; however, Spreen and Gaddes's data are given for combined groups of right- and left-handed children and are not separated according to preferred and non-preferred handedness.

When each of the hands is considered separately, several trends emerge from the studies. First, performance tends to be better with the preferred than the nonpreferred hand. Strength is related to sex, with males being stronger than females. There is a positive correlation between grip strength and height and weight, and between grip strength and education. Better-educated individuals score higher than less-educated subjects. Finally, strength is also related to age. Longitudinal assessments of age changes in physical strength suggest that the decline in the older age groups is greater than is indicated by cross-sectional comparisons of different age groups. The underestimation of strength loss in cross-sectional estimates probably occurs because relatively fewer weak individuals are

Table 14—3. Mean Performance of Adults for Grip Strength in kg

Age group	Education <grade 12			Education ≥grade 12		
	n	M	SD	n	M	SD
Males						
Preferred hand						
20–39	21	50.8	11.5	86	49.9	8.4
40–59	13	39.8	6.0	17	48.2	7.3
60–69	16	38.7	5.9	22	44.5	5.6
Nonpreferred hand						
20–39	21	47.7	11.7	86	46.4	7.6
40–59	13	38.2	6.5	17	46.4	9.1
60–69	16	37.2	5.4	22	39.3	5.5
Females						
Preferred hand						
20–39	13	32.7	8.7	50	31.0	5.4
40–59	22	27.7	5.9	43	29.8	5.8
60–69	22	25.6	5.3	34	25.0	4.9
Nonpreferred hand						
20–39	13	31.2	8.0	50	28.7	5.0
40–59	22	24.9	6.7	43	26.9	5.4
60–69	22	24.0	6.0	34	22.8	4.8

Note: The sample consisted of 365 healthy individuals from the general population of a large Western Canadian city.

Source: Bornstein (1985).

represented in older healthy samples (Clement, 1974).

Age and education do not affect the magnitude of intermanual differences (Bornstein, 1986a; Ernst, 1988). The findings regarding sex differences in intermanual difference scores are inconsistent; some studies find sex-related differences (i.e., greater between-hand differences for males than for females) (Bornstein, 1986a), and others do not (Ernst, 1988; Fromm-Auch & Yeudall, 1983; Thompson et al; 1987). There is also some evidence

Table 14—4. Mean Performance of Children for Grip Strength in kg

Age	n	Male				Female			
		Right hand		Left hand		Right hand		Left hand	
		M	(SD)	M	(SD)	M	(SD)	M	(SD)
6	20	10.40	(2.80)	9.45	(2.87)	9.05	(2.50)	7.90	(2.34)
7	20	11.95	(2.10)	11.10	(2.27)	9.30	(1.75)	8.80	(1.80)
8	20	12.25	(2.36)	11.40	(2.08)	11.55	(2.36)	10.15	(2.46)
12	20	21.95	(3.10)	19.55	(3.88)	23.05	(5.36)	19.10	(5.04)
13	20	28.30	(4.15)	27.55	(5.47)	25.00	(5.21)	23.25	(4.29)
14	20	35.25	(8.95)	33.80	(7.29)	28.30	(2.98)	25.65	(4.30)

Note: The data were derived from 120 normal right-handed children, 20 at each of six age levels, with boys and girls being equally represented.

Source: Finlayson & Reitan (1976).

that right-handers show larger intermanual differences than left-handers (Thompson et al., 1987).

References

Benton, A.L., Meyers, R., & Polder, G.J. (1962). Some aspects of handedness. *Psychiatrica et Neurologica Basel, 144,* 321–337.

Bornstein, R.A. (1985). Normative data on selected neuropsychological measures from a nonclinical sample. *Journal of Clinical Psychology, 41,* 651–659.

Bornstein, R.A. (1986a). Normative data on intermanual differences on three tests of motor performance. *Journal of Clinical and Experimental Neuropsychology, 8,* 12–20.

Bornstein, R.A. (1986b). Consistency of intermanual discrepancies in normal and unilateral brain lesion patients. *Journal of Consulting and Clinical Psychology, 54,* 719–723.

Brown, S.J., Rourke, B.P., & Cicchetti, D.V. (1989). Reliability of tests and measures used in the neuropsychological assessment of children. *The Clinical Neuropsychologist, 3,* 353–368.

Clement, F.J. (1974). Longitudinal and cross-sectional assessments of age changes in physical strength as related to sex, social class, and mental ability. *Journal of Gerontology, 29,* 423–429.

Crews Jr., W.D., & Harrison, D.W. (1994). Functional asymmetry in the motor performances of women: Neuropsychological effects of depression. *Perceptual and Motor Skills, 78,* 1315–1322.

Dodrill, C.B. (1978). The hand dynamometer as a neuropsychological measure. *Journal of Consulting and Clinical Psychology, 46,* 1432–1435.

Dodrill, C.B., & Troupin, A.S. (1975). Effects of repeated administrations of a comprehensive neuropsychological battery among chronic epileptics. *Journal of Nervous and Mental Disease, 161,* 185–190.

Dunn, J.M. (1978). Reliability of selected psychomotor measures with mentally retarded adult males. *Perceptual and Motor Skills, 46,* 295–301.

Ernst, J. (1988). Language, grip strength, sensory-perceptual, and receptive skills in a normal elderly sample. *The Clinical Neuropsychologist, 2,* 30–40.

Finlayson, M.A., & Reitan, R.M. (1976). Handedness in relation to measures of motor and tactile-perceptual functions in normal children. *Perceptual and Motor Skills, 43,* 475–481.

Finlayson, M.A., & Reitan, R.M. (1980). Effect of lateralized lesions on ipsilateral and contralateral motor functioning. *Journal of Clinical Neuropsychology, 2,* 237–243.

Fromm-Auch, D., & Yeudall, L.T. (1983). Normative data for the Halstead-Reitan Neuropsychological Tests. *Journal of Clinical Psychology, 5,* 221–238.

Haaland, K.Y., & Delaney, H.D. (1981). Motor deficits after left or right hemisphere damage due to stroke or tumor. *Neuropsychologia, 19,* 17–27.

Haaland, K.Y., Temkin, N., Randahl, G., & Dikmen, S. (1994). Recovery of simple motor skills after head injury. *Journal of Clinical and Experimental Neuropsychology, 16,* 448–456.

Hom, J., & Reitan, R.M. (1982). Effect of lateralized cerebral damage upon contralateral and ipsilateral sensorimotor performances. *Journal of Clinical Neuropsychology, 4,* 249–268.

Koffler, S.P., & Zehler, D. (1985). Normative data for the hand dynamometer. *Perceptual and Motor Skills, 61,* 589–590.

Lewandowski, L., Kobus, D.A., Church, K.L., & Van Orden, K. (1982). Neuropsychological implications of hand preference versus hand grip performance. *Perceptual and Motor Skills, 55,* 311–314.

Lewis, R., & Kupke, T. (1990). Intermanual differences on skilled and unskilled motor tasks in nonlateralized brain dysfunction. *The Clinical Neuropsychologist, 6,* 374–382.

Matarazzo, J.D., Wiens, A.N., Matarazzo, R.G., & Goldstein, S. (1974). Psychometric and clinical test–retest reliability of the Halstead Impairment Index in a sample of healthy, young, normal men. *Journal of Nervous and Mental Disease, 158,* 37–49.

Montazer, M.A., & Thomas, J.G. (1992). Grip strength as a function of 200 repetitive trials. *Perceptual and Motor Skills, 75,* 1320–1322.

Provins, K.A., & Cunliffe, P. (1972). The reliability of some motor performance tests of handedness. *Neuropsychologia, 199–206.*

Reddon, J.R., Stefanyk, W.O., Gill, D.M., & Renney, C. (1985). Hand dynamometer: Effects of trials and sessions. *Perceptual and Motor Skills, 61,* 1195–1198.

Reitan, R.M., & Davison, L.A. (1974). *Clinical Neuropsychology: Current Status and Applications.* Washington, D.C.: V.H. Winston.

Reitan, R.M.., & Wolfson, D. (1985). *The Halstead-Reitan Neuropsychological Test Battery: Theory and Interpretation.* Tucson, AZ: Neuropsychology Press.

Sappington, J.T. (1980). Measures of lateral dominance: Interrelationships and temporal stability. *Perceptual and Motor Skills, 50,* 783–790.

Satz, P., Achenbach, K., & Fennel, E. (1967). Correlations between assessed manual laterality and predicted speech laterality in a normal population. *Neuropsychologia, 5,* 295–310.

Smiljanic-Colanovic, V. (1974). The measurement of different aspects and degrees of hand dominance. *Studiae Psychologica, 16,* 204–208.

Spreen, O., & Gaddes, W.H. (1969). Developmental norms for 15 neuropsychological tests age 6 to 15. *Cortex, 5,* 170–191.

Strauss, E., & Wada, J. (1988). Hand preference and proficiency and cerebral speech dominance determined by the carotid amytal test. *Journal of Clinical and Experimental Neuropsychology, 10,* 169–174.

Sunderland, A., Tinson, D., Bradley, L., & Langton-Hewer, R. (1989). Arm function after stroke. An evaluation of grip strength as a measure of recovery and a prognostic indicator. *Journal of Neurology, Neurosurgery, and Psychiatry, 52,* 1267–1272.

Thompson, L.L., Heaton, R.K., Mathews, C.G., & Grant, I. (1987). Comparison of preferred and nonpreferred hand performance on four neuropsychological motor tasks. *The Clinical Neuropsychologist, 1,* 324–334.

PURDUE PEGBOARD TEST

Purpose

The purpose of this test is to measure finger and hand dexterity.

Source

The pegboard, manual, and record forms can be ordered from Lafayette Instrument Co., Inc., P.O. Box 5729, Sagamore Parkway, Lafayette, Indiana 47903, at a cost of $109 US or from Technolab Industries Ltd., 5757 Decelles Ave. Suite 329, Montreal, Quebec H3S 2C3, at a cost of $134 Cdn.

Description

The Purdue Pegboard was developed in the 1940s as a test of manipulative dexterity for use in personnel selection (Tiffin & Asher, 1948; Tiffin, 1968). In addition to its use in personnel selection, the Purdue Pegboard has been used in neuropsychological assessment to assist in localizing cerebral lesions and deficits (Reddon et al., 1988). The board consists of two parallel rows of 25 holes each. Pins (pegs) are located at the extreme right-hand and left-hand cups at the top of the board. Collars and washers occupy the two middle cups. In the first three subtests, the subject places as many pins as possible in the holes, first with the preferred hand, then with the non-preferred hand, and finally with both hands, within a 30-second time period. To test the right hand, the subject must insert as many pins as possible in the holes, starting at the top of the right-hand row. The left-hand test uses the left row. Both hands then are used together to fill both rows top to bottom. In the fourth subtest, the subject uses both hands alternately to construct "assemblies," which consist of a pin, a washer, a collar, and another washer. The subject must complete as many assemblies as possible within one minute.

Administration

The instructions are described in the test manual. Briefly, the subject is required to take pins with the preferred (e.g., right) hand from the right-hand cup and place them as quickly as possible in the right column of holes, during a 30-second period. The pins are allowed to remain in the holes and the same procedure is repeated with the nonpreferred hand. The pins are then removed and the test is repeated with the subject using both hands simultaneously. Again the trial period is 30 seconds. The pins are then removed and the subject is asked to form "assemblies." The subject is asked to use continuous alternating movements of the right and left hands, one picking up a pin, one a washer, one a collar, and so on. The time allowed is 60 seconds. Demonstration and practice are provided prior to each subtest. Examiners may repeat each task three times; however, most of the recent normative data are based on a single-trial administration.

Table 14—5. Performance of Children on Purdue Pegboard (One trial per subtest):
Means and Standard Deviations

Age	n	Preferred hand		Nonpreferred hand		Both hands		Assembly	
		M	SD	M	SD	M	SD	M	SD
Boys									
5:0–5:5	30	9.33	1.81	8.40	1.33	6.73	1.17	14.10	3.29
5:6–5:11	30	9.93	1.51	8.83	1.95	6.97	1.54	15.57	3.56
6:0–6:5	30	9.77	1.57	9.13	1.83	7.30	1.53	15.93	2.94
6:6–6:11	30	11.57	1.45	10.17	2.17	8.23	1.77	19.20	3.84
7:0–7:5	30	11.67	1.67	11.00	1.70	8.77	1.41	19.23	4.95
7:6–7:11	30	12.07	1.95	11.23	1.68	9.57	1.59	20.40	4.10
8:0–8:5	30	12.70	1.60	12.17	1.51	9.83	1.51	22.20	3.80
8:6–8:11	30	13.90	2.19	12.57	1.85	10.90	1.73	24.47	5.35
9:0–9:5	30	13.33	1.60	12.43	1.59	10.50	1.48	24.57	3.75
9:6–9:11	30	13.87	1.91	12.87	2.05	11.33	1.65	27.37	4.55
10:0–10:5	30	14.03	1.88	12.87	1.72	10.93	1.84	26.37	6.15
10:6–10:11	30	14.93	1.51	13.90	1.84	11.77	1.65	28.17	5.38
11:0–11:5	30	14.93	1.86	14.00	1.98	11.30	1.68	29.53	6.19
11:6–11:11	30	14.83	1.60	13.93	1.60	12.27	1.41	31.13	5.19
12:0–12:5	30	14.83	1.78	13.67	2.02	11.67	1.52	31.13	5.78
12:6–12:11	30	15.37	2.81	14.00	2.38	11.87	1.87	30.13	6.08
13:0–13:5	40	15.15	1.92	13.90	2.00	11.85	1.58	33.73	5.00
13:6–13:11	30	14.87	1.72	14.10	1.47	11.53	1.80	34.57	5.88
14:0–14:5	30	15.67	1.47	14.40	1.57	12.03	1.67	33.97	6.58
14:6–14:11	30	14.70	1.49	14.33	1.65	12.20	1.61	31.37	7.24
15:0–15:5	30	15.57	1.50	14.87	1.50	12.57	1.48	32.20	6.21
15:6–15:11	23	15.09	1.50	14.30	1.61	12.65	1.30	33.04	6.24
Girls									
5:0–5:5	30	10.00	1.53	8.50	1.36	6.97	1.25	14.70	2.55
5:6–5:11	30	9.30	1.73	9.13	1.59	6.77	1.28	14.37	4.02
6:0–6:5	30	11.43	1.33	10.23	1.52	8.53	1.46	18.03	3.54
6:6–6:11	30	11.87	1.68	10.47	1.38	8.67	1.79	20.63	4.27
7:0–7:5	30	12.03	1.65	10.47	2.08	8.83	1.80	19.77	4.49
7:6–7:11	30	12.47	1.53	11.50	1.80	9.50	1.70	20.20	4.61
8:0–8:5	30	13.07	1.78	12.03	1.40	10.10	1.81	21.93	4.31
8:6–8:11	30	13.77	1.63	12.30	1.26	10.43	1.59	24.50	5.83
9:0–9:5	30	13.37	1.79	11.83	2.12	9.83	1.62	24.97	6.81
9:6–9:11	30	14.40	1.52	13.03	1.67	11.60	1.65	29.07	6.01
10:0–10:5	30	15.13	1.48	13.20	1.35	11.33	1.42	27.90	5.10
10:6–10:11	30	15.47	1.59	13.63	1.33	12.27	1.46	31.70	6.02
11:0–11:5	30	14.90	1.79	14.00	2.00	11.67	1.63	32.77	5.50
11:6–11:11	30	15.70	1.84	13.83	1.88	12.00	1.82	33.47	7.24
12:0–12:5	30	15.57	1.65	14.20	1.73	12.00	1.23	34.57	5.20
12:6–12:11	30	15.40	1.96	14.07	1.66	12.03	1.65	34.70	7.52
13:0–13:5	40	15.55	1.69	14.15	1.64	12.03	1.44	34.85	5.57
13:6–13:11	32	15.38	1.58	14.09	1.44	12.13	1.31	37.40	5.34
14:0–14:5	30	16.33	1.73	14.93	1.78	12.63	1.61	36.43	6.76
14:6–14:11	30	16.03	1.77	14.83	1.66	12.40	1.94	34.17	6.62
15:0–15:5	28	16.68	1.49	14.89	1.40	12.89	1.64	36.89	7.75
15:6–15:11	31	16.42	1.84	15.29	2.04	12.77	1.45	37.35	8.24

Note: Data were derived from 1,334 normal schoolchildren.

Source: Gardner & Broman (1979).

Table 14—6. Performance of Children on Purdue Pegboard: Percentiles

Age	n	10	20	30	40	50	60	70	80	90
Percentiles for boys: Preferred hand										
5:0–5:5	30	7.0	8.0	8.0	9.0	9.0	10.0	10.0	11.0	11.0
5:6–5:11	30	8.0	9.0	9.0	10.0	10.0	10.0	11.0	11.8	12.0
6:0–6:5	30	7.1	9.0	9.0	9.0	9.5	10.0	11.0	11.0	11.9
6:6–6:11	30	9.1	10.2	11.0	11.0	12.0	12.0	12.0	13.0	13.0
7:0–7:5	30	9.1	10.2	11.0	11.4	12.0	12.0	12.7	13.0	13.9
7:6–7:11	30	9.0	10.0	11.0	12.0	12.0	12.6	13.0	14.0	14.0
8:0–8:5	30	11.0	12.0	12.0	12.0	13.0	13.0	14.0	14.0	14.0
8:6–8:11	30	11.1	12.0	12.3	13.0	14.0	15.0	15.0	16.0	17.0
9:0–9:5	30	11.0	12.0	12.0	13.0	13.0	14.0	15.0	15.0	15.0
9:6–9:11	30	12.0	12.0	13.0	13.0	14.0	14.6	15.0	15.0	15.9
10:0–10:5	30	11.1	12.2	13.0	14.0	14.0	15.0	15.0	15.8	16.9
10:6–10:11	30	13.0	13.2	14.0	14.0	15.0	15.0	15.0	16.0	17.0
11:0–11:5	30	13.0	13.0	13.0	14.0	14.5	16.0	16.0	16.8	17.0
11:6–11:11	30	13.0	14.0	14.0	14.0	15.0	15.0	15.0	16.8	17.0
12:0–12:5	30	13.0	13.0	14.0	14.0	14.5	15.0	15.7	16.0	17.9
12:6–12:11	30	13.0	13.2	15.0	15.0	15.0	15.0	16.0	17.0	18.9
13:0–13:5	40	12.1	14.0	14.0	15.0	15.0	15.0	16.0	16.8	18.0
13:6–13:11	30	13.0	13.0	14.0	14.4	15.0	15.0	16.0	16.0	17.0
14:0–14:5	30	14.0	14.0	14.3	15.0	16.0	16.0	17.0	17.0	17.9
14:6–14:11	30	13.0	13.0	14.0	14.4	15.0	15.0	15.0	16.0	16.9
15:0–15:5	30	14.0	14.0	14.0	15.0	15.5	16.0	16.7	17.0	18.0
15:6–15:11	23	13.0	14.0	14.0	15.0	15.0	15.0	16.0	17.0	17.0
Percentiles for boys: Nonpreferred hand										
5:0–5:5	30	6.1	7.0	8.0	8.0	8.5	9.0	9.0	9.0	10.0
5:6–5:11	30	6.1	8.0	8.0	8.0	9.0	9.6	10.0	10.0	11.0
6:0–6:5	30	6.0	8.0	9.0	9.0	9.0	10.0	10.0	10.0	12.0
6:6–6:11	30	7.1	8.2	9.0	10.0	10.5	11.0	11.7	12.0	13.0
7:0–7:5	30	9.0	10.0	10.0	11.0	11.0	11.0	12.0	12.0	12.9
7:6–7:11	30	9.1	10.0	10.0	11.0	11.0	11.0	12.0	13.0	13.9
8:0–8:5	30	10.0	11.0	11.0	12.0	12.5	13.0	13.7	13.0	15.9
8:6–8:11	30	10.1	11.0	11.0	12.0	12.0	13.0	13.7	14.0	15.9
9:0–9:5	30	10.0	11.0	11.3	12.0	13.0	13.0	13.7	14.0	14.0
9:6–9:11	30	10.0	11.2	12.0	12.0	12.0	13.0	14.0	15.0	16.0
10:0–10:5	30	10.1	12.0	12.0	13.0	13.0	13.6	14.0	14.0	15.0
10:6–10:11	30	11.0	12.2	13.0	13.0	14.0	14.0	15.0	15.8	17.0
11:0–11:5	30	12.0	13.0	13.0	13.0	13.5	14.0	15.0	15.8	16.9
11:6–11:11	30	11.1	13.0	13.0	14.0	14.0	14.0	15.0	15.0	16.0
12:0–12:5	30	12.0	13.0	13.0	13.0	14.0	14.0	15.0	16.0	16.0
12:6–12:11	30	11.0	12.2	13.0	13.4	14.0	14.0	15.0	16.0	16.9
13:0–13:5	40	11.0	11.2	13.0	14.0	14.0	15.0	15.0	16.0	16.0
13:6–13:11	30	12.0	13.0	13.0	14.0	14.0	14.0	15.0	15.8	16.0
14:0–14:5	30	12.1	13.0	14.0	14.0	14.5	15.0	15.7	16.0	16.0
14:6–14:11	30	11.2	13.2	14.0	14.0	14.5	15.0	15.0	15.8	16.0
15:0–15:5	30	13.0	14.0	14.3	15.0	15.0	15.0	16.0	16.0	16.9
15:6–15:11	23	12.0	13.0	13.0	14.0	15.0	15.0	15.0	16.0	16.6

(*continued*)

Scoring

Scores are derived for each part of the test. The scores for the pin (peg) placement subtests consists of the number of pins inserted in the time period for each hand. The score for the bimanual condition consists of the total number of pairs of pins inserted. The assembly score refers to the number of parts assembled (see source).

Table 14—6. Performance of Children on Purdue Pegboard: Percentiles (*Continued*)

Age	n	10	20	30	40	50	60	70	80	90
Percentiles for boys: Both hands										
5:0–5:5	30	5.1	6.0	6.0	6.0	7.0	7.0	7.0	8.0	8.0
5:6–5:11	30	5.0	6.0	6.0	6.4	7.0	7.0	8.0	8.0	9.0
6:0–6:5	30	5.0	6.0	6.3	7.0	7.0	7.6	8.0	9.0	9.0
6:6–6:11	30	6.0	7.0	8.0	8.0	9.0	8.6	9.0	9.0	10.9
7:0–7:5	30	7.0	8.0	8.0	8.0	8.0	9.0	10.0	10.0	10.0
7:6–7:11	30	8.0	8.0	8.0	9.0	9.5	10.0	10.7	11.0	12.0
8:0–8:5	30	8.0	8.0	9.0	9.0	10.0	10.0	11.0	11.0	12.0
8:6–8:11	30	9.0	9.2	10.0	10.0	11.0	11.0	12.0	12.8	13.0
9:0–9:5	30	8.1	9.0	10.0	10.0	10.0	11.0	11.0	12.0	12.0
9:6–9:11	30	9.1	10.0	10.0	11.0	11.0	11.6	12.0	13.0	13.9
10:0–10:5	30	9.0	9.0	10.0	10.4	11.0	11.0	11.0	12.8	13.9
10:6–10:11	30	10.0	10.2	11.0	11.0	12.0	12.0	12.0	13.0	14.0
11:0–11:5	30	9.0	10.0	10.3	11.0	11.0	12.0	12.7	13.0	13.0
11:6–11:11	30	11.0	11.0	12.0	12.0	12.0	13.0	13.0	13.8	14.0
12:0–12:5	30	9.1	11.0	11.0	11.0	12.0	12.0	12.0	12.8	14.0
12:6–12:11	30	9.1	10.2	11.0	12.0	12.0	12.6	13.0	13.8	14.0
13:0–13:5	40	9.1	11.0	11.0	11.4	12.0	12.0	13.0	13.0	14.0
13:6–13:11	30	9.1	10.0	11.0	11.0	11.0	12.0	12.0	13.0	14.0
14:0–14:5	30	10.1	11.0	11.0	11.0	12.0	12.0	13.0	14.0	14.0
14:6–14:11	30	10.0	11.0	11.0	12.0	12.0	12.0	13.0	14.0	15.0
15:0–15:5	30	10.1	11.0	12.0	12.0	13.0	13.0	13.0	14.0	14.9
15:6–15:11	23	11.0	11.8	12.0	12.0	13.0	13.0	13.0	14.0	14.0
Percentiles for boys: Assembly										
5:0–5:5	30	10.0	11.2	12.0	13.0	14.0	14.6	16.0	16.0	17.0
5:6–5:11	30	10.1	12.2	14.0	15.0	16.0	16.0	17.7	18.0	20.0
6:0–6:5	30	12.1	14.0	15.0	15.0	16.0	16.0	17.0	19.0	20.0
6:6–6:11	30	14.0	16.2	18.0	18.0	19.5	20.6	22.0	22.8	24.0
7:0–7:5	30	12.1	16.0	17.3	18.4	19.0	20.6	21.7	23.0	26.7
7:6–7:11	30	16.0	17.2	18.3	19.4	21.0	22.0	22.7	24.0	25.0
8:0–8:5	30	19.0	20.2	21.0	22.4	23.5	24.0	24.0	26.8	28.9
8:6–8:11	30	18.0	20.0	20.3	23.4	24.0	25.0	27.1	30.0	32.0
9:0–9:5	30	20.0	21.2	23.0	24.0	24.0	26.0	26.0	27.0	28.0
9:6–9:11	30	21.1	24.0	24.3	25.4	26.0	29.2	30.7	31.8	32.0
10:0–10:5	30	19.1	20.2	24.0	25.0	26.0	26.0	28.7	30.0	35.7
10:6–10:11	30	22.0	24.0	25.3	28.4	29.0	30.0	30.0	31.0	33.8
11:0–11:5	30	22.0	22.2	26.0	27.4	28.0	31.0	32.0	34.6	39.9
11:6–11:11	30	25.1	27.0	28.6	30.0	31.0	32.6	33.7	35.0	39.0
12:0–12:5	30	25.0	26.0	27.0	29.0	29.0	32.6	35.4	36.0	40.9
12:6–12:11	30	23.1	25.4	28.0	29.0	30.5	32.2	34.0	35.8	37.0
13:0–13:5	40	27.0	30.0	31.0	32.0	34.0	34.8	36.0	37.0	40.9
13:6–13:11	30	27.1	30.0	30.0	33.0	34.5	35.6	36.7	39.8	43.8
14:0–14:5	30	26.1	29.2	31.0	32.0	34.0	36.0	38.7	40.0	41.0
14:6–14:11	30	23.0	25.2	26.3	29.0	30.5	32.0	34.7	35.8	45.4
15:0–15:5	30	24.0	26.0	28.0	31.4	33.5	35.6	36.0	37.8	39.9
15:6–15:11	23	24.4	26.8	29.4	32.0	33.0	34.4	35.8	39.0	42.0

(*continued*)

Comment

In normal people, moderate test–retest reliabilities, ranging from .63 to .82, have been obtained by correlating the scores for one trial on each of the subtests with the one-trial scores obtained by giving the subtests 1–2 weeks later (Reddon et al., 1988; Tiffin, 1968). There are, however, practice effects, with scores improving on subsequent trials (Fein-

Table 14—6. (*Continued*)

Age	n	10	20	30	40	50	60	70	80	90
Percentiles for girls: Preferred hand										
5:0–5:5	30	8.0	8.2	9.3	10.0	10.0	10.6	11.0	11.0	12.0
5:6–5:11	30	7.0	8.0	8.0	9.0	9.5	10.0	11.0	11.0	11.0
6:0–6:5	30	9.1	10.2	11.0	11.0	11.5	10.0	12.0	12.0	13.0
6:6–6:11	30	10.1	11.0	11.0	11.0	11.0	12.0	3.0	14.0	14.0
7:0–7:5	30	10.0	11.0	11.0	12.0	12.0	12.0	13.0	13.0	14.9
7:6–7:11	30	10.1	11.0	12.0	12.0	13.0	13.0	13.0	14.0	14.0
8:0–8:5	30	11.0	12.0	12.0	12.4	13.0	13.0	14.0	14.8	15.9
8:6–8:11	30	12.0	12.0	13.0	13.0	14.0	14.0	14.7	15.0	16.9
9:0–9:5	30	10.1	12.0	13.0	13.0	13.0	14.0	14.0	15.0	16.0
9:6–9:11	30	12.0	13.0	14.0	14.0	14.0	15.0	15.0	16.0	16.9
10:0–10:5	30	13.0	14.0	14.0	15.0	15.0	15.0	16.0	16.0	17.9
10:6–10:11	30	13.1	14.0	14.8	15.0	15.5	16.0	16.0	16.8	17.9
11:0–11:5	30	12.0	13.2	14.0	15.0	15.0	15.0	15.7	16.8	17.0
11:6–11:11	30	14.0	14.0	15.0	15.0	16.0	16.0	17.0	17.0	18.0
12:0–12:5	30	14.0	14.0	14.0	15.0	15.0	16.0	17.0	17.0	17.9
12:6–12:11	30	12.1	13.2	15.0	15.0	16.0	16.0	16.0	17.0	18.0
13:0–13:5	40	14.0	14.0	15.0	15.0	16.0	16.0	16.0	17.0	18.0
13:6–13:11	30	13.3	14.0	14.0	15.0	15.0	15.0	16.0	17.0	18.0
14:0–14:5	30	14.1	15.0	15.0	16.0	16.0	16.0	17.0	17.8	19.0
14:6–14:11	30	14.0	14.0	15.0	15.0	16.0	16.6	17.0	17.0	18.9
15:0–15:5	30	15.0	15.0	16.0	16.0	17.0	17.0	18.7	18.0	19.0
15:6–15:11	23	14.0	15.0	15.6	16.0	16.0	17.0	17.4	18.0	19.0
Percentiles for girls: Nonpreferred hand										
5:0–5:5	30	7.0	7.0	8.0	8.0	9.0	9.0	9.0	10.0	10.0
5:6–5:11	30	7.0	7.2	8.0	8.4	9.0	10.0	10.0	11.0	11.0
6:0–6:5	30	8.0	8.2	9.3	10.0	10.0	11.0	11.0	11.8	12.0
6:6–6:11	30	9.0	9.2	10.0	10.0	10.0	11.0	11.0	12.0	12.0
7:0–7:5	30	8.0	9.0	10.0	10.0	11.0	11.0	11.0	12.0	13.0
7:6–7:11	30	9.0	10.0	10.3	11.0	11.0	12.0	13.0	13.0	14.0
8:0–8:5	30	10.0	11.0	11.0	12.0	12.0	12.0	12.7	13.0	14.0
8:6–8:11	30	11.0	11.0	12.0	12.0	12.0	12.6	13.0	13.8	14.0
9:0–9:5	30	9.0	10.0	11.0	11.0	11.5	12.6	13.0	14.0	14.9
9:6–9:11	30	11.0	11.0	12.0	12.0	13.0	13.6	14.0	14.8	15.0
10:0–10:5	30	11.0	12.0	13.0	13.0	13.0	13.6	14.0	14.8	15.0
10:6–10:11	30	11.2	13.0	13.0	13.4	14.0	14.0	14.0	14.8	15.0
11:0–11:5	30	10.2	12.4	14.0	14.0	14.0	15.0	15.0	15.0	16.8
11:6–11:11	30	11.0	12.0	13.0	14.0	14.0	14.0	15.0	15.0	16.0
12:0–12:5	30	12.0	13.0	13.3	14.0	14.0	14.0	15.0	16.0	16.9
12:6–12:11	30	12.0	13.0	13.0	13.0	14.0	14.0	15.0	15.0	16.9
13:0–13:5	40	12.1	13.0	13.0	13.4	14.0	14.0	15.0	16.0	16.0
13:6–13:11	30	12.0	13.0	14.0	14.0	14.0	15.0	15.0	15.0	16.0
14:0–14:5	30	13.0	13.0	14.0	15.0	15.0	15.0	15.7	16.0	17.0
14:6–14:11	30	13.0	13.2	14.0	14.0	15.0	15.0	16.0	16.8	17.0
15:0–15:5	30	12.9	14.0	14.0	14.6	15.0	15.4	16.0	16.0	17.0
15:6–15:11	23	13.0	13.0	14.0	14.0	15.0	16.0	16.4	17.8	18.0

(*continued*)

stein et al., 1994; Reddon et al., 1988; Wilson et al., 1982). For example, Feinstein et al. (1994) examined the effects of practice in healthy volunteers tested at 2- to 4-week intervals over eight test sessions. Performance improved with time and was still discernible at the eighth session. The improvement was more marked for younger subjects, aged 25–33 years, who performed better than older subjects, aged 41–57 years, and who contin-

Table 14—6. Performance of Children on Purdue Pegboard: Percentiles (*Continued*)

Age	n	10	20	30	40	50	60	70	80	90
Percentiles for girls: Both hands										
5:0–5:5	30	5.0	6.0	6.0	7.0	7.0	7.6	8.0	8.0	8.0
5:6–5:11	30	5.0	6.0	6.0	6.4	7.0	7.0	7.7	8.0	8.0
6:0–6:5	30	6.1	7.2	8.0	8.0	9.0	9.0	9.0	10.0	10.0
6:6–6:11	30	6.1	8.0	8.0	8.0	8.0	8.6	9.7	10.0	12.0
7:0–7:5	30	6.0	7.2	8.0	9.0	9.0	9.0	10.0	10.8	11.0
7:6–7:11	30	7.0	8.0	9.0	9.0	9.5	10.0	10.7	11.0	11.0
8:0–8:5	30	8.0	8.2	9.0	10.0	10.0	11.0	11.0	11.0	12.0
8:6–8:11	30	8.0	9.0	10.0	10.0	10.5	11.0	11.0	12.0	12.9
9:0–9:5	30	8.0	8.0	9.0	9.4	10.0	10.0	11.0	11.0	12.0
9:6–9:11	30	9.0	10.0	11.0	12.0	12.0	12.0	13.0	13.0	13.0
10:0–10:5	30	10.0	10.0	11.0	11.0	11.0	11.6	12.0	12.0	13.0
10:6–10:11	30	11.0	11.0	11.3	12.0	12.0	12.0	13.0	13.8	14.9
11:0–11:5	30	9.1	10.0	11.0	11.4	12.0	12.0	12.7	13.0	13.0
11:6–11:11	30	9.1	10.2	11.0	11.0	13.0	13.0	13.0	14.0	14.0
12:0–12:5	30	10.0	11.0	12.0	12.0	12.0	12.0	12.0	13.0	14.0
12:6–12:11	30	10.0	10.2	11.0	12.0	12.0	12.0	13.0	13.8	14.0
13:0–13:5	40	10.0	11.0	11.0	12.0	12.0	12.0	13.0	13.0	14.0
13:6–13:11	30	10.3	11.0	11.9	12.0	12.0	12.0	13.0	13.0	13.7
14:0–14:5	30	11.0	11.0	12.0	12.0	12.0	13.0	13.0	14.8	15.0
14:6–14:11	30	9.1	11.0	11.3	12.0	12.0	13.0	13.7	14.0	15.0
15:0–15:5	30	11.0	11.0	12.0	12.0	13.0	13.0	14.0	14.0	16.0
15:6–15:11	23	11.0	11.0	12.0	13.0	13.0	13.0	13.4	14.0	14.0
Percentiles for girls: Assembly										
5:0–5:5	30	11.1	13.0	13.0	14.0	15.0	15.6	16.0	17.0	18.0
5:6–5:11	30	9.0	11.0	12.3	13.4	14.0	15.6	16.0	17.0	20.0
6:0–6:5	30	14.0	16.0	16.0	16.0	17.0	18.0	20.0	22.0	23.9
6:6–6:11	30	16.0	17.0	18.0	19.0	20.0	21.0	22.7	25.6	27.8
7:0–7:5	30	14.0	15.2	17.0	18.0	19.5	21.6	22.0	24.0	24.9
7:6–7:11	30	14.0	16.0	17.0	18.4	19.5	21.6	23.4	25.8	26.9
8:0–8:5	30	16.0	17.0	20.0	21.0	22.0	23.0	23.0	24.8	28.9
8:6–8:11	30	18.0	19.2	20.3	21.4	23.0	24.6	27.4	31.8	32.0
9:0–9:5	30	18.0	19.0	20.3	22.0	23.5	26.0	29.0	31.8	16.0
9:6–9:11	30	22.1	23.2	26.0	27.0	28.0	31.0	32.0	34.8	37.9
10:0–10:5	30	20.3	23.2	26.0	27.0	28.0	29.0	29.7	30.8	35.8
10:6–10:11	30	24.1	27.0	28.3	29.4	30.5	31.6	35.7	37.8	39.8
11:0–11:5	30	25.1	28.0	29.3	31.4	32.5	34.0	35.7	37.0	40.9
11:6–11:11	30	22.2	25.4	28.3	31.0	34.5	37.0	39.0	40.0	41.0
12:0–12:5	30	28.0	31.0	32.0	34.0	34.0	34.6	36.7	39.0	43.6
12:6–12:11	30	24.0	28.0	30.3	32.8	35.0	36.0	38.7	41.7	45.7
13:0–13:5	40	27.0	31.2	32.3	33.4	35.0	37.6	38.0	39.0	41.9
13:6–13:11	30	29.5	33.0	34.9	36.4	38.0	38.0	40.0	42.0	44.1
14:0–14:5	30	25.3	30.2	34.0	34.0	36.0	38.0	40.7	43.0	45.9
14:6–14:11	30	27.1	28.2	30.3	32.0	33.0	35.2	37.7	40.8	44.9
15:0–15:5	30	28.7	29.8	31.7	33.6	35.5	38.4	41.3	43.2	50.2
15:6–15:11	23	23.2	29.4	33.0	36.8	39.0	40.0	41.0	43.0	47.8

Note: Data were derived from 1,334 normal schoolchildren.

Source: Gardner & Broman (1979).

ued to improve for a greater length of time. It is important to note that right-left difference scores or ratios tend not to be very reliable, with correlations ranging from .22 to .61 (Reddon et al., 1988; Sappington, 1980).

Factor-analytic studies (Fleishman & Ellison, 1962; Fleishman & Hempel, 1954) have shown that the Purdue Pegboard loads on a finger dexterity factor defined as "the ability to make rapid, skillful, controlled manipulative movements of small objects, where the fingers are primarily involved." However, the Assembly test appears to measure something in addition to finger dexterity and also loads on a manual dexterity factor defined as "the ability to make skillful, controlled arm-hand manipulations of larger objects."

Schmidt et al. (1993) reported that normal individuals, without neuropsychiatric or other disease, who showed MRI white matter hyperintensities (WMH), performed worse on the Assemblies subtest than did patients without WMH. Brown et al. (1993) noted impaired execution of bimanual movements on the Purdue test in patients with Parkinson's disease, in patients with cerebellar disease, and in Huntington's disease. Further, the peg placement portion of the Purdue Pegboard Test appears to be sensitive to the presence of brain damage and may provide information of lateralizing significance (Costa et al., 1983; Gardner & Broman, 1979; Rapin et al., 1966; Vaughan & Costa, 1962). Because changes in performance occur over time, however, right-left differences (or ratios) on the Purdue Pegboard Test may only have diagnostic value when differences are also found on other tests (Reddon et al., 1988).

Table 14—7. Mean Performance of Young Adults for the Purdue Pegboard (one Trial per Subtest)

	Age groups				
	15–20	21–25	26–30	31–40	15–40
Females					
n	30	36	16	16	98
Preferred hand	16.69	16.64	17.25	15.94	16.64
SD	2.16	2.31	1.88	1.61	2.10
Nonpreferred hand	16.10	15.89	16.13	15.63	15.95
SD	1.57	1.79	1.50	1.89	1.68
Both hands	13.76	13.75	13.31	13.13	13.58
SD	1.41	1.54	1.45	1.31	1.45
Assemblies	41.83	42.47	40.44	41.44	41.77
	5.08	5.43	5.90	5.75	5.42
Males					
n	32	37	32	26	127
Preferred hand	15.56	15.44	16.22	15.35	15.65
SD	1.52	1.71	1.81	1.72	1.71
Nonpreferred hand	15.09	15.08	15.41	15.12	15.17
SD	1.42	1.98	2.08	1.77	1.82
Both hands	12.59	12.97	12.94	12.42	12.75
SD	1.56	1.18	1.29	1.65	1.42
Assemblies	40.25	38.89	39.13	37.50	39.01
SD	4.64	6.60	3.58	3.64	4.92

Note: Data were compiled from 225 healthy adults, largely right-handed (87.7%), with above average IQ, residing in a large city in Western Canada.

Source: Yeudall et al. (1986).

Table 14—8. Mean Performance of Older Adults for the Purdue Pegboard (one Trial per Subtest)

	Age Groups		
	50–59	60–69	70+
Males			
n	10	12	8
Preferred hand	14.7	14.2	11.4
SD	2.2	2.8	2.0
Nonpreferred hand	14.4	13.6	10.9
SD	2.0	2.8	1.5
Both hands	12.1	10.1	8.4
SD	1.9	.7	1.5
Assemblies	30.6	27.2	21.9
SD	6.7	5.9	5.4
Females			
n	11	10	15
Preferred hand	14.5	14.4	13.2
SD	1.9	1.3	1.5
Nonpreferred hand	14.0	13.6	12.6
SD	2.1	2.2	2.0
Both hands	11.3	11.1	9.4
SD	1.5	1.7	1.6
Assemblies	28.3	28.2	24.9
SD	5.1	7.0	3.2

Note: Data were compiled from healthy volunteers living in Victoria, British Columbia.
Source: Strauss & Spreen (1990).

Table 14—9. Mean Performance of Adults for the Purdue Pegboard (three trials per subtest)

	Age Groups				
	40–49	50–59	60–69	70–79	80–89
Males					
n	19	20	24	17	11
Preferred	14.6	14.4	13.6	13.0	10.8
SD	2.08	2.15	1.74	1.90	1.33
Nonpreferred hand	14.4	13.9	13.1	12.4	10.6
SD	2.35	2.19	1.56	1.48	1.84
Both hands	12.2	11.9	10.9	10.4	8.5
SD	2.43	2.22	1.46	1.27	1.21
Purdue Assembly	34.9	33.8	28.0	27.5	21.5
SD	7.66	9.66	5.06	5.06	4.81
Pref. minus nonpref.	0.16	0.23	0.44	0.59	0.18
SD	1.19	1.21	1.86	0.93	1.46
Females					
n	21	27	29	31	13
Perferred hand	15.9	15.0	14.6	13.8	12.9
SD	1.45	1.56	2.03	1.27	1.80
Nonpreferred hand	15.2	14.4	13.9	12.9	11.3
SD	1.48	1.69	1.78	1.52	2.05
Both hands	13.1	12.1	11.6	10.5	9.2
SD	1.56	1.30	1.87	1.19	1.92
Purdue Assembly	39.8	34.6	31.7	29.1	21.9
SD	4.54	8.21	6.83	4.85	4.54
Pref. minus nonpref.	0.73	0.63	0.71	0.94	1.56
SD	1.05	1.31	1.23	1.39	1.24

Source: Agnew et al., 1988. Reprinted with permission.

Normative Data

In general, performance is better with the preferred than the nonpreferred hand; females perform better than males, and performance slows with advancing age (Agnew et al., 1988; Gardner & Broman, 1979; Mathiowetz et al., 1986; Peters, 1990; Sattler & Engelhardt, 1982; Wilson et al., 1982; Yeudall et al., 1986; but see Costa et al., 1963, who did not find sex-related differences). Sex differences in fine manual dexterity may be confounded by sex differences in finger size. Peters et al. (1990) have reported that when measures of index finger and thumb thickness were used as covariates, sex differences in performance disappeared. Further, negative correlations between performance and finger size were observed in both men and women. The implication is that for most men, the fingers are of a size that is relatively unsuitable for this task. With larger-sized pegs, men may no longer be at a disadvantage. Education appears to be unrelated to performance (Costa et al., 1963; Yeudall et al., 1986).

Tables 14–5 through 14–7 provide normative data for children and adults, stratified on the basis of age (5–40) and sex (Gardner & Broman, 1980; Yeudall et al., 1986). Table 14–8 provides normative data (Strauss & Spreen, 1990, unpublished data) for healthy, well-educated (mean = 13.2 years), older adults, ages 50–85. These tables are based on an administration of one trial per subtest. Nielsen et al. (1989) provide data (for dominant, nondominant, and both hands) using a sample of 101 nonneurological patients, aged 20–54 years, tested following discharge from hospital. The data, however, are not broken down by gender. Mathiowetz et al. (1986) give normative data, based on a three-trial administration, for 176 subjects 14–19 years of age. The scores are higher than those reported here, perhaps reflecting the influence of practice afforded by additional trials. Their sample is also smaller than that of Gardner and Broman (1979). Agnew et al. (1988) provide data based on a sample of 212 healthy, well-educated, 40- to 85-year-olds. Subtest scores consist of the average of three trials per subtest. Differences between dominant and nondominant hands

were also calculated. The manual difference was greater for women than for men. There was a trend for this difference to become greater with increasing age, but the effect did not prove statistically significant. The data, derived from this relatively large sample of older adults, are shown in Table 14–9. Wilson et al. (1982) modified the pegboard by shortening the board so that it could be used with preschoolers. They compiled data on right-handed children, ages 2.5–6 years, for the peg placement portions only.

References

Agnew, J., Bolla-Wilson, K., Kawas, C.H., & Bleeker, M.L. (1988). Purdue Pegboard age and sex norms for people 40 years old and older. *Developmental Neuropsychology, 4*, 29–35.

Brown, R.G., Jahanshahai, M., & Marsden, D.C. (1993). The execution of bimanual movements in patients with Parkinson's, Huntington's, and cerebellar disease. *Journal of Neurology, Neurosurgery and Psychiatry, 56*, 295–297.

Costa, L.D., Vaughan, H.G., Levita, E., & Farber, N. (1963). Purdue Pegboard as a predictor of the presence and laterality of cerebral lesions. *Journal of Consulting Psychology, 27*, 133–137.

Costa, L.D., Scarola, L.M., & Rapin, I. (1983). Purdue Pegboard scores for normal grammar school children. *Perceptual and Motor Skills, 18*, 748.

Feinstein, A., Brown, R., & Ron, M. (1994). Effects of practice of serial tests of attention in healthy subjects. *Journal of Clinical and Experimental Neuropsychology, 16*, 436–447.

Fleishman, E.A., & Ellison, G.D. (1962). A factor analysis of fine manipulative tests. *Journal of Applied Psychology, 46*, 96–105.

Fleishman, E.A., & Hempel, W.E., Jr. (1954). A factor analysis of dexterity tests. *Personnel Psychology, 7*, 15–32.

Gardner, R.A., & Broman, M. (1979). The Purdue Pegboard: Normative data on 1334 school children. *Journal of Clinical Child Psychology, 8*, 156–162.

Mathiowetz, V., Rogers, S.L., Dowe-Keval, M., Donahoe, L., & Rennels, C. (1986). The Purdue Pegboard: Norms for 14- to 19-year-olds. *The American Journal of Occupational Therapy, 40*, 174–179.

Nielsen, H., Knudsen, I., & Daugbjerg, O. (1989). Normative data for eight neuropsychological tests based on a Danish sample. *Scandinavian Journal of Psychology, 30,* 37–45.

Peters, M. (1990). Subclassification of non-pathological left-handers poses problems for theories of handedness. *Neuropsychologia, 28,* 279–289.

Peters, M., Servos, P., & Day, R. (1990). Marked sex differences on a fine motor skill task disappear when finger size is used as a covariate. *Journal of Applied Psychology, 75,* 87–90.

Rapin, I., Tourk, L.M., & Costa, L.D. (1966). Evaluation of the Purdue Pegboard as a screening test for brain damage. *Developmental Medicine and Child Neurology, 8,* 45–54.

Reddon, J.R., Gill, D.M., Gauk, S.E., & Maerz, M.D. (1988). Purdue Pegboard: Test–retest estimates. *Perceptual and Motor Skills, 66,* 503–506.

Sappington, T.J. (1980). Measures of lateral dominance: Interrelationships and temporal stability. *Perceptual and Motor Skills, 50,* 783–790.

Sattler, J.M., & Engelhardt, J. (1982). Sex differences on Purdue Pegboard norms for children. *Journal of Clinical Child Psychology, 11,* 72–73.

Schmidt, R., Fazekas, F., Offenbacher, H., Dusek, T., et al. (1993). Neuropsychologic correlations of MRI white matter hyperintensities: A study of 150 normal volunteers. *Neurology, 43,* 2490–2492.

Strauss, E., & Spreen, O. (1990). Unpublished data.

Tiffin, J. (1968). *Purdue Pegboard: Examiner Manual.* Chicago: Science Research Associates.

Tiffin, J., & Asher, E.J. (1948). The Purdue Pegboard: Norms and studies of reliability and validity. *Journal of Applied Psychology, 32,* 234–247.

Vaughan, H.G., & Costa, L.D. (1962). Performance of patients with lateralized cerebral lesions: II. Sensory and motor tests. *Journal of Nervous and Mental Disease, 134,* 237–243.

Wilson, B.C., Iacovello, J.M., Wilson, J.J., & Risucci, D. (1982). Purdue Pegboard performance of normal preschool children. *Journal of Clinical Neuropsychology, 4,* 19–26.

Yeudall, L.T., Fromm, D., Reddon, J.R., & Stefanyk, W.O. (1986). Normative data stratified by age and sex for 12 neuropsychological tests. *Journal of Clinical Psychology, 42,* 918–946.

15

Adaptive Behavior and Personality

Although an accurate description of a patient's abilities based on test results is of primary importance for the neuropsychologist in the diagnostic and rehabilitation process, relatively little can be inferred from such tests about the ability of the patient to function in the daily living situation at home, in new situations, or even in hospital or long-term care facilities. For the assessment of such abilities, other factors such as the functional capability to dress, eat, and cook for oneself, as well as personality variables including premorbid personality features, the reaction to illness and disability, and direct personality alteration as a result of the brain lesion must be taken into account.

Adaptive behavior assessment is frequently (and expertly) done informally by the occupational therapist who relies on home visits, observation of the patient's behavior, and information provided by the primary caretaker (spouse, nurse, group home staff, etc.). In addition, occupational therapists make use of one of the many "Activities of Daily Living" scales to monitor patients' abilities and progress during therapy (e.g., Klein & Bell, 1982; see reviews by Eakin, 1989a, 1989; and Law & Letts, 1989). The development of more comprehensive, formal instruments to assess adaptive behavior was first started in the field of mental retardation (Doll, 1935), and has more recently resulted in the development of relatively sophisticated instruments: for example, the American Association on Mental Retardation (AAMR) Adaptive Behavior Scale

(Lambert et al., 1993; Nihira et al., 1992, also available with computer scoring and interpretation); the revised Vineland Adaptive Behavior Scales (Sparrow et al., 1984); an Adaptive Behavior Inventory (Brown & Leigh, 1986); a short Adult Functional Adaptive Behavior Scale (Pierce, 1989); the Comprehensive Test of Adaptive Behavior (Adams, 1984); the Minnesota Child Development Inventory (MCDI, Ireton & Thwing, 1974; Byrne et al., 1995) and the revised Child Development Inventory (CDI, Ireton, 1992), specifically designed for children between the age of 6 months and 6 years 6 months; and the System of Multicultural Pluralistic Assessment (SOMPA) (Mercer & Lewis, 1978) and the related Adaptive Behavior Inventory for Children (Mercer & Lewis, 1982), a comprehensive system of assessment stressing culture–fairness. For school-age children and adolescents (grades K–12), Gresham and Elliott (1990) developed a brief Social Skills Rating System that focuses mainly on interaction with others.

The importance of adaptive behavior is stressed in all recent definitions of mental retardation, which require significantly subnormal functioning in both intelligence and adaptive behavior (American Association on Mental Retardation, 1991; Grossman, 1983; Heber, 1959). Similar weight of adaptive behavior has only recently been placed on definitions of dementia and other neurological disorders by neuropsychologists although it is of crucial importance in making recommendations about appropriate settings of care, in rehabilitative efforts, and in compensation litigation as well as in rating the severity of dementia. We recommend the use of the Vineland or the Activities of Daily Living scales when such questions arise.

The assessment of the personality and affect of the brain-damaged patient, on the other hand, has a long history in neuropsychology, dating back to descriptions of the "frontal lobe syndrome," the "catastrophic reactions of patients with missile wounds," or the search for "the epileptic personality." The need to consider the premorbid personality and the emotional reaction to the handicap (which is often related to premorbid personality features) has been recognized for some time. The need to make a distinction between the superficially similar behavior of patients with depression and dementia has lead to further work in this field in more recent years. Yet, no generally accepted instrument covering these specific neuropsychological problems has been developed. Our selection covers the most useful instruments currently available, ranging from the traditional Rorschach Test, the Thematic Apperception Test (TAT), the Minnesota Multiphasic Personality Inventory (MMPI-2), the Profile of Mood States (POMS), to two specific depression scales (Beck Depression Scale, Geriatric Depression Scale).

Some clinicians may prefer the relatively new Personality Assessment Inventory (PAI, Morley, 1991) over the MMPI because of its brevity (344 items), its inexpensive computer administration/scoring/interpretation support, and its low demands on reading skills. The PAI is similar to the MMPI in that it provides four validity, 11 clinical, five treatment considerations, and two interpersonal scales, although the construction principles differ. The PAI scales were developed from an impressive normative and clinical data base. However, we do not provide a full description of the PAI because independent research and studies of neuropsychological applications are as yet not available.

Two new instruments specifically designed for neuropsychological assessment are also included: the Neuropsychology Behavior and Affect Profile (Nelson et al., 1989), which is designed to measure both pre- and postmorbid neuropsychological features as seen by a person close to the patient, and the Neurobehavioral Rating Scale (NRS, Levin et al., 1987), which provides the clinician with a comprehensive rating of the patient's disabilities. Such instruments based on alternative reporting sources rather than the patient him/herself are a relatively recent addition to the neuropsychological assessment (Nelson & Cicchetti, 1995). Some clinicians may wish to use the newly revised Neuropsychological Impairment Scale (NIS, O'Donnell et al., 1994), which has two forms, one to be given to the patient and one for the "observer." It is relatively lengthy (95 items) and, in addition to a global impairment rating, includes four validity check scales, a critical items list, and six subscales for various areas of impairment. The NIS is not described in detail because not enough independent research is available. We did include a description of the new Penn Inventory for Posttraumatic Stress Disorder (Hammarberg, 1992) because of its obvious relevance to the assessment of accident victims.

Other inventories and scales, developed along psychiatric-diagnostic lines (Millon Clinical Multiaxial Inventory-III, Millon, 1993; Coolidge Axis II Inventory, Coolidge, 1983) or for specific symptoms in a psychiatric context (Beck Anxiety Inventory, Beck & Steer, 1990; Beck Hopelessness Scale, Beck & Steer, 1988; Beck Scale for Suicidal Ideation, Beck & Steer, 1991; State-Trait Anxiety Inventory, Spielberger, 1983) are not described because they offer little additional information in a neuropsychological setting. None of the scales is administered routinely; rather, a selection is made based on the nature of the presenting problem and the complaints and behavior of the patient during testing and interview.

For children, we included the Personality Inventory for Children (PIC) and the Child Behavior Checklist (CBCL). Not discussed here, but preferred by some clinicians because of its brevity (93 items for parents, 48 items for teachers), is the Conner's Rating Scale (CRS, including hyperactivity scales) for parents and for teachers (Conners, 1990). The CRS provides nine scales, and even shorter versions (48, 39, or 28 items) of the same instrument, as well as computer administration, scoring, and interpretation. Similarly, the Children's Depression Inventory (CDI, Kovacs, 1992), a 27-item self-rated symptom-oriented scale for 7- to 17-year-olds, may be of interest in some child-service settings.

Reynolds (1987a, 1989) designed the Reynolds Adolescent and Child Depression scales, which can be given directly to the client. These scales were designed for group administration ("screening for depression") in schools but can also be given to individual clients. Because of their limited usefulness in neuropsychology, we do not review these and other scales developed by Reynolds (Suicidal Ideation Inventory, Reynolds, 1987b) and others (Adolescent Drinking Index, Harrell et al., 1989). Such scales may at times be useful because they do not rely on parent or teacher reports, and they may provide useful information preliminary to the interview of the child or adolescent.

References

Adams, G.L. (1984). *Comprehensive Test of Adaptive Behavior*. San Antonio, TX: The Psychological Corporation.

American Association of Mental Retardation. (1991). *Manual on Terminology and Classification in Mental Retardation*. Washington, D.C.: American Association on Mental Retardation.

Beck, A., & Steer, R.A. (1988). *Beck Hopelessness Scale*. San Antonio, TX: The Psychological Corporation.

Beck, A., & Steer, R.A. (1990). *Beck Anxiety Inventory*. San Antonio, TX: The Psychological Corporation.

Beck, A., & Steer, R.A. (1991). *Beck Scale for Suicidal Ideation*. San Antonio, TX: The Psychological Corporation.

Brown, L., & Leigh, J.E. (1986). *Adaptive Behavior Inventory*. Austin, TX: Pro-Ed.

Byrne, J.M., Backman, J.E., & Bawden, H.N. (1995). Minnesota Child Development Inventory: A normative study. *Canadian Psychology*, 35, 115–130.

Conners, C.K. (1990). *Conners' Rating Scales Manual*. North Tonawanda, NY: Multi-Health Systems.

Coolidge, F.L. (1993). *Coolidge Axis II Inventory*. Clermont, FL: Synergistic Office Solutions.

Doll, E.A. (1935). A genetic scale of social maturity. *American Journal of Orthopsychiatry*, 5, 180–188.

Eakin, P. (1989a). Assessments of activities of daily living: A critical review. *British Journal of Occupational Therapy*, 52, 11–15.

Eakin, P. (1989b). Problems with the assessment of activities of daily living. *British Journal of Occupational Therapy*, 52, 50–54.

Gresham, F.M., & Elliott, S.N. (1990). *Social Skills Rating System*. Manual. Circle Pines, MN: American Guidance Service.

Grossman, H.J. (1983). *Manual on Terminology and Classification in Mental Retardation* (1983 revision). Washington, D.C.: American Association on Mental Retardation.

Hammarberg, M. (1992). Penn Inventory for Posttraumatic Stress Disorder: Psychometric properties. *Psychological Assessment*, 4, 67–76.

Harrell, A.V., & Wirtz, P.W. (1989). *Adolescent Drinking Index*. Odessa, FL: Psychological Assessment Resources.

Heber, R. (1959). *A Manual on Terminology and Classification in Mental Retardation*. Monograph Supplement. *American Journal of Mental Deficiency*.

Ireton, H. (1992). *Child Development Inventory*. Minneapolis: Behavior Science Systems.

Ireton, H., & Thwing, E. (1974). *Manual for the Minnesota Child Development Inventory*. Minneapolis, MN: Behavior Science Systems.

Klein, R.M., & Bell, B. (1982). Self-care skills: Behavioral measurement with the Klein-Bell ADL scale. *Archives of Physical Medicine and Rehabilitation*, 63, 335–338.

Kovacs, M. (1992). *Children's Depression Inventory*. North Tonawanda, NY: Multi-Health Systems.

Lambert, N., Nihira, K., & Leland, H. (1993). *AAMR Adaptive Behavior Scales, School* (2nd ed.) (ABS-S:2). Austin, TX: Pro-Ed.

Law, M., & Letts, L. (1989). A critical review of scales of activities of daily living. *American Journal of Occupational Therapy*, 43, 522–528.

Levin, H.S., High, W.M., Goethe, K.E., Sisson, R.A., Overall, J.E., Rhoades, H.M., Eisenberg, H.M., Kalisky, Z., & Gary, H.E. (1987). The neurobehavioral rating scale: Assessment of the behavioural sequelae of head injury by the clinician. *Journal of Neurology, Neurosurgery, and Psychiatry*, 50, 183–193.

Mercer, J.R., & Lewis, J.F. (1978). *System of Multicultural Pluralistic Assessment*. New York: Psychological Corporation.

Mercer, J.R., & Lewis, J.F. (1982). *Adaptive Behavior Inventory for Children.* San Antonio, TX: Psychological Corporation.

Millon, T. (1993). *Millon Clinical Multiaxial Inventory* (4th ed.). Minneapolis, MN: National Computer Systems.

Morley, L.C. (1991). *Personality Assessment Inventory.* Odessa, FL: Psychological Assessment Resources.

Nelson, L.D., & Cicchetti, D.V. (1995). Assessment of emotional functioning in brain-impaired individuals. *Psychological Assessment, 7,* 404–413.

Nelson, L.D., Satz, P., Mitrushina, M., van Gorp, W., Cicchetti, D., Lewis, R., & Van Lancker, D. (1989). Development and validation of the neuropsychology behavior and affect profile. *Psychological Assessment: A Journal of Consulting and Clinical Psychology, 1,* 266–272.

Nihira, K., Leland, H., & Lambert, N. (1992). *Adaptive Behavior Scale—Residential and Community* (2nd ed.) (ABS-RC:2). Odessa, FL: Psychological Assessment Resources.

O'Donnell, W.E., DeSoto, C.B., DeSoto, J.L., & Reynolds, D.M. (1994). *The Neuropsychological Impairment Scale.* Manual. Los Angeles: Western Psychological Services.

Pierce, P.S. (1989). *Adult Functional Adaptive Behavior Scale.* Manual of Directions (Rev. Ed.). Togas, ME: Veteran's Administration Medical and Regional Office Center.

Reynolds, W.M. (1987a). *Reynolds Adolescent Depression Scale.* Odessa, FL: Psychological Assessment Resources.

Reynolds, W.M. (1987b). *Suicidal Ideation Questionnaire.* Odessa, FL: Psychological Assessment Resources.

Reynolds, W.M. (1989). *Reynolds Child Depression Scale.* Odessa, FL: Psychological Assessment Resources.

Sparrow, S.S., Balla, D.A., & Cicchetti, D.V. (1984). *Vineland Adaptive Behavior Scales.* Circle Pines, MN: American Guidance Service.

Spielberger, C.D. (1983). *State-Trait Anxiety Inventory.* Palo Alto, CA: Mind Garden.

BECK DEPRESSION INVENTORY (BDI)

Purpose

The purpose of this test is to screen for depression by self-report statements.

Source

The test can be ordered from Psychological Corporation, P.O. Box 39954, San Antonio, TX 78283-3954; or 55 Horner Ave., Toronto, Ont. M8Z 4X6, Canada. The manual and 25 forms cost $49.50 US or $82 Cdn. A Spanish version is available.

The newly available BDI-II contains several item changes to bring the scale in line with the DSM-IV criteria of depression, and costs $53.00 US. This review follows the first edition.

Description

The patient checks 21 four-choice statements presented on a single page [or on a 13-item short form (items with asterisk [*]) by Beck & Beck, 1972] for the choice or choices most appropriate to him or her. The statements refer to the following areas:

1. Sadness*
2. Pessimism/discouragement*
3. Sense of failure*
4. Dissatisfaction*
5. Guilt*
6. Expectation of punishment
7. Self-dislike*
8. Self-accusation
9. Suicidal ideation*
10. Crying
11. Irritability
12. Social withdrawal*
13. Indecisiveness*
14. Unattractiveness*
15. Work inhibition*
16. Insomnia
17. Fatigability*
18. Loss of appetite*
19. Weight loss
20. Somatic preoccupation
21. Loss of libido

An example of the four-choice items* follows:

0   I don't have any thoughts of killing myself.
1   I have thoughts of killing myself, but I would not carry them out.
2   I would like to kill myself.
3   I would kill myself if I had the chance.

Administration

Say to the patient: *"This questionnaire consists of 21 groups of statements. After reading each group of statements carefully, circle the number (0, 1, 2 or 3) next to the one statement in each group which best describes the way you've been feeling in the* past week, *including today. If several statements within a group seem to apply equally well, circle each one. Be sure to read all the statements in each group before marking your choice"*.

At this point, hand a copy of the questionnaire to the patient and say: *"Here is a copy for you, so that you can follow along as I read."* Read the entire group of statements in the first category (do not read the numbers appearing before the statements); then say: *"Now, which one of the statements best describes the way you have been feeling in the* past week, *including today?"*

If the patient indicates her or his choice by responding with a number, read back the statement corresponding to the number given by the patient, to clarify exactly which statement the examinee has selected. When the patient says, *"The first statement,"* he or she may mean (0) or (1). After it is apparent that the patient understands the numbering system, the numerical answer should be sufficient to indicate her or his choice.

The BDI may be given to the patient for self-administration or group administration, but it should be verified that the patient understands the purpose and the answering method for the test as outlined above.

Approximate Time for Administration

The time required is 5–10 minutes.

Scoring

The total score is obtained by adding the highest score circled for each of the 21 items. The maximum score is 63. Item 19 (weight loss) was designed to assess anorexic symptoms. If the patient responds affirmatively to the supplementary question, "Are you trying to lose weight by eating less?" the score on that group is *not* added to the total score.

Computer administration, scoring, and interpretation in combination with other Beck scales (Hopelessness, Anxiety, Suicide Ideation Scales) with use-charges are also available (Beck, 1992). Again, the warnings about computer interpretation (see Chapter 4) apply.

Comment

Test–retest reliability with 38 patients was above .90; changes in scores tended to follow changes in depth of depression for the individual patient (Beck, 1970). Spearman-Brown reliability was .93, and internal consistency for test items .86 (Reynolds and Gould, 1981); other authors reported a coefficient alpha of .88 (Steer et al., 1989), and of .91 for elderly patients (.71 for elderly patients with depression; Gallagher et al., 1982). The short form correlates .94 with the BDI (Gould, 1982).

Depression has been recognized as a multidimensional disorder. Bolon and Barling (1980), for example, extracted three factors (ideational depression, physiological depression, behavioral depression) from the BDI; and Reynolds and Gould (1981) and Brown et al. (1995) both found five (Brown's factors: Negative Self-Focus, Anhedonia/Functional Impairment, Sleep/Hypochondriasis, Weight Loss, Decreased Libido). Byrne et al. (1993) also confirmed three similar factors (negative attitude, performance difficulty, somatic concerns), which showed only minimal variance between genders in adolescents. Louks et al. (1989) conducted a major study of the factor structure of the BID with 777 consecutive admissions to a Veterans Hospital (mean age = 50.5 years), including 17 percent with major mental illness and a 72 percent incidence of alcoholism. A factor analysis ($n = 407$) yielded a cognitive-depression first factor and a vegetative-symptom second factor. There was good replication ($r = .94$) of the first in the second sample ($n = 370$), but only a weak replication ($r = .58$) for the second factor; additional factors were only found in the second analysis. The authors concluded that the BDI is most useful as a measure of the cognitive aspects of severity of depression (represented mostly in items 1–13), but that because of the limited number of items, no other dimensions of depression can be reliably measured.

Concurrent validity coefficients with Lubin's Depression Adjective Checklist range from .38 to .50 for psychiatric patients and .66 in normal subjects; .79 in psychiatric patients and .54 in college students (Kerner & Jacobs, 1983), and .57 in a 30-year-old methadone treatment group (Reynolds & Gould, 1981) with the Zung Self-Rating Depression scale; with the MMPI D-Scale .75; with the MMPI-PK scale (posttraumatic stress disorder, Sutker et al., 1995) .72; and with the Hamilton Rating Scale between .70 and .85 (Brown et al., 1995; Schwab et al., 1967; Williams et al., 1973). Marsella et al. (1974) described correlations ranging from .32 to .74 with four other depression scales including the MMPI D-Scale (.63 in male, .73 in female Caucasian students). Beck (1970) also reports correlations of .66 between the BDI and psychiatric ratings of university students. The test also overlapped with the Beck anxiety checklist (.60) and the Maudsley obsessive-compulsive index (.49; Dent & Salkovskis, 1986) in nonclinical populations. It has only a modest negative correlation ($-.41$) with Rotter's (1966) Internalizing-Externalizing Scale and with Duttweiler's (1984) Internal Control Index ($-.37$), suggesting less depression in persons with internal control (Meyers & Wong, 1988). Ehrenberg (1990, personal communication) reported a strong correlation (.68) with scales of self-efficacy in adolescents; Garske and Thomas (1992) found strong correlations with emotional security, physiological perception

of physical health, and economic security, three subscales of the Rosenberg (1965) Self-Esteem Scale. Discriminant validity between depression and other psychiatric disorders in adolescents was high for both males and females (Marton et al., 1991). Ambrosini et al. (1991) reported sensitivity of 89 percent, specificity of 82 percent, and positive predictive power of 83 percent in a similar population.

One disadvantage of the test is its obvious face validity, which is also apparent to the patient and hence makes dissimulation easy. This was suggested in a study by Dahlstrom et al. (1990), who found that a large sample of college students scored higher when benign and distressed items were presented in randomized order as compared to the standard order of presentation. On the other hand, a group of students instructed to simulate depression because of exposure to a toxic waste dump managed to score in the severe depression range; only a few made scores so high as to be suspect (Lees-Haley, 1989). It is not clear whether self-administration or administration by an examiner leads to different results.

The BDI has been used in 47 individuals (mean age = 22.9 years) with severe closed-head injury approximately 50 months post injury (Garske & Thomas, 1992); the authors found that 55 percent of this sample showed some degree of depression according to BDI scoring guidelines. Severity of depression was not directly related to length of coma. Test scores did not discriminate between right- and left-sided strokes in two studies (Gordon, 1990; Ng et al., 1995), whereas another (Schramke et al., 1996) found significantly higher depression scores in left-hemisphere stroke patients. Ng et al. also found that depression was significantly associated with degree of functional impairment in stroke patients. Levin et al. (1988) studied 119 adult Parkinson's disease patients and found that the BDI is a reliable measure of depression in this population despite the inclusion of somatic items that may be endorsed because of the disease. Taylor et al. (1986) also found that the BDI does not reflect disease severity in

Short / Long form		
0–4	0–9	Normal range
5–7	10–15	Minimal depression (cutoff = 10.9, SD = 8.1)
8–11	16–19	Mild–moderate depression (cutoff = 18.7, SD = 10.2)
11–15	20–29	Moderate-to-severe depression (cutoff = 25.4, SD = 9.6)
16+	30–63	Severe depression (cutoff = 30.0, SD = 10.4)

Figure 15—1. Interpretation guidelines for the BDI. Cutoff points are based on Marsella et al. (1974) and Beck (1987). From the Beck Depression Inventory. Copyright © 1987 by Aaron T. Beck. Reproduced by permission of the Publisher, The Psychological Corporation. All rights reserved.

Parkinson's disease patients. A study of 109 patients before and after open-heart surgery found only mild elevation of depression scores at both times; BDI scores did not correlate significantly with a variety of cognitive tests (Vingerhoets et al., 1995). Schramke (1996) also found that measures of depression including the Beck scale tend to measure "distress" rather than anxiety in stroke patients because of lack of specificity (poor correlation between three different anxiety scales) in such patients, whereas specificity was high in non-neurologic psychiatric patients. In AD patients, depression is usually not severe and is unrelated to severity of dementia and the patient's self-awareness of illness (Cummings et al., 1995).

For use in a neuropsychological setting, it should be noted that the BDI is not specifically designed to evaluate depression in elderly populations, and its value for the differential diagnosis of dementia vs. depression has not been established. Plumb and Holland (1977) and Cavenaugh et al. (1983) recommend the use of the first 13 items as a cognitive affective subscale for estimating depression in patients with vegetative/somatic complaints, whereas the remaining eight items tend to measure somatic/performance complaints.

The BDI is just one of several depression scales (e.g., Hamilton, 1967; Lubin, 1965; Radloff, 1977; Schwab et al., 1973; Zung, 1965) developed to detect depression in routine screening or research. It was selected because of its simplicity of administration, scoring, and interpretation. Since the items are

very similar to many MMPI items, it need not be given if the MMPI is administered.

We recommend the use of the Geriatric Depression Scale (Brink et al., 1982) for elderly subjects (see following description). A report comparing the Geriatric Depression Scale with the BDI in 68 geriatric medical outpatients (Norris et al., 1987) and a study of depression in alcoholics (Tamkin et al., 1987) suggested that both instruments accurately identified patients with depression. However, it was noted that the BDI's multiple-choice format makes it more difficult for elderly patients to respond, that some somatic content items* make the BDI less suitable for them, and that neither instrument has been validated in patients with cognitive or sensory impairment.

Normative Data

There are no arbitrary scores that can be used for all purposes to classify different degrees of depression. However, Figure 15–1 provides suggested guidelines to interpret the full scale (Beck, 1978, slightly revised by Beck & Steer, 1993) and the short form (Beck & Beck, 1972). Some confirmation for these norms comes from a study with Dutch students (Bosscher, 1986) and British nonclinical populations (Dent & Salkovskis, 1986). For an unbiased estimate of depression for epidemiological purposes along DSM-III lines, a cutting score of 18/19 has been recommended (Oliver & Simmons, 1984).

*Some of these items have been changed in the new second edition.

The BDI has not been used with children, but a well-researched, separate Children's Depression Inventory is available (Finch et al., 1985; Kovacs, 1983). In adolescents, an increase in scores for the long form of the BDI from 8.9 to 12.3 between age 13 to 17 has been reported (Baron et al., 1986; Ehrenberg, 1990); scores for females were consistently higher than for males. An inference from a study by Kerner and Jacobs (1983) suggests that scores drop gradually with increasing age (mean for college freshmen = 8.8; seniors = 6.5). Knight (1984) reported significant increases of the short form BDI scores with age in males, but not in females in their 70s and 80s, based on a survey of a small New Zealand community; Talbott (1990) described a similar age bias. Marsella et al. (1974) report similar values for college students, which remained consistently higher for females; they were also consistently higher for Japanese and Chinese than for Caucasian students.

References

Ambrosini, P.J., Metz, C., Bianchi, M.D., & Rabinovich, H. (1991). Concurrent validity and psychometric properties of the Beck Depression Inventory in outpatient adolescents. *Journal of the American Academy of Child and Adolescent Psychiatry, 30,* 51–57.

Baron, P. (1986). Sex differences in the Beck Depression Inventory scores of adolescents. *Journal of Youth and Adolescence, 15,* 165–171.

Beck, A.T. (1970). *Depression: Causes and Treatment.* Philadelphia: University of Pennsylvania Press.

Beck, A.T. (1978; Beck, A.T., & Steer, R.A., 1993). *Beck Depression Inventory.* Manual. San Antonio, TX: Psychological Corporation.

Beck, A.T. (1992). *Beck Computer Scoring.* San Antonio, TX: Psychological Corporation.

Beck, A.T., & Beck, R.W. (1972). Screening depressed patients in family practice. *Postgraduate Medicine, 52,* 81–85.

Bolon, K., & Barling, J. (1980). The measurement of self-rated depression: A multidimensional approach. *Journal of Genetic Psychology, 137,* 309–310.

Bosscher, R.J. (1986). Reliability and validity of the BDI in a Dutch college population. *Psychological Reports, 58,* 696–698.

Brink, T.L., Yesavage, J.A., Owen, L., Heersema, P.H., Adey, M., & Rose, T.L. (1982). Screening tests for geriatric depression. *Clinical Gerontology, 1,* 37–43.

Brown, C., Schulberg, H.C., & Madonia, M.J. (1995). Assessing depression in primary care practice with the Beck Depression Inventory and the Hamilton Rating Scale for Depression. *Psychological Assessment, 7,* 59–65.

Byrne, B.M., Baron, P., & Campbell, T.L. (1993). Measuring adolescent depression: Factorial validity and invariance of the Beck Depression Inventory across gender. *Journal of Research on Adolescence, 3,* 127–143.

Cavenaugh, S.V., Clark, D.C., & Gibbons, R.D. (1983). Diagnosing depression in the hospitalized medically ill. *Psychosomatics, 24,* 809–815.

Cummings, J.L., Ross, W., Absher, J., & Gornbein, J. (1995). Depressive symptoms in Alzheimer disease: Assessment and determinants. *Alzheimer Disease and Associated Disorders, 9,* 87–93.

Dahlstrom, W.G., Brooks, J.G., & Petersen, C.D. (1990). Item order and the impact of response set. *Journal of Personality Assessment, 55,* 224–233.

Dent, H.R., & Salkovskis, P.M. (1986). Clinical measures of depression, anxiety, and obsessionality in non-clinical populations. *Behavioral Research and Therapy, 24,* 689–691.

Duttweiler, P.C. (1984). The Internal Control Index: A newly developed measure of locus of control. *Educational and Psychological Measurement, 44,* 209–221.

Ehrenberg, M. (1990). Personal communication.

Finch, A.J., Saylor, C.F., & Edwards, G.L. (1985). Children's depression inventory: Sex and grade norms for normal children. *Journal of Consulting and Clinical Psychology, 53,* 424–425.

Gallagher, D., Nies, G., & Thompson, L.W. (1982). Reliability of the Beck Depression Inventory with older adults. *Journal of Consulting and Clinical Psychology, 50,* 152–153.

Garske, G.G., & Thomas, K.R. (1992). Self-reported self-esteem and depression: Indexes of psychosocial adjustment following severe traumatic brain injury. *Rehabilitation Counseling Bulletin, 36,* 44–52.

Gordon, H.W. (1990). The neurobiological basis of hemisphericity. In C. Trevarthen (Ed.), *Brain Functions and Circuits of the Mind: Essays in honor of Roger W. Sperry.* Cambridge: Cambridge University Press.

Gould, J. (1982). A psychometric investigation of the standard and short form Beck Depression Inventory. *Psychological Reports, 51,* 1167–1170.

Hamilton, M (1967). Development of a rating scale for primary depressive illness. *British Journal of Social and Clinical Psychology, 6,* 278–296.

Kerner, S.A., & Jacobs, K.W. (1983). Correlation between scores on the Beck Depression Inventory and the Zung Self-Rating Depression Scale. *Psychological Reports, 53,* 969–970.

Knight, R.G. (1984). Some general population norms for the short form Beck Depression Inventory. *Journal of Clinical Psychology, 40,* 751–753.

Kovacs, M. (1983). *The Children's Depression Inventory:* A self-rated depression scale for school-aged youngsters. Unpublished manuscript. University of Pittsburgh.

Lees-Haley, P.R. (1989). Malingering traumatic mental disorder on the Beck Depression Inventory: Cancerphobia and toxic exposure. *Psychological Reports, 65,* 623–626.

Levin, B.E., Llabre, M.M., & Weiner, W.J. (1988). Parkinson's disease and depression: Psychometric properties of the Beck Depression Inventory. *Journal of Neurology, Neurosurgery and Psychiatry, 51,* 1401–1404.

Louks, J., Hayne, C., & Smith, J. (1989). Replicated factor structure of the Beck Depression Inventory. *Journal of Nervous and Mental Disease, 177,* 473–479.

Lubin, B. (1965). Adjective check lists for the measurement of depression. *Archives of General Psychiatry, 12,* 57–62.

Marsella, A.J., Sanborn, K.O., Kamboka, V., Shizuri, L., & Brennan, J. (1974). Cross-validation of self-report measures of depression among normal populations of Japanese, Chinese, and Caucasian ancestry. *Journal of Clinical Psychology, 30,* 281–287.

Marton, P., Churchard, M., Kutcher, S., & Kornblum, M. (1991). Diagnostic utility of the Beck Depression Inventory with adolescent outpatients and inpatients. *Canadian Journal of Psychiatry, 36,* 428–431.

Meyers, L.S., & Wong, D.T. (1988). Validation of a new test of locus of control: The Internal Control Index. *Educational and Psychological Measurement, 48,* 753–761.

Ng, K.C., Chan, K.L., & Straughan, P.T. (1995). Depression and functional impairment in stroke victims. *Acta Psychiatrica Scandinavica, 92,* 75–79.

Norris, J.T., Gallagher, D., Wilson, A., & Winograd, C.H. (1987). Assessment of depression in geriatric medical outpatients: The validity of two screening measures. *Journal of the American Geriatrics Society, 35,* 989–995.

Oliver, J., & Simmons, M. (1984). Depression as measured by the DSM-III and the Beck Depression Inventory in an unselected adult population. *Journal of Consulting and Clinical Psychology, 52,* 892–898.

Plumb, M.M., & Holland, J. (1977). Comparative studies of psychological function in patients with advanced cancer. I: Self-reported depressive symptoms. *Psychosomatic Medicine, 30,* 264–279.

Radloff, L.S. (1977). The CES-D scale: A new self-report depression scale for research in the general population. *Applied Psychological Measurement, 1,* 385–401.

Reynolds, W.M., & Gould, J.W. (1981). A psychometric investigation of the standard and short form Beck Depression Inventory. *Journal of Consulting and Clinical Psychology, 49,* 306–307.

Rosenberg, M. (1965). *Society and the Adolescent Self-Image.* Princeton, NJ: Princeton University Press.

Rotter, J.B. (1966). Generalized expectancies for internal versus external control of reinforcement. *Psychological Monographs, 80* (Whole No. 609).

Schramke, C., Stowe, R., Ratcliff, G., & Goldstein, G. (1996). Depression and anxiety following stroke: Separating distress from affective and anxiety disorders. Paper presented at the meeting of the International Neuropsychological Society, Chicago.

Schwab, J.J., Bialow, M.R., & Holzer, C.E. (1967). A comparison of two rating scales for depression. *Journal of Clinical Psychology, 23,* 45–46.

Schwab, J.J., Holzer, C.E., & Warheit, G.J. (1973). Depressive symptomatology and age. *Psychosomatics, 14,* 135–141.

Steer, R.A., Beck, A.T., & Brown, G. (1989). Sex differences on the revised Beck Depression Inventory for outpatients with affective disorders. *Journal of Personality Assessment, 53,* 693–702.

Sutker, P.B., Vasterling, J.J., Brailey, K., & Allain, A.N. (1995). Memory, attention, and executive deficits in POW survivors: Contributing biological and psychological factors. *Neuropsychology, 9,* 118–125.

Talbott, M.M. (1990). Age bias in the Beck Depression Inventory: A proposed modification for use with older women. *Clinical Gerontologist, 9,* 23–35.

Tamkin, A.S., Carson, M.F., Nixon, D.H., & Hyer, L.A. (1987). A comparison among some measures of depression in male alcoholics. *Journal of Studies on Alcohol, 48,* 176–178.

Taylor, A.E., Saint-Cyr, J.A., Lang, A.E., & Kenny, F.T. (1986). Parkinson's disease and depression: A critical reevaluation. *Brain, 109,* 279–292.

Vingerhoets, G., De Soete, G., & Jannes, C. (1995). Relationship between emotional variables and cognitive test performance before and after open-heart surgery. *Clinical Neuropsychologist, 9,* 198–202.

Williams, J.G., Barlow, D.H., & Agras, W.S. (1973). Behavioral measurement of severe depression. *Archives of General Psychiatry, 16,* 321–325.

Zung, W.W.K. (1965). A self-rating depression scale. *Archives of General Psychiatry, 12,* 63–70.

CHILD BEHAVIOR CHECKLIST (CBCL)

Purpose

The purpose of this test is to obtain a personality assessment of the child through parent or teacher ratings.

Source

The Child Behavior Checklist is published in two forms, with the 1992 profile for ages 2–3 (CBCL/2–3), and with 1991 profile for ages 4–18 (CBCL/4–18). The two forms and four related forms, a Teacher's Report Form (TRF) with 1991 profile for ages 5–18, a Youth Self-Report (YSR) with 1991 profile for ages 11–18, a Direct Observation Form (DOF) with profiles for ages 5–14, and the 1994 Semistructured Clinical Interview for Children and Adolescents (SCICA), together with separate manuals for each form are available from the University of Vermont, Department of Psychiatry, Burlington, VT 05401; in Canada from the Guidance Center, Ontario Institute for Studies in Education, 712 Gordon Baker Road, Toronto, Ont. M2H 3R7, at a price of $31.00 Cdn for the sample package, and approximately $80.00 Cdn for each form, including manual and hand-scoring templates. The package comes with a 862-item bibliography (also available on computer disk), compiled in 1995, for $69.95 Cdn. Note, however, that this list includes many references not directly related to the CBCL. Computer scoring programs for Apple or IBM for each form are available from the source for $299.00 Cdn each.

Description

This test has evolved over a 20-year period (Achenbach & Edelbrock, 1986) and is popular, compared to the PIC, because of its brevity. The CBCL/4–18 (Achenbach, 1991a), for example, presents 113 statements (e.g., "Would rather be alone than with others"), which are rated by the parent or other principal caregiver on a three-point scale. The CBCL/2–3 has 100 items. There is considerable overlap of items between forms (CBCL/4–18, YSR, and TRF have 89 items in common), but the scoring follows factor-analytically derived scales that differ from one age group to the other. For example, for children age 6–11 years, nine "syndrome" scales are available: Schizoid or Anxious, Depressed, Uncommunicative, Obsessive-Compulsive, Somatic Complaints, Social Withdrawal, Hyperactive, Aggressive, and Delinquent. These scales are grouped into two broad-band factors, Internalizing and Externalizing. In addition, three Competency Scales, a Total Competence Scale, and a Total Problem Scale are available; these scales were not developed by factor analysis, but by a listing of functioning during normal daily activities. The TRF (Achenbach, 1991c) has eight slightly different "syndrome" scales plus four scales for academic and adaptive functioning ("working hard, behaving appropriately, learning, happy"). The Direct Observation Form uses four-point rating scales geared to 10-minute samples of behavior as well as a section for scoring on-task behavior at one-minute intervals.

Administration

The CBCL is filled out by the parent or caregiver by marking each statement as "very true or often true" (2), "somewhat or sometimes true" (1), or "not true" (0). For some items, the opportunity to provide additional descriptive information is available. A reading level of at least grade 5 is required for the semistructured interview, and if there is a question about the respondent's reading skills, the test is administered by giving one form to the client and reading along with him or her on a second copy. Preceding the test questions, basic information about the child and competence items (sports, hobbies, organizations and clubs, jobs and chores, etc.) is requested on the form.

Approximate Time for Administration

Approximately 10–15 minutes are required for each form. The TRF takes about 10 minutes. The semi-structured interview takes between 60 and 90 minutes.

Scoring

Each scale is scored by using the hand-scoring key template and summing the item point score for each scale. The sum of each scale is transformed into an age-appropriate T-score and is entered into a profile. A T-score of 67–70 (60–63 for internalizing and externalizing scales) is considered to be in the "borderline clinical" range.

Comment

The CBCL, the most frequently cited measure in studies of child psychopathology, is very similar to the Revised Behavior Problem Checklist (Quay & Peterson, 1987), although the latter has somewhat different scales and only one form. Each of the CBCL forms comes with a manual that describes in detail construction and revision of the scale, normative, reliability, and validity data, practical application information, and research use, with detailed explanations of each term and of statistical procedures. In addition, the Integrative Guide repeats much of the information on the CBCL/4–18, the YSR, and the TRF and can be used as a joint manual.

One-week retest reliability for the CBCL/4–18, the core instrument, is good (mean r = .90 for boys, .88 for girls), with minimal variability of correlations across scales. One-year and two-year stabilities were high (mean r = .72 and .71, respectively). Interparent agreement ranged from a mean r of .75 for younger boys to .69 for older girls. One-week reliability for the YSR averaged .72, and 7-months reliability averaged .49 (Achenbach, 1991b); i.e., both were considerably lower than for the CBCL and the TRF.

Validity for the CBCL is demonstrated by the factor-analytic scale construction described above and is generally good, especially for the externalizing-internalizing dimension. However, Externalization and Internalization are not orthogonal since they are correlated highly in the normative sample (Achenbach, 1991d); hence these two "broad band" scales, resulting from a second-order factor analysis, may not provide additional information beyond the more content-specific scales from which they are constructed, except for a gross index of habitual behavioral tendencies. Individual "syndrome" scales do not necessarily correspond to diagnostic groups. Validity or "lie" scales are not included.

Concurrent validity was established by correlations with similar scales on the Conners Parent Questionnaire and the Quay-Peterson Revised Behavior Problem Checklist (RBPC, n = 60, correlations ranging from .67 to .88). For example, the correlation of the externalizing scale with the conduct disorder scale of the RBPC was .84 in boys and .77 in girls. Discriminant validity, tested by comparison of 2,064 boys and 2,147 girls nonreferred or referred for mental health services, accounted for 26–37 percent of the variance. One item ("unhappy, sad, depressed") was among the best discriminators between referred and nonreferred children.

Partial validation of the Hyperactive scale was found by Massman et al. (1988), who correlated CBCL scores with performance on tests that included a strong attentional component (WISC-R Coding, WRAT Arithmetic, Benton VRT). A significant correlation was found in older children (ages 9 years to 12 years 11 months, n = 90), but not in younger children (6 years to 8 years 11 months, n = 92). The authors speculated that the attentional deficit is not manifest at the younger age, but that attentional skills lag behind as hyperactive children grow older.

The TRF-1991 correlates with pre-1991 TRF at .9 or better. Reliability for the scales after 15 days was between .83 and .99 (mean = .90), 2- to 4-months stability for 19 clinic-referred boys was between .47 and .89, and agreement between teachers was between .41 and .89, between teachers and teacher's aides between .35 and .71 (mean for academic/adaptive scales .60, for problem scores .55). Correlations between the TRF and CBCL and YSR ranged from .71 to .15, and were, as expected, highest for academic performance and delinquent behavior. The relatively low agreement between the two parents, teachers, and self-report suggests that the respondents may see somewhat different aspects of the behavior of the individual from his or her point of view; this emphasizes the need to examine cross-informant information and to resolve differences between sources in follow-up discussions.

TRF correlational validity was established using the Conners scales (Goyette, Conners, & Ulrich, 1978); correlations were .67 for aggressive, .71 for externalizing, and .80 for attentional behavior. External validity rests on the finding of significant differences between 2,550 demographically matched clinic-referred and nonreferred groups: "Clinical range" scores were found in approximately 65 percent of referred cases. Discriminant function analysis classified 78.3 percent of the subjects correctly, mainly based on Academic, Adaptive, Anxious/Depressed, and Delinquent scales.

The YSR correlates .27 (boys, .25 for girls) with the TRF and .36 (boys, girls .40) on average with the CBCL/4–18; the highest correlations were obtained for delinquent behavior and social problems.

The test is designed for school and child mental health settings. A handful of studies of neuropsychological interest have been published. Sollee and Kindlon (1987) found that children with lesions of the nondominant hemisphere had higher Internalizing scores than those with dominant–hemisphere lesions. They attributed this finding to difficulties in processing nonverbal cues and emotionally laden stimuli, which in turn lead to difficulties in interpersonal relationships, resulting in being ostracized, withdrawn, and socially isolated. The authors also claimed higher Externalizing scores for children with lesions of the dominant hemisphere, but this interpretation is questionable because both dominant and nondominant lesion groups had Externalizing scores in the clinical range, and the difference between groups was not significant. Fletcher et al. (1990) found lower competency scores on the CBCL/4–18 in 45 severely head-injured children 6- and 12-months post-injury as compared to those with mild or moderate injury. In this study, the Competence Scales correlated .46 (at 6 months) and .67 (at 12 months) with the Vineland Adaptive Behavior Scales, indicating correlational validity; the authors did not find correlations with cognitive tests.

Severity of tics in Tourette's syndrome was correlated with somatic complaints on the CBCL, and inversely related to social competency ($r = .39$) and activities scales ($-.38$ and $-.43$ respectively; Rosenberg et al., 1984). In a study of children who had overcome meningitis 6–8 years earlier (Taylor et al., 1984) as compared to their siblings, the CBCL indicated increased behavior problems that were not related to IQ and neuropsychological status, even though the post-meningitis group did show significant differences from their siblings in both IQ and neuropsychological tests.

In our experience, the test shows real peaks rarely, and in an inpatient psychiatric population often shows elevations on most or all behavior scales; however, the CBCL is useful as an adjunct to the parent and child interview, particularly if the responses to specific items are reviewed prior to the interview. Translations into 33 different languages are available (Achenbach, 1991c), although the generalizability of the norms to other languages or other countries remains inconclusive (Bird et al., 1991).

The term *multiaxial* used in the manuals does not refer to DSM-IV dimensions; rather, the term is used to indicate that the CBCL measures just one "axis" of child assessment, which should be complemented by the "axes" of school reports and records, cognitive assessment, physical assessment, self- and teacher reports, direct observation (DOF), and personality tests.

Normative Data

The CBCL/4–18 is well standardized on a sample of 2,368 normal and 4,455 clinic-referred children, stratified by age, sex, SES (predominantly middle and upper socioeconomic status), ethnicity, and region in the United States. Norms are provided for ages 4–5 years, 6–11 years, and 12–16 years, separately by sex.

The CBCL/2–4 was normed on 368 non-referred children.

The TRF norms are based on the responses of teachers and counselors for 1,391 subjects who were predominantly white and from upper socioeconomic classes.

YSR norms are based on 1,315 nonreferred youths, representative of the U.S. population, compared to 1,272 clinically referred youth.

The DOF was normed on 287 normal children observed in the classroom.

References

Achenbach, T.M. (1991a). *Manual for the Child Behavior Checklist/4–18 and 1991 Profile.* Burlington, VT: University of Vermont, Department of Psychiatry.

Achenbach, T.M. (1991b). *Manual for the Youth Self-Report and 1991 Profile.* Burlington, VT: University of Vermont, Department of Psychiatry.

Achenbach, T.M. (1991c). *Manual for the Teacher's Report Form and 1991 Profile.* Burlington, VT: University of Vermont, Department of Psychiatry.

Achenbach, T.M. (1991d). *Integrative Guide for the 1991 CBCL/4–18, YSR, and TRF Profiles.* Burlington, VT: University of Vermont, Department of Psychiatry.

Achenbach, T.M., & Edelbrock, C.S. (1986). *Child Behavior Checklist and Youth Self-Report.* Burlington, VT: Author.

Bird, V.R., Gould, M.S., Rubio-Stipec, M., Staghezza, B.M., & Canino, G. (1991). Screening for childhood psychopathology in the community using the Child Behavior Checklist. *Journal of the American Academy of Child and Adolescent Psychiatry, 30,* 116–123.

Fletcher, J.M., Ewing-Cobbs, L., Miner, M.E., Levin, H.S., & Eisenberg, H.M. (1990). Behavior changes after closed head injury in children. *Journal of Consulting and Clinical Psychology, 58,* 93–98.

Goyette, C.H., Conners, C.K., & Ulrich, R.F. (1978). Normative data on revised Connors Parent and Teacher Rating Scales. *Journal of Abnormal Child Psychology, 6,* 221–236.

Massman, P.J., Nussbaum, N.L., & Bigler, E.D. (1988). The mediating effect of age on the relationship between Child Behavior Checklist Hyperactivity scores and neuropsychological test performance. *Journal of Abnormal Child Psychology, 16,* 89–95.

Quay, H.C., & Peterson, D.R. (1987). *Revised Behavior Problem Checklist.* H.C. Quay.

Rosenberg, L.A., Harris, J.C., & Singer, H.S. (1984). Relationship of the Child Behavior Checklist to an independent measure of psychopathology. *Psychological Reports, 54,* 427–430.

Sollee, N.D., & Kindlon, D.J. (1987). Lateralized brain injury and behavior problems in children. *Journal of Abnormal Child Psychology, 15,* 479–490.

Taylor, H.G., Michaels, R.H., Mazur, P.M., Bauer, R.E., & Liden, C.B. (1984). Intellectual, neuropsychological, and achievement outcomes in children six to eight years after recovery from *Homophilus influenzae meningitis. Pediatrics, 74,* 198–205.

GERIATRIC DEPRESSION SCALE (GDS)

Other Test Name

Another test name is the Mood Assessment Scale.

Purpose

The test is a screening instrument to measure depression in the elderly.

Source

There is no commercial source for this test. The questions are included in this volume (Brink et al., 1982; Yesavage, 1983).

Description

The GDS consists of 30 yes/no questions designed for self-administration. The directionality of answers scored for depression changes randomly. The purpose of the scale is partially disguised by the title "Mood Assessment Scale" at the top of the questionnaire. An Italian translation was presented by Ferrario et al. (1990). A short (15-item) screening test has been found satisfactory (Baker & Miller, 1991; Burke et al., 1991), but Alden et al. (1989) warn that it is not an appropriate substitute for the long form.

Administration

The examiner requests the patient to complete a simple questionnaire (Fig. 15–2) referring to changes in mood, and to answer these questions by circling yes or no, whichever appropriately describes his or her feelings at that time. Alternatively, the questions can be read to the patient if there is any concern about his or her ability to read or comprehend written material.

Mood Assessment Scale

1.	Are you basically satisfied with your life?	Yes/**No**
2.	Have you dropped many of your activities and interests?	**Yes**/No
3.	Do you feel that your life is empty?	**Yes**/No
4.	Do you often get bored?	**Yes**/No
5.	Are you hopeful about the future?	Yes/**No**
6.	Are you bothered by thoughts that you can't get out of your head?	**Yes**/No
7.	Are you in good spirits most of the time?	Yes/**No**
8.	Are you afraid that something bad is going to happen to you?	**Yes**/No
9.	Do you feel happy most of the time?	Yes/**No**
10.	Do you often feel helpless?	**Yes**/No
11.	Do you often get restless and fidgety?	**Yes**/No
12.	Do you prefer to stay home rather than go out and doing new things?	**Yes**/No
13.	Do you frequently worry about the future?	**Yes**/No
14.	Do you feel you have more problems with memory than most?	**Yes**/No
15.	Do you think it is wonderful to be alive now?	Yes/**No**
16.	Do you often feel downhearted and blue?	**Yes**/No
17.	Do you feel pretty worthless the way you are now?	**Yes**/No
18.	Do you worry a lot about the past?	**Yes**/No
19.	Do you find life very exciting?	Yes/**No**
20.	Is it hard for you to get started on new projects?	**Yes**/No
21.	Do you feel full of energy?	Yes/**No**
22.	Do you feel that your situation is hopeless?	**Yes**/No
23.	Do you think that most people are better off than you are?	**Yes**/No
24.	Do you frequently get upset about little things?	**Yes**/No
25.	Do you frequently feel like crying?	**Yes**/No
26.	Do you have trouble concentrating?	**Yes**/No
27.	Do you enjoy getting up in the morning?	Yes/**No**
28.	Do you prefer to avoid social gatherings?	**Yes**/No
29.	Is it easy for you to make decisions?	Yes/**No**
30.	Is your mind as clear as it used to be?	Yes/**No**

Figure 15—2. Geriatric Depression Scale. (*Source:* Brink et al., 1982; Yesavage et al., 1983.)

Approximate Time for Administration

About 5–10 minutes are required.

Scoring

One point is given for each of the answers marked in bold in Fig. 15–2.

Comment

The original item pool also included 12 items focusing on psychosomatic complaints that were dropped because of poor item-total correlation. As Parmelee et al. (1989) point out, items such as "My appetite is poor," "My sleep was restless," "Everything I do is an effort," may be a fact of life for elderly people with chronic functional limitations independent of any real depressive affect. The item-total correlations of the current scale range from .32 to .83 with a mean of .56; internal consistency (alpha) was .94, and split-half reliability was .94 (Brink et al., 1982). Abraham (1991) reports an internal consistency between .69 and .88 over 18 occasions during a 39-week period in frail, multiply impaired nursing home patients, aged 71–97 years. Retest reliability after one week was .85 (Koenig et al., 1988). Lyons et al. (1989) reported a reliability of .92 between postsurgery testing and discharge 15 days later in patients with hip replacement surgery. Parmelee et al. (1989) reported very similar internal consistency and reliability values in a group of 806 institutionalized persons between 61 and 99 years. In a study of 585 psychiatric patients (age 17–99 years) Rule et al. (1989) found good internal consistency and convergent validity for the full age range, although correlations were somewhat lower in the age group below 55 years.

Factor analysis established a major factor of dysphoria (unhappiness, dissatisfaction with life, emptiness, downheartedness, worthlessness, helplessness) and minor factors of worry/dread/obsessive thought, and of apathy/withdrawal (Parmelee et al., 1989). As pointed out for the BDI, the test is therefore almost unidimensional because additional minor factors lack replicability and do not meet Cattell's (1966) scree criterion.

Concurrent validity was established by correlations of .73 with the BDI (Hyer & Blount, 1984), of .84 with the Zung scale, and of .83 with the Hamilton scale (Yesavage et al., 1983, 1986). Similar correlations were found in 65- to 89-year-olds, using the Zung (.86) and the Gilleard scale (.89; Gilleard et al., 1981) although the wording of the GDS was found less confusing than that for the other two scales (Hickie & Snowdon, 1987). Dunn and Sacco (1989) found a correlation of .82 with the Depression Symptom Checklist (Sacco, 1983) and of .59 with the Zung scale in 439 community-dwelling 60- to 97-year-olds. Bielauskas and Lamberty (1992) reported 72–77 percent agreement of the GDS with the MMPI Mini-Mult-Depression Scale and the DSM-based Symptom Checklist for Major Depressive Disorders. Staff rating of depression correlated only moderately (.34; Parmelee et al., 1989).

Criterion validity was measured against the Research Diagnostic Criteria and reported as .82 (Yesavage & Brink, 1983). The age range for the populations studied by the authors of the scale have not been reported, except that subjects were specified as over 55 years old. Parmelee et al. (1989) found good agreement with ratings of major, minor, and no depression that were based on clinical diagnosis and symptom checklists, although the false-negative rate in minor depression was fairly high (17.4 percent).

Yesavage et al. (1981) found the GDS useful in elderly subjects with physical illness (arthritis; mean for depressed subjects = 13.1, for nondepressed subjects = 5.1). Discrimination between mildly demented depressed and nondepressed subjects was satisfactory in three studies (Snowdon & Donnelly, 1986; Stebbins & Hopp, 1990; Yesavage et al., 1983). Age and length of institutionalization did not affect the GDS scores (Parmelee et al., 1989). Discriminant validity for dementia vs. depression was investigated in a study by Folstein et al. (1975). Depressed demented elderly subjects showed a mean score of 14.72 (SD = 6.13), while nondepressed demented elderly subjects had a mean score of only 7.49 (SD = 4.26). The difference between the two groups was significant ($p < .001$). Burke et al.

(1989, 1992) found good agreement between clinical diagnosis and GDS scores even in mildly cognitively impaired patients, but not in patients with dementia of the Alzheimer's type. Brink et al. (1984) admit that the test loses some validity in patients with severe dementia.

Bohac et al. (1996) used the short form with 413 community-dwelling elderly patients with cognitive impairment, including 37 diagnosed as suffering from depression. They found that a cutoff score of 5 points resulted in a sensitivity of 65 percent and a specificity of 76 percent.

O'Neill et al. (1992) found significant differences between scores resulting from a self-administered and staff-administered GDS in 100 elderly medical patients, and they recommend that in similar populations the test should routinely be staff- rather than self-administered.

The GDS was developed specifically for elderly subjects. It deliberately omits items dealing with guilt, sexuality, and suicide, which the authors considered inappropriate for elderly subjects. It includes items dealing with perceived locus of control that makes this test more suitable for hospitalized and long-term care subjects. The yes/no format makes fewer demands on the cognitive skills of the patient and leads to better completion rates than point-scales like the BDI in clinical populations with mild cognitive impairment (Dunn & Sacco, 1989; Hickie, 1987; Norris et al., 1987). Obviously, the test cannot be used if comprehension is seriously impaired.

Normative Data

Table 15–1 lists normative data for the GDS, including sensitivity (correct classification of depressives) and specificity (correct classification of normals). Shah et al. (1992) found similar values with a cutoff of 10/11 points; they reported that sensitivity (75 percent) and specificity (73 percent) was optimal at a cutoff of 12/13. The means for normal, healthy elderly subjects were confirmed in a study by Rich (1993), who found means of 4.45 (SD = 4.97) for 20 young adult (age 18–38) subjects, of 2.25 (SD = 2.29) for 20 young-old (age 60–

Table 15—1. Geriatric Depression Scale: Normative Data for Elderly Subjects

Subjects	n	M	SD
Mild depression	26	15.05	4.34
Severe depression	34	22.85	5.07
Controls	40	5.75	4.34

	Cutoff scores		
	>8	>10	>13
Sensitivity	90	84	80
Specificity	80	95	100

Note: The distinction between mild and severe depression is based on Research Diagnostic Criteria (Spitzer et al., 1978).

Sources: Brink et al. (1982); Yesavage et al. (1983).

72) subjects, and of 3.20 (SD = 3.67) for 20 old-old (age 73–85) subjects; in contrast, 20 patients with AD (ages 58–83) showed a mean of 5.30 (SD = 5.98).

It should be remembered that the GDS, like the BDI, is a screening instrument, not a diagnostic tool. The following cutoff points are recommended: normal, 0–9; mild depressives, 10–19; severe depressives, 20–30. These values agree with those published by Hickie and Snowdon (1987).

References

Abraham, I.L. (1991). The geriatric depression scale and hopelessness index: Longitudinal psychometric data on frail nursing home residents. *Perceptual and Motor Skills, 72,* 875–880.

Alden, D., Austin, C.N., & Sturgeon, R. (1989). A correlation between the Geriatric Depression Scale long and short form. *Journal of Gerontology, 44,* 124–125.

Baker, F.M., & Miller, C.L. (1991). Screening a skilled nursing home population for depression. *Journal of Geriatric Psychiatry and Neurology, 4,* 218–221.

Bielauskas, L.A., & Lamberty, G.J. (1992). Assessment of depression in elderly patients. *Clinical Neuropsychologist, 6,* 322 (abstract).

Bohac, D.L., Smith, G.E., & Rummans, T.R. (1996). Sensitivity, specificity, and predictive value of the Geriatric Depression Scale—Short Form (GDS-SF) among cognitively impaired elderly. *Archives of Clinical Neuropsychology, 11,* 370 (abstract).

Brink, T.L., Yesavage, J.A., Lum, O., Heersema, P.H., Adey, M., & Rose, T.S. (1982). Screening tests for geriatric depression. *Clinical Gerontologist, 1*, 37–43.

Brink, T.L. (1984). Limitations of the GDS in cases of pseudodementia. *Clinical Gerontology, 2*, 60–61.

Burke, W.J., Nitcher, R.L., Roccaforte, W.H., & Wengel, S.P. (1992). A prospective evaluation of the Geriatric Depression Scale in an outpatient geriatric assessment center. *Journal of the American Geriatrics Society, 40*, 1227–1230.

Burke, W.J., Houston, M.J., Boust, S.J., & Roccaforte, W.H. (1989). Use of the Geriatric Depression Scale in dementia of the Alzheimer type. *Journal of the American Geriatrics Society, 37*, 856–860.

Burke, W.J., Roccaforte, W.H., & Wengel, S.P. (1991). The short form of the Geriatric Depression Scale: A comparison with the 30-item form. *Journal of Geriatric Psychiatry and Neurology, 4*, 173–178.

Cattell, R.B. (1966). The scree test for number of factors. *Multivariate Behavioral Research, 1*, 245.

Dunn, V.K., & Sacco, W.P. (1989). Psychometric evaluation of the Geriatric Depression Scale and the Zung Self-Rating Depression Scale using an elderly community sample. *Psychology and Aging, 4*, 125–126.

Ferrario, E., Cappa, G., Bertone, O., Poli, L., & Fabris, F. (1990). Geriatric Depression Scale and assessment of cognitive-behavioural disturbances in the elderly: A preliminary report on an Italian sample. *Clinical Gerontologist, 10*, 67–73.

Folstein, M.F., Folstein, S.E., & McHugh, P.R. (1975). Mini Mental State: A practical method for grading the cognitive state of patients for the clinician. *Journal of Psychiatric Research, 12*, 189–198.

Gilleard, C.J., Willmott, M., & Vaddadi, K.S. (1981). Self-report measures of mood and morale in elderly depressives. *British Journal of Psychiatry, 138*, 230–235.

Hickie, C., & Snowdon, J. (1987). Depression scales for the elderly: GDS, Gilleard, Zung. *Clinical Gerontologist, 6*, 51–53.

Hyer, L., & Blount, J. (1984). Concurrent and discriminant validities of the GDS with older psychiatric patients. *Psychological Reports, 54*, 611–616.

Koenig, H.G., Meador, K.G., Cohen, H.J., & Blazer, D.G. (1988). Self-rated depression scales and screening for major depression in older hospitalized patients with medical illness. *Journal of the American Geriatrics Society, 36*, 699–796.

Lyons, J.S., Strain, J.J., Hammer, J.S., Ackerman, A.D., & Fulop, G. (1989). Reliability, validity, and temporal stability of the Geriatric Depression Scale in hospitalized patients. *International Journal of Psychiatry in Medicine, 19*, 203–209.

Norris, J.T., Gallagher, D., Wilson, A., & Winograd, C.H. (1987). Assessment of depression in geriatric medical outpatients: The validity of two screening measures. *Journal of the American Geriatrics Society, 35*, 989–995.

O'Neill, D., Rice, I., Blake, P., & Walsh, J.B. (1992). The Geriatric Depression Scale: Rater-administered or self-administered? *International Journal of Geriatric Psychiatry, 7*, 511–515.

Parmelee, P.A., Lawton, M.P., & Katz, I.R. (1989). Psychometric properties of the Geriatric Depression Scale among the institutionalized aged. *Psychological Assessment, 1*, 331–338.

Rich, J.B. (1993). Pictorial and verbal implicit and recognition memory in aging and Alzheimer's disease: A transfer-appropriate processing account. Ph.D. dissertation. University of Victoria.

Rule, B.G., Harvey, H.Z., & Dobbs, A.R. (1989). Reliability of the Geriatric Depression Scale for younger adults. *Clinical Gerontologist, 9*, 37–43.

Sacco, W.P. (1983). The Depression Symptom Checklist. Unpublished manuscript. University of South Florida.

Shah, A., Phongsathorn, V., George, C., Bielawska, C., & Katona, C. (1992). Psychiatric morbidity among continuing care geriatric inpatients. *International Journal of Geriatric Psychiatry, 7*, 517–525.

Snowdon, J., & Donnelly, N. (1986). A study of depression in nursing homes. *Journal of Psychiatric Research, 20*, 327–333.

Spitzer, R.L., Edicott, J., & Robins, E. (1978). Research diagnostic criteria: rationale and reliability. *Archives of General Psychiatry, 35*, 773–782.

Stebbins, G., & Hopp, G. (1990). Elderly residents' depression levels at admission and post admission to a long-term care facility. Unpublished manuscript. University of Victoria.

Yesavage, J. (1987). The use of self-rating depression scales in the elderly. In L.W. Poon (Ed.), *Handbook of Clinical Memory Assessment of Older Adults*, pp. 213–217. Washington, D.C.: American Psychological Association.

Yesavage, J.A., Brink, T.L., Rose, T.L., & Adey, M. (1986). The geriatric depression rating scale:

Comparison with other self-report and psychiatric rating scales. In L.W. Poon (Ed.), *Handbook of Clinical Memory Assessment of Older Adults*, pp. 153–167. Washington, D.C.: American Psychological Association.

Yesavage, J.A., Brink, T.L., Rose, T.L., Lum, O., Huang, V., Adey, M.B., & Leirer, V.O. (1983).

Development and validation of a geriatric depression rating scale: A preliminary report. *Journal of Psychiatric Research, 17*, 37–49.

Yesavage, J.A., Rose, T.L., & Lapp, D. (1981). *Validity of the Geriatric Depression Scale in Subjects with Senile Dementia*. Palo Alto, CA: Veterans Administration Medical Clinic.

MINNESOTA MULTIPHASIC PERSONALITY INVENTORY—2 (MMPI-2) AND MINNESOTA MULTIPHASIC PERSONALITY INVENTORY—ADOLESCENT (MMPI-A)

Purpose

This test is designed for general personality assessment with true-false questions.

Source

The MMPI-2 and the MMPI-A (manual, reusable booklets, scoring keys for basic and supplementary scales, and answer sheets) are available from National Computer Systems (NCS), P.O. Box 1416, Minneapolis, MN 55343, at a cost of approximately $300 US each for the complete set; in Canada from Multi-Health Systems, Inc., 65 Overlea Blvd., Suite 210, Toronto, Ont. M4H 1P1, for $426.25 Cdn (MMPI-2), and $457.25 Cdn (MMPI-A). NCS also offers mail-in or on-site computer scoring and interpretation. Computer interpretation programs are also available from Western Psychological Services (12031 Wilshire Blvd., Los Angeles, CA 90025), Psychological Assessment Resources (P.O. Box 998, Odessa, FL 33556), and Behaviordyne (P.O. Box 10994, Palo Alto, CA 94303-0992). NCS also offers a Spanish version, designed for Spanish speakers in North America.

The original MMPI is also still available and can be ordered from National Computer Systems for approximately $70 US, or from the Institute of Psychological Research, Inc., 34 Fleury Street West, Montreal, P.Q., Canada H3L 1S9, for approximately $100 Cdn. Tape-recorded questions and hand-scoring keys for 76 supplementary scales are also available.

Description

The MMPI-2 is a self-administered test consisting of 567 true/false questions, first published by Hathaway and McKinley in 1943, and revised by Hathaway et al. in 1989. The patient marks his or her answers on the standard answer sheet, which is then scored by overlay scoring keys or by computer entry for a variety of scales. The revision uses the same (slightly revised) validity and clinical scales and the critical item list of the original MMPI, but adds a second F-scale (Fb, backpage infrequency scale, using only the second half of the answer sheet to check on the possibility of a change in response attitude), two new validity scales (VRIN and TRIN, variable response inconsistency and true response inconsistency), and a new set of 15 content scales (107 items; see comment section). It eliminates 13 duplicate, nonworking, objectionable, or outmoded items, and rewords 14 percent of the items in more modern, simplified language, eliminating potential sexist wording and grammatical ambiguities (Graham, 1993). Three hundred and ninety-four items of the MMPI were left unchanged. A computerized scoring and reporting system (The Minnesota Report, Butcher et al., 1989) is available. Greene et al. (1990) and Marks et al. (1993a, 1993b) also offer a computerized interpretative system, and Greene (1992) offers an interpretative manual.

Numerous subscales and new scales have been developed for the original MMPI over the years; the MMPI Handbook (Dahlstrom et al., 1975) lists over 550 scales, including some with neuropsychological content. For the new content scales, two separate profiles are available in addition to the traditional profile sheet. A number of the additional scales (e.g., ASP antisocial practices, Type-A personality) have been adopted for the MMPI-2 with the assumption that the actual content of the test has not been changed.

The MMPI-A (Butcher et al., 1992a, 1992b), designed for age 14–18, contains 478 items, mostly culled from the MMPI-2, but includes items written or rewritten for adolescent development or psychopathology. It retains all validity and clinical scales of the original MMPI and many of its subscales and additional scales. As on the MMPI-2, the F-scale has been broken down into two scales (F1, F2), one each for the first and the second half of the test to detect changes in test-taking attitude. The response inconsistency scales described for the MMPI-2 have also been added to the MMPI-A. In addition, a separate profile sheet is provided for content and supplementary scales: acting-out and antisocial attitudes (A-con, A-cyn), negative treatment indicator (A-trt), anxiety (A-anx), obsessiveness (A-obs), depression (A-dep), health concerns (A-hea), alienation (A-ain), bizarre mentation (A-biz), anger (A-ang), low self-esteem (A-lse), low aspirations (A-las), social discomfort (A-sod), family problems (A-fam), school problems (A-sch); supplementary scales include anxiety (A), repression (R), the revised McAndrew alcoholism scale (MAC-R), alcohol and drug problem acknowledgement (ACK), alcohol and drug problem proneness (PRO), and immaturity (IMM). Archer (1993) and Williams et al. (1992) provide guides to the MMPI-A for the assessment of adolescent psychopathology, and Butcher and Williams (1992) cover both the MMPI-2 and the MMPI-A in their book.

Administration

Instructions are printed on the front of the booklet. Briefly, the patient is instructed to read each statement and to decide whether it is true or false as applied to him/her. The patient is then asked to mark his/her answer on the answer sheet and is encouraged to answer all items. Reassurance may be given by stating that there are no right or wrong answers, and that the patient should answer each statement spontaneously and without lengthy deliberation. It is recommended that the test administrator check during the initial 45 items and, if necessary, later during the test, to determine whether the patient follows the item numbering correctly, since skipping items may invalidate the whole test. The test can also be given by personal computer with software available from the source. Allowing the client to complete the MMPI at home is not recommended because norms were generated under carefully controlled conditions, circumstances during test-taking that may affect validity cannot be observed, and responses may be influenced by others at home, and indeed someone else may have completed the instrument (Butcher & Pope, 1992).

For poor readers, tape-recorded versions are available. Generally, a grade 6 reading ability (grade 7 for the MMPI) is considered minimal (Butcher & Pope, 1992; Paolo, Ryand, & Smith, 1991; Ward & Ward, 1980).

For the MMPI-A, a grade 6 reading level is considered minimal.

Approximate Time for Administration

Approximately 40–90 minutes are required.

Scoring

The test comes complete with overlay scoring keys for the original four validity, 10 clinical, and 15 content scales. Additional scoring keys for various subscales and newly developed research and clinical scales can be obtained (see source; also, Psychological Assessment Resources Inc., P.O. Box 98, Odessa, FL 33556) or made up by the user. Each scale produces the sum of answers relevant to that scale. These raw scores can then be transferred to the standard profile sheet, which also provides corrections for some scales that are affected by a concealing attitude or by attempting to appear in a favorable light (K-Scale). Corrected scores can then be plotted on the profile sheet, which directly translates into T-scores. In addition, a "critical items" check is provided. High scores on the clinical scales are usually expressed in a one-, two-, or three-point "high-point-code" (Welsh code), listing scale elevations above a T-score of 65 (70 for the old MMPI). Users often also continue the Welsh code with the number of scales expressing lower elevations and scales that are 15 or more T-score points below the norm.

Considering the large number of scales, computer scoring is usually preferable; this is available on disk or through a PC-attached Scorbox from the source, using the examiner's personal computer (paid on a per-use basis), or by professional scoring services (see source).

Comment

The original MMPI with its T-score profile has set a standard for personality tests of this type, used by generations of clinicians, and has continued to remain the most widely used personality test (Piotrowski & Lubin, 1990) in the world, as documented by over 9,000 publications in 1977 (Graham, 1977) and 140 foreign-language adaptations. It has been criticized because of outdated and limited standardization, lack of regard for age effects, poor item selection and phrasing, redundancy and heterogeneity of scales, as well as overlap in item content. The group-contrast method used to develop the original scales has been especially criticized (Helmes & Reddon, 1993). While some reviewers consider the MMPI "suboptimal" and would prefer to use other personality tests, others agree that with adequate safeguards in interpretation, the test remains useful, particularly if the newer scales, not based on group contrasts, are used.

The MMPI-2 was published in 1989, and many clinicians have adopted it as more and more studies about its use have become available. The revisions of the original MMPI have been relatively minor (rewriting of 82 items for clarity and current language usage, deletion of duplicated or noncontributing items), and all validity and clinical scales have been reverently maintained (including the now rather obsolete Kraepelinian terminology, e.g., "hysteria"); it was obviously the intent of the developers of the MMPI-2 to make only very conservative, necessary revisions to the test in order to maintain the validity of published research as far as possible. Test manuals published for the MMPI-2 tend to take such transfer of validity of MMPI studies for granted, although this is not necessarily true (Duckworth, 1991); a more fundamental revi-

sion may have been more appropriate (Horvath, 1992). The restandardization, however, and the addition of the new content scales are welcome improvements. Profile differences for the MMPI between black and white subjects have been described by Lachar et al. (1986). The Spanish version has yet to be fully validated (Fantoni-Salvador & Rodgers, 1997).

It has been noted that the means for the clinical scales were 5–7 points higher than after restandardization. This is ascribed to differences of test administration: In the original sample for the MMPI, clients were allowed to omit items they were unsure of or felt did not apply to them; this resulted in an average of 30 omissions and lowered scale means. For the restandardization sample, omissions were discouraged (average: fewer than two omissions, Butcher & Pope, 1992).

Administration and interpretation of the MMPI-2 require considerable training and reasonable familiarity with the literature. Books for introduction and reference (e.g., Graham, 1993) have been published. For the user of the original MMPI, several books and updated norms are available (Dahlstrom et al., 1960, 1975; Colligan & Offord, 1992; Colligan et al., 1989; Lanyon, 1968; Graham, 1977; Greene, 1980; Gilberstadt & Duker, 1965). For computer interpretations, the warnings expressed in the section of this book on report writing (Chapter 4) apply.

Reliability varies from scale to scale, but test–retest reliability of the MMPI has been reported as ranging from .50 to .90 (Buros, 1978), depending on whether they are reflecting "mood" or more "characterological" content, and depending on the time elapsed between testing (Fekken & Holden, 1987; Hunsley et al., 1988). Retest reliability for the MMPI-2 scales after 7 days is reported as ranging from .51 for Pa to .92 for Si; internal consistency estimates range from .34 for Pa to .87 for Si (Hathaway et al., 1989). Test–retest reliability of the MMPI-A ranges from .55 to .84, internal consistency from .43 to .90. Internal consistency coefficients range from .34 (Pa in men) to .87 (Pt in women) (Butcher et al., 1989).

The likelihood that the single high-point code of the MMPI remains the same on retest after one week or more ranged from 44 to 90 percent in nine studies summarized by Graham et al. (1986). On the MMPI-2, two studies of high-point code stability after 1–2 days reported only between 50 and 63 percent agreement; the agreement of the two- or three-point codes on retest ranged from 20 to 90 percent (two-point), and from 23 to 28 percent (three-point) (Graham, 1993). However, if a discrepancy of at least five T-score points is used to define the code, two-point congruence increased to 93 percent for both men and women (Graham, 1993). The congruence of high-point and two-point codes between MMPI and MMPI-2 in psychiatric patients ranges from 60 to 93 percent, depending on the level of scale elevation.

Validity has been investigated in numerous studies and also varies from scale to scale. The original validation of the MMPI was based on the discrimination between various psychiatric groups and normal subjects in the Minnesota area. However, discriminant validity for individual scales cannot be assumed; Davies et al. (1987), for example, found that Scale 8 (Sc) did not show significant differences between psychotic and normal adolescents. Instead, the profile as a whole is usually considered for interpretation. Subscales and new scales were in part based on construct (factor-analytic) as well as criterion validity. Recent studies showed good discriminant validity for the MMPI-2 between DSM-III diagnosed schizophrenia, major depression, and paranoid disorders (Patrick, 1988) and DSM-III diagnosed personality disorders (Morey et al., 1988). Other extra-test correlates are listed by Graham (1993).

Rather than using the test for assigning diagnostic labels, most users interpret the high-point scales descriptively. DeMendonca and colleagues (1984) summarized the most commonly used descriptor terms* for the clinical scales:

*The full names of the scales are: (1) hypochondriasis, (2) depression, (3) hysteria, (4) psychopathic deviance, (5) male-female scale, (6) paranoia, (7) psychasthenia, (8) schizophrenia, (9) mania, (0) social introversion. The validity scales are: L, lie scale; K, correction scale; F, conformity. These terms are somewhat misleading and outdated—the scales are usually referred to only by number, abbreviation, or letter.

Scale 1 (Hs): Immature, self-centered, complaining, demanding.

Scale 2 (D): Pessimistic, withdrawn, slow, timid, shy.

Scale 3 (Hy): Immature, egotistical, suggestible, friendly.

Scale 4 (Pd): Rebellious, resentful, impulsive, energetic, irresponsible.

Scale 5 (MF, male): Fussy, idealistic, submissive, sensitive, effeminate.

Scale 5 (MF, female): Aggressive, dominant, masculine.

Scale 6 (Pa): Suspicious, hostile, rigid, distrustful.

Scale 7 (Pt): Worrying, anxious, dissatisfied, sensitive, rigid.

Scale 8 (Sc): Confused, imaginative, individualistic, impulsive, unconventional.

Scale 9 (Ma): Energetic, enthusiastic, active, sociable, impulsive.

Scale 0 (Si): Aloof, sensitive, inhibited, timid.

In addition, the author lists possible descriptors for high scores on the three validity scales as follows:

L-Scale: Conventional, rigid, self-controlled.

F-Scale: Restless, changeable, dissatisfied, opinionated.

K-Scale: Defensive, inhibited.

Subscales for the clinical scales have been in use for some time (Harris & Lingoes, 1955) and are also scored for the MMPI-2. For example, Scale 2 (Depression) is broken down into D1 (Subjective depression), D2 (Psychomotor retardation), D3 (Physical malfunctioning), D4 (Mental dullness), and D5 (Brooding).

Clinical scales 2, 3, 4, 6, 8, and 9 were broken down into "obvious" (items with clearly recognizable face validity) and "subtle" scales by Wiener (1948). These subscales are still scorable, although Graham (1993) does not recommend their use because they fail to discriminate subjects instructed to fake good from those instructed to fake bad; because nontest behavior has been shown to be best predicted by the obvious items of these scales; and because the standard validity scales of the MMPI are better in detecting a deviant response set. However, two scales (Social Desirability Scale, Wiggins, 1959; Superlative Scale, Butcher & Han, 1993) have been shown to have significant incremental validity over the L and K scales in detecting underreporting of symptoms (Baer et al., 1995).

New content scales replace the Wiggins content scales of the old MMPI and cover the following areas: anxiety (ANX), fears (FRS), obsessiveness (OBS), depression (DEP), health concerns (HEA), bizarre mentation (BIZ), anger (ANG), cynicism (CYN), antisocial practices (ASP), type A behavior (TPA), low self-esteem (LSE), social discomfort (SOD), family problems (FAM), work interference (WRK), and negative treatment indicators (TRT). These scales are thought to be homogenous in content, show little item overlap, and therefore are relatively easy to interpret. However, Jackson et al. (1997) argue that convergent and discriminant validity of the MMPI-2 content scales are seriously compromised by the presence of substantial general variance attributable to response style. The supplementary scales also appear to provide little new information when compared to the MMPI-2 basic scales, at least in a psychiatric population (Archer et al., 1997). Kohutek (1992) also provided item location, means, and standard deviations for the Wiggins content scales (Social Maladjustment, Depression, Feminine Interest, Poor Morale, Psychoticism, Organic Symptoms, Family Problems, Manifest Hostility, Phobias, Hypomania, Poor Health) on the MMPI-2, so that readers familiar with these scales can score them on the revised test. Recently, Harkness et al. (1995) presented five new personality scales for the MMPI-2 that are based on the PSY-5 construct model with a deductive process of item selection rather than group contrasts. The five constructs are Aggressiveness, Psychoticism, Constraint, Negative Emotionality/Neuroticism, and Positive Emotionality/Extraversion.

Another clinical use frequently recommended is an item-by-item check of 73 "Critical Items" developed by Koss and Butcher, and by Lachar and Wrobel (see manual and Graham, 1993), which require follow-up in subsequent interviews since they bear on serious symptoms, impulses, or experiences. A guide for the use of the MMPI, MMPI-2, and MMPI-A in forensic testimony is provided by Pope et al. (1993).

In clinical use, higher elevations on each of the scales and on scale combinations have shown validity for various forms of abnormal and pathological traits and as indicators for treatment (e.g., Scale 1 elevation: "Not very good candidates for psychotherapy and counseling"). We deal with these scales only briefly and focus on the use of the MMPI in neuropsychology. A full listing of all scales can be found in Graham (1993).

Neuropsychological Studies. Within the context of the neuropsychological examination, many clinicians avoid routine administration of the MMPI-2 because of its length and consequent demands on attention, concentration, and comprehension. A recent study by Mittenberg and colleagues (1996) suggests that because of accompanying deficits in these areas, neuropsychological patients with a loss of 20 or more IQ points below the estimated premorbid IQ or with IQs below 70 tend to produce invalid scores on the MMPI-2 independent of level of education and reading ability. Shorter measures can be used for the measurement of depression (e.g., Beck, GDI). The most frequent indications for the use of the MMPI are differential diagnostic considerations (e.g., between psychosis and organic disorder), the question of functional disorders accompanying or resulting from brain damage, personality alterations after brain damage, issues of motivation, and questions relating to the personality that may be relevant to the design of rehabilitation programs. Considerable research on these questions has been published. Unfortunately, neither the manual nor Graham (1993) provide coverage of this topic. Graham merely notes that 1-9 / 9-1 high-point codes are sometimes found in individuals with brain injury who have difficulty coping with their limitations, and that 2-9 /

9-2 codes are found in patients with brain injury who try to cope with their deficits through excessive activity or who have lost emotional control. A study by Alfano et al. (1992) with 102 patients with closed-head injury found general elevations of all scales of the MMPI except 0, with high-points of Scale 8 for males and 2 for females. In addition, Scales 1 and 3 showed frequent elevations, although no single high-point was characteristic for this patient group. Elevations on Scales 1 and 3 and on the Health Concerns contents scale of the MMPI-2 were found in patients with traumatic brain injury (TBI) and loss of consciousness (Kelland et al., 1995). Artzy (1995) found elevations for Scales 1, 2, 3, 7, and 8, and lower scores for Es and Do (reflecting lack of assertiveness) in both male and female clients referred for evaluation of possible head injury. Putnam et al. (1995) reported that in 426 valid MMPI-2 protocols, patients with moderate-to-severe head injury showed a high prevalence of single-point codes on Scales 8 and 9, whereas patients with mild head injury tended to show elevations on Scales 1, 2, and 3; they ascribed this to the ambiguity of the patient's injury and the intrusion of external influences, including litigation. Miller and Paniak (1995) found that high points for brain-injured subjects on the MMPI were similar to those on the MMPI-2, but that two-point codes agreed only moderately; they recommend caution in the interpretation of 2-point codes. A study by Goldstein and Primeau (1995) found that, in a multivariate analysis with TBI patients, elevations on Scale 1 and low scores on Scale 5 were predictors of poor resumption of employment after recovery, with a 91 percent correct classification rate (post-injury neuropsychological variables had a 92 percent correct classification rate).

In the earlier literature, Gass and Russell (1986) found that elevation of the MMPI depression scale did not affect performance on the WAIS Digit Span subtest or on the Wechsler Memory Scale, while brain damage did. Similarly, Query and Megran (1984) found that MMPI-defined depression only affected the first trial of the Rey Auditory-Verbal Learning Test, but not subsequent recall and

recognition. A recent study of Gass (1996) with 80 male psychiatric inpatients and 48 male patients with closed head injury confirmed that, in both samples, MMPI-2 measures of depression, anxiety, and psychotic thinking (Scales 2, 7, and 8) were related to poor attention span, but independent of list learning performance.

Diagnosis of "organicity," though attempted by some authors, is not a question that can or should be answered by the MMPI or the MMPI-2. For example, Hovey's (1964) five-item scale failed to discriminate between organic impairment, functional disorder, schizophrenics, alcoholics, and normal subjects (Chaney et al., 1977; Maier & Abidin, 1967; Watson, 1971; Weingold et al., 1965). The "pseudoneurologic scale" (Shaw & Matthews, 1965), designed to identify patients with neurological complaints not supported by neurological findings, also failed to show adequate discriminating power (Watson, 1971). Similarly, the P-O scale (Watson & Plemel, 1978) did not sufficiently discriminate between patients with functional and those with organic disorders (Golden et al., 1979). Limited support for the validity of the P-O scale and Russell's MMPI key (Russell, 1975) in differentiating brain-damaged and schizophrenic patients has been described (Carpenter & LeLieuvre, 1981; Horton & Wilson, 1981; Trifiletti, 1982).

Discrimination between anterior and posterior lesions has been attempted with the Parietal-Frontal (Pf) (Friedman, 1950) and the Caudality Scale (Williams, 1952), but a study by Reitan (1976) found inadequate support for this claim. More recently, however, Black and Black (1982) found qualified support for the "caudality" hypothesis of increased MMPI abnormality in posterior lesions if the study controls for cognitive, motor, and sensory defects. Moehle and Fitzhugh-Bell (1988) confirmed two earlier studies indicating that the MMPI is not sensitive to lateralization of lesion in brain-injured adults. Trenerry et al. (1996) found no MMPI-2 elevations specific to right ($n = 79$) or left ($n = 96$) temporal lobe seizure activity or to temporal lobectomy. However, Cullum and Bigler (1988) found somewhat higher D-scale scores in adults with lesions in the left hemisphere and in the posterior right hemisphere, and Gass and Russell (1987) found mild elevations of the MMPI D-scale in patients with right-hemisphere lesions, although no left-hemisphere control group was used in this study. In a subsequent study, Gass and Ansley (1994) confirmed that higher anxiety and distress (Pt-scale) is associated with sensorimotor difficulties in left-hemisphere, but not in right-hemisphere CVA patients. Verbal deficits were more strongly associated with limited social facility (Hy-scale) and greater openness in reporting emotional difficulties (F-scale). Such unsatisfactory findings led Lezak (1995) to the statement that "the MMPI was not constructed for neuropsychological assessment and may be inherently inappropriate for this purpose." However, we feel that the MMPI does contribute to the study of personality changes and deficits in neuropsychological populations and can be used with caution. Moreover, it is superior to other comprehensive inventories, e.g., the MCMI-II (Millon, 1987), which are computer-bound (and therefore less accessible to independent research) and primarily constructed for the purpose of psychiatric classification.

A feature of interest to neuropsychologists is the development of a scale for posttraumatic stress disorder (PTSD, PK-scale, Keane et al., 1984), which was retained in the MMPI-2. It has good internal consistency, and reliability and has mainly been validated in combat-related PTSD, but it may also be valid in cases of civilian trauma (Graham, 1993). A recent study of 108 survivors of POW camps (Sutker et al., 1995) found that the PK-scale (as well as weight loss during internment) highly correlated with the BDI ($r = .72$) as well as with a learning/memory factor extracted from neuropsychological tests. If given as a stand-alone version, the PK scale results are quite comparable to those obtained if the scale is embedded in the MMPI (Herman et al., 1996).

Forty-five items of the PK-scale overlap with another posttraumatic stress disorder scale (PS scale, 60 items) developed by Schlenger and Kulka (1989). Sloan et al. (1996) reported that both PK and PS were significantly related to symptoms of posttraumatic stress in participants of the Persian Gulf war without combat exposure. Shepard (1995) examined 50 adults referred for evaluation of possible head injury with both the MMPI-2 and Penn PTSD inventory. The PK and PS scale, were highly correlated (.94) with each other, and correlated moderately with the Penn PTSD scale (.63 and .67). PK and PS scales showed a modest relation with the WAIS-R PIQ ($r = .45$).

Neurocorrections. A frequent criticism of the use of the MMPI and MMPI-2, especially in forensic testimony, is that scale elevations may be caused by valid neurological damage or dysfunction and therefore should not be considered a reflection of a patient's emotional state. Meyerink et al. (1988) isolated MMPI items that are affected by the physical symptoms of multiple sclerosis and pointed out that the neurological disease process can artificially inflate four of the clinical scales (Scales 1, 2, 3, and 8). Alfano et al. (1990) suggested that 44 MMPI items be deleted when scoring the results in neurologically impaired clients. These items had been identified for neurological content by at least 12 out of 18 expert physicians. The resulting "neurocorrected MMPI-NC44" showed somewhat lower clinical and F-scales in neurological patients; the high point remained unchanged in 46 percent, but the two-point code remained the same in only 29 percent, suggesting that the full-length MMPI should be interpreted with caution when given to neurological patients. They also constructed four neurobehavioral factor-analytic scales for the MMPI, reflecting attention/concentration/memory, somatic complaints, emotionality, and behavioral disturbances (Alfano et al., 1991). A later paper (Alfano et al., 1993) suggests that only 14 items of the MMPI-2 need to be deleted in patients with closed-head injury. Gass and Russell (1991) developed a similar list of 42 items of the MMPI, based on endorsement frequencies of 58 patients with long-term effects of CHI. Later, working with the MMPI-2, Gass (1991, 1992a) developed a list of 22 items endorsed by patients with CHI. These items had been identified by the judgement of 3 board-certified neurologists. A cross-validation (Gass and Wald, 1997) based on 54 patients with recent mild head injury identified 15 items that were endorsed significantly more frequently compared to endorsement in the normal standardization sample or in a psychiatric group. They suggested that both the uncorrected and the neurocorrected scores be calculated and considered for interpretation, and proposed a correction for neurologic-related items proportionate to the ratio of endorsement of non-neurologic-related items on a given scale. In contrast, Dunn and Lees-Haley (1995) found that only 5 of the 15 items showed a significantly different response frequency in 59 CHI patients involved in litigation, as compared to 102 patients evaluated for physical injury other than head injury. The authors found that the effect of subtracting these 5 items on the scoring of the MMPI-scales was negligable, and, as a result, do not recommend a correction. Rayls et al. (1997) reported a higher endorsement of correction items only during the early period (1 to 15 days) after mild CHI, but not when tested an average of 7.7 months post-injury. Another list of 42 MMPI-2 items was compiled by Artzy (1995), based on response frequencies of 170 patients with CHI assessed during the process of litigation for compensation. The items and scales for the MMPI-2 listed in at least two of these studies are tabulated in Table 15–2. Seven items overlap in all four lists. The differences in items may be due to differences between population bases and in the method of defining them.

A recent study by Brulot et al. (in press) found that the CHI neurocorrection scales by

Table 15—2. Correction Table for Computing Adjusted MMPI-2 Raw Scores for Patients with Closed Head Injury

	Item No.			
Source	MMPI-2	MMPI	Scoring	MMPI/MMPI-2 Scales
*	31	32	T	2, 3, 4, 7, 8, 0
A, AR	38	41	T	2, 7, 8
A, AR	53	52	T	1
GH, GH2, AR*	101	114	T	1, 3
*	106	119	F	8, 9, 0
A, AR	146	158	T	2, 6
*	147	159	T	2, 7, 8
GH, A, AR*	149	161	T	1
A, AR	164	174	F	L, F
GH, GH2	165	178	F	2, 7, 8
A, AR	168	156	T	F, 8, 9
GH, GH2	170	182	T	2, 7, 8
GH, GH2, AR*	172	186	T	2, 7, 8
GH, GH2, AR*	175	189	T	1, 2, 3, 7
A, AR	177	187	F	5, 8
*	179	192	F	1, 3, 8
*	180	168	T	F, 8
*	247	273	T	1, 8
*	295	330	F	8
A, AR	299	335	T	8
GH, GH2, A	325	356	T	7, 8

Total: 21 items with at least 2 sources in agreement

Sources: A = Alfano, 1993, closed head injury only (22 items)

AR = Artzy, 1995, head injury with litigation (42 items)

GH = Gass, 1992b, chronic closed head injury (14 items)

GH2 = Gass, 1996, acute mild closed head injury (15 items)

* = three or all of 4 sources in agreement (11 items)

Table 15—3. Correction Table for Computing Adjusted MMPI-2
Raw Scores for Patients with Cerebrovascular Accidents

Item No.			
MMPI-2	MMPI	Scoring	Other MMPI/MMPI-2 Scales
10	9	F	1, 2, 3
31	32	T	2, 3, 4, 7, 8, 0
45	51	F	1, 2, 3
47	55	F	1, 3
53	52	T	1
106	119	F	8, 9, 0
141	153	F	1, 2, 3
147	159	T	2, 7, 8
148	160	F	2, 3
152	163	F	1, 3
164	174	F	L, F
168	156	T	F, 8, 9
172	186	T	2, 7, 8
173	188	F	1, 3
175	189	T	1, 2, 3, 7
177	187	F	5, 8
182	194	T	8, 9
224	243	F	1, 3
229	251	T	8, 9
247	273	T	1, 8
249	274	F	1, 3
Total: 21			

Sources: Gass, 1992a, 1995.

Alfana, Gass, and Artzy did not correlate with measures of loss of consciousness, length of posttraumatic amnesia, or a number of measures of neuropsychological deficit; instead, they correlated significantly with the depression content scale, suggesting that these scales measure emotional distress rather than neurological disturbance. Obviously, further research is needed to develop an appropriate neurocorrection.

Gass (1992b) also produced a list of 21 items frequently endorsed by patients with cerebrovascular accident (CVA) (Table 15–3). A cross-validation study (Gass, 1996a) showed that these items were endorsed significantly more frequently by CVA patients compared to the normal standardization sample. The CVA and the CHI lists overlap, but also contain unique items; this may be based on differences in symptomatology. However, age differences (mean for CHI 38.2, for CVA 62.4) may also contribute, since mild nonspecific physical complaints (e.g., "I have few or no pains" - F, "I have never felt better in my life than I do now" - F) may be more common in elderly subjects.

Exaggeration, Simulation, and Malingering. Simulation of psychopathology is mainly explored by "Infrequence of Response" scales (F, F(b)) based on the principle that items in different content areas which are only rarely answered in a positive direction, are unlikely to be scored more than a few times. For their interpretation, random responding, poor comprehension or poor reading must be excluded first.

Simulation of psychopathology is relatively easy to detect; however, many disturbed subjects can simulate normal profiles (Archer et al., 1987). Gillis et al. (1990) examined the "faking bad" response style in a community sample of 80 subjects, half of whom were instructed to answer untruthfully, and reported that they had a lot of problems faking in a convincing and believable manner. The cutting scores for the F-scale (raw score < 23) and for F-K (raw score < + 17) successfully discriminated between this group and a community outpatient sample (n = 33) referred to the Clark Institute of Psychiatry. Similar results were obtained by Austin (1992) and Rothke et al. (1994). Wetter et al. (1992) used 172 university students, some of whom were instructed to answer truthfully, to mark the answer sheet randomly, to malinger a moderate psychological disturbance, and to malinger a severe disturbance. Both random and malingered response sets produced significant elevations on the F- and Fb-scales, random responding led to significant elevations of VRIN as well as F; both F-K and Ds2 (Dissimulation scale) increased significantly as degree of simulated disturbance increased. A study of prison inmates instructed to malinger as compared to other inmates and psychiatric inpatients showed good discrimination between groups on all standard validity scales (Iverson et al., 1995). This is confirmed in another study with college students by Bagby et al. (1995); these authors found the F-scale superior in detecting faking bad, and the Obvious-Subtle index and the Fb- and L-scales equally effective in detecting faking good. Gallen and Berry (1996) found that random responding was optimally (with up to 98 percent accuracy) detected by a combination of the VRIN, F, and Fb scales (VRIN + [F - Fb]).

Arbisi and Ben-Porath (1995) noted that elevations of the validity scales occur fairly frequently in patients with psychopathology because such items can often be endorsed in the presence of severe pathology. The authors constructed a new F(p) scale,* which is based on items that are rarely endorsed by either healthy individuals or psychiatric patients. A follow-up study (Arbisi & Ben-Porath, 1997) confirmed that T-scores for patients with PTSD, major depression, substance abuse, and bipolar disorders were in the low 60s range, and showed a mean T-score of 70.2 in schizophrenics—in contrast to the F and F(b) scales which showed considerably higher elevations.

In comparison, studies of malingering of head injury have shown quite variable results. In a recent study (Lamb et al., 1994), detailed instructions were given to 179 undergraduate

students: One group was instructed to fake closed-head injury believably, based on a handout with the most common symptoms. One group also received information on typical questions contained in the validity scales. Compared to a group answering the MMPI-2 honestly, the experimental malingerers showed elevations of both clinical and validity scales; those with information about the validity scales showed lowered scores on clinical and validity scales. The authors concluded that "coaching may have an impact on the veracity of simulation on the MMPI-2." Cullum et al. (1991) compared two actual head-trauma groups, one of which appeared to have made good effort on neuropsychological tests and one which had not: The two groups were not distinguishable on the MMPI-2. However, Youngjohn et al. (1995) found that patients with functional complaints who were under litigation after concussion differed significantly from patients with documented brain damage on Scales 1 and 3, but not on the validity scales. Berry et al. (1995) found that the MMPI-2 overreporting scales distinguished well between nonclinical participants instructed to fake closed-head injury, and between compensation-seeking and noncompensation-seeking closed-head injury patients. In contrast, Smith and Frueh (1996) examined 145 U.S. veterans with PTSD and found that patients with an F-K > 13 ("apparent exaggeration") were not more likely to seek compensation. However, comorbidity, especially with affective disorders, was high in this group. Also, Wetter and Deitsch (1996) found that subjects instructed to fake PTSD or closed-head injury were able to do so consistently on retest. Greiffenstein et al. (1995) examined three groups referred to a forensic clinic: 53 post-concussion patients who had returned to full-time work and whose litigation involved only past medical bill payment, 68 patients who had sustained very mild head injury but were still pursuing continuing compensation claims ("probable malingerers"), and 56 medically stable patients with established traumatic head injury. Of the MMPI-2 scales, only the sum of obvious scales and Sc contributed to the discrimination of the malingering group. The authors recommend caution in the use of the MMPI-2 to detect malin-

---

*True: 66, 114, 162, 193, 216, 228, 252, 270, 282, 291, 294, 322, 323, 336, 371, 387, 478, 555
False: 51, 7, 90, 93, 102, 126, 192, 276, 501.
Raw scores of 11 or higher receive a T-score of 120; a score of 6 represents a T-score of 84 in men and 89 in women; a score of 2 corresponds to a T-score of 56 in men and 57 in women.

gering of head injury because most of the validity scales are designed to detect exaggeration or malingering of psychopathology other than head injury. It should be noted that almost all studies of the detection of malingering rely on group differences. Actual sensitivity and specificity data are rarely reported.

Two studies of malingerers (pseudo-PTSD patients) by Lees-Haley (1991, 1992) suggested that the Es (ego-strength) scale tends to be low, that F and F-K tend to be high, and that a newly developed Fake-Bad scale helps in correctly identifying malingerers.* The second study (Lees-Haley, 1992) found good sensitivity and specificity for the FBS. Millis et al. (1995) reported that the Fake-Bad scale was most successful in separating a group of suspected malingerers with mild head injury from a severe head-injury group. There is also some evidence (Slick et al. 1996) that FBS correlates with symptom validity tests such as the VSVT. Of note, the VSVT did not show a meaningful correlation with the F(p) scale.

In short, while the validity scales and various indices have been reasonably successful in detecting simulation and dissimulation of psychopathology on the MMPI-2, these measures have not always been adequate for the detection of malingered head injury. Clinicians still await the development of suitable scales and require, in addition, the use of more direct methods of symptom validity testing, described in Chapter 17 of this book.

Normative Data

The MMPI-2 has been restandardized for a randomly chosen sample of 2,600 adults between 18 and 90 years of age, which was representative of the 1980 U.S. census in terms of age, ethnic origin, sex, education, socioeconomic status, and geographical distribution. Uniform T-scores were prepared for all scales, but age-appropriate norms are not available. A study by Butcher et al. (1991) sug-

gests that differences between younger and older age groups are minimal and that, at least for men, age-related norms are not needed. Comparability with the original MMPI has been maintained as far as possible.

The norms for the MMPI-A are based on a random sample of 1,620 adolescents from eight U.S. states, providing a representative sampling along gender, socioeconomic, and ethnic distributions. A clinical sample of 713 adolescents was tested in the validation process.

The norms for the original MMPI are based on data collected from friends and relatives of patients at the University of Minnesota as well as high school graduates, workers employed in the U.S. work program in the late 1930s, and general medical patients in the early 1940s. No allowance for age or education corrections is made. Traditionally, clinicians have learned to modify their interpretation of the profile on the basis of books, publications, teaching, and experience. For example, elevated clinical scales are quite common in 20- to 25-year-old college students. Colligan et al. (1989) published new norms based on 1,408 usuable MMPIs collected in the 1980s from randomly selected households in Minnesota, Iowa, and Wisconsin. From these, 335 females and 305 males, age 18–99 years, were drawn to constitute a census-matched subsample. The authors published new norms broken down by sex and age groups (18–19, 20–29, 30–39, 40–49, 50–59, 60–69, 70+). In general, the new T-scores are two to seven points above the original means. In normal elderly subjects, increases in Hs, D, and L were noted. Previous studies had shown these elevations, but had also shown elevations in the K, Hy, and Sc scales (Lezak, 1987). Even larger changes were observed in a recent restandardization of the MMPI for teenagers (age 13–17) based on 691 girls and 624 boys (Archer, 1987; Colligan & Offord, 1989, 1992; Colligan et al., 1988). Norms for 15- and 18-year-olds were also recently published by Gottesman et al. (1987). While far from ideal because of the geographic and ethnic (predominantly white) restrictions, these norms are preferable and can and should be plotted by users of the MMPI. Colligan and Offord

---

*The scale contains the following items: True: 11, 18, 28, 30, 31, 39, 40, 44, 59, 111, 252, 274, 325, 339, 464, 469, 505, 506. False: 12, 41, 57, 58, 81, 110, 117, 152, 164, 176, 224, 227, 248, 249, 250, 255, 264, 284, 362, 373, 374, 419, 433, 496, 561.

(1987, 1988a, 1988b) also updated norms for Barron's Ego-Strength scale, McAndrew's Alcoholism scale, the A-scale (anxiety/maladjustment), the R-scale (repression/control), and the Wiggin Content Scales. Gapinski et al. (1987) provided updated norms for the Augmented Purdue Content Scales; these are 10 scales that represent direct item content in the following areas:

1. anxiety/tension
2. somatic complaints
3. cognitive/sensory deficits
4. paranoid ideation
5. sensorimotor disturbance
6. emotional lability
7. interpersonal conflicts
8. personal/social inadequacy
9. stereotypic feminine interests
10. brooding/distractibility.

They also updated norms for 30 direct-content subscales within the validity and clinical scales. Normative data for other scales and subscales often remain unreplicated and have not been updated.

References

Alfano, D.P., Finlayson, M.A.J., Stearns, G.M., & MacLennan, R.N. (1991). Dimensions of neurobehavioral dysfunction. *Neuropsychology, 5,* 35–41.

Alfano, D.P., Finlayson, M.A.J., Stearns, G.M., & Neilson, P.M. (1990). The MMPI and neurologic dysfunction: Profile configuration and analysis. *The Clinical Neuropsychologist, 4,* 69–79.

Alfano, D.P., Neilson, P.M., Paniak, C.E., & Finlayson, M.A.J. (1992). The MMPI and closed head injury. *The Clinical Neuropsychologist, 6,* 134–142.

Alfano, D.P., Paniak, C.E., & Finlayson, M.A.J. (1993). The neurocorrected MMPI for closed head injury. *Neuropsychiatry, Neuropsychology, and Behavioral Neurology, 6,* 111–116.

Arbisi, P.A., & Ben-Porath, Y.S. (1995). An MMPI-2 infrequent response scale for use with psychopathological populations: The infrequency-psychopathology scale, F(p). *Psychological Assessment, 7,* 424–431.

Arbisi, P.A., & Ben-Porath, Y.S. (1997). Characteristics of the MMPI-2 F(p) scale as a function of diagnosis in an inpatient sample of veterans. *Psychological Assessment, 9,* 102–105.

Archer, R.P. (1987). *Using the MMPI with Adolescents.* Hillsdale, N.J.: Lawrence Erlbaum.

Archer, R.P. (1993). *MMPI-A: Assessing Adolescent Psychopathology.* Hillsdale, NJ: Lawrence Erlbaum.

Archer, R.P., Elkins, D.E., Aiduk, R., & Griffin, R. (1997). The incremental validity of MMPI-2 supplementary scales. *Assessment, 4,* 193–205.

Archer, R.P., Gordon, R.A., & Kirchner, F.H. (1987). MMPI response-set characteristics among adolescents. *Journal of Personality Assessment, 51,* 506–516.

Artzy, G. (1995). Correction factors for the MMPI-2 in head injured men and women. Ph.D. dissertation. University of Victoria.

Austin, J.S. (1992). The detection of fake good and fake bad on the MMPI-2. *Educational and Psychological Measurement, 52,* 669–674.

Baer, R.A., Wetter, M.W., Nichols, D.S., Greene, R., & Berry, D.T.R. (1995). Sensitivity of MMPI-2 validity scales to underreporting of symptoms. *Psychological Assessment, 7,* 419–423.

Bagby, R.M., Buis, T., & Nicholson, R.A. (1995). Relative effectiveness of the standard validity scales in detecting fake-bad and fake-good responding: Replication and extension. *Psychological Assessment, 7,* 84–92.

Berry, D.T.R., Wetter, M.W., Baer, R.A., Youngjohn, J.R., Gass, C.S., Lamb, D.G., Franzen, M.D., MacInnes, W.D., & Buchholz, D. (1995). Overreporting of closed-head injury symptoms on the MMPI-2. *Psychological Assessment, 7,* 517–523.

Black, F.W., & Black, I.L. (1982). Anterior-posterior locus of lesion and personality: Support for the caudality hypothesis. *Journal of Clinical Psychology, 38,* 468–477.

Brulot, M.M., Strauss, E.H., & Spellacy, F.J. (in press). The validity of MMPI-2 correction factors for use with patients with suspected head injury. *The Clinical Neuropsychologist.*

Buros, O.K. (1978). *The Eighth Mental Measurement Yearbook.* Highland Park, NY: Gryphon Press.

Butcher, J.N., Aldwin, C.M., Levenson, M.R., & Ben-Porath, Y.S. (1991). Personality and aging: A study of the MMPI-2 among older men. *Psychology and Aging, 6,* 361–370.

Butcher, J.N., Dahlstrom, W.G., Graham, J.R., Tellegen, A.M., & Kaemmer, B. (1989). *MMPI-2, Minnesota Multiphasic Personality Inventory—2.* Manual for Administration and

Scoring. Minneapolis, MN: University of Minnesota Press.

Butcher, J.M., & Han, K. (1993). Development of an MMPI-2 scale to assess the presentation of self in a superlative manner: The S scale. Paper presented at the 28th symposium on recent developments in the use of the MMPI/MMPI-2/MMPI-A. St. Petersburg, FL.

Butcher, J.N., & Pope, K.S. (1992). The research base, psychometric properties, and clinical uses of the MMPI-2 and MMPI-A. *Canadian Psychology, 33,* 61–78.

Butcher, J.N., & Williams, C.L. (1992). *Essentials of MMPI-2 and MMPI-A Interpretation.* Minneapolis: University of Minnesota Press.

Butcher, J.N., Williams, C.L., Graham, J.R., Archer, R.P., Tellegan, A., Ben-Porath, Y.S., & Kaemmer, B. (1992a). *MMPI-A: Manual for Administration, Scoring, and Interpretation.* Minneapolis: University of Minnesota Press.

Butcher, J.N., & Williams, C.L. (1992b). *MMPI-A: User's Guide for the Minnesota Report: Adolescent Interpretative System.* Minneapolis: University of Minnesota Press.

Butcher, J.N., & Hostetler, K. (1990). Abbreviating MMPI administration: What can be learned from the MMPI for the MMPI-2? *Psychological Assessment: A Journal of Consulting and Clinical Psychology, 2,* 12–21.

Carpenter, C.B., & LeLieuvre, R.B. (1981). The effectiveness of three MMPI scoring keys in differentiating brain damaged women from schizophrenic women. *Clinical Neuropsychology, 3,* 18–20.

Chaney, E.F., Erickson, R.C., & O'Leary, M.R. (1977). Brain damage and five MMPI items with alcoholic patients. *Journal of Clinical Psychology, 33,* 307–308.

Colligan, R.C., Greene, R.L., Gapinski, M.P., Archer, R.P., & Lingoes, J.C. (1988). MMPI subscales and profile interpretation: Harris and Lingoes revisited. Symposium, 96th Annual APA Convention (mimeo).

Colligan, R.C., Osborne, D., Swenson, W.M., & Offord, K.P. (1989). *The MMPI: A Contemporary Normative Study of Adults* (2nd ed.). Odessa, FL: Psychological Assessment Resources.

Colligan, R.R., & Offord, K.P. (1987). Resilience reconsidered: Contemporary MMPI normative data for Barron's ego strength scale. *Journal of Clinical Psychology, 43,* 467–472.

Colligan, R.C., & Offord, K.P. (1988a). Changes in MMPI factor scores: Norms for the Welsh A and R dimensions from a contemporary sample. *Journal of Clinical Psychology, 44,* 142–148.

Colligan, R.C., & Offord, K.P. (1988b). Contemporary norms for the Wiggins Content Scales: A 45-year update. *Journal of Clinical Psychology, 44,* 23–32.

Colligan, R.C., & Offord, K.P. (1989). The aging MMPI: Contemporary norms for contemporary teenagers. *Mayo Clinic Proceedings, 64,* 3–27.

Colligan, R.C., & Offord, K.P. (1992). *The MMPI: A Contemporary Normative Study of Adolescents.* Norwood, N.J.: Ablex.

Cullum, C.M., & Bigler, E.D. (1988). Short-form MMPI findings in patients with predominantly lateralized cerebral dysfunction: Neuropsychological and computerized axial tomography-derived parameters. *Journal of Nervous and Mental Disease, 176,* 332–342.

Cullum, C.M., Heaton, R.K., & Grant, I. (1991). Psychogenic factors influencing neuropsychological performance: Somatoform disorders, factitious disorders, and malingering. In H.O. Doerr & A.S. Carlin (Eds.), *Forensic Neuropsychology: Legal and Scientific Bases.* New York: Guilford.

Dahlstrom, W.G., & Welsh, G.S. (1960, 1975). *An MMPI Handbook: A Guide to Use in Clinical Practice and Research.* Vol. 1, 2. Minneapolis, MN: University of Minnesota Press.

Davies, A., Lachar, D., & Gdowski, C. (1987). Assessment of PIC and MMPI scales in adolescent psychosis: A caution. *Adolescence, 22,* 571–577.

DeMendonca, M., Elliott, L., Goldstein, M., McNeill, J., Rodriguez, R., & Zelkind, I. (1984). An MMPI based behavior descriptor/personality trait list. *Journal of Personality Assessment, 48,* 483–485.

Duckworth, J.C. (1991). The Minnesota Multiphasic Personality Inventory—2: A review. *Journal of Counseling and Development, 69,* 564–567.

Dunn, J.T. & Lees-Haley, P.R. (1995). The MMPI-2 correction factor for closed-head-injury: A caveat for forensic cases. *Assessment, 2,* 47–51.

Fantoni-Salvador, P., & Rogers, R. (1997). Spanish version of the MMPI-2 and PAI: An investigation of concurrent validity with Hispanic patients. *Assessment, 4,* 29–39.

Fekken, G.C., & Holden, R.R. (1987). Assessing the person reliability of an individual MMPI protocol. *Journal of Personality Assessment, 51,* 123–132.

Friedman, S.H. (1950). Psychometric effects of frontal and parietal lobe damage. Unpublished Ph.D. dissertation. University of Minnesota.

Gallen, R.T., & Berry, D.T.R. (1996). Detection of random responding on MMPI-2 protocols. *Assessment, 3,* 171–178.

Gapinski, M.P., Colligan, R.C., & Offord, K.P.

(1987). A new look for the old MMPI scales: Contemporary norms for the augmented Purdue subscales. *Journal of Clinical Psychology, 43,* 669–682.

Gass, C.S. (1991). MMPI-2 interpretation and closed head injury: A correction factor. *Psychological Assessment, 3,* 27–31.

Gass, C.S. (1992). MMPI-2 interpretation of patients with cerebrovascular disease: A correction factor. *Archives of Clinical Neuropsychology, 7,* 17–27.

Gass, C.S. (1996a). MMPI-2 interpretation and stroke: Cross-validation of a correction factor. *Journal of Clinical Psychology, 52,* 1–4.

Gass, C.S. (1996b). MMPI-2 variables in attention and memory test performance. *Psychological Assessment, 8,* 135–138.

Gass, C.S., & Ansley, J. (1994). MMPI correlates of poststroke neurobehavioral deficits. *Archives of Clinical Neuropsychology, 9,* 461–469.

Gass, C.S., & Russell, E.W. (1986). Differential impact of brain damage and depression on memory test performance. *Journal of Consulting and Clinical Psychology, 54,* 261–263.

Gass, C.S., & Russell, E.W. (1987). MMPI correlates of performance intellectual deficits in patients with right hemisphere lesions. *Journal of Clinical Psychology, 43,* 484–489.

Gass, C.S., & Russell, E.W. (1991). MMPI profiles of closed head trauma patients: Impact of neurological complaints. *Journal of Clinical Psychology, 47,* 253–260.

Gass, C.S., & Wald, H.S. (1997). MMPI-2 interpretation and closed-head trauma: Cross-validation of a correction factor. *Archives of Clinical Neuropsychology, 12,* 199–205.

Gilberstadt, H., & Duker, J. (1965). *A Handbook for Clinical and Actuarial MMPI Interpretation.* Philadelphia: Saunders.

Gillis, J.R., Rogers, R., & Dickens, S.E. (1990). The detection of faking bad response style on the MMPI. *Canadian Journal of Behavioural Science, 22,* 408–416.

Golden, C.J., Sweet, J.J., & Osmon, D.C. (1979). The diagnosis of brain damage by the MMPI: A comprehensive evaluation. *Journal of Personality Assessment, 43,* 138–142.

Goldstein, D., & Primeau, M. (1995). Neuropsychological and personality predictors of employment after traumatic brain injury. *Journal of the International Neuropsychological Society, 1,* 370 (abstract).

Gottesman, I.I., Hanson, D.R., Kroeker, T.A., & Briggs, P.F. (1987). New MMPI normative data and power-transformed T-score tables for the Hathaway-Monachesi Minnesota cohort of 14,019 15-year-olds and 3,674 18-year-olds. In R.P. Archer (Ed.), *Using the MMPI with Adolescents,* pp. 241–297. Hillsdale, N.J.: Erlbaum.

Graham, J.R. (1977). *The MMPI: A Practical Guide.* New York: Oxford University Press.

Graham, J.R. (1993). *MMPI-2: Assessing Personality and Psychopathology* (2nd ed.). New York: Oxford University Press.

Graham, J.R., Smith, R.L., & Schwartz, G.F. (1986). Stability of MMPI configurations for psychiatric inpatients. *Journal of Consulting and Clinical Psychology, 54,* 375–380.

Grayson, H.M. (1951). *A Psychological Admissions Testing Program and Manual.* Los Angeles: Veterans' Administration Center, Neuropsychiatric Hospital.

Greene, R.L. (1980). *The MMPI: An Interpretive Manual.* New York: Grune & Stratton.

Greene, R.L. (1992). *The MMPI-2/MMPI: An Interpretative Manual.* Odessa, FL: Psychological Assessment Resources.

Greene, R.L. (1990). *MMPI-2 Adult Interpretive System.* Odessa, FL: Psychological Assessment Resources.

Greiffenstein, M.F., Gola, T., & Baker, W.J. (1995). MMPI-2 validity scales versus domain specific measures of detection of factitious traumatic brain injury. *The Clinical Neuropsychologist, 9,* 230–240.

Harkness, A.R., McNulty, J.L., & Ben-Porath, Y.S. (1995). The personality psychopathology five (PSY-5): Constructs and MMPI-2 scales. *Psychological Assessment, 7,* 104–114.

Harris, R., & Lingoes, J. (1955). Subscales for the Minnesota Multiphasic Personality Inventory. Mimeo. Langley Porter Clinic.

Hathaway, S.R., & McKinley, J.C. (1943). *Booklet for the Minnesota Multiphasic Personality Inventory.* New York: The Psychological Corporation.

Hathaway, S.R., McKinley, J.C., with Butcher, J.N., Dahlstrom, W.G., Graham, J.R., Tellegen, A., & Kaemmer, B. (1989). *Minnesota Multiphasic Personality Inventory 2: Manual for Administration and Scoring.* Minneapolis: University of Minnesota Press.

Helmes, E., & Reddon, J.R. (1993). A perspective on developments in assessing psychopathology: A critical review of the MMPI and MMPI-2. *Psychological Bulletin, 113,* 453–471.

Herman, D.S., Weathers, F.W., Litz, B.T., & Keane, T.M. (1996). Psychometric properties of the embedded and stand-alone versions of the MMPI-2 Keane PTSD scale. *Assessment, 3,* 437–442.

Horton, A.M., & Wilson, F.M. (1981). Cross-validation of the Psychiatric-Organic (P-O) special role of the MMPI. *Clinical Neuropsychology, 3,* 1–3.

Horvath, P. (1992). The MMPI-2 considered in the contexts of personality theory, external validity, and clinical utility. *Canadian Psychology, 33,* 79–83.

Hovey, H.B. (1964). Brain lesions and five MMPI items. *Journal of Consulting Psychology, 28,* 78–79.

Hunsley, J., Hanson, R.K., & Parker, K.C. (1988). A summary of the reliability and stability of MMPI scales. *Journal of Clinical Psychology, 44,* 44–46.

Iverson, G.L., Franzen, M.D., & Hammond, J.A. (1995). Examination of inmates' ability to malinger on the MMPI-2. *Psychological Assessment, 7,* 118–121.

Jackson, D.N., Fraboni, M., & Helmes, E. (1997). MMPI-2 content scales: How much content do they measure? *Assessment, 4,* 111–117.

Keane, T.M., Malloy, P.F., & Fairbank, J.A. (1984). Empirical development of an MMPI subscale for the assessment of combat related post-traumatic stress disorder. *Journal of Consulting and Clinical Psychology, 52,* 888–891.

Kelland, D.Z., Bennett, J.M., Mercer, W.N., Caroselli, J.S., & DelDotto, J.E. (1995). A comparison of MMPI-2 profiles in TBI and non-TBI patients. *Archives of Clinical Neuropsychology, 10,* 349 (abstract).

Kohutek, K.J. (1992). The location of items of the Wiggins Content Scales on the MMPI-2. *Journal of Clinical Psychology, 48,* 617–620.

Lachar, D., Dahlstrom, W.G., & Moreland, K.L. (1986). Patterns of item endorsement on the MMPI. In W.G. Dahlstrom, D. Lachar, L.A. Dahlstrom (Eds.), *MMPI Patterns of American Minorities,* pp. 179–189. Minneapolis: University of Minnesota Press.

Lamb, D.G., Berry, D.T.R., Wetter, M.W., & Baer, R.A. (1994). Effects of two types of information on malingering of closed head injury on the MMPI-2: An analog investigation. *Psychological Assessment, 6,* 8–13.

Lanyon, R.I. (1968). *A Handbook of MMPI Group Profiles.* Minneapolis: University of Minnesota Press.

Lees-Haley, P.R. (1991). Ego strength denial on the MMPI-2 as a clue to simulation of personal injury in vocational neuropsychological and emotional distress evaluations. *Perceptual and Motor Skills, 72,* 815–819.

Lees-Haley, P.R. (1992). Efficacy of the MMPI-2 validity scales and MCMI-II modifier scales for detection of spurious PTSD claims: F, F-K, Fake-Bad scale, ego strength, subtle-obvious subscales, Dis, and Deb. *Journal of Clinical Psychology, 48,* 681–689.

Lees-Haley, P.R., English, L.T., & Glenn, W.G. (1991). A Fake-Bad-Scale for personal injury claimants. *Psychological Reports, 68,* 203–210.

Lezak, M.D. (1987). Norms for growing older. *Developmental Neuropsychology, 3,* 1–12.

Lezak, M.D. (1995). *Neuropsychological Assessment* (3rd ed.). New York: Oxford University Press.

Maier, L.R., & Abidin, R.R. (1967). Validation attempt of Hovey's five-item MMPI index for central nervous system disorder. *Journal of Consulting Psychology, 31,* 542.

Marks, P.A., Lewak, R.W., & Nelson, G.E. (1993a). *The Marks MMPI and MMPI-2 Adult Clinical Report.* Los Angeles, CA: Western Psychological Services.

Marks, P.A., Lewak, R.W., & Nelson, G.E. (1993b). *The Marks MMPI and MMPI-2 Adult Feedback and Treatment Report.* Los Angeles, CA: Western Psychological Services.

Meyerink, L.H., Reitan, R.M., & Selz, M. (1988). The validity of the MMPI with multiple sclerosis patients. *Journal of Clinical Psychology, 44,* 764–769.

Miller, H.B., & Paniak, C.E. (1995). MMPI and MMPI-2 profile and code type congruence in a brain-injured sample. *Journal of Clinical and Experimental Neuropsychology, 17,* 58–64.

Millis, S.R., Putnam, S.H., & Adams, K.M. (1995). Neuropsychological malingering and the MMPI-2: Old and new indicators. Paper presented at the 30th Annual Symposium on the use of the MMPI, MMPI-2, and MMPI-A. St. Petersburg, FL.

Millon, T. (1987). *Manual for the MCMI-II* (2nd ed.). Minneapolis, MN: National Computer Systems.

Mittenberg, W., Tremont, G., & Rayls, K.R. (1996). Impact of cognitive function on MMPI-2 validity in neurologically impaired patients. *Assessment, 3,* 157–163.

Moehle, K.A., & Fitzhugh-Bell, K.B. (1988). Laterality of brain damage and emotional disturbance in adults. *Archives of Clinical Neuropsychology, 3,* 137–144.

Morey, L.C., Blashfield, R.K., Webb, W.W., & Jewell, J. (1988). MMPI scales for DSM-III personality disorders: A preliminary validation study. *Journal of Clinical Psychology, 44,* 47–50.

Paolo, A.M., Ryan, J.J., & Smith, A.J. (1991). Reading difficulty of the MMPI-2 subscales. *Journal of Clinical Psychology, 47*, 529–533.

Patrick, J. (1988). Concordance of the MCMI and the MMPI in the diagnosis of three DSM-III Axis I disorders. *Journal of Clinical Psychology, 44*, 186–190.

Piotrowski, C., & Lubin, B. (1990). Assessment practices of health psychologists: Survey of APS division 38 clinicians. *Professional Psychology: Research and Practice, 21*, 99–106.

Pope, K.S., Butcher, J.N., & Seelen, J. (1993). *The MMPI, MMPI-2, and MMPI-A in Court: A Practical Guide for Expert Witnesses and Attorneys.* Washington, D.C.: American Psychological Association.

Putnam, S.H., Kurtz, J.E., Millis, S.R., & Adams, K.M. (1995). Prevalence and correlates of MMPI-2 codetypes in patients with traumatic brain injury. Unpublished manuscript.

Query, W.T., & Megran, J. (1984). Influence of depression and alcoholism on learning, recall, and recognition. *Journal of Clinical Psychology, 40*, 1097–1100.

Rayls, K., Mittenberg, W.B., Williams, J. & Theroux, S. (1997). Longitudinal analysis of the MMPI-2 neurocorrection factor in mild head trauma.

Reitan, R.M. (1976). Neurological and physiological basis of psychopathology. *Annual Review of Psychology, 27*, 189–216.

Rothke, S.E., Friedman, A.F., Dahlstrom, W.G., Greene, R.L., Arredondo, R., & Mann, A.W. (1994). MMPI-2 normative data for the F-K index: Implications for clinical, neuropsychological, and forensic practice. *Assessment, 1*, 1–15.

Russell, E.W. (1975). Validation of a brain-damage vs. schizophrenia MMPI key. *Journal of Clinical Psychology, 31*, 659–661.

Schlenger, W.E., & Kulka, R.A. (1989). *PTSD scale development for the MMPI-2.* Research Triangle Park, NC: Research Triangle Institute.

Shaw, D.J., & Matthews, C.G. (1965). Differential MMPI performance of brain-damaged vs. pseudo-neurologic groups. *Journal of Clinical Psychology, 21*, 405–408.

Shepard, J. (1995). *Posttraumatic Stress Disorder and Head Injury.* MA Thesis, University of Victoria.

Slick, D.J., Hopp, G., Strauss, E., & Spellacy, F.J. (1996). Victoria Symptom Validity Test: Efficiency for detecting feigned memory impairment and relationship to neuropsychological tests and MMPI-2 validity scales. *Journal of Clinical and Experimental Neuropsychology, 18*, 911–922.

Sloan, P., Arsenault, L., Hilsenroth, M., & Harvill, L. (1996). Assessment of noncombat, war-related posttraumatic stress symptomatology: Validity of the PK, PS, and IES scales. *Assessment, 3*, 37–41.

Smith, D.W., & Frueh, B.C. (1996). Compensation seeking, comorbidity, and apparent exaggeration of PTSD symptoms among Vietnam combat veterans. *Psychological Assessment, 8*, 3–6.

Sutker, P.B., Vasterling, J.J., Brailey, K., & Allain, A.N. (1995). Memory, attention, and executive deficits in POW survivors: Contributing biological and psychological factors. *Neuropsychology, 9*, 118–125.

Trenerry, M.R., Hermann, B.P., Barr, W.B., Chelune, G.J., Loring, D.W., Perrine, K., Strauss, E., & Westerveld, M. (1996). MMPI scale elevations before and after right and left temporal lobectomy. *Assessment, 3*, 307–315.

Trifiletti, R.J. (1982). Differentiating brain damage from schizophrenia: A further test of Russell's MMPI key. *Journal of Clinical Psychology, 38*, 39–44.

Ward, L.C., & Ward, J.W. (1980). MMPI readability reconsidered. *Journal of Personality Assessment, 44*, 387–389.

Watson, C.G. (1971). An MMPI scale to separate brain-damaged from schizophrenics. *Journal of Consulting and Clinical Psychology, 36*, 121–125.

Watson, C.G., & Plemel, D. (1978). An MMPI scale to separate brain-damaged from functional psychiatric patients in neuropsychiatric settings. *Journal of Consulting and Clinical Psychology, 36*, 121–125.

Weingold, H.P., Dawson, J.G., & Kael, H.C. (1965). Further examination of Hovey's "index" of identification of brain lesions: Validation study. *Psychological Reports, 16*, 1098.

Wetter, M.W., Baer, R.A., Berry, D.T.R., Smith, G.T., & Larsen, L.H. (1992). Sensitivity of the MMPI-2 validity scales to random responding and malingering. *Psychological Assessment, 4*, 369–374.

Wetter, M.W., & Deitsch, S.E. (1996). Faking specific disorders and response consistency on the MMPI-2. *Psychological Assessment, 8*, 39–47.

Wiener, D.N. (1948). Subtle and obvious keys for the MMPI. *Journal of Consulting Psychology, 12*, 164–170.

Wiggins, J.S. (1959). Interrelationship among MMPI measures of dissimulation under standard and social desirability instructions. *Journal of Consulting Psychology, 23*, 419–427.

Williams, C.L., Butcher, J.N., Ben-Porath, Y.S., &

Graham, J.R. (1992). *MMPI-A Content Scales: Assessing Psychopathology in Adolescents.* Minneapolis: University of Minnesota Press.

Williams, H.L. (1952). The development of a caudality scale for the MMPI. *Journal of Clinical Psychology, 8,* 293–297.

Youngjohn, J.R., Burrows, L., & Erdal, K. (1995). Brain damage or compensation neurosis? The controversial post-concussion syndrome. *Clinical Neuropsychologist, 9,* 112–123.

NEUROPSYCHOLOGY BEHAVIOR AND AFFECT PROFILE (NBAP)

Purpose

The purpose of this test is to assess personality and emotional changes frequently encountered after brain damage through self- or other-related questionnaires.

Source

Forms S (self-rating) and O (rating by others) are available in a "sampler" (including manual and scoring instructions) from Mind Garden, P.O. Box 60669, Palo Alto, CA 94306, for $25 US. "Permission" to reproduce 200 copies of the NBAP with the sampler in an "easy to reproduce format" costs $90 US. A Canadian source is not available.

Description

The NBAP, developed by Nelson et al. (1994), consists of 106 statements phrased either directly (Form S; e.g., "I have periods of over-exuberance") or in the third-person format (Form O; e.g., "The patient has periods of over-exuberance") that should be marked "agree" or "disagree." The test assesses five scales relevant to neuropsychological complaints: Indifference (anosognosia and denial of illness; "a tendency to minimize disability or current condition, an indifference to or denial of an illness"), Mania (impulsivity, irritability, euphoria; "elevated, expansive, or irritable mood, sustained high energy, and high levels of activity"), Depression (apathy, withdrawal, crying behavior, and profound sadness; "dysphoric mood and/or loss of interest or pleasure in most usual activities"), Inappropriateness (unusual or bizarre behavior; "behavior that is inappropriate to the context in which it is occurring or to an outside event"), and Prognosia (defect in the pragmatics of communicative style). Four validity scales ("Atypical Post-Injury Symptom Scale", "Infrequency", "Contradictory Responses", "Complementary Responses") have been added recently (Satz et al., 1996). A special feature of the NBAP is that it is given in the "before" (onset of symptoms) and "after" condition by phrasing it in the past or present tense.

Administration

For Form O, the closest relative or caregiver is asked to fill in the questionnaire by marking either A (agree) or D (disagree) on the answer form. Form S is administered to the patient directly if he or she has adequate reading and comprehension. The "before" form is given together with the "after" form on different sides of the page.

Approximate Time for Administration

Approximately 20–30 minutes are required.

Scoring

Scoring keys for each of the five scales are used, and the sum of A (agree) responses is counted for each scale on the "before" and "after" responses. The appendix allows both percentile-rank and T-score conversions of the raw scores.

Comment

Eighty-one test items were selected from a large item pool to represent the five categories of behavior and affect. Fifteen neutral items were created to break the tendency of a yes-response pattern. Forced sorting into the categories by six judges showed that only 66 of the 81 items showed 80 percent interjudge agreement (Nelson et al., 1989). Internal consistency for the 66-item set for "before" ratings for 39 outpatients of a dementia clinic ranged from .78 for Depression to .49 for Prognosis; for "now" responses from .82 for Indifference to .68 for Inappropriateness. Inclusion of the 25 items that did not meet the sorting criteria improved internal consistency minimally. Internal consistency in 70 stroke patients ranged from .82 for Indifference to .70 for Pragnosia for the "before" set of 66 items, and from .82 to .77 for the "now" set; this increased slightly when the full 91-item set was used (Nelson, 1993). Test–retest reliability (after one month) ranged from .92 to .97 for "now" and from .97 to .99 for "before" responses. Four items did not meet an item-consistency criterion of greater than 75 percent.

Discriminant validity between a dementia group and a group of 88 healthy volunteers from a retirement center showed, as expected, nonsignificant differences for the "before" responses, and significant differences for the "after" (retirement) responses for all but the Mania scale. A comparison of the patient group divided into mild and moderate-to-severe impairment (based on the MMSE) showed no significant differences except for Inappropriateness (Nelson et al., 1989). A cross-validation with 70 stroke patients (2 weeks post-stroke) compared to the same control group showed significant differences on three scales, but not on Mania and Inappropriateness (Nelson et al., 1993). A study of 19 patients 2 weeks, 2 months, and 6 months after stroke (Nelson et al., 1994) found increased Indifference, Inappropriateness, and Depression, which decreased over time, suggesting a slow rate of recovery after left-hemisphere stroke; in contrast, a worsening of emotional functioning in right-hemisphere stroke patients at the 6-month follow-up was observed. The authors noted that right-hemisphere stroke patients tend to deny emotional factors and are thus less motivated to engage in treatment.

A comparison of 23 closed-head injury survivors with their siblings (Drebing et al., in press) showed no significant differences for the "before" responses, and significant differences for the "after" responses for all scales except Mania. The same study compared a matched control group with the closed-head injury group: again, all scales except Mania were significantly elevated in the closed-head injury group. It was noted, however, that relatives tended to rate their closed-head injury family member more positively for the "before" set than did controls—an indication of a possible tendency to view the time before the injury in more positive terms.

The new validity scales showed promising discriminative validity between groups with mild and with moderate head trauma and all three groups (licensed clinical psychologists with low training, medium training or high training in the neuropsychology of head trauma) of subjects instructed to fake mild head trauma, although the clinical scales also contributed to the discrimination (Satz et al., 1996).

This is one of the few personality/affect inventories developed specifically for neurological patients and evaluates five domains of personality change of interest to neuropsychologists. So far, all studies of the NBAP have come from the test authors. Four of the five scales have shown differences expected for brain-damaged populations. Validating evidence for the Mania scale may be found if specific populations (e.g., frontal lobe lesions) are studied.

Normative Data

No general norms are yet available, but the manual provides data on the control groups used in validation studies. These consist of 88 well-off elderly retirees (mean age = 70 years), 37 siblings of closed-head injury patients, and university students (age 16–60 years) rating their relatives. "Before" and "after" ratings for the older control group refer to before and after retirement, assumed to be a major life stress. Controls who have undergone severe life stress, who are socioeconomically representative for the population at large, and who provide sufficient coverage of the age ranges have yet to be investigated. Normative data are also provided in the manual for post-stroke and dementia patients.

References

Drebing, C., Dyer-Kline, A., Satz, P., Mitrushina, M., van Gorp, W.G., Holston, S., Foster, J., Nelson, L.D., Forney, D., & Cannon, B. (in press). Personality change in head trauma: A validity study of the Neuropsychology Behavior and Affect Profile.

Nelson, L.D., Cicchetti, D., Satz, P., Sowa, M., & Mitrushina, M. (1994). Emotional sequelae of stroke: A longitudinal perspective. *Journal of Clinical and Experimental Neuropsychology, 16,* 796–806.

Nelson, L.D., Mitrushina, M., Satz, P., Sowa, M., & Cohen, S. (1993). Cross-validation of the Neuropsychology Behavior and Affect Profile in stroke patients. *Psychological Assessment, 5,* 374–376.

Nelson, L., Satz, P., & D'Elia, L.F. (1994). *Neuropsychology Behavior and Affect Profile.* Palo Alto, CA: Mind Garden.

Nelson, L.D., Satz, P., Mitrushina, M., van Gorp, W., Cicchetti, D., Lewis, R., & van Lancker, D. (1989). Development and validation of the Neuropsychology Behavior and Affect Profile. *Psychological Assessment, 1,* 266–272.

Satz, P., Holston, S.G., Uchiyama, C.L., Shimahara, G., Mitrushina, M., et al. (1996). Development and evaluation of validity scales for the Neuropsychology Behavior and Affect Profile: A dissembling study. *Psychological Assessment, 8,* 115–124.

NEUROBEHAVIORAL RATING SCALE (NRS)

Purpose

The purpose of this scale is to assess behavioral sequelae of head injury.

Source

No commercial source exists for this scale. It is reproduced here with the permission of the authors (Levin et al., 1987, 1990).

Description

This scale was developed from the Brief Psychiatric Rating Scale (Overall & Gorham, 1962) to focus more specifically on behavioral sequelae of brain damage rather than on general psychiatric disorders. It is specifically designed for patients who are unable to complete valid self-report scales (e.g., the MMPI). A clinician or other interviewer familiar with the patient fills in seven-point ratings on 27 items as shown in Figure 15–3. The scale is also available in Spanish (Pelegrin Valero, Martin Carrasco, and Tirapu Usteroz, 1995). The somewhat similar Portland Adaptability Inventory is reproduced and described in Lezak (1995).

Administration

Prior to filling in the rating scale, the authors recommend the use of a brief structured interview, including a brief test of orientation and memory for recent events, a review of postconcussional symptoms and emotional state, questions pertaining to proverbs, focused attention and information processing (serial 7s), attitude towards hospital staff (irritability, hostility, misinterpretation of actions of others, suspiciousness), capacity for self-insight and long-range planning, and delayed recall of three objects presented at the beginning of the interview. The examiner also records observations during the examination pertaining to the patient's alertness, distractibility, intrusions of irrelevant material, coherence of conversation, physical signs and verbal expressions of anxiety, visible signs of tension, disinhibitory behavior or agitation, disturbances of mood, motor behavior, and expressive/receptive language. Stamina and apparent effort on mental status tasks are also rated.

Scoring

As mentioned, items are scored on a seven-point scale ("not present" to "extremely severe"), and a total NRS score (Maximum = 189) can be calculated. The items appear in random order on the scale list, but they can be meaningfully grouped by area (factor scores, see below) for profiling as follows:

Factor 1, Cognition/energy: 3, 6, 7, 10, 17, 19, 21.

Directions: Place an x in the appropriate box to represent level of severity of each symptom.

	not present	very mild	mild	moderate	moderately severe	severe	extremely severe
1. Inattention/Reduced Alertness—fails to sustain attention, easily distracted, fails to notice aspects of environment, difficulty directing attention, decreased alertness.	☐	☐	☐	☐	☐	☐	☐
2. Somatic Concerns—volunteers complaints or elaborates about somatic symptoms (e.g., headaches, dizziness, blurred vision) and about physical health in general.	☐	☐	☐	☐	☐	☐	☐
3. Disorientation—confusion or lack of proper association for person, place, or time.	☐	☐	☐	☐	☐	☐	☐
4. Anxiety—worry, fear, overconcern for present or future.	☐	☐	☐	☐	☐	☐	☐
5. Expressive Deficit—word-finding disturbance, anomia, pauses in speech, effortful and agrammatic speech, circumlocution.	☐	☐	☐	☐	☐	☐	☐
6. Emotional Withdrawal—lack of spontaneous interaction, isolation, deficiency in relating to others.	☐	☐	☐	☐	☐	☐	☐
7. Conceptual Disorganization—thought processes confused, disconnected, disorganized, disrupted; tangential social communication; perseverative.	☐	☐	☐	☐	☐	☐	☐
8. Disinhibition—socially inappropriate comments and/or actions, including aggressive/sexual content, or inappropriate to the situation, outbursts of temper.	☐	☐	☐	☐	☐	☐	☐
9. Guilt Feelings—self-blame, shame, remorse for past behavior.	☐	☐	☐	☐	☐	☐	☐
10. Memory Deficit—difficulty learning new information, rapidly forgets recent events, although immediate recall (forward digit span) may be intact.	☐	☐	☐	☐	☐	☐	☐
11. Agitation—motor manifestations of overactivation (e.g., kicking, arm flailing, picking, roaming, restlessness, talkativeness).	☐	☐	☐	☐	☐	☐	☐
12. Inaccurate Insight and Self-Appraisal—poor insight, exaggerated self-opinion, overrates level of ability and underrates personality change in comparison with evaluation by clinicians and family.	☐	☐	☐	☐	☐	☐	☐
13. Depressive Mood—sorrow, sadness, despondency, pessimism.	☐	☐	☐	☐	☐	☐	☐
14. Hostility/Uncooperativeness—animosity, irritability, belligerence, disdain for others, defiance of authority.	☐	☐	☐	☐	☐	☐	☐
15. Decreased Initiative/Motivation—lacks normal initiative in work or leisure, fails to persist in tasks, is reluctant to accept new challenges.	☐	☐	☐	☐	☐	☐	☐
16. Suspiciousness—mistrust, belief that others harbor malicious or discriminatory intent.	☐	☐	☐	☐	☐	☐	☐
17. Fatigability—rapidly fatigues on challenging cognitive tasks or complex activities, lethargic.	☐	☐	☐	☐	☐	☐	☐
18. Hallucinatory Behavior—perceptions without normal external stimulus correspondence.	☐	☐	☐	☐	☐	☐	☐
19. Motor Retardation—slowed movements or speech (excluding primary weaknesses).	☐	☐	☐	☐	☐	☐	☐
20. Unusual Thought Content—unusual, odd, strange, bizarre thought content.	☐	☐	☐	☐	☐	☐	☐
21. Blunted Affect—reduced emotional tone, reduction in normal intensity of feeling, flatness.	☐	☐	☐	☐	☐	☐	☐
22. Excitement—heightened emotional tone, increased reactivity.	☐	☐	☐	☐	☐	☐	☐
23. Poor Planning—unrealistic goals, poorly formulated plans for the future, disregards prerequisites (e.g., training), fails to take disability into account.	☐	☐	☐	☐	☐	☐	☐
24. Lability of Mood—sudden change in mood which is disproportionate to the situation.	☐	☐	☐	☐	☐	☐	☐
25. Tension—postural and facial expression of heightened tension, without the necessity of excessive activity involving the limbs or trunk.	☐	☐	☐	☐	☐	☐	☐
26. Comprehension Deficit—difficulty in understanding oral instructions on single or multistage commands.	☐	☐	☐	☐	☐	☐	☐
27. Speech Articulation Defect—misarticulation, slurring or substitutions of sounds which affect intelligibility (rating is independent of linguistic content).	☐	☐	☐	☐	☐	☐	☐

Figure 15—3. Neurobehavioral Rating Scale (Levin et al., 1987). Reproduced with permission of Dr. H. Levin and the BMJ Publishing Group. All rights reserved.

Factor 2, Metacognition: 8, 11, 12, 20, 22, 23.

Factor 3, Somatic/anxiety: 2, 4, 13, 14, 16, 25.

Factor 4, Language: 5, 26.

Items not appearing on factors: 1, 9, 15, 18, 24, 27.

Comment

Interrater reliability for the total NRS score for 101 patients was reported as .90 and .88 between two pairs of raters (Levin et al., 1987). Disagreement between one pair of raters by one category of disability was 6.4 percent on average, and disagreement by two categories was 2.7 percent; for the second pair only 3.9 percent disagreement by one category was found. A replication study on 44 head-injured patients (Corrigan et al., 1990) produced an interrater reliability of .78; a week later, readministration of the scale resulted in an interrater reliability of .76. Reliability in patients with dementia was .93, and correlations for individual factors were also satisfactory (Sultzer et al., 1995). Corrigan et al. also found internal consistency satisfactory (Cronbach's alpha = .88–.90). Investigating reliability of individual scales for a French version, Levin et al. (1990) found coefficients ranging from .23 to .95. Reliabilities for items 2, 4, 6, and 17 were not significant. Reliability would seem heavily dependent on the availability of all information described by the authors.

A principal component analysis resulted in four major factors: (1) cognition/energy, (2) metacognition (insight, planning, disinhibition), (3) somatic concern/anxiety, and (4) language (Levin et al., 1987). Inattention loaded on both Factors 1 and 2, and decreased initiative on Factors 1 and 3.

Groups of patients with mild, moderate, and severe head injury (based on Glasgow Coma Scale ratings) differed significantly from one another on Factor scores 1, 2, and 4, but not on Factor 3. Severity of head injury also showed significant differences on individual ratings, except those for Factor 3. Further validity studies were conducted by comparing the NRS during acute hospitalization with those obtained one month or more later during rehabilitation; significant differences were found (Levin et al., 1987). The comparison of matched nonfrontal and frontal groups of patients showed a nonsignificant trend for more abnormal scores on Factors 1, 2, and 3 for frontal lobe injuries; however, the difference score between Factor 1 and Factor 2 (cognition/energy minus metacognition) was significantly greater in the nonfrontal group, suggesting a different pattern of impairment. A study of 37 survivors of severe head trauma in the home setting after an average of 2.5 years used ratings based on observation and interviews of both patients and relatives (Douglas, 1994); memory, disinhibition, and increased fatiguability formed the most severely impaired deficit triad. Vilkki et al. (1994) found that psychosocial outcome one year after closed-head injury was best predicted by the cognition/energy factor of the NRS, administered 4 months after the injury.

Patients with Alzheimer's disease showed a somewhat different factor structure: cognition/insight, agitation/disinhibition, behavioral retardation, anxiety/depression, verbal output disturbance, and psychosis (Sultzer et al., 1992). Sultzer et al. (1993) found patients with vascular dementia more impaired and depressed on the NRS than patients with Alzheimer's disease.

The validity of scales of this type can also be inferred from other studies. High scores on the Brief Psychiatric Rating Scale (on which this scale was based), for example, have been found to be related to computed tomography and EEG abnormalities in head-injured patients (Levin & Grossman, 1978). The similarly constructed Blessed Dementia Scale (Blessed et al., 1968) was found to be moderately (.64) correlated with counts of senile plaques in the brains of demented patients (Blessed et al., 1968). The NRS was recommended for behavioral outcome assessment by Clifton et al. (1992).

Normative Data

Norms are not applicable, because in normal, healthy subjects none of the scales are expected to be elevated except for minor elevations in the somatic-anxiety factor area. The clinician using this scale can interpret elevations on individual items or on subscales (factors). The authors note that women with head injury score slightly higher for depression, but that on all other scales sex differences are minimal.

References

Blessed, G., Tomlinson, B.E., & Roth, M. (1968). The association between quantitative measures of dementia and of senile changes in the cerebral grey matter of elderly subjects. *British Journal of Psychiatry, 114*, 797–811.

Clifton, G.L., Hayes, R. L., Levin, H.S., Michel, M.E., & Choi, S.C. (1992). Outcome measures for clinical trials involving traumatically brain-injured patients: Report of a conference. *Neurosurgery, 31*, 975–978.

Corrigan, J.D., Dickerson, J., Fisher, E., & Meyer, P. (1990). The Neurobehavioral Rating Scale: Replication in an acute, inpatient rehabilitation setting. *Brain Injury, 4*, 215–222.

Douglas, M.J. (1994). Indicators of long-term family functioning following severe traumatic brain injury in adults. Ph.D. dissertation: University of Victoria.

Levin, H.S. (1990). Predicting the neurobehavioral sequelae of closed head injury. In R.I. Wood (Ed.), *Neurobehavioral Sequelae of Traumatic Head Injury.* Bristol, PA: Taylor & Francis.

Levin, H.S., High, W.M., Goethe, K.E., Sisson, R.A., Overall, J.E., Rhoades, H.M., Eisenberg, H.M., Kalisky, Z., & Gary, H.E. (1987). The neurobehavioral rating scale: Assessment of the behavioural sequelae of head injury by the clinician. *Journal of Neurology, Neurosurgery, and Psychiatry, 50*, 183–193.

Levin, H.S., & Grossman, R.G. (1978). Behavioral sequelae of closed head injury: A quantitative study. *Archives of Neurology, 35*, 720–727.

Levin, H.S., Mazaux, J.M., Vanier, M., Dartigues, J.F., Giriore, J.M., Davaret, P., Pilon, M., Hebert, D., Johnson, C., Fournier, G., & Barat, M. (1990). Evaluation des troubles neuropsychologiques et comportementaux des traumatises craniens par le clinicien: Proposition d'une echelle neurocomportementale et premier resultats de sa version francaise. *Annales de Readaptation et de Medicine physique, 33*, 35–40.

Lezak, M.D. (1995). *Neuropsychological Assessment* (3rd ed.). New York: Oxford University Press.

Overall, J.E., & Gorham, D.R. (1962). The Brief Psychiatric Rating Scale. *Psychological Reports, 10*, 799–812.

Pelegrin Valero, M., Martin Carrasco, M., & Tirapu Usterroz, J. (1995). La Escala NRS: La version espanola de la Neurobehavioral Rating Scale. *Anales de Psichiatria, 11*, 88–98.

Sultzer, D.L., Berisford, M.A., & Gunay, I. (1995). The Neurobehavioral Rating Scale: Reliability in patients with dementia. *Journal of Psychiatric Research, 29*, 185–191.

Sultzer, D.L., Levin, H.S., Mahler, M.E., & High, W.M. (1992). Assessment of cognitive, psychiatric, and behavioral disturbance in patients with dementia: The Neurobehavioral Rating Scale. *Journal of the American Geriatric Society, 40*, 549–555.

Sultzer, D.L., Levin, H.S., Mahler, M.E., & High, W.E. (1993). A comparison of psychiatric symptoms in vascular dementia and Alzheimer's disease. *American Journal of Psychiatry, 150*, 1806–1812.

Vilkki, J., Ahola, K., Holst, P., Ohman, J., Servo, A., & Heiskanen, O. (1994). Prediction of psychosocial recovery after head injury with cognitive tests and neurobehavioral ratings. *Journal of Clinical and Experimental Neuropsychology, 16*, 325–338.

PENN INVENTORY FOR POSTTRAUMATIC STRESS DISORDER (PTSD)

Purpose

The purpose of this test is to determine the presence of a posttraumatic stress disorder (PTSD) by means of a questionnaire.

Source

The inventory is available from Dr. Melvyn Hammarberg, Department of Anthropology, 325 Museum, University of Pennsylvania, Philadelphia, PA 19104-6398, for a one-time fee of $35.

Description

This is a 26-item self-report questionnaire (Hammarberg, 1992) modeled after the Beck Depression Scale. The items were chosen to represent all aspects of the DSM-IV definition of PTSD (experience of intense fear, helplessness, or horror). Each item allows four choices with increasing weight, for example:

0   I have not experienced a major trauma in my life.
1   I have experienced one or more traumas of limited intensity.
2   I have experienced very intense and upsetting traumas.
3   The traumas I have experienced were so intense that memories of them intrude on my mind without warning.

Another self-report measure of PTSD is the 17-item Purdue Posttraumatic Stress Disorder scale (PPTSD) revised recently by Lauterbach and Vrana (1996). For suitable subscales of the MMPI-2 refer to the description of the MMPI in this volume.

Administration

The subject is instructed to read each group of statements carefully and to circle the number beside the statement that applies to him or her during the past week, including today. The instrument is self-administered and can be given in group settings or (according to the author) by mail.

Approximate Time for Administration

Approximately 5–10 minutes are required for completion of the inventory.

Scoring

The points circled on the 26 items of the inventory are summed to obtain a total score. Maximum score = 78.

Comment

The current inventory was selected from an original pool of 80 items for clarity, sensitivity, and meaning (Hammarberg, 1989). A first study with 28 Vietnam veterans diagnosed by psychiatrists according to DSM-III standards and in treatment for PTSD, 24 post-treatment veterans, 15 veterans without PTSD, and 16 nonveterans without PTSD (mean age = 42 years for all groups) resulted in an internal consistency of .94. Test–retest reliability after a minimum of 2 and a mean of 5 days was .96. The item test–retest reliability ranged from .58 to .87. A replication study with 39, 26, 17, and 16 subjects respectively produced very similar results.

Group mean scores were 52.4 for veterans in treatment, 48.1 for post-treatment veterans, 16.9 for non-PTSD veterans, and 15.6 for non-PTSD civilians. Using a cutoff score of 35, the test provided a predictive power (sensitivity) of 94 percent in the first study, and of 97 percent in the replication study. Specificity is reported as 85 percent.

A third study (Hammarberg, 1992) compared 22 Vietnam veterans in treatment for PTSD, 18 veterans with general psychiatric admission but no PTSD, and 17 civilian subjects with PTSD who were survivors of the Piper oilrig explosion. Means for these groups were 57.1, 28.2, and 48.8, respectively. Three Piper explosion survivors without PTSD had a mean of 23.3. The predictive power in this study was 95 percent. An outcome study after 90-day inpatient treatment (Hammarberg & Silver, 1994) showed improvement on the Penn scale for 48 percent of their subjects, but a follow-up one year later indicated a return to pretreatment levels on the PTSD symptom measures employed.

Concurrent validity was demonstrated by a correlation of .40 with a combat exposure scale, and of .85 with the Mississippi PTSD scale (Keane et al., 1988). The test correlated positively with the Beck Depression Scale (.74), the Beck Anxiety Scale (.52), and state anxiety as measured with the Spielberger Trait-State Anxiety scale (.77).

A study by Shepard (1995) with 50 patients referred for evaluation of possible head injury found correlations of .5 to .6 between the Penn and the PK and PS scales of the MMPI-2. The test does show promise as a short scale for use with non-combat-related PTSD in neuropsychological practice. Although Sbordone & Liter (1995) argue that PTSD is rarely found in patients with mild traumatic head injury, Shepard reported that 58 percent of her sample scored above the clinical cut-off on the Penn Inventory.

Engdahl et al. (1996) compared the Mississippi PTSD scale, the MMPI-PK scale and the Impact-of-Events scale in 214 community-dwelling WWII veterans who had been prisoners of war and 114 veterans who were not. They found that all three scales showed good sensitivity (.6 to .78) and specificity (.82 to .93), but noted that "the simultaneous use of two or all three self-report instruments does not seem justified by our data" (p. 448).

Normative Data

Only the norms on small groups of male non-PTSD veterans and nonveterans by Hammarberg (1992) are available so far. They suggest an optimal cutoff point of 35 points. No significant differences due to race, religion, or education are reported.

References

Engdahl, B.E., Eberly, R.E., & Blake, J.D. (1996). Assessment of posttraumatic stress disorder in World War II veterans. *Psychological Assessment, 8,* 445–449.

Hammarberg, M. (1989). Outcome of inpatient treatment for posttraumatic stress disorder among Vietnam combat veterans. Ph.D. dissertation: University of Pennsylvania.

Hammarberg, M. (1992). Penn inventory for posttraumatic stress disorder: Psychometric properties. *Psychological Assessment, 4,* 67–76.

Hammarberg, M., & Silver, S.M. (1994). Outcome of treatment for post-traumatic stress disorder in a primary care unit serving Vietnam veterans. *Journal of Traumatic Stress, 7,* 195–216.

Keane, T.M., Caddell, J.M., & Taylor, K.L. (1988). The Mississippi scale for combat-related PTSD. Three studies in reliability and validity. *Journal of Consulting and Clinical Psychology, 56,* 85–90.

Lauterbach, D., & Vrana, S. (1996). Three studies on the reliability and validity of a self-report measure of posttraumatic stress disorder. *Assessment, 3,* 17–25.

Sbordone, R.J., & Liter, J.C. (1995). Mild traumatic head injury does not produce post-traumatic stress disorder. *Brain Injury, 9,* 405–412.

Shepard, L. (1995). PTSD in patients referred for evaluation of closed head injury. M.A. Thesis. University of Victoria.

PERSONALITY INVENTORY FOR CHILDREN (PIC)

Purpose

The test provides a personality evaluation through a parent questionnaire.

Source

Revised manuals, administration booklets, answer sheets, and scoring keys can be obtained from Western Psychological Services, 12031 Wilshire Blvd., Los Angeles, CA 90025, at a cost of about $175 US. Computer scoring and interpretation disks are available from the same source. A young children's version (ages 3–6 years; Keenan & Lachar, 1988) and a self-report version (Personality Inventory for Youth, PIY; Lachar & Gruber, 1995; $160, computerized test report $17.50, disk for 25 interpretations $295) are also available from the same source.

Description

The PIC (Wirt et al., 1984) is a true/false statement questionnaire for the parent, modeled along lines similar to the MMPI. It can be applied to children and adolescents, ages 6–16, and to preschoolers, ages 2–6. The full-length version contains 600 statements (e.g., "My child has little self-confidence", "Other children look upon my child as a leader"). The revised format booklet allows the scoring of four broad factor dimensions of childhood psychopathology (externalizing behavior, internalizing behavior, social incompetence, cognitive dysfunction), based on the first 131 items (Part I) only. The first 280 items (Part I and II) allow scoring of abbreviations of the four dimensions and 12 clinical scales (achievement, intellectual skills, development, somatic concerns, depression, family relations, delinquency, withdrawal, anxiety, psychosis, hyperactivity, social skills). The first 421 items (Parts I, II, and III) allow scoring of all scales in full, whereas the 600-item version is needed if scoring of research scales is desired.

The new PIY consists of 270 items, mostly drawn from PIC items and rephrased in the first person. It is designed for 6- to 18-year-olds and requires only a grade 3 reading level. An 80-item short form and a 32-item screening version of this test are described by the authors.

Administration

Since the PIC is designed for self-administration by the parent, instructions are presented on the front of the question booklet. Briefly, the test is introduced as an inventory of statements about children and family relationships. The parent or primary caregiver is asked to read each statement and decide if it is true or false as applied to the child, and to mark the answer sheet accordingly. On the PIY the student answers questions about himself or herself.

Approximate Time for Administration

The test requires 60–90 minutes unless one of the shortened versions is used. The full-length PIY takes 30–60 minutes.

Scoring

The 12 clinical scales, the four validity scales (assessing dimensions of underreporting, random reporting, or exaggeration), the one

screening scale ("adjustment," for any type of psychopathology) and four factor scales can be scored by using overlay templates and counting the total number of items of each scale marked in the appropriate direction. Alternatively, computerized scoring is available (see source). The clinical scales reflect concern on the part of the parent about the following areas: (1) Achievement, (2) Intellectual Screening (separately scored for ages 6–10+), (3) Development, (4) Somatic Concern, (5) Depression, (6) Family Relations, (7) Delinquency, (8) Withdrawal, (9) Anxiety, (10) Psychosis, (11) Hyperactivity, (12) Social Skills. The factor scales represent "broad bands" of (1) Externalization, (2) Social Orientation and Skills, (3) Internalization, and (4) Cognitive Achievement Status (Lachar et al., 1984). The totals for each scale are inserted into the profile form, which automatically converts the scores into T-scores similar to those of the MMPI. Code types, based on the single highest or two highest scores, similar to the MMPI-codes, can be determined (DeHorn et al., 1979). Seventeen supplemental scales are also available.

The PIY covers nine similar basic areas and includes four validity scales (endorsement of very unusual items, inconsistency, dissimulation, and defensiveness) but also offers a breakdown into subscales; for example, the Delinquency scale contains subscales for antisocial behavior, dyscontrol, and noncompliance.

Comment

The PIC should be filled out by both parents independently. Use of the 421- or the 280-item version is recommended. Use of the full-length version allows the scoring (also computer scoring) of several supplemental scales that may be of interest in individual cases: ACDM (Assessment of Career Decision Making), BCAS (Barclay Classroom Assessment System), DP-II (Developmental Profile II), ISI (Interpersonal Style Inventory), LBC (Louisville Behavior Checklist), MSI (parental Marital Satisfaction Inventory), MDQ (Menstrual Distress Questionnaire), MKAS (Meyer-Kendall Assessment Survey), MDI

(Multiscore Depression Inventory), PHCSC (Piers-Harris Children's Self-Concept Scale), TSCS (Tennessee Self-Concept Scale), TSCS:DC (Tennessee Self-Concept Scale—Diagnostic Classification Report), VII (Vocational Interest Inventory). An interpretative guide is available (Lachar & Gdowski, 1979).

The reliability, reported in the manual, is adequate (mean alpha of .74 in a heterogenous clinic sample of 1,226 clients) and does not drop seriously when the short form is used. The average retest correlation after 4–72 days was .86 (lowest correlation of .46 for Defensiveness); the values were similar for the shortened versions. Retest reliability in normal subjects after 2 weeks was .89 (range .70 to .93); for preschoolers with the short form, retest reliability after 2 weeks ranged from .77 to .92 with the exception of Somatic Concerns (.59) and Defensiveness (.31) (Keenan & Lachar, 1988). Between-parents agreement defined as scores within 10 T-scale points was 75 percent for normals, but less in parents of clinical cases. Father-produced profiles appear to have limited validity. However, psychopathology of the mother (as measured by the MMPI) does not appear to limit the predictive accuracy of the PIC (Lachar et al., 1987). The PIY has a similarly strong data base and good reliability. Cross-informant agreement (e.g., parent's PIC vs. students' PIY) is not reported, but is likely to be only marginal (see CBCL).

Validity of the PIC was originally established by selecting items that correlated highly with criterion group membership, then further refined to achieve maximum correlation. Sex effects on 18 of the scales led to the construction of separate profiles for males and females. Since its first publication in 1977, numerous studies have supported the validity of the PIC. Davies et al. (1987), however, point out that the profile as a whole should be considered for interpretation since the psychosis scale alone did not significantly discriminate between psychotic and normal adolescents. Nor should the other clinical scales be interpreted as diagnostic for specific types of pathology. T-scores of 79 and higher are considered as indicating significant concern in the respective area. Lachar et al. (1978) described

scale correlations for a variety of child psychopathologies, and LaCombe et al. (1991) provided interpretation rules for 12 specific types of profiles. However, DeMoor-Peal and Handal (1983, 1985) found statistical, but not clinical-diagnostic support for the clinical scales in preschool children, and they warn against the use of fixed "cook-book" cutoff scores (T-score of > 60) as suggested in the interpretative manual (Lachar & Gdowski, 1979).

Correlations between parent checklists of behavioral observations and PIC scales are generally good, whereas those with checklists filled out by professionals and teachers tend to be poorer. Correlational validity with other instruments, such as the Child Behavior Checklist and the MMPI, is high for several of the PIC scales. Discrimination between impaired and normal preschoolers was high (91 percent correct classifications, Keenan & Lachar, 1988). Kline et al. (1987b) and Clark et al. (1987) reported good discriminant validity when the PIC was used to predict intellectual, academic, and classroom placement, as well as attentional deficit and emotional impairment. Similarly, Clark et al. (1987) reported good identification of salient personality and cognitive features in learning-disabled, emotionally disturbed, and intellectually handicapped children. Fuerst and Rourke (1995) used PIC data for 728 7- to 13-year-old children with learning disability in a subtype/cluster analysis, and they found that at all ranges seven subtypes of psychosocial behavior could be distinguished that resembled subtypes found in other studies: normal, hyperactive, mild anxiety, somatic concern, conduct disorder, internalized psychopathology, and externalized psychopathology.

Lachar et al. (1984) used a factor analysis of home, clinic, and school ratings for 691 children aged 2–18 years as "external validation" for the development of their factor scales. However, Cornell (1985) questioned this method of external validation because the ratings contained wordings very similar to the PIC items; he argued that this would create artificial correlations based on rater reliability rather than external validity.

Whether the cognitive scales of the PIC are

an adequate measure of intelligence remains controversial. Beck and Spruill (1987) found in 79 children referred to a university clinic because of academic, behavior, or emotional problems only minimal correlations with the WISC-R (.24 to .46) and with the Arithmetic score on the Wide Range Achievement Test (WRAT; .06 to .29), although correlations with WRAT Reading and Spelling were significant (.29 to .41). On the other hand, Bennett and Welsh (1981), using 100 children from a clinic-referred population, found correlations of the Achievement Scale with the WISC-R of .56 to .61; with WRAT-Spelling of .55; with WRAT-Reading of .53; and with WRAT-Arithmetic of .43; the corresponding correlations with the Intellectual Screening scale were .46, .52, .43, .44, and .53, respectively.

DeMoor-Peal and Handal (1983, Handal & DeMoor-Peal, 1985) reported a correlation of .74 between WPPSI IQ and Intellectual Screening in preschool children. Cognitive impairment in preschoolers was detected with some success (correlation with the McCarthy Scales .38 to .59), but correct classification of normal preschoolers was poor (Byrne et al., 1987). On the other hand, Kline et al. (1987a) reported 90 percent correct classification between groups of school-age children with autism, mental retardation, and pervasive developmental disorder, and Clark et al. (1987) found in learning-disabled children correlations of .56, .49, and .56 between the Wechsler Intelligence Scale for Children—Revised (WISC-R) and the achievement, intellectual screening, and development scales, respectively. The contradictory results may be due to the wide range of age, intelligence, and pathology sampled in these studies.

Kline et al. (1985) investigated the effects of gender and ethnicity in 329 children and adolescents referred to a child guidance facility. They found that even though the WISC-R, PIAT, and PPVT showed expected differences of gender and race, the PIC showed only minimal bias on selected scales (white > black on ADJ; black > white on SOM; girls > boys on DLQ). An attempt to discriminate between groups of normal children and children with somatoform, neurological, and chronic medical disorders on the PIC (Pritchard et al.,

1988) found significant group differences in comparison to controls, but failed to distinguish among the three clinical groups. De-Horn et al. (1979) included a cerebral dysfunction group in their study of profile classification strategies: This group showed high elevations, mainly on the Intellectual Screening and Development scales cluster, similar to that found in children with mental retardation.

The PIY was validated against the MMPI and other scales as well as behavior dimensions derived from medical records. Other external validation studies are not yet available.

In neuropsychological settings, it is important to remember that, like the MMPI, the PIC and the PIY are not designed to detect neurological impairment in children. The PIC also, of course, reflects only the parent's perception of their child's problems, while the PIY measures the problems as perceived by the child or adolescent. The PIC should therefore be used as a supplement to the parent interview, and both the PIC and PIY as screening instruments to point to areas of concern and potential emotional and behavioral problems. PIC profiles based on mother's and father's responses frequently differ; however, it is useful to be aware of the respective bias of each parent.

The PIC hyperactivity scale is an adequate substitute for specific questionnaires for attention deficit syndrome with hyperactivity (e.g., Conners, 1973); in fact, it may be superior to such scales because of the availability of validity scales in the PIC.

Normative Data

The normative data from which the profiles were created are based on 2,600 normal children 6–16 years old; these data take into account the U.S. census in terms of race and socioeconomic status.

References

Beck, B.L., & Spruill, J. (1987). External validation of the cognitive triad of the Personality Inventory for Children: Cautions on interpretation. *Journal of Consulting and Clinical Psychology, 55,* 441–443.

Bennett, T.S., & Welsh, M.C. (1981). Validity of a configurational interpretation of the intellectual screening and achievement scales of the Personality Inventory for Children. *Educational and Psychological Measurement, 41*, 863–868.

Byrne, J.M., Smith, D.J., & Backman, J.E. (1987). Cognitive impairment in preschoolers: Identification using the Personality Inventory for Children. *Journal of Abnormal Child Psychology, 15*, 239–246.

Clark, E., Kehle, T.J., Bullock, D., & Jenson, W.R. (1987). Convergent and discriminant validity of the Personality Inventory for Children. *Journal of Psychoeducational Assessment, 2*, 99–106.

Conners, C.K. (1973). Rating scales for use in drug studies with children. *Psychopharmacology Bulletin, 3*, 24–29.

Cornell, D.G. (1985). External validation of the Personality Inventory for Children—Comment on Lachar, Gdowski, and Snyder. *Journal of Consulting and Clinical Psychology, 53*, 273–274.

Davies, A., Lachar, D., & Gdowski, C. (1987). Assessment of PIC and MMPI scales in adolescent psychosis: A caution. *Adolescence, 22*, 571–577.

DeHorn, A.B., Lachar, D., & Gdowski, C.J. (1979). Profile classification strategies for the Personality Inventory for Children. *Journal of Consulting and Clinical Psychology, 47*, 874–881.

DeMoor-Peal, R., & Handal, P.J. (1983). Validity of the Personality Inventory for Children with four-year-old males and females: A caution. *Journal of Pediatric Psychology, 8*, 261–271.

Fuerst, D.R., & Rourke, B.P. (1995). Psychosocial functioning of children with learning disabilities at three age levels. *Child Neuropsychology, 1*, 38–55.

Handal, P.J., & DeMoor-Peal, R. (1985). Validity of the Personality Inventory for Children with four-year-old males and females: A reanalysis. *Journal of Pediatric Psychology, 10*, 355–358.

Keenan, P.A., & Lachar, D. (1988). Screening preschoolers with special problems: Use of the Personality Inventory for Children (PIC). *Journal of School Psychology, 26*, 1–11.

Kline, R.B., Lachar, D., & Sprague, D.J. (1985). The Personality Inventory for Children (PIC): An unbiased predictor of cognitive and academic status. *Journal of Pediatric Psychology, 10*, 461–477.

Kline, R.B., Maltz, A., Lachar, D., Spector, S., & Fischhoff, J. (1987a). Differentiation of infantile autistic, child-onset pervasive developmental disorder, and mentally retarded children with the Personality Inventory for Children. *American Journal of Child Psychiatry, 15*, 839–843.

Kline, R.B., Lachar, D., & Boersma, D.C. (1987b). A personality inventory for children (PIC) profile typology: III. Relationship to cognitive functioning and classroom placement. *Journal of Psychoeducational Assessment, 4*, 327–339.

Lachar, D., Butkus, M., & Hryhorczuk, L. (1978). Objective personality assessment of children: An exploratory study of the Personality Inventory for Children (PIC) in a child psychiatric setting. *Journal of Personality Assessment, 42*, 529–537.

Lachar, D., & Gdowski, C.L. (1979). *Actuarial Assessment of Child and Adolescent Personality: An Interpretive Guide for the Personality Inventory for Children.* Los Angeles, CA: Western Psychological Services.

Lachar, D., Gdowski, C.L., & Snyder, D.K. (1984). External validation of the Personality Inventory for Children (PIC) profile and factor scales: Parent, teacher, and clinician ratings. *Journal of Consulting and Clinical Psychology, 52*, 155–164.

Lachar, D., & Gruber, C.P. (1995). *Personality Inventory for Youth.* Los Angeles, CA: Western Psychological Services.

Lachar, D., Kline, R.B., & Gdowski, C.L. (1897). Respondent pathology and interpretive accuracy of the Personality Inventory for Children: The evaluation of a "most reasonable" assumption. *Journal of Personality Assessment, 51*, 165–177.

LaCombe, F., Kline, R.B., Lachar, D., Butkus, M., & Hillman, S. (1991). Case history correlates of a Personality Inventory for Children (PIC) profile typology. *Psychological Assessment, 3*, 678–687.

Pritchard, C.T., Ball, J.D., Culbert, J., & Faust, D. (1988). Using the Personality Inventory for Children to identify children with somatoform disorders: MMPI findings revisited. *Journal of Pediatric Psychology, 13*, 237–245.

Wirt, R.D., Lachar, D., Klinedinst, J.K., & Seat, P.D. (1984). *Multidimensional Description of Child Personality: A Manual for the Personality Inventory for Children, Revised.* Los Angeles, CA: Western Psychological Services.

PROFILE OF MOOD STATES (POMS)

Purpose

Assessment of transient affective states through rating of adjectives or short phrases.

Source

The test can be obtained from the Educational and Industrial Testing Service, P.O. Box 7234, San Diego, CA 92167.

Description

The test, developed in an earlier version in the early 1960s (McNair et al., 1981; Lorr et al., 1961), consists of 65 adjectives (e.g., tense, miserable, muddled, listless) or short phrases (e.g., sorry for things done, ready to fight, uncertain about things), which are rated by the patient on a five-point scale (0 = not at all, 1 = a little, 2 = moderately, 3 = quite a bit, 4 = extremely). The items are scored for seven "transient, fluctuating affective states" (McNair et al., 1981): Fatigue-Inertia, Anger-Hostility, Vigor-Activity, Confusion-Bewilderment, Depression-Dejection, Tension-Anxiety, Friendliness. Because of poor subscale reliability for the Friendliness scale, the items of this scale are frequently omitted, reducing the test to 55 items. An investigation of 705 pregnant older women (33–44 years) replicated the factors of vigor, fatigue, and depression, and found additional factors of sociability, being relaxed-unafraid, not being angry or irritable, negative regard for self and others, and distractibility (Tunis, 1990). A shortened 40-item version is described by Grove and Prapavessis (1992), and a 37-item version is reported by Shacham (1983).

Administration

The patient is asked to rate each of the items on a five-point scale as they experienced it during the past week. If patients have difficulty remembering their mood during the past week, they can be instructed to report how they feel "right now." If questions arise concerning the meaning of a given word or phrase, Albrecht and Ewing (1989) suggest that a first and/or second alternative be offered orally. The alternatives have been standardized and show a sufficient alpha level of internal consistency.

Approximate Time for Administration

The test can be administered in approximately 5 minutes.

Scoring

The six factor scores and a total distress score can be easily calculated with a scoring key. The manual provides T-score conversions for each of the six subscales.

Comment

Retest reliability ranged from .65 for Vigor to .74 for Depression-Rejection during an intake to pretherapy interval for 100 outpatients; from intake to 6 weeks into therapy, reliability coefficients were between .43 for Vigor and .52 for Confusion-Bewilderment, reflecting both the longer time span and the effect of treatment. Internal consistency was between .84 and .95.

Validity rests on studies investigating the effect of short-term psychotherapy with and without a variety of tranquilizers, drug trials, emotion-inducing conditions (e.g., viewing a film of an autopsy, public speaking), marijuana use, and alcoholism. Concurrent validity was established by computing correlations with the Manifest Anxiety Scale (.36 to .80), therapist ratings on the Interpersonal Behavior Inventory (.18 to .32), ratings on the Inpatient Multidimensional-Psychiatric Scale (.30), observer rating for interview anxiety (.38), and other measures for substantial groups of patients (n = 60–500+). Social desirability (role playing, defensiveness) is relatively independent from POMS factor scores, except for Anger ($r = -.52$) (source).

Reddon et al. (1985) found no male/female differences in 261 college students, and they found only insufficient support for the six scales. These authors, based on the analysis of three actual populations and three Monte

Carlo simulations, recommend using only the overall distress score. A group of 257 prison inmates differed from the college population by showing poorer adjustment on all scales except Fatigue-Inertia, a result that was independent of differences in intelligence.

Kay et al. (1988) examined 505 older (> 65 years, mean age = 83.4) adult volunteers and found that they appeared relatively healthier than the original sample except on Vigor. Factor analysis confirmed and showed high internal consistency for five of the six original factors; the Confusion factor extracted in this study matched only three of the original items ("muddled, efficient, uncertain"), but included two new items ("clearheaded, alert"), apparently specific to the elderly.

Norcross et al. (1984) examined the factor structure of the POMS with 165 psychiatric outpatients and 298 smokers. Three scales emerged as independent factors (Anger-Hostility, Vigor-Activity, and Fatigue-Inertia), while the other three were highly correlated and may have been affected by social desirability (not wanting to admit psychopathology) or may represent overall distress levels.

A modest correlation ($r = .38$) of the POMS with measures of locus of control was found in patients with moderate and severe closed-head injury (Moore et al., 1991). Lowick (1995) found a modest correlation between accuracy in recognizing emotions and total POMS score in 24 head-injured patients during a rehabilitation program, but no significant increase in scores compared to a control group. In a large group of closed-head injury patients, Stambrook et al. (1990) found a low but significant correlation between employment status and Tension, Confusion, and Depression. In studies of patients exposed to environmental and industrial toxins, four scales (Vigor, Tension, Confusion, and Fatigue) were higher than in a carefully matched control group (Morrow et al., 1993). A large-scale study of epileptic patients before and one month after being put on anticonvulsant medication showed medication effects: The Tension score dropped, but scores for Anger and Fatigue increased (Smith et al., 1986).

The short form of the POMS was investigated by Curran et al. (1995) with 600 subjects

(five clinical samples with severe non-neurological physical diseases and a control group); they found correlations between subscales of the short and long form ranging from .81 to .95. Internal consistency was reported as .93 (Malouff et al., 1985).

Normative Data

The manual presents norms for the seven factor scores based on the responses from 856 college men and women in the Boston area separately; these norms are considered "very tentative" by the authors. In addition, the manual describes norms based on 650 female and 350 male psychiatric outpatients, aged 17–80 years (half of them between 17 and 25 years old), from a broad, but not necessarily representative sample. They are also presented separately by "no treatment," "psychotherapy," and "hospitalized" status, and in five diagnostic groups (psychoneurosis, personality disorder, psychosis, psychophysiologic, no disorder). Moore et al. (1990) found higher scores than those presented in the manual for DSM-III-R diagnosed depressed and anxious Australian women on all scales except Vigor, while the control group means were lower than those presented in the manual. Tunis et al. (1990) published norms for 705 pregnant women, aged 33–44 years.

Age showed a minor negative correlation with all scales in the outpatient standardization sample, and education showed a minor significant correlation only in women; white males, but not females, had significantly higher scores than blacks.

References

Albrecht, R.R., & Ewing, S.J. (1989). Standardizing the administration of the Profile of Mood States (POMS): Development of alternative word lists. *Journal of Personality Assessment, 53,* 31–39.

Curran, S.L., Andrykowski, M.A., & Studts, J.L. (1995). Short form of the Profile of Mood States (POMS-SF): Psychometric information. *Psychological Assessment, 7,* 80–83.

Grove, J.R., & Prapavessis, H. (1992). Preliminary evidence for the reliability and validity of an abbreviated Profile of Mood States. *International Journal of Sport Psychology, 23,* 93–109.

Kay, J.M., Lawton, M.P., Gitlin, L.N., Kleban, M.H., Windsor, L.A., & Kaye, D. (1988). Older people's performance on the Profile of Mood States. *Clinical Gerontologist, 7,* 35–56.

Lorr, M., McNair, D.M., Weinstein, G.J., Michaux, W.W., & Raskin, A. (1961). Meprobamate and chlorpromazine in psychotherapy. *Archives of General Psychiatry, 4,* 381–389.

Lowick, B. (1995). The Victoria Emotion Recognition Test: Validation with a head-injured population. Ph.D. dissertation. University of Victoria.

Malouff, J.M., Schutte, N.S., & Ramerth, W. (1985). Evaluation of a short form of the POMS-depression scale. *Journal of Clinical Psychology, 41,* 389–391.

McNair, D.M., Lorr, M., & Droppleman, L.F. (1981). *Manual for the Profile of Mood States.* San Diego: Educational and Industrial Testing Service.

Moore, A.D., Stambrook, M., & Wilson, K.G. (1991). Cognitive moderators in adjustment to chronic illness: Locus of control beliefs following traumatic head injury. *Neuropsychological Rehabilitation, 1,* 185–198.

Moore, K., Stanley, R., & Burrows, G. (1990). Profile of Mood States: Australian normative data. *Psychological Reports, 66,* 509–510.

Morrow, L.A., Kamis, H., & Hodgson, M.J.

(1993). Psychiatric symptomatology in persons with organic solvent exposure. *Journal of Consulting and Clinical Psychology, 61,* 171–174.

Norcross, J.C., Guadagnoli, E., & Proschaska, J.O. (1984). Factor structure of the Profile of Mood States (POMS): Two partial replications. *Journal of Clinical Psychology, 40,* 1270–1277.

Reddon, J.R., Marceau, R., & Holden, R.R. (1985). A confirmatory evaluation of Mood States: Convergent and discriminant item validity. *Journal of Psychopathology and Behavioral Assessment, 7,* 243–259.

Shacham, S. (1983). A shortened version of the Profile of Mood States. *Journal of Personality Assessment, 47,* 305–306.

Smith, D.B., Craft, B.R., & Collins, J. (1986). Behavioral characteristics of epilepsy patients compared with normal controls. *Epilepsia, 27,* 760–768.

Stambrook, M., Moore, A.D., & Peters, L.C. (1990). Effects of mild, moderate, and severe closed head injury on long-term vocational status. *Brain Injury, 4,* 183–190.

Tunis, S.L., Golbus, M.S., Copeland, K.L., & Fine, B.A. (1990). Normative scores and factor structure of the Profile of Mood States for women seeking prenatal diagnosis for advanced maternal age. *Educational and Psychological Measurement, 50,* 309–324.

RORSCHACH TEST

Purpose

This is a projective test requiring interpretation (free association to) of black and colored inkblots.

Source

The boxed plates can be ordered from Hogrefe & Huber publishers (North American office: P.O. Box 2487, Kirkland, WA 98083-2487) for $75 US or from Psychological Assessment Resources, Inc., P.O. Box 998, Odessa, FL 33556 for $95 US. Pads of 100 location charts are available for $30 (black and white) or $38 (colored). A Canadian source (Hogrefe & Huber, 12 Bruce Park Ave., Toronto, Ont. M4P 2S3) offers the plates for $97 Cdn, and black and white location chart pads for $20 Cdn. A three-plate form designed

for children, the Zulliger-Rorschach Test, is available from Hogrefe & Huber publishers.

Description

This "classic" test, first published in 1921 by Hermann Rorschach, consists of 10 stimulus cards. Each card contains symmetrical "inkblot" shapes in black, black and red, or several colors. We prefer this test over similar tests with larger numbers of cards in which only one response per card is allowed (Holtzman et al., 1972).

Administration

Administration of the Rorschach test should not be attempted without previous instruction and supervised experience with the test. Various authors differ slightly in their administration procedure. Our administration generally follows Exner (1993). Other manuals are by Aaronow and Reznikoff (1984), Klopfer (1954), Klopfer and Davidson (1977), Phillips and Smith (1980), and Ulett and Silverton (1993). The test administration is deliberately unstructured, forcing the individual to deal with the situation in his or her own manner. After some rapport has been established with the patient, a brief introductory statement is made, for example: *"I will show you some cards and I would like you to tell me what you see. There are no right or wrong answers on this test. Just tell me everything you see."* The first card is presented and the subject is asked: *"Tell me what you see on this card. Tell me what this could be. Tell me everything you see"*. Questions by the subject should be answered as noncommittally as possible ("That is entirely up to you," Klopfer, 1954, p. 7), and conversations and discussions during testing should be avoided. For anxious subjects, some reassurance ("good," "fine") may be given. During the presentation of the first three cards, the subject should be encouraged to give as many responses as possible, and to rotate the plates. If the subject produces a very large number of responses, it should be pointed out that it is not important to see how many responses the individual can produce. Occasionally, it may be necessary actually to limit the number of responses. Some examiners (Exner, 1993) suggest that protocols of less than 14 responses be discarded or readministered.

After completion of the last card, the examiner should explain to the subject that the cards will be presented again to allow the examiner to see exactly where on the card each response of the subject was seen. Repeat the response to the subject and inquire by asking the subject to outline the figure with the finger on the card (e.g., "You said this was a pretty bear rug. Please show me where on the card you saw this"). Additional scoring sheets with all 10 cards in miniature form are available from the source and allow the examiner to make notations, circle the parts outlined by the subject, etc. At the same time, the inquiry subtly extends to the determinants of each response (i.e., form, color, etc.) unless it is quite clear from the first answer (e.g., "What made it look like a bear rug? Does this also belong to it? What makes it look pretty?").

Approximate Time for Administration

The time required is 15–30 minutes.

Scoring

The examiner should prepare recording sheets (standard size paper held sideways not lengthwise) by folding (or dividing by lines down the page) blank paper into three approximately equal sections. The left-hand section is used to keep a protocol of everything said by the subject, the time in minutes and seconds at the presentation of each card, and the time when the first response (R) is given, the rotated position of the card ($\uparrow$, $\rightarrow$, $\leftarrow$, $\downarrow$), as well as any interjections or instructions made by the examiner. The second column is used for recording the responses given during the inquiry. A simple example (Figure 15–4) illustrates the method of recording.

The third column of the page is used for scoring the responses. For an experienced practitioner, a preliminary scoring can be combined with the inquiry process; the attempted scoring may lead to additional questions during the inquiry (e.g., "Is it moving? What makes you think of a butterfly"), particularly when the possibility of color, shading, texture, movement, or unusual (original) responses or response combinations needs to be explored. Formal scoring includes the summation of various types of responses and response characteristics as well as the preparation of several percentage scores (e.g., animal percentage, F+ [good form] percentage, popular response percentage) and indices (e.g., for suicide potential, depression, isolation, hypervigilance, schizophrenia, coping deficit, and obsessive style). Each index is based on up to 12 different "signs," such as CF + C > FC (color-form plus color greater than form-color responses) or R < 17. As an aid for formal scoring, Hertz (1992) offers frequency tables based on responses from 1,000 11- to 19-year-olds; other authors have similar frequency tables. Although formal scoring of the protocol

Response Record	Inquiry	Explanation of Response Record (Col. 1)	Scoring
I. 8.50–20"		I = Card 1	
1.∧ 20" The wings of a bat.	At first I saw only those wings, but then the whole thing seemed like a bat.	8.50–20" Card 1 was presented at 8:50 a.m. + 20 seconds. 1. First response. 20" It took 20 seconds before participant responded to this card. ∧ Card in upright position	D > W F+ A p
2.>	Just this upper part, wings and head raised, claws down here.	A large-winged animal ready to pounce down on its prey. 2. Second response > Card in rotated position	D F+ m pers
II. 8.52–10"		II. 8.52–10" Time when second card was presented	
3.∧ 45" There are two red things,	They are here on the side, just blotches, I can't think of what it could be.	3. ∧ 45" It took 45 seconds to produce first response. (consecutively numbered #3) to this card.	D C color CS
4.	Two black things, and	4. No upright signs needed if patient does not rotate card.	D FC A
5.	Another red thing. Like shadow images of people. Could be a butterfly.		D FC A p

Figure 15—4. Rorschach Test sample response record/scoring sheet.

with either Klopfer's, Beck's (1961) or Exner's (1993, 1991, 1982) system is desirable, many practitioners have abandoned the practice of calculating the many totals, percentage, and index values, which are highly dependent on the total number of responses (Meyer, 1993; for a proposed adjustment, see Morey, 1982). Instead, they view the Rorschach protocol as a reflection of the cognitive processes of the individual (Frank, 1991), observing rather than calculating cognitive flexibility or rigidity, perseverative tendencies, emotional reaction to color or shading, the ability to recoup after a delayed color response (see responses 3, 4, and 5 in Figure 15–4), to free-associate some of the more common responses, the accuracy of form, especially in novel ("original") responses, and the presence of responses suggestive of psychopathology.

At least five different computer scoring (e.g., Exner et al., 1990) and Rorschach Interpretation Programs (e.g., Exner, 1995) are available. The warnings about the use of interpretative computer programs (see Chapter 4) apply.

Comment

Interscorer agreement was reported as .87 (De Cata, 1983, 1984). Retest reliability for 6-year-old children after 24 months ranged from .86 for active movement to .13 for inanimate movement; for adults after 36–39 months from .87 for human movement to .31 for inanimate movement; for adults after 7 days, from .91 for active movement to .28 for inanimate movement; and for 8-year-olds after 3–4 days from .94 for active movement to .27 for inanimate movement (Exner, 1980; Haller & Exner, 1985). Odd-even split-half reliabilities ranged from .89 for the total number of responses to .39 for form/movement (Wagner et al., 1986, 1990).

A meta-analysis by Parker (1983) reported predictive and correlational validity coefficients of .45 to .50 and higher. Garwood (1978) reports good predictive validity for success in psychotherapy within 30 weeks. Wenar and Curtis (1991) review Exner's norms for children in the context of child development theory and confirm the predicted increases in cognitive complexity, integration, and precision of thinking; richness of ideas; conformity to socially acceptable ways of thinking; and the concomitant decrease in unrealistic, egocentric ideas.

The long history of this test has led to many suggested usages, including Rorschach's (1921, 1951) own observation that cerebrally impaired patients show (1) illogical combinatory responses, (2) inconsistent succession of form level and area used, (3) a tendency to give A (animal), Hd (human detail), and o (original) responses, and (4) only 30–60 percent F+ (good form) responses. Further "screening for organicity" was developed by Oberholzer (1931) and Piotrowski (1937). Most recently, Perry et al. (1996) developed a new scale, which significantly separated AD patients from normal controls. Many of these indices have fallen into disuse. Numerous publications have dealt with the application of the test for its original purpose: usage in personality and psychiatric diagnosis, in psychoanalytic therapy, and for the detection of specific organic disorders. Norms for "organic," schizophrenic, normals, and even for reading-disabled children (Alheidt, 1980, Fuller & Lovinger, 1980) and adult offenders (Prandoni & Swartz, 1978) have been published. For example, Spreen (1955, 1956) found differences between 50 patients with verified lesions in the dorsolateral-frontal and 50 patients with orbito-frontal lesions; while both groups showed poor form perception, the latter produced many more small detail and color responses, suggesting "disinhibition," while the former were considerably more perseverative.

Exner et al. (1996) examined 60 CHI patients, and found that they showed impoverishment in terms of available resources, simplistic ways of attending to details, inconsistency in coping and decision making, unwillingness or inability in dealing with feelings and emotional stimulation, and lack of common social skills for promoting and maintaining meaningful relationships, as compared to matched healthy individuals. Bartell and Solanto (1995) examined children diagnosed with ADHD and found fewer human movement (M) responses, poorer form quality (percentage of F− responses), and a lower ratio of human movement and whole figure responses.

Because of the multiple determination of the responses, the open-ended, free-association response form, and the deliberate ambiguity of the stimuli, severe criticism has been expressed about the validity of the test in terms of strict psychometric standards, and about its suitability for statistical analysis. One particular problem is that many Rorschach "signs," especially those based on raw scores, are highly dependent on R, the total number of responses produced by the patient (Meyer, 1993). However, Weiner (1996) presented good stability coefficients (between .82 and .94) after retest intervals of 7 days, 3 weeks, 1 year, and 3 years for a number of "trait" personality measures (e.g., M, FC, SumC, D) and maintained that the Rorschach test is psychometrically sound, valid, and useful. He also cited four articles which indicate that veterans with posttraumatic stress disorder tend to show a high distress (D) score, an index of the relationship between a number of coded scores, and responses with morbid thematic imagery (MOR).

However, some view the test as a sensitive measure of clinical interaction, which may be an indispensible tool in the hands of the skilled clinician and which may be suitable for research with both a psychometric and a cognitive approach (Weiner, 1977) or as a "type of structured interview" (Howes, 1981). A meta-analysis by Atkinson (1986) of studies with the Rorschach and the MMPI suggested that there is no difference between the two tests in conceptually designed validity studies.

In relation to neuropsychological assessment, Lezak (1995) mentions that the test can be evaluated as a measure of the patient's perceptual abilities, as a test of processing and integrating multiple stimuli, as a measure of the patient's certainty of his or her own perceptions, and as a measure of reaction time. Although all of these factors are aspects of the Rorschach protocol, many other neuropsychological tests provide more specific and more accurate measures of these abilities.

We use the test only secondarily for the measurement of these basic features, and, instead, treat it as a measure of changes of cognitive style and personality as well as an indicator of primary or secondary functional disorders of personality. For example, impoverished thinking in dementia frequently results in very few, poorly perceived, perseverative responses; linguistic errors and perseverations are common (Perry et al., 1996). Neurotic or psychotic intrusions are frequently noted in unusual reactions to some of the plates and "poor original" responses on many cards or even in an isolated response or two. Disinhibition and other frontal lobe disorders may be evident in inappropriate or overly aggressive or destructive responses or in numerous small detail responses, which often bear no resemblance to the stimuli presented.

Normative Data

Normative data for pre-school (Takeuchi, 1986) and for inner-city children from age 3–12 years (Krall et al., 1983), college-student twin pairs and sex differences (Rice et al., 1976), and numerous other groups have been published. Although such norms show trends, they are of limited value for the interpretation of individual cases because of the large variability of Rorschach responses. However, textbook authors such as Beck, Exner, and Klopfer list both age-appropriate responses and response summaries for children as well as "optimal" response patterns (including "popular" responses) for healthy adults and for elderly subjects that may serve as a guide. Lezak (1987) notes that in the few studies with normal elderly subjects, fewer responses, decreased creativity (more stereotyped content, fewer complex and original perceptions), and constriction (fewer movement and color responses) have been noted, although this may be partly due to the institutional status of subjects in these studies.

References

Aaronow, E., & Reznikoff, M. (1984). *A Rorschach Introduction: Content and Perceptual Approaches.* Los Angeles: Western Psychological Services.

Aldheidt, P. (1980). The effect of reading ability on Rorschach performance. *Journal of Personality Assessment, 44*, 3–10.

Atkinson, L. (1986). The comparative validity of the Rorschach and the MMPI: A meta-analysis. *Canadian Psychology, 27*, 238–249.

Bartell, S.S., & Solanto, M.V. (1995). Usefulness of the Rorschach inkblot test in assessment of attention deficit hyperactivity disorder. *Perceptual and Motor Skills, 80*, 531–541.

Beck, S.J., Beck, A.G., Levitt, E.E., & Molish, H.B. (1961). *Rorschach's Test: Basic Processes.* New York: Grune & Stratton.

DeCato, C.M. (1983). Rorschach reliability: Cross validation. *Perceptual and Motor Skills, 56*, 11–14.

DeCato, C.M. (1984). Rorschach reliability: Toward a training model for interscorer agreement. *Journal of Personality Assessment, 48*, 58–64.

Exner, J.E. (1993, 1991, 1982). *The Rorschach: A Comprehensive System*, Vol. 1, 3rd ed., 2, 2nd ed., 3. New York: Wiley.

Exner, J.E. (1980). But it's only an inkblot. *Journal of Personality Assessment, 44*, 563–576.

Exner, J.E. (1995). *Rorschach Interpretative Assistance Program.* Version 3 (RIAP3) Odessa, FL: Psychological Assessment Resources.

Exner, J.E., Cohen, J.B., & McGuire, H. (1990). *Exner's Rorschach Scoring Program.* San Antonio, TX: Psychological Corporation.

Exner, J.E., Colligan, S.C., Boll, T.J., & Stircher, B. (1996). Rorschach findings concerning closed head injury patients. *Assessment, 3*, 317–326.

Frank, G. (1991). Research on the clinical usefulness of the Rorschach: II. The assessment of cerebral dysfunction. *Perceptual and Motor Skills, 72*, 103–111.

Fuller, G.B., & Lovinger, S.L. (1980). Personality characteristics of three sub-groups of children with reading disability. *Perceptual and Motor Skills, 50*, 303–308.

Garwood, J. (1978). Six-month prognostic norms derived from studies of the Rorschach prognostic rating scale. *Journal of Personality Assessment, 42*, 22–26.

Haller, N., & Exner, J.E. (1985). The reliability of Rorschach variables for inpatients presenting symptoms of depression and/or helplessness. *Journal of Personality Assessment, 49*, 516–521.

Hertz, M.R. (1992). *Frequency Tables for Scoring Rorschach Responses* (5th ed.). Los Angeles, CA: Western Psychological Services.

Holtzman, W.H., Thorpe, J.S., Swartz, J.D., & Herron, E.W. (1972). *Inkblot Perception and Personality: Holtzman Inkblot Technique* (4th ed.). Austin: University of Texas Press.

Howes, R.J. (1981). The Rorschach: Does it have a future? *Journal of Personality Assessment, 45*, 339–351.

Klopfer, B. (1954). *Developments in the Rorschach Technique.* Vol. 1, 2, 3. Yonkers-on-Hudson: World Book Company.

Klopfer, B., & Davidson, H.H. (1977). *The Rorschach Technique: An Introductory Manual.* Los Angeles: Western Psychological Services.

Krall, V., Sachs, H., Lazar, B., Rayson, B., Growe, G., Novar, L., & O'Connell, L. (1983). Rorschach norms for inner-city children. *Journal of Personality Assessment, 47*, 155–157.

Lezak, M.D. (1995). *Neuropsychological Assessment* (3rd ed.). New York: Oxford University Press.

Lezak, M.D. (1987). Norms for growing older. *Developmental Neuropsychology, 3*, 1–12.

Meyer, G.J. (1993). The impact of response frequency on the Rorschach constellation indices and on their validity with diagnostic and MMPI-2 criteria. *Journal of Personality Assessment, 60*, 153–180.

Morey, L.C. (1982). An adjustment for protocol length in Rorschach scoring. *Journal of Personality Assessment, 46*, 286–288.

Oberholzer, E. (1931). Zur Differentialdiagnose psychischer Folgezustände nach Schädeltraumen mittels des Rorschachschen Formdeutversuchs (On differential diagnosis of psychological sequelae after head trauma by means of the Rorschach form interpretation experiment). *Zeitschrift für die gesamte Neurologie und Psychiatrie, 136*, 596–629.

Parker, K. (1983). A meta-analysis of the reliability and validity of the Rorschach. *Journal of Personality Assessment, 47*, 227–230.

Perry, W., Potterat, E., Auslander, L., & Kaplan, E. (1996). A neuropsychological approach to the Rorschach in patients with dementia of the Alzheimer type. *Assessment, 3*, 351–363.

Phillips, L., & Smith, J.G. (1980). *Rorschach Interpretation: Advanced Technique.* Los Angeles: Western Psychological Services.

Piotrowski, Z. (1937). The Rorschach inkblot method in organic disturbances of the central nervous system. *Journal of Nervous and Mental Diseases, 86*, 525–537.

Prandoni, J.R., & Swartz, C.P. (1978). Rorschach protocols for three categories of adult offenders: Normative data. *Journal of Personality Assessment, 42*, 115–120.

Rice, D.G., Greenfield, N.S., Alexander, A.A., & Sternbach, R.A. (1976). Genetic correlates and sex differences in Holtzman inkblot technique responses of twins. *Journal of Personality Assessment, 40*, 122–129.

Rorschach, H. (1921, 1951). *Psychodiagnostics.* New York: Grune & Stratton.

Spreen, O. (1955). Stirnhirnverletzte im Rorschach-Versuch. *Zeitschrift für diagnostische Psychologie und Persönlichkeitsforschung, 3*, 3–23.

Spreen, O. (1956). Stirnhirnverletzte im Rorschach-Versuch II. *Zeitschrift für diagnostische Psychologie und Persönlichkeitsforschung, 4*, 146–173.

Tacheuki, M. (1986). Educational productivity and Rorschach location responses of pre-school Japanese and American children. *Psychology in the Schools, 23*, 368–373.

Ulett, G., & Silverton, L. (1993). *Rorschach Introductory Guide.* Los Angeles, CA: Western Psychological Services.

Wagner, E.E., Adair, H.E., & Alexander, R.A. (1990). An empirical demonstration of the stability of the maximized correlation as an internal-consistency reliability estimate for tests of small item size. *Educational and Psychological Measurement, 50*, 539–544.

Wagner, E.E., Alexander, R.A., Roos, G., & Adair, H. (1986). Optimum split-half reliabilities for the Rorschach: Projective techniques are more reliable than we think. *Journal of Personality Assessment, 50*, 107–112.

Weiner, I. (1977). Approaches to Rorschach validation. In M.A. Rickers-Ovsiankina (Ed.), *Rorschach Psychology.* Huntington, N.Y.: R.E. Krieger.

Weiner, I.B. (1996). Some observations on the validity of the Rorschach Inkblot method. *Psychological Assessment, 8*, 206–213.

Wenar, C., & Curtis, K.M. (1991). The validity of the Rorschach for assessing cognitive and affective changes. *Journal of Personality Assessment, 57*, 291–308.

THEMATIC APPERCEPTION TEST (TAT)

Purpose

This is a projective test of thought content, emotions, and conflicts through story-telling based on pictures.

Source

The manual and 31 cards can be ordered from Psychological Assessment Resources, P.O. Box 998, Odessa, FL 33556, for $47 US. The children's version (CAT) with manual is available from the same source for $39 US. A supplementary form (CAT-S) with manual is also available from the same source for $39 US.

Description

The TAT consists of individual pictures about which the client is instructed to make up a story. The basic set includes 10 pictures. The remaining set contains 10 pictures designated for children, males, and females, and one "picture" as a blank page, resulting in a total of 31 pictures. A separate "Children's Apperception Test" (CAT) and a supplementary CAT-S (Bellak & Bellak, 1974) are also available.

Administration

Adequate rapport and knowledge of some basic personal data are required prior to administration. The full test is normally given in two sessions (pictures 1–10, 11–20) on separate days, although many examiners prefer to make a selection of only a few pictures, which may be presented in one session; in this case, however, the examiner should be very familiar with the client so that pictures relevant to the client's problem areas can be selected in advance. Typical general selections recommended for all clients are cards 1, 2, 3BM,* 4MF, 6BM, 7BM, 8BM, 10, 11, 13MF, 14, 16, 20 (Arnold, 1962); cards 2, 3GF, 4, 6GF, and 7GF for females; and 2, 3BM, 4, 6BM, and 7BM for males (Dana, 1956). Keiser and Prather (1990) list the cards used most frequently in recent research in rank order: 1, 2, 6BM, 13MF, 3BM, 16, 4, 7BM, 8BM, 10.

Instruction A for adolescents and adults with at least average intelligence are as follows: *"We have here a test to study fantasy. I will show you some pictures, and for each picture I want you to make up as dramatic a story as you can. Please look at the picture and tell*

*M and F refer to male and female, B and G to boys and girls.

me what happens in the picture at the moment, what the people in the picture are thinking, feeling, planning to do. Please make a complete story, inventing how it came to this situation, what happened before, how it developed further, and how it came out in the end. You cannot make a mistake in this test; it is only necessary to let your fantasy play and to invent a dramatic story. You can take about 5 minutes for each story. Here is the first picture."

Instruction B for children and adults with low intelligence or education is: "*I have here a story-telling test. I will show you some pictures; and for each picture you make up a story. Tell me what is happening in the picture, and what happened before. Then tell me also how the story goes on and how it ended. You can tell any story you like, just as it comes to your mind.*"

If the client does not observe all parts of the instruction, the client should be told what he or she did right, and what she or he has not done yet (e.g., "Tell me how it came out in the end"). Otherwise, the test administrator should interfere as little as possible, except for occasional encouraging remarks when the client hesitates or long pauses occur. Neutral questions (avoiding any suggestions) may be asked during the test to encourage continuity and to avoid awkward pauses. If the client asks what a particular part of the picture is, he or she should be informed that that is entirely up to him- or herself, that the client can make out of it whatever he or she wishes.

Scoring

The examiner tries to keep a verbatim protocol of everything that was said during the test, including exclamations and other initial reactions that are not part of the story, and the "response latency," that is, the time from card presentation to first response. This should be done unobtrusively in a note-taking manner, although in some cases tape-recording may be necessary to keep pace with the client's story. Most authors agree that asking the client to write the stories reduces productivity and should be avoided.

A supplementary interview ("inquiry") is often recommended: In this case, the examiner reads the story back to the client and asks the client to elaborate, and to explain whether the story is based on or reminiscent of personal experiences, books, or shows. If such sources are mentioned, details should be noted carefully. Frequently, the examiner will ask the client to point out the most and least favorite card. Finally, the inquiry can be used as a base for free associations by the examiner who is trained in psychotherapy.

The evaluation of the protocol is a complex process that requires considerable training and experience. As a guide to interpretation, Murray (1943) suggests noting the following "press" and "need" factors (rated from 1 to 5) for each of the stories:

1. Affiliation
   a. Social
   b. Emotional
2. Aggression
   a. Affective or verbal
   b. Physical and social
   c. Physical and asocial
   d. Destruction of property
3. Dominance
   a. External force
   b. Interference by others
   c. Influence or persuasion
4. Nurturance—includes feeding, protecting, encouragement, consolation, help or forgiving.
5. Rejection
6. Lack or loss
   a. Lack of recognition, happiness, success, family, poverty, etc.
   b. Loss as in (a)
7. Physical damage by nonhuman factors
   a. Active
   b. Loss of solid foundation (drowning, ship or airplane accident, etc.)
8. Physical injury

For each story, the key figure ("hero")—which is most likely the one with whom the client identifies—should be established. Other "figures" (father, mother, sibling, teacher) should be noted for each story.

The stimulus value of each card is different and has been discussed by several authors. Since this is of importance for both card selection and interpretation, the following list (abbreviated from Murray, 1943) may be useful:

Card 1: *Young boy contemplating violin on table:* need for achievement, autonomy, particularly with respect to parents and authorities, self- versus other-motivation.

Card 2: *Country scene:* family relations, separation and individuation, achievement values and aspirations, pregnancy issues.

Card 3BM: *Boy huddled on floor and revolver:* depression, helplessness, suicide, guilt, impulse control, handling of aggression.

Card 3GF: *Woman standing with downcast head:* depression, loss, suicide, guilt.

Card 4: *Woman clutching shoulders of man:* male-female relationships, sexuality, infidelity, interpersonal control, dominance, and conflict.

Card 5: *Middle-aged woman looking into a room:* attitude towards mother or wife, guilt, autonomy issues, fear of intruders, paranoia.

Card 6BM: *Elderly woman with back towards young man:* mother-son relations, loss and grief, separation-individuation.

Card 6GF: *Young woman sitting, looking at older man with pipe:* daughter-father or male-female relationships, heterosexual relationships, interpersonal trust, employer-employee relationship.

Card 7BM: *Grey-haired man looking at younger man:* father-son relationship, employer-employee relationship, authority issues.

Card 7GF: *Older woman sitting close to young girl:* mother-daughter relationship, rejection issues, child-rearing attitudes and experiences.

Card 8BM: *Adolescent boy with rifle and surgery in background:* aspirations and achievement, handling of aggression, guilt, fears of being harmed, oedipal issues.

Card 8GF: *Young woman looking off into space:* diverse themes, aspirations, thoughts of future.

Card 9BM: *Four men lounging on grass:* homosexuality, male-male relationship, work attitude, social prejudice.

Card 9GF: *Young woman observing woman in party dress:* female-female relationships, rivalry, jealousy, sexual attack, trust versus suspicion, suicide.

Card 10: *Young woman resting head against man's shoulder:* marital or parents' relationship, intimacy, loss or grief.

Card 11: *Road between cliffs and dragon:* unknown, threatening forces, attack and defense, aggression.

Card 12M: *Young man on couch and elderly man stretching out hands above:* health, homosexuality, father-son relationship, issues of control, response to psychotherapy.

Card 12F: *Young woman and weird old woman grimacing in background:* mother and mother-in-law relationship, guilt and superego conflict, good and evil.

Card 12BG: *Rowboat drawn up on river bank:* loneliness, nature, peace, imaginal capacities, suicide.

Card 13MF: *Young man with head downcast and woman lying on bed:* sexual conflict and attitude, heterosexual relations, guilt, handling of provocative stimuli, aggression.

Card 13B: *Boy sitting on doorstep of log cabin:* loneliness, abandonment, childhood memories.

Card 13G: *Little girl climbing winding stairs:* childhood memories, loneliness.

Card 14: *Silhouette of man or woman against bright window:* wishes and aspirations, depression, suicide, loneliness, burglary, intrapersonal concerns.

Card 15: *Gaunt man among gravestones:* death, religion, fantasy, aggression.

Card 16: *Blank card:* varied themes, handling of unstructured situations, imaginal capacities, optimism vs. pessimism.

Card 17BM: *Naked man clinging to rope:* achievement and aspirations, homosexuality, optimism and pessimism, danger, escape, competitiveness.

Card 17GF: *Female leaning over river bridge railing:* loneliness, suicide, intrapersonal concerns.

Card 18BM: *Man clutched from behind by three hands:* alcoholism, drunkenness, homosexuality, aggression, paranoia, helplessness.

Card 18GF: *Woman with hands squeezed around throat of another woman:* aggression, particularly mother-daughter, rivalry, jealousy, conflict.

Card 19: *Cloud formations overhanging snow-covered cabin:* varied themes, imaginal capacities.

Card 20: *Figure of man or woman at night leaning against lamppost:* loneliness, fears, aggression.

A variety of scoring methods (reviewed by Vane, 1981) including quantitative and non-quantitative systems and rating scales have been developed. Experienced clinicians frequently prefer to review the stories without quantitative evaluation, keeping in mind the "normal" responses to each card based on stimulus properties.

Comment

Despite Murray's (1938) somewhat outdated personality theory underlying the construction of the TAT, the test has found continuing use up to today, with more than 2,000 papers and books published. Validity and reliability data are scarce, leading Swartz (1978) to remark that "if the TAT were published today with the same amount of information on its reliability, validity, and standardization, it is very doubtful that it would ever attain anywhere near its present popularity" (p. 1127). He adds, however, that Murray described the test as "an aid to the exploration of personality, and as such, of course, it must be rated an overwhelming success" (p. 1127). Boyvin and Begin (1982) report interjudge scoring agreement between .87 and .96; Squyres and Craddick (1982) report agreements of .77 and .82. A study by Langenmeyr and Schlag (1981) reported some correlational validity of TAT fac-

tor scores with MMPI scores. Black and white subjects showed little difference when presented with cards containing persons with either white or black features, nor did race of the examiner produce differences in the results (Lefkowitz & Fraser, 1980). However, a review of 69 studies published between 1978 and 1988 (Keiser & Prather, 1990) comments on the high variability of card usage, which makes generalizations about the validity and reliability difficult; and Vane (1981) blames the paucity of reliability and validity data on the lack of usage of a standardized administration and scoring method.

The TAT is not a diagnostic instrument, but a projective technique suitable for the exploration of specific problems, conflicts, fears, and needs of the individual at the conscious and at a more subliminal level. Stories may reflect more recent experiences at a superficial level (e.g., recently viewed movies), the current situational problems of the individual at work or at home, as well as more persistent personal motivation, needs, fears, etc., and even more subliminal (i.e., to the individual not immediately apparent) past experiences and other personality features. For these reasons, thorough training of the interpreter of the test and the person conducting the inquiry as well as a background in personality theory and psychotherapy are necessary.

In the context of a neuropsychological examination, the TAT can be used in a manner similar to the Rorschach Test or other story-telling techniques; that is, it provides information about (1) general response-time delays in brain-damaged patients; (2) ability to organize a story sequentially; (3) paucity of ideas (concrete description of picture rather than making up a story, or stories with few characters and little action); (4) misinterpretation of pictures or parts of pictures due to confusion, simplification, or vagueness (Lezak, 1995); (5) perseveration of content or phrasing; (6) word-finding difficulties; and (7) inability to interpret the picture as a whole. In addition, the TAT may reflect the personal reaction to injury or deficit, "catastrophic reactions," indications of a posttraumatic stress disorder, feelings of failure, as well as insights into premorbid or postmorbid reactive mechanisms, and it may guide the examiner into current problem content.

Normative Data

Although the most common themes for each picture and the qualitative aspects of normal and abnormal performance have been described above, no normative data in the usual sense exist for this test because of the large variety and the personal nature of possible responses ("projections"). Subjects with low education level and elderly subjects (Fogel, 1967) tend to produce shorter and less elaborate stories. Hayslip and Lowman (1986) and Kahana (1978) also report less emotional expression and themes reflecting increasing social isolation and passivity in the elderly.

References

Arnold, M.B. (1962). *Story Sequence Analysis.* New York: Columbia University Press.

Bellak, L., & Bellak, S. (1974). *Children's Apperception Test.* Los Angeles, CA: Western Psychological Services.

Boivin, M., & Begin, G. (1982). Comparison of interjudge reliabilities in scoring TAT protocols as a measure of NACH. *Perceptual and Motor Skills, 54,* 59–62.

Dana, R.H. (1956). Selections of abbreviated TAT sets. *Journal of Clinical Psychology, 12,* 36–40.

Fogel, M.L. (1967). Picture description and interpretation in brain-damaged subjects. *Cortex, 3,* 433–448.

Hayslip, B., & Lowman, R.L. (1986). The clinical use of projective techniques with the aged. In T.L. Brink & L. Terry (Eds.), *Clinical Gerontology: A Guide to Assessment and Intervention.* New York: Hayworth Press.

Kahana, B. (1978). The use of projective techniques in personality assessment of the aged. In M. Storandt, I. Siegler, & M. Ellis (Eds.), *The Clinical Psychology of Aging.* New York: Plenum Press.

Keiser, R.E., & Prather, E.N. (1990). What is the TAT? A review of ten years of research. *Journal of Personality Assessment, 55,* 800–803.

Langenmayr, A., & Schlag, B. (1981). Objektive Auswertungskriterien im TAT: Die Überprüfung ihrer Aussagekraft anhand des MMPI und sozialstatistischer Daten. *Psychologie und Praxis, 25,* 166–182.

Lefkowitz, J., & Fraser, A.W. (1980). Assessment of achievement and power motivation of blacks and whites, using black and white TAT, with black and white administrators. *Journal of Applied Psychology, 65,* 685–696.

Lezak, M.D. (1995). *Neuropsychological Assessment* (3rd ed.). New York: Oxford University Press.

Murray, H.A. (1938). *Explorations in Personality.* New York: Oxford University Press.

Murray, H.A. (1943). *Thematic Apperception Test.* Manual. Cambridge, MA: Harvard University Press.

Squyres, E.M., & Craddick, R.A. (1982). A measure of time perspective with the TAT and some issues of reliability. *Journal of Personality Assessment, 46,* 257–259.

Swartz, J.D. (1978). Thematic Apperception Test. In O.K. Buros (Ed.), *The Eighth Mental Measurement Yearbook.* Vol. 1, pp. 1127–1130. Highland Park, N.J.: Gryphon Press.

Vane, J.R. (1981). The Thematic Apperception Test: A review. *Clinical Psychology Review, 1,* 319–336.

VINELAND ADAPTIVE BEHAVIOR SCALES

Purpose

The purpose of this test (Sparrow et al., 1984) is to assess social and personal adaptive abilities in daily living.

Source

The complete set can be ordered from American Guidance Service, Inc., Circle Pines, MN 55014-1796, for $95 US. Also available are cassette training tape, computer program for scoring and interpreting (ASSIST), technical and interpretative manual, and a Spanish test version.

Description

The survey form consists of 297 items; the expanded form includes an additional 280 items, which are presented to the primary caretaker in a semistructured interview similar to Doll's original Vineland Social Maturity Scales. The test is not administered directly to the subject, but rather to the person most familiar with him or her. The items cover four domains: communicative, daily living skills, socialization, and motor skills. There are subdomains within domains: for communicative—receptive, expressive, and written communication; for daily living—personal, domestic, and community; for socialization—interpersonal relationships, play and leisure time, and coping skills; for motor skills—gross and fine. In addition, an optional set of items covers maladaptive behavior (e.g., bedwetting, inappropriate impulsiveness, crying, or laughing). The scales are designed to cover ages 3 years to 18 years 11 months (when presumably an adult ceiling is reached). The expanded form is designed to serve as a systematic basis for preparing educational, habilitative, and treatment programs by means of a separate booklet ("Program Planning Report"). A "Classroom Edition" of 244 items, which is to be completed by the teacher, differs considerably from the interview edition and has been criticized because it requires "guesstimates" on many items that are not known to the teacher (Kamphaus, 1987).

Administration

The approximate age starting points for non-handicapped individuals are indicated in the record booklet for each domain. Considerable time can be saved by beginning the interview at a level estimated as appropriate for the patient's estimated "adaptive age" equivalent. After establishing rapport with the respondent, the examiner explains that the purpose of the interview is to determine what the client does to take care of himself or herself and to get along with others, and what others usually do for the client. Then begin with the items, for example "speaks in full sentences," uses "a" and "the" in phrases or sentences, follows instructions in "if-then" form, etc. The items are presented in general form but are followed by probe questions for clarification as needed. Extensive training in administration is essential since many items may require probing. Refer to the manual for details.

Approximate Time for Administration

The time required is approximately 20–60 minutes for the survey form, or 60–90 minutes for the expanded form.

Scoring

A simple scoring system of 2 points (activity performed satisfactorily and habitually), 1 point (emerging or sometimes correctly performed skill), and 0 points is used for each item, following the criteria appended to the manual. Sums of total raw scores for each subdomain and domain are calculated. These can be transferred into standard scores appropriate for age (SAS; with confidence interval), percentile ranks, adaptive levels, and age equivalents by the use of tables in the manual; they may then be plotted in a standard score profile.

Comment

This "revision" of the Doll scales, the most frequently used test of adaptive behavior (Wodrich & Barry, 1991), resulted in a virtually new test, although the interview technique remained the same. The standardization is based on 3,000 normal individuals chosen from all parts of the country to represent the 1980 U.S. census. However, Evans and Bradley-Johnson (1988) point out weaknesses in the number of subjects used to represent socioeconomic status, geographic distribution, and urban-rural residence. Interrater reliabilities are .74 for the composite score, and between .62 and .78 for domain scores (see source); this has been criticized as inadequate (Oakland & Houchins, 1987). Split-half reliability for a variety of handicapped groups ranges from .83 for the Motor Skill domain to .94 for the Adaptive Behavior composite (see source). Retest reliability after an interval of 2–4 weeks (based on 484 subjects) was .90 for children up to age 6, .80 for older subjects, and .98 for the whole age range across domains (see source).

Construct validity is documented by satisfactory increase with age in each domain, and by the extraction of one significant factor, accounting for 55–70 percent of the variance, dependent on age level. The test also correlates only .12 to .37 with the Peabody Picture Vocabulary Test (PPVT), indicating its relative independence from measures of verbal ability. The correlation of the Communications Domain with the Kaufman Assessment Battery for Children (Kaufman & Kaufman, 1983) was highest with the Achievement portion of that test (.52). Correlation with the WISC-R was .37, with the Stanford-Binet (Form L-M) between .44 for the communication domain to .16 for the motor domain (Douthitt, 1992). This suggests that adaptive behavior and intelligence are related but separate constructs (Platt et al. 1991). Because the scales are designed to provide a profile of developmental delay, criterion validity relies on the quality of standardization. Correlational validity with the original Vineland is reported as .55, with the Minnesota Child Development Inventory as .62 (Brodsky, 1990), with the Adaptive Behavior Inventory for Children (Mercer & Lewis, 1978) as .58, with the Scales of Independent behavior as .83 (Middleton et al., 1990), with the shorter Adult Functional Adaptive Behavior Scale .72 (Kerby et al., 1989), and with the AAMD Adaptive Behavior Scale as between .40 and .70 (Perry & Factor, 1989).

The test showed highly significant differences between gifted (Binet IQ 132–164+) and average (IQ 96–131) children between 3 and 16 years of age, suggesting that the scales are sensitive in the upper as well as the lower ranges of intelligence. A study by Douthitt (1992) showed higher scores on communication, socialization, and daily living skills, but not on motor skills for gifted as compared to nongifted children.

Few systematic investigations of patients with dementia or other forms of brain damage are available. Dammers et al. (1995) stress that poor adaptive functioning is part of the diagnosis of dementia, but that in a survey of 500 psychologists relatively few reported formally assessing adaptive functioning in one or more areas. Fletcher et al. (1990) used the VABS in a follow-up of 45 children (mean age = 8 years 6 months) with mild, moderate, and severe closed-head injury. At 6- and 12-months follow-up, the group with severe head injury showed continuing decline in the composite score, whereas the mild- and moderate-head-injury group showed progress, unrelated to age at time of injury. In particular, severely injured children had more school problems and engaged in fewer social activities. These effects were stronger than those reported by parents in the Child Behavior Checklist, although the two scales correlated (.46 at 6 months, .67 at 12 months) with each other. The VABS scores also correlated with the length of impaired consciousness ($-.42$ and $-.47$) as well as with the Continuous Recognition Memory Test ($-.66$) and the Selective Reminding Test ($-.41$). Morris et al. (1993) examined 25 children between 21 and 179 months of age who had survived cardiac arrest and found VABS scores in the low or deficient range, correlating with duration of cardiac arrest and medical risk scores. A study of 28 children with hydrocephalus and spina bifida without mental retardation (Holler et al., 1995) showed mild impairment of communication and daily-living skills in the younger (age 5–7 years) group, and more severe impairment in both areas as well as in socialization in the older (age 9 years to 12 years 6 months) group.

Its tendency toward "statistical overkill"—provision of too many different scores (Holden, 1984)—can easily be avoided by using the score that is most familiar to the examiner and that is comparable to other scores used in testing.

As discussed for other tests with multiple subtests and area scores like the WPPSI-R, WISC-III, and Stanford-Binet, the significance of differences between domains and subdomains is dependent on the standard error of measurement and must be interpreted with great caution. Although such differences may be suitable for generating hypotheses of relative strength and weaknesses of an individual, they do not constitute "proof" unless they are quite large (2–3 SDs). Because of the two-part definition of mental retardation, differences between intelligence tests (IQ) and adaptive behavior scores, Atkinson (1990) provided tables for the interpretation of differences between all three forms of the VABS on the one hand, and the WPPSI, the WISC-R, the WAIS-R, the Stanford-Binet, the Bayley, and the McCarthy scales at various levels of confidence. For example, at the .01 level of significance, the required difference between the VABS survey form SAS and the WISC-R IQ ranges from 12 to 15 points, dependent on age.

Normative Data

As mentioned above, the test was standardized on 1,500 males and 1,500 females fairly representative of the geographic and racial composition of the United States. The manual presents detailed domain standard scores and bands of error from age 0 to 18 years 11 months and older in increments of 3 months or less, as well as supplementary norms for maladaptive behavior in seven handicapped groups.

References

Atkinson, L. (1990). Intellectual and adaptive functioning: Some tables for interpreting the Vineland in combination with intelligence tests. *American Journal on Mental Retardation, 95,* 198–203.

Brodsky, M.E. (1990). Measuring adaptive behavior: The relationship between the Minnesota Child Development Inventory and the Vineland Adaptive Behavior Scale. M.A. thesis, University of Victoria.

Dammers, P.M., Bolter, J.F., Todd, M.E., Gouvier, W.D., Batiansila, B., & Adams, S.G. (1995). How important is adaptive functioning in the diagnosis of dementia? A survey of practicing clinical psychologists. *Clinical Neuropsychologist, 9,* 27–31.

Doll, E.A. (1935). A genetic scale of social maturity. *American Journal of Orthopsychiatry, 5,* 180–188.

Douthitt, V.L. (1992). A comparison of adaptive behavior in gifted and nongifted children. *Roeper Review, 14,* 149–151.

Evans, L.D., & Bradley-Johnson, S. (1988). A review of recently developed measures of adaptive behavior. *Journal of Clinical Psychology, 44,* 276–287.

Fletcher, J.M., Ewing-Cobbs, L., Miner, M.E., Levin, H.S., & Eisenberg, H.M. (1990). Behavioral changes after closed head injury in children. *Journal of Consulting and Clinical Psychology, 58,* 93–98.

Holden, R.H. (1984). Vineland Adaptive Behavior Scales. In D.J. Keyser & R.C. Sweetland (Eds.), *Test Critiques.* Vol. 1. Kansas City, MO: Test Corporation of America, pp. 715–719.

Holler, K.A., Fennell, E.B., Crosson, B., Boggs, S.R., & Mickle, J.P. (1995). Neuropsychological and adaptive functioning in younger versus older children shunted for early hydrocephalus. *Child Neuropsychology, 1,* 63–73.

Kamphaus, R.W. (1987). Critiques of school psychological materials. *Journal of School Psychology, 25,* 97–98.

Kaufman, A.S., & Kaufman, N.L. (1983). *Kaufman Assessment Battery for Children.* Circle Pines, MN: American Guidance Service.

Kerby, D.S., Wentworth, R., & Cotten, P.C. (1989). Measuring adaptive behavior in elderly developmentally disabled clients. *Journal of Applied Gerontology, 8,* 261–267.

Mercer, J.R., & Lewis, J.F. (1978). *Adaptive Behavior Inventory for Children.* New York: Psychological Corporation.

Middleton, H.A., Keene, R.G., & Brown, G.W. (1990). Convergent and discriminant validities of the scales of independent behavior and the revised Vineland Adaptive Behavior Scales. *American Journal on Mental Retardation, 94,* 669–673.

Morris, R.D., Krawiecki, N.S., Wright, J.A., & Walter, L.W. (1993). Neuropsychological, academic, and adaptive functioning in children who survive in-hospital cardiac arrest and resuscitation. *Journal of Learning Disabilities, 26,* 46–51.

Oakland, T., & Houchins, S. (1987). A rejoinder to a misguided attack on the bearer of some good news and some bad news. *Journal of Counselling and Development, 65,* 575–576.

Perry, A., & Factor, D.C. (1989). Psychometric validity and clinical usefulness of the Vineland Adaptive Behavior Scales and the AAMD Adaptive Behavior Scale for an autistic sample. *Journal of Autism and Developmental Disorders, 19,* 41–55.

Platt, L.O., Kamphaus, R.W., Cole, R.W., & Smith, C.I. (1991). Relationship between adaptive behavior and intelligence: Additional evidence. *Psychological Reports, 68,* 139–145.

Sparrow, S.S., Balla, D.A., & Cicchetti, D.V. (1984). *Vineland Adaptive Behavior Scales.* Circle Pines, MN: American Guidance Service.

Wodrich, D.L., & Barry, C.T. (1991). A survey of school psychologists' practices for identifying mentally retarded students. *Psychology in the Schools, 28,* 165–171.

16

Occupational Interests and Aptitude

Neuropsychological assessment has gradually shifted its emphasis from purely neurodiagnostic purposes to more prognostic, consulting, and rehabilitation roles. Retraining of the brain-damaged patient for a suitable occupation is one of the purposes of many assessments, as is the formulation of realistic occupational goals for the brain-damaged child. The actual abilities and skills of the individual can be judged to some extent from test performance, but a full assessment of occupational abilities is best left to specialized settings that use aptitude testing and provide hands-on tryout information and basic training.

We describe two of the more popular tests for this area, the Career Assessment Inventory and the General Aptitude Test Battery. Other well-designed tests that may be promising for use in rehabilitation are the Strong Interest Inventory (Hammer & Kummerow, 1990), the Kuder Occupational Interest Survey, and the Jackson Vocational Interest Survey.

References

Hammer, A.L., & Kummerow, J.M. (1990). *Strong and MBTI Career Development Guide and Workbook*. Palo Alto, CA: Consulting Psychologists Press.

CAREER ASSESSMENT INVENTORY (CAI)

Purpose

This instrument is a detailed vocational interest inventory, originally designed in 1973, revised in 1986, designed for the high school to adult range, including retraining for a new career.

Source

The CAI (Advanced version) and the CAI (Vocational version) are available from National Computer Systems Inc., P.O. Box 1416, Minneapolis, MN 55440, for a price of approximately $30 US, or from Multi-Health Systems Inc., 65 Overlea Blvd., Toronto, Ont. M4H 1P1, for $46.50 Cdn each (Manual and Software). A Hispanic version and computer software for profiles and interpretative reports are available on a pay-per-use basis.

Description

The Career Assessment Inventory (Johansson, 1986) consists of 305 items in three sections: Activities (151 items), School Subjects (43 items), and Occupations (111 items). For each item, the subject marks a circle indicating "like very much," "like somewhat," "indifferent or undecided," "dislike somewhat," or "dislike very much." The Inventory has an enhanced and a vocational version and is designed for career exploration and for assistance in making career decisions in grades 10–

12, for community college students considering continued studies in a specialized field, for adults considering mid-career changes, as well as for "vocational rehabilitation settings where retraining is a vital concern" (p. 7). Males and females take the same test.

Administration

The inventory can be administered individually or in groups. The client should be instructed as to the meaning of the five choices for each item, that there are no correct or incorrect answers, and that there is no time limit. A grade 8 reading proficiency is required.

Approximate Time for Administration

The inventory takes about 35–40 minutes, but administration may take longer for clients unfamiliar with psychological inventories.

Scoring

Scoring is done with the aid of a personal computer and a scorebox from National Computer Service on a pay-per-use basis. Hand-scoring is possible, but the test material does not provide keys, although the items for each scale are listed. Scoring includes six "general theme" (realistic, investigative, artistic, social, enterprising, conventional), 22 "basic interest" (ranging from mechanical/fixing, electronics, carpentry to mathematics, community service, public speaking, food services) and 42 occupational (e.g., aircraft mechanic, caterer, bank teller) scales. The response range for an individual can be compared with the average response range for males or females on each scale. A choice of a computer-generated profile and/or of an interpretative narrative report is offered. Response percentage, response consistency, response variability, and infrequent response index are also scored; these allow a check on random responding and validity.

Comment

The CAI is a well-developed instrument and is similar to the older Strong-Campbell Interest Inventory. It is longer than other inventories, but short enough to maintain the interest of the average client. Test–retest correlations for the general theme scales range from .91 to .96, for the basic interest scales from .88 to .95, and for the occupational scales from .81 to .96 after one week; even after 2–3 months, reliabilities are quite high (Zarrella & Schuerger, 1990).

Content validity was established by high item-total correlations with internal consistency coefficients between .89 and .92. Correlational validity with similar scales on the Strong-Campbell Interest Inventory, with the Kuder Occupational Interest Survey, and with the Jackson Vocational Interest Survey were satisfactory.

Unfortunately, only one study of the application of this inventory in rehabilitation settings for persons with disabilities is available (Jagger et al., 1992), nor does the manual provide case studies or other references pertinent to rehabilitation. The use of the CAI for patients with neurological impairment will have to be approached with caution, and, in particular, the computer-generated narrative report will have to be carefully edited in order to provide meaningful information for the neuropsychological assessment report.

It should be noted that this inventory measures vocational interests, not aptitudes. For aptitude testing, the GATB may be more appropriate.

Normative Data

Norms are based on the responses of 450 males and 450 females established in the various occupations, with similar representation on the general theme scales, taken "from a broad occupational spectrum." Geographic representativeness of the normative sample has apparently not been attempted, and age varies from 26 to 49 years.

References

Jagger, L., Neukrug, E., & McAuliffe, G. (1992). Congruence between personality traits and chosen occupation as a predictor of job satisfaction for people with disabilities. *Rehabilitation Counseling Bulletin, 36,* 53–60.

Zarrella, K.L., & Schuerger, J.M. (1990). Temporal stability of occupational interest inventories. *Psychological Reports, 66,* 1067–1074.

GENERAL APTITUDE TEST BATTERY (GATB)

Purpose

The GATB measures a selection of job-related aptitudes for vocational and educational counseling.

Source

The test is available from the U.S. Government Printing Office through the Superintendent of Documents, P.O. Box 371954, Pittsburgh, PA 15250-7954 for approximately $110 US. A Spanish-language version, a version for the deaf, and a Nonreading Aptitude Test Battery (NATB) are available from the same source. A GATB Test Scoring System for the PC ($1,000 US) as well as narrative report programs are available through National Computer Systems Interpretative Scoring Service, P.O. Box 1416, Minneapolis, MN 55435. Hand-scoring answer sheets and keys are also available. The battery is also available in French and Spanish translations. A slightly modified Canadian version (General Aptitude Test Battery, 1986) is available from Nelson Canada, 1120 Birchmount Road, Scarborough, Ont. M1K 5G4, for approximately $460 Cdn. A software package for scoring and interpretation ("Profile"), comparing the profile against a database organized according to the Canadian National Occupation Classification, is available from Nelson for $650 Cdn.

Description

This test battery was developed by the U.S. Department of Labor in 1945 and has been widely used with minor modifications. The 1986 Canadian edition includes a 1985 renorming of all paper-and-pencil tests and a revision of part 6 (Arithmetic Reasoning) to eliminate all references to imperial or metric measurements (because of the changeover to metric measures in the Canadian school curriculum).

The manual comes in four parts: I. Administration and Scoring, II. Norms and Occupational Aptitude Patterns, III. Development (1970, no further revision), and IV. Norms for Specific Occupations. Bezanson (1984; Bezanson & Monsebraaten, 1984) provides an introduction to the test. In addition, the scoring booklets 1 and 2 come in two equivalent forms (A and B). For the administration of parts 9–12, a manual dexterity board and a finger dexterity board are required.

The test battery consists of:

1. Name Comparison: decide if name pairs are the same or different, e.g., C.G. Jones & Co.—G.C. Jones & Co.

2. Computation: arithmetic exercises requiring addition, subtraction, multiplication, and division of whole numbers.

3. Three-Dimensional Space: viewing a two-dimensional drawing of a stimulus figure that can be rolled or bent along dotted lines. The subject must select one of four three-dimensional figures that corresponds to the stimulus figure.

4. Vocabulary: the subject selects two of four words that have either the same or opposite meaning.

5. Tool Matching: the subject looks at a black-and-white drawing of a shop tool (e.g., hammer) and then selects one out of four tools with the same shape and shading.

6. Arithmetic Reasoning: Verbally enclosed arithmetic; e.g., Jill can walk twice as fast as Jack. Jack walks to the park in two hours. How much time will Jill need to get to the park? Choice of one out of five answers.

7. Form Matching: Stimulus line drawings of various shapes must be matched with identical shapes contained in 10 drawings below.

8. Mark Making: two vertical and one horizontal pencil mark must be made in a series of squares as rapidly as possible.

9. Place: Cylindrical pegs must be transferred from the upper to the lower part of the 48-peg board. Three 15-second trials.

10. Turn: On the same board, pegs must be turned (inverted) and transferred to the lower board. Three 30-second trials with the preferred hand.

11. Assemble: A different pegboard with two sections of 50 holes is used. Subject must take a washer from a rod at the side of the

board and place it on each rivet while transferring it to the lower board.

12. Dissemble: Rivet is transferred to the upper board and the washer is removed and placed on a rod at the side of the board.

Administration

The administration of all parts is described in detail in the source. The battery is designed for group administration but can be given individually. All parts of the battery are timed.

Approximate Time for Administration

Actual test time is 48 minutes. The battery takes approximately 2.5 hours to administer.

Scoring

Raw scores can be obtained by use of a plastic handscoring stencil or through the optical scanning machine-scoring service. Raw scores are recorded for each test and can be used as an individual score or summed for nine aptitudes as follows:

1. General Learning Ability (G): Vocabulary, Arithmetic Reasoning, and Three-dimensional Space.
2. Verbal Aptitude (V): Vocabulary.
3. Numerical Aptitude (N): Computation, Arithmetic Reasoning.
4. Spatial Aptitude (S): Three-dimensional Space.
5. Clerical Perception (Q): Name Comparison.
6. Form Perception (P): Tool Matching and Form Matching.
7. Motor Coordination (K): Mark Making.
8. Manual Dexterity (M): Place and Turn.
9. Finger Dexterity (F): Assemble and Dissemble.

Each individual or summed score is transferred into standard scores with a mean of 100 and a SD of 20 by the use of conversion tables found in Part I of the manual. Combinations of the nine standard scores have been used to create Specific Aptitude Test Batteries and 66 Occupational Aptitude Patterns that have pass-fail cutoff scores.

Comment

Test–retest reliability with the same or with the alternate form ranges from .80 to .90. Aptitude scores remain highly stable over retest periods ranging from one day to 26 weeks (U.S. Department of Labor, 1982).

Validity has been established by comparing the scores of successful and unsuccessful students and workers in numerous occupations selected with and without GATB scores. Validity coefficients for students majoring in various areas are also provided. It should be noted, however, that aptitude profiles for 66 specific occupations provide only a general guide and are not necessarily occupation-specific. Gibson and Siefker (1989) also noted disagreement between GATB occupational aptitude patterns and those based on the U.S. Dictionary of Occupational Titles, and they provide corrections. Validity was established by the analysis of correlations between supervisors' rating and G, V, and N scores in 24,219 individuals and found satisfactory (.30) (Baydown & Neuman, 1992) across the full range of possible scores (Waldman & Avolio, 1989).

Although the nine aptitudes were derived from factor-analytic studies (U.S. Department of Labor, 1982), more recent studies have concluded that the GATB measures three major abilities: cognitive (G, V, and N), perceptive (S, Q, and P), and psychomotor (K, M, and F) (Avolio & Waldman, 1990). Hammond (1983) described four factors: symbolic (V, N, P, Q), perceptual (S, P), manual dexterity (M), and finger dexterity (F, K). Using profile analysis through multidimensional scaling (PAMS), Davison et al. (1996) found on data from 23,428 workers a two-dimensional solution, with dimension 1 characterized by V, G, and N, and its mirror image; dimension 2 was characterized by K, Q, and V, and its mirror image S, F, and P. These dimensions are viewed as the most frequently occurring patterns in this population.

Concurrent validity with more than 90 other tests is reported in Part III of the manual. Correlations with other aptitude tests are satisfactory (e.g., .68 to .84 with the Occupational Aptitude and Interest Survey, Parker et al.,

1990), but correlations with vocational interest tests such as the Kuder Preference Record are only marginal.

The G-score correlates strongly with general intelligence measures (e.g., .71 with the WAIS, .81 with the California Test of Mental Maturity); for this reason, the test authors have designated this score as a measure of general intelligence.

The test has found only limited application in disabled populations. Part III of the manual reports scores for emotionally disturbed, mentally retarded, and deaf populations. Few specific applications in neuropsychological rehabilitation have been published; Lacroix (1992) provides an annotated bibliography. Tellegen (1965) found in 90 young adults with epilepsy a pattern of low motor aptitude, especially in the unemployed subgroup; this subgroup, however, also had more frequent seizures and received more medication. Clemmons et al. (1987) reported that adults with epilepsy had mean GATB scores that were lower than the published norms, and lower than scores of job applicants in the local general labor force, especially in dexterity and motor speed. Nevertheless, the GATB scores were not highly predictive of employment outcome, although unemployed subjects tended to have lower scores. No age effects were found, but this is probably due to the fact that the impairment obscured any potential age effects. The authors also observed discrepancies of more than 2 SD between V- and S- or P-scores in subjects with right or left lateralized foci, but no statistical data on this difference was presented. A study by Lacroix (1992) in our laboratory examined 60 patients at least one year after traumatic brain injury between 18 and 54 years of age. Compared to the general working population, these subjects scored lower on G, V, N, K, F, and M, with the lowest scores usually obtained on motor tests. The author concluded that these subjects will likely experience substantial difficulties in the competitive labor market. Indeed, the rate of unemployment for this group had risen from 7 percent prior to the accident to 55 percent one year after the accident. In addition, age effects were also noted. The author recommended that in a rehabilitation set-ting alternative administrations for the speeded motor and other tests be used to distinguish between the ability of the individual to perform correctly and the ability to perform rapidly. She also concluded that the GATB is useful for job-fit matching with traumatically brain-injured individuals; 78 percent correct classification of the ability or inability to do a specific job was obtained, mostly based on cognitive and perceptual aptitude composites. The usefulness of motor aptitude and composite was found to be questionable.

The battery is of potential use in rehabilitation settings. The overlap of some of the tests of the battery with tests frequently used in neuropsychology (Perdue Pegboard, WAIS-R Arithmetic, Visual Form Discrimination) suggests that it may provide information on neuropsychological deficits in addition to its role as an aptitude test. A dissertation by Cole (1984) examined this relationship in 113 patients with a variety of neurological conditions. The author found strong correlations between GATB-Q (perceptive) and Trails-C and WAIS PIQ. Correlations between GATB-K (coordination) and Trails A, B, C were between .53 and .57; between GATB-F (finger dexterity) and the Tactual Performance Test (TPT time and blocks) −.61 and .51; between GATB-M (manual dexterity) and TPT (time) −.55.

Normative Data

Numerous studies have provided general population norms and norms for trainees and experienced workers in a large number of occupations, ranging from medical students to asparagus sorters. The standard scores refer to 4,000 people between 18 and 54 years of age, representative of the general U.S. population in 1940. A Canadian study in 1964 showed little difference from the U.S. norms, and the 1986 version was renormed on 1,000 working Canadians.

Although performance on all GATB subtests declines with age (less so on measures of "crystallized" intelligence, Fozard et al., 1972), adjustments for sex and age differences or for ethnic minority status are not made because, in the opinion of the test developers, this would defeat the purpose of testing aptitudes. The use of differential norms (or race group norms) for hiring purposes has been extremely controversial (Baydoun & Neuman, 1992; Gottfredson, 1994) and has led to a temporary suspension of the use of the GATB by the U.S. Department of Justice.

A four-state study of age effects with 2,439 subjects ranging in age from 18 to 74 years showed significant age effects for eight of the nine aptitudes (with the exception of V), and sex effects for Q, K, and F. Another study with 21,646 individuals in the same age range (Avolio & Waldman, 1990) showed only a modest correlation with age for G ($-.16$), V ($-.12$) and N ($-.13$) across 10 different job types, and no differential effects of the interaction between job complexity and age.

References

Avolio, B.J., & Waldman, D.A. (1990). An examination of age and cognitive test performance across job complexity and occupational types. *Journal of Applied Psychology, 75,* 43–50.

Baydoun, R.B., & Neuman, G.A. (1992). The future of the General Aptitude Test Battery (GATB) for use in public and private testing. *Journal of Business and Psychology, 7,* 81–91.

Bezanson, L. (1984). *Using Tests in Employment Counselling.* Part I. Theory. Scarborough, Ont.: Nelson.

Bezanson, L., & Monsebraaten, A. (1984). *Using Tests in Employment Counselling.* Part II: Interpretation. Scarborough, Ont.: Nelson.

Clemmons, D.C., Fraser, R.T., & Trejo, W. (1987). The General Aptitude Test Battery: Implications for vocational counseling and employment in epilepsy rehabilitation. *Journal of Applied Rehabilitation Counseling, 18,* 33–38.

Cole, J.C. (1984). An investigation into the interrelationship between neuropsychological and vocational assessments in the neurologically impaired. Ph.D. dissertation, Memphis State University.

Davison, M.L., Gasser, M., & Ding, S. (1996). Identifying major profile patterns in a population: An exploratory study of WAIS and GATB patterns. *Psychological Assessment, 8,* 26–31.

Fozard, J.L., Nuttall, R.L., & Vaugh, N.C. (1972). Age-related differences in mental performance. *Aging and Human Development, 3,* 19–24.

Gibson, G.G., & Siefker, J.M. (1989). Discrepancies between DOT aptitudes and GATB OAP cutoff scores. *Vocational Evaluation and Work Adjustment Bulletin, 22,* 25–30.

Gottfredson, L.S. (1994). The science and politics of race-norming. *American Psychologist, 49,* 955–963.

Hammond, S.M. (1983). An investigation into the factor structure of the General Aptitude Test Battery. *Journal of Occupational Psychology, 5,* 43–48.

Lacroix, J. (1992). The GATB's contribution to the vocational rehabilitation of adults with traumatic brain injuries. Innovations Program, Employment and Immigration Canada, Ottowa: Queens Printer (Serial #1242 IX3, 2nd ed.).

Manual for the General Aptitude Test Battery (1986). Section 1, 2, 4. Scarborogh, Ont: Nelson Canada.

Parker, R.M., Chan, F., & Carter, H.S. (1990). Concurrent validity study of the OASIS Aptitude Survey. *Educational and Psychological Measurement, 50,* 209–212.

Tellegen, A. (1965). The performance of chronic seizure patients on the General Aptitude Test Battery. *Journal of Clinical Psychology, 22,* 180–184.

U.S. Department of Labor. (1982). *Manual for the USES General Aptitude Test Battery.* Section III: Development. Washington, D.C.: Government Printing Office.

Waldman, D.A., & Avolio, B.J. (1989). Homogeneity of test validity. *Journal of Applied Psychology, 74,* 371–374.

17

Malingering and Symptom Validity Testing

According to the American Psychiatric Association (APA, 1994), malingering is "the intentional production of false or grossly exaggerated physical or psychological symptoms, motivated by external incentives such as avoiding military duty, avoiding work, obtaining financial compensation, evading criminal prosecution, or obtaining drugs." Complicating this diagnosis is the fact that it is often difficult to assess patients' internal states and that both conscious and unconscious motivations may contribute to a patient's behavior. Further, although various legal and nosological systems encourage black-and-white diagnostic decisions, fabricated or exaggerated deficits may coexist with real impairments.

The detection of feigned or exaggerated deficits is a complex diagnostic process that rests on a combination of thorough record review, interviews of the patient and other informants, psychological tests, and behavioral observation (Slick, 1996). It becomes a diagnostic consideration whenever (1) readily identifiable and commonly recognized incentives for exaggeration or fabrication exist, (2) subjective complaints or test results are not consistent with neurological or functional status, (3) symptoms and complaints do not make medical sense, (4) there is a history of emotional/personality disorder (e.g., sociopathic behavior), and (5) patient cooperation is questionable.

Two approaches are available to assess feigning or exaggeration of symptoms. In one approach, validity scales are developed for use with conventional clinical measures. The other approach involves the use of specially designed instruments for detecting dissimulation.

Conventional Measures

Studies that detail reliable presentations of malingering on conventional neuropsychological or psychological tests can be found in the Comment section of relevant measures elsewhere in this book, and only a brief overview is provided here.

The best example of this first approach is probably the MMPI and its successor, the MMPI-2. The MMPI was designed to include a set of validity scales, and a number of additional scales have subsequently been developed. These scales include F, F-K, Obvious minus Subtle (for recent reviews see Berry et al., 1994; Graham, 1992; Greiffenstein et al., 1995), Lees-Haley Fake Bad Scale (FBS) (Lees-Haley et al., 1991) and the F(p) scale (Abrisi & Ben-Porath, 1995).

Researchers have also attempted to derive cutoff scores on conventional neuropsychological tests (see Nies & Sweet, 1994, for a recent review). Although studies have found that some malingerers overplay their brain-injured role, producing readily identifiable deficits, other malingerers are often able to simulate realistic overall levels of impairment that cannot easily be distinguished from those produced by actual brain-damaged patients (Tenhula & Sweet, 1996). Consequently, investigators have begun to employ more sophisticated techniques, looking for patterns of performance that can distinguish between groups. For example, potentially useful malingering indices have been developed by evaluating serial position effects on list learning tests such as the Rey Auditory Verbal Learning Test (e.g., Bernard, 1991 but see Iverson et al., 1991), by evaluating recognition hits on the Rey Auditory Verbal Learning Test and the California Verbal Learning Test (e.g., Bernard, 1991; Binder et al., 1993; Millis, 1994; Millis et al., 1995; Trueblood, 1994), by examining performance on implicit memory tests (e.g., Davis et al., 1997), by comparing performance on easy and hard items on measures such as the Category Test (e.g., Tenhula & Sweet, 1996) and the PASAT (Strauss et al., 1994), by comparing performance on obvious (e.g., categories achieved) versus subtle (e.g., perseverative errors) items on tasks such as the Wisconsin Card Sorting Test (Bernard et al., 1996), by evaluating digit span (Reliable Digit Span; Greiffenstein et al., 1994) by comparing indices of attention to indices of memory on tests such as the WMS-R (Mittenberg et al., 1993), by evaluating the configuration of motor skills scores (e.g., Greiffenstein et al., 1996), and by combining multiple sources of data in statistical procedures such as discriminant function analysis (e.g., Bernard et al., 1996, Iverson & Franzen, 1996; Mittenberg et al., 1996).

Overall, attempts to develop malingering indices for conventional neuropsychological tests have met with varying degrees of success. Clinicians should note, however, that although studies using these tests show promise, they require independent cross-validation and further research in various clinical populations to ensure that these patterns are reliable and would not be produced under special circumstances with legitimate patients (Nies & Sweet, 1994).

Specific Tests To Detect Malingering

Several tests have been devised specifically to detect enhanced complaints of memory impairment. Rey's 15-Item Visual Memory Test, introduced initially in 1964 (reported in Lezak, 1983) and described here, remains popular, despite mixed opinion about its utility. More useful measures are symptom validity tests.

First introduced by Lezak (1976), the term *symptom validity testing* (SVT) refers to a method for detecting poor effort or malingering. Essentially, SVT is a probabilistic analysis of patient performance on forced-choice tests. Most use a two-choice response format. For example, in two-choice recognition tests, the probability of responding correctly on all items by chance alone (that is, guessing) is 50 percent. Overall performance should therefore approximate 50 percent correct in the most severe cases of memory impairment. Assuming random responses to a given number of two-choice items, confidence intervals for chance-level performance can be calculated. Scores within the confidence interval about chance-level performance are assumed to reflect either severe impairment or possibly exaggeration of deficits. High or low scores that are outside this large confidence interval are highly unlikely by chance alone. Such scores are assumed to be the product of purposeful selection of correct or incorrect answers (in either case depending on intact memory), with the latter being suggestive of exaggerated or faked memory deficits. A number of researchers have developed forced-choice tests (e.g., Binder, 1990; Davis et al., 1995; Hiscock & Hiscock, 1989; Iverson et al., 1991; Rosenfeld et al., 1996; Slick et al., in press). We describe here the Victoria Symptom Validity Test (VSVT; Slick et al., in press), a forced-choice technique that is based on the Hiscock and Hiscock (1989) method but is less time-consuming, assesses both accuracy and response latency, and includes a normative-based scoring system since the diagnostic criterion of significantly below-chance performance may be too stringent, and therefore less sensitive to more sophisticated forms of malingering. It also includes a classification confidence matrix for given scores with varying base rates. Binder (1990, 1993) has developed a similar forced-choice procedure. Rosenfeld et al. (1996) adapted the Hiscock and Hiscock procedure to involve recording of the P300 event-related brain potential in response to the match probe. Davis et al. (1995) have provided a software package that includes a forced choice recognition test, similar to Binder's Portland Digit Recognition Test, as well as tests of malingering that rely on measures of lexical priming, free recall of word lists and of prose, category classification, and semantic knowledge. These tasks are of potential utility but require additional development (e.g., to date, the authors have relied on students instructed to fake memory deficit, not head-injured patients or patients with an extrinsic motivation to malinger).

The dichotomous forced-choice format has also been applied to list learning tasks. Iverson et al. (1991) devised the 21-Item Test composed of two word lists containing nouns. Following presentation of the target list, patients are given a two-alternative, forced-choice recognition task that requires selection of the previously presented word. The 21-Item Test is also described here.

Although not originally designed to assess motivation, the Recognition Memory Test (Warrington, 1984), which uses a forced-choice recognition format with words and faces as stimuli, has been adapted for assessment of the validity of memory complaints (Millis, 1994). It is described in the section on memory. We describe here The TOMM (Tombaugh, 1996) which is similar to the Recognition Memory Test and requires forced-choice recognition of 50 common objects.

It is worth bearing in mind that scores that fall in the normal range on the tests discussed above do not rule out malingering. The individual may have been feigning symptoms that he or she perceives to be unrelated to performance on memory tests (e.g., attention, motor or sensory deficit). Additional SVT tests relevant to domains other than memory need to be developed.

Note too that, to date, no single methodology has proven sufficient. Accordingly, the use of several measures (e.g., VSVT, RMT, Portland Digit Recognition Test, Recognition Memory Test, Rey 15 Item, 21-Item Test, TOMM, examination of serial position effects, recognition hits, scores on tests of attention

and response latencies) is recommended. In addition, independent information on the patient's report of limited success in coping with everyday living and work activities should be sought. Given the current state of affairs, it is our view that multiple approaches must be used in the diagnostic process and that statements regarding incomplete effort should not be based on a single test score (see fig. 17–1).

Recently, Greiffenstein, Baker, and Gola (1994) introduced criteria for the classification of overt malingering for use with litigating post-concussive patients. Probable malingerers are those who meet two or more of the following four criteria: (a) two or more impairment ratings of severe on neuropsychological tests in comparison to appropriate age and education standardization groups, (b) an improbable symptom history contradicted by records or surveillance films, (c) total disability in work or in a major social role after one year, and (d) claims of remote memory loss. Greiffenstein and his colleagues (1994, 1995) have shown significant associations between classifications made by their index and scores on malingering measures, such as the Portland Digit Recognition Test (PDRT). These results demonstrate the value of Greiffenstein's heuristic criteria and also reveal the important link between performance on some measures of malingering and the patient's functioning outside the test situation.

As noted above, there is no method that can definitively detect simulation, despite the availability of sophisticated techniques. There is some evidence that warning individuals of the possibility of detection of exaggeration on neuropsychological tests may reduce malingering behavior (Johnson & Lesniak-Karpiak, 1997). Provision of a warning may augment these techniques in order to reduce the probability of malingering behavior, as opposed to detecting malingering when it occurs. Provision of a warning is unlikely, by itself, to be sufficient in decreasing malingering behavior.

Communication of findings can be difficult, given the pejorative overtones associated with the term malingering, the substantial consequences that such diagnosis can have for an individual's life, the difficulty in confirming its presence, and the complex motivations that

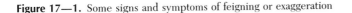

1. A disability that is disproportionate with the severity of the illness of injury.
2. Symptoms and complaints that do not make medical or neuropsychological sense.
3. An improbable symptom history contradicted by records.
4. Inconsistencies between complaints and behavior observed during the test or outside the test situation.
5. Claims of remote memory loss.
6. Suppression of first half of items on list learning tasks.
7. Unusually low recognition scores on list learning tasks and Symptom Validity Tests.
8. Abnormally slowed response latencies.
9. Failing easy or obvious items, passing hard or subtle items (e.g., Wechsler Test, Category Test, WCST, Paired-Associate task).
10. Unusually low digit span.
11. Disproportionately impaired attention relative to vocabulary, learning or memory scores (e.g., Vocabulary minus Digit Span, Attention/Concentration Index lower than General Memory Index).
12. Absurd or grossly illogical responses and approximate answers (e.g., on Wechsler Test).
13. Discrepancies between scores on tests measuring similar processes.
14. Abnormal scores on validity scales (e.g., MMPI-2 F, F-K, Obvious minus Subtle, Less-Haley Fake Bad Scale, F(p) scale).
15. Unusual configuration on motor skills (e.g., poor grip strength relative to measures of speed and dexterity).
16. Impaired performance on implicit memory tasks.

Figure 17—1. Some signs and symptoms of feigning or exaggeration

underlie a person's behavior. Accordingly, the report should be written in a manner that is factual rather than accusatory. It should provide a detailed description of how the patient was responding, indicate how this relates to both diagnostic issues and the referral question and acknowledge any limitations in interpretation (Binder & Thompson, 1994; Tombaugh, 1996). For example, the examiner might state the following: "Results from the neuropsychological examination raise the concern that Ms. Jones may be exaggerating her memory complaints. Thus, her scores on a number of forced-choice recognition tests (e.g., VSVT, 21-Item, TOMM) were significantly lower than expected. While such low scores can occur in severely demented individuals, they are rarely, if ever, obtained by normal people or individuals suffering from mild brain injury. In addition, Ms. Jones. . . ."

In some cases, rather than stating that the person is malingering, the most appropriate conclusion (Binder & Thompson, 1994; Tombaugh, 1996) where malingering is suspected is merely to comment on the invalidity of the testing and make no diagnosis. The examiner might state that "the inconsistency of the results preclude a diagnosis at this time," or "the results are not consistent with any known diagnosis" or "the results are not consistent with the presenting complaint."

Finally, clinical reports are most useful when they contain some information about the motivation that prompted the dissimulation. Such reasons may reflect a desire to avoid responsibility, a plea for acknowledgement of an injury or an attempt to obtain medical or special care services. The report should also include suggested therapeutic interventions.

References

Abrisi, P.A., & Ben-Porath, J.S. (1995). An MMPI-2 infrequent response scale for use with psychopathological populations: The Infrequency-Psychopathology Scale F(p). *Psychological Assessment, 7*, 424–431.

American Psychiatric Association (1994). *Diagnostic and Statistical Manual of Mental Disorders* (4th ed.). Washington: American Psychiatric Association.

Bernard, L.C. (1991). The detection of faked deficits on the Rey Auditory Verbal Learning Test: The effect of serial position. *Archives of Clinical Neuropsychology, 6*, 81–88.

Bernard, L.C., McGrath, M.J., & Houston, W. (1996). The differential effects of simulating malingering, closed head injury, and other CNS pathology on the Wisconsin Card Sorting Test: Support for the "Pattern of Performance" hypothesis. *Archives of Clinical Neuropsychology, 11*, 231–245.

Berry, D.T.R., Baer, R., & Harris, M. (1994). Detection of malingering on the MMPI: A meta-analysis. *Clinical Psychology Review, 11*, 585–598.

Binder, L.M. (1990). Malingering following minor head trauma. *The Clinical Neuropsychologist, 4,* 25–36.

Binder, L.M. (1993). An abbreviated form pf the Portland Digit Recognition Test. *The Clinical Neuropsychologist, 7,* 104–107.

Binder, L.M., Villaneuva, M.R., Howieson, D., & Moore, R.T. (1993). The Rey AVLT Recognition Memory Task measures motivational impairment after mild head trauma. *Archives of Clinical Neuropsychology, 8,* 137–149.

Binder, L.M., & Thompson, L.I. (1994). The ethics code and neuropsychological assessment practices. *Archives of Clinical Neuropsychology, 10,* 27–46.

Davis, H.P., King, J.K., Bajszar Jr. J.H., & Squire, L.R. (1995). *Colorado Malingering Test Package, Version 2.0.* Colorado Springs, CO: Colorado Neuropsychology Tests Co.

Davis, H.P., King, J.H., Bloodworth, M.R., Spring, A., & Klebe, K.J. (1997). The detection of simulated malingering using a computerized category classification test. *Archives of Clinical Neuropsychology, 12,* 191–198.

Graham, J.R. (1992). *MMPI-2: Assessing Personality and Psychopathology* (2nd ed.). New York: Oxford University Press.

Greiffenstein, M.F., Baker, W.J., & Gola, T. (1994). Validation of malingered amnesia measures with a large clinical sample. *Psychological Assessment, 6,* 218–224.

Greiffenstein, M.F., Gola, T., & Baker, W.J. (1995). MMPI-2 validity scales versus domain specific measures in detection of factitious traumatic brain injury. *The Clinical Neuropsychologist, 9,* 230–240.

Greiffenstein, M.F., Baker, W.J., & Gola, T. (1996). Motor dysfunction profiles in traumatic brain injury and postconcussion syndrome. *Journal of International Neuropsychological Society, 2,* 477–485.

Hiscock, M., & Hiscock, C.K. (1989). Refining the forced-choice method for the detection of malingering. *Journal of Clinical and Experimental Neuropsychology, 11,* 967–974.

Iverson, G.L., Franzen, M.D., & McCracken, L.M. (1991). Evaluation of a standardized instrument for the detection of malingered memory deficits. *Law and Human Behavior, 15,* 667–676.

Iverson, G.L., & Franzen, M.D. (1996). Using multiple objective memory procedures to detect simulated malingering. *Journal of Clinical and Experimental Neuropsychology, 18,* 38–51.

Johnson, J.L., & Lesniak-Karpiak, K. (1997). The effect of warning on malingering on memory and motor tasks in college samples. *Archives of Clinical Neuropsychology, 12,* 231–238.

Lees-Haley, P.R., English, L.T., & Glenn, W.J. (1991). A fake bad scale on the MMPI-2 for personal injury claimants. *Psychological Reports, 68,* 203–210.

Lezak, M.D. (1976). *Neuropsychological Assessment.* New York: Oxford University Press.

Lezak, M.D. (1983). *Neuropsychological Assessment* (2nd ed.). New York: Oxford University Press.

Millis, S.R. (1994). Assessment of motivation and memory with the Recognition Memory Test after financially compensable mild head injury. *Journal of Clinical Psychology, 50,* 601–605.

Millis, S.R., Putnam, S.H., Adams, K.M., & Ricker, J.H. (1995). The California Verbal Learning Test in the detection of incomplete effort in neuropsychological evaluation. *Psychological Assessment, 7,* 463–471.

Mittenberg, W., Azrin, R., Millsaps, C., & Heilbronner, R. (1993). Identification of malingered head injury on the Wechsler Memory Scale—Revised. *Psychological Assessment, 5,* 34–40.

Mittenberg, W., Rotholec, A., Russell, E., & Heilbronner, R. (1996). Identification of malingered head injury on the Halstead-Reitan Battery. *Archives of Clinical Neuropsychology, 11,* 271–281.

Nies, K.J., & Sweet, J.J. (1994). Neuropsychological assessment and malingering: A critical review of past and present strategies. *Archives of Clinical Neuropsychology, 9,* 501–552.

Rosenfeld, J.P., Sweet, J.J., Chuang, J., Ellwanger, J., & Song, L. (1996). Detection of simulated malingering using forced choice recognition enhanced with event-related potential recording. *The Clinical Neuropsychologist, 10,* 163–179.

Slick, D.J. (1996). The Victoria Symptom Validity Test: A new clinical measure of response bias. Ph.D. dissertation, University of Victoria.

Slick, D., Hopp, G., & Strauss, E. (in press). *Victoria Symptom Validity Test.* Odessa, Fl: Psychological Assessment Resources.

Strauss, E., Spellacy, F., Hunter, M., & Berry, T. (1994). Assessing believable deficits on measures of attention and information processing capacity. *Archives of Clinical Neuropsychology, 9,* 483–490.

Tenhula, W.N., & Sweet, J.J. (1996). Double cross-validation of the Booklet Category Test in detecting malingered traumatic brain injury. *The Clinical Neuropsychologist, 10,* 104–116.

Tombaugh, T.N. (1996). *Test of Memory Malingering*. New York: Multi Health Systems.

Trueblood, W. (1994). Qualitative and quantitative characteristics of malingered and other invalid WAIS-R and clinical memory data. *Journal of* Clinical and Experimental Neuropsychology, 16, 597–607.

Warrington, E.K. (1984). *Recognition Memory Test Manual*. Windsor, England: NFER-NELSON.

REY FIFTEEN ITEM MEMORY TEST (FIT)

Other Test Names

The test is also called Fifteen Item Test, Rey's Memory Test, or Rey's 3 × 5 Test.

Purpose

This test is used to assess effort on memory tests and exaggeration or feigning of memory complaints.

Source

The test can be made, using the description provided below.

Description

The FIT (see Figure 17–2), developed by Rey (1964), consists of 15 items that are arranged in three columns by five rows. Patients are shown a card (21.5 cm in width and 28 cm in height) containing the 15 items for 10 seconds and then asked to draw the items from memory. In the instructions, the number "15" is stressed to make the test appear difficult (Lezak, 1995). In reality, because this is primarily a test of immediate memory and attention and because of item redundancy (i.e., ABC, 123, abc, etc.), the FIT is actually rather easy and patients need recall only three or four ideas to recall most of the items. Malingerers are thought to misjudge the difficulty of the task and thus perform more poorly than all but the patients with severe intellectual impairment. In her discussion of the FIT, Lezak (1983) felt that anyone who was not significantly impaired could recall at least three of the five character sets, or nine of the 15 items.

Administration

Provide the patient with a blank sheet of paper and instruct as follows (Arnett et al., 1995): "*This is a memory test. It is a very difficult memory test, but I want you to give it your best. What I am going to do is show you a card with <u>fifteen different</u> (emphasized) designs. You will get 10 seconds to study the card, then I will take the card away. After I take the card away, please draw as many of the designs as you can remember and arrange them in the same way as they were on the card. Again, this is a <u>hard</u> (emphasized) test, but do the best you can. Here is the card.*" Griffin et al. (1996) suggest that the effectiveness of the test can be increased by requesting that subjects record the 15 items "just as they appear on the card" (see comment).

Approximate Time for Administration

About 5 minutes are required for the entire test.

Scoring

A number of scores can be computed. Record the total number of items recalled correctly, regardless of their spatial location, range 0–15. Also record the number of correct rows in proper sequence; that is, the number of rows that are in the correct place in the 3 × 5 matrix and that contain all of the correct items arranged in the right order. The range is 0–5. One can also sum the number of symbols placed within a row. Thus ACB would receive a score of 1. The range of scores is 0–15. Analysis of type of error may also be of some use

Figure 17—2. Rey's Fifteen Item Test.

(Greiffenstein et al. 1996; Griffen et al. 1996) (see comment section).

Comment

Goldberg and Miller (1986) reported that independent raters showed 95 percent agreement in items correct and 97 percent agreement in rows correct scores. Information regarding test–retest reliability is not available. However, Paul et al. (1992) devised a 16-item version of the FIT consisting of four rows and four items (A B C D, 1 2 3 4, a b c d, I II III IIII) and gave the task to community volunteers. On retesting following a 2-week interval, community dwellers achieved a reliability coefficient of .48 (due to the fact that normal subjects typically obtain perfect scores on both tests) which rose to .88 under simulation conditions.

Ideally, a test designed to detect malingered memory defects should be sensitive to faking but insensitive to genuine memory disturbance. However, the FIT appears to fall far short of this ideal. Bernard (1990) gave the test to 28 healthy controls and 58 individuals simulating memory deficits. The FIT did not distinguish between groups. Schretlen et al. (1991) gave the test to 76 subjects faking various mental disorders, 148 patients with amnesia, dementia, severe mental illness, or other neuropsychiatric disorder, and 80 normal controls. They reported that 27 percent of the patients scored in the "malingering" range, and only 15 percent of the subjects instructed to fake impairment were detected as malingerers with the FIT. Similarly, Morgan (1991) examined 60 nonlitigating subjects with mild-to-severe memory impairment and found that 12 of the 60 subjects "failed" the FIT when a criterion of three rows or nine items was utilized. Adjusting the cutoff score to 7 has been recommended to improve diagnostic efficiency (Lee et al., 1992). Lee et al. gave the FIT to 100 temporal lobe epilepsy inpatients, 56 nonlitigating outpatients, and 16 outpatients who were in litigation and whose optimal performance could not be assumed. They found that a score of 7 items recalled was at or below the 5th percentile for each reference group except the outpatient group in litigation. Guilmette et al. (1994), however, used this

modified cutoff score and found that the FIT was overly sensitive to genuine memory impairment and not sensitive enough to identify individuals feigning brain damage. Using a cutoff of 7 or less items correct, 40 percent of nonlitigating patients with moderate-to-severe brain damage and 20 percent of depressed psychiatric inpatients would have been classified as possible malingerers. In contrast, only 5 percent of a group of normals asked to feign believable deficits fell in the "malingering" range. They also found that a version of the Hiscock and Hiscock (1989) forced-choice procedure was superior to the FIT as a malingering detection procedure within neuropsychological assessment (see the Victoria Symptom Validity Test for an adaptation of Hiscock and Hiscock's procedure). Using a cutoff of 90 percent or less correct as suggesting malingering on the Hiscock and Hiscock forced-choice procedure, all of the brain-damaged subjects and all but 15 percent of the simulators were correctly classified. Iverson and Franzen (1996) evaluated students, psychiatric patients, and a mixed group of memory-impaired patients on a number of tasks, including the 16-item version of the FIT. The 16-item version was not effective in classifying individuals instructed to malinger (22.5 percent) although forced-choice procedures had relatively high rates of correct classification. Greiffenstein et al. (1994) tested a sample of 106 postconcussive patients with and without overt signs of malingering (e.g., improbable poor performance on two or more neuropsychological measures, contradiction between collateral sources and symptom history) on a battery of neuropsychological tests (e.g., RAVLT, WMS, WMS-R) and a number of malingered amnesia measures, including the FIT. Probable malingerers could not be differentiated from seriously brain-injured patients on free-recall measures from the Wechsler scales and the RAVLT. In contrast, probable malingerers performed poorly on the malingering measures, including the FIT, although the Portland Digit Recognition Test achieved a better hit rate. Greiffenstein et al. (1995) noted, however, that malingered amnesia measures, including the FIT, were generally more sensitive to noncompliance than were MMPI-2 measures. Moreover, factor analysis suggested independent psychiatric (containing MMPI-2 measures) and memory (containing memory measures including the FIT, Portland Digit Recognition Test, RAVLT Recognition condition, and Reliable Digit Span) malingering factors. Recently, Millis and Kler (1995) gave the FIT to seven individuals claiming to have severe cognitive deficits as a result of closed-head injuries but who were judged to be malingerers because of significantly below-chance performance on the Recognition Memory Test, a forced-choice memory measure. A reference group of seven patients with acute moderate-to-severe traumatic brain injuries was also given the FIT. The brain-injured subjects recalled significantly more items on the FIT than the malingering subjects. Using a cutoff score of seven, the FIT was able to detect only about half of the malingerers but did not misclassify any brain-injured subjects.

Not only do some patients with focal memory disturbance do poorly on this test, but those with more diffuse cognitive impairment may perform poorly as well. Goldberg and Miller (1986) gave the task to 50 adult psychiatric inpatients of average intelligence (mean = 101.1, SD = 12.5) and 16 retarded adults (WAIS-R IQs ranged from 40 to 69, mean = 63.4, SD = 7.54). They found that all of the psychiatric patients recalled at least 9 of the 15 items while over 37 percent of retarded subjects recalled fewer than 9 items. Nine of the 16 retarded adults failed to recall at least three of the five rows. The typical errors made by the retarded subjects were perseverations and reversals, as opposed to omissions. They also found that in the psychiatric sample, the number of rows recalled correctly was negatively correlated with the MMPI Infrequency (F) scale ($r = -.31$) and the Wiggins Organicity scale ($r = -.42$), but positively correlated with IQ ($r = .38$). Performance on the FIT showed no relation to Gough's F-K index. Schretlen et al. (1991) also found moderate-to-high correlations ($r = .55$ to $.81$) between general intellectual status and FIT performance. Philpott and Boone (1994) gave the test to patients with probable dementia of the Alzheimer's type (AD) who varied with respect to level of cognitive impairment (from mild to severe according to scores on the MMSE) and to

healthy adults, aged 46–80 years. They found that performance on the FIT varied with severity of dementia. Only two of the 49 patients with AD obtained a FIT score greater than 9. Even patients with mild cognitive decline exhibited a high rate of "failure" on this test. Back et al. (1996) reported that in a sample of 30 patients with schizophrenia, 13% obtained a score less than 9.

Application of a different criterion may yield somewhat better results, at least with regard to specificity. Arnett et al. (1995) compared the performance of a mixed sample of neurological patients (predominantly traumatic brain-injured patients with intracerebral hemorrhage) to normal individuals instructed to simulate impairment on several quanittate and qualitative variables derived from the FIT. They found that a cutoff of <2 rows in proper location provided the best discrimination of groups (in comparison to a cutoff of <3 rows correct, <9 items correct, <2 rows correct), producing sensitivity of 47 percent and specificities of 97 percent. The same cutoff applied to a replication study yielded a sensitivity of 64 percent and specificity of 96 percent. Note, however, that their group of brain-damaged patients was not ideal since they suffered moderate-to-severe damage. Patients with minor traumatic brain injuries would provide a more appropriate comparison. Nonetheless, the finding that patients with documented evidence of cerebral damage can achieve two or more correct rows on the FIT suggests that performance below this cutoff in the context of minor head injury should be considered as suspect.

Griffin et al. (1996) recommend altering the administration by requesting that subjects record the fifteen items *just as they appear on the card*. They suggested, based on a study of psychiatrically disabled and normal nonmalingerers, as well as possible malingerers, that both quantitative and qualitative analysis should be used. Possible malingerers made significantly more gestalt (failure to reproduce the 3×5 configuration), row sequence, dyslexic (character reversal), and embellishment errors than did nonmalingerers.

Greiffenstein et al. (1996) examined the utility of some other scoring modifications. In 60 patients with severe traumatic brain injury and 90 litigating postconcussion patients who were probably malingering, hit rates (64 percent sensitivity, 72 percent specificity) with Rey's original scoring method (9 items or less) could be improved (69 percent sensitivity, 77 percent specificity) with a spatial scoring system in which the correct within-row reproductions are computed. Note that the specificity levels are quite low, with a false-positive error rate of about 33 percent. A 15-word forced-choice recognition memory test proved to be more effective than the FIT.

Morgan (1991) found that the five rows that comprise the FIT differ in degree of difficulty. In nonlitigating brain-damaged individuals, recall of the three capital letters is best, followed by arabic numerals, lower case letters, geometric figures, and Roman numerals. The most frequent qualitative error was misordering of geometric shapes. Repetition and perseveration occurred both in individuals who "passed" or "failed" the FIT.

The FIT is quick to administer and easy to score. It is more useful than personality measures such as the MMPI-2 in the detection of exaggerated traumatic brain injury (Greiffenstein et al., 1995). On the other hand, it appears sensitive to genuine cognitive dysfunction (including dementia, amnesia, visual-spatial problems) and insufficiently sensitive to malingering (e.g., Arnott et al., 1995; Beetar & Williams, 1994; Greiffenstein et al., 1996; Guilmette et al., 1994; Iverson & Franzen, 1996; Morgan, 1991; Schretlen et al., 1991). If poor scores occur on the FIT, clinicians should first consider the possibility of severe neurological disturbance before drawing conclusions about the validity of malingering scores (Greiffenstein et al., 1994, 1996). We, like others (Greiffenstein et al., 1994; Guilmette et al., 1994; Iverson & Franzen, 1996; Millis & Kler, 1995), prefer forced-choice procedures. If clinicians choose to use the FIT in combination with other measures, the FIT's greatest utility may be in detecting blatant malingering strategies following mild brain injury (Millis & Kler, 1995; Palmer et al., 1995). In such cases, the test should be given at the very beginning of the evaluation, before the patient is exposed to more difficult tests and subsequently understands the sim-

plicity of the procedure (Iverson & Franzen, 1996). The use of the test in patients with severe cerebral dysfunction is not recommended.

The question arises as to what makes the task somewhat effective in the separation of real from fabricated memory problems. Greiffenstein et al. (1996) note that the task measures short-term memory since the 15 items can be easily chunked into five ideational units, well within the capacity of the short-term buffer. They suggest that malingerers may perform poorly on both short-term and long-term memory tasks, not knowing that short-term memory is intact in nondemented amnesiacs.

Normative Data

With regard to number of items correct, a cutoff score of 7 is recommended (Lee et al., 1992). Adjusting the cutoff score higher may increase the FIT's sensitivity but decreases its specificity (Lee et al., 1992; Schretlen et al., 1991). Alternatively, examiners can use a cutoff of <2 rows in proper location (Arnett et al., 1995) or <9 symbols accurately placed within rows (Greiffenstein et al., 1996).

Schretlen et al. (1991) found that the number of items recalled is inversely related to age ($r = -.25$). Others have also reported that scores on the FIT decline with advancing age (Philpott & Boone, 1994), suggesting that, in combination with other nonmotivational factors, older adults may be erroneously classified as malingering. Intellectual level is also related (.38 to .81) to performance on the test (Goldberg & Miller, 1986; Schretlen et al., 1991; but see Back et al. 1996 who failed to find a relation between MMSE and FIT scores in schizophrenic patients). Back et al. (1996) reported that level of education affects scores. Thus, the FIT may be inappropriate for individuals with less than average IQ/education.

References

Arnett, P.A., Hemmeke, T.A., & Schwartz, L. (1995). Quantitative and qualitative performance on Rey's 15-Item Test in neurological patients and dissimulators. *The Clinical Neuropsychologist, 9,* 17–26.

Back, C., Boone, K.B., Parks, C., Burgoyne, K., & Silver, B. (1996). The performance of schizophrenics on three cognitive tests of malingering, Rey 15-Item Memory Test, Rey Dot Counting, and Hiscock forced-choice method. *Assessment, 3,* 449–457.

Beetar, J.T., & Williams, J.M. (1994). Malingering response styles on the Memory Assessment Scales and symptom validity tests. *Archives of Clinical Neuropsychology, 10,* 57–72.

Bernard, L.C. (1990). Prospects for faking believable memory deficits on neuropsychological tests and the use of incentives in simulation research. *Journal of Clinical and Experimental Neuropsychology, 12,* 715–728.

Goldberg, J.O., & Miller, H.R. (1986). Performance of psychiatric inpatients and intellectually deficient individuals on a task that assesses the validity of memory complaints. *Journal of Clinical Psychology, 42,* 792–795.

Greiffenstein, M., Baker, W.J., & Gola, T. (1994). Validation of malingered amnesia measures with a large clinical sample. *Psychological Assessment, 6,* 218–224.

Greiffenstein, M.F., Gola, T., & Baker, W.J. (1995). MMPI-2 validity scales versus domain specific measures in detection of factitious traumatic brain injury. *The Clinical Neuropsychologist, 9,* 230–240.

Greiffenstein, M.F., Baker, W.J., & Gola, T. (1996). Comparison of multiple scoring methods for Rey's malingered amnesia measures. *Archives of Clinical Neuropsychology, 11,* 283–293.

Griffin, G.A.E., Normington, J., & Glassmire, D. (1996). Qualitative dimensions in scoring the Rey Visual Memory Test of malingering. *Psychological Assessment, 8,* 383–387.

Guilmette, T.J., Hart, K.J., Giuliano, A.J., & Leininger, B.E. (1994). Detecting simulated memory impairment: Comparison of the Rey Fifteen-Item Test and the Hiscock Forced-Choice Procedure. *The Clinical Neuropsychologist, 8,* 283–294.

Hiscock, M., & Hiscock, C.K. (1989). Refining the forced choice method for the detection of malingering. *Journal of Clinical and Experimental Neuropsychology, 11,* 967–974.

Iverson, G.L., & Franzen, M.D. (1996). Using multiple object memory procedures to detect simulated malingering. *Journal of Clinical and Experimental Neuropsychology, 8,* 1–14.

Lee, G.P., Loring, D.W., & Martin, R.C. (1992). Rey's 15-Item Visual Memory Test for the detection of malingering: Normative observations on patients with neurological disorders. *Psychological Assessment, 4,* 43–46.

Lezak, M.D. (1983). *Neuropsychological Assessment* (2nd ed.). New York: Oxford University Press.

Lezak, M.D. (1995). *Neuropsychological Assessment* (3rd ed.). New York: Oxford University Press.

Millis, S.R., & Kler, S. (1995). Limitations of the Rey Fifteen-Item test in the detection of malingering. *The Clinical Neuropsychologist, 9,* 241–244.

Morgan, S.F. (1991). Effect of true memory impairment on a test of memory complaint validity. *Archives of Clinical Neuropsychology, 6,* 327–334.

Palmer, B.W., Boone, K.B., Allman, L., & Castro, D.B. (1995). Co-occurrence of brain lesions and cognitive deficit exaggeration. *The Clinical Neuropsychologist, 9,* 68–73.

Paul, D.S., Franzen, M.D., Cohen, S.H., & Fremouw, W. (1992). An investigation into the reliability and validity of two tests used in the detection of dissimulation. *International Journal of Clinical Neuropsychology, 14,* 1–9.

Philpott, L.M., & Boone, K.B. (1994). The effects of cognitive impairment and age on two malingering tests: An investigation of the Rey Memory Test and Rey Dot Counting Test in Alzheimer's patients and normal middle aged/older adults. Paper presented to the International Neuropsychological Society, Cincinnati, Ohio.

Rey, A. (1964). *L'examen clinique en psychologie.* Paris: Presses Universitaires de France.

Schretlen, D., Brandt, J., Krafft, L., & Van Gorp, W. (1991). Some caveats using the Rey 15-Item Memory Test to detect malingered amnesia. *Psychological Assessment, 3,* 667–672.

TEST OF MEMORY MALINGERING (TOMM)

Purpose

This test is used to assess effort on memory tests and exaggeration or feigning of memory complaints in adults.

Source

The complete kit (including two stimulus booklets, 25 score sheets, and manual) can be ordered from Multi Health Systems (MHS), Inc., 65 Overlea Blvd, Suite 210, Toronto, Ontario, M4H 1P1 or from MHS, 908 Niagara Falls Blvd, North Tonawanda, NY, 14120-2060, at a cost of $95 US or $135 Cdn.

Description

The TOMM (Tombaugh, 1996) is similar to the Recognition Memory Test (Warrington, 1984). It consists of a 50-item recognition test that includes two learning trials and a retention trial. On each learning trial, the patient is shown 50 line drawings (target pictures) of common objects for 3 seconds each, at 1-second intervals. The patient is then shown 50 recognition panels, one at a time. Each panel contains one of the previously presented target pictures and a new picture. On this forced-choice recognition task, the patient is required to select the previously shown target picture. Explicit feedback on response correctness is given on each item. The same fifty pictures are used on each trial. However, they are presented in a different order during the second learning trial. There is an optional retention trial about fifteen minutes after Trial 2. This is similar to the previous trials except that the target pictures are not readministered. Tombaugh suggests that the two learning trials are usually sufficient to assess malingering. However, use of the retention trial helps corroborate results.

Administration

See Source. Briefly, the patient is told that the examiner will test the patient's ability to remember 50 pictures of common objects and will then test how many of them the patient can remember. The examiner then presents the test stimuli, records responses on the record sheet for the two-choice recognition test and provides feedback regarding the correctness of the response.

Approximate Time for Administration

About 15 minutes are required for the test.

Scoring

One point is given for each correct answer provided by the patient on the recognition and retention trials. Thus, the maximum score on each trial is 50.

Comment

Tombaugh (personal communication November 1996) reported that coefficient alphas ($n = 40$) were high for each trial (Trial 1 = .94. Trial 2 = .95, Retention Trial = .94). With regard to validity, Tombaugh (1996) reports that in normal individuals, perceived difficulty exceeds the demonstrated difficulty. That is, it gives the impression of being more difficult than it really is, supporting its potential usefulness in the detection of poor effort. The test was given to 158 in- and outpatients seen for neuropsychological assessment. Performance appeared relatively insensitive to neurological impairment although profound cognitive impairment appears to affect performance; that is, highly accurate performance occurred with a clinical sample of cognitively impaired, aphasic and non-compensation seeking TBI patients. Scores, however, were lower in those with dementia, with about 27 percent obtaining scores below 45 on Trial 2. Further, performance on the TOMM appears only modestly related to measures of learning and memory. Scores showed only a modest relation (r's ranging from .20 to .35) to free recall measures of visual and verbal learning (Visual Reproduction from the WMS-R, CVLT, and Word-List subtest from the LAMB). In short, patients who score in the impaired range on standardized tests of learning and retention generally perform well on the TOMM.

The TOMM appears sensitive to motivational defects (see source). A battery of neuropsychological tests, including the TOMM, was given to a group of 27 undergraduate students asked to simulate symptoms following head injury and to 22 controls. Simulating participants demonstrated lower scores than controls. On Trial 2 in particular, all controls achieved a score of 49 or greater (100% specificity), while 93 percent of the simulators scored lower than 49 (93% sensitivity). Further, analysis of debriefing questionnaires revealed that participants did not distinguish the TOMM from other tests as a measure of malingering. In a subsequent study, the performance of litigating TBI patients ($n = 11$) was contrasted with that of a non-litigating control group ($n = 17$), a group of cognitively intact normal subjects ($n = 11$) and a group of patients with focal neuropsychological impairment recruited from a neurological unit ($n = 12$). On Trial 1, TBI patients "not-at-risk" for malingering performed slightly lower than either normals or patients with focal impairment, but performed at comparable levels on the other two trials. This was in marked contrast to the substantially lower performance of the "at-risk" TBI group. On all three trials, the scores from the "at-risk" TBI group were significantly lower than those from the other groups, which did not differ from one another. Sensitivity and specificity, however, were not reported.

Tombaugh cautions that interpretation of the TOMM involves many factors and that diagnosis of malingering should not be made on the basis of the test score itself. The score on the TOMM only addresses whether the results reflect the patient's optimal performance. It does not, however, address issues of intentionality and the motivational basis of the behavior. Adequate diagnosis requires examination of information from additional sources (e.g., performance on other neuropsychological tests, information about the onset, duration and severity of the injury, level of pre- and post-injury functioning). It is also worth bearing in mind that scores that fall in the normal range on the TOMM do not rule out malingering. For example, a person feigning motor or sensory deficits may perceive the TOMM to be unrelated to her/his symptoms and perform normally on it.

The TOMM appears to be a useful, new measure to detect motivational difficulties with respect to memory. However, there are some limitations. The influence of psychological distress is not known. Further, additional studies of reliability and validity (e.g., its utility with respect to other measures to detect malingering) are needed.

Normative Data

The test was developed on a sample of 475 community-dwelling individuals, ranging in age from 16 to 84 years and on a sample 161 patients referred for neuropsychological evaluations. Tombaugh (1996; in press) reports that performance on Trial 2 is very high for non-malingerers regardless of neurological dysfunction. More than 95 percent of adults living in the community obtained a score of 49 or 50 on the second trial. Moreover, scores for different clinical samples showed that most non-demented individuals obtained a perfect score on Trial 2. Accordingly, Tombaugh (see source) recommends that any score lower than 45 on Trial 2 or on the Retention Trial should raise concern that the individual is not putting forth maximum effort. Rather than using the score of 45 as a rigid cutoff, it should be viewed as a guideline, with the likelihood of malingering increasing as the score deviates further from the performance of specific clinical samples (see Tables 3–5 and 3–7 in source).

Age and education have little impact on performance. The influence of IQ is not reported although moderate to severe cognitive deficit appears to have an impact.

References

Tombaugh, T. (in press). The Test of Memory Malingering (TOMM): Normative data from cognitively intact and cognitively impaired individuals. *Psychological Assessment.*

Tombaugh, T.N. (1996). *Test of Memory Malingering (TOMM)* New York: Multi Health Systems.

Warrington, E. (1984). *Recognition Memory Test.* Windsor, England: NFER-Nelson.

21 ITEM TEST

Purpose

This test is designed to identify negative response bias.

Source

The manual and test protocols can be ordered from Grant Iverson, Ph.D., Department of Psychiatry; 2255 Wesbrook Mall, University of British Columbia, Vancouver, British Columbia, Canada V6T 2A1, at a cost of $15 US or $20 Cdn.

Description

The 21 Item Test was designed as a rapid screen for nonoptimal effort (Iverson, Franzen, & McCracken, 1991). The test is a refinement of the symptom validity paradigm that was popularized by Pankratz (1983; Pankratz, Fausti, & Peed, 1975). It is composed of a target list of 21 nouns that are read to the subject (see fig. 17–3). Following presentation of the list, the patient is instructed to freely recall as many words as possible. A second list of 21 nouns is used as foils in a recognition task. Immediately following the free-recall trial, the patient is given the two-alternative forced-choice recognition task and is instructed to select the word that had previously been presented from the target list.

Administration

The patient is told that the examiner will present a list of words and that the patient is to remember as many as possible. The examiner then reads the list of words at a rate of one word per 1.5 seconds (about 30–33 seconds for the entire list). Immediately after the last word is read, the patient is asked to recall all the words heard. After the patient has recalled the last word, the examiner reads a list of word pairs and the patient is asked to choose the word on the original list. On both the free-recall and forced-choice trials, the examiner records the patient's responses on the answer form.

Approximate Time for Administration

The entire test takes about 5 minutes to administer and score.

Scoring

The primary score derived from the test is the total number correct on the forced-choice task. Additional scores include the total number correct on free recall that are subsequently missed on forced choice (inconsistency score), and the greatest number of consecutive misses on the forced-choice task.

Comment

Information regarding test–retest reliability is currently not available.

The test appears sensitive to less than optimal effort. In their initial study with this task, Iverson et al. (1991) found that college students instructed to malinger memory impairment could be differentiated from students performing their best and from a mixed group of neurological patients with evidence of memory impairment. Applying a cutting

---

```
1. Hat
2. House
3. Table
4. Door
5. Dish
6. Clock
7. Oil
8. Snow
9. Road
10. Plane
11. Boys
12. Ball
13. Station
14. Arms
15. Wood
15. Chart
17. Stone
18. Hand
19. Nose
20. City
21. Sugar
```

Figure 17—3. Target Words on the 21 Item Test. *Source:* Copyright Grant Iverson & Michael Franzen (1989).

score that eliminated false positives on the forced-choice component of the task resulted in a correct classification rate of 100 percent for normal controls and memory-impaired patients, 65 percent for experimental malingerers, and 88 percent overall. In a subsequent study, Iverson, Franzen, and McCracken (1994) gave the 21 Item Test to a heterogenous group of 60 psychiatric inpatients, 60 community volunteers, and a heterogeneous sample of 60 patients seen for neuropsychological examination. None of the patients in this latter group were involved in forensic or disability evaluations. Half of the samples of community and psychiatric subjects were given instructions to malinger memory impairment. The remaining subjects were given instructions to do their best. The neuropsychological patients were sorted into normal and impaired-memory subgroups on the basis of their performance on objective memory tests. Discriminant function analysis, using free-recall and recognition memory scores as predictor variables, correctly classified 90 percent of the subjects into malingering/nonmalingering groups. In a third study (Iverson & Franzen, 1996), the 21 Item Test was one of several measures (Personal History/Orientation Questionnaire, Modification of Rey's 15 Items Test, Digit Span, WMS-R Logical Memory with Forced-Choice Supplement) given to evaluate the efficacy for detecting malingered memory deficits. Twenty undergraduates and 20 psychiatric inpatients were given the procedures twice in a repeated-measures, counterbalanced design. In one condition, subjects were instructed to try their best, and in the other condition they were instructed to malinger memory impairment. Malingering subjects performed worse on both free-recall and forced-choice recognition than did the control and memory-impaired participants. The forced-choice procedure was, however, more sensitive to the effects of dissimulation. Applying a cutting score of 9 that eliminated false positives on the forced-choice component resulted in a correct classification rate of 100 percent for normal control and memory-impaired subjects, 22.5 percent for experimental malingerers, and 69 percent overall. A cutoff score of 13 resulted in

a much higher classification rate but resulted in some false positives. The cutting score of 9, although identifying a lower number of experimental malingerers, was recommended since it seemed to approximate a lower limit of performance for actual memory-impaired patients. Subjects' performances were also compared to chance. On the forced-choice component, individuals employing a random response strategy would score between 7 and 15 correct 95 percent of the time. Subjects scoring 6 or below are performing below chance, suggesting that they are providing nonoptimal effort. No control or memory-impaired subjects in the three studies performed below chance, whereas 10 to 60 percent of the experimental malingerers scored in this range (Iverson & Franzen, 1993).

Two additional scores on the 21 Item Test have shown promise as indicators of biased responding. The inconsistency score represents the number of words recalled on free recall that are subsequently missed on forced-choice recognition. This finding is rare in control samples and in patients giving full effort. The second score represents the greatest number of consecutive misses. A large number of consecutive misses on the forced-choice task is both clinically unlikely and statistically improbable. Iverson, Wilhelm, and Franzen (1992) combined nonmalingering samples of community volunteers ($n = 31$), inpatients from a substance abuse program ($n = 60$), inpatients from a psychiatric unit ($n = 18$), and patients seen for neuropsychological evaluation ($n = 56$) and found that they obtained an average inconsistency score of .4 (SD = .8) and a greatest-consecutive-misses score of 1.5 (SD = .9). Experimental malingerers ($n = 133$) obtained an average inconsistency score of 1.4 (SD = 1.6) and a greatest-consecutive-misses score of 3.7 (SD = 2.2).

Financial incentives, however, may decrease sensitivity in the detection of response bias. Frederick, Sarfaty, Johnston, and Powel (1994) evaluated the 21 Item Test along with other measures of response bias. College students were offered financial incentives if they could convincingly suppress their actual cognitive abilities. A cutting score of 13 on the forced-choice task resulted in excellent speci-

Table 17—1. 21 Item Test Data

	Forced-Choice Score		
	n	M	SD
Control Subjects			
Undergraduates[a]	20	18.75	1.6
Undergraduates[b]	20	18.6	1.1
Undergraduates[c]	20	18.5	1.5
Psychiatric Inpatients[d]	30	17.7	2.3
Psychiatric Inpatients[a]	20	18.3	1.6
Federal Inmates[b]	20	17.4	2.0
Community Volunteers[c]	30	17.9	2.3
Mixed Patient Sample[c] (no memory impairment)	30	17.1	2.5
Memory Impaired Subjects			
Mixed Patient Sample[e]	20	16.10	2.7
Mixed Patient Sample[c]	30	15.8	2.9
Mixed Patient Sample[a]	20	16.0	3.0
Patients with Mod/Severe CHI[b]	20	16.61	1.4
Experimental Malingerers			
Undergraduates[e]	20	6.85	3.3
Undergraduates[a]	20	11.3	3.7
Psychiatric Inpatients[c]	30	9.8	3.2
Psychiatric Inpatients[a]	20	10.2	2.5
Community Volunteers[c]	30	9.5	4.9

[a] Iverson et al. (1991)

[b] Iverson & Franzen (1996)

[c] Iverson & Franzen (1994)

[d] Iverson et al. (1994)

[e] Reprinted with permission of the authors.

ficity but only limited sensitivity. Somewhat better sensitivity and specificity were obtained by a forced-choice test of nonverbal ability.

The 21 Item Test is best used at the very beginning of a neuropsychological examination, as a rapid screen for less than optimal effort. While the test is highly sensitive to blatant exaggeration, it is considerably less sensitive to more subtle or sophisticated response bias. The test likely is even less sensitive to exaggeration if it is used reactively; that is, if it is used mid-way through the evaluation after suspicions of biased effort have been raised. The subject will have been exposed to a variety of difficult neuropsychological measures so that the 21 Item Test will appear relatively simple and straightforward.

Normative Data

Comparison data were derived from a series of studies (Iverson et al., 1991, 1994; Iverson & Franzen, 1994, 1996) and combined in Table 17–1. Random responding on the forced-choice component of the test would result in a score between 7 and 14.

Iverson et al. (1994) found a modest negative relation between free recall scores and age ($r = -.38$) among nonmalingering individuals. Education was not related to free-recall performance. Neither age nor education correlated with forced-choice performance in non-malingering subjects.

References

Frederick, R.I., Sarfaty, S.D., Johnston, J.D., & Powel, J. (1994). Validation of a detector of response bias on a forced-choice test of nonverbal ability. *Neuropsychology, 8*, 118–125.

Iverson, G.L., Franzen, M.D., & McCracken, L.M. (1991). Evaluation of an objective assessment technique for the detection of malingered memory deficits. *Law and Human Behavior, 15*, 667–676.

Iverson, G.L., Franzen, M.D., & McCracken, L.M. (1994). Application of a forced-choice memory procedure designed to detect experimental malingering. *Archives of Clinical Neuropsychology, 9*, 437–450.

Iverson, G.L., & Franzen, M.D. (1996). Using multiple objective memory procedures to detect simulated malingering. *Journal of Clinical and Experimental Neuropsychology, 18*, 38–51.

Iverson, G.L., & Franzen, M.D. (1994). The Recognition Memory Test, Digit Span, and Knox Cube Test as markers of malingered memory impairment. *Assessment, 1*, 323–334.

Iverson, G.L., & Franzen, M.D. (1993). A brief assessment instrument designed to detect malingered memory deficits. *The Behavior Therapist*, May, 134–135.

Iverson, G.L., Wilhelm, K., & Franzen, M.D. (1992). Objective assessment of simulated memory deficits: Additional scoring criteria for the 21 Item Test. Paper presented to the National Academy of Neuropsychology, Pittsburgh, PA.

Pankratz, L. (1983). A new technique for the assessment and modification of feigned memory deficit. *Perceptual and Motor Skills, 57*, 367–372.

Pankratz, L., Fausti, S.A., & Peed, S. (1975). A forced-choice technique to evaluate deafness in the hysterical or malingering patient. *Journal of Consulting and Clinical Psychology, 433*, 421–422.

VICTORIA SYMPTOM VALIDITY TEST (VSVT)

Purpose

This test is used to assess effort on memory tests and exaggeration or feigning of memory complaints.

Source

The computerized version of this test (including disk and manual) can be ordered from Psychological Assessment Resources, Inc., P.O. Box 998, Odessa, Florida 33556. A flip-card version can be made, using the description provided below, when a computer is not available.

Description

In order to assess memory complaints, Hiscock and Hiscock (1989) developed a two-alternative forced-choice recognition task. In their task, a five-digit number is presented on a card for a 5-second study period, followed after a brief delay by another card containing the correct choice and a foil. The correct answers can always be distinguished from foils by recognizing the first or last digit. In order to increase the face validity of the task, the period between study and recognition is overtly increased to 10, then 15 seconds. Malingering subjects are cued to perform poorly by being told that the test is difficult for those with memory problems, and that the level of difficulty increases with retention interval. Because all items have two response possibilities, overall error rates should be approximately 50 percent under conditions of random responding. That is, scores in this range would result from either (a) severe disturbances in attention and/or memory, or (2) symptom exaggeration. Error rates that depart from 50 percent are less likely to have occurred by chance alone, with an associated probability that is easily calculated. Performance below chance at a low probability (e.g., $p < .05$) is indicative of deliberate choice of incorrect answers (that is, malingering). Protocols where the number of correct items are above chance are considered valid.

Slick et al. (1994, 1996; in press) modified the task in a number of ways. First, the administration time of the original task was quite lengthy, about 30–40 minutes. The number of items was therefore reduced from 72 to 48, halving administration time. Second, item difficulty was manipulated, making items appear more difficult than in fact they are. *Easy* items are those in which the foil and study number share no common digits (e.g., 34092 and 56187) so that recognition of first, last, or any other digit or pattern of digits from the study number will facilitate a correct choice. *Hard* items are those in which the foil is identical to the study number with the exception of a transposition of the second and third, or third and fourth digits (e.g., 46923 and 46293). To choose correctly on hard items, the order of the middle digits must be remembered; recognition of the first or last digit of the study number will not aid in making a correct choice. Like the increase in retention intervals, the difference in actual difficulty between easy and hard items is assumed to be small. Third, response time is also recorded. Finally, because probabilistic analysis may be ineffective for detecting all but the most overt attempts at simulation, normative data are provided allowing for interpretation of scores that do not differ from chance. Thus, below-chance performance at $p < .05$ is still labeled as unequivocally invalid/malingered, and performance significantly above chance at $p < .05$ is labeled as unequivocally valid. A new third category, labeled "questionable," consists of scores that fall within the remaining 90 percent confidence interval of chance performance.

The VSVT includes a total of 48 items, presented in three blocks of 16 items each. In each block, a five-digit number is presented at the center of a computer monitor, followed by a blank screen retention interval, after which the previously shown study number and a five-digit foil are displayed, one to each side of center screen. Subjects respond by striking one of two keys (left or right shift) on the keyboard. Side of correct choices and foils are counterbalanced and pseudorandomized. The retention interval is 5 seconds in the first block, and then increases to 10, and then 15 seconds in the second and third blocks respectively.

All three sections contain an equal number (eight each) of easy and difficult items. Within sections, the order of easy and difficult items and screen location (left or right) of foils is pseudorandomized.

Administration

Test presentation is controlled by the computer program. The examiner should ensure that the patient is properly oriented to the monitor and keyboard. The examiner may input responses for clients who are unable to use both hands for the keyboard. Additionally, we suggest that all patients undergoing a symptom validity assessment should be informed at the beginning of the assessment that the instruments employed are sensitive to failure to provide good effort.

Approximate Time for Administration

About 15–20 minutes are required for the test.

Scoring

Test scoring is provided by the computer program. Results are printed for the test as a whole (i.e., out of 48), as well as for each section. The following summary information is provided.

1. The number of correct trials for each block and item difficulty level, along with the maximum number of correct items (e.g., 6/8);

2. Z-scores derived from a binomial probability curve centered at chance-level performance (50 percent correct). Thus, a z-score of 0 indicates exact chance-level performance with half of the items passed. Z-scores are translated directly to p values, indicating the likelihood of a patient's obtaining a particular score by chance alone (that is, responding randomly). High positive scores ($z > 1.65$) indicate better than chance performance, and low negative scores ($z < -1.65$) represent worse than chance performance;

3. Bias is a measure of the tendency to use one hand more than the other. Scores can

range from −1 (using only the left hand) to +1 (using only the right hand). High scores (<.6) raise the question of a perceptual (e.g., visual field defect) or motoric defect or some other unusual response set.

4. Mean response latency (and standard deviation) to easy and hard items in milliseconds.

Comment

Slick (1996) reported that alphas for the 24 easy, 24 hard, and the entire set of 48 items were .82, .87, and .89, respectively. The VSVT was administered twice to 30 healthy participants and 27 compensation-seeking patients. Test–retest correlations for selected measures from the VSVT ranged from .53 (Hard RT) to .73 (Total Correct). The moderate magnitude of the test–retest correlations likely reflect restriction in ranges, particularly among the control sample. All of the control participants obtained the same classification at retest (valid) as they did at first testing. Among the compensation-seeking patients, 86 percent obtained the same classification at retest.

The VSVT appears sensitive to motivational defects (for a discussion of the original Hiscock and Hiscock procedure [1989], see Binder, 1990; Guilmette et al., 1993, 1994). Slick et al. (1994; Slick et al., 1996) gave the task to healthy adults (n = 43), normal individuals instructed to simulate postconcussion symptoms (n = 42), compensation-seeking patients (n = 121), and patients not seeking compensation (n = 26). They found that simulating participants demonstrated lower scores on hard items. Adoption of a three-category classification system (below chance, above chance, questionable) showed excellent specificity, producing zero false-positive rates, and very good sensitivity. All control and noncompensation-seeking participants performed above chance. About 83 percent of individuals simulating impairment fell within the questionable or invalid range. Approximately 83 percent of the compensation-seeking patients achieved above-chance scores. Further, individuals who produced invalid protocols took

about twice as long to respond as those who produced valid protocols, suggesting that response time may be a useful adjunct to measures of symptom validity.

Berry and colleagues (personal communication, July 1995) also found a low false-positive rate when the VSVT was given to a group of 30 moderately to severely head-injured adults (mean number of days of unconsciousness = 21, SD = 29) who were not seeking compensation at the time of assessment. Twenty-nine (97 percent) of the patients obtained scores in the valid range while only one patient (3 percent) obtained a score in the questionable range. These data further demonstrate that scores in the questionable range are unlikely in patients who do not have obvious, grossly impaired function (e.g., severe attentional disturbance or impaired consciousness).

In short, even the presence of profound cognitive impairment only affects performance on the VSVT minimally. In contrast, the forced-choice procedure employed by Binder and Willis (1991) creates a more difficult task in which even nonpatients putting forth their best effort make a number of errors. Depression also has little impact on VSVT performance (Slick et al., 1996; see also Guilmette et al., 1994, with regard to an abbreviated version of the Hiscock and Hiscock procedure).

Divergent validity has been demonstrated by small correlations between the VSVT and scores on tests designed to measure dissimilar constructs. Slick et al. (1996) reported that no memory test (e.g., RAVLT, Rey Figure) shared more than 5 percent of its variance with easy- or hard-item scores from the VSVT, indicating that the VSVT is largely unaffected by level of cognitive function. The implication is that scores in the questionable range, especially those at the low end, likely reflect some degree of exaggeration. Response times to easy and hard items, however, showed considerably less divergent validity, being moderately correlated (.32 to .53) with digit span and measures with heavy processing-speed components (e.g., Stroop, Trails), suggesting caution in the interpretation of response times.

Correlations between MMPI-2 validity

Table 17—2. Classification of Subject Performance by Scores on the VSVT

	Valid Above Chance	Questionable At Chance	Invalid/Malingering Below Chance
Total Correct	29 or above	20–28	19 and lower
Easy Correct	16 or above	9–15	8 or lower
Hard Correct	16 or above	9–15	8 or lower

scales and VSVT scores were in the small-to-medium range. However, when participant classifications from the two tests were compared, a low rate of agreement was found between the two measures. This is perhaps not a surprising finding because the tests differ considerably in task (self-report vs. actual performance) and domain (memory vs. personality assessment) (see also Greiffenstein et al., 1995, with regard to a number of other malingered amnesia measures and the MMPI-2).

Although the VSVT procedure is useful, several limitations should be noted. First, perfect performance does not definitively rule out fabrication or exaggeration of symptomatology (Guilmette et al., 1993, 1994). Second, Slick et al. (1996) caution that symptom validity tests such as the VSVT are at best only capable of indicating that factors other than, or perhaps in addition to, certain forms of cognitive impairment may be influencing client performance (see also Palmer et al., 1995). Even in cases where financial or other incentives exist, and the patient's performance is suspect, the patient may be legitimately impaired and/or acting without conscious intent. For example, patients with impaired judgment (perhaps reflecting executive dysfunction) may exhibit chance-level performance. In cases where suspect performance is detected, the use of multiple measures (see Figure 17–1) is recommended to clarify whether poor performance is intentional and to evaluate alternative explanations for questionable or invalid scores.

Normative Data

Scores for the total, easy, and hard items can be evaluated with reference to Table 17–2. Slick et al. (1996) found that no healthy individual or noncompensation-seeking patient obtained a score of 15 or less on the hard items. It is important to note that cutoff scores do not make allowances for differing base-rate conditions. Accordingly, a classification confidence matrix is available (see source) so that scores on hard items can be evaluated with respect to various base-rate conditions.

Slick et al. (1996) noted that steep drops in scores across retention intervals were unusual in bona fide brain-damaged individuals. They also suggested that average response times in excess of 4 seconds in patients who do not appear confused or disoriented may be indicative of motivational problems.

Preliminary data suggest that age and years of education do not influence accuracy scores on the VSVT (Slick et al., in press).

References

Binder, L.M. (1990). Malingering following minor head trauma. *The Clinical Neuropsychologist, 4,* 25–36.

Binder, L.M., & Willis, S.C. (1991). Assessment of motivation after financially compensable minor head trauma. *Psychological Assessment: A Journal of Consulting and Clinical Psychology, 3,* 175–181.

Greiffenstein, M.F., Gola, T., & Baker, W.J. (1995). MMPI-2 validity scales versus domain specific measures in detection of factitious traumatic brain injury. *The Clinical Neuropsychologist, 9,* 230–240.

Guilmette, T.J., Hart, K.J., & Giuliano, A.J. (1993). Malingering detection: The use of a forced-choice method in identifying organic versus simulated memory impairment. *The Clinical Neuropsychologist, 7,* 59–69.

Guilmette, T.J., Hart, K.J., Giuliano, A.J., & Leininger, B.E. (1994). Detecting simulated memory impairment: Comparison of the Rey Fifteen-Item Test and the Hiscock Forced-Choice Procedure. *The Clinical Neuropsychologist, 8,* 283–294.

Hiscock, M., & Hiscock, C.K. (1989). Refining the forced choice method for the detection of malingering. *Journal of Clinical and Experimental Neuropsychology, 11*, 967–974.

Palmer, B.W., Brauer Boone, K., Allman, L., & Castro, D.B. (1995). Co-occurrence of brain lesions and cognitive deficit exaggeration. *The Clinical Neuropsychologist, 9*, 68–73.

Slick, D. (1996). The Victoria Symptom Validity Test: A new clinical measure of response bias. Ph.D. dissertation, University of Victoria.

Slick, D., Hopp, G., Strauss, E., Hunter, M., & Pinch, D. (1994). Detecting dissimulation: Profiles of simulated malingerers, traumatic brain-injury patients, and normal controls on a revised version of Hiscock and Hiscock's forced choice memory test. *Journal of Clinical and Experimental Neuropsychology, 16*, 472–481.

Slick, D., Hopp, G., & Strauss, E. (in press). *Victoria Symptom Validity Test*. Odessa, Fl: Psychological Assessment Resources.

Slick, D., Hopp, G., Strauss, E., & Spellacy, F. (1996). Victoria Symptom Validity Test: Efficiency for detecting feigned memory impairment and relationship to neuropsychological tests and MMPI-2 validity scales. *Journal of Clinical and Experimental Neuropsychology, 18*, 911–922.

Name Index

Test and Subject Index

Page references in italics are for main test entries.